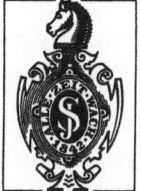

# ATHERO-SCLEROSIS VI

Proceedings of the
Sixth International Symposium

Edited by
F. G. Schettler  A. M. Gotto
G. Middelhoff  A. J. R. Habenicht
K. R. Jurutka

With 264 Figures and 214 Tables

Springer-Verlag
Berlin Heidelberg New York 1983

Proceedings of the
Sixth International Symposium
on Atherosclerosis
Held in Berlin, June 13–17th, 1982

In cooperation with the International Society
and Federation of Cardiology

Prof. Dr. Dr. F. Gotthard Schettler
Priv.-Doz. Dr. Gert Middelhoff
Dr. Andreas J. R. Habenicht
Klara R. Jurutka

Medizinische Klinik, Bergheimer Str. 58
6900 Heidelberg (Germany)

Antonio M. Gotto, Jr., M.D., Ph.D.

Baylor College of Medicine, Department of Medicine
Houston, Texas 77030 (USA)

ISBN-13:978-3-642-81819-6     e-ISBN-13:978-3-642-81817-2
DOI: 10.1007/978-3-642-81817-2

The Library of Congress Cataloged The First Issue Of This Work As Follows: RC 692 15a.
International Symposium on Atherosclerosis. Atherosclerosis. New York [etc.] Springer-Verlag.
v. ill. 25 cm. "Proceedings of the International Symposium." Key title: Atherosclerosis (Berlin),
ISSN 0170-0626. 1. Atherosclerosis—Congresses. I. Title. II. Key title.
RC692.15a   616.1'36   80-646682   MARC-S

2127/3140-543210

# ACKNOWLEDGMENT

Bundesministerium für Jugend, Familie und Gesundheit
Senat der Stadt Berlin
American Heart Association
British Atherosclerosis Discussion Group
European Atherosclerosis Group
International Society of Cadiology
National Institutes of Health, Bethesda, Maryland USA
Ontario Heart Foundation

Abbott Laboratories, North Chicago, Illinois
American Cynamid, Pearl River, New York
Astra Chemicals
Ayerst Laboratories
Ayerst Laboratories, New York, N.Y.
Bayer AG, 5090 Leverkusen
Beecham Wülfing GmbH & Co. KG, 4040 Neuss
Alfred Benzon
Bristol-Myers Co. Pty. Ltd.
Boehringer Mannheim GmbH, 6800 Mannheim
Burroughs Wellcome Co., Research Triangle Park, N.C.
Canadian Heart Foundation, Ottawa, Ontario
Chemiewerk Homburg, Zweigniederlassung der Degussa, 6000 Frankfurt/Main
Ciba-Geigy GmbH, 7867 Wehr/Baden
Corby Distilleries Ltd., Montreal, Quebec
Council on Arteriosclerosis of the American Heart Association
Deutsche Wellcome GmbH, 3006 Burgwedel
Dome Petroleum Limited, Calgary, Alberta
Dow Chemical, Houston, Texas

Dupont & de Nemours and Co.
E. I. Dupont, Wilmington, Delaware
Dr. Falk GmbH. & Co. Pharm. Präparate KG. 7800 Freiburg
Farmitalia Carlo Erba (Montedison group)
Forschungsgesellschaft Rauchen und Gesundheit mbH. 2000 Hamburg
General Foods Inc., Toronto, Ontario
Glaxo Holdings
Gödecke A. G., 7800 Freiburg-Berlin
Gulf Canada Limited, Toronto, Ontario
Henning Berlin GmbH, 1000 Berlin
Hoechst Aktiengesellschaft, Frankfurt/Main
Hoechst Fennica
Hoechst Roussel Pharmaceuticals, Inc.
Hoechst-Roussel Pharmaceuticals, Sommerville, New Jersey
Hoffmann-La Roche AG., 7889 Grenzach-Wyhlen
Hoffmann-La Roche, Nutley, New Jersey
IC-Pharma Arzneimittelwerk Plankstadt, 6900 Heidelberg
ICI Americas, Inc.
I. C. I. Americas, Inc., Stuart Pharmaceuticals
Wilmington, Delaware
ICI Australia Ltd.
Imasco Limited, Montreal, Quebec
Jansen Düsseldorf
Japanese Atherosclerosis Society
Johnson and Johnson
Jon & Johnson, New Brunswick, New Jersey
Kaufman Footwear, Kitchener, Ontario
Klinge Pharma
Heinrich Mack Nachf. 7918 Illertissen
Dr. Madaus & Co. 5000 Köln
Maizena GmbH
McNeil Laboratories

McNeil Pharmaceutical, Spring House, Pennsylvania

E. Merck, 6100 Darmstadt

Merck & Company, Rahway, New Jersey

Merck Frosst Laboratories, Dorval, Quebec

L. Merckle GmbH u. Co. 7902 Blaubeuren

Merrell Pharma, Rüsselsheim

Merrill Dow Pharmaceutical Company, Indianapolis, Indiana

MPS - Medizinisch Pharmazeutische Studiengesellschaft e. V., 6500 Mainz

The National Heart Foundation of Australia

Nattermann – Arzneimittel GmbH, Köln

Nattermann & Cie

Nova An Alberta Corporation, Calgary, Alberta

Ontario Heart Foundation, Ontario

Pfitzer GmbH, 7500 Karlsruhe

Pfizer Pharmaceuticals and Diagnostic Products

Procter & Gamble Company, Cincinnati, Ohio

Rhone Poulenc

A. H. Robbins, Richmond, Virginia

Robco Inc., Montreal, Quebec

Roussel Uclaf

Sandoz AG, 8500 Nürnberg

Sandoz Pharmaceutical Co.

Sandoz France

Sandoz Inc., East Hanover, New Jersey

Searle & Company, Chicago, Illinois

Sharp & Dohme

Shell Oil, Houston, Texas

Smith Kline

Smith Kline Corp.

Smith Kline, Philadelphia, Pennsylvania

Squibb Corporation, New York, New York

Suncor Inc., Toronto, Ontario

Schenley Canada Inc., Montreal, Quebec

Schering AG Berlin/Bergkamen, 1000 Berlin

Dr. Wilmar Schwabe, 7500 Karlsruhe 41

Standard Brands Limited, Westmount, Quebec

Texaco Canada Inc., Don Mills, Ontario

Dr. Karl Thomae GmbH, 7950 Biberach an der Riß

V.-Unilever Research Laboratorium, Vlaardingen

Unilever Australia Pty. Ltd.

Upjohn Pty. Ltd.

The Upjohn Company, Kalamazoo, Michigan

Warner-Lambert Company, Morrist Plains, New Jersey

Warner Lambert/Parke Davis Research

J. A. Wülfing

# INTRODUCTION

In 1982 Berlin was host for the second time to the International Symposium on Atherosclerosis. In 1973 the third symposium was held there, following the first in Athens – opened by the unforgettable Paul D. White – and the second in Chicago, where the great gentlemen of atherosclerosis research – Louis Katz and Irving Page – left their special imprint on the meeting.

Since the third symposium in Berlin impressive advances have been made in the field of atherosclerosis. The symposia in Tokyo in 1976 and in Houston in 1979 introduced important new knowledge from current research, stimulating worldwide interest; Berlin highlighted the latest developments.

The International Atherosclerosis Society (IAS) provides an international forum for the entire field of atherosclerosis research. Its main purpose is to apply the results of basic research to clinical medicine, and thereby to benefit the practitioner. Prevention and rehabilitation are of special importance. Intensified international cooperation is urgently needed at all levels. A declared goal of the IAS is contact between young investigators and between international research and work groups.

Participating in the Berlin meeting were 1400 researchers from 42 nations. This illustrates the growing interest in atherosclerosis as the leading cause of death in „developed" societies. However, the incidence of atherosclerosis is increasing worldwide, although there are national differences in the pattern and appearance of the disease; this was documented at the Berlin Symposium.

We still lack a definite solution to the problem of atherosclerosis; however, we have obtained new insights into the pathogenesis, etiology, clinical aspects, and prognosis of the disease. The recent conclusions published by the World Health Organization and the American Heart Association demonstrate the many efforts to stop the spread of the disease. Meetings such as the Symposium in Berlin contribute new ideas for research; they are also useful in drawing conclusions from the work that has been done.

It is my special pleasure to thank all who were involved in the organization of the Symposium. I deeply appreciate not only the help of the team responsible for editing the proceedings but also the efforts of many assistants and sponsors in accomplishing a symposium that truly reflects the dynamic growth of atherosclerosis research today.

German researchers have contributed significantly to the concepts of pathogenesis and morphology of atherosclerosis. This is particularly true of Rudolf Virchow, whose early ideas are still very much valid. One of his successors, Robert Rössle, once said: „The human being is as old as his blood vessels." We can say more positively: „The human being is as young as his blood vessels."

We appreciate the rapid publication by Springer-Verlag of the Proceedings, which will serve as a record of the manifold results that were presented in Berlin.

We look forward to the Seventh Symposium, which will be held in Melbourne, Australia, in 1985.

G. Schettler

# TABLE OF CONTENTS

XIV

XX

# LIST OF SENIOR AUTHORS

Adams, CWM, M.D., Department of Pathology, Guy's Hospital, Medical School, London SE1 9RT, United Kingdom

Alaupovic, P, M.D., Laboratory Lipid and Lipoprotein Studies, Oklahoma Medical Research Foundation, 825 N.E. 13th Street, Oklahoma City, OK 73104, USA

Antoniades, HN, Ph.D., Harvard University School of Public Health, Department of Nutrition, Huntington Avenue, Boston, MA 02115, USA

Arntzenius, AC, M.D., Department of Cardiology, University Hospital Leiden, Rijnsburgerweg 10, 2333 AA Leiden, Netherlands

Assmann, G, Prof. Dr., Westfälische Wilhelms-Universität, Medizinische Einrichtungen, Zentrallaboratorium, Westring 3, 4400 Münster/Westf., West Germany

Astrup, P, M.D., „Vildtfogedhus", Rude Skov, 2840 Holte, Denmark

Augustin, J, Priv.-Doz. Dr., Medizinische Klinik der Universität Heidelberg, Bergheimer Straße 58, 6900 Heidelberg, West Germany

Avogaro, P, Prof., Department of Internal Medicine, Unit for Atherosclerosis and Hyperlipemias, Ospedale Regionale, 30100 Venezia, Italy

Azen, SP, M.D., University of Southern California School of Medicine Los Angeles, Ca., USA

Barter, PJ, M.D., The Flinders University of South Australia, Clinical Biochemistry, Bedford Park, South Australia 5042, Australia

Baumgartner, HR, Dr., Hoffmann-La Roche & Co., Abteilung Pharma Forschung, 4002 Basel, Switzerland

Beisiegel, U, Dr., Institut für Humangenetik und Genetische Poliklinik, Philipps-Universität Marburg, Bahnhofstraße 7a, 3550 Marburg, West Germany

Bensadoun, A, Ph.D., Professor on sabbatical leave at Baylor College of Medicine and The Methodist Hospital MS/A601, Department of Medicine, 6565 Fannin Street, Houston, TX 77030, USA

Berenson, GS, M.D., Section of Cardiology, Department of Medicine, Louisiana State University Medical Center, 1542 Tulane Avenue, New Orleans, LA 70112, USA

Bertrand, ME, Prof. Dr., Service de Cardiologique et Hemodynamique, Hôpital Cardiologique, 59037 Lille, France

Bierman, E, M.D., Medicine/Metabolism RG-20, University of Washington, Seattle, WA 98195, USA

Björntorp, P, M.D., University of Göteborg, Department of Medicine I, Sahlgrenska Sjukhuset, 41345 Göteborg, Sweden

Blackburn, H, M.D., University of Minnesota Twin Cities, Laboratory of Physiological Hygiene, School of Public Health, 611 Beacon Street S.E., Minneapolis, MN 55455.USA

Blackshear, PL, Jr., M.D., University of Minnesota Twin Cities, Department of Mechanical Engineering, 125 Mechanical Engineering Bldg., 111 Church Street S.E., Minneapolis, MN 55455, USA

Blankenhorn, DH, M.D., Cardiology Section LAC, USC School of Medicine, 2025 Zonal Avenue, Los Angeles, CA 90033, USA

Born, GVR, Prof., F.R.C.P., F.R.S., University of London, King's College, Department of Pharmacology, Strand London WC2R 2LS

Bowyer, DE, M.D., University of Cambridge, Department of Pathology, Tennis Court Road, Cambridge, CB2 1QP, United Kingdom

Breddin, HK, Prof. Dr., Zentrum der Inneren Medizin, Klinikum der Johann-Wolfgang-Goethe-Universität, Theodor-Stern-Kai 7, 6000 Frankfurt, West Germany

Calvert, GD, M.D., F.R.A.C.P., Unit of Clinical Biochemistry, Flinders Medical Center, Bedford Park, S.A. 5042, Australia

Caro, CG, M.D., Imperial College of Science and Technology, Department of Aeronautics, Physiological Flow Studies Unit, Prince Consort Road, London SW7, United Kingdom

Carroll, K, Dr., University of Western Ontario, Department of Biochemistry, 561 St. George, London, Ontario N6A 5C1, Canada

Chakravarti, RN, DR., Department of Experimental Medicine, Postgraduate Institute of Medical Education and Research, Chandigarh 160 023, India

Chaldakov, G, Dr., Department of Anatomy and Histology, Medical Institute, 9002 Varna, Bulgaria

Chan, L, M.D., Baylor College of Medicine, Department of Cell Biology, Texas Medical Center, 1200 Moursund Avenue, Houston, TX 77030, USA

Chen, HW, Dr., The Jackson Laboratory, Box 258, Bar Harbor, ME 04609, USA

Chesterman, CN, M.D., University Department of Medicine and St. Vincent's School of Medical Research, St. Vincent's Hospital, Melbourne, Australia

Crepaldi, G, Prof., M.D., Istituto de Medicina Clinica dell' Università di Padova, Cattedra di Gerontologia, Via Giustiniani, 2, 35100 Padova, Italy

Daoud, AS, M.D., Veterans Administration Laboratory Service, Albany Medical Center, Albany, NY 12208, USA

Davies, PF, Vascular Pathophysiology Unit, Department of Pathology, Brigham and Women's Hospital, Havard Medical School, Boston, MA 02115, USA

Day, AJ, Dr.,Department of Physiology, University of Melbourne, Parkville, Victoria 3052, Australia

DeGennes, JL, M.D., Service Endoctrinologie-83, Hôpital la Pitie, 75013 Paris, France

Duffield, RGM, M.D., Department of Chemical Pathology and Metabolic Disorders, St. Thomas's Hospital, Medical School,, London SE1 7EH, United Kingdom

Eisenberg, S, M.D., Lipid Research Laboratory, Department of Medicine B, Hadassah University Hospital, P.O. Box 1172, Jerusalem, Israel

Epstein, FH, Prof., Dr., Institut für Sozial- und Präventivmedizin der Universität Zürich, Gloriastraße 32B, 8006 Zürich, Switzerland

Erikson, U, M.D., University Hospital, Department of Diagnostic Radiology Fack, 75014 Uppsala 14, Sweden

Feinleib, M, M.D., Dr. P.H., Epidemiology Branch, Division of Heart and Vascular Diseases, National Heart, Lung, and Blood Institute, NIH, Bethesda, MD 20205, USA

Fellin, R, Prof., M.D., Istituto di Medicina Clinica dell' Università di Padova, Divisione di Gerontologia e Malattie del Ricambio, Via Guistiniani, 2, 35100 Padova, Italy

Fidge, NH, M.D., Baker Medical Research Institute, Commerical Road, Prahran, Victoria 3181, Australia

Förster, W, Prof., Dr. sc. med., Institut für Pharmakologie und Toxikologie, Leninallee 4, 4020 Halle/Saale, German Democratic Republic

Fowler, S, M.D., University of South Carolina, Department of Pathology, School of Medicine, Electron Microscope Laboratory, Booker T. Washington Medical Center, Columbia, SC 29208, USA

Franke, WW, Dr., Deutsches Krebsforschungszentrum, Im Neuenheimer Feld, 6900 Heidelberg, West Germany

Fritz, KE, Ph.D., Albany Medical College, Atherosclerosis Research Laboratory, Veterans Administration Hospital, Albany, NY 12208, USA

Fuster, V, M.D., Division of Cardiology, Cardiovascular Diseases and Internal Medicine, Mayo Clinic, 1st Street, S.W., Rochester, MN 55905, USA

Gerrity, RG, M.D., Department of Atherosclerosis and Thromb. Research, The Cleveland Clinic, 9500 Euclid Avenue, Cleveland, OH 44106, USA

Glueck, CJ, M.D., University of Cincinnati, College of Medicine, Department of Internal Medicine, Div. Lipid Research and the General Clinical Research Center, 234 Goodman Street (Rm. C2.2), Cincinnati, OH 45267, USA

Goldberg, IJ, M.D., (Brown, WV,) The Mount Sinai Medical Center, Department of Medicine, One Gustave L. Levy Place, New York, NY 10029, USA

Gotto, AM, Jr., M.D., Department of Medicine, The Methodist Hospital, Baylor College of Medicine, 6516 Bertner Boulevard, Houston, TX 77030, USA

Gries, FA, Prof., Dr., Klinische Abteilung, Diabetes-Forschungsinstitut der Universität Düsseldorf, Auf'm Hennekamp 65, 4000 Düsseldorf 1, West Germany

Gutzwiller, F, PD Dr., PH Dr. med., Kantonsspital Basel, Universitätskliniken, 4031 Basel, Switzerland

Habenicht, AJR, Dr., Medizinische Klinik der Universität Heidelberg, Bergheimer Straße 58, 6900 Heidelberg 1, West Germany

Haller, H, OMR Prof., Dr. sc. med., Medizinische Klinik, Medizinische Akademie „Carl Gustav Carus", Fetscherstraße 74, 8019 Dresden, German Democratic Republic

Hammarström, S, Dr., Karolinska Institute, Institutionen för Medisinsk Kemie, Box 60400, S-10401 Stockholm, Sweden

Hanefeld, M, Doz. Dr. sc. med., Medizinische Akademie „Carl Gustav Carus", Fetscherstraße 74, 8019 Dresden, German Democratic Republic

Hatano, S, M.D., Department of Epidemiology, Tokyo Metropolitan Institute of Gerontology, Tokyo, Japan

Haust, MD, M.D., F.R.C.P.(C), The University of Western Ontario, Health Sciences Centre, Department of Pathology, London, N6A 5C1, Canada

Havel, RJ, M.D., Cardiovascular Research Institute, University of California, San Francisco, CA 94143, USA

Henze, K, Dr., Medizinische Poliklinik der Universität München, Pettenkoferstraße 8a, 8000 München 2, West Germany

Heyden, S, Prof., Dr., Duke University Medical Center, Department of Community and Family Medicien, Box 29 14, Durham, NC 27710, USA

Holme, I, M.D., (Hjermann I,), Medical Out-Patient Clinic, Oslo Study, Ullevaal Hospital, Oslo 1, Norway

Howard, AN, Prof., University of Cambridge Clinical School, Department of Medicine, Level 5, Addenbrooke's Hospital, Hills Road, Cambridge CB2 2QC, United Kingdom

Hudon, G, M.D., F.R.C.P.(C), Institut de Cardiologie de Montréal, 5000 est, rue Bélanger, Montréal, Québec H1T 1C8, Canada

Illingworth, DR, M.D., Ph.D., Division of Endocrinology, Metabolism and Clinical Nutrition, Department of Medicine, Oregon Health Sciences University, Portland, OR 97201, USA

Jackson, RL, Ph.D., University of Cincinnati, College of Medicine, Department of Pharmacology and Cell Biophysics, Division of Lipoprotein Research, 231 Bethesda Avenue, Cincinnati, OH 45267, USA

Julien, P, Ph.D., Department of Medicine, University of Toronto, 1 King's College Circle, Medical Sciences Bldg., Room 7302, Toronto, Ontario M5S 1A8, Canada

Kádár, A, Dr., 2nd Department of Pathology, Semmelweis Medical University, Üllöi-ut 93, 1091 Budapest, Hungary

Kannel, WB, M.D., Section of Preventive Medicine and Epidemiology, Boston University School of Medicine, Doctor's Office Building, 720 Harrison Avenue, Suite 1105 Boston, MA 02118, USA

Kappert, A, Prof., Dr., Spezialarzt für Innere Medizin bes. Herz- und Kreislaufkrankheiten, FMH, Schwanengasse 9, 3000 Bern, Switzerland

Kesaniemi, YA, M.D., Department of Medicine, Veterans Administration Hospital, University of California, 3350 La Jolla Village Drive, La Jolla, CA 92161, USA

Klimov, AN, Prof., M.D., Institute for Experimental Medicine, Acad. Med. Sci. USSR, Kirovsky 69/71, Leningrad 197022, USSR

Knuiman, JT, M.D., (Hautvast J,), Department of Human Nutrition, Agricultural University, De Dreijen 11, 6703 BC Wageningen, Netherlands

Kornitzer, M, Dr., Université Libre de Bruxelles, Faculte de Medecine et de Pharmacie, Laboratoire d'Epidemiologie et de Medecine Sociale, Campus Erasme CP.590/5,808, route de Lennik, 1070 Bruxelles, Belgium

Koschinsky, T, Dr., Diabetes-Forschungsinstitut an der Universität Düsseldorf, Klinische Abteilung, Auf'm Hennekamp 65, 4000 Düsseldorf 1, West Germany

Kostner, GM, Prof., Dr., Institut für Medizinische Biochemie, Universität Graz, Harrachgasse 21, 8010 Graz, Austria

Kral, JG, Dr., St. Luke's Roosevelt Hospital Center, Amsterdam Avenue at 114th Street, New York, NY 10025, USA

Kramsch, DM, Prof., Dr., M.D., Senior Director, Cardiovascular/Renal Group, Clinical Research International, Merck & Co., Inc., R86-218, P.O. Box 2000, Rahway, NJ 07065 USA

Kritsikis, SP, Prof., Clinicoepidemiological Section, University of Athens, Medical Center, Department of Cardiology, 38, Kifisias Avenue, Athens, 608, Greece

Kübler, W, Prof., Dr., Medizinische Klinik der Universität Heidelberg, Bergheimer Straße 58, 6900 Heidelberg 1, West Germany

Kupke, I, Prof., Dr., Laboratorium für Pädiatrische Klinische Chemie und Lipidforschung, Zentralinstitut für Klinische Chemie und Laboratoriumsdiagnostik, Universität Düsseldorf, Moorenstraße 5, 4000 Düsseldorf 1, West Germany

Kuusi, T, Dr., Third Department of Medicine, University of Helsinki, 00290 Helsinki 29, Finland

Lamm, G, Dr., WHO, z. Z. Medizinische Universitätsklinik, Abt. Prof., Dr., E. Nüssel, Bergheimer Straße 58, 6900 Heidelberg 1, West Germany

Lapetina, EG, Dr., Wellcome Research Laboratories, Department of Molecular Biology, 3030 Cornwallis Road, Research Triangle Park, NC 27709, USA

Larrue, J, Dr., Unité de Recherches de Cardiologie, U8, INSERM, Avenue du Haut-Lévêque, 33600 Pessac, France

Laustiola, K, Dr., University of Tampere, Department of Biomedical Sciences, Box 607, 33101 Tampere 10, Finland

Lee, KT, M.D., Ph.D., Department of Pathology, The Albany Medical College of Union University, Albany, NY 12208, USA

Lehtonen, A, Dr., Department of Medicine, University of Turku, Kiinanmyllynkatu 4–8, 20520 Turku 52, Finland

Levy, RI, M.D., Vice President for Health Sciences, Medical School, Tufts University, 193 Harrison Avenue, Boston, MA 02111, USA

Lewis, B, Prof., Department of Chemical Pathology and Metabolic Disorders, St. Thomas's Hospital, Medical School, London SE1 7EH, United Kingdom

Lichtlen, P, Prof., Dr., Medizinische Hochschule Hannover, Abteilung für Kardiologie, Karl-Wiechert-Allee 9, 3000 Hannover, West Germany

Long, JM, Dr., Department of Surgery, University of Minnesota Medical School, Mayo Memorial Building, Minneapolis, MN 55455, USA

Mahley, RW, M.D., Ph.D., Gladstone Foundation Laboratories for Cardiovascular Disease, University of California, San Francisco, CA 94110, USA

Malinow, MR, M.D., Cardiovascular Diseases, Oregon Regional Primate Research Center, 505 N.W. 185th Avenue, Beaverton, OR 97006, USA

Mancini, M, Prof., M.D., Semeiotica Medica, Universitá di Napoli, II Facoltá di Medicina e Chirurgia, Nuovo Policlinico, Via Sergio Pansini, 80131 Napoli, Italy

Marcus, AJ, M.D., Hematology – Oncology, 13 West, New York Veterans Administration, Medical Center, 408 First Avenue, New York, NY 10010, USA

Marenah, CB, M.D., Department of Chemical Pathology, St. Thomas's Hospital, London SE1 7EH, United Kingdom

Marmot, MG, Dr., Department of Medical Statistics and Epidemiology, London School of Hygiene and Tropical Medicine, Keppel Street (Gower Street), London WC1E 7HT, United Kingdom

Marshall, J, Prof., Institute of Neurology, National Hospital, Queen Square, London WC1, United Kingdom

Middelhoff, G, Priv.-Doz. Dr., Medizinische Klinik der Universität Heidelberg, Bergheimer Straße 58, 6900 Heidelberg 1, West Germany

Miettinen, TA, M.D., Second Department of Medicine, University of Helsinki, 00290 Helsinki 29, Finland

Miller, NE, M.D., Department of Chemical Pathology, St. Thomas's Hospital, London SE1 7EH, United Kingdom

Moore, S, M.B., F.R.C.P.(C), McMaster University, Department of Pathology, 1200 Main Street West, Hamilton, Ontario L8N 3Z5, Canada

Mordasini, R, Dr., Institut für klinische Eiweißforschung, Tiefenauspital, 3004 Bern, Switzerland

Nerem, RM, University of Houston, Central Campus, Department of Mechanical Engineering, Houston, TX 77004, USA

Nestel, PJ, M.D., F.R.A.C.P. Cardiovascular Metabolism and Nutrition Research Unit, Baker Medical Research Institute, Commercial Road, Prahran, Victoria 3181, Australia

Newman III, WP, M.D., Department of Pathology, Louisiana State University Medical Center, 1901 Perdido Street, New Orleans, LA 70112, USA

Nüssel, E, Prof., Dr., Medizinische Klinik der Universität Heidelberg, Bergheimer Straße 58, 6900 Heidelberg 1, West Germany

Nugteren, DH, Dr., Unilever Research Laboratory, P.O. Box 114, 3130 AC Vlaardingen, Netherlands

Numano, F, M.D., Department of Internal Medicine (3), Tokyo Medical and Dental University, 5-45, Yushima, 1-chome, Bunkyo-ku, Tokyo 113, Japan

Oster, P, Priv.-Doz. Dr., Medizinische Klinik der Universität Heidelberg, Bergheimer Straße 58, 6900 Heidelberg 1, West Germany

Packard, S, Dr., Department of Pathological Biochemistry, University of Glasgow, Royal Infirmary, Glasgow G4 OSF, United Kingdom

Paffenbarger, Jr., RS, M.D., Dr. P.H., Stanford University School of Medicine, Department of Family, Community and Preventive Medicine, Stanford, CA 94305, USA

Paul, O, M.D., Harvard Medical School, Office of Admission, 25 Shattuck Street, Boston, MA 02115, USA

Postiglione, A, M.D., Semeiotica Medica, II Facoltá di Medicina e Chirurgia, Universitá di Napoli, Nuovo Policlinico, Via Sergio Pansini 5, 80131 Napoli, Italy

Pyörälä, K, M.D., Department of Medicine, University of Kuopio, P.O. Box 138, 70210 Kuopio 21, Finland

Rauramaa, R, Dr., Kuopio Institute of Exercise Medicine, Puistokatu 20, P.O. Box 138, 70100 Kuopio 10, Finland

Renaud, S, M.D., Unité de Recherches de Physiopathologie vasculaire, INSERM, Unité 63, 22, avenue du Doyen Lépine, 69500 Lyon-Bron, France

Rhomberg, HP, Dr., Medizinische Klinik der Universität Innsbruck, Anichstraße 35, 6020 Innsbruck, Austria

Richard, JL, Dr., Equipe de Recherche Cardiologie, INSERM, 15, rue de l'Ecole de Médécine, 75006 Paris, France

Rifkind, BM, Dr., National Heart, Lung and Blood Institute, National Institutes of Health, Fed. Bldg. Rm. 401, 9000 Rockville Pike, Bethesda, MD 20205, USA

Robert, L, Dr., Laboratoire de Biochimie du Tissu Conjonctif, Faculté de Médecine, Université Paris Val de Marne, 8, rue du General Sarrail, 94010 Créteil Cedex, France

Rosenhamer, G, M.D., King Gustav V Research Institute, Karolinska Hospital, Box 60004, 10401 Stockholm, Sweden

Ross, R, M.D., Ph.D., Department of Pathology, SM-30, School of Medicine, University of Washington, Seattle, WA 98195, USA

Russel, MAH, Dr., Addiction Research Unit, Institute of Psychiatry, 101 Denmark Hill, London, SE5 8AF, United Kingdom

Scanu, AM, M.D., University of Chicago, Department of Medicine, 950 East 59th Street, Box 231, Chicago, IL 60637, USA

Scott, RF, M.D., Department of Pathology, The Albany Medical College of Union University, Albany, NY 12208, USA

Simons, LA, M.D., F.R.A.C.P., Medical Professorial Unit, The University of New South Wales, St. Vincent's Hospital, Darlinghurst, NSW 2010, Australia

Sinzinger, H, Prof., Dr., Dep. Med. Physiologie, Forschergruppe für Atherosklerose, Universität Wien, Schwarzspanierstraße 17, 1090 Wien, Austria

Sirtori, CR, Dr., Center E. Grossi Paoletti, University of Milano, Via A. del Sarto 21. Milano, Italy

Smith, EB, Dr., Department of Chemical Pathology, University of Aberdeen, Forester-hill, Aberdeen AB9 1ZD, United Kingdom

Smith, LC, Ph.D., Department of Medicine, The Methodist Hospital, MS/A601, Room A 654 A, Alkek Tower, 6565 Fannin Street, Houston, TX 77030, USA

Schettler, G, Prof., Dr. Dr. h. c. mult., Medizinische Klinik der Universität Heidelberg, Bergheimer Straße 58, 6900 Heidelberg 1, West Germany

Schievelbein, H, Prof. Dr. med., Institut für Klinische Chemie, Deutsches Herzzentrum München, Lothstraße 11, 8000 München 2, West Germany

Schotz, MC, Ph.D., Veterans Administration, Wadsworth Medical Center, Wilshire and Sawtelle Boulevards, Los Angeles, CA 90073, USA

Schwartz, SM, M.D., Ph.D., Department of Pathology SM-30, Biophysics Section, University of Washington, Medical School, Seattle, WA 98195, USA

St. Clair, RW, Ph.D., Department of Pathology, Wake Forest University, Bowman Gray School of Medicine, 300 South Hawthorne Road, Winston-Salem, NC 27103, USA

Stange, EF, M.D., Department of Internal Medicine, The University of Texas, Health Science Center at Dallas, Southwestern Medical School, 5323 Harry Hines Boulevard, Dallas, TX 75235, USA

Stary, HC, M.D., Department of Pathology, Louisiana State University, Medical Center, 1901 Perdido Street, New Orleans, LA 70112, USA

Stein, O, M.D., Department of Experimental, Medicine and Cancer Research, Hebrew University, Hadassah Medical School, P.O. Box 1172, Jerusalem, Israel

Steiner, G, Dr., Room 7302, Medical Science Bldg., University of Toronto, Toronto M5S 1A8, Canada

Stoffel, W, Prof. Dr. Dr., Physiologisch-Chemisches Institut der Universität Köln, Joseph-Stelzmann-Straße 52, 5000 Köln 41, West Germany

Strasser, T, M.D., Cardiovascular Diseases, World Health Organization, 1211 Geneva 27, Switzerland

Strong, JP, M.D., Department of Pathology, Louisiana State University, Medical Center, 1901, Perdido Street, New Orleans, LA 70112, USA

Taylor, JM, M.D., Gladstone Foundation Laboratories for Cardiovascular Disease, 2550 – 23rd Street, B.O. Box 40608, San Francisco, CA 94140, USA

Thompson, GR, M.D., F.R.C.P., Medical Research Council, Lipid Metabolism Unit, Hammersmith Hospital, Ducane Road, London W12 OHS, United Kingdom

Till, U, Doz. Dr. sc. med., Medizinische Akademie Erfurt, Abteilung Pathobiochemie, Nordhäuser Straße 74, 5060 Erfurt, German Democratic Republic

Tremoli, E, M.D., Institute of Pharmacology and Pharmacognosy, University of Milan, Via A. Del Sarto, 21, 20129 Milano, Italy

Tyroler, HA, M.D., The School, of Public Health, Department of Epidemiology, The University of North Carolina, Rosenau Hall 201 H, Chapel Hill, NC 27514, USA

Utermann, G, Prof., Dr., Institut für Humangenetik, Bahnhofstraße 7 A, 3550 Marburg, West Germany

VanItallie, TB, M.D., Department of Medicine and Institute of Human Nutrition, College of Physicians and Surgeons, Columbia University, St. Luke's Hospital Center, Amsterdam Avenue at 114th Street, New York, NY 10025, USA

Vergroesen, AJ, M.D., Unilever Research Laboratorium, Olivier van Noortlaan 120, Postbus 114, 3133 AT Vlaardingen, Netherlands

Vesselinovitch, D, D.V.M., M.Sc., The University of Chicago, Department of Pathology, 950 East 59th Street, Chicago, IL 60637, USA

Walli, AK, Dr., Abteilung Klinische Chemie, Universitätsklinik Göttingen, Robert-Koch-Straße 40, 3400 Göttingen, West Germany

Walton, KW, Prof., Department of Pathology, Rheumatism Research Wing, The University of Birmingham, Birmingham B15 2TJ, United Kingdom

Watanabe, Y, D.V.M., Ph.D., Experimental Animal Laboratory, Kobe University School of Medicine, 12 Kusunoki-cho, 7-chome, Ikuta-ku, Kobe, 650, Japan

Weber, G, Prof., M.D., Istituto Anatomia e Istrologia Pathologia, Via Laterino 8, 53100 Siena, Italy

Weber, PC, Prof., Dr., Medizinische Klinik Innenstadt der Universität München, Ziemssenstraße 1, 8000 München 2, West Germany

Weinstein, DB, M.D., Department of Medicine, M-O13D, University of California, San Diego, La Jolla, CA 92093, USA

Weisgraber, KH, M.D., Gladstone Foundation Laboratories for Cardiovascular Disease, University of California, San Francisco, CA 94110, USA

Widmer, LK, Prof., Dr., Leiter der Angiologischen Abteilung, Departement für Medizin, Kantonsspital Basel, CH-4031 Basel

Wilhelmsen, L, Dr., Department of Medicine, University of Göteborg, Östra Hospital, CK Plan 2, 41685 Göteborg, Sweden

Williams, RS, M.D., Duke University Medical Center, Department of Medicine, Cardiovascular Division, P.O. Box 3945, Durham, NC 27710, USA

Wirth, A, Dr., Medizinische Klinik der Universität Heidelberg, Bergheimer Straße 58, 6900 Heidelberg 1, West Germany

Wissler, RW, M.D., Specialized Center of Research in Atherosclerosis, The University of Chicago, The Division of the Biological Sciences and the Pritzker School of Medicine, 950 East 59th Street, Chicago, IL 60637, USA

Witte, LD, Ph.D., College of Physicians and Surgeons, Columbia University, Department of Medicine, 630 West 168th Street, New York, NY 10032, USA

Wolfe, BM, F.R.C.P.(C), Department of Medicine, University Hospital, University of Western Ontario, 339 Windermere Road, London, Ontario N6A 5A5, Canada

Wood, PD, D.Sc., Ph.D., Stanford University Medical Center, Stanford Heart Disease Prevention Program, 730 Welch Road, Palo Alto, CA 94304, USA

Yamori, Y, M.D., Shimane Medical University, Department of Pathology, Japan Stroke Prevention Center, Izumo 693, Japan

Yasugi, T, M.D., 2nd Department of Internal Medicine, Nihon University School of Medicine, 30-1 Oyaguchi-Kamimachi, Itabashi-ku, Tokyo, Japan

Zanchetti, A, M.D., (Magrini F.) Istituto di Ricerche Cardiovasc., Via F. Sforza 35, 20122 Milano, Italy

# 1 Clinical Aspects of Atherosclerosis

# Atherosclerosis. The Major Problem in Man

G. Schettler

Fatal incidences of stroke and heart infarctions in countries with high initial rates have decreased in the last decades. The higher the initial rate, the greater the reduction. This applies to Australia, Canada, South Africa and the USA; as well as the European countries of Belgium, Finland and Norway. Even some countries with low initial rates, such as Israel and Japan show a decline.

No changes were evidenced in Austria, Italy, Holland, Switzerland and Great Britain. On the other hand, mortality continues to increase in Bulgaria, German Democratic Republic, Denmark, France, Hungary, Ireland, Poland, Romania, Sweden and Yugoslavia. In our country death rates of stroke are decreasing but myocard infarcts still increase. Some countries such as Italy, France and Japan had lower death rates to start with. In 1975 the highest mortality rates were registered in Finland, Sweden, Scotland, Denmark, England, Northern Ireland and the Irish Republic in contrast to France, Poland, Portugal, Romania, Yugoslavia and Spain, which reported the lowest.

Unfortunately, we have no morbidity statistics suitable for intercountry comparisons. Advances in treatment of transient cerebral ischemia, stroke, heart infarctions and the subsequent shock, arrhythmias and sudden death confound the prevalence figures; and therefore good morbidity data is required to get a true picture of the incidence of arteriosclerotic events. The number of silent infarctions, which are only accidentally discovered are also important. The true prevalence of damaged kidney and intestinal arteries, the aorta and arteries of the extremities remain unfortunately unknown. Nevertheless, it is significant that vessels of the heart and brain are by far the most prevalent site of arteriosclerotic deaths.

Statistics on arteriosclerotic disease should take into account the total mortality rates of the population in question; a perspective which is often not accounted for in global comparisons.

## What is responsible for the decline in fatal arteriosclerotic events?

Cerebrovascular diseases and ischemic heart diseases, such as heart attacks, angina pectoris, arrhythmias, cardiac insufficiency as well as sudden unexpected death can be prevented and overcome to a large extent through the adoption of a three-pronged approach to the problem:

first of all, we can influence and modify the way of life of whole ethnic groups by changing their ecological, social and economic environment;
secondly, we can detect and control high-risk individuals, and
thirdly, we can supplement this primary program with a secondary effort by intensifying the care and treatment of those persons already afflicted.

Primordial prevention deals with populations not yet burdened with high rates of coronary disease.

Over the past twelve years the World Health Organization (WHO) has instituted a series of international programs. Five of these I have listed below:
first:   the AMI Community Register Program with 19 centers in Europe which records the incidence and ultimate outcome of myocardiac attacks.
second: the much-discussed Primary Prevention Program of IHD employing clofibrate in Edinburgh, Budapest and Prague.

4

third: the Multifactor Prevention Program initiated in 1942 in Great Britain, which
now has additional centers in Belgium, Italy, Poland and Spain
fourth: the self-explanatory Coronary Care and Rehabilitation Program.
fifth: the Comprehensive Community Cardiovascular Control Program with its 23
centers in Europe and one in Israel, which concern themselves with physical
fitness training, changes in smoking habits, normalizing blood pressure,
dietary advice and solution of psychosociological problems. In this connection
reference is made to the publication PUBLIC HEALTH IN EUROPE and the
report "The Cardiovascular Disease Program of WHO in Europe."

These programs are comparable with those of the National Heart, Lung, and Blood
Institute in the USA and others worldwide (Australia, Canada, Europe, Japan, Israel,
etc.). Examples of others include:
Hypertension Detection and Follow-up program (HDFP)
Lipid Research Clinics Coronary Primary Prevention Trial (LRC-CPPT)
Multiple Risk Factor Intervention Trial (MRFIT)
Primary Prevention of Hypertension
Control of High Blood Pressure by Non-Pharmacologic Means
Systolic Hypertension in the Elderly
Coronary Drug Project (CDP)
NHLBI Type II Coronary Intervention Study
Surgical Control of Hypercholesterolemia

A WHO Expert Committee released a report in December 1981 on the prevention of
coronary heart disease which addresses the risk factor concept of arteriosclerosis.
According to this report hypertension, hypercholesterolaemia, cigarette smoking and
diabetes mellitus are considered the primary and most dangerous risk factors, while
overweight, lack of exercise and stress in its many forms are regarded as secondary,
less pernicious risks. This total regression program should cover the industrialized
and primarily endangered populations from childhood to late middle age – around 60.
The Committee of Experts knows of no population with high rates of coronary disease
which do not also have relatively high blood levels of cholesterol. They classify as
"high blood levels" those exceeding 200 mg/dl. The nutrition of these groups is characterized by an excessive caloric intake caused by a high consumption of saturated
fats and cholesterol as well as sodium. Populations with total cholesterol levels between 160 and 200 mg/dl found throughout the world, for example, around the Mediterranean Sea and in the Orient, have low rates of coronary disease. There is no
evidence that such dietary habits lead to an increase in noncoronary mortality and
life expectancy in all age groups is comparatively good. Up to now, there is no causal
relationship of low cholesterol and cancer (NIH-Symposium 1981).

Specifically, a reduction in cholesterol intake by substituting mono- and polyunsaturated fats for saturated fats is recommended. A further recommendation is an increase
in the consumption of foods providing intestinal bulk and complex carbohydrates.
However, the portion of caloric intake provided by polyunsaturated fats should not
exceed ten percent. In most industrialized nations the percentage of polyunsaturated
fats in the diet is far below this figure at the present time. Populations with cholesterol
readings of 160 mg/dl and lower have little or no coronary disease or serious forms
of arteriosclerosis. This same relative "immunity" is also generally exhibited by
groups with average levels ranging between 160 and 200 mg/dl.

The International Society and Federation of Cardiology adopted identical recommendations for postinfarct secondary prevention at a symposium held on the 1st and 2nd
of May 1980 in Kronberg/Taunus. Practically identical recommendations have been
published by the Nutrition Committee of the American Heart Association this year
(Rationale of the Diet-Heart Statement of the AHA).

An expert committee of the Deutsche Forschungsgemeinschaft has prepared recommendations about the importance of fat in nutrition which agree with the recommendations

of the WHO. It goes further in describing the physiological significance of polyunsaturated fatty acids. The recommendations state that plant fats and oils are critically important in supplying essential fatty acids (linoleic and linolenic acids) to animals and man. A daily intake of 3 - 10 % of the daily energy intake is recommended and the significance of linoleic and linolenic acid in the synthesis of prostaglandin and its derivatives is emphasized.

This report concerns itself with the role these substances play in vessel tone, platelet aggregation and disaggregation as well as the interaction with the endothelium of the vessels. Through these mechanisms essential fatty acids play a direct role in arteriosclerosis. The finding of the expert committee of the Deutsche Forschungsgemeinschaft that trans fatty acids, which are sometimes considered dangerous, and come from hydrogenization of plant fats, have no different metabolic effects than the cis-forms is worthy of note. Previous implications and conclusions are thus proven wrong.

The International Atherosclerosis Society (IAS) has initiated through its member organizations a worldwide questionnaire; some of whose results I would like to cite here. Almost all the scientists responding agree with the risk factor concept of coronary heart disease. Approximately 90 % believe high cholesterol and LDL values are etiological factors. The intake of cholesterol and saturated fats should be reduced. Two thirds of those recommended an increased intake of linoleic as a protective measure. The total fat content of the diet should be 30 % of calories, with 10 % saturated, 9.1 % as polyunsaturated fatty acids. The cholesterol intake should not be greater than 200 mg. The opinions of the questioned arteriosclerosis researchers, not only the lipid specialists, were remarkably consistent.

Early diagnosis of arteriosclerosis for those cases is extremely important. Before organic damage due to inadequate blood circulation sets in, we must try to determine the patient's angiological status. The use of scanners which permit non-invasive examinations have contributed greatly to progress in the field and we can expect to obtain still better results as time goes on. Selective and specific angiographic procedures which serve to simplify decision-making regarding local fibrinolysis are indeed a significant therapeutic advance. The same can be said for the use of streptokinase and urokinase in the emergency treatment of myocardial infarcts as well as other vascular impediments, for example in renal, peripheral and cerebral arteries. In the hands of experts the percutaneous transluminal angioplastic procedure can prove to be a valuable supplement to surgery. In my opinion too little application of these possibilities has been made up to now.

Blood circulation problems can be alleviated by improving the fluidity of the blood, a therapeutic measure which has also been somewhat neglected up to now. Finally, attention should be called to the fact that hypotension can also represent a risk for organs threatened by blood deficiency. Furthermore, mention must be made of those methods of treatment which can improve the functions of ischemic organs, namely calcium antagonists and the beta blockers. Lastly, we cannot overlook the enormous progress which has been made in the differentiation and therapy of highly dangerous arrhythmias. Antiplatelet drugs and anticoagulants have also shown promising results. Here, however, the positive and negative aspects of such medication must be carefully weighed. Further evidence, especially in the field of platelet suppressive therapy, from studies still in progress is in the offing. For patients with high risk thrombotic complications prolonged therapy with anticoagulants is indicated.

Of course, we must realize that the risk concept is not the whole etiological story. We encounter quite a few patients in whom such factors are not perceptible. In the future we shall have to pay special attention to such cases. Research to determine whether or not negative conditions foster the development of arteriosclerosis must also be continued. Since the thirties we have known that patients suffering from chronic anemia, for example through an iron deficiency, or those afflicted with pernicious anemia are seldom troubled with arteriosclerosis and, if so, only in its mildest forms. The same is typical for the emaciating, consumptive diseases, especially cancer. This would seem to indicate that arteriosclerosis can be manipulated and indeed within relatively

6

short periods of time, which tends to confirm our observations made in times when
extreme hunger prevailed. The relationship between cancer on the one hand and
cholesterol metabolism on the other should also be a subject for further research.
However, for the present we can refer to the conclusion reached at the NIH symposium
which states that up to now a causal relationship between low levels of cholesterol
in the blood and cancer is not evident. This does not free us from the responsibility
of testing carefully the effects of cholesterol-reducing drugs, with special emphasis
on their influence on bile acid metabolism.

The strategy of the future will be characterized by the concept of life-time care provided by the community. I would like to give you some examples from our own studies,
undertaken in the areas of Eberbach and Wiesloch.

15 to 30 % of the children were overweight and 10 % had blood pressure values necessitating medical control or/and specific preventive action. These findings originate
from weight and blood pressure control of 1,000 kindergarten- and 7,000 school children,
where the children themselves were taught to measure these parameters. This active
arousal of interest in important health indices resulted in favourable changes of their
health related behaviour.

A further step in the right direction is our endeavour to prevent - and not to correct -
bad health habits. In the field of smoking-prevention we have a strong collaboration
between children, kindergarten-and school personnel, parents and local medical practitioners. The success of our interpersonal community prevention approach is reflected
by the nearly full - 98 % - participation in the total screening of the two towns. Its
results confirmed the high-risk status of the population, i.e. only approximately 1/3
were "free" of the seven main risk factors in the age group 30 - 60 years (1). What
"free" means is open to debate, however. In relation to cholesterol for instance 44 %
have values over 220 mg%, and 25 % over 260 mg% (Fig. 1). In view of the multiple
risk theory, who is now "free" from the risk factor cholesterol?

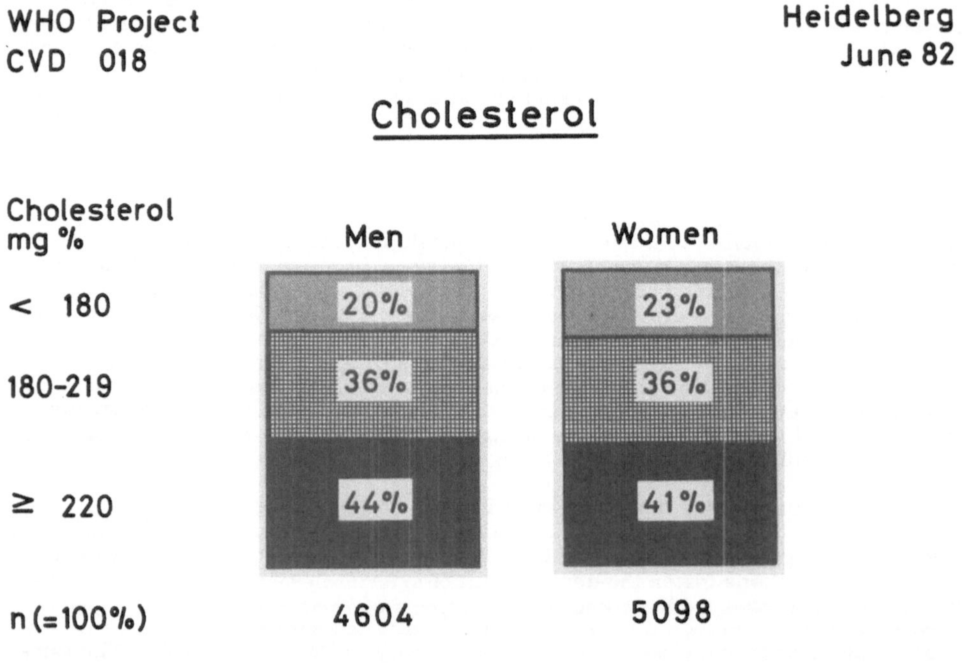

WHO Project
CVD 018

Heidelberg
June 82

## Cholesterol

| Cholesterol mg % | Men | Women |
|---|---|---|
| < 180 | 20% | 23% |
| 180-219 | 36% | 36% |
| ≥ 220 | 44% | 41% |
| n (=100%) | 4604 | 5098 |

Fig. 1

E. Nüssel

The second screening after three years wanted to establish only baseline variability and shifts in subgroups. Cigarette smoking is a potent risk factor for coronary heart disease and peripheral arterial occlusion, altough there are individuals and populations who, despite heavy smoking, remain free of complications. It is possible that triggers exist which are required to induce the damage.

Dietz and Schömig have suggested that the increase in heart rate and in blood pressure during cigarette smoking may be due to a stimulation of sympathetic activity as a possible mechanism of the observed hemodynamic changes (2).

Sympathetic activity is stimulated markedly during a submaximal physical exercise (150 W, bicycle ergometry for 3 min.). Plasma noradrenaline rose from basal values of about 180 pg/ml to 1000 pg/ml and plasma adrenaline from 40 pg/ml to 170 pg/ml. This stimulation of sympathetic activity was accompanied by an increase in heart rate and in blood pressure.

In comparison, smoking of 5 cigarettes (1.3 mg nicotine) within a period of 50 min. (5 min. smoking, 5 min. recovery) also induced a rise in heart rate from 64 to 90 beats/min.) and in blood pressure (from 119/81 to 130/89) (Fig. 2).

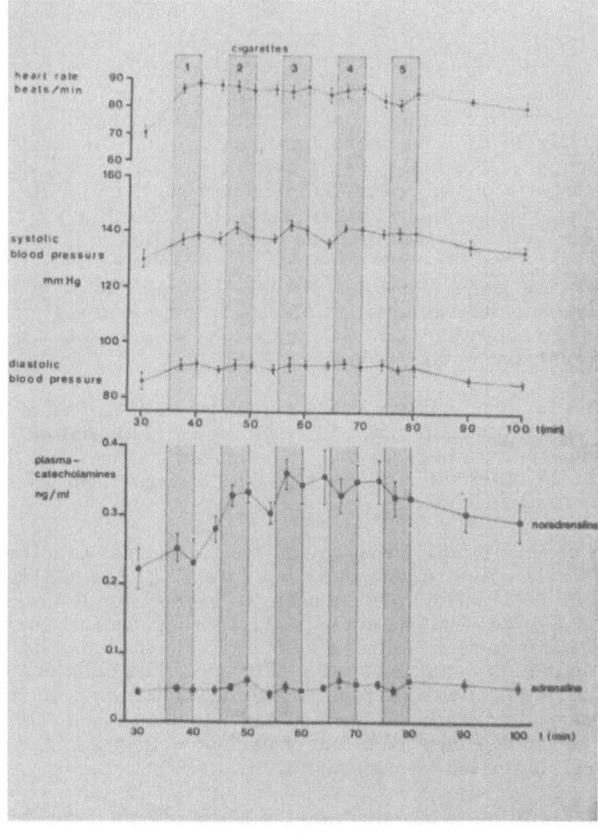

Fig. 2

Despite these hemodynamic changes neither plasma noradrenaline or adrenaline rose significantly during the observation period. Blockade of cardiac beta receptors by 200 mg of the ß$_1$ selective antagonist metoprolol resulted in a fall in heart rate and in blood pressure. When full beta blockade was established 60 min. after the administration of the tablets, cigarette smoking again induced a rise in heart rate and blood pressure. Plasma concentrations of noradrenaline and adrenaline, however, remained unchanged again.

Thus it's rather unlikely that the smoking associated acute hemodynamic changes can be explained solely by sympathetic stimulation. The long term harmful effects of smoking on the cardiovascular system may also not be related to sympathetic stimulation alone, since sympathetic activity is activated much more by moderate physical activity, a procedure which is commonly recommended for protection against cardiovascular diseases.

Lipoproteins and Smoking

In one study young smokers inhaled the smoke of two cigarettes within 15 min. During and up to 60 min. after the procedure, plasma nicotine levels, free fatty acids and hepatic triglyceride lipase rose tremendously (3). At the same time plasma triglycerides and especially VLDL triglycerides decreased significantly. LDL components, mainly triglycerides, phospholipids and apo B increased. HDL phospholipids and HDL cholesterol decreased considerably. The data demonstrate that smoking leads to a stimulated interconversion of triglyceride-rich lipoproteins. In addition considerable effects of smoking on lipoproteins in the density range 1.063 - 1.21 g/ml could be shown in this study.

A further investigation was performed to see whether nicotine is responsible for the effects of smoking on lipoprotein metabolism. In this study young volunteers chewed nicotine-containing gums. Again plasma nicotine levels, free fatty acids and hepatic triglyceride lipase rose significantly (3). In parallel we found a decrease in plasma triglycerides and phospholipids and even more prominent in VLDL-triglycerides. LDL-cholesterol and -phospholipids increased and HDL-cholesterol and HDL-phospholipids decreased. These data indicate that the influence of smoking on lipoprotein lipids is due to the effect of nicotine with activation of intravascular lipolysis and degradation of triglyceride-rich lipoproteins, which are then found in the LDL-density range. Furthermore, important changes in the HDL composition could be demonstrated. Simultaneous determination of plasma epinephrine and norepinephrine revealed that under these conditions circulating catecholamines are of minor importance in the regulation of intravascular lipolysis.

The arterial endothelial is apparently affected most by smoking. Drs. Jellineck, Augustin and Haberbosch incubated endothelial cell cultures from normal persons with plasma from persons who had smoked 2 cigarettes 10 min. earlier. Remarkable changes in the cultured cells can be seen. Plasma from the same individuals before smoking served as controls.

Phasecontrast microscopy shows the normal endothelial cells in culture to have a polygonal structure with clear borders (Fig. 3). On the second day after administration of a 10 % smoker plasma changes in the endothelial cells are seen (Fig. 4). The cells are longer and the nucleus is hyperchromatic. On the 4th day a 3 times higher rate of mitosis is seen. After 6 days of treatment the cells become polymorphic and lose their endothelial characteristics (Fig. 5). The cells are greatly enlarged, with enlarged nucleus and a light plasma, which contains no detectable fat. Many of these cells show necrotic changes. Studies with electron microscopy and freeze fractioning are underway to compare the effect of various concentrations of pure nicotine on endothelial cell cultures.

In addition to our work on the acute effects of smoking on plasmalipoproteins we are conducting an epidemiological study on the influence of chronic cigarette exposure on plasma lipoproteins. This research is supported by the Forschungsrat Rauchen und Gesundheit. The screening is based on the communities of Eberbach and Wiesloch with a 10 % random sample. In 1976 these included 122 men and 97 women between the age of 30 - 44 years in the city of Eberbach (Table 1). Preliminary data are now available for Eberbach where this study has just been completed.

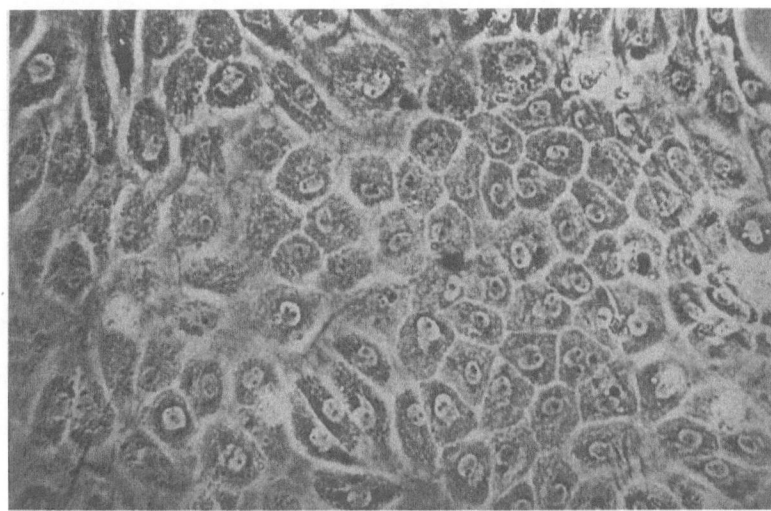

<u>Fig. 3.</u> Phasecontrast microscopy of normal human endothelial cell linings in culture

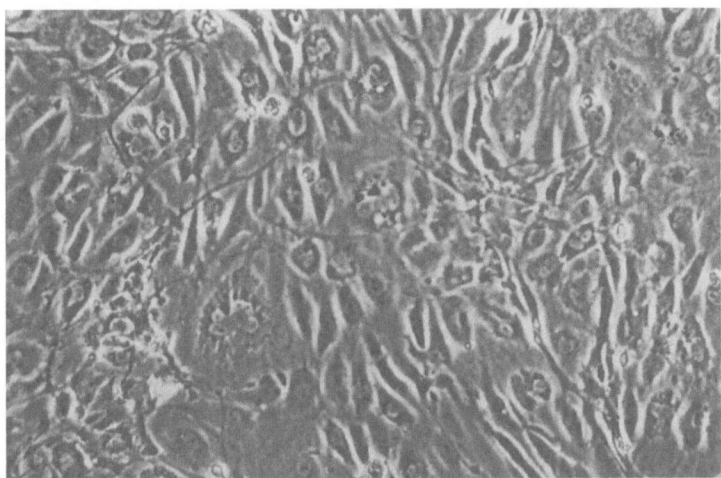

<u>Fig. 4.</u> Human endothelial cell linings 2 days after incubation with plasma obtained from a smoker 10 min. after smoking

Five years later, in the summer of 1981, when we started the study 33 % of the men but only 8 % of the women had stopped smoking (Table 2). The reliability of these data was tested with the determination of cotinine in plasma, a rather stable metabolite of nicotine.

The following preliminary data of this random sample divided into two groups, non- and exsmokers together, compared with smokers, are given on Table III for men. The level of significance has not been reached in some results because the sample is yet too small and will be completed when the study is also finished in Wiesloch. There is strong evidence that VLDL triglycerides, LDL-cholesterol and Apo B in the LDL fraction are higher in smokers compared to non- and exsmokers. Total HDL-cholesterol is 2.5 mg% lower in smokers but these data did not reach significance.

10

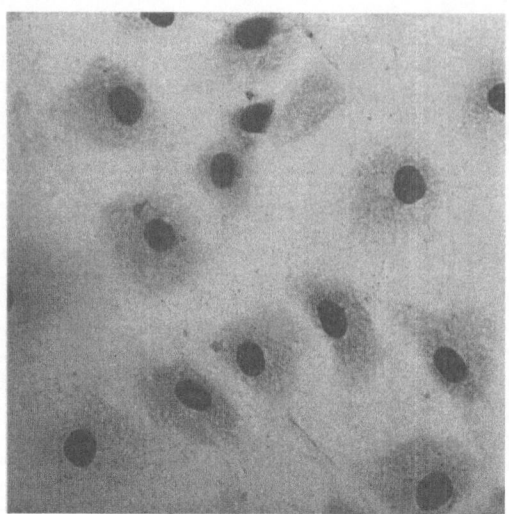

Fig. 5. Human endothelial cell linings 6 days after incubation with plasma obtained from a smoker 10 min. after smoking

Table 1. WHO Project CVD 018 - Eberbach/Wiesloch. First screening random sample 1976 Eberbach.

| Age | Male | | Female | | Σ | |
|---|---|---|---|---|---|---|
| | n | % | n | % | n | % |
| 30 – 34 | 19 | 16 | 26 | 27 | 45 | 21 |
| 35 – 39 | 56 | 46 | 35 | 36 | 91 | 42 |
| 40 – 44 | 47 | 38 | 36 | 37 | 82 | 37 |
| Σ | 122 | 100 | 97 | 100 | 219 | 100 |

Table 2. WHO Project CVD 018 - Eberbach/Wiesloch. The influence of smoking on plasmalipoproteins. Screening random sample 1981/82 Eberbach.

| | Male | | Female | | Σ | |
|---|---|---|---|---|---|---|
| | n | % | n | % | n | % |
| Smokers | 35 | 29 | 26 | 27 | 61 | 28 |
| Ex-smokers | 40 | 33 | 8 | 8 | 48 | 22 |
| Non-smokers | 45 | 38 | 63 | 65 | 108 | 50 |
| Σ | 120 | 100 | 97 | 100 | 217 | 100 |

The same is true for women with a difference of 3.1 mg% in total HDL-cholesterol (Table 4). In women total cholesterol and LDL-cholesterol are about 15 mg% higher in smokers than in nonsmokers.

These preliminary data indicate that smoking has a significant effect on plasma lipoprotein levels. In addition these results support our data obtained from the exposure to cigarette smoke or nicotine since several data are comparable.

In conclusion, these experiments favour the hypothesis that cigarette smoking and nicotine lead to damages of the endothelial lining of the arterial wall. In conjunction with this, increase in atherogenic LDL might lead to a further hazardous situation for

Table 3. The influence of smoking on plasmalipoproteins. Screening 1981/82
Eberbach (mg% $\pm$ SEM)  Males (107/120).

|  | Non/Ex-Smokers | | Smokers | |
|---|---|---|---|---|
| Plasma-cholesterol | 232.9 | ( 5.1) | 242.6 | ( 8.7) |
| Plasma-triglycerides | 205.1 | (17.6) | 229.0 | (38.9) * |
| VLDL-triglycerides | 136.8 | (14.4) | 173.0 | (39.1) * |
| LDL-cholesterol | 121.5 | ( 3.7) | 131.5 | ( 6.8) * |
| LDL-apolipoprotein B | 81.9 | ( 2.6) | 93.3 | ( 4.9) |
| Total HDL-cholesterol | 51.2 | ( 1.6) | 48.7 | ( 2.7) |

* $p < 0.05$

Table 4. The influence of smoking on plasmalipoproteins. Screening 1981/82
Eberbach (mg% $\pm$ SEM)  Females (88/97).

|  | Non-/Ex-Smokers | | Smokers | |
|---|---|---|---|---|
| Plasma-cholesterol | 203.5 | ( 4.1) | 218.3 | ( 6.9) * |
| Plasma-triglycerides | 98.6 | ( 6.8) | 102.3 | ( 8.1) |
| VLDL-triglycerides | 47.7 | ( 4.9) | 53.3 | ( 7.5) * |
| LDL-cholesterol | 113.5 | ( 3.3) | 128.8 | ( 7.2) |
| LDL-apolipoprotein B | 71.7 | ( 2.9) | 76.6 | ( 6.1) |
| Total HDL-cholesterol | 61.7 | ( 2.0) | 58.6 | ( 3.4) |

* $p < 0.05$

the vessel. This might be even aggravated by the fact that HDL as a scavenger of
tissue cholesterol changes in composition and decreases in concentration.

## References

1. Schömig A, Dietz R, Strasser R, Rascher W, Kübler W (1981) Noradrenaline metabolism during smoking before and after beta-blockade. Circulation A2804
2. Nüssel E (1982) Intervention - Das Modell Eberbach-Wiesloch. In: Risikofaktoren -
   Medizin - Fortschritt oder Irrweg? Bock KD, Hofmann L (eds) Vieweg, p. 180-191
3. Augustin J, Beedgen B, Buchholz L, Gnasso A, Haberbosch W, Spohr U, Schettler
   G (1982) The influence of smoking on plasmalipoproteins. In: Proceedings of
   VIth International Symposium on Atherosclerosis. Schettler FG, Gotto AM, Middelhoff G, Habenicht AJR (eds) Springer-Verlag Berlin Heidelberg New York,
   in press

# Clinical Aspects of Atherosclerosis –
# Recent Advances in Diagnosis and Evaluation of Coronary Heart Disease

P. R. Lichtlen and W. Rafflenbeul

## A. Introduction

Death rate of acute myocardial infarction and the rate of incapaci-
tated patients due to coronary artery disease is still increasing in
many of the western countries; further developments of techniques
allowing early detection of coronary artery disease would therefore
be of utmost importance.

### a) Advances in the Early Diagnosis of Coronary Artery Disease

In order to embrace a large population, techniques to recognize coronary lesions should be simple, easily applicable and not too costly.
This request is in conflict with the fact that obstructions in the
coronary arteries usually progress to an advanced stage (f.i. up to
75 % luminal narrowing) without becoming clinically manifest. Therefore, all non-invasive techniques, by the fact that they do not detect
the vascular alterations themselves but their results, i.e. the ensuing ischemia, cannot be used for early recognition of the vascular
damage, i.e. in the pre-clinical stage of the disease (Table 1). Early
detection of the beginning atherosclerotic process in the pre-clinical
non-ischemic stage is only possible by coronary angiography, which,
however, at this time usually is not indicated and performed for other
reasons (f.i. in case of cardiomyopathy or severe valvular disease).
All non-invasive techniques such as exercise electrocardiography with
or without additional assessments of coronary perfusion by 201-Thallium
scintigraphy or left ventricular angiography during exercise either
using contrast medium or nuclear isotopes have to rely on the presence
of high-grade, greater than 75 % obstructions in major epicardial coronary arteries, inhibiting a sufficient increase in coronary blood flow
during stress and by this resulting in ischemia. Unfortunately, in the
pre-clinical stage of silent ischemia (=ischemia only demonstrated by
ECG-changes or wall motion abnormalities during exercise, however, not
accompanied by anginal pain), these techniques have a rather low sensitivity (Table 2) and, therefore, are often not conclusive. This is
due to the fact that usually the disease is still located on a single
coronary artery (single vessel disease), often the left circumflex or
the right coronary artery being involved rather than the left anterior
descending branch. Hence, also at this pre-clinical stage of the disease, detection of the underlying coronary artery alterations by non-
invasive means is still difficult. Nevertheless, as there is a 50 %
chance for early demonstration of ischemia at least in patients with
advanced lesions, these tests should be used more frequently in the
situation of asymptomatic patients with a high risk for coronary artery disease or patients above a certain age (more than 50 years).

In the clinical stage, i.e. in the presence of <u>manifest coronary disease,</u> of overt signs of ischemia, a history of angina pectoris or myocardial infarction (= coronary heart disease), non-invasive and invasive techniques both have a high sensitivity in objectivating the disease either by demonstrating signs of ischemia or directly objectivating the underlying atherosclerotic process. However, also in this advanced stage the various techniques differ widely with regard to their sensitivity (Table 3). Furthermore, when overt signs of coronary disease are present, methods allowing its quantification are more important than those leading only to a qualitative diagnosis. If invasive therapy, that is revascularization by bypass surgery or balloon dilatation is envisaged, quantitative techniques are indispensable (see below).

Hence, at the present time, no new techniques allowing an early diagnosis of the underlying coronary process and especially leading to a quantitative judgement with regard to the extent of the disease are available. Several groups are, however, working today on improvements of angiography by digital substraction techniques in the hope to increase the sensitivity to the point where by means of intravenous injections of contrast medium the lumen of coronary arteries could be visualized to an extent allowing a precise and at least semiquantitative diagnosis. However, these techniques, though promising, are still far away from practical clinical use (BOGREN 1981, NORRIS 1982).

b) Advances in the Evaluation of Coronary Heart Disease

Recently significant advances were made both with non-invasive and invasive techniques in quantitating coronary artery disease and myocardial ischemia. The non-invasive study of left ventricular function during exercise induced ischemia, using nuclear left ventricular angiography and analyzing global and regional ejection fraction as well as wall motion, allows a precise recognition of both the location and extent of the area of ischemia and their functional consequences (BORER 1979). Left ventricular function analysis during exercise proved to be more sensitive than perfusion studies by 201-Thallium scintigraphy which, by the understanding of most investigators, is difficult to quantify with regard to the extent of perfusion defects, especially in multivessel disease (STEINGART 1982). Twodimensional echocardiography also seems to allow a fairly good analysis of the extent and location of the ischemic or infarcted area by non-invasive means. However, at the present, twodimensional echocardiography during exercise or other techniques provoking ischemia is still difficult to perform and therefore of limited use.

Coronary Angiography

Selective coronary angiography remains the most essential tool in evaluating coronary artery disease. For many years, quantification of coronary obstructions was regarded as being of little value and therefore the problem was approached only by few centers (GENSINI 1972), (RAFFLENBEUL 1975). During the last years, however, important progress was achieved in quantifying coronary obstructions employing coronary angiography. Furthermore, quantification of the size and degree of coronary stenoses as well as of the most narrow stenotic diameter has become extremely important for various reasons summarized in Table 4. Our method developed since 1974, consists in the use of a vernier caliper with an accuracy of 0.05 mm as measuring device, connected to a digital converter for reading, and to a table computer allowing calculations of the smallest diameters from various projections as well as of the degree of obstruction. Obstructions are always measured in several projections (2 to 7, average 4) using 35 mm cinefilms, projected onto the screen of a Tage-Arno projector, the tip of the catheter (approximate diameter both for the SONES and JUDKINS catheter = 1.8 mm) being used for calibration. Intraobserver variability was found to be in the range of approximately 10 %. Comparison with postmortem analysis of obstructions revealed an acceptable correlation (RAFFLENBEUL 1979). In addition, there exist today several computerized video systems where the measurement of the obstruction is fully automatic, employing either various edge detection or video techniques (BROWN 1977, REIBER 1980). The results of these systems are comparable to the direct measurements although subjected to errors often due to inadequate contrast media in the area of the stenosis. - Some of our own findings using the exact quantitation of obstructions are presented here:

## 1. Progression of Coronary Artery Disease Based on Quantitative Analysis of Obstructions

Only few prospective studies on the progression of coronary artery disease, using a quantitative approach are available (RAFFLENBEUL 1979); in contrast, most of the investigations in this field, also our earlier ones (LICHTLEN 1979), are based on qualitative, approximative assessments of obstructions and are retrospective in nature (BEMIS 1973; LICHTLEN 1979, BRUSCHKE 1981, KRAMER 1981). In a study of 25 patients with unstable angina pectoris and 69 obstructions restudied after one year, RAFFLENBEUL et al. (1979) were able to show 1. that progression occured in only 11 of 56 lesions after an interval of one year and 2. that progression to total occlusion occured in all cases with obstructions greater than 90 %, yet in only one case with a lower degree, i.e. a 60 % narrowing; patients with obstructions of less than 90 % progressed from an average of 38.6 % to 82.8 %, and 3. that 3 obstructions were newly formed from 0 to 73, 75 and 81 %. The high tendency for greater than 90 % obstructions to occlude completely within a short period of time is regarded as the result of the critical reduction in coronary blood flow, the "low flow phenomenon", due to the obstruction and in some cases the additional presence of scar tissue with a low oxygen demand, further reducing flow and by this enhancing the tendency to progressive thrombotic occlusion (for typical examples see Figures 1, 2).

## 2. Influence of Intracoronary Administration of Streptokinase on Coronary Obstructions (Fig. 3)

The reopening of thrombotically occluded arteries by intracoronary administration of streptokinase (250.000 U for one hour) with the aim to reduce infarct size has become popular during the last two years (RENTROP 1980). Here, exact measurements of the rest-occlusion are extremely helpful, especially in the decision for further surgical revascularization (FELDMAN 1981). Usually, in these cases, the most narrow diameter is below 1.5 mm and has a high tendency to reocclude.

## 3. Influence of Percutaneous Transluminal Coronary Angioplasty on Coronary Obstructions (Fig. 4)

PTCA has found a definite indication in the treatment of angina pectoris (GRÜNTZIG 1978). However, its results have to be objectivated by
exact measurements of the most narrow diameter and calculations of the
degree of obstruction before and after PTCA. Usually, clinically critical diameters, necessitating the procedure are smaller than 1.5 mm
and often dilated to 2 and more millimeters by PTCA; a further spontaneous dilatation often occurs in the following month, sometimes
leading to an almost normal situation after one year (ENGEL 1980)
(Fig. 4). Therefore, especially for PTCA objective measurements of
obstructions today are indispensable.

## 4. Influence of "Vasodilating" Drugs on Coronary Obstructions

During the last years, coronary artery spasm was found to be an important cause for angina at rest (MASERI 1977) i.e. transmural ischemia
and sometimes even of acute myocardial infarction. Extensive studies
have shown that rather than spastic occlusion an increase in vasomotor
tone takes place in the normal smooth muscle still present within eccentric obstructions, leading to further narrowing of the rest lumen.
The anatomical correlate was found in the normal wall segment of various extent, observed in eccentric obstructions by postmortem histological studies (FREUDENBERG 1981). Nitrates and especially calcium-antagonists, f.i. nifedipine, were found to be able to release the increased
vasomotor tone and to dilate eccentric obstructions to various degrees,
especially if both drugs are given simultaneously (LEUTENEGGER 1980,
RAFFLENBEUL 1980, 1982) (Figures 5, 6). Furthermore, it was found that
in patients with stable, exercise-induced angina, this increase in
vasomotor tone in high-grade eccentric coronary obstructions can persist for a long period of time (weeks to months), even in the presence
of ischemia. This indicates that profound differences must exist between the poststenotic coronary arteriolar system and the extramural
coronary artery segment with regard to their reaction to ischemia,
the latter obviously not following a feedback mechanism and not dilating during ischemia.

All these studies, especially the ones on the progression of coronary
artery disease, lead to the conclusion that basically two types of
"progression" of coronary lesions can be observed: Typ I, primary progression, takes place over months and years and represents either the
formation of new or the growth of already existing plaques through the
basic atherosclerotic process. This, as shown by angiography, can either be a continously ongoing process or one of various steps, quiescent phases being followed by phases of further rapid growth. The second type (Type II) is characterized by secondary progression which
usually takes place more rapidly, over minutes, hours or days and often
concerns the transition from a subtotal, 90 % obstruction to total
occlusion. Pathophysiologically, this often involves the formation of
a platelet thrombus provoked by the rupture of an artheriosclerotic
plaque, or a sudden increase in vasomotor tone of the remaining vascular smooth muscle within an eccentric obstruction, often also leading to secondary thrombus formation. This change in the degree of obstruction by both mechanisms most often results in attacks of transient
ischemia, clinically corresponding to the picture of unstable angina
pectoris, rather than in the development of acute myocardial infarction.

Clinically and especially angiographically it is today possible in most of the cases to distinguish between the primary and secondary progress of coronary artery disease. This distinction, however, is often of minor importance as the secondary progression often seems to enhance the primary process (Figures 1, 2), the low flow phenomenon predisposing for the progression of the underlying disease.

Hence, coronary angiography, if properly applied, contributes substantially to the understanding of the atherosclerotic process in man, especially to its evolution and correlation to the clinical aspects of the disease. Unfortunately, although several hundred thousands of patients undergo coronary angiography every year, very few studies were performed so far in this field, rendering our picture of the anatomical progression of coronary artery disease in man still very inprecise.

## References

1. Bemis CE, Gorlin R, Kemp HG, Herman MV: Progression of coronary artery disease: A clinical angiographic study. Circulation 47, 455, 1973
2. Bogren HG, Bürsch JH, Brennecke R, Heintzen PH: Intravenous angiocardiography using digital image processing: Experience with axial projections in normal pigs. Circulation 64, Suppl IV-220, 1981
3. Borer JS, Kent KM, Bacharach SL, Green MV, Rosing DR, Seides SF, Epstein SE, Johnson GS: Sensitivity, specificity and predictive accuracy of radionucleide cineangiography during exercise in patients with coronary artery disease; comparison with exercise electrocardiography. Circulation 60, 572, 1979
4. Brown BG, Bolson E, Frimer M, Dodge HT: Quantitative coronary arteriography: Estimation of dimensions, hemodynamic resistance and atheroma mass of coronary artery lesions using the arteriogram and digital computation. Circulation 55, 329, 1977
5. Bruschke AVG, Wijers TS, Kolsters W, Landmann J: The anatomic evolution of coronary artery disease demonstrated by coronary arteriography in 256 nonoperated patients. Circulation 63, 527, 1981
6. Engel HJ, Kaltenbach M, Kober G, Scherer D, Lichtlen PR: Spontaneous regression of coronary obstructions after transluminal dilatation. Circulation 62, III-159, 1980
7. Feldman RL, Crick WF, Pepine CJ, Conti CR: Quantitative coronary angiography during intracoronary Streptokinase in acute myocardial infarction: How long to continue thrombolytic therapy? Circulation 64, IV-9, 1981
8. Freudenberg H, Lichtlen PR: Das normale Wandsegment bei Koronarstenosen - eine postmortale Studie (The normal wall segment in coronary stenosis - a postmortal study). Z. Kardiol. 70, 863-869, 1981
9. Gensini GG, Kelly AE: Incidence and progression of coronary artery disease: An angiographic correlation in 1263 patients. Arch.Int. Med. 129, 814, 1972
10. Grüntzig A, Hirzel H, Gattiker R, Turina M, Myler R, Kaltenbach M: Die perkutane transluminale Dilatation chronischer Koronarstenosen. Schweiz.Med.Wschr. 108, 1721, 1978
11. Kramer JR, Matsuda Y, Mulligan JC, Aronow M, Proudfit WL: Progression of coronary atherosclerosis. Circulation 63, 519, 1981
12. Leutenegger F, Rafflenbeul W, Gahl K, Walpurger G, Engel HJ, Lichtlen P: Quantitative Koronarangiographie: Dilatation von Koronarstenosen nach Nifedipin. Schweiz.Med.Wschr. 110, 1703, 1980 (Abstr.)

13. Lichtlen P: Koronarangiographie und Prognose der koronaren Herz-krankheit. In: Koronarangiographie, edited by P. Lichtlen, Verlag Straube, Erlangen, 1979, p. 375
14. Maseri A, Severi E, L'Abbate A, Pesola A: Variant angina: One aspect of a continuous spectrum of vasospastic angina. Circulation 55/56, III-33, 1977
15. Norris S, Higgins ChB, Haigler FH, Werner FG: Comparison of intravenous versus left ventricular contrast injection on left ventricular function. Am.J.Cardiol. 49, 965, 1982
16. Rafflenbeul W, Dzuiba M, Henkel B, Lichtlen P:Morphometric analysis of coronary obstructions during life. Circulation 51/52, II-27, 1975
17. Rafflenbeul W, Lichtlen P: Intravitale Morphometrie. In: Koronarangiographie, edited by P. Lichtlen, Verlag Straube, Erlangen, 1979, p. 325
18. Rafflenbeul W, Smith LR, Rogers WJ, Mantle JA, Rackley CE, Russel RO: Quantitative coronary arteriography. Coronary anatomy of patients with unstable angina pectoris reexamined 1 year after optimal medical therapy. Am.J.Cardiol. 43, 699, 1979
19. Rafflenbeul W, Urthaler F, Russel RO, Lichtlen P, James TN: Dilatation of coronary artery stenosis after isosorbide'dinitrate in man. Br.Heart J. 43, 546, 1980
20. Rafflenbeul W, Lichtlen P, Kaltenbach M, Kober G: Zur dilatierenden Wirkung von Nitroglycerin und Nifedipin auf hochgradige Koronarstenosen. Z. Kardiol. 71, 166, 1982
21. Reiber JHC, Rafflenbeul W, Booman F, Serruys PW, Brand Mvd, Lichtlen P, Meester GT: Quantitative coronary angiography: Effect on interpretation accuracy. European Society of Cardiology, Congress VIII, Paris 1980 (Abstract)
22. Rentrop P, Blanke H, Köstering H, Karsch KR: Intrakoronare Streptokinase: Applikation beim akuten Infarkt und instabiler Angina pectoris. Dtsch.Med.Wschr. 105, 221, 1980
23. Steingart RM, Bontemps R, Scheuer J, Yipintsoi T: Gamma camera quantification of Thallium-201 redistribution at rest in a dog model. Circulation 65, 542, 1982

Table 1

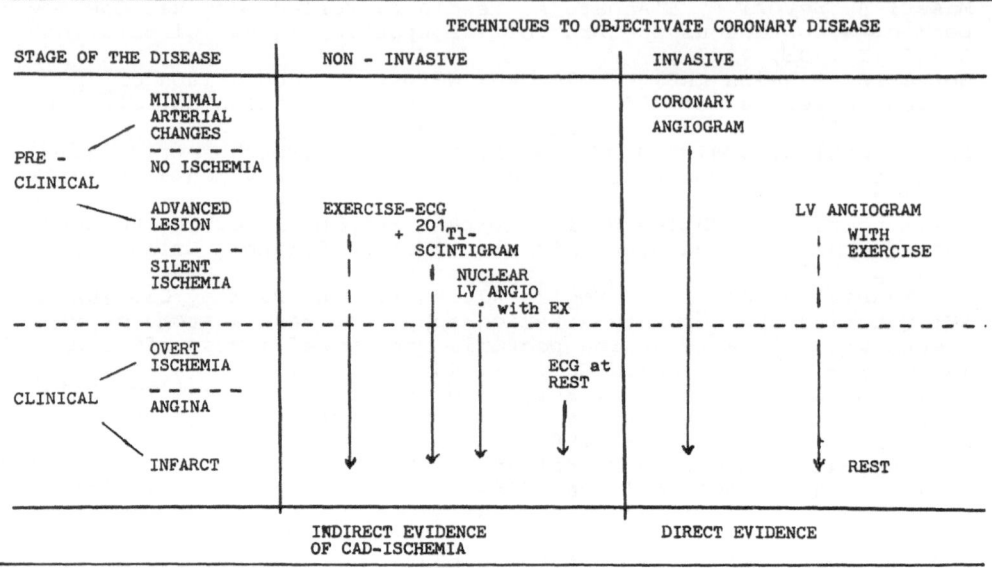

TECHNIQUES TO OBJECTIVATE CORONARY DISEASE

| STAGE OF THE DISEASE | | NON - INVASIVE | INVASIVE |
|---|---|---|---|

PRE - CLINICAL
- MINIMAL ARTERIAL CHANGES
- - - - - -
- NO ISCHEMIA
- ADVANCED LESION
- - - - -
- SILENT ISCHEMIA

CLINICAL
- OVERT ISCHEMIA
- - - - -
- ANGINA
- INFARCT

CORONARY ANGIOGRAM

EXERCISE-ECG
+ 201Tl-SCINTIGRAM
NUCLEAR LV ANGIO with EX

LV ANGIOGRAM WITH EXERCISE

ECG at REST

REST

INDIRECT EVIDENCE OF CAD-ISCHEMIA

DIRECT EVIDENCE

Table 2

DETECTION OF LATENT CAD
   SILENT ISCHEMIA
ASYMPTOMATIC PATIENTS

| TECHNIQUE | SENSITIVITY |
|---|---|
| ECG - EXERCISE - TEST | 40% |
| + 201-Tl-SCINTIGRAM | 50-60% |
| 24 HOUR AMBULATORY ECG | 30% |
| CORONARY ANGIOGRAM | 90% |
| CONTRAST - LV ANGIOGRAM | |
|      REST | 30% |
|      EXERCISE | 60% |
| NUCLEAR LV ANGIOGRAM | |
|      REST | 20% |
|      EXERCISE | 40% |

Table 3

DETECTION OF MANIFEST CAD
SYMPTOMATIC PATIENTS

| TECHNIQUE | SENSITIVITY |
|---|---|
| CORONARY ANGIOGRAPHY | 95-100% |
| ECG - EXERCISE - TEST | 75- 80% |
| + 201-Tl-SCINTIGRAM | 80- 90% |
| 24 HOUR AMBULATORY ECG | 60- 70% |
| CONTRAST - LV ANGIOGRAM | |
|      REST | 50% |
|      EXERCISE | 80- 90% |
| NUCLEAR LV ANGIOGRAM | |
|      REST | 40% |
|      EXERCISE | 60- 75% |
| ECHOCARDIOGRAPHY 2 - D | 50% |
|      M—MODE | 25% |

Table 4

QUANTIFICATION OF CORONARY OBSTRUCTIONS
WHERE TO APPLY

IN THE ASSESSMENT OF   .......

- PROGRESSION, REGRESSION OF CAD
- CHANGES AFTER "DILATING" PROCEDURES
        TRANSLUMINAL ANGIOPLASTY
        INTRACORONARY STREPTOKINASE
        DRUGS (NITRATES, CA-BLOCKERS)
- INDICATIONS FOR BYPASS SURGERY
- PHYSIOLOGY OF OBSTRUCTIONS
      SPONTANEOUS CHANGES IN VASOMOTOR TONE
      RELATION BETWEEN DEGREE OF OBSTR. and
            CORONARY BLOOD FLOW, WALL MOTION
            during ISCHEMIA etc.

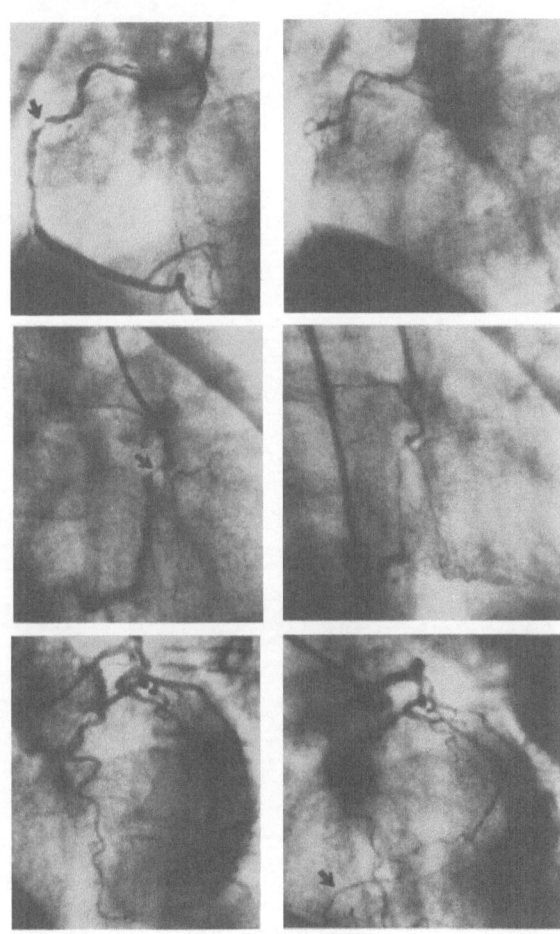

Fig. 1. Progression of CAD:
left: RCA (upper and middle
panel) March, 7, 1980, demonstrating a> 90 % proximal
obstruction (arrow) ; right:
RCA, December 22, 1980. Note
the total occlusion of the
RCA, the distal portions
being now filled through
collaterals from the LCA
(arrow) (lower panel at
right). The patient, at this
moment, experienced unstable
angina

7.3.80
♂ geb. 1923                22.12.80

20

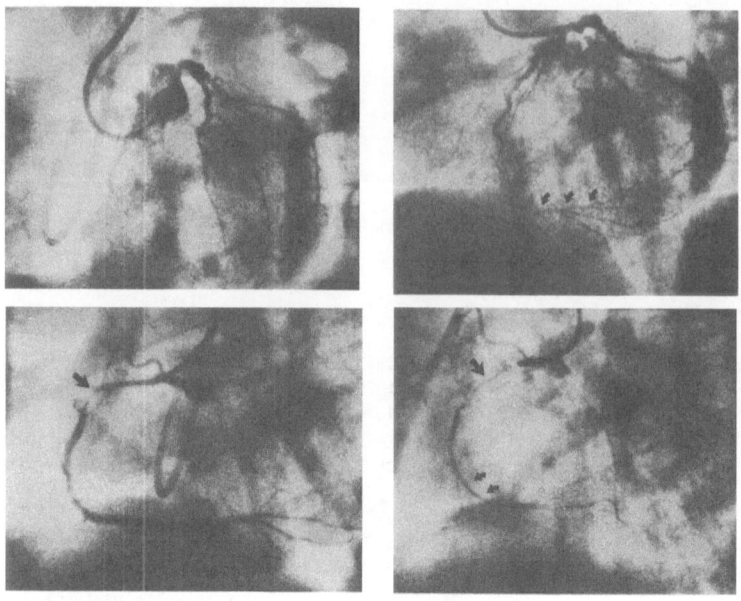

**FEBRUARY 2,1978**
**B.W., m,1936**

**JUNE 2,1982**

<u>Fig. 2.</u> Progression of CAD: Within 4 years further occlusion of the
RCA occured without a clinical correlate

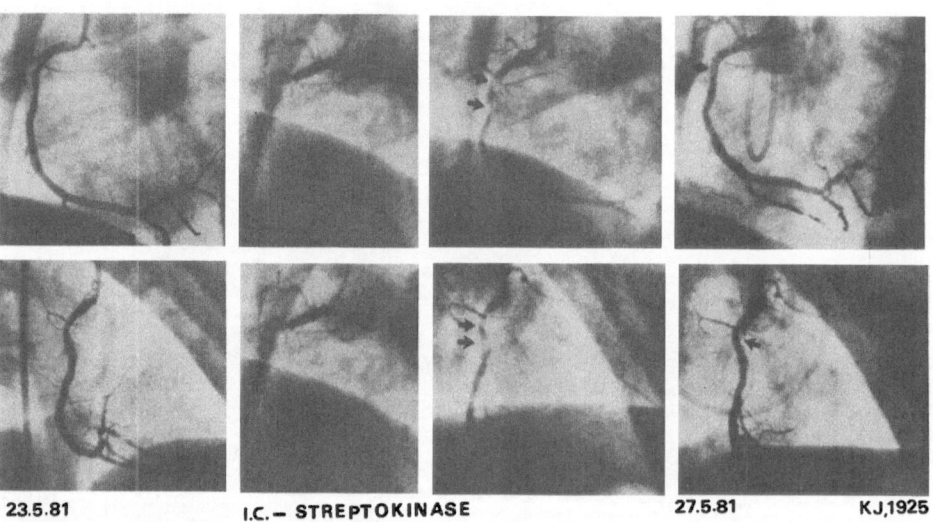

**23.5.81**          **I.C.— STREPTOKINASE**          **27.5.81**          **KJ,1925**

<u>Fig. 3.</u> Sudden occlusion of the RCA during coronary angiography
(panels on the left before and after occlusion). Immediate infusion
of 250.000 U Streptokinase led to complete reopening of the vessel.
On the beginning of intracoronary SK a typical thrombus formation
could be observed (arrows)

**PTCA** ▼                                                    PA ,1927

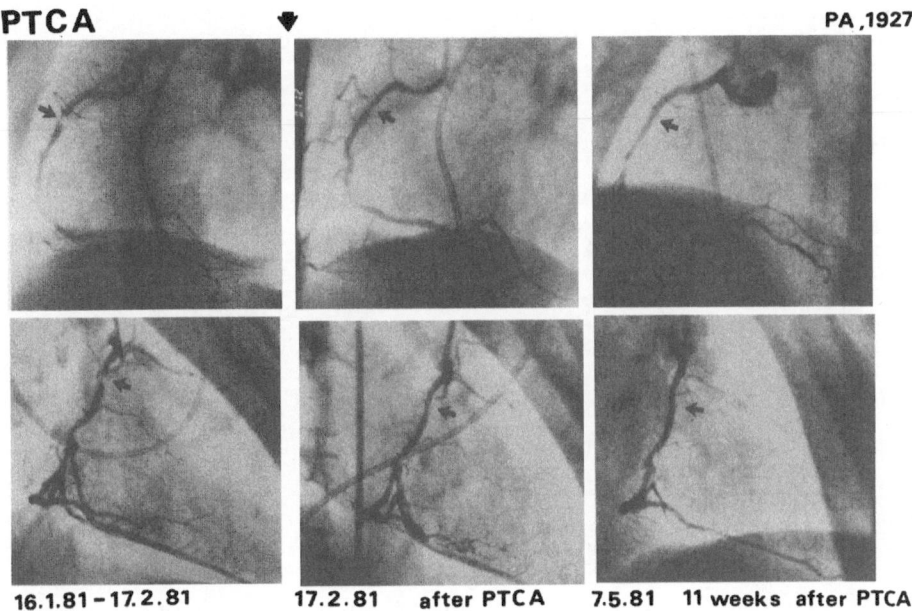

16.1.81 – 17.2.81          17.2.81   after PTCA      7.5.81   11 weeks after PTCA

Fig. 4. Balloon dilatation (PTCA) of a highgrade proximal obstruction of the RCA, panels on the left: immediately before PTCA; in the middle: after PTCA; on the right: 4 months after PTCA

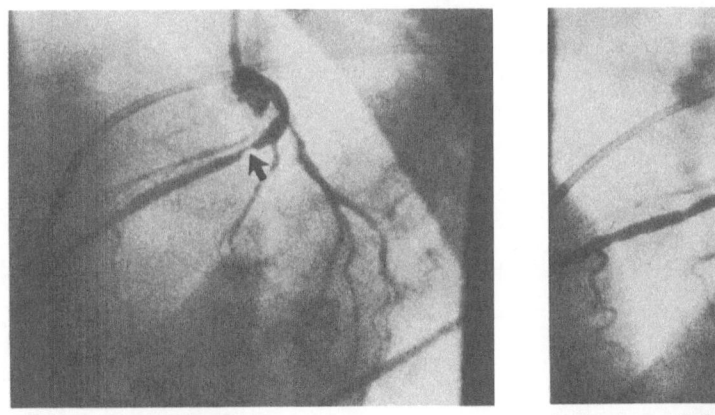

D$_{sten}$ = 1.40 mm                     D$_{sten}$ = 1.96 mm

Fig. 5. Highgrade obstruction of the proximal LAD, smallest diameter 1.4 mm (on the left). 10 min after combined administration of .8 mg NTG s.l. and 20 mg Nifedipine s.l. dilatation of the obstruction to a diameter of 1.96 mm

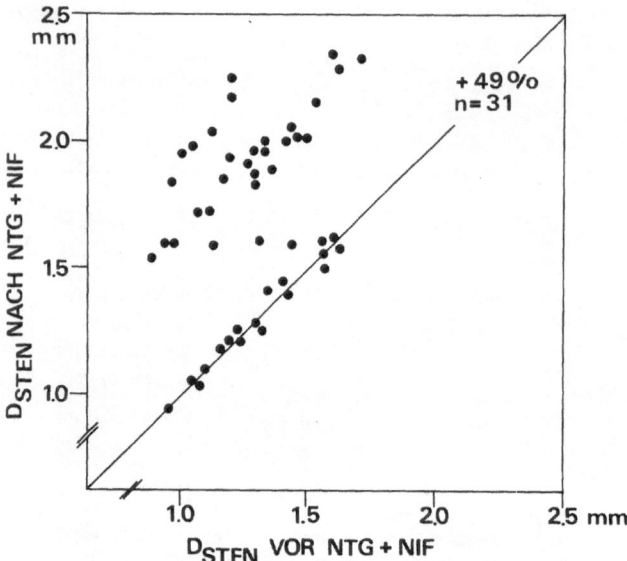

<u>Fig. 6.</u> Pharmacological dilatation of coronary stenoses by combined administration of NTG .8 mg s.l. and Nifedipine 20 mg s.l. Horizontal axis: the most narrow diameter of 50 obstructions before, vertical axis: 15 min after drug administration. Note that approx. half of the obstructions were dilated, at an average of 49 %

# Recent Advances in Diagnosis and Evaluation.
# Peripheral Artery Disease

D. H. Blankenhorn, H. P. Chin, and J. D. Hestenes

New non-invasive procedures for peripheral atherosclerosis evaluation which
are now available include ultrasound imaging, digital subtraction angiography,
and imaging with isotope labelled low density lipoprotein (LDL) or platelets (1).
These techniques provide information which cannot be obtained from traditional
procedures to assess peripheral blood flow, such as plethysmography, oscilo-
metry, rheography, phonoangiography, and oculoplethysmography. Ultrasound
imaging and digital angiography produce morphologic images of vessels and
atherosclerotic lesions. Isotope imaging with labelled LDL and platelets
probe normal and abnormal functions of the vessel wall and have great
promise for contributing to our knowledge of development of atherosclerotic
plaques.

If an arterial evaluation procedure is to be used in randomized clinical
trials or epidemiologic studies of atherosclerosis prevalence, desirable
features are:

1.  The procedure should be easy to replicate and have no cumulative toxicity.
2.  The procedure should be standardized against test objects and/or autopsy
material.
3.  The instruments should be reasonably portable and obtained at reasonable
cost.

Among the new diagnostic procedures ultrasound imaging most nearly meets
these requirements; the carotid artery is the target of choice for ultrasound imaging because it has clinical importance and is well visualized.
Two ultrasound techniques which provide carotid arterial images are widely
known. The first was developed in 1971 by Hokanson and Strandness (2). A
pulsed doppler transducer is moved in various positions along a single axis
in one plane close to the neck recording the position and range of any
ultrasound signal which detects a doppler shift. This produces a two-
dimensional map of moving blood and outlines the inner contour of blood
vessel walls. The procedure has potential for producing three-dimensional
images, but this use has not been reported. In 1972, Reid and Spencer reported a two-dimensional ultrasound imaging procedure which uses a continuous
wave doppler flow detector (3). The flow detector is moved in two directions
in a single plane near the vessel. An image is formed by recording every
point in the plane where moving blood is detected. Continuous wave doppler
flow detection is a dimensionless parameter, but three-dimensional images
could potentially be obtained by moving the detector along two perpendicular
planes. Three-dimensional procedures using this principle have been reported
for cardiac continuous wave ultrasound doppler scanning, but not for peripheral
vessels.

The procedures of Hokanson and Strandness and Reid and Spencer both involve
free motion of the scanning head. The scanning head is hand held and its
movement is recorded through a coupling arm to a motion detector. In

contrast, the three-dimensional imaging procedure developed at the University of Southern California/Jet Propulsion Laboratory (USC/JPL) uses a scanning head held by a rigid external support arm. This technique obtains reflected B-mode ultrasound images to create a three-dimensional reconstruction of vessel lumen and lesions. We currently employ a commercial production line 8-10 MHz scanner (BioDynamics Inc., Indianapolis, IN). The scanning head is held by an extension arm with two ball and socket joints which can be locked into a rigid position. We scan patients lying supine with feet elevated several degrees. This position is used to fill the jugular vein because we believe that fluid in the vein improves transmission of ultrasound energy from the scanning head to the carotid artery. The ball and socket joints are first loosened to allow the operator to move the head freely until a vessel image is located. Then the joints are fixed and a micrometer screw is used to move the head measured distances back and forth along one axis over the vessel (Figure 1).

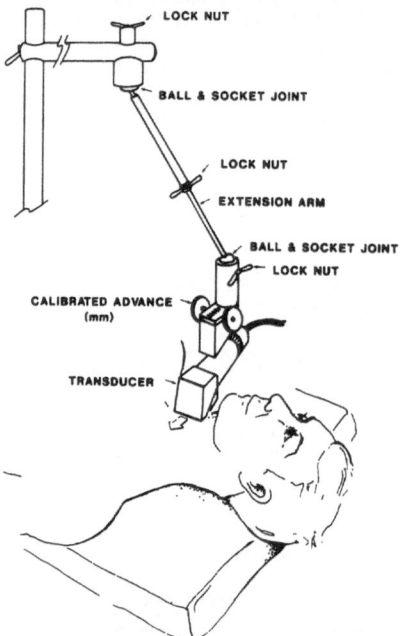

Fig. 1. Ultrasound carotid scanning procedure

A series of parallel two-dimensional images is obtained and assembled into a three-dimensional construction of the vessel with its lesions. The parallel two-dimensional image planes can be positioned either at right angles to the vessel (cross-sectional scanning) or parallel with the vessel (longitudinal scanning). A three-dimensional reconstruction is obtained from either type of scan when the three available measurements are combined. The three measurements are ultrasound azimuth, ultrasound range, and head traverse. Figure 2 illustrates cross-sectional scanning.

25

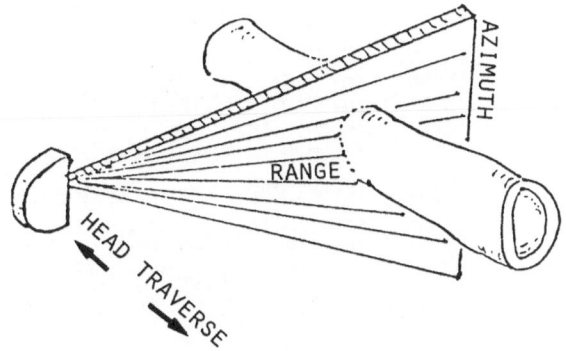

CROSS-SECTIONAL

Fig. 2. Cross-sectional ultrasound scanning

Another new feature of the USC/JPL procedure is the standardization of measurements by scanning test objects with simulated vessels of known size. Ultrasound phantoms which contain vessels 1 cm in diameter can be purchased
(Radiation Measurements Inc., Middleton, WI). In these phantoms the characteristics of ultrasound transmission through living tissue are reproduced with
a mixture of agar, propanol, and graphite. The apparent size of vessels in
an ultrasound image is influenced by many variables, including the motion of
the scanning beam, how the beam is focused, and the degree of amplification of
returned ultrasound energy. The performance of a scanning instrument can be
calibrated under conditions of use by comparing images obtained with the
size of simulated vessels in tissue phantoms. Calibration can also be based
on the micrometer scale in the head advance mechanism of the USC/JPL scanning
arm; to do this the ultrasound beam is moved through a longitudinal scan from
a position where one side of the simulated vessel just becomes visible to
a position where the opposite side of the simulated vessel just disappears.
The distance of head traverse between these two positions is compared with
known dimensions of the simulated vessel.

The precision and accuracy of the USC/JPL three-dimensional reconstruction
procedure has been tested in agar, graphite, and propanol phantoms containing
vessels with simulated lesions. For these studies the simulated vessels were
filled with thorium dioxide to make them radiopaque for exact determination
of vessel width and lesion size from contact radiograms. A phantom with two
different sized vessels and a variety of lesion shapes is shown in Figure 3.
A typical cross-sectional scan between the two arrows is shown in Figure 4,
cross-sectional images were recorded at 1 mm intervals and every fourth image
is illustrated.

Accuracy of vessel width determination by ultrasound in the phantom shown in
Figure 3 as compared with size determination by contact radiograms is given
in Table 1. Table 1 also includes estimates of the coefficient of variation
of a single measurement of vessel width as determined by each of the three
ultrasound dimensions -- range, azimuth, and head traverse. An inherent
problem in ultrasound imaging and vessel reconstruction is that the

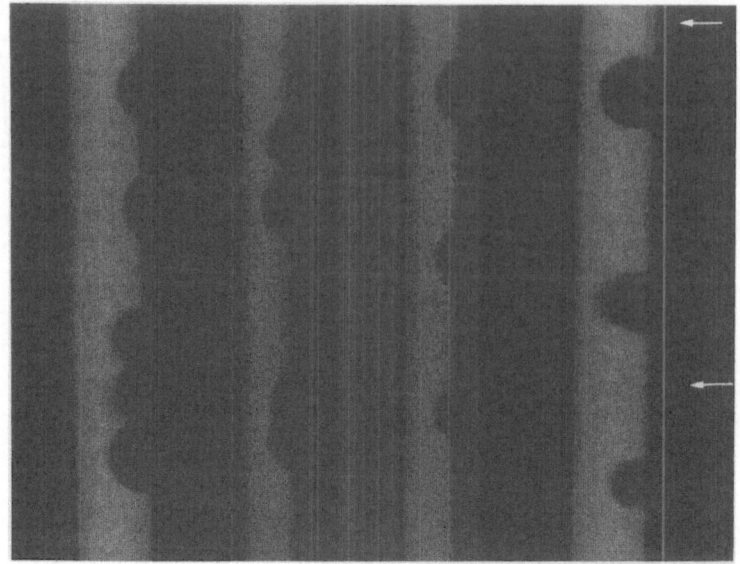

Fig. 3. Contact radiogram of an ultrasound phantom containing vessels
with simulated lesions

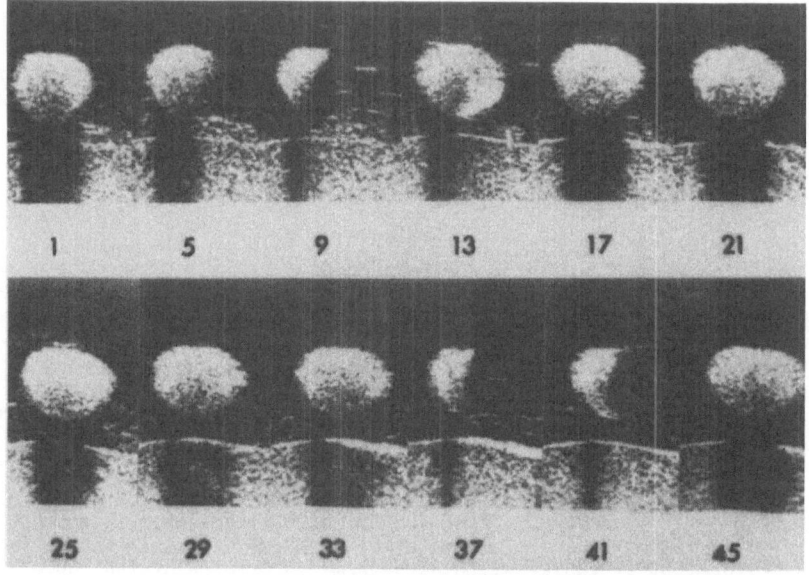

Fig. 4. A typical cross-sectional scan between the two arrows in
Figure 3

resolution of the ultrasound beam is not the same for all three dimensions. Ultrasound range measurements are more accurate than measurements made in the other two dimensions.

Table 1. Accuracy and precision of vessel width determination by ultrasound
Accuracy: Comparison with contact radiograms

|  | Large Vessel<br>mm | Small Vessel<br>mm |
|---|---|---|
| X-ray | 11.40 | 7.90 |
| Ultrasound | 11.18 | 7.89 |

Precision: Coefficient of variation of a single measurement

| Azimuth | 5.7% |
|---|---|
| Head Traverse | 4.5% |
| Range | 3.0% |

Table 2 compares ultrasound estimates of lesion size in the phantom shown in Figure 3 with estimates of lesion size made on contact radiograms. The correlation coefficient between ultrasound and X-ray estimates of lesion size is $r^2 = 0.86$.

Table 2. Comparison of lesion size estimates: Ultrasound versus contact radiograms

| Lesion | Ultrasound, mm | X-ray, mm |
|---|---|---|
| 1 | 8.05 | 8.20 |
| 2 | 4.92 | 4.10 |
| 3 | 5.82 | 6.10 |
| 4 | 5.82 | 6.80 |
| 5 | 5.27 | 5.50 |
| 6 | 4.48 | 4.50 |
| 7 | 3.58 | 4.00 |
| 8 | 5.37 | 4.90 |

The performance of three-dimensional scanning and reconstruction is now under test with tissue specimens obtained at autopsy. For this, the carotid artery, jugular vein, and sternocleidomastoid muscle are removed en bloc from a cadaver. The ends of both vessels are cannulated and major branches are ligated. The specimen is wrapped in a vinyl plastic sheath and immersed in ultrasound coupling gel. The artery is inflated to 80 mmHg pressure with saline, the vein is inflated to approximately 30 mmHg. Under these conditions, cross-sectional and longitudinal scans which are quite similar to scans obtained in living subjects can be obtained. Vessels in these specimens can be made to pulsate, but our current studies are made with no vessel motion. Our preliminary results suggest that a single measurement of vessel width in tissue specimens may have a coefficient of variation between 5 and 10 percent and a single measurement of lesion size a coefficient of variation between 10 and 15 percent. The images used for these estimates have been obtained with a production model scanner which is also in daily use for routine clinical examination of patients. The performance of the scanning head and of the signal processing electronics have not been specially tuned. We believe measurements made after specially tuning the scanner would show improved precision. We also feel that redesign of our extension arm could improve the precision of measurements.

Our current procedure for reconstructing carotid profiles in living subjects where pulsation changes vessel size is to measure maximum size during arterial systole. This is a first approach to the problem and does not take advantage of information which is potentially available from study of vessel wall motion. Our images are recorded on video tape and we observe them frame by frame to find maximum vessel size. Vessel pulsation in many patients has at least two components -- a lateral expansion and a simultaneous cephalad thrust. We are assembling a timing device which records the electrocardiogram on video tape with vessel images and plan to study vessel motion by constructing a series of vessel profiles during cardiac systole and diastole.

Our experience with carotid ultrasound scanning in living subjects is principally in men known to have coronary atherosclerosis because they have required coronary artery bypass surgery. Later, at this Symposium, Dr. Azen will describe the USC randomized angiographic study of lipid lowering in men who have had coronary bypass surgery. We scan the right carotid artery in these patients and compare results with carotid angiograms obtained by an aortic arch injection at the time of coronary angiography. All subjects are men between 40 and 59 years of age who are non-smokers or ex-smokers. In 108 consecutive men, scanned by the same operator, right carotid lesions were visible in 46. This experience is in agreement with the distribution of atherosclerosis found at autopsy (4,5,6). There is significant correlation between the degree of involvement of cervical and cerebral vessels with the amount of coronary atherosclerosis found at autopsy. The first appearance of raised carotid lesions is delayed until after the first appearance of raised coronary lesions, but when this lag is taken into account, coronary atherosclerosis and carotid atherosclerosis progress in parallel.

*Acknowledgments.* The authors wish to acknowledge and thank the following individuals for their assistance in this work. Sipke Strikwerda, Joyce C. Pinckard, and C. Joan Darnall.

This work was supported by NHLBI Program Project Grant HL 23619.

## References

1. Noninvasive Diagnosis of Atherosclerotic Lesions: Quantitative Evaluation of Morphology, Biochemistry, and Pathophysiology. Bond MG, Insull W Jr., Glagov S, Cornhill JF, Chandler AB (editors) Springer-Verlag, New York, publishers, in press
2. Hokanson DE, Mozersky D, Sumner DS, Strandness DE Jr. (1971) Ultrasonic arteriography: A new approach to arterial visualization. Biomed Eng 6: 420
3. Reid JM, Spencer MP (1972) Ultrasonic doppler techniques for imaging blood vessels. Science 176: 1235-1236
4. Solberg LA, McGarry PA (1972) Cerebral atherosclerosis in Negroes and Caucasians. Atherosclerosis 16: 141-154
5. Sternby NH (1968) Atherosclerosis in a defined population. An autopsy survey in Malmo, Sweden. Acta Path Microbiol Scan Supplementum 194
6. Young W, Gofman JW, Tandy R, Malamud N, Waters ESG (1960) The quantitation of atherosclerosis III. The extent of correlation of degrees of atherosclerosis within and between the coronary and cerebral vascular beds. Am J Card 6: 300-308

# Atherosclerosis.
## Recent Advances in Diagnosis and Evaluation – Cerebrovascular Disease

J. Marshall

Atheroma of the cerebral circulation and of its major arteries of supply is a frequent cause of stroke and transient ischaemic attacks (TIAs). For this reason these events are often used as measures of atheroma. This paper poses the question, 'Is this approach justified?' 'Is the incidence of strokes and the increasing or decreasing frequency of TIAs an adequate measure of atheroma in the cerebral arteries? If it is not, what alternatives have we?'

## Atheroma and completed strokes

Pathological observations lead us to equate cerebral haemorrhage with hypertensive vascular disease which produces fibrinoid necrosis of arterioles and the formation of miliary aneurysms of Charcot-Bouchard type. Cerebral infarction on the other hand is usually thought to be associated with thrombosis which in turn takes place against a background of atheroma. Distinction between haemorrhage and infarction as a cause of stroke would therefore be a first step towards evaluation of atheroma. Unfortunately as DALSGAARD-NIELSEN[1] showed many years ago this differential diagnosis when based on clinical criteria alone is very unreliable. He followed 1000 cases of stroke to autopsy and found that the clinical diagnosis of haemorrhage was confirmed in only 65 per cent and of infarction in only 58 per cent.

Happily CT scanning has dramatically changed this. Haemorrhage can be distinguished from infarct with complete confidence providing - and this is an important proviso - the scan is performed at the correct time. Because of the high density image caused by blood haemorrhage can be detected immediately after its occurrence; the earliest an infarct can be seen is about 6 hours after onset and many will not become apparent until 24 hours. If a positive diagnosis is wanted, rather than an assumption that there must be an infarct because of the absence of blood, scanning must be delayed for 24 to 48 hours. Likewise after 10 to 14 days it may be very difficult to determine whether an abnormality is a resolving haemorrhage or infarct. Serial scanning during the first two weeks has shown that haemorrhage and infarct may become indistinguishable from about 10 days onwards. However if these limitations of time are borne in mind it is now possible to distinguish haemorrhage from infarction with a high degree of confidence.

Though certain diagnosis of infarction by CT scan has been a major advance recent pathological observation has somewhat diminished its importance vis a vis atheroma. Large cerebral infarcts were generally accepted as being the result of thrombosis, this in turn being a consequence of atheroma. Pathological studies[2,3,4] have shown that as many as 45 per cent or more of large cerebral infarcts may be embolic in origin. The emboli may in some instances arise from atheromatous lesions in proximal large vessels and travel distally to occlude a vessel and so be some reflection of atheroma. But in many instances the emboli come from the heart and from lesions in the heart which were not associated with atheroma.

In this context there have been tremendous developments in cardiology, the end result being that a wide spectrum of cardiac conditions which may give rise to cerebral emboli is now recognized. Cardiomyopathy, atrial myxoma, prolapsed mitral valve and various forms of dysrhythmia are now recognized to be capable of producing emboli. Hence recognition of cerebral infarction albeit with great confidence in the CT scan cannot be taken as a good measure of the presence or progress of atheroma.

There is one type of infarct - the lacunar infarct - which, as a result of a series of careful studies by MILLER FISHER[5] was previously thought to be closely related to hypertensive vascular disease and so not to be a marker for atheroma. However a recent CT scan study of lacunar infarcts showed that lacunes may also be associated with emboli.  In a series of 312 stroke patients, 37 had presented with a clinical picture usually associated with a lacunar infarct; in 18 of the 37 the lacune was demonstrated on the CT scan.  Whilst many of the patients were hypertensive, some were not and there were possible sources of emboli present.[6] A lacune cannot therefore be taken as necessarily indicative of hypertensive vascular disease, some may be embolic.  The fact that a lacune is embolic does not mean it is a consequence of atheroma; some embolic infarcts will be associated with atheroma, some will not.

## Atheroma and transient ischaemic attacks

If strokes cannot readily be equated with atheroma what of transient ischaemic attacks (TIAs)?  Here again there has been a tendency to equate TIAs with atheroma of the internal carotid artery.  The association is frequent but by no means exclusive.  If we leave aside diagnostic difficulties posed by migraine with marked vasospastic manifestations but little headache, sensory focal epilepsy and by the fact that neoplasms may present with transient focal neurological deficits there are still formidable problems in correlating TIAs with atheroma.

When interest in TIAs was first aroused it was thought that they were due to haemodynamic changes.[7]  This was subsequently shown not to be the case[8] and that the majority are caused by emboli of various kinds arising from atheromatous lesions at the origin of the internal carotid artery.[9]  Nevertheless, haemodynamic TIAs do occur and must be taken into account.  Then there are general causes of TIAs such as anaemia, polycythaemia and cardiac dysrhythmia. TIAs may also occur in the premalignant phase of hypertension.

There are therefore a number of possibilities apart from atheroma.  Even when atheroma is present and responsible, the actual mechanism of the TIAs is more related to thrombus formation with embolisation which in turn may reflect changes in the coagulation and fibrinolytic systems of the blood rather than changes in the atheroma.  Waxing and waning of TIAs is not therefore a good measure of atheroma.

## Multi-infarct dementia

Dementia in older age groups was commonly thought to be the result of ischaemia, the term cerebral arteriosclerosis frequently being used as a clinical diagnosis. As with stroke so with dementia, diagnostic difficulties abound.  Clinico-pathological studies[10,11] have shown that the commonest cause of dementia in later life is Alzheimer's disease which can occur in both the presenium and senium.  The general attribution of dementia in later life to ischaemia was not therefore justified.

In those whose dementia is on a vascular basis the relationship to atheroma is tenuous.  The striking pathological change in this type of dementia is a multiplicity of small infarcts.  Cerebral blood flow (CBF) though slightly reduced, is not profoundly depressed.[12]  Moreover, CBF can be increased by increasing $pCO_2$ indicating that the arteries are not so 'hardened' as to be incapable of responding.  For these reasons the term multi-infarct dementia was coined[13] to express better the underlying problem.  This type of change is usually associated with hypertensive vascular disease rather than with atheroma.

## The clinical assessment of cerebral atheroma

The evidence so far presented indicates that the clinical end-points stroke, TIAs or the development of multi-infarct dementia are not reliable measures of cerebral atheroma. Diagnostic difficulties in each of these categories is the first source of inaccuracy. Even when the phenomenon is correctly diagnosed it may be associated with vascular disturbance other than that caused by atheroma.

This does not mean that nothing can be gleaned clinically about the presence or absence of cerebral atheroma. Some assessment can be made first by the absence of hypertension in what is clearly a cerebrovascular event. This negative evidence makes it more likely that the event is associated with atheroma. Secondly, repeated events such as TIAs, provided a non-atheromatous cardiac source of trouble has been carefully excluded by appropriate means, are likely to be associated with atheroma.

A more positive indication of cerebral atheroma is provided by the presence of a bruit over the origin of the internal carotid artery. There are other sources of bruits in the neck but the clinical characteristics of a carotid bruit are well defined and not easily confused. This remains the best clinical measure of atheroma.

## Investigations

Because of the unreliability of clinical measures of cerebral atheroma investigative procedures play an important role in the assessment.

### Cerebral angiography

First among these is cerebral angiography which provides a picture of the carotid, vertebral and intracranial vessels and will demonstrate occlusion, stenosis, irregularities and ulceration. Magnification angiograms can provide a wealth of detail. The problem about routine use of angiography to diagnose and assess cerebral atheroma is that it is invasive and carries a morbidity in the form of strokes and even on occasion mortality. The risks of angiography in skilled hands is small but cannot be ignored. Angiographic investigation on one occasion or sometimes on more than one occasion can be justified and is indeed required in order to manage the patient. Repeated angiography to assess the progress of atheroma could not be justified.

This difficulty may be solved by the introduction of Digital Vascular Imaging. With this technique contrast medium is injected intravenously thus avoiding the major source of hazard namely intra-arterial catheterisation. Adequate images are obtained by digital subtraction of the films. The toxic effects of contrast medium will remain but these are minimal and it seems likely that serial studies of patients will become possible.

### Doppler studies

A non-invasive technique which has proved of value is the use of the Doppler effect. As originally employed it proved reliable in detecting occlusion and severe stenosis of the carotid artery.[14,15] Lesser degrees of stenosis were not detectable. A more sophisticated Continuous Wave (CW) Doppler Technique with spectrum analysis of the signals and real time B-scan imaging promises to give a detailed assessment of the state of the neck vessels. With this technique the incidence of asymptomatic extracranial disease has been assessed,[16] an important factor which hitherto escaped the clinical net. In a series of 604 patients good correlation between CW Doppler and angiography was obtained in 97 per cent. There is no hazard to the procedure which does not take long to perform and promised to be a valuable method of assessing serially atheroma of the carotid arteries in the neck.

## Radioactive isotope imaging

Another promising development has been to label fibrinogen and study its uptake
in the neck. Its incorporation into the thrombus on plaques at the origin of
the internal carotid artery can be recorded by a radioactive imaging technique.
Its serial use would be limited by the need to avoid excessive radiation but
the technique promises to have a role in the assessment of carotid atheroma.[17,18]

## Conclusion

It must be recognized that the diagnosis and evaluation of cerebral atheroma is
as yet very imperfect. The relative inaccessibility of the vessels involved
makes the task more difficult than in the peripheral circulation. Likewise,
the frequency of alternative vascular pathology makes the problem more complex
than in the coronary circulation. Clinical assessment gives only the crudest
estimate. Investigative procedures are more informative but limited at present
by risk but recent developments suggest that these difficulties may well be
overcome.

## References

1 Dalsgaard-Nielsen T  (1956) Some clinical experience in the treatment of cerebral
  apoplexy (1000 cases).  Acta psychiat Scand Suppl 108: 101-19
2 Blackwood W, Hallpike JF, Kocen RS, Mair WGP (1969)  Atheromatous disease of the
  carotid arterial system and embolism from the heart in cerebral infarction: a
  morbid anatomical study.  Brain 92: 897-910
3 Jorgensen L, Torvik A (1966)  Ischaemic cerebrovascular diseases in an autopsy
  series.  Part I. Prevalence, location and predisposing factors in verified
  thrombo-embolic occlusions, and their significance in the pathogenesis of
  cerebral infarction.  J neurol Sci 3: 490-509
4 Jorgensen L, Torvik A (1969)  Ischaemic cerebrovascular diseases in an autopsy
  series.  Part 2. Prevalance, location, pathogenesis and clinical course of
  cerebral infarcts.  J neurol Sci 9: 285-320
5 Fisher CM (1965)  Lacunes: small, deep cerebral infarcts.  Neurology (Minneap)
  15: 774-84
6 Nelson RF, Pullicino P, Kendall BE, Marshall John (1980)  Computed tomography in
  patients presenting with lacunar syndromes.  Stroke 11: 256-61.
7 Denny-Brown D, Meyer JS (1957)  The cerebral collateral circulation. 2. Production of cerebral infarction by ischemic anoxia and its reversibility in
  early stages.  Neurology (Minneap) 7: 567-79.
8 Kendell RE, Marshall J (1963)  Role of hypotension in the genesis of transient
  focal cerebral ischaemic attacks.  Brit med J 2: 344-8.
9 Gunning AJ, Pickering GW, Robb-Smith AHT, Ross Russell R (1964)  Mural thrombosis
  of the internal carotid artery and subsequent embolism.  Quart J Med 33: 155-95.
10 Corsellis JAN (1962)  Mental illness and the ageing brain.  Oxford University
  Press, London
11 Tomlinson BE, Blessed G, Roth M (1970)  Observations on the brains of demented
  old people.  J Neurol Sci 11: 205-42
12 Hachinski VC, Iliff LD, Zilkha E, Du Boulay GH, McAllister VL, Marshall J,
  Ross Russell RW, Symon L (1975)  Cerebral blood flow in dementia.  Arch Neurol
  32: 632-7.
13 Hachinski VC, Lassen NA, Marshall J (1974)  Multi-infarct dementia.  A cause of
  mental deterioration in the elderly.  Lancet ii: 207-10.
14 Maroon JC, Campbell RL, Dyken ML (1970)  Internal carotid artery occlusion
  diagnosed by Doppler ultrasound.  Stroke 1: 122-7.

15 Muller HR (1973) Directional Doppler senography. A new technique to demonstrate flow reversal in the ophthalmic artery. Neuroradiology 5: 91-4.
16 Hennerici M, Aulich A, Sandmann W, Freund H-J (1981) Incidence of asymptomatic extracranial arterial disease. Stroke 12: 750-8.
17 Mettinger KL, Ericson K, Larsson S, Casseborn S (1978) Detection of atherosclerotic plaques in carotid arteries by the use of $^{123}$I-fibrinogen. Lancet i: 242-244.
18 Davis HH, Siegel BA, Joist JH, Heaton WA, Mathias CJ, Sherman LA, Welch MJ (1978) Scintigraphic detection of atherosclerotic lesions and venous thrombi in man by indium-III-labelled autologous platelets. Lancet i: 1185-1187.

# Clinical Aspects of Atherosclerosis. Role of Coronary Artery Spasm

M. E. Bertrand

Over the past several years, pathological and pathophysiological studies suggested that fixed coronary artery stenosis due to atherosclerosis were responsible
for myocardial ischemia and infarction. Most physicians had been taught in medical school that the coronary narrowing was the cause of angina and that pain occured as a result of an imbalance of myocardial oxygen supply and demand. However in the 18's many authors have postulated that spasm was the likely cause of
angina. In fact, like many concepts in medicine the idea of spasm, once popular, was subsequently rejected and is now being rediscovered. In 1959 Prinzmetal (1) revived interest in coronary artery spasm when he described a group
of patients with "variant angina" and postulated that this clinical syndrome
could be related to an increased vascular tonus superimposed on fixed proximal
atherosclerotic narrowing. In 1962 Gensini (2) was able to document the appearance of spontaneous coronary artery spasm. Subsequent developments including
coronary arteriography, hemodynamic and electrocardiographic monitoring, isotope studies provided important evidence concerning the existence of coronary
artery spasm in man. Maseri and colleagues (3) have provided very elegant physiopathologic investigations in patients with angina at rest. These developments have implicated coronary artery spasm in the pathophysiology of many
other ischemic syndromes in addition to Prinzmetal's variant angina. More recently provocative testing (4-7) provided some more lights on the possible role of
coronary spasm in heart disease in general.

## Definition - Characteristics and frequency of coronary arterial spasm

Coronary arterial spasm could be defined as a transient reversible total or subtotal occlusion of a major epicardial coronary artery associated with objective
evidence for myocardial ischemia. Most often the spasm is recognized during coronary arteriography and the angiographical criterias have been edicted in 1975
by Chahine (8) : (1) Appearance of transient narrowing in a coronary segment
that initally or subsequently appeared to be angiographically normal. (2) Occurrence of transient total obstruction in a normal coronary segment or at the site of a partial atherosclerotic narrowing. (3) Prompt response of the narrowing
or obstruction to the administration of nitroglycerin or its spontaneous relief, documented upon subsequent arteriograms.

Cather induced spasm (located within 1 or 2 cm of the catheter tip) is usually
considered as a iatrogenic phenomenon resulting of the contact of the catheter
with arterial wall. However some authors considering the incidence of associated spontaneous spasm, suggested that it may indicate a predisposition to spasm

Usually spasm involves only one vessel (92.1 %). The right coronary artery is
the most common location (50.3 %) followed by the left anterior descending coro
nary artery (31 %) and the circumflex branch (10.3 %). Moreover spasm can involved 2 or even the three main coronary branches. Usually, spontaneous spasm
is not frequently observed during coronary arteriography (18.8 % in a personal
serie of 165 cases of documented spasm). This results of the standard coronary
angiography techniques reducing the likehood of spasm (vasodilator effects of
contrast media, premedication or nitroglycerin given routinely or at the begin-

ning of the procedure). This leads to the development of various provocative testing (ergonovine maleate, cold pressor test, alkalinisation, etc...). The most utilized is the ergonovine or ergometrine provocative test and Curry et al. (9) have demonstrated the similarities of spontaneous and ergonovine provoked coronary artery spasm.

The wide use of this test has allowed Bertrand et al. (7) to perform a kind of epidemiological study and to establish the frequency of coronary arterial spasm in a group of 1 089 patients undergoing coronary arteriography (the patients with several vessel disease i.e. left main stenosis or severe triple vessel obstructions or heart failure were excluded).

Table 1 . Frequency of provoked spasm in 1 089 consecutive patients undergoing coronary arteriography

| Group | n | Vessel disease | | | | Spasm |
|---|---|---|---|---|---|---|
| Atypical chest pin | 248 | 221 | 22 | 5 | | 3(1.2 %) |
| Exert AP | 117 | 23 | 38 | 26 | 30 | 5(4.3 %) |
| AP ou effort at rest | 138 | 58 | 22 | 34 | 24 | 9(13.8 %) |
| AP at rest | 203 | 93 | 55 | 29 | 26 | 7(38 %) |
| Recent M.I. | 116 | 7 | 54 | 31 | 24 | 3(20 %) |
| "Old" M.I. | 64 | 3 | 26 | 20 | 15 | 4(6.2 %) |
| Valvular dis. | 154 | 132 | 16 | 5 | 1 | 3(2 %) |
| Cardiomyopathy | 49 | 44 | 4 | 1 | | 0(0 %) |
| | 1089 | 581 | 237 | | 120 | 134 |

Table 1 demonstrated that the incidence of false positive tests in control group (patients with valvular disease or cardiomyopathy) is very low. The frequence of coronary spasm in patients with exertional angina pectoris was very low and was not significantly different from the control group. However if angina on effort was associated with episodes of pain at rest the frequency reached 14 %. The highest incidence of coronary arterial spasm was observed in patients who complained of angina pain at rest and in patients with asymptomatic, recent ( 6 weeks) transmural myocardial infarction (20 %). In patients (n = 78) with angina at rest and ST segment changes during the attacks (ST or ST or T wave changes) spasm was documented in 60 cases (77 %) and mainly in patients with Prinzmetal's variant angina (85 %). In asymptomatic patients with recent transmural myocardial infarction coronary spasm was demonstrated in 10 % on the infarction related vessel and in 10 % on another vessel. Finally if one consider the incidence of coronary artery spasm in a group of 462 patients with significant vessel disease but without evidence of Prinzmetal's variant angina the incidence of spasm was 11.7 %.

II Clinical syndromesin which coronary artery spasm may be involved

    A -  Ischemic heart disease.

The role of spasm had to be discuss in angina pectoris, myocardial infarction and sudden death. Table 2 summarizes our experience and shows the clinical expression of 165 cases of angiographically documented coronary spasm. Most often the patients were admitted in the hospital with the diagnosis of angina at rest, alone or associated with exertional angina pectoris.

Table 2 . Clinical syndromes in 165 patients with documented coronary arterial spasm

|  | n | % |
|---|---|---|
| Angina at rest | 92 | 55.7 % |
| Angina at rest and on effort | 37 | 22.5 % |
| Myocardial infarction | 23 | 14 % |
| Syncopes | 6 | 3.6 % |
| Exertional angina | 5 | 3 % |
| Atypical chest pain | 2 | 1.2 % |
| Total | 165 |  |

## 1. Angina pectoris at rest

In this section, one can describe a first group of patients with the syndrome delineated by Prinzmetal. This syndrom consisted of generally severe chest pain at rest, unrelated to effort, and associated with ST-segment elevation. Dysrythmias especially ventricular can occur and in many instances patients have thought to have a myocardial infarction. However, spontaneously or with the treatment, E.C.G. changes and pain disappeared. A large serie of studies led to the conclusion that coronary arterial spasm in Prinzmetal's angina was a "proved hypothesis" (Meller) (10) and spasm can be detected in 87 to 92 % of cases of variant angina.

However Maseri (1) came to the conclusion that variant angina represents only one extreme aspect of a continuous spectrum of acute vasospastic myocardial ischemia. In the Maseri's (11) view, vasospasm can also be demonstrated during episodes of pain at rest with ST segment depression or T wave changes. The direction of the ST segment changes appears only to indicate the degree of ischemia related to different severity and extension of vasospasm. However it is unclear if rest angina associated with only ST-segment depression is also due to spasm. Some patients of the Maseri's series had either ST segment elevation or ST segment depression but the extrapolation of these observations cannot be done to patients with only ST segment depression. Continuous hemodynamic monitoring demonstrated that some of these patients have no change in hemodynamic determinants of myocardial oxygen consumption before the onset of ischemic E.C.G. changes (implying a mechanism of spasm) but some others patients increased these determinants of myocardial oxygen consumption. In our experience provoked spasm was induced in only 47 % of patients with ST segment depression during pain at rest. Thus it is clear that rest angina associated with ST segment elevation is due to spasm but the role of spasm in angina at rest with only ST-segment depression is not certain.

## 2. Exertional angina pectoris

Usually exertional angina is considered as resulting of an increase in myocardial oxygen demand above the supply allowed by atherosclerotic narrowings. However, Angoli (12), Yasue (13) presented evidence of coronary artery spasm during angina on effort. Yasue (13) observed that coronary artery tone was high in the early morning in opposition to a low vasomotor tone in the afternoon.

In fact, if the concept of effort angina entirely related to increased myocardial oxygen requirements should be reassessed, the incidence of spasm in a large population is low. Thus, we have observed only a very small incidence of provoked spasm in a large group of patients with exertional angina pectoris alone (7). We can suspect the role of spasm in exertional angina pectoris in the fol-

lowing conditions. (1) High sensitivity to cold (2) Large variations of the
threshold of ischemia during repeated exercises (3) ST segment elevation in the
abscence of previous myocardial infarction (4) ST segment elevation during the
exercise recovery (5) Walk through phenomenon.

## 3. Myocardial infarction

Previous studies presented evidence suggesting a role for spasm in the pathophysiology of myocardial infarction : Maseri et al. (14) noted that in a group of
187 patients with angina at rest, 37 had myocardial infarction in the same area
corresponding to previous E.C.G. changes during resting angina attacks. Moreover in 6 patients with recurrent angina at rest, where infarction occurred immediately after (n = 4) or during hemodynamic or angiographic studies, the onset
of the infarction could not be discerned from a usual attack. Prinzmetal's variant angina, where spasm is the most important factor is complicated by myocardial infarction in a rate of 10 to 38 %.

During the acute phase of myocardial infarction, Oliva and Breckenridge (15) have been able to reopen 40 % of the occluded vessels by intracoronary injections
of nitroglycerin in a group of 12 patients who were studied within twelve hours
after the onset of infarction. More recently, Rentrop (16) in a group of 29 patients with evolving myocardial infarction who underwent intracoronary thrombolysis was able to relieve vasoconstriction or spasm in 5 cases (17 %), the total occlusion, being transformed into narrowing by injection of nitroglycerin.
However Mathey (12) observed this phenomenon in only one out of 41 cases.

Recent studies by Dewood (18) demonstrated that in the first hours of myocardial infarction, there is a very high percentage of total occlusion. Thus, 87.3
% of the vessels related to the area of the infarction were totally occluded
within the 4 first hours. This percentage declines to 85.3 % between 4 ans 6
hours and to 65 % during the period of 12 to 24 hours. In an earlier study of a
group of patients who underwent coronary arteriography at an average of 16 days
after infarction, we noted that 56 % of patients had total occlusion of the corresponding vessel. Thus, these changes observed during the acute phase of myocardial infarction could be related either to the recanalization of a thrombus or
to the relief of a severe spasm superimposed on an organic narrowing. In fact,
these two mechanisms could be interrelated. One patient of Maseri et al. (14)
developped infarction and died shortly after the coronary angiography which documented coronary spasm. The autopsy showed a fresh thrombus at the site of the
spasm. In animals, Folts et al (15) demonstrated a cyclic decrease of coronary
flow induced by platelet agregation on a stenosis. More recently, Gertz et al.
(20) have demonstrated that partial constriction of a coronary artery could result in endothelial cell damage and subsequent thrombosis. Thus a vicious circle could be established involving coronary spasm, endothelial cell damage and
thrombosis with platelet agregation and the released thromboxane $A_2$ sustaining
the cycle.

## 4. Sudden death

It is well known that patients with Prinzmetal's variant angina can have episodes of complete heart block, ventricular tachycardia and fibrillation. Thus it
is not unreasonable to assume that coronary artery spasm could lead to sudden
death. Curry (21) and Conti have suggested that the risk of sudden death could
reach 21 % of the patients with Prinzmetal's angina. Conti observed 5 episodes
of cardiac arrest in a total of 36 patients with proved coronary artery spasm
who were followed for 1-30 months. It is very difficult to assess the exact in-

cidence of spasm in the pathogenesis of sudden death but this mechanism should not be underestimated.

B - Association of peripheral vasospasm and coronary arterial spasm

Some authors have pointed out that coronary artery spasm could be associated with peripheral vasospasm. Arciniegas (22) observed that Raynaud's phenomenon was more frequent in a group of patients with ergonovine induced spasm than in other patients. However Raynaud's phenomenon is only observed in 5.5 % of our patients with documented spasm. Some authors have also brought attention to the association with headache and eclampsia (23).

C - Nitrate withdrawal in munitions workers

Lange (24) et al. reported 9 cases of ischemic heart disease non related to atherosclerosis following withdrawal from chronic industrial nitroglycerin exposure. One patient died and 4 others had clinical evidence of myocardial infarction without evidence of coronary artery disease. The authors assumed that chronic vasodilatation could lead to homeostatic vasoconstriction inducing ischemia during withdrawal period.

III Relationship between atherosclerosis and coronary artery spasm

In 57.6 % of our 165 cases, coronary spasm occurred and was superimposed on a site of preexisting organic stenosis. In 40 % spasm was observed on a "angiographically" normal vessel. In fact these data are biased by inclusion of patients with mild grade (25-30 %) of organic narrowing or small irregularities. The consistent occurence of spasm in the vicinity of atherosclerotic lesions (Mc Alpin (25) sharpens the focus on the intimate association between the fixed lesions and coronary artery spasm. Thus, figure 1 offers a schematic representation of the contribution of coronary atherosclerosis and coronary spasm to myocardial ischemia. At one end are the patients with severe fixed organic atherosclerotic narrowing. The major mechanism for ischemia is the unability of the vessels to supply the myocardial oxygen demand (Secondary angina pectoris (26).

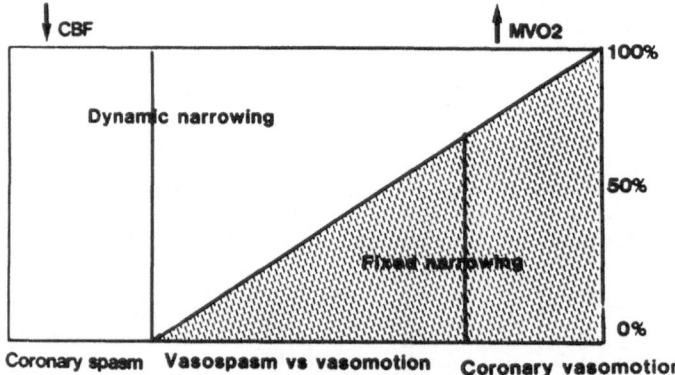

Fig. 1

At the other extreme are the patients with normal or near normal coronary arteries. Angina, in these patients, occurred as a result of coronary artery spasm decreasing coronary blood flow ((primary angina pectoris). The patients in the mid part of the diagram have either severe or moderate fixed organic narrowing with superimposition of various degrees of excess coronary vasomotion. The mechanism for ischemia combine increased myocardial oxygen demand and decreased coronary blood flow secondary to excessive vasomotion. This classification has not only been of pathophysiological interest but also has therapeutic implications because certain drugs (betablockers) used routinely may not always be appropriate.

Just before to conclude, it is also interesting to note that some authors postulate an evolutionary relationship between coronary spasm and fixed coronary atherosclerosis. Marzilli and colleagues (29) suggested that coronary artery spasm could be a possible antecedent leading to the later development of fixed atherosclerotic coronary arterial obstruction. This provocative theory opens new avenues for investigating atherosclerosis but the paucity of direct evidence requires further confirmation.

Conclusions : Over the past ten years it has been demonstrated that coronary artery spasm may have a far more important role in the pathogenesis of ischemic heart disease than was previously thought possible. However there is a great deal of speculation but little data to document the pathophysiologic mechanisms triggering the spasm and this opens a large and fascinating view for clinical and experimental research.

## References

1. Prinzmetal M, Kenamer R, Merliss R, Wada T, Bor N (1959) Angina pectoris I - A
   variant from of angina pectoris. Preliminary report. Am. J. Med. 27 : 375-388
2. Gensini GG, Di Giorgi S, Murao Netto S (1962) Arteriographic demonstration of coronary artery spasm and its release after the use of a vasodilatàtor in a case of angina pectoris and in the experimental animal. Angiology 13 : 550-553
3. Maseri A, Nimmo R, Chierchia S, Marchesi C, Pesole A, l'Abbate A (1975) The ergoCoronary artery spasm as a cause of acute myocardial ischemia in man. Chest 68 625
4. Heupler F, Proutfit W, Siegel W, Shirey E, Razavi M, Sones M (1975) The ergonovine maleate for the diagnostic of coronary spasm. Circulation 51, suppl. 2, 11
5. Bertrand ME, Rousseau MF, Lablanche JM, Warembourg Jr H, Carre AG, Lekieffre J, (1979) La détection du spasme des artères coronaires par le test à la méthylergométrine. Technique, Résultats. Indications. Arch. Mal. Coeur 72 : 123
6. Bertrand ME, Lablanche JM, Tilmant PY (1980) Use of provocative testing in angina pectoris. Herz 5 : 65
7. Bertrand ME, Lablanche JM, Tilmant PY, Thieuleux FA, Delforge MR, Carre AG, Asseman Ph, Berzin B, Libersa C, Laurent JM (1982). Frequency of provoked coronary arterial spasm en 1 089 consecutive patients undergoing coronary arteriography. Circulation 42 : 605
8. Chahine RA, Raizner AE, Ishimori T, Luchi RJ, Mc Intosh MD (1975) The incidence and clinical implications of coronary artery spasm. Circulation 52 : 972.

9. Curry JR, Pepine CJ, Sabomi MB, Conti CR (1979). Similarities of ergonovine induced and spontaneous attacks of variant angina. Circulation 59 : 307
10. Meller J, Pichard A, Dack S (1976) Coronary arterial spasm in Prinzmetal's angina. A proved hypothesis. Am. J. Cardiol. 37 : 938
11. Maseri A, Severi S, De Nes M, L'Abbate A, Chierchia S, Marzilli M, Ballestra AM, Parodi O, Biagini A, Distante A (1978) "Variant" angina : One aspect of a continuous spectrum of vasospastic myocardial ischemia. Pathogenetic mechanisms. Estimated incidence and clinical and coronary arteriographic findings in 138 patients. Am. J. Cardiol. 42 : 1 019.
12. Angoli L, Marinoni GP, Palcone C, Bramucci E, De Servi S, Specchia G, Montemartini C (1977) Spasme coronaire à l'effort. Démonstration coronarographique d'un cas. Arch. Mal. Coeur 71 : 823.
13. Yasue H, Omote S, Takizana A, Nagao M, Miwa K, Tanaka S (1979) Exertional angina pectoris caused by coronary arterial spasm : effects of various drugs. Am. J. Cardiol. 43 : 647.
14. Maseri A, L'Abbate A, Baroldi G, Chierchia S, Marzilli M, Ballestra AM, SeveriS, Parodi O, Biagini A, Distante A, Pesola A (1978) Coronary vasospasm as a possible cause of myocardial infarction : a conclusion derived from the study of pre-infarction angina. N. Engl. J. Med. 299 : 1271-77.
15. Oliva PB, Breckinridge JC (1977)Arteriographic evidence of coronary arterial spasm in acute myocardial infarction. Circulation 56 : 366-74000.
16. Dewood MA, Sporess J, Notske R, Mouser MT, Burroughs R, Galden M, Lang HT (1980). Prevalence of total coronary occlusion during the early hours of transmural myocardial infarction. N. Engl. J. Med. 303 : 897-903.
17. Rentrop P, Blanke H, Karsch KR, Kaiser H, Kostering H, Leitz K (1981). Selective intracoronary thrombolysis in acute myocardial infarction and unstable angina pectoris. Circulation 63 : 307-17.
18. Mathey DE, Kuck KH, Tilsner V, Krebber HJ, Bleifeld W (1981). Non surgical coronary artery recanalization after acute transmural myocardial infarction. Circulation 63 : 489-97.
19. Folts JD, Crowell EB, Rowe GG (1976). Platelet aggregation in partially obstructed vessels and its elimination with aspirin. Circulation 54 : 365-70.
20. Gertz SD, Vretsky G, Wainberg S, Navot N, Gotsman MS (1981). Endothelial cell damage and thrombus formation after partial constriction : relevance to the role of coronary artery spasm in the pathogenesis of myocardial infarction. Circulation 63 : 476-86.
21. Curry RC Jr, Pepine CJ, Feldman RL, Whittle JL, Conti CR (1980). Frequency of myocardial infarction and sudden death in 44 variant angina patients. A high risk ischemic heart disease subset. Proc. of VII European Congress of Cardiol. Paris p. 6.
22. Arciniegas J, Little WC, Coghlan HC, Russell RO, Rackley CE, Mantle JA (1981). Coronary artery spasm : an isolated phenomenon or one manifestation of a more diffuse hyperreactivity (abst.). Am. J. Cardiol. 47 : 450.
23. Bauer TW, Moore GW, Hutchins GM (1982). Morphologic evidence for coronary artery spasm in eclampsia. Circulation 65 : 255.
24. Lange R, Reid M, Tresch D, Keelan M, Bernhard V, Coolidge G (1972). Non atheromatous ischemic heart disease following withdrawal from chronic industrial nitroglycerin exposure. Circulation 46 : 666.
25. Mc Alpin R (1980). Coronary arterial spasm to sites of organic narrowing. Am. J. Cardiol. 46 : 143.
26. Maseri A, Severi S, Chierchia S, Parodi O, Biagini A (1978). Characteristics and pathogenetic mechanism of "primary" angina at rest. In "primary and secondary angina pectoris". (Maseri A, Klassen GA, Lesch M édit.) Grune et Stratton, New York, p. 265.
27. Marzilli M, Goldstein S, Trivella M, Palumbo C, Maseri A (1980). Some clinical considerations regarding the relation of coronary vasospasm to coronary atherosclerosis. A hypothetical pathogenesis. Am. J. Cardiol. 45 : 882.

# Conservative Treatment of Coronary Heart Disease

W. Kübler

For the medical treatment of coronary heart disease - i.e. unsufficient myocardial oxygen supply - 3 groups of drugs are nowadays widely used: nitrates, beta-blocking agents and calcium antagonists.

For coronary dilators, such as e.g. dipyridamole, which increase coronary blood flow in a dose dependent manner, no therapeutic benefit has been demonstrated. These drugs induce a reduction of vascular component of coronary resistance. This, however, is in an ischemic myocardial area already at its lowest level as hypoxia is the strongest stimulus for coronary dilatation (for references see KÜBLER 1969, 1).

The drugs effective in angina act predominantly by reduction in myocardial energy demands.

## 1. The nitrates

The drugs most widely used for the interruption of an anginal attack are the nitrates. They reduce myocardial oxygen consumption due to a decrease in preload achieved by venous pooling and due to a less pronounced reduction in afterload. In addition the nitrates improve especially subendocardial perfusion, which is predominantly affected during an anginal attack. This is achieved by reduction in extravascular or myocardial component of coronary resistance and by dilatation of large so-called "conductance" arterioles (2, 3), which predominantly regulate subendocardial blood flow. In contrast to coronary dilators, such as dipyridamole, small arterioles are not affected by nitrates.

The beneficial effects of nitrates in treating angina is, therefore, explained by the combination of reduction in myocardial energy demands and increase in perfusion, especially in the subendocardial layers.

## 2. The beta-blocking agents

In contrast to the nitrates, which predominantly act on the peripheral circulation, the beta-blockers act on the myocardium itself by inhibition of sympathetic activity, i.e. by a negative chronotropic and negative inotropic effect.

Among the beta-blockers different groups can be differentiated: $beta_1$-blocking agents, with some cardioselectivity, and non-selective beta-blocking agents acting on both $beta_1$- and $beta_2$-receptors. Some beta-blockers have intrinsic sympathomimetic activity leading - apart

---

[1] Own investigations mentioned in this paper were performed with support from the Deutsche Forschungsgemeinschaft, Bad Godesberg - within the SFB 90 - cardiovascular system - University of Heidelberg

from the inhibiting effect – to some stimulation of beta-receptors. In addition to specific binding to the beta-receptors non-specific binding sites exist, which, however, are only saturated with doses usually not reached under clinical conditions.

The cardioselective beta$_1$-blockers are preferentially recommended for diabetics, as the antihypoglycaemic effect of catecholamines is still preserved, and for patients with obstructive airways disease, as the bronchi are predominantly supplied with beta$_2$-receptors. The difference between beta$_1$- and beta$_2$-blocking agents, however, is only relative and, therefore, great care is necessary, if beta-blockers are used under these conditions mentioned above.

Beta-blockers with intrinsic sympathetic activity are especially recommended for patients with bradycardia and/or conduction defects. Generally, however, the beta-blocking quality overcomes intrinsic sympathetic activity, so that again great care is mandatory.

Newer findings of our group (4) indicate, that some beta-blockers, such as sotalol, have additional group III antiarrhythmic effects, in otherwise therapy-resistant cases these beta-blockers may well be of special use in the treatment of supraventricular and especially of ventricular tachyarrhythmias.

Beta-blockers block by definition beta-receptors, which are coupled via the coupling factor to the enzyme adenylate-cyclase, which ultimately catalyzes the formation of the second messenger c-AMP. This receptor-enzyme-system is modulated by several factors, such as e.g. GTP/GDP, which act on the coupling factor. Beta-blockers, too, modulate this system by increasing the number of beta-receptors. Sympathetic overactivity observed in some patients after acute beta-blocker withdrawal can be attributed to this increase in receptors. Hence, withdrawal of beta-blockers should be achieved, if possible, stepwise.

Beta-blockers are competitive inhibitors, their action depends on the ratio of beta-blocker concentration to noradrenaline concentration in the synaptic cleft. Under clinical conditions the action of beta-blockers can easily be evaluated by determination of the inhibition of the increase in heart rate and/or blood pressure during exercise or during the administration of beta-stimulants. Using the bicycle stress test it could be shown that the inhibitory effect of beta-blockers on the rise in heart rate stays constant, whereas the inhibitory effect on exercise induced rise in systolic blood pressure decreases with time (5). This is most likely due to counteraction by other pressure systems, allowing in practice a marked reduction in heart rate without pronounced fall in blood pressure and coronary perfusion pressure in the normotensive.

From these data it follows, that the instantaneous action of beta-blockers depends: 1. on the drug concentration at the receptor site, 2. on the sympatho-neuronal and sympatho-adrenal activity, 3. on the number of beta-receptors present, 4. possibly on the modulation of the receptor-adenylate-cyclase complex and 5. on the counteraction, especially by other pressor systems.

## 3. The calcium-antagonists

This new group of drugs acts by inhibition of the slow inward current (6), i.e. the $Ca^{2+}$-inward or in some tissues the slow $Na^+$-current. The calcium-antagonists, therefore, reduce heart rate, they depress conduction in the A-V node. On the myocardium the calcium-antagonists have a mild negative inotropic action. The coronary arteries are dilated, this applies less to the arterioles but more to the large epicardial vessels, on which a predominant spasmolytic effect is exerted. Hence, the calcium-antagonists are drugs of choice for the treatment of spastic PRINZMETAL- or variant angina. Due to relaxation of smooth muscles the calcium-antagonists induce a slight reduction in preload and in afterload.

Probably due to reduction in blood pressure via stimulation of the baroreceptor reflex sympatho-neuronal activity is increased which counteracts the reduction in heart rate, the negative inotropy and the reduction in blood pressure.

The action of the calcium-antagonists is probably not yet fully understood, there are marked differences between different drugs: whereas e.g. verapamil has a marked effect in reducing heart rate and A-V conduction, this effect is not present for nifedipine under therapeutic dosages (7).

These differences, which might be attributed to different affinities to different sites of the calcium-channel, have serious clinical implications: Verapamil is the drug to interrupt A-V nodal reentry tachycardia, whereas nifedipine has no effect. Nifedipine, on the other hand, has a synergistic effect to beta-blockers in treating angina, whereas the combination of beta-blockers and verapamil can induce serious side-effects.

Apart from the administration of drugs the non-surgical treatment of coronary heart disease has been extended by 2 new methods:
- angioplasty of coronary stenosis, and
- reperfusion of infarcting myocardium by reopening of the occluded coronary vessel due to intracoronary application of streptokinase.

## Percutaneous transluminal coronary angioplasty (PTCA)

By application of a balloon catheter, developped by GRÜNTZIG (8) localized coronary stenoses can be dilated, in this way myocardial oxygen supply is improved.

Till now, the following results could be obtained: About 1500 interventions were registered by the National Institute of Health, the successrate is about 60 - 80 %. Fatal complications occurred in 16 cases = 1 %. Myocardial infarcts were observed in 2 % of all cases. Recurrence of the stenosis within 1 year occurred in about 15-20 %. In most of these cases, however, a successful second angioplasty is possible.

## Intracoronary thrombolysis in acute myocardial infarction

The beneficial effects of percutaneous transluminal coronary angioplasty can be easily documented by coronary angiography and/or exercise testing. The results obtained by reperfusion due to intracoronary thrombolysis in acute myocardial infarction, however, are more difficult to evaluate. The main aim of this procedure does not consist solely in the reopening of an occluded vessel, but in salvage of infarcting, jeopardized myocardium. In this way early and late prognosis of the patient could be improved due to reduction in infarct size.

In order to demonstrate in an individual patient a reduction in in-farct size due to successful intracoronary thrombolysis, in own experiments tomographic Tl.-scintigrams were obtained immediately before the intervention and after 24 hrs. In this way after success-ful thrombolysis an almost complete normalization of the preexisting myocardial perfusion defect could be demonstrated, whereas in pa-tients with an unsuccessful thrombolytic intervention or a too long ischemic period the myocardial perfusion defect was virtually un-changed.

In order to evaluate the factors, which might be responsible for a beneficial effect of this procedure - i.e. salvage of infarcting myocardium - the patients were allocated to 3 groups:

Group A: patients with successful thrombolysis and a peak plasma CK-activity ≤1000 IU.

Group B: patients with successful thrombolysis and a peak plasma CK-activity >1000 IU.

Group C: patients with unsuccessful thrombolysis

In group A with successful thrombolysis plasma CK-activity is by definition only moderately elevated. The scintigraphic Tl-perfusion-defect is significantly reduced, and regional ejection fraction in the infarcted area significantly increased. Also global ejection fraction is significantly augmented, indicating a good functional result.

In group B, also with successful thrombolysis but high plasma CK-activity, there is a small also significant reduction of the Tl-per-fusion-defect, but no significant change in regional ejection frac-tion of the infarcted area and in global ejection fraction.

In group C, with unsuccessful thrombolytic intervention, high plas-ma CK-activities were observed, but as may be expected, no change in the Tl-perfusion defect and in the regional or global ejection fraction.

The 2 groups with successful thrombolysis: group A with good func-tional result and group B with questionable result differ in the extent of ischemic damage, which had occurred in the myocardium and which depends on:

1. The ischemic period - defined from the beginning of symptoms up to re-opening of the occluded coronary vessel. This ischemic period is significantly shorter in group A compared with group B.

2. Compared with group B in group A significantly more collaterals can bei observed, which supply the infarcting myocardial area. In this way the tolerable ischemic period of infarcting myocar-dium is prolonged.

This can be explained by biochemical findings obtained in ischemic canine hearts. Under conditions of still maintained coronary per-fusion, although unsufficient to cover oxygen demands, i.e. low flow ischemica, the myocardial energy deficit - characterized by the breakdown of the high energy phosphates CP and ATP - develops more slowly compared with conditions of total or stop flow ische-mia (9).

As the salvage of myocardial tissue by thrombolytic reperfusion depends on both, the ischemic period and the presence of collaterals, no fixed time limit for thrombolytic therapy in acute myocardial infarction can be given. In practice, however, beyond an ischemic period of 4 - 6 hrs a satisfactory functional result cannot be expected. In the various studies on the effect of systemic thrombolysis in acute myocardial infarction this critical time lag  has been greatly exceeded with 12 - 72 hrs (10).

Up to the 31st December 1981 in 9 out of 50 patients with successful thrombolysis a reocclusion of the vessel supplying the infarcting area could be observed. This reocclusion rate of about 20 % would favour early revascularisation of the reopened but still stenosed coronary artery either by bypass- surgery or by angioplasty.

As revascularisation should only be performed when viable myocardial tissue is present in the poststenotic myocardial area, the following criteria can be considered as arguments for early revascularisation: Recurrence of anginal pain, no Q-waves in the ECG, only moderate elevation of CK-activity in plasma ($\leqslant$1000 IU), marked reduction in the Tl-perfusion-defect.

As revascularisation of irreversibly damaged myocardial tissue or even of scar tissue cannot be recommended, it should not be performed under the following conditions: no further anginal pain, marked Q-waves with loss of R-waves in the ECG, marked elevation of plasma CK-activity ($>$1500 IU) and no reduction of the Tl-perfusion-defect.

In our own series up to the 31st of December 1981 thrombolysis in acute myocardial infarction was successful in 70 %. Early revascularisation either by angioplasty or by bypass-surgery was performed in about 30 % of these patients. The hospital mortality was extremely low in the groups with successful thrombolysis, independent whether early revascularisation or only medical treatment were performed with no death during the first 4 weeks. It has, however, to be mentioned, that hospital mortality in the group with unsuccessful thrombolytic intervention reached the rather high value of 27 %. Therefore, the favourable result in the groups with successful thrombolysis can be due to the intervention itself and to some selection of patients with better prognosis.

## In conclusion

Also the clinical cardiologists have achieved some progress during the past years: A better understanding of the mode of action of antianginal drugs contributes to the safety of the treatment and to a more rational and more effective approach based on a better insight into the underlying mechanisms of coronary heart disease.

Percutaneous transluminal coronary angioplasty and intracoronary thrombolysis in acute myocardial infarction offer new perspectives in the conservative treatment of coronary heart diesease.

References

1. Kübler W (1969) Tierexperimentelle Untersuchungen zum Myokard-
   stoffwechsel im Angina-pectoris-Anfall und beim Herzinfarkt.
   Bibliotheca Cardiologica No. 22, Karger, Basel, New York
2. Tillmanns H, Steinhausen M, Leinberger H, Thederan H (1979)
   Different response of the ventricular microcirculation to coronary vasodilators. Circulation 59/60 Suppl. II, 11-142
3. Tillmanns H, Leinberger H, Thederan H, Steinhausen M (1980)
   Einfluss von Nitroglycerin auf die Mikrozirkulation des Katzen-
   und Rattenherzens. In: Lichtlen P, Engel J (Eds.) Nitrate III.
   Urban und Schwarzenberg, München, p. 119
4. Senges J, Lengfelder W, Jauernig R, Czygan E, Rizos J, Cobbe S,
   Kübler W (1982) Differenzierte Wirkung der Betablocker Sotalol
   und Metroprolol bei Patienten mit chronisch rezidivierenden
   ventrikulären Tachykardien. Ztschr. Kardiol. 71 (in press)
5. Krämer B, Krämer G, Hausen M, Mäurer W, Kübler W (1981) Beziehung
   zwischen ß-Blockerkonzentration im Plasma und Plasmakatechola-
   minen bei ergometrischer Belastung. Ztschr. Kardiol. 70:275 (P75)
6. Fleckenstein A (1977) Specific pharmacology of calcium in myocardium, cardiac pacenmakers, and vascular smooth muscles. Ann.
   Rev. Pharmacol. Toxicol. 17:149
7. Jauernig R, Senges J, Rizos J, Anders G, Uckuns F, Kübler W
   (1981) Unterschiedliche Wirkung der Ca-Antagonisten Verapamil,
   AQ-A 39 und Nifedipin bei AV-junktionaler Reentry-Tachykardie.
   Ztschr. Kardiol 70:294 (P144)
8. Grüntzig A (1976) Perkutane Dilatation von Koronarstenosen. Be-
   schreibung eines neuen Kathetersystems. Klin. Wschr. 54:543
9. Kübler W (1974) Glycolytic pathway in the myocardium. In: Muir
   JR: Prospects in the management of ischaemic heart disease.
   Ciba-Symposium p. 161
10. Kübler W, Röhrig D, Schuler G, Schwarz F (1982) Der akute Myo-
    kardinfarkt. Grundlagen der medikamentösen Therapie. Verh. Dtsch.
    Ges. Inn. Med., in press

# Conservative Treatment of Peripheral Artery Disease

A. Kappert

## A. Introduction

From the historical point of view many errors in the concepts of
treatment of peripheral arterial diseases have to be noted. They are
based on uncomplete knowledge about the pathophysiology of oblitera-
tive arteriopathies of the extremities and on misinterpretation of
the pharmacological effects. Forty years ago and in the following decades an analysis of the peripheral blood flow under clinical conditions was not possible. Thermometric methods were widely in use, but
gave only a limited information over the skin circulation. It could
even happen that the sensation of heat after the intraarterial injection of calcium was interpretated as a marked improvment of the peripheral blood flow. But it has to be said that even in our days the
analysis of drug effects on the arterial circulation of the limbs is
still a difficult task.

Ever since the introduction of vasoactive drugs in the treatment of
arterial occlusive diseases, consideration of their efficacy has been
based on the law of HAGEN-POISEUILLE (HAGEN 1839, POISEUILLE 1846).
This law maintains that blood flow through an artery is directly related to the perfusion pressure in the vessel and to the radius in
its fourth power; the flow rate is in inverse proportion to the length
of the artery, viscosity, and factor 8

$$Q = \frac{r^4 \cdot P \cdot \pi}{l \cdot \eta \cdot 8}$$

Fig. 1. Law of Hagen-Poiseuille: Q = Blood flow, r = Radius of the
vessel, P = Perfusion pressure, l = Length of the vessel, $\eta$ = Viscosity of the blood, $\pi$ = Constant

It seems logical that an augmentation of the radius would have marked
effects on a pathologically reduced blood flow, and to this end many
vasodilating drugs have been introduced over the years. From the beginning some authors have been sceptical about the effectiveness of
such drugs, and it was debate on this point which lead GILLESPIE
(1967) to write of "the use and abuse of vasodilators". The complexity of the pathophysiology of obliterating arteriopathies causes many
difficulties including the phenomenon of hemometakinesis and various
forms of steal effects. Today the use of vasodilators in arterial occlusive diseases is usually confined to stage II (according to the
classification of FONTAINE (1980), a stage characterized by intermittent claudication, and they are best prescribed in combination with

exercise.

In the last ten years, interest in the evolution of the medical treatment of arterial occlusive diseases has focussed on the viscosity factor of the law of HAGEN-POISEUILLE. Analysis of the microcirculation
has brought many important facts to light, and, in the field of rheo-
logy, microrheology has gained increasing theoretical and practical
importance. It is indeed clear that the flow properties of blood have
a great influence on arterial circulation. Four parameters are of particular importance: the flexibility of the red cells, the viscosity of
the plasma, the viscosity of the whole blood, and the aggregation tendency of the platelets.

The program for the conservative treatment of peripheral arterial disease depends of the stage of the clinical manifestations of the vascular alterations according to the four stages of FONTAINE: Stage I:
asymptomatic, detected by imaging methods like arteriography and ultrasonic tomography, auscultation and Doppler analysis ecc. Stage II:
dominated by the symptom of intermittent claudication; here several
diagnostical procedures are standardizised and serve also as parameters for the efficacy of the used treatment: determination of the
claudication distance, oscillography at rest and after exercise, measurement of the systolic ankle pressure at rest and after exercise,
determination of the pressure gradient arm - ankle, values of the segmental oscillography and the pulse volume recorder ecc. - Stage III:
rest pain and beginning trophic changes of the skin. - Stage IV: necrosis and gangrene.

I. <u>Stage I</u>: The symptomless stage I of peripheral occlusive arterial
diseases is seldom an indication for a systematic treatment. The exploration of one lower extremity, e. g. after a trauma, may show by
a vascular imaging technique like arteriography the existence of
plaques and stenoses without hemodynamic consequences. In such a case
a program which should stop the further evolution or even forces the
regression of the vascular alterations is indicated. It concerns mainly the elimination of risk factors. For arteriopathies of the limbs,
smoking is in first position. It is well known that in Buerger's disease the vascular progress can really "burn out" after complete stop
of smoking. In arteriosclerosis the effects may be less impressive.
But a rigorous program with elimination of other risk factors like
hypertension and hyperlipidemia, systematic treatment of diabetes,
infections, overweight and physical inactivity and perhaps reduction
of platelet aggregation may at least stabilize the hemodynamic conditions. The disapparance of plaques is possible but the application of
drugs for such a mean is still in the experimental phase. Under the
program outlined above between 60 - 85 % of the patients may show a
stationary state or even an improvement 3 - 6 years after the discovery of the disease. The risk of later amputation in such patients is
not higher than 1 - 2 % per year. (KANNEL and SHURTLEFF 1971).

II. <u>Stage II</u>: In a case of intermittent claudication in stage II a
(walking distance higher than 50 - 100 m) systematic walking training
including special exercises like knee bending ecc. is the base of the
treatment. Here again the whole program mentioned above including the
elimination of the risk factors is essential. Favourable results may

be seen in 82 % of cases at early or moderate stage II. At later stage II a stabilization of the situation is possible in 69 % (CLOAREC 1981). In stage II b with a claudication distance under 50 m a combination with a rheologically active drug like pentoxyfilline, isoxsuprine, cinnarizine and bencyclane is recommended (DORMANDY 1981). The controversal opinions about the efficacy of vasodilators has be mentioned before. In stage II b the indication for angioplasty or reconstructive surgery may be evaluated if the clinical course shows a trend for progression of the disease. The natural history depends although on the site of the lesions. A distal process, alone or in combination with proximal stenoses or obliterations is especially dangerous. Here a continous careful hemodynamic control is very important.

III. <u>Stage III</u>: The pain at rest forces the patient to spend a part of the night out of bed. During the day the symptom of intermittent claudication with a rather short claudication distance of 50 to 100m or less may be of minor importance. Beginning trophic changes of the skin and the nails may show the danger of necrosis or gangrene. Good care to the feet which evitates any traumatisation by pressure of the shoes, manipulation on corns ecc., application of aggressive ointments ecc. is very important to prevent those events. Even small surgical interventions may turn the situation to stage IV with necrosis and gangrene. An interdigital mycosis has to be treated. The skin care includes daily cleaning and application of talk powder. Exposition to cold or heat has to be avoided. Both factors may provoke an ischemic reaction with subsequent necrosis. During the night the feet should be placed low to facilitate blood perfusion. Slight exercises in bed to stimulate reactive hyperemia are allowed but forced walking and other formes of physical training are contraindicated. Analgetic drugs are sometimes unevitable but morphine and similar agents have to be excluded. One of the rheologically active agents is indicated. Vasodilators are contraindicated. Some authors applie intraarterial infusions in the femoral artery with 250 to 500 ml of rheomacrodex and triphosadenine combined with adapted exercise under the supervision of a trained physiotherapist.

With the beginning of resting pain a first period of bed rest over two to three weeks may be helpful. During this time a careful exploration has to decide if a surgical reconstructive intervention, a sympathectomy or an angioplasty have to be performed. It has to be repeated that surgery has no place in stage II eccept with a very short claudication distance of 50 and less. Systematic treatment of heart insufficiency, diabetes and other risk factors is essential. Special therapeutical approaches like hemodilution and artificial hypertension are only indicated in cases which resist to the program described here. They are discussed below. Anticoagulants although have a very small place in stage III like in cases of arterio-arterial emboli.

IV. <u>Stage IV</u>: In Stage IV necrosis and gangrene are the dominant problems beside resting pain and practical minimal walking distance. The treatment is mostly a combination of surgical intervention and conservative measures which are described under stage III. Infected necroses and gangrene need antibiotics locally and systematically. They may be added to intraarterial infusions with rheomacrodex and tri-

phosadenine (antibiogram!). Bed rest is compulsery. There are specific indications for anticoagulants (ectatic-aneurysmatic arteririosccle-
rosis with arterio-arterial emboli, by-pass-operations, fibrinolysis,
stenosis of critical sites like popliteal artery, combination of coronary heart disease with peripheral alterations on multiple levels) and
inhibitors of platelet aggregation (endarterectomy and angiplasty, essential thrombocytosis). Those methods are called secondary prophylaxis compared with the primary prophylaxis against risk factors. - Prostacycline is still in the experimental phase.

The local treatment includes wet dressings with methylene blue, chlo-
razodine ecc. and application of powders with trypsine, miconazole,
clotrimazole ecc. Small surgical interventions to clean the necrotic
areas may be necessary. All has to be done to evitate an major amputation but on the other side the intervention has not to be postponed
if the necrotic process shows steady progression (KAPPERT 1981).

Three methods may overbridge critical hemodynamic situations: 1. Hemodilution which reduces blood viscosity by lowering the hematocrit value from 45 to 30 % by taking step by step up to 1500 ml of blood and
replacing it by rheomacrodex 10 % or human serum albumine 5 %. This is
the form of isovolemic hemodilution. The hypervolemic form with infusions of 500 ml rheomacrodex daily can only be applied over a short
period and is contraindicated in cardiac and renal insufficiency as
well as in coronary heart disease. - 2. An artificial systemic hypertension provoked by fludrocortisone and salt rich diet (LASSEN et. al
1968) has a limited indication because of the danger of heart insuf-
fiency. - 3. Lowering the viscosity of the blood by a decrease of the
fibrinogene level of normally 200 - 450 mg% to 50 - 100 mg% which can
be realized by injections of snake poison (arwin ecc.). This method
has lost somebit its importance.

The treatment of the various forms of arteriitis cannot be discussed
in detail. Antibiotics, prednisone, azathioprine, cyclophosphamide and
thioamphenicole may be indicated.


V. Conclusions


Before the beginning of the conservative treatment of peripheral artery disease history and hemodynamic evaluation have to determine the
stage of the disease, the site of the alterations and the eventual
combination with coronary and cerebral vascular manifestations. The
natural course of the disease has to be considered when the efficacy
of any kind of treatment is evaluated. Without elimination of existing
risk factors, especially smoking, most therapeutical efforts are of
doubtful value.

References

1. Cloarec M., Cristol R., Graisely B., Dumas JR., Coel MC., Pedri-
   set G., Tuot (1981). In: Balas P., Kappert A. (ed): Progress in
   the medical treatment of arterial occlusive diseases. Suppl. Folia
   Angiologica, Vol. VII, p. 57 - 71.

2. Dormandy JA, Yates CJP, Bennett D. (1981), Angiology 32: 236 - 241.

3. Fontaine R.; cited in Kappert A. (ed): Lehrbuch und Atlas der Angiologie. Tenth edition, p. 65. Bern/Stuttgart/Wien, Hans Huber (1980).

4. Gillespie JA (1967). Vasodilator properties of alcohol. Brit. med.
   J. 2: 27 - 31.

5. Hagen GHL (1839). Ueber die Bewegung des Wassers in engen cylind-
   rischen Röhren. Ann. Phys. u. Chem. 46: 423 - 442.

6. Kannel MB, Shurtleff D. (1971). The natural history of arteriosclerosis obliterans. Peripheral vascular disease. Cardiosvascular
   Clinics, vol 3, nr. 1, p. 38 - 44.

7. Kappert A. (1981). Lehrbuch und Atlas der Angiologie. H. Huber,
   Bern/Stuttgart/Wien, p. 370.

8. Lassen NA., Larsen DA., Sørensen AWS., Hallböök T., Dann I., Nilsen
   R., Westling H. (1968). Conservative treatment of gangrene using
   mineralcorticoid-induced moderated hypertension. Lancet 606, I:
   69 - 81.

9. Poiseuille JLM (1846). Rècherches expérimentales sur le mouvement
   des liquides dans les tubes de très petits diamètres. Mém. Svants
   Etrangers (Paris) 9: 433 - 543.

# 1.1 Atherosclerosis in Childhood

# An Introduction to Atherosclerosis in Children[1]

J. P. Strong

The late RUSSELL L. HOLMAN(1) in 1961 raised the question,
"Atherosclerosis--a Pediatric Nutrition Problem?" Holman's
colleagues, J.P. STRONG and H.C. MCGILL, JR,(2) eight years later
attempted to answer this provocative question in a paper concerning the pediatric aspects of atherosclerosis. They indicated
that the atherosclerotic process was not inevitable but at least
in part environmentally determined. They suggested that preventive measures undertaken before fibrous plaques become extensive
should control permanently the epidemic of heart disease. In 1978
a volume entitled "Atherosclerosis: Its Pediatric Aspects" edited by WILLIAM B. STRONG (3) was published. This volume summarized the status of knowledge concerning atherosclerosis in children at that time.

## A LITTLE HISTORY

Long before Holman and his colleagues asked and addressed the
question of atherosclerosis as a pediatric problem there was concern with the very early lesions of atherosclerosis. In 1911,
KLOTZ and MANNING(4) introduced their study of the aortas from 90
cases between 1 and 73 years of age with this statement: "It is
quite useless to argue the questions concerning the development
of intimal sclerosis if we study and discuss the late stages of
the disease alone...if we wish to gain a true insight into the
complex question of arteriosclerosis we must attempt to follow the
lesion from its earliest beginning." These authors found a high
incidence of fatty streaks (which they considered the earliest
lesions of arteriosclerosis) without using any gross staining
technique.

SALTYKOW(5) in 1915, in attempting to differentiate normal de-
velopmental and degenerative changes in the aorta, concluded "the
so-called fatty changes in the arteries of childhood and youth,
especially in the aorta, are nothing else but the beginning of
atherosclerosis."

MÖNCKEBERG(6) in 1921, in reporting aortic findings in war dead,
found 5 of 14 cases (36 percent) under 20 years of age with
"atheromatosis" of the aortic intima. The percentages increased
in the older age groups, i.e., 76 percent from the 20- to 25-year
group; 80 percent, 30-35 years; and 100 percent of 16 cases 35-
40 years. These and the observations of ASCHOFF(7) reveal that
pathologists were aware of the presence of fatty streaks in the
aortas of young persons early in the twentieth century.

---

[1] Supported by grant HL-08974 NHLBI, NIH, USPHS.

ZINSERLING(8) in 1925 examined 320 aortas from children up to 15
years of age after gross staining with Sudan III. He graded
these specimens into five groups on the basis of extent of surface involved, and he found that gross staining not only enhanced the detection of lesions in the younger ages, but also increased the estimation of the extent of intimal surface involved
by fatty streaks. He found that sudanophilic deposits were present in some cases before the age of four years, and he found a
steady rise in the severity of lesions with age. When he analyzed the data on aortic lesions with respect to cause of death
and the state of nutrition, he could find no single cause of
death that was associated with significantly more extensive or advanced lesions. There was no difference between well-nourished
individuals and those severely emaciated as a result of starvation
during the postwar famine.

ZEEK(9) in 1930 made an exhaustive and critical review of the
literature pertaining to juvenile arteriosclerosis, defined as
"lesions believed to begin in the intima with lipoid degeneration"
and concluded that arteriosclerosis may occur at any age. Most
of the cases she reviewed had a history of renal disease and many
had elevated blood pressure. These cases were those in which
lesions were easily visible even without the gross staining of
arterial specimens with fat stains.


## THE DISEASE

The importance of atherosclerosis is in direct proportion to its
disease-producing potential. There is abundant evidence that the
arterial lesions of atherosclerosis are pathogenetically related
to coronary occlusion and myocardial infarction, cerebral infarction, and ischemic damage to other organs. There is still uncer-
tainity about the interrelationships of the different steps of the
atherosclerotic process--a process known to begin in childhood but
which does not become clinically manifest until later life.

The simple fatty streak is considered to represent the earliest
lesion of atherosclerosis that can be easily recognized either
grossly or histologically. The fatty streak is gradually converted into a fibrous plaque, in which there is abundant connective
tissue as well as lipid. A fibrous plaque may become sufficiently
large to cause slowly progressive stenosis of the lumen of a vessel. It may undergo sufficiently enlargement by accretion of additional lipid, connective tissue, or mural thrombus on the surface so as to produce a similar effect; or it may become vascu-
larized and undergo hemorrhage, or ulcerated and be covered by a
thrombus. In the latter instances rapid occlusion of the artery
may result. Rarely, the lesion may so weaken the underlying media that an aneurysm is produced; or it may become calcified, a
change possibly representing a healing process but, nevertheless,
reflecting an advanced stage of the atherosclerotic process.

## NOMENCLATURE

Arteriosclerosis is a general term that includes practically any arterial disease that leads to thickening and hardening of arteries.

Atherosclerosis is a specific form of arteriosclerosis. The most distinctive feature of atherosclerosis is the accumulation of lipid in the intima of large elastic arteries (aorta) and medium-sized muscular arteries (coronary, femoral, carotid, and others). In addition to lipid, cells, connective tissue fibers, and various blood products accumulate in the lesions. Complications, including thrombosis, hemorrhage into a plaque, and ulceration, can also occur in the lesions. The hallmarks of atherosclerosis are its intimal location in the initial stage, involvement of large and medium-sized arteries, and the accumulation of lipid. Atherosclerosis is the form of arteriosclerosis that most frequently causes clinically significant disease.

Mönckeberg's medial calcific sclerosis is a form of medial disease characterized by calcification of the muscular arteries. Arteriolsclerosis (or arteriolar sclerosis) is a form of arteriolar disease characterized by thickening, fibrosis, hyalinization, and narrowing of arterioles. These are subtypes of arteriosclerosis quite distinct from atherosclerosis and are beyond the scope of this report.

Investigations of prevalence and extent of human atherosclerosis have predominantly been based on the gross appearance and on the physical characteristics of lesions in sampled arteries. The following operational definitions are used.

Fatty streak. A fatty intimal lesion that is stained distinctly by Sudan IV and shows no other underlying change. Fatty streaks are flat or only slightly elevated and do not significantly narrow the lumina of blood vessels.

Fibrous plaque. A firm, elevated intimal lesion which in the fresh state is gray-white, glistening, and translucent. The surface of the lesion may be sudanophilic, but usually is not. Human fibrous plaques characteristically contain fat. A thick fibrous connective tissue cap containing varying amounts of lipid usually covers a more concentrated "core" of lipid. If a lesion also contains hemorrhage, thrombosis, ulceration, or calcification, that lesion is classified according to one of the following two categories.

Complicated lesion. An intimal plaque in which there is hemorrhage, ulceration, or thrombosis with or without calcification.

Calcified lesion. An intimal plaque in which insoluble mineral salts of calcium are visible or palpable without overlying hemorrhage, ulceration or thrombosis.

The term <u>raised</u> <u>atherosclerotic</u> <u>lesion</u> is sometimes used to include the sum of fibrous plaques, complicated lesions, and calcified lesions.  Raised lesions are contrasted with fatty streaks,
which typically show little or no elevation above the adjacent
intimal surface.

Use of the word <u>atheroma</u> is not consistent among investigators
and authors.  Some use it for the lesion described earlier--a
plaque with a pool of degenerated or necrotic lipid-rich debris.
Others use atheroma to refer to the process of atherosclerosis or
arteriosclerosis.  Still others have used the term to refer to
various lesions, from a fatty streak to a complicated lesion.  To
avoid ambiguity when one uses the term, it should be qualified or
modified so that its meaning is perfectly clear.  We do not use
it here.

Certain other intimal lesions are sometimes considered as subtypes
of atherosclerosis or as lesions predisposing to atherosclerosis.
These include <u>musculoelastic</u> or <u>fibromuscular</u> <u>intimal</u> <u>thickening</u>,
<u>gelatinous</u> or <u>edematous</u> <u>lesions</u>, and organizing mural thrombi on
an otherwise normal intima.  The pathogenetic relationship of
atherosclerosis and its clinical manifestations is less well
established for these lesions, and quantitative information related to the natural history, topography, and geographic photography is not available.  "Rhythmic" or <u>periodic</u> <u>wrinkling</u> of the
intimal surface of the aortas of children and adolescents is
another change whose relationship to atherosclerosis has not been
established.

<u>GOALS OF THIS WORKSHOP</u>

This workshop on atherosclerosis in children is designed to shed
more light on the development of arterial lesions of atherosclerosis in children and to provide information concerning present
state of knowledge concerning CHD risk factors as they occur in
children.  This VIth International Symposium in Berlin provides an
outstanding opportunity to expand our knowledge of atherosclerosis
in children.

<u>Acknowledgments</u>  We gratefully acknowledge the assistance of Rhea
Dupeire and Charlotte Swain in preparing this manuscript.

References

1.  Holman RL (1961) Atherosclerosis -A pediatric nutrition
    problem.  Am J Clin Nutr 9: 565

2.  Strong JP, McGill HC Jr (1969) Pediatric aspects of
    atherosclerosis.  J Atheroscler Res 9: 25-65

3.  Strong WB (ed) (1978) Atherosclerosis: Its Pediatric Aspects.
    Grune & Stratton, New York

4.  Klotz O, Manning MF (1911) Fatty streaks in the intima of
    arteries.  J Pathol Bacteriol 16: 211

5.  Saltykow S (1915) Jugendliche und beginnende Atherosklerose.
    Cor.-Bl. f. schweiz. Aertze 45:  1057-1089

6.  Mönckeberg JG (1921) Das Gefäßsystem und seine Erkrankungen.
    Handb. ärztl. Erfahr. Weltkr. 8:  8-18

7.  Aschoff L (1924) Atherosclerosis in Lectures on Pathology.
    Hoeber, New York, 131-153

8.  Zinserling WD (1925) Untersuchungen über Atherosklerose.
    I. Über die Aortaverfettung bei Kindern.  Virchows Arch
    Pathol Anat 255: 677-705

9.  Zeek P (1930) Juvenile arteriosclerosis.  Arch Pathol 10:
    417-466

# Clinical and Anatomic Correlates of Cardiovascular Disease in Children from the Bogalusa Heart Study

G. S. Berenson, A. W. Voors, P. Gard, W. P. Newman, III, and R. E. Tracy

## Introduction

During the past 10 years, much clinical information has been obtained on cardio-vascular (C-V) risk factors in pediatric populations. Impetus to study C-V risk in children for adult heart diseases evolved naturally from adult population studies, i.e., Framingham, Tecumseh, Evans County and others. The major medical advance was made in documenting clinical parameters that predict morbid C-V events. It became apparent that similar clinical parameters could be observed in children. Equally important to the clinical observations has been recognition that atherosclerotic lesions are already present in early life. ZEEK (1), HOLMAN et al. (2) noted athero-sclerotic lesions developed early, even in infancy. Findings of coronary artery lesions in soldiers necropsied in the Korean War (3), and later in Vietnam (4), were impressive. The nature of coronary artery lesions, occurring early and gradually increasing during a subclinical phase, is now well recognized. As an outgrowth to this history, it became important as part of an epidemiology program, to study the early natural history of coronary artery disease in children (5) and to correlate anatomic changes along with clinical C-V risk factors.

Although extensive clinical data have been obtained in several childhood populations around the world, a major limitation exists in understanding what constitutes abnor-mal levels of risk factors. A major advantage of the adult studies is the occurrence of endstage disease or morbid events that are lacking in childhood. Since noninva-sive methods have not yet reached a state-of-the-art to quantitate the extensiveness of C-V disease in large populations of asymptomatic individuals, it is not possible to equate anatomic changes with clinical risk factors. Autopsy studies are obviously needed as a component of the extensive clinical C-V risk factor surveys. The close association of hypertension with coronary artery disease, the high prevalence of essential hypertension in adults, and the recognition of the onset of essential hypertension in early life (6) show our need to understand the early natural history of essential hypertension and to obtain anatomic correlates with the early onset of hypertension as well.

A prospective study correlating clinical risk and anatomic C-V changes associated with atherosclerosis and hypertension provides an opportunity to examine questions important to adult C-V diseases, e.g., "What is the relationship between early ath-erosclerotic lesions in coronary vessels and the clinical C-V risk factor variables?" "How do C-V risk factor variables relate to the transition of fatty streaks, early fibromuscular lesions and the lumen occupying raised lesions?" "What is the temporal relationship between growth and development, blood pressure levels, heart weight and small artery changes?" Obviously there are many other possible questions.

## Population and Methods of Study

Population - The Bogalusa Heart Study, for the past 10 years, has been describing C-V risk factor variables in children of a biracial (black-white), semi-rural popu-lation of 5,000 children in a geographically defined area containing 22,000 people

(5). The observations include anthropometric and growth characteristics, blood pressure levels, serum lipids and lipoproteins, dietary studies, and biobehavioral observations such as Type A behavior. Similar risk factor information is being obtained on an adjacent community, Franklinton, Louisiana, with approximately 9,000 people. With cooperation of local resources, a local information system was developed to let us obtain family consent and to necropsy any resident, age 3 to 24 years, dying in our community. This system has been in operation for 4 years, and approximately 90% of all deaths occurring during this time (N=54) were studied. Strategic aspects of this organization are the cooperation of the local pathologist and coroner and the 24-hour communication with physicians, hospitals, and funeral homes maintained by Bogalusa Heart Study staff nurses. Autopsies are conducted in local hospitals or funeral homes, and selected tissues are sent to the Department of Pathology, LSU Medical Center in New Orleans, for examination. Anatomic studies are conducted by a standard protocol (7).

## Anatomic Observations

General - For all autopsy studies body length, weight, organ weights, and a set of macro and microscopic C-V measurements are recorded. Cardiac weight is noted, and the aorta and coronary arteries are graded for atherosclerosis according to the percent surface involvement by fatty streaks and fibrous plaque raised lesions. The grading is conducted by 3 pathologists blindly using standard techniques.

Methods to develop wall-lumen ratios of small renal arteries, based on studies of FURUYAMA (8) and FOLKOV (9), were developed in our laboratory. Small renal arteries, 200 to 1000 μ, are being studied in one kidney perfused under 125 mmHg pressure during fixation and in the other kidney, which is left unperfused. Measurements of artery diameter and medial thickness are taken using an electronic digitizer superimposed on camera lucida images of vessels projected from microscopic slides.

Heart weights were compared with published standards for age and sex (10). These show an observed excess of heart weight, possibly due to a secular increase of body weight at the adolescent age in our population. When heart weights are compared to reported weight for height and sex groups, boys in our study appear to have greater heart weights, and girls smaller weights than previously published (11).

The percent of abdominal aorta surface area covered by atherosclerotic lesions (nearly all of which are fatty streaks) by age, race and sex are presented in Figure 1. Around the period of maturation, a sudden and consistent increase in involvement with atherosclerosis occurs. A marked individual variability of involvement is apparent. The thoracic aorta surface area also shows wide individual distributions of lesions but generally less surface involvement than in the abdominal portion. As expected, even less area is involved in the coronary system, although lesions are noted. The average percent aorta surface area covered by atherosclerotic lesions adjusted to age showed a strong and statistically significant correlation with serum β-lipoprotein levels (Figure 2). These are preliminary observations and more samples must be completed to amplify relationships with serum lipoproteins and other risk factors.

In the studies of vessel wall thickness, we observed a significant correlation between wall-to-lumen ratio and a blood pressure index (R=0.71, N=14) (Figure 3) (12, 13). These observations suggest thickening of the arterial media begins in childhood in a relationship to blood pressure levels; excessive thickness (relative) may be a manifestation of early hypertension.

## Discussion

These observations show that it is feasible to conduct a necropsy study of C-V

**BOGALUSA NECROPSY STUDY, 1978-1981**

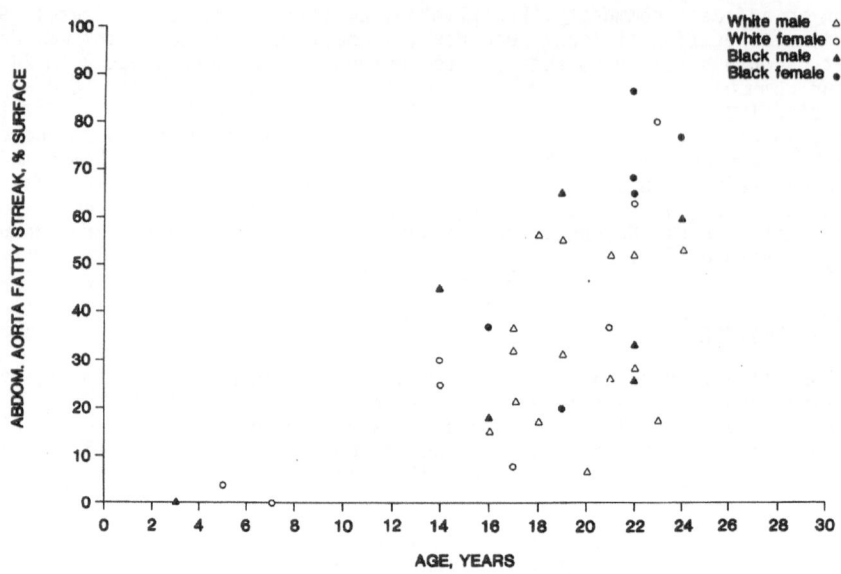

Figure 1. Area of abdominal aorta covered by fatty streak by age, race and sex. At the age of sexual maturation, a sharp increase occurs

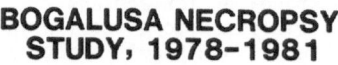

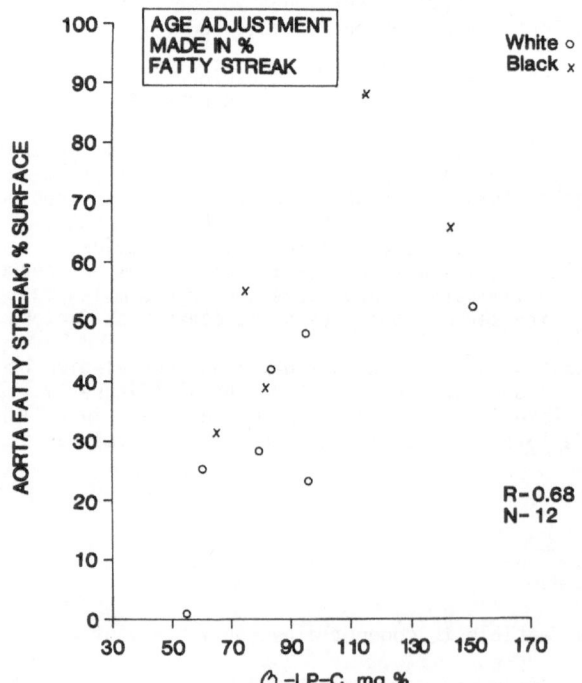

Figure 2. Scatter plot of aortic area (mean of abdominal and thoracic) covered by fatty streak versus fasting serum β-lipoprotein cholesterol level. R=0.68, N=12, p<0.02

## WALL-TO-LUMEN RATIO OF PRESSURE - FIXATION SMALL RENAL ARTERIES VS BLOOD PRESSURE INDEX (HRT WT/BLD VOL) BOGALUSA NECROPSY STUDY, 1978-1980

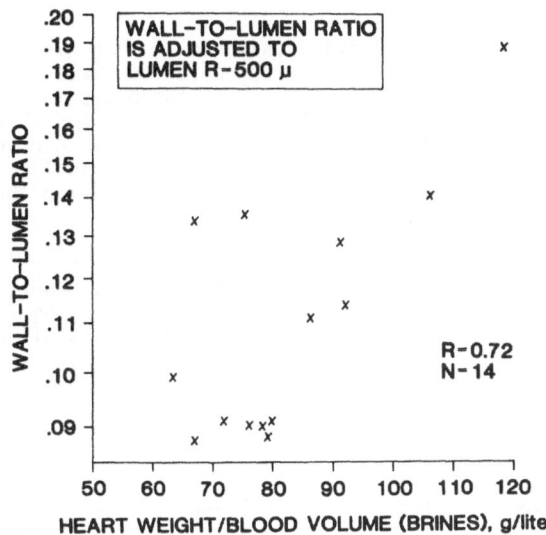

Figure 3. Scatter plot of wall-to-lumen ratio of renal small arteries versus an index of blood pressure. This index is the ratio of heart weight to blood volume estimated according to BRINES et al. (12) and CROPP (13). R=0.73, N=14, p<0.005

changes along with a C-V risk factor survey of children within a community. Documentation of anatomic substrates for known C-V risk factor variables is needed as an important component of the early natural history of coronary artery disease and essential hypertension. Surveys of risk factors in pediatric populations are limited in clarifying the etiology of arteriosclerosis because biological endpoints are ill-defined, deaths are infrequent, and there is an inability to observe and describe anatomic changes occurring in the C-V system in life. Noninvasive methods are beginning to provide evidence that changes are occurring with early hypertension. Upper arm arterial blood flow, under maximal dilatation as measured by plethysmography, differs in young adults with hypertension (14) and echocardiographic measurements show an increased left ventricular posterior wall thickness in children with elevated blood pressure levels (15,16,17). These findings and clinical risk factor observations obtained over time ("tracking") are consistent with the hypothesis that essential hypertension occurs early in life and target organ damage occurs during the gradual subclinical phase of disease. The link between clinical and anatomic C-V changes has implications for intervention at an early stage of the natural course of essential hypertension.

With regard to early atherosclerotic disease, in contrast to the importance of the onset of fibromuscular intimal thickening, the significance of the fatty streak remains controversial. Although fatty streaks are noted in populations even without a high incidence of coronary heart disease, it is generally accepted as the earliest identifiable lesion of atherosclerosis. The importance of such lesions in the aorta is debatable, but coronary lesions appearing in the second and third decades of life are the hallmarks of more advanced disease. It is presumed that transition from the ubiquitous fatty streak to the more significant fibromuscular lesion occurs in the late second and early third decades of life when considerable changes of clinical risk factors occur (18). Further observations are needed to understand formation of lesions in early adulthood. Even the preliminary findings of this pathology study of Bogalusa children are indicating a high correlation with risk factors, such as serum β-lipoproteins.

## Conclusion

Although a large amount of clinical data on free-living children at high risk for coronary artery disease and essential hypertension is being collected, reliable follow-ups by standard autopsy methods are needed to complement these studies. Anatomic observations are an important aspect of research on the pathogenesis of atherosclerosis and primary hypertension. Studies on the young are strategic in providing clues to these diseases; understanding the association of clinical C-V risk factors and anatomic lesions in the C-V system will provide information that will guide optimum aspects of prevention.

*Acknowledgments* This research was supported by funds from the National Heart, Lung, and Blood Institute of the United States Public Health Service, HL15103, Specialized Center of Research-Arteriosclerosis (SCOR-A) and HL08974, Natural and Experimental Atherosclerosis.

## References

1. Zeek P (1930) Juvenile atherosclerosis. Arch Path 10:417-446
2. Holman RL, McGill HC, Strong JP, Geer JC (1958) The natural history of athero-sclerosis: The early aortic lesions as seen in New Orleans in the middle of the 20th century. Am J Path 34:209-235
3. Enos WF, Holmes RH, Beyer J (1953) Coronary disease among United States sol-diers killed in action in Korea. JAMA 152:1090-1093
4. McNamara JJ, Molot MA, Stremple JF, Cutting RT (1971) Coronary artery disease in combat casualties in Vietnam. JAMA 216:1185-1187
5. Berenson GS, McMahan CA, Voors AW, Webber LS, Srinivasan SR, Frank GC, Foster TA, Blonde CV (1980) Cardiovascular risk factors in children--The early natural history of atherosclerosis and essential hypertension. New York, Oxford Univer-sity Press, pp. 450
6. Voors AW, Webber LS, Berenson GS (1977) A consideration of essential hyperten-sion in children. Prac Cardiol 3:29-40
7. International Atherosclerosis Project (1962) Standard Operating Protocol. New Orleans, Louisiana State University Medical Center, pp. 43
8. Furuyama M (1962) Histometrical investigations of arteries in reference to arterial hypertension. Tohoku J Exper Med 76:388-414
9. Folkov B (1978) Cardiovascular structural adaptation: Its role in the initia-tion and maintenance of primary hypertension. Clin Sci Molec Med 55:3S-22S
10. Bardeen CR (1948) Determination of the size of the heart by means of the x-rays. Am J Anat 23:423-484
11. Zeek PM (1942) Heart weight. I. The weight of the normal human heart. Arch Path 34:820-832
12. Brines JK, Gibson JG, Kunkel P (1941) The blood volume in normal infants and children. J Pediatr 18:447-457
13. Cropp GJA (1971) Changes in blood and plasma volumes during growth. J Pediatr 78:220-229
14. Takeshita A, Mark AL (1980) Decreased vasodilator capacity of forearm resistance vessels in borderline hypertension. Hypertension 2:610-616
15. Riopel DA, Hohn AR, Taylor AB, Leadholt BC (1980) Echocardiographic variables in

progeny of hypertensive and normotensive patients. Circulation 62(suppl 3): 270
16. Schieken RM, Clarke WR, Lauer RM (1981) Left ventricular hypertrophy in children with blood pressures in the upper quintile of the distribution. Hypertension 3:669-675
17. Laird WP, Fixler DE (1981) Left ventricular hypertrophy in adolescents with elevated blood pressure: Assessment by chest roentgenography, electrocardiography. Pediatrics 67:255-259
18. Berenson GS, Srinivasan SR, Cresanta JL, Foster TA, Webber LS (1981) Dynamic changes of serum lipoproteins in children during adolescence and sexual maturation. Am J Epidemiol 113:157-170

# Dietary Prevention of Atherosclerosis in Childhood

J. T. Knuiman, S. Westenbrink, L. van der Heijden, C. E. West,
and G. A. J. Hautvast

## A. Introduction

Despite the enormous body of knowledge that has accumulated on the
relationship between nutrition, atherosclerosis and coronary heart
disease (CHD), the results of nutritional intervention studies
aimed at reducing the incidence of CHD (1,2) have been somewhat
disappointing. Although significant reductions in death from CHD
have been reported, there has been no significant reduction in
total mortality. It is possible that intervention earlier in life
would be more effective. Studies in non-human primates have shown
that experimentally induced fatty streaks and fibrous plaques can
be made to regress by feeding diets low in cholesterol and saturated
fat (3). However, only the simplest fatty streaks appear to be truly
reversible. It may well be, that two populations of fatty streaks
exist: one destined, perhaps by its location or risk factors, to
develop into fibrous plaques; and a second which remains as fatty
streaks and never goes on to become fibrous plaques (4).

Fibrous plaques can already be found in the coronary artieries of
persons in their early twenties (5,6) and even in children between
10 and 14 years of age (7). The concept that atherosclerosis possibly
already begins in childhood probably dates from the paper of HOLMAN
in 1961 (8) in which he drew attention to the pathology of atherosclerosis in children. As a result of this early work, several studies
on the risk factors for CHD in children have already been carried
out or have commenced.

## B. Objectives for research in children

Studies in children should try to provide answers to the following
questions (9):
- What is the magnitude of the risk indicators for CHD in children
  living in different biological, social and cultural environments?
- How does the magnitude of the risk indicators in young children
  relate to the magnitude of the risk indicators and to the disease
  itself in their parents and grandparents?
- At what time and under what circumstances does an increased level
  of the risk indicator appear and what is the cause of this increase?
- What can be done to prevent an increased level of risk indicators
  from developing, and more importantly, to prevent the onset of
  severe CHD and its complications?

## C. Results of earlier studies

Many studies in children have been carried out in the last 20 years especially in the more affluent countries in the developed world (10-20). From 1974 to 1976, VAN DER HAAR and KROMHOUT (10) from our department carried out a regional comparative study in the Netherlands in children aged 6 to 10 years in three towns with populations from 25,000 to 40,000. The mean serum cholesterol concentrations was found to be 4.5 mmol/l and the HDL-cholesterol concentration was 1.4 mmol/l. We felt the need to compare these results with those from children in other countries. However, relatively little was known about the concentration of total- and HDL-cholesterol in the serum of children living in countries differing in their rates of mortality from CHD. In addition, it is also difficult to compare published data on serum total and HDL cholesterol concentrations, because of variations not due to the true biological variation of the actual concentrations. Apparent concentrations may vary up to 40% by the use of different methods or by the use of similar methods not only by different people but also by the same person under different conditions or at a different time (21). Variability may also arise from differences in the methods of blood sampling, storage of serum, etc.

Therefore, in order to obtain reliable data on the concentration of total- and HDL-cholesterol in the serum of 7- and 8-year old boys from populations with different rates of coronary heart disease, a study was designed using a standardised protocol for the collection of samples with the analyses being carried out in a single laboratory (22,23).

The concentrations of HDL cholesterol appeared to be linearly related to the concentration of total cholesterol in serum between populations (r=0.90; n=26). This suggests that a 'Western' type of diet with a relatively high intake of fat especially saturated fat intake, is responsible for the higher concentrations of both serum total cholesterol and HDL-cholesterol in the more developed countries. This is in line with results obtained in controlled dietary trials in healthy volunteers (24-26), studies in Masai men (27) and also in vegetarians (28). Perhaps an even more important result of this study is that it clearly demonstrated that marked differences exist in the serum concentrations of total- and HDL-cholesterol between populations already by the age of 7 or 8 years. The importance of this result is highlighted even more when it is taken into account that higher concentrations were found in those countries with higher rates of mortality from CHD. Of course, the crucial question is whether these results mean that children with elevated serum cholesterol concentrations are already at risk at such an early age. Further studies on the relationship between environmental factors such as diet and the level of risk indicators together with tracking studies, familial studies and controlled dietary trials may provide an answer to this question. Preliminary data obtained in our earlier study revealed strong relationships between the mean serum total cholesterol concentrations and the availability of several items between the populations

## D. Results of recent studies

However, as the reliability of food availability data is often questioned, the relationship, of dietary parameters with total- and HDL-cholesterol concentrations in serum have been examined in more detail in five countries: Finland, Ghana, Italy, the Netherlands and the Philippines (29). These countries were selected because they represent a wide range of total- and HDL-cholesterol concentrations and dietary intake patterns. The study was carried out in cooperation with  Dr. Räsänen and Dr. Viikari and Mrs. Virkkunen from  Finland, with  Mrs. Lokko and Prof. Pobee from Ghana, Prof. Ferro-Luzzi and Dr. Ferrini from Italy and Dr. Bulatao-Jayme and Mrs. Villavieja from the Philippines. Before the study was commenced in the five countries a training period was held in the Netherlands for the leaders of the teams of nutritionists from the five countries in order to enhance the comparability of the data collected in the food consumption survey. The study was carried out in 120 boys aged 8 and 9 years in each of the five countries. The intakes of energy, macronutrients and choles-terol were measured on 7 days spread over a period of 15 days by the use of the record and recall method. In addition the body mass index was calculated and a physical activity score was estimated through a questionnaire on weekly activity patterns in leisure time.

Differences in the mean concentrations of total cholesterol between the groups correlated well with the predicted differences calculated by the formula of Keys: $\Delta = 1.35 \ (2S-P + 1.5\sqrt{Z}$ with $r = 0.98$, although the actual differences in the concentrations of total cholesterol were more than twice as high as were predicted by this formula. Within 4 out of 5 populations there were statistically significant relation-ships between the intake of energy from saturated fatty acids and the concentration of total cholesterol.

In a multiple regression analysis allowing for a country specific intercepts, the energy percentage from saturated fat was the only dietary variable that was positively related with the concentration of total cholesterol. Physical activity score was negatively related with the concentration of total cholesterol but this was only of borderline significance. The energy percentage from carbohydrates and the body mass index (weight/height$^2$) were negatively related with the concentration of HDL-cholesterol, while the energy percentage of polyunsaturated fatty acids and the physical activity score were positively related with the ratio of HDL-cholesterol/total choles-terol.

The results of our study suggest that the concentrations of total- and HDL-cholesterol of young children are influenced by dietary factors, physical activity and body mass index. The results also suggest that the intake of saturated fatty acids should be decreased as this will have a favourable influence on the concentration of total cholesterol. Saturated fatty acids can be exchanged for mono-unsaturated and polyunsaturated fatty acids and carbohydrates. Although the energy percentage from carbohydrates is negatively related with the concentration of HDL-cholesterol there is evidence that on population level the concentration of total cholesterol is the major determinant of coronary heart disease (30).

Therefore, in practical terms, we suggest that for the prevention of CHD a diet with a relatively large contribution of vegetable products be recommended. Such a recommendation is supported by studies recently carried out in vegetarian children and adults which have shown that a more vegetarian way of life is compatible with good health (31,32). Thus we support those who recommend restriction of the percentage of energy from saturated fat and cholesterol in the diet and increasing the percentage of energy from carbohydrates in the diet. From our data, there is no support for the recommendation that the percentage of energy from polyunsaturated fats in the diet should be increased to ten energy percent.

## References

1. Miettinen M, Turpeinen O, Karvonen MJ, Elosuo F, Paavilainen E (1972) Effect of cholesterol-lowering diet on mortality from coronary heart disease and other causes. Lancet 2: 835-838.
2. Dayton S, Pearce ML, Goldman H, Harnish A, Plotkin D, Shickman M, Winfield M, Zager A, Dixon W (1968) Controlled trial of a diet high in unsaturated fat for prevention of atherosclerotic complications  Lancet 2: 1060-1062.
3. Armstrong ML (1976) Regression of atherosclerosis. In: Raven Press, New York. Paoletti R, Gotto AM (eds) Atherosclerosis Reviews 1: 137.
4. Pearson TA, Dillman JM, Solez K, Heptinstall RH (1980) Evidence for two populations of fatty streaks with different roles in the atherogenetic process  Lancet 2: 496-498.
5. Enos WJ, Beijer JC, Holmes FH (1955) Pathogenesis of coronary disease in American soldiers killed in Korea  JAMA 158: 912-917.
6. McNamara J, Malot MA, Stremple JF, Cutting RT (1971) Coronary artery disease in combat  casualties in Vietnam  JAMA 216: 1185-1187.
7. Vihert AM (1976) Atherosclerosis of the aorta in five towns. Bull World Health Org 53: 501-508.
8. Holman RL (1961) Atherosclerosis - a pediatric nutrition problem? Am J Clin Nutr 9: 565-569.
9. WHO/ISFC meeting on precursors of atherosclerosis in children (1977) CVD/78.1, WHO, Geneva.
10. Van der Haar F, Kromhout D (1978) Food intake, nutritional anthropometry and blood chemical parameters in 3 selected Dutch schoolchildren populations. Med Landbouwhogeschool, Wageningen, The Netherlands.
11. Räsänen L, Wilska M, Kantero R, Näntö V, Ahlström A, Hallman N (1978) Nutrition survey of Finnish rural children. IV. Serum cholesterol values in relation to dietary variables. Am J Clin Nutr 31: 1050-1056.
12. Frank GC, Berenson GS, Webber LS (1978) Dietary studies and the relationship of diet to cardiovascular disease risk factor variables in 10-year old children. Am J Clin Nutr 31: 328-340.
13. Nichols AB, Ravenscroft C, Lamphear DE, Ostrander L (1976) Daily nutritional intake and serum lipid levels. The Tecumseh study. Am J Clin Nutr 29: 1384-1392.
14. Askevold R, Høstmark AT, Vellar OD, Von Kraemer Bryn M, Glattre E (1978) Serum cholesterol and triglyceride levels in Norwegian adolescent schoolchildren. Acta Paed Scand 67: 157-160.

15. Dyerberg J, Hjörne N (1973) Plasma lipid and lipoprotein levels in childhood and adolescence. Scand J Clin Lab Invest 31: 473-479.
16. Golubjatnikov R, Paskey T, Inhorn SL Serum cholesterol levels of Mexican and Wisconsin schoolchildren. Am J Epid 1972; 96: 36-9.
17. Lauer RM, Connor WE, Leaverton PE, Reiter MA, Clarke WR (1975) Coronary heart disease risk factors in schoolchildren. The Muscatine Study. J Pediatr 86: 679-706.
18. Antonini AC, Dal Palù C (1980) Pordenone study on the precursors of atherosclerosis in childhood. Savioprint, Italy.
19. Tamir I, Heiss G, Glueck CJ, Christensen B, Kwiterovich P, Rifkind BM (1980) Lipid and lipoprotein distributions in white children ages 6-19 yr. The Lipid Research Clinics Program Prevalence Study. J Chron Dis 34: 27-39.
20. Weidman WH, Elveback LR, Nelson RA, Hodgson PA, Ellefson RD (1978) Nutrient intake and serum cholesterol levels in normal children 6 to 16 years of age. Pediatrics 61: 354-359.
21. Whitehead TP, Brownings DM, Gregory A (1973) A comparative survey of the results of analysis of blood serum in clinical chemistry laboratories in the U.K. J Clin Path 26: 435-445.
22. Knuiman JT, West CE, Hermus RJJ, Hautvast JGAJ (1979) Is serum cholesterol outmoded? Lancet 2: 1183-1184.
23. Knuiman JT, Hermus RJJ, Hautvast JGAJ (1980) Serum total and high density lipoprotein (HDL) cholesterol concentrations in rural and urban boys from 16 countries. Atherosclerosis 36: 529-537.
24. Shepherd J, Packard CJ, Patsch JR, Gotto AM, Taunton OD (1978) Effects of dietary polyunsaturated and saturated fat on the properties of high density lipoproteins and the metabolism of apoprotein A-1. J Clin Invest 61: 1582-1592.
25. Schaefer EJ, Levy RI, Ernst ND, Van Sant D, Brewer B (1981) The effects of low cholesterol, high polyunsaturated fat, and low fat diets on plasma lipid and lipoprotein cholesterol levels in normal and hypercholesterolemic subjects. Am J Clin Nutr 34: 1758-1763.
26. Brussaard JH, Katan MB, Groot PHE, Havekes LMH, Hautvast JGAJ (1982) Serum lipoproteins of healthy persons fed a low-fat diet or a polyunsaturated fat diet for three months. A comparison of two cholesterol-lowering diets. Atherosclerosis 42:205-219.
27. Robinson D, Williams P (1979) High density lipoprotein cholesterol in the Masai of East Africa - A cautionary note. Brit Med J 1: 1249.
28. Burslem J, Schonfeld G, Howald MA, Weidman SW, Miller JP (1978) Plasma apoprotein and lipoprotein lipid levels in vegetarians. Metabolism 27: 711-719.
29. Knuiman JT, Westenbrink S, Van der Heijden L, West CE, Hautvast JGAJ (1981) International study on food consumption and serum lipids in boys. Department of Human Nutrition, Agricultural University, Wageningen, The Netherlands.
30. Knuiman JT, West CE, Burema J (1982) Serum total and high density lipoprotein (HDL) cholesterol concentrations and body mass index in adult men from 13 countries. Am J Epid: in press.
31. Dwyer JT, Dietz WH, Andrews EM, Suskind RM (1982) Nutritional status of vegetarian children. Am J Clin Nutr 35: 204-216.
32. Sanders TAB, Purves R (1981) An anthropometric and dietary assessment of the nutritional status of vegan preschool children. J Hum Nutr 35: 349-357.

# Early Indicators for the Risk of Atherogenesis.
# A Field Test of a New Methodology on German and
# Japanese Kindergarten Children in Düsseldorf

I. R. Kupke, F. Wellern, and S. Zeugner

Among several approaches to the early detection of atherogenesis -
related risk indicators, one is the screening of pediatric popula -
tions (1). Procedures adequate for this purpose, should be simple
and precise, yet inexpensive and applicable to the examination of
large groups of children outside the clinic. As the blood lipids
and lipoproteins (LPs) have been found to play a key role in atherogenesis, assay of these metabolites is certainly meaningful. In
order to meet these requirements, we have developed new micromethods
which have proved to be adequate for this purpose: A total of 31 µl
capillary blood serum is sufficient for analyzing various serum
lipids together with the cholesterol in LP fractions ( $\alpha$ -, pre- $\beta$ -,
$\beta$ -LP) (2-4). Results obtained by these methods were found to be
in good agreement with those obtained by current methods.

The aim of a recent study (5) was to provide a field test of a methodology which includes the new analytical procedures just mentioned.
This methodology (described in detail below) has proved to be appropriate for the screening of a pediatric population (6). In this field
test, we have examined kindergarten children living in an industrialized city such as Duesseldorf. Several groups could be discerned
among 566 children (3-7 yr) in 17 kindergartens. According to anthropometric criteria, one group (n=335) was classified as a reference
sample group. The blood serum of these children served for the evaluation of reference values. Another group (n=22) was overweight.
Furthermore, children from 5 kindergartens lived in a district classified by the local authorities as socially underprivileged. Among these
children, 96 were anthropometrically normal, while 14 exhibited retarded growth. The decrease of $\beta$ -LP observed in overweight children,
was interpreted as an early indicator of metabolic disorders in obesity, which in turn may lead to atherosclerosis. The socially underprivileged children-normal with respect to height and weight-showed
metabolic disorders which followed a pattern similar to that observed
in protein malnutrition syndromes. In growth-retarded children, the
levels of total cholesterol (TC) were comparable to those in the former group; however, a pronounced predominance of $\beta$ -LP over $\alpha$ -LP
was seen. These data on socially underprivileged children suggest that
poor living conditions might also favor development of the disease(7).

Modified metabolic patterns have also been shown to result from environmental influences. A Westernized life style of Japanese men living
in Hawaii and California (8), as well as of Greenlandic Eskimos living
in Denmark (9), has been reported to shift the metabolic patterns
toward those of the Western natives associated with an increased risk
of coronary heart disease (CHD). On the other hand, in subjects from
the Western countries living in Japan and adjusting to a Japanese
life style, the metabolic patterns were also shifted toward those of
the natives (10). Obviously, environmental changes are diminishing
racial differences (11).

Since the Duesseldorf area has developed during the last 2 decades into the largest commercial center of Japanese industry in Europe, it is of considerable interest to study Japanese children who have been living in Duesseldorf for a period of time. Using the same methodology as described for the investigation of German children, we have examined a group of 78 Japanese children (3-7 yr) and compared them with the German reference sample group. Since metabolic patterns have also been shown to depend on sex and race, even in childhood (12), we differentiated the data from both groups of children on this basis.

## Subjects and Methods

Japanese children investigated belonged to families of middle and higher industrial managment; they live in Germany for 3-4 years. The young children may go to the Misono-en kindergarten, which is re - served for Japanese children, but most go to German kindergartens together with German children. Provided permission was given by the head nurse, written information in Japanese on the content and goals of the examination was given to the nurses and parents at least one week beforehand. It was clearly pointed out that the examination would be performed on a voluntary basis and that only those children whose parents had given written consent would be examined. About 95 % par- ticipated in the examination. The children were in the fasting state. Blood pressure, height and weight were measured. For blood sampling, hyperemization of one finger tip was induced by applying an analgesic cream for 10 min, followed by another 10-15 min of bathing the entire hand in warm water. During the bathing procedure children were re - quested to squeeze colored foam rubber sponges; not only did this promote hyperemization, it also created a relaxed atmosphere. 0.5 - 1.0 ml capillary blood could then be easily obtained by lancing the finger tip.

The lipid profiles (free and esterified cholesterol (C,CE), triacyl- glycerols (TG), phosphatidylcholine (PC), and phosphatidylethanol - amine (PE), were analyzed by high-performance thinlayerchromatography (HPTLC): After direct application of 0.5 µl capillary serum to the silica-gel layer, the lipids were separated and quantitated by fluo- rescence measurement. The coeeficients of variation (CV) were < 2.8 % for all lipids tested, and recovery of known amounts of lipid was 96-100 %. There was close correlation between data obtained by current methods and HPTLC (2).

The following procedure was used for the determination of LP -chole- sterol without ultracentrifugation: The LP fractions of 15 µl cap. serum were separated on the same day by electrophoresis on agarose gel. The samples were dried, dissolved in HCl and neutralized with a saturated Tris-solution producing a Tris-buffer system at pH 7. This system was found to be highly suitable for enzymatic determination of LP-cholesterol. The kinetic properties and the linear range of this reaction system, the precision (CV: 1-3 %)and recovery of TC (100 %) were found to be optimal. This microprocedure gave nearly identical results to those obtained with ultracentrifugation (3,4).

## Results and Discussion

The average age of the German and Japanese groups was only moderately different (5.0 and 5.4 yr). Although Japanese school children are the tallest in Asia (13), our Japanese children were shorter than German children (107 and 113 cm), respectively, but they had the same weight

Table 1.  Comparison of German and Japanese children

| Variable (mmol/l) | | German children (n=335) | | | | Japanese children (n=78) | | | | |
|---|---|---|---|---|---|---|---|---|---|---|
| | | 10 | M | 90 | p | 10 | M | 90 | p | P |
| G L U C | Total | 4.50 | 5.06 | 5.88 | | 4.59 | 5.18 | 5.77 | | |
| | Boys | 4.56 | 5.25 | 6.04 | <.0005 | 4.62 | 5.15 | 5.75 | | |
| | Girls | 4.40 | 4.92 | 5.71 | | 4.43 | 5.19 | 5.77 | | |
| U A | Total | 0.15 | 0.22 | 0.28 | | 0.16 | 0.21 | 0.26 | | |
| | Boys | 0.17 | 0.22 | 0.28 | | 0.16 | 0.21 | 0.25 | | |
| | Girls | 0.13 | 0.22 | 0.29 | | 0.15 | 0.22 | 0.27 | | |
| T G | Total | 0.44 | 0.83 | 1.22 | | 0.52 | 0.76 | 1.13 | | |
| | Boys | 0.39 | 0.77 | 1.15 | <.01 | 0.48 | 0.78 | 1.13 | | |
| | Girls | 0.51 | 0.87 | 1.23 | | 0.52 | 0.68 | 1.13 | | |
| P C | Total | 1.90 | 2.33 | 2.84 | | 1.85 | 2.19 | 2.68 | | <.01 |
| | Boys | 1.91 | 2.30 | 2.86 | | 1.89 | 2.20 | 2.64 | | |
| | Girls | 1.89 | 2.36 | 2.79 | | 1.83 | 2.17 | 2.68 | | |
| P E | Total | 0.39 | 0.49 | 0.61 | | 0.40 | 0.54 | 0.66 | | <.0005 |
| | Boys | 0.39 | 0.49 | 0.59 | | 0.41 | 0.54 | 0.68 | | |
| | Girls | 0.40 | 0.50 | 0.62 | | 0.36 | 0.53 | 0.64 | | |
| C | Total | 0.92 | 1.21 | 1.56 | | 0.91 | 1.18 | 1.51 | | |
| | Boys | 0.86 | 1.16 | 1.50 | <.01 | 0.92 | 1.17 | 1.48 | <.10 | |
| | Girls | 0.95 | 1.24 | 1.62 | | 0.87 | 1.21 | 1.56 | | |
| C E | Total | 2.70 | 3.39 | 4.05 | | 2.66 | 3.15 | 3.71 | | <.0005 |
| | Boys | 2.70 | 3.37 | 3.90 | | 2.73 | 3.15 | 3.64 | | |
| | Girls | 2.68 | 3.42 | 4.13 | | 2.59 | 3.10 | 3.86 | | |
| T C | Total | 3.70 | 4.56 | 5.40 | | 3.56 | 4.24 | 5.11 | | <.0005 |
| | Boys | 3.66 | 4.52 | 5.32 | <.10 | 3.56 | 4.20 | 4.86 | | |
| | Girls | 3.72 | 4.60 | 5.61 | | 3.55 | 4.40 | 5.23 | | |
| $\alpha$ -LP | Total | 0.98 | 1.34 | 1.74 | | 1.06 | 1.36 | 1.80 | | |
| | Boys | 0.97 | 1.35 | 1.78 | | 1.04 | 1.35 | 1.85 | | |
| | Girls | 0.98 | 1.32 | 1.66 | | 1.06 | 1.37 | 1.75 | | |
| Pre- $\beta$ -LP | Total | 0.33 | 0.58 | 0.90 | | 0.17 | 0.31 | 0.58 | | <.0005 |
| | Boys | 0.33 | 0.58 | 0.93 | | 0.16 | 0.33 | 0.59 | | |
| | Girls | 0.32 | 0.57 | 0.90 | | 0.17 | 0.30 | 0.46 | | |
| $\beta$ -LP | Total | 1.86 | 2.50 | 3.24 | | 1.93 | 2.53 | 3.23 | | |
| | Boys | 1.79 | 2.35 | 3.07 | <.0005 | 1.83 | 2.41 | 3.13 | <.10 | |
| | Girls | 1.91 | 2.58 | 3.43 | | 2.03 | 2.62 | 3.40 | | |
| $\beta : \alpha$ -LP | Total | 1.21 | 1.87 | 2.64 | | 1.21 | 1.80 | 2.56 | | |
| | Boys | 1.18 | 1.79 | 2.54 | <.005 | 1.19 | 1.73 | 2.45 | | |
| | Girls | 1.36 | 1.93 | 2.76 | | 1.28 | 1.89 | 2.47 | | |

Concentrations refer to capillary blood serum. Data are expressed as percentiles; M = median; level of significance (Mann-Whithney-test):  p = between sexes,  P  = between races. The remaining differences were not significant. GLUC = glucose, UA = uric acid

(18 kg). Systolic and diastolic blood pressure was significantly higher in Japanese than in German children (96/69 and 90/57 mm Hg); however, these measurements were not made under standardized condi- tions, and will not be discussed further. German boys were taller and heavier than girls (114 and 112 cm; 19 and 18 kg); there was no unequivocal difference in the Japanese group.

As shown in Table 1, the concentrations of TC were markedly lower in Japanese than German children ( 9 %), but they were higher than in Japanese children (12 %) living in Tokyo (14). In accordance with observations on Japanese men living in Hawaii and California (8), Japanese people living in Duesseldorf are adapting to German in - fluences: They eat more meat and milk products, but less soy protein and fish. However, the basicdiet of Japanese men in Duesseldorf is still a Japanese diet (15) rich in soy protein and fish, which have been found to reduce TC as well as pre- $\beta$ -LP (16-18). Interestingly, TC was reduced at the expense of pre- $\beta$ -LP in our Japanese group.

Furthermore, in Japanese children, significantly lower levels of PC and higher levels of PE were observed (Table 1). Since both variables are related to each other by transmethylation processes dependent on the availability of methionine, a relative deficiency of this amino- acid in Japanese children might be the cause, again explicable by differences in German and Japanese diets: In the latter, total protein intake is comprised to a considerable extent by soy protein, which is relatively poor in methionine (19,20).

Table 2. Population comparisons of venous serum lipids [+]

| City | | TG | TC | $\alpha$ -LP/HDL | $\beta$-LP/LDL | $\beta$: $\alpha$ |
|---|---|---|---|---|---|---|
| Duesseldorf (Germans) | Boys | 0.86±0.36 | 4.94±0.73 | 1.44 ±0.31 | 2.54±0.55 | 1.8 |
| | Girls | 0.95±0.33 | 5.12±0.88 | 1.41 ±0.31 | 2.77±0.66 | 2.0 |
| Duesseldorf (Japanese) | Boys | 0.92±0.28 | 4.62±0.57 | 1.48 ±0.33 | 2.61±0.52 | 1.8 |
| | Girls | 0.86±0.31 | 4.87±0.85 | 1.49 ±0.28 | 2.87±0.67 | 1.9 |
| Tokyo (14) | Boys | - | 4.15±0.57 | - | - | - |
| | Girls | - | 4.28±0.66 | - | - | - |
| Geneva (21) | Boys | 0.57 | 4.80±0.70 | 1.66 ±0.24 | 2.64±0.56 | 1.6 |
| | Girls | 0.60 | 5.06±0.80 | 1.61 ±0.33 | 2.72±0.61 | 1.9 |
| Rochester (22) | Boys | 0.59±0.25 | 4.12±0.52 | 1.37 ±0.15 | 2.69±0.47 | 2.0 |
| | Girls | 0.65±0.29 | 4.15±0.62 | 1.30 ±0.21 | 2.77±0.40 | 2.1 |
| Cincinnati (23) | Boys | 0.57±0.18 | 4.09±0.54 | 1.45 ±0.28 | 2.44±0.54 | 1.7 |
| | Girls | 0.81±0.40 | 4.17±0.41 | 1.27 ±0.23 | 2.62±0.49 | 2.1 |
| Bogalusa (24) | Boys | 0.72±0.30 | 4.01±0.62 | 1.56 ±0.47 | 2.28±0.53 | 1.5 |
| | Girls | 0.79±0.35 | 4.09±0.65 | 1.55 ±0.50 | 2.38±0.50 | 1.5 |

Data are expressed as mmol/l ($\bar{x} \pm s_x$).    [+] Data obtained on children in Duesseldorf were extrapolated for venous serum concentrations (25)

Several sex differences in the variables tested were observed (Table 1). The levels of $\beta$ -LP were found to be markedly higher in German girls than in boys. Since TG and TC in $\beta$ -LP/LDL are directly related to each other (26), the augmented serum-TG levels found in German girls might reflect the correspondingly high levels of $\beta$ -LP cholesterol, which in turn elevates the $\beta$ : $\alpha$ -LP ratio. This inherent factor should be considered when using the ratio as an atherogenic index. In parallel to German girls, Japanese girls also tended to have higher $\beta$ -LP levels. Note that this sex difference exists as the same tendency in the other pediatric populations as well (Table 2).

## Conclusions

The entire procedure in the kindergartens was orientated at ethical considerations and its adequacy for children was confirmed by all parents and nurses. Furthermore, the advantage of our new micro - methods lies in being able to analyze several variables in serum of capillary blood, since this can be easily obtained outside the clinic, even from neonates.

Among numerous results on German children, reference values of various metabolites were evaluated. In a further study on Japanese children living in Duesseldorf, these values served for comparative purposes. Sex differences so far observed were more pronounced in the German group. The differences between the German and Japanese groups suggest that environmental influences are more important than racial differences.

## References

1.  Kwiterovich, P.O. (1979) Pediatric lipoprotein metabolism and atherosclerosis: A prospectus. In: Gotto, M., Smith, L.C., Allen, B. (eds) Atherosclerosis V. Springer- Verlag New York, Heidelberg, Berlin, pp 286 - 293
2.  Kupke, I.R., Zeugner, S. (1978) Quantitative high-performance thin-layer chromatography of lipids in plasma and liver homogenates after direct application of 0.5 ul samples to the silica-gel layer. J. Chromatogr. 146: 261 - 271
3.  Kupke, I.R. (1979) Enzymatic microdetermination of plasma lipoprotein cholesterol without ultracentrifugation. Clin. Chim. Acta 95: 123 - 127
4.  Kupke, I.R., Zeugner, S., Gottschalk, A. (1979) Comparison of two micromethods for determination of lipoprotein cholesterol in plasma. Clin. Chem. 25: 1795 - 1798
5.  Kupke, I.R., Heller, B., Weiss, P. (1982) Early indicators for the risk of atherogenesis. A field test of a new methodology on kindergarten children in Duesseldorf. Atheroscl. (in press)
6.  WHO workshop on pilot projects for the study and control of atherosclerosis precursors in childhood and youth. CVD/80.2
7.  Kupke, I.R., Heller, B., Weiss, P. (1978) Plasma lipids, lipoproteins and other factors related to atherosclerosis: A pediatric study in Duesseldorf. In: Hayase, S., Murao, S. (eds) Proceedings of the VIII World Congress of Cardiology. Exerpta Medica 90219, 9021903946, ISBN Elsevier North-Holland 0444900713, pp 394-399
8.  Tillotson, J.L., Kato, H., Nichiman, M.Z., Miller, D.C., Gay,M.L., Johnson, K.G., Rhoads, G.G. (1973) Epidemiology of coronary heart disease and stroke in Japanese men living in Japan, Hawaii, and California: Methodology for comparison of diet. J. Clin. Nutr. 26: 177 - 184
9.  Bang, H.O., Dyerberg, H.O. (1972) Plasma lipids and lipoproteins in Greenlandic West Coast Eskimos. Acta med. Scand. 192: 85 - 94
10. Yano, Y., Irie, N., Homma, Y., Tsushima, M., Takeuchi, I., Nakaya, N., Goto, Y. (1980) High density lipoprotein cholesterol levels in the Japanese. Atheroscl. 36: 173 - 181
11. Strong, J.P. (1976) An introduction to the epidemiology of athero-

sclerosis. In: Schettler, G., Goto, Y., Hata, Y., Klose, G. (eds) Atherosclerosis IV. Springer-Verlag, New York, Heidelberg, Berlin, pp 92 - 98

12. Berenson, G.S., Srinivasan, S.R., Voors, A.W., Webber, L.S. (1979) Clues to mechanisms of cardiovascular disease from an epidemiologic study of children - The Bogalusa Heart Study. In: Ref. 1, pp 272 - 277

13. Innami, S. (1970) Nutritional status - Japan. Nutr. Rev. 27: 275 - 278

14. Okuni, M., Kiryu, H.S., Yamauchi, K. (1980) Risk factors of atherosclerosis in Japanese children. Jap. Circul.J.44: 69 - 75

15. Keys, A., Kimura, N. (1970) Diets of middle-aged farmers in Japan. Am. J. Clin. Nutr. 23: 212 - 223

16. Carrol, K.K., Giovannetti, P.M., Moase, O., Robert, D.C.K., Wolfe, B.M. (1978) Hypocholesterolemic effect of substituting soy bean protein for animal protein in the diet of healthy young women. Am. J. Clin. Nutr. 31: 1312 - 1321

17. Holmes, W.L., Rubel, G.B., Hood, S.S. (1980) Comparison of the effect of dietary meat versus dietary soybean protein on plasma lipids of hyperlipidemic individuals. Atheroscl. 36: 379 - 387

18. Lossonczy, T.O., Ruiter, A., Bronsgeest-Schoute, H.C., Gent,C.M., Hermus, R.J.J. (1978) The effect of a fish diet on serum lipids in healthy human subjects. Am. J. Clin. Nutr. 31: 1340 - 1346

19. Huff, M.W., Hamilton, R.M.G., Carrol, K.K. (1977) Plasma chole- sterol levels in rabbits fed low fat, cholesterol-free, semi - purified diets: Effects of dietary proteins, protein hydrolysates and amino acid mixtures. Atheroscl. 28: 187 - 195

20. Oiso, T., Suzue, R. (1970) Topics of nutrition in Japan. Am. J. Clin. Nutr. 23: 1096 - 1098

21. Pometa, D., Micheli, H., Raymond, L., Oberhaensli, I., Suenram,A. (1980) Decreased HDL cholesterol in prepubertal and pubertal children of CHD patients. Atheroscl. 36: 101 - 109

22. Elleffson, R.D., Elveback, L.R., Hodgson, P.A. (1978) Cholesterol and triglycerides in serum lipoproteins of young persons in Rochester, Minnesota. Mayo Clin. Proc. 53: 307 - 320

23. Morrison, J.A., deGroot, I., Edwards, B.K., Kelly, K.A., Mellies, M.J., Khoury, P., Glueck, Ch.J. (1978) Lipids and lipoproteins in 927 schoolchildren, ages 6-17 years. Pediatrics 62: 990 - 995

24. Berenson, G.A., Foster, T.A., Frank, G.C., Frerichs, R.R., Srinivasan, S.R., Voors, A.W., Webber, L.S. (1978) Cardiovascular disease risk factor variables in the preschool age. The Bogalusa Heart Study. Circulation 57: 603 - 612

25. Kupke, I.R., Zeugner, S., Gottschalk, A., Kather, B. (1979) Differences in lipid and lipoprotein concentrations of capillary and venous blood samples. Clin. Chim. Acta 97: 279 - 283

26. Carlson, L.A., Ericsson, M. (1975) Quantitative and qualitative serum lipoprotein analysis. Part 1. Studies in healthy men and women. Atheroscl. 21: 417 - 433

# Morphologic Changes in Coronary Arteries of Children in Different Geographic Locations

R. F. Scott and A. S. Daoud

The study of coronary atherosclerosis in children has at least two general objectives. One is to learn more about the natural history of the early development of the disease. Another, in comparing coronaries from geographic areas with differing severity of atherosclerosis in adults, is to learn at what time the disease begins to progress rapidly in the high risk group, and to determine if there are qualitative differences in early lesions from different locations.

In reporting on different studies, immediate problems are encountered because of different methods used to quantitate and describe the lesions, and the differing terminology used. Nevertheless, useful comparisons can be made. In this report we will describe some microscopic features of coronary atherosclerosis in children and young adults from Albany, NY and New Orleans, LA in the U.S.; Uganda in East Africa; Santiago, Chile; Costa Rica; Guatamala; Durban, South Africa; and Bucharest, Romania.

The impetus for the first study to be described (1) was a report by Daoud et al. (2) showing that at autopsy coronary atherosclerosis was much more severe in 16-40 year old males in Albany, New York than in age matched males from Uganda in East Africa (Fig. I). New Yorkers had more, and thicker, atheroma lesions than East Africans. Furthermore, by fifty years, myocardial infarcts are common in New York males, while they are virtually unknown in East Africa at any age.

To follow up on Daoud's findings, we carried out a histologic study of New Yorker and East African coronary arteries from newborn to age 20, and a lipid analysis of coronaries from newborn to age 40. There were 109 New Yorker newborn to 39 years (60 male and 49 females) and 137 East African arteries (95 male and 42 females) available for chemical analysis. In the newborn to 19 year old group, where alternate arterial segments were used for chemical and histologic analysis, there were 35 New Yorkers (24 male and 11 females) and an equal number of age and sex matched East Africans. The tissue for microscopic study was fixed in Carbowax, cut and stained with H & E, oil Red 0, and Verhoef-Van Giesin. Lesions were graded as atheroma if they had necrosis or calcification; non-atheroma lesions were classified as being with and without stainable lipid. The thickness of all lesions was measured with a micrometer. The lipids measured were cholesterol, phospholipid and their esterified fatty acids. Complete details of the methodology are given in the original publication.

AMERICANS

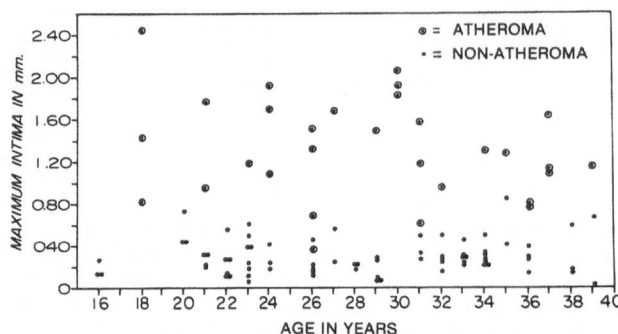

AFRICANS

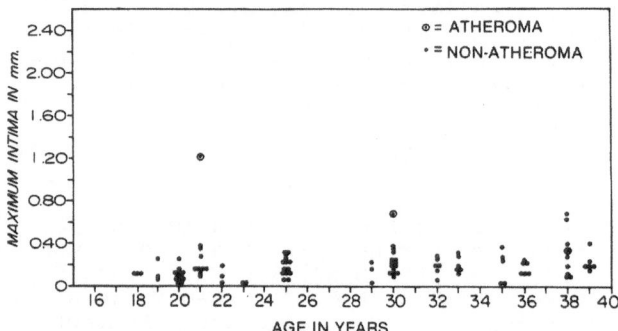

<u>Figure I</u> - A comparison of the number of non-atheroma and atheroma lesions in the coronary arteries of New Yorker and East African males 16-40 years. The atheroma lesions (those with necrosis) are obviously greater in number and are thicker in the New Yorkers

The number and kinds of lesions and their thickness in New York and East African male coronary arteries, newborn to 19 years, is shown in Figure II. There were few atheroma lesions in either group (3 New Yorker and 1 East African), but non-atheroma lesions were found in both groups at all ages; there was no difference in the thickness of the lesions in the two groups. The only striking histologic difference before age 20 in the coronary arteries of the two groups was the increased number of non-atheroma lesions containing lipid in the New Yorker compared to the East African group in the second decade.

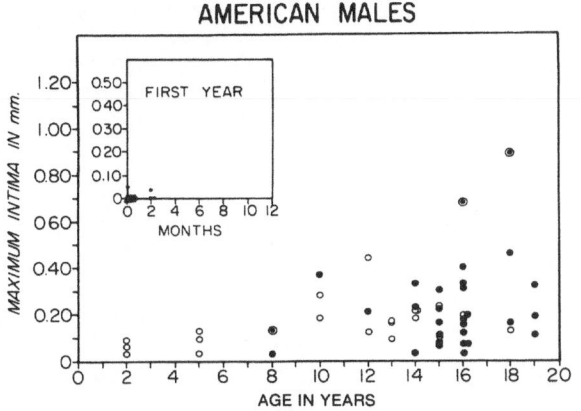

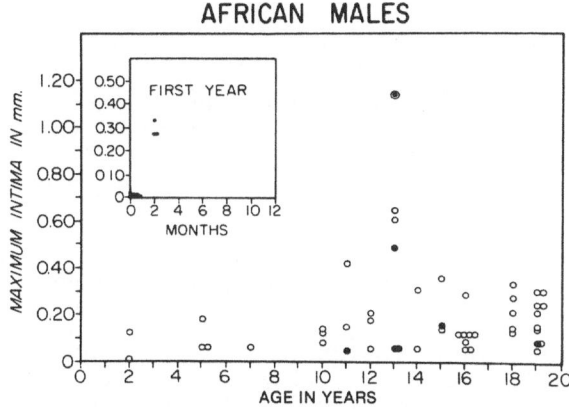

Figure II - Atheroma, non-atheroma with fat, and non-atheroma without
fat lesions in New Yorker and East African coronary arteries newborn
to age 20 years

_____//_____

The values for total and ester cholesterol in the coronary arteries
are shown in Figure III.  No difference was found till the 3rd decade
and no statistically significant differences were present until the
fourth decade.  The analysis of phospholipid and esterified fatty acids
in the arteries of the two groups showed no striking differences.  The
quantitative similarity of types of lipid is in keeping with the similar
histological appearance of lesions in the two groups as seen by light
microscopy.

This study shows that in two population groups with greatly differing
amounts of coronary atherosclerosis by the fourth decade, there is a
slight increase in stainable lipid within the coronary lesions as early
as the second decade in the higher risk New Yorker group, but that it
was not until the third decade that New Yorkers showed appreciably more
atherosclerotic lesions and lipid in their coronary arteries.  The kinds
of lipid present in the arteries and the histology of the lesions in
the two groups was generally similar, suggesting that the disease, at

80

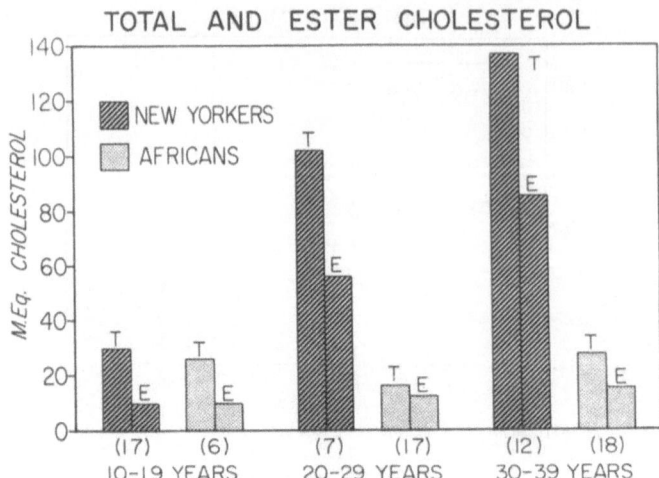

Figure III - Both total and ester cholesterol as measured chemically
increase in New Yorkers' arteries in the third decade
_____//_____

least as far as could be determined by the methods used, is the same
in both groups.

In a histologic study only, Geer et al. (3) used a standard site from
the left anterior descending to compare coronary arteries in 10 to 40
year old subjects from different geographic areas.  These areas, in
order of decreasing severity of atherosclerosis, were New Orleans,
Jamaica, Santiago (Chile), Lima (Peru), Guatamala and South Africa.
The most positive finding was that even as early as 10-19 years, the
amount of intimal lipid predicted the disposition to develop severe
atherosclerosis later in life.  The findings parallelled those in the
study of New Yorkers and East Africans.  Interestingly, Geer's study
showed that increased intimal thickness alone did not predict the severity of subsequent atherosclerosis.

The recent series of papers by Velican and Velican (4,5) examining
young coronary arteries in Bucharest, Romania has provided insight into
the natural history of the disease.  Non-raised fibrous plaques were
found in 2% of 6-10 year olds and 4% of 11-15 year olds.  Fatty streaks
and gelatinous plaques were seen in 6% of the 11-15 year age group,
appearing later than the non-raised fibrous plaques seen in the 6-10
year old group.  There was considerable evidence that pads or cushions
at vessel branching were the source of fibrous plaques.  As in other
parts of the world, fatty streaks did not appear until the second decade,
and followed the appearance of earlier lesions.

They pointed out then that fatty streaks are not the initial lesion in
the coronaries of children, a finding also true to the Albany and East
African studies.  They did not rule out the possibility, however, that
fatty streaks in the second decade could be the impetus to develop a
large number of lesions in adult life.

References

1.  Scott, RF, Florentin, RA, Daoud, AS, Morrison, ES, Jones, RM, Hutt, MSR (1966) Coronary arteries of children and young adults:  A comparison of lipids and anatomic features in New Yorkers and East Africans.  Exp. Mol. Pathol. 5: 12-42.
2.  Daoud, AS, Jarmolych, J, Zumbo, O, Fani, K, Florentin, RA (1964) "Pre-atheroma" phase of coronary atherosclerosis in man.  Exp. Mol. Pathol. 3: 475-484.
3.  Geer, JC, McGill, HC, Robertson, WB, Strong, JP (1968) Histologic characteristics of coronary artery fatty streaks.  Lab. Invest. 18(5): 565-570.
4.  Velican, D, Velican, C (1979)  Study of fibrous plaques occurring in the coronary arteries of children.  Athero. 33: 201-215.
5.  Velican, C, Velican, D (1980)  The precursors of coronary atherosclerotic plaques in subjects up to 40 years old.  Athero. 37: 33-46.

Figures 1, 2 and 3 originally appeared in the journal Experimental and Molecular Pathology published by Academic Press.

# Structure and Ultrastructure of the Coronary Artery Intima in Children and Young Adults Up to Age 29[1]

H. C. Stary

## Introduction

This paper describes the intima of the coronary arteries of young
human subjects as it develops and changes during maturation.  The
work represents a preliminary report of one part of a continuing study
of the coronary arteries and aortas of the population of New Orleans
in the first 29 years of life.  Investigators who studied human coronary intima in the past found that it was thickened and that there
was regional variation in thickness and structure.  A thick intima
was also reported for other arteries.  Thoma (1) who studied human
aortic intima with the light microscope, a century ago described and
illustrated areas in which the intima was consistently thicker.  He
stated that the thick segments were a universal feature in human
aortic development.  Awareness of the fact that human arterial intima
is far more than a thin and nondescript space between the basement
membrane of the endothelial cells and the internal elastic lamina has,
however, not been general.

The present study of coronary artery intima differs from the ones that
preceded it in that the coronary arteries we studied and measured were
fixed under pressures similar to those existing during life, that light
microscopy was on 1-$\mu$m plastic-embedded sections which allow a resolution far superior to that of traditional 5-$\mu$m sections, that the 1-$\mu$m
sections were complete cross-sections, and that we used semiserial
sectioning and electron microscopy.  The reason for this study was
not only the wish to add to the basic knowledge about human coronary
intima by using improved methods but the hope that we could answer
some questions about the development of atherosclerotic lesions in
some preferred coronary segments.  The incidence of coronary atherosclerotic lesions in the young population and the mechanism of their
development and progression will be the subject of subsequent reports.

## Methods

The data in this report are on the coronary arteries of 276 black and
white, male and female subjects aged up to 29 years.  These were selected from more than 400 autopsy cases obtained so far for this project and from 50 autopsy cases used in a feasibility study preceding
the project.  The 276 cases were chosen for pressure-perfusion and
morphological studies because of a shorter interval between death and
autopsy.  Most of the subjects died in accidents or homicides.  As

[1] This work was supported by the National Institutes of Health,
Grant HL-22739

soon after death as possible, we perfusion-fixed the coronary arteries
under a pressure of 100 mm Hg by connecting the ascending aorta by
plastic tube to a container with 3% glutaraldehyde, elevated 135 cm
above the level of the heart.  The fixative drained through the coronary sinus and through a small peripheral artery incised at the apex
of the heart.  The pressure within the coronary arteries was not monitored during perfusion and some variation in the contour of the internal elastic lamina from case to case suggests that variation in
the actual intracoronary pressure occurred.  Variation was within
limits and we are confident that the comparisons which we base on our
measurements are nevertheless valid.

Although a thick intima occurs in all coronary artery branches, we
confined our coronary studies to a detailed investigation of a precisely defined segment of the left coronary artery, consisting of the
main stem, the main bifurcation, and the proximal left anterior descending (LAD) branch.  We already knew that intimal thickening is
prominent in these segments, and that coronary artery disease, if it
will occur at all, will develop preferentially in this location.
Limiting the study to a precisely defined segment made study in depth
feasible.  We studied the same coronary segment in several nonhuman
primate species also.  We cut the segment into five consecutive tube-
like blocks (main, bifurcation, LAD 1, 2, and 3), each measuring 2
to 3 mm in length, and embedded these in the epoxy resin Maraglas or,
in some instances, in water-soluble methacrylate.  Measurements were
made on the 1-μm thick cross-sections of the plastic-embedded coronary
segments.  For comparative measurements of intimal and medial thickness we used only the three blocks of the proximal LAD branch, because
media and intima are well defined in the LAD.  While we did also measure the intima and its points of emphasis in the main stem and in
the bifurcation, we used the results of these measurements with reservation since the intimal-medial boundary is often ill defined in the
left main segment and at the bifurcation.  We also did not use for
comparisons of intimal thickness coronary arteries that had developed
atherosclerosis.  The three LAD blocks of twenty five cases were sectioned and measured semiserially.  Thus in each one of 25 cases,
measurements were made in about 30 complete cross-sections of the
proximal LAD.  Four separate measurements were made of each coronary
cross-section, the thickest part of the wall constituting the first
measurement, the other three measurements being at right angles to
the first one.  For measurement we used the light microscope containing an eyepiece disk with a scale subdivided into 100 segments.  The
eyepiece segments were converted into μm with a stage micrometer.

## Definition of Coronary Artery Intima

The term coronary artery intima as we use it in this report refers to
an intima in which one or more layers of intimal smooth muscle cells
and a variable amount of glycosaminoglycan (GAG)-rich extracellular
martix separate the endothelial basement membrane from the internal
elastic lamina or, in the absence of an internal elastic, from the
first lamina of the media.  Terms that are being frequently used for
the thick intima of human coronary (and other) arteries and for the
less severely and less extensively thick coronary artery intima of
other species are diffuse intimal thickening (DIT) and nonatherosclerotic intimal thickening.  Since it is established that the

coronary intima is, in every human being, a substantial structure
which rivals the media in thickness from birth, a special term to
emphasize this point seems unnecessary.  Furthermore, a term like
diffuse intimal thickening might suggest that a pathological process
rather than human development has caused the intima to be thick.

Special terms such as intimal cushion, intimal pad, and intimal cell
mass are in use for the particularly thick segments of intima that
are related more closely to arterial branch points where hemodynamic
shear stresses and turbulence may be greater, particularly in arteries
with great pulse differentials.  Cushions and pads are not separate
structures but rather local points of special emphasis in the intima.
Under systolic pressure they are crescent-shaped accentuations of the
intima, but at or below diastolic pressure they become apparent as
cushions, pads, or humps that protrude into the lumen of arteries.
They jut forth especially prominently in collapsed arteries not under
any pressure at all.

Some writers who have studied the coronary arteries of young people
without fixation under pressure have used the term plaque, fibrous
plaque, and obstructive plaque for local points of intimal emphasis.
Most writers, including ourselves, prefer to reserve the terms plaque,
and fibrous plaque, for the even more prominent and histologically
distinct intimal thickening caused by pathological processes, in particular by atherosclerotic disease.  Although points of intimal emphasis and atherosclerotic fibrous plaques have certain components
in common, the two are entirely distinct in structure and ultrastructure.  Furthermore, fibrous plaques can eventually develop into a
thickness that is not achieved by normal points of intimal emphasis.

## Results

The intima of every coronary artery was at least several cell layers
thick throughout the segment we studied.  The degree of intimal thickness was, however, not uniform in its circumferential and longitudinal
distributions, nor did the number of cell layers express the real
thickness since the extracellular GAG matrix varied considerably in
degree within the coronary segment we studied.  In the posterolateral
quadrant of the LAD, opposite to the flow divider, the intima was
thicker than elsewhere.  This posterolateral prominence extended into
the LAD from the bifurcation of the main stem.  The intima of the
circumflex had a similar posterolateral prominence opposite the flow
divider.  Under systolic pressure, this posterolateral prominence
appeared as a crescent-shaped emphasis of the diffusely thick intima.
Under lower pressures, the crescent changed from concave to convex,
protruding into the lumen and forming a ridge which extended along
the length of the segment, from the distal main into the proximal
LAD branch.  The degree of the luminal bulge increased with the degree
of loss in the intracoronary pressure.  In coronary arteries not fixed
under pressure, the ridge projected into the lumen prominently, simulating severe obstruction to flow.

The topograpy of the distribution of intimal thickness within the
coronary artery was similar in all individuals, but the degree of the
thickness varied in individuals of identical age, sex and race.  Intimal thickness equaled or exceeded medial thickness in one half of

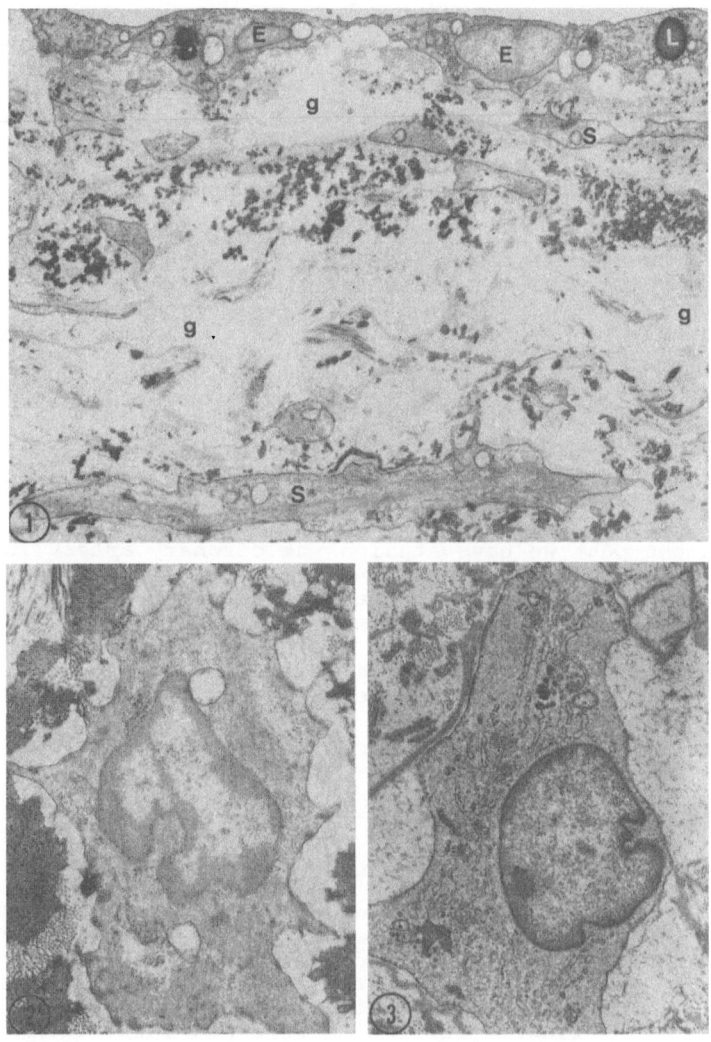

Figure 1.  GAG-rich part of the left main coronary intima of a
5-year-old girl (Case P-1133).
Figure 2. Myofilament-rich intimal smooth muscle cell (SMC)
in same artery as in Fig. 1.
Figure 3.  RER-rich intimal SMC in the bifurcation of a 9-year-old boy
(Case C-38).  Endothelial cell (E); SMC (S); lipid droplet (L); GAG (g)
the male and female cases within any age group.  The thickness of the
posterolateral prominence in the proximal LAD always at least matched
the thickness of the media, measuring up to four times the media in
some cases.  With increasing age the degree of intimal thickness, the
degree of the posterolateral prominence, and the degree of medial
thickness, all increased.  Their proportions to each other remained
the same, however.  Toward the end of the second decade the posterolateral prominence became a preferred location for the development
of fibrous plaques in the coronary arteries of those individuals with
atherosclerotic lesions.

Ultrastructurally, smooth muscle cells of two types of morphological expression were the principal cell component of human coronary intima. These were smooth muscle cells rich in thick (myosin) filaments (Figs. 1 and 2), and smooth muscle cells rich in rough-surfaced endoplasmic reticulum (RER) (Fig. 3).  RER-rich smooth muscle cells had less thick filaments and some may have lacked thick filaments completely.  RER-rich smooth muscle cells were more frequent in the GAG-rich extracellular matrix of the upper, subendothelial, part of the intima which was especially thick in posterolateral intimal accentuations.  The proportion of cells that were RER-rich smooth muscle cells was greater in the intima of children which also contained proportionately more GAG than adults.  The proportion of RER-rich cells decreased as myofilament-rich smooth muscle cells and the degree of cellular and fibrillar density of the intima increased during maturation.  However, the proportion of the two cell types to each other began to change again in favor of the RER-rich type in those segments of the intima in which atherosclerotic plaques developed.

Macrophages were the only additional cell type we noticed in coronary artery intima.  We report details about the macrophage population of the intima elsewhere in this volume (2).

In the past we have studied the coronary artery intima of several nonhuman primate species.  In relation to the media, the coronary intima of nonhuman primates is far less thick than that of man, although a basic similarity exists in composition.  In the young humans we are also studying the aorta.  There is a resemblance between segments of the intima of the abdominal aorta and the posterolateral emphasis of the proximal LAD.  The resemblance lies in the thickness of the GAG-rich intimal component.

References

1.  Thoma R (1883) Über die Abhängigkeit der Bindegewbsneubildung in der Arterienintima von den mechanischen Bedingungen des Blutumlaufs.  Virchows Arch path Anat Phsyiol 93: 443-505
2.  Stary HC (1982) Macrophages in coronary artery and aortic intima and in atherosclerotic lesions of children and young adults up to age 29.  Proc 6th Int Symp Atherosclerosis, Springer-Verlag, Berlin-Heidelberg-New York (this volume)

# The Natural History of Aortic Atherosclerosis in Children, Adolescents and Young Adults

J. P. Strong

EARLY QUANTITATIVE STUDIES OF THE NATURAL HISTORY OF AORTIC
ATHEROSCLEROSIS

HOLMAN et al. (1) in 1958 examined aortas from 526 necropsied individuals between 1 and 40 years of age obtained at a large general
hospital and a medicolegal laboratory in New Orleans. These specimens were examined before and after gross staining with Sudan IV,
and the extent of fatty streaks, fibrous plaques, and complicated
lesions (hemorrhage, ulceration, thrombosis, or calcification) was
estimated for each aorta in terms of percentage of intimal surface
affected by each type of lesion. Gross Sudan staining increased the
ability to detect fatty streaks, and thus increased their incidence
and extent, particularly in the younger age groups.

Fatty streaks did not seem to be precipitated by terminal acute ill-
nesses, for comparison of the average extent of lesions in cases dying
suddenly as a result of trauma or poisoning with the average of lesions in natural deaths, disclosed no significant difference.

All patients 3 years of age or older had at least minimal sudanophilic
intimal deposits. Minimal lesions were found so frequently that some
question was raised as to the significance of gross Sudan staining,
i.e., whether it actually indicated an early lesion of atherosclerosis. Histologic sections were examined with this particular question in mind, and in every instance there were histologic alterations
in the intima corresponding to the macroscopic sudanophilia. These
alterations consisted of both intracellular and extracellular glob-
ules of lipid (as indicated by the application of Sudan IV), and a
slight increase in interstitial mucinous material. The intima in
these early lesions was not always elevated, and there was little
cellular reaction.

The percentage of surface involved rose slowly until the 6- to 10-
year age group at which time the extent of lesions began to rise
precipitously in the black. Five years later, the extent of fatty
streaks began to rise in the white, but did not reach a peak as high
as in the black. The patterns in the black male and female were very
much alike, with more severe involvement in females than in males at
some ages. White females were consistently the group least affected.

Fibrous plaques began to appear in the second decade but did not increase appreciably until the fourth decade. They paralleled the
development of fatty streaks but lagged about 15 years, and the relative decree of involvement of white and black was reversed as compared
to fatty streaks. By 40 years of age, only about 20 percent of the
area covered by fatty streaks had been converted into fibrous plaques.
Additional complications in the lesions were rarely seen in this
series.

The aortic ring was the first region of the aorta to be the seat of
fatty streaks, but it was the descending thoracic and particularly
the abdominal portions which gave the distinctive pattern of increasing lesions between 5 and 20 years. Fibrous plaques also developed
most extensively in the abdominal portion.

There was sufficient fatty change to serve as a basis for all the
fibrous plaques encountered at later ages, and the data indicated
that it requires at least 15 years for the conversion to take place.
The rate of development of fibrous plaques and fatty streaks was
reversed in the white as compared to the black, leading these authors
to suggest that whatever initiates the atherosclerotic process differs
from whatever carries it on to produce clinical manifestations.


EARLY GEOGRAPHIC STUDIES


Data from the more than 1600 autopsied persons in New Orleans which
were studied prior to 1960 revealed, after gross staining of specimens, that aortic fatty streaks were present in many children under
age 3 and in all children over age 3(2). Fatty streaks of coronary
arteries were rare before age 10, but were more frequent in the second decade of life and were almost universal after age 20. These
data were compared with similar data from autopsied young persons in
other locations--Guatemala, Costa Rica(3) and Durban, South Africa(4).
Fatty streaks began in the first decade of life in these populations
also. The earliest lesions were located in the aortic ring and aortic
arch, and lesions soon began to appear in the thoracic and abdominal
aortic segments.

After 10 years of age the extent of aortic intimal surface involved
by fatty streaks increased rapidly in succeeding age groups from
all locations. There was no striking or consistent difference in
aortic fatty streaks among groups from different geographic locations,
but there was a racial difference. The black groups between ages 15
and 25 years from New Orleans, and Durban had more extensive fatty
streaks than the other groups. Aortic fibrous plaques, complicated
plaques, and clacified plaques tended to parallel differences in
incidence of coronary heart disease in middle-aged adults from the
same populations. New Orleans white cases were most extensively
involved with fibrous plaques.

## INTERNATIONAL ATHEROSCLEROSIS PROJECT

These studies stimulated the development of the International Atherosclerosis Project (IAP), an extensive study of the geographic pathology of atherosclerosis(5).  In this study, aortas, coronary arteries,
and (in some locations) cerebral arteries were collected from autopsied persons in 14 countries and systematically examined and evaluated
by a group of cooperating pathologists.  The IAP data are based on
quantitative grading of over 23,000 sets of coronary arteries and
aortas.  Geographic, racial, and other comparisons have been reported
in detail(5) and have been reviewed extensively(6-8).

## PEDIATRIC ASPECTS OF ATHEROSCLEROSIS

Because of special interest in the pediatric aspects of atherosclerosis, STRONG AND MCGILL(9) studied aortic and coronary artery lesions
in 4737 autopsied cases of both sexes, ages 10-39, from six location-
race groups in the IAP.  These cases represented a subsample of the
IAP material.  The six geographic and ethnic groups were selected
because they represented populations in which the extremes of average
involvement of advanced atherosclerosis were found in older persons.
The six groups were New Orleans, white, New Orleans black, Santiago,
Costa Rica, Guatemala, and Durban Bantu.

NEWMAN AND STRONG(10) summarized the findings concerning atherosclerosis in children based on the IAP material and previous studies in New
Orleans.  The essentials of that geographic comparison of lesions in
young persons are described in the next sections of this report.

## METHODOLOGY FOR COLLECTING AND EVALUATING SPECIMENS

In each laboratory, coronary arteries and aortas were dissected "uniformly" at necropsy, labeled with coded numbered tags, and shipped to
a central laboratory.  The central laboratory staff stained the specimen grossly with Sudan IV and packed them in plastic bags identified
by code numbers.  A team of five pathologists estimated the percentage of intimal surface area covered by different types of lesions as
defined at the beginning of this chapter.  Interobserver variation was
reduced by developing explicit criteria and by training.

RESULTS OF STUDY OF 10- TO 39-YEAR AGE GROUPS

Table 1 compares the percentage of aortas positive for fatty streaks
in these six location-age groups. By age 10, almost all aortas from
these groups were positive for aortic fatty streaks.

Coronary fatty streaks (data not shown here) were not as frequent as
aortic fatty streaks, but they occurred in some cases from each loca-
tion-race group even in the 10-14 age group. Fatty streaks of some
degree were present in the coronary arteries of practically all persons over age 20 in New Orleans, and were present in approximately
90 percent of persons in the other age groups by age 30.

Table 2 shows the percentages of aortas positive for any of the raised
atherosclerotic lesions. Raised lesions began in some cases from each
group before age 20, and the frequency involved with raised lesions
increased rapidly in the two decades following. New Orleans cases
were most frequently involved with raised lesions in most age groups.
Raised lesions were much more frequent in men than in women in the
New Orleans white and in the cases from Santiago and Costa Rica
(both predominantly white racial groups).


EXTENT OF LESIONS


The mean percentage of aortic intimal surface involved by fatty streaks
and raised atherosclerotic lesions is shown for males in Table 3. On
the average fatty streaks involved from 7 to 19 percent of the aortic
intima in cases 10-14 years of age, and from 20 to 38 percent in cases
20-24 years of age. Aortic fatty streaks showed no clear pattern of
geographic or ethnic differences except for the greater than average
involvement of the New Orleans black.

Aortic raised lesions showed geographic and ethnic differences by age
30 with New Orleans white most extensively involved and with slightly
less involvement in New Orleans black and Durban Bantu.

Aortic Atherosclerosis in New Orleans in the 1960's

STRONG, RESTREPO AND GUZMÁN(11) reported comparisons of coronary and
aortic atherosclerosis in New Orleans by age, sex and race for 2,700
autopsied subjects during the 1960's. This study included subjects
10 to 64 years of age. Aortic fatty streaks were present in all of
the youngest age group (10 to 14 years) and in this age group were
more extensive in blacks than whites as reported in previous studies.
The only other consistent differences in aortic lesions in the relatively young individuals was greater involvement with fatty streaks
in black females than in white females. Fatty streaks in the aorta
were replaced by fibrous plaques and more advanced lesions in subsequent decades. In the older age groups the more advanced lesions
of aortic atherosclerosis were more extensive in white men. The
differences among the remaining 3 subgroups of white women, black
men and black women were not striking or consistent.

**Table 1.**

Percentage of Cases Positive for Fatty Streaks in the Aorta by Location–Race Group, Age, and Sex

| Location–Race Groups | 10–14 | | 15–19 | | 20–24 | | 25–29 | | 30–34 | | 35–39 | |
|---|---|---|---|---|---|---|---|---|---|---|---|---|
| | Male | Female | Male | Female | Male | Female | Male | Female | Male | Female | Male | Female |
| New Orleans, white | 100 | 100 | 100 | 100 | 100 | 100 | 100 | 100 | 100 | 100 | 100 | 100 |
| New Orleans, black | 94 | 90 | 100 | 100 | 100 | 100 | 100 | 100 | 100 | 100 | 100 | 100 |
| Santiago | 100 | 100 | 100 | 100 | 100 | 100 | 100 | 100 | 100 | 100 | 100 | 100 |
| Costa Rica | 100 | 100 | 100 | 100 | 100 | 100 | 100 | 100 | 100 | 100 | 100 | 100 |
| Guatemala | 100 | 100 | 100 | 100 | 100 | 100 | 100 | 100 | 100 | 100 | 100 | 100 |
| Durban Bantu | 95 | 100 | 100 | 100 | 100 | 100 | 100 | 100 | 100 | 100 | 100 | 99 |

Strong and McGill[9]

**Table 2.**

Percentage of Cases Positive for Raised Atherosclerotic Lesions in the Aortas by Location–Race Group, Age, and Sex

| Location–Race Groups | 10–14 | | 15–19 | | 20–24 | | 25–29 | | 30–34 | | 35–39 | |
|---|---|---|---|---|---|---|---|---|---|---|---|---|
| | Male | Female | Male | Female | Male | Female | Male | Female | Male | Female | Male | Female |
| New Orleans, white | 0 | 0 | 7 | 0 | 5 | 5 | 40 | 38 | 67 | 76 | 80 | 71 |
| New Orleans, black | 6 | 0 | 0 | 6 | 9 | 14 | 26 | 42 | 47 | 59 | 76 | 76 |
| Santiago | 0 | 7 | 3 | 1 | 7 | 3 | 11 | 15 | 29 | 20 | 39 | 38 |
| Costa Rica | 3 | 14 | 2 | 11 | 2 | 13 | 8 | 23 | 36 | 26 | 40 | 49 |
| Guatemala | 0 | 3 | 2 | 2 | 9 | 17 | 17 | 15 | 26 | 17 | 36 | 48 |
| Durban Bantu | 0 | 4 | 12 | 9 | 19 | 10 | 26 | 19 | 52 | 36 | 56 | 45 |

Strong and McGill[9]

**Table 3.**

Mean Percentage of Intimal Surface Involved with Aortic Fatty Streaks (FS) and Raised Atherosclerotic Lesions (RL) in Males by Location–Race Group and Age

| Location–Race Groups | 10–14 | | 15–19 | | 20–24 | | 25–29 | | 30–34 | | 35–39 | |
|---|---|---|---|---|---|---|---|---|---|---|---|---|
| | FS | RL | FS | RL | FS | RL | FS | RL | FS | RL | FS | RL |
| New Orleans, white | 7 | 0 | 17 | 1 | 25 | 0 | 28 | 3 | 27 | 8 | 25 | 17 |
| New Orleans, black | 19 | 0 | 31 | 0 | 28 | 1 | 27 | 2 | 24 | 5 | 25 | 10 |
| Santiago | 9 | 0 | 15 | 0 | 18 | 0 | 20 | 1 | 21 | 2 | 20 | 3 |
| Costa Rica | 9 | 0 | 15 | 1 | 19 | 0 | 23 | 0 | 22 | 2 | 24 | 3 |
| Guatemala | 12 | 0 | 16 | 0 | 21 | 1 | 24 | 0 | 24 | 2 | 25 | 3 |
| Durban Bantu | 9 | 0 | 16 | 1 | 21 | 1 | 25 | 2 | 26 | 6 | 26 | 6 |

Strong & McGill[9]

## Current Studies of Aortic Atherosclerosis

STARY and STRONG are restudying the natural history of coronary and aortic atherosclerotic lesions in young individuals - infants children, and young adults. In regard to aortic lesions, they have evaluated the grossly visible lesions in over 400 aortas in autopsied individuals from the newborn period through 29 years of age. They are also studying the microscopic and ultrastructural features of these lesions. The preliminary findings in this ongoing study indicate that, as in previously reported studies, grossly visible aortic fatty streaks are frequently found in young children in the second and third year of life and are almost universally present to some extent after that time. STARY is reporting on preliminary findings in the coronary arteries elsewhere in this volume(12 and 13). The details of gross microscopic and ultrastructural features of the aortic lesions will be the subject of a future report.

## SUMMARY

The following statements are based on some of the principal findings and conclusions from our studies pertaining to the natural history, geographic pathology, and epidemiology of atherosclerotic lesions.

Fatty streaks begin in childhood. Fibrous plaques develop in early adult life. Complicated lesions leading to arterial occlusion and ischemia occur in later adult life, years after the initial intimal lesions. Aortic fatty streaks are present in practically all individuals from every human population that has been studied. The aortic intimal surface involved with fatty streaks is not very different among different populations. Coronary fatty streaks begin to form in adolescence. With some exceptions, the extent of coronary fatty streaks in a population tends to be related to the extent of more advanced atherosclerotic lesions and to the risk of developing coronary heart disease (CHD). Fatty streaking is clinically harmless and potentially reversible; the progression of fatty streaks to fibrous, calcified, and complicated plaques is a critical stage of the atherosclerosis process. The extent of these more advanced lesions in both aorta and coronary arteries varies greatly among different human populations. The development of advanced lesions occurs much more rapidly in populations with much CHD than in populations with little CHD.

Comparisons among populations from the same broad ethnic groups reveal much variation in average extent of atherosclerosis. The large variation in atherosclerosis among white and black populations suggests that environmental conditions are important determinants of the prevalence and extent of atheroslcerotic lesions.

The progression of atherosclerosis is not inevitable but is, to an important degree, environmentally determined. Programs to control atherosclerosis, including changes in dietary patterns and other lifetime habits, should be directed toward children, adolescents, and young adults. These beneficial patterns should be established in childhood.

*Acknowledgments*  We gratefully acknowledge the assistance of Rhea Dupeire, Terry Grimes, and Charlotte Swain in preparing this manuscript.

Supported by grant HL-08974 NHLBI, NIH, USPHS.

References

1.  Holman R, McGill HC Jr., Strong JP, Geer JC (1958)  The natural
    history of atherosclerosis:  The early aortic lesions as seen
    in New Orleans in the middle of the 20th century.  Am J Pathol
    34: 209-235

2.  Strong JP, McGill HC Jr (1962) The natural history of coronary
    atherosclerosis.  Am J Pathol 40: 37-49

3.  Strong JP, McGill HC Jr, Tejada C, Holman, RL (1958) The
    natural history of atherosclerosis.  Comparison of the early
    aortic lesions in New Orleans, Guatemala, and Costa Rica.
    Am J Pathol 34: 731-744

4.  Strong JP, Wainwright J, McGill HC Jr (1959) Atherosclerosis
    in the Bantu.  Circulation 20(6): 1118-1127

5.  McGill HC Jr (ed) (1968) The Geographic Pathology of Athero-
    sclerosis.  Williams & Wilkins, Baltimore, or Lab Invest
    18(5): 463-635

6.  Strong JP, Eggen DA, Oalmann MC, Richards ML, Tracy RE, (1973)
    Pathology and epidemiology of atherosclerosis.  J Am Diet
    Assoc 62(3): 262-268

7.  Strong JP (1972) Atherosclerosis in human populations.
    Atherosclerosis 16: 193-201

8.  Strong JP, Eggen DA, Tracy RE (1978) The geographic pathology
    and topography of atherosclerosis and risk factors for athero-
    sclerotic lesions.  Chandler, Eurenius, McMillan, Nelson,
    Schwartz, Wessler (eds)  The Thrombotic Process in Athero-
    genesis.  Plenum Publishing Corp. 11-31

9.  Strong JP, McGill HC Jr (1969) Pediatric aspects of athero-
    sclerosis.  J Atheroscler Res 9: 25-65

10. Newman WP III, Strong JP (1978) Natural history, geographic
    pathology and pediatric aspects of atherosclerosis.  Strong
    WB (ed) Atherosclerosis: Its Pediatric Aspects, Grune & Stratton
    15-40

11. Strong JP, Restrepo C, Guzmán M (1978) Coronary and aortic
    atherosclerosis in New Orleans.  II. Comparison of lesions by
    age, sex, and race.  Lab Invest 39(4): 364-369

12. Stary HC (1982a) Macrophages in coronary artery and aortic
    intima of children and young adults up to age 29.  Proc 6th
    Int Symp Atherosclerosis, Springer-Verlag, Berlin-Heidelberg-
    New York (this volume)

13. Stary HC (1982b) Structure and ultrastructure of the coronary
    artery intima in children and young adults up to age 29.  Proc
    6th Int Symp Atherosclerosis, Springer-Verlag, Berlin-Heidelberg-
    New York (this volume)

# Immunohistology of Aortic Fatty Streaks in Children and Adults

K. W. Walton

## INTRODUCTION

The W.H.O. Study Group on the Classification of Atherosclerotic Lesions
in 1958 defined the term "fatty streak or spot" as one applied "to
superficial yellow or yellowish-grey intimal lesions which are stained
selectively by fat stains" (1).  The Group did not attempt to reach
an agreement on the stages of progression of various changes from the
earliest recognisable lesions to the onset of clinical disease.
Perhaps because of this, the origin, fate and significance in relation
to the development of atherosclerosis of these lesions is still a
matter of controversy.

On the one hand, it was for a long time thought (2) that they are an
early stage in the development of later raised lesions (plaques) and
therefore the characteristic atherosclerotic lesion of childhood and
adolescence.  On the other hand, small, flat, lipid-containing lesions
are often present (especially in the ascending aorta) in individuals
late in life and these, in terms of the definition quoted above,might
still be regarded as "fatty spots or streaks".  But there is no means
of knowing whether these were initially formed early or late in life.

It has been noted that, from the statistical viewpoint, the topographic
distribution of fatty streaks and spots in childhood differs from the
distribution of plaques in later life and also that fatty streaks are
prevalent in the ascending aorta in children of ethnic groups in which
raised lesions at the same site are relatively rare.  Such observations
have been interpreted as evidence that fatty streaks and spots are
unrelated to later lesions (for discussion, see Refs. 3,4).

The term "fatty streak or spot" is essentially a naked-eye description
of a lesion.  There is even some disagreement about the characteristic
histological appearance of fatty streaks and spots.  Many authors have
stressed that these lesions (especially in children and young adults)
often contain large numbers of fat-filled cells and have suggested a
possible origin of such cells from smooth-muscle cells (but see Ref.4).
In contrast, it has been pointed out (5) that, even the fatty streaks
and spots of childhood usually contain, not only fat-filled cells, but
in addition show the presence of extracellular lipid identifable as
apolipoprotein B-containing lipoproteins (LpB), resembling in this
respect, the structure of the raised lesions of adult life (6).  Childhood lesions have also been shown ·to contain fibrinogen-related antigen
(FRA) like adult lesions (7) and both LpB and FRA are also present in
fatty streaks in adolescence (8).

These observations have now been extended by comparing fatty spots and
streaks in the ascending aorta in children with morphologically similar
flat or slightly raised circumscribed lesions at the same anatomical

site in older age-groups using histological and immunohistological
methods.  As a control, sections were examined from the same aortic
region but from areas where the intima was free from visible or
discrete lesions, in the same age-groups.  For comparative purposes,
observations were also made on fatty spots and streaks encountered in
the trunk of the pulmonary artery in subjects of various ages.


## MATERIALS and METHODS

The material examined was derived from Coroner's autopsies from cases
of sudden and unexpected death.  In the case of the youngest subjects,
death had invariably been due to accidental causes (road traffic
accidents, falls or accidental burns) and the subjects had previously
been in good health.  Material from subjects of this kind was obtained
from 7 boys aged 4 to 13 years and from 5 girls aged 6 to 15 years.
Material from essentially similarly healthy subjects was obtained from
4 young men aged 17 to 25 years and 3 young women, aged 17 to 23 years,
except that in 3 instances (1M, 2F) the cause of death was suicide.
The 50 older subjects ranged in age between 32 and 84 years (26 men
and 24 women) and had died not only from accidents but also from a
variety of natural causes (mainly acute cardiovascular deaths).

For the present purpose, attention was confined to the arterial tissue
comprising the first $2\frac{1}{2}$ in. of the ascending aorta and the corresponding portion of the pulmonary trunk.  Conventional histological and
immunohistological examination was carried out on fresh frozen sections,
and on sections of fixed tissues, using the reagents, methods and
apparatus described in detail in previous communications (5-9).


## RESULTS

### Aortic lesions in children and adolescents

In confirmation of previous observations, scanty fatty streaks and
spots were seen in the ascending aorta in some of the youngest
subjects examined which, microscopically, showed the presence of fat-
filled cells in the superficial intima but also of extracellular
lipid in the deeper intima (and sometimes in the subjacent muscular
coat) in sections stained with Oil red O.

The fat-filled cells, in corresponding sections examined immunohisto-
logically, reacted with variable intensity, some failing to react and
appearing as 'black holes' following treatment of the sections with
fluorescein-labelled anti-apolipoprotein B (apo B).  In contrast, there
was precise co-distribution of lipid-staining and of immunohistological
localisation of apo B in areas where extracellular lipid was present
as fine droplets on intimal collagen and elastic fibres.  In sections
treated with labelled anti-fibrinogen, specific fluorescence was seen
diffusely distributed in the superficial intima and as irregular dots
and blobs in the deeper intima, in the muscular coat and as streaks
in the adventitia.  The appearances seen with anti-apo B and with anti-
FRA were esentially similar to those previously reported and illustrated
(see Refs. 5-8).


### Aortic lesions in older subjects

Discrete, flat, lipid-containing lesions were infrequently seen in the
ascending aorta in subjects in their twenties and thirties but became
progressively commoner with advancing age.  In the oldest age-groups

examined, multiple and sometimes coalescent fatty spots and streaks were seen. In these age-groups (seventh and eighth deciles) it was also found that even apparently 'normal' areas of intervening thickened and slightly pigmented intima showed diffuse lipid infiltration. This was sometimes in the form of fat-filled cells but more frequently as lipid droplets on the surface of collagen and elastic fibrils. Similar droplets were often seen on the underlying smooth muscle cells of the muscular coat. This intimal extracellular lipid in localised lesions and in 'normal' intima reacted with anti-apo B but it was observed that the material in or on smooth muscle cells in the muscular coat (in contradistinction to the intracellular material in the intimal fat-filled cells) was also immuno-reactive for apo B.

## Fatty spots in the pulmonary artery

These were only occasionally observed in routine autopsies, occurring especially in subjects with evidence suggestive of pulmonary hypertension. Their histological and immunohistological characteristics were essentially similar to those of aortic fatty spots.

## DISCUSSION

The occurrence of apo B in a precise similar distribution to that of extracellular lipid allows the inference (for reasons previously discussed, see Refs. 6-9) that intact LpB occurs in fatty streaks and spots, as it does in raised lesions. The presence of LpB and of FRA in the lesions suggest that they originate by an insudative process of the kind suggested for plaque formation (6). The close morphological similarity between fatty spots in the pulmonary artery and those in the aorta suggests that blood-pressure may be an important factor at either site. Studies on the entry of plasma proteins (including plasma lipoproteins) into arterial intima have suggested that there is a gradient of intimal permeability and of plasma protein concentration in aortic intima with distance from the aortic valve (9.10). But, if the epidemiological evidence on the subject is accepted, it is not easy to understand why the fatty spot lesions of childhood in the proximal aorta form early but also regress early. In this latter connection, it is possible that the marked prevalence of fat-filled cells in childhood lesions is, indeed, an indication of an active cellular removal mechanism for the disposal of lipid and lipoprotein, as previously suggested (11).

The other distinguishing characteristic of childhood fatty spots, as opposed to adult ones, is that they occur as circumscribed areas of lipid infiltration surrounded by areas of normal intima. This suggests they may arise from localised areas of altered intimal permeability, perhaps due to localised haemodynamic factors.

In contrast, adult fatty spots and streaks frequently arise as areas of even more intense fatty infiltration arising within areas of thickened and diffusely lipid-infiltrated intima. The close similarity in structure of lesions in the pulmonary artery suggests that more generalised factors (hypertension, hyperlipidaemia, and perhaps the generalised alteration of permeability of membranes, all of which accompany ageing) may play a significant role.

It is therefore possible that childhood fatty spots are not the direct fore-runners (in the sense of being the early stages ) of the lesions of later life and that most childhood lesions do undergo regression, as has been suggested (12). However it also seems possible that their occurrence at particular sites in the proximal aorta may indicate "sites of predeliction" at which morphologically similar lesions recur later in life. Such lesions may progress to form plaques but many appear to persist unaltered as others have also reported (13).

REFERENCES

1. World Health Organisation (1958) Classification of atherosclerotic lesions. Wld Hlth Org techn Rep Ser No: 143
2. Geer JC, McGill HC, Strong JP (1961) The fine structure of human atherosclerotic lesions. Amer J Pathol 38: 263-288
3. Haust MD (1971) The morphogenesis and fate of potential and early atherosclerotic lesions in man. Hum Pathol 2: 1-30
4. Schaffner T, Taylor K, Bartucci EJ, Fischer-Dzoga K, Beeson JH, Glagov S, Wissler RW (1980) Arterial foam cells with distinctive immunomorphologic and histochemical features of macrophages. Amer J Pathol 100: 57-74
5. Walton, KW (1972) The role of serum lipoproteins in very early and in late atherosclerosis. In: Connective Tissue and Ageing (Vogel HC, ed) Excerpta Medica, Amsterdam, pp34-37
6. Walton KW, Williamson N (1968) Histological and immunofluorescent studies on the evolution of the human atheromatous plaque. J Atheroscler Res 8: 599-624
7. Walton KW (1975). Pathogenetic mechanisms in atherosclerosis. Amer J Cardiol 35: 542-558
8. Walton KW (1978) Atherosclerosis and aging. In: Brocklehurst JC(ed) Textbook of geriatric medicine and gerontology 2nd edn Chap 5, Churchill Livingstone Edinburgh
9. Bradby GVH, Walton KW, Watts R (1979) The binding of total low-density lipoproteins in human arterial intima affected and un-affected by atherosclerosis. Atherosclerosis 32: 403-422
10. Duncan LE, Cornfield J, Buck K (1962) The effect of blood pressure on the passage of labelled plasma albumin into canine aortic wall. J Clin Invest 41: 1537-1545
11. Walton KW. The role of lipoproteins in human atherosclerosis In: Peeters H (ed) The Lipoprotein Molecule, Plenum Press, New York
12. Mitchell JRA, Schwartz CJ (1965) Arterial Disease, Blackwell, Oxford
13. Pearson TA, Dillman JM, Solez K, Hepinstall RH (1980) Evidence for two populations of fatty streaks with different roles in the atherogenic process. Lancet 2: 496-498

# 1.2  Diseases of Lipid Metabolism

# Heterogeneity of Genetic Transmission of Familial Hypercholesterolemia (F.H.) from Direct Parents in 20 Families of Homozygotes Type IIa

J. L. de Gennes, F. Dairou, and G. Luc

(Paris - France)

On the basis of classical criteria of homozygotism of familial hypercholesterolemia (F.H.) type IIa, we have revised, among 20 distinct families, genetic transmission from direct parents, father and mother, by using the generally accepted index of clearcut elevation of level of Serum Total Cholesterol (TC) and/or LDL cholesterol.

According to these criteria, heterogeneity of this genetic background has clearly appeared, allowing to separate three distinctive groups, with a different pattern of direct parental genetic transmission. All individual details concerning these three groups, including age, clinical and biologic characteristics for both homozygote patients and their own parents are included in the respective tables for each group : tables I, II and III.

- The group I (cf table I) is the most prevalent group, and represents 11 families (out of 20) in which both parents of homozygote patients, as well fathers as mothers, exhibit clearly an abnormally high level of Cholesterol and/or LDL cholesterol. However, already many of these parents do not exhibit the full expected picture of heterozygote F.H., as well at the clinical standpoint as at the biological standpoint.

At the clinical standpoint definitive tendinosum xanthomatosis is present in less of 50% of cases as well in mothers (5/11) as in fathers (5/11). Cardiovascular symptoms of premature atherosclerosis, chiefly coronary heart disease (CDH), are absent in all mothers, and only present two times in fathers (one angina at the age of 48, one myocardial infarction at the age of 50).

At the biological standpoint, the mean level of serum total cholesterol and LDL cholesterol are only slightly elevated at the respective levels for fathers of 362 mgs and 244 mgs/dl, and for mothers of 354 mgs/dl and 232 mgs/dl, compared with mean levels in heterozygote FH with tendinous xanthomas of 445 mgs/dl (LDL C 370 mgs/dl) and 414 mgs/dl (LDL C 334 mgs/dl) for men and women of same ages. As for as the Apo B measurements were available, the levels in fathers and mothers of this group I were also less elevated than the mean level of Apo B in men or women with heterozygote FH with tendinosum xanthomas.

Therefore it already appears that a mild degree hypercholesterolemia is able to generate an hypermajor grade of familial hypercholesterolemia, as defined by classical criteria of homozygote type IIa.

Among this group I, 9 homozygote propositi (out of 12) were available for quantitative studies of LDL receptor of cultured fibroblasts from skin biopsy, performed by Dr J. GOLDSTEIN et M. BROWN (1). Most of these patients (8/9) were receptor negative with less of 2% of receptors ; only one (case n° 4) has 15% of receptors).

- The group II : includes 6 families with only one parent clearly hypercholesterolemic, while the other remains apparently normal as well in level of total cholesterol, as in the level of LDL cholesterol. Among the 6 normocholesterolemic parents, mothers were always concerned.

In this group, a study of blood compatibility between the homozygote children and fathers has led to exclude father of n° 5. Moreover the prevalence of normocholesterolemic mothers, not only excludes such a risk of wrong filiation, but also indicates that the genic biological expression of LDL hypercholesterolemia is more prone to be hindered or latent in women than it is in men. Interesting also is the fact that, in at least in 2 cases of these mothers, hypercholesterolemia was not always absent or latent, but rather intermittent, and occasionnally revealed either following use of contraceptive pills or following marked change in body weight or dietary intake (n° 5 and 6 ).

Anyway, this situation indicates that the slighest degree of hypercholesterolemia, specially in mothers, is susceptible to generate, in combination with a patent hypercholesterolemia in the other parent, the homozygote state of F.H. Among this group, 5 homozygote children have been able to be checked for LDL receptors owing to the collaboration of Dr GOLDSTEIN and M. BROWN. Only 1 was receptor negative (case 6 table II), and the remaining cases were only receptor defective with 15 to 35% of LDL receptors. Other characteristics of these homozygote patients were the relative easiness of response to a pure medical drug treatment such as Clofibrate derivative in 3 cases out of 9 (n° 2, 4 and 5). So it seems quite possible that the inherited metabolic defect is not the same from both parents, and could combine an heterozygote state for receptor defect and an other metabolic impairment (perhaps on apoproteins) enhancing the level of LDL hypercholesterolemia (2)(3).

- The last group III, seems exceptional, but exceedingly interesting for covering the whole picture of homozygotes type IIa. Up to now we have only met 3 families, with 2 homozygote children in the first, 1 in the second  and the third, with both parents without any abnormality of LDL cholesterol (cf table III). In the first family, parents are first cousins without any biological evidence, checked by ultracentrifugation and apoprotein B measurements, of LDL disturbance. However, it must be noticed that the father had intermittent VLDL rise, and had sudden myocardial infarction at the age of 30. In the two homozygote children, LDL membrane cell receptors were checked quite normal around 100%. The HMG coenzyme A reductase activity, was shown repressed in the first child, either by its own LDL or by LDL of control normal subjects. Thus this family, unique up to now in the world litterature, demonstrates clearly that some homozygote type IIa are not explained by the LDL receptor pathway, and that it does necessarily exist one or more  other metabolic origin for Essential Familial Hypercholesterolemia.

In the second family, the propositus girl 9 years old, has 40% of LDL receptors on cultured fibroblasts from skin biopsy. So she seems heterozygote for the LDL receptor BROWN and GOLDSTEIN disease,despite of normal LDL C and Apo B levels of her both parents. But, for not understood reasons, this girl shares with her parents a defect in postheparin lipolytic activity as well in vivo (strip test) as in vitro, without any rise of Triglyceride levels in any member of the family. The propositus girl responds dramatically to Clofibrate treatment with a fall of more 50% of TC falling from 565 mgs/dl to 250 mgs/dl. Obviously this is a metabolic situation quite distinct of that of the previous family, but which reflects again how a transmitted gene of familial hypercholesterolemia can be completely biologically unexpressed, and then latent even in both direct parents of homozygote type IIa. The additional third family still requires further investigations not yet available, but is similar for absence of LDL abnormality in both parents. The concept of latent hypercholesterolemia, and the need of further studies on this line as already engaged previously by HIGGINS and coworkers (4) and by ZOLLNER and coll (5) is well documented from these reported family studies focused on direct parents of type IIa homozygote.

REFERENCES

1 - Goldstein JL, Brown MS (1974) Binding and degradation of low density lipoproteins by cultured human fibroblasts comparison of cells from a normal subject with homozygous familial hypercholesterolemia. J Biol Chem 249 : 51-53

2 - Breslow JL, Spaulding DR, Lux SE, Levy RI and Lees RS (1975) Homozygous familial hypercholesterolemia : a possible biochemical explanation of clinical heterogeneity. The New Engl 900-903

3 - Higgins MJP, Lecamwasam DS and Galton DJ (1975) A new type of familial hypercholesterolemia. The Lancet i: 737-740

4 - Hazzard WR, Miller N, Albers JJ, Russel Warnick G, Baron P and Lewis B (1981) Association of isoapolipoprotein E3 deficiency with heterozygous familial hypercholesterolemia. Implication for lipoprotein physiology. The Lancet, i : 298-301

5 - Keller Ch, Harders-Spengel K, Spengel F, Wilczorek A, Wolfram G and Zollner N (1981) Serum cholesterol levels in patiens with familial hypercholesterolemia confirmed by tissue culture. Atherosclerosis 39: 51-59

104

## Table I Group I

| Family | Sex | Age Years | PROPOSITUS TC | LDL C | CX | TX | CV | LDL receptor | FATHER Age | TC | LDL C | TX | CV | MOTHER Age | TC | LDLC | TX | CV |
|---|---|---|---|---|---|---|---|---|---|---|---|---|---|---|---|---|---|---|
| 1 | M | 1 | 980 | 870 | + | - | - | <2% | 28 | 290 | 220 | - | - | 27 | 355 | 250 | + | - |
| 2 | M | 5 | 635 | 384 | + | + | - | <2% | 34 | 440 | 216 | + | - | 36 | 360 | 173 | - | - |
| 3a | M | 9 | 615 | 559 | + | + | - | <2% | 50 | 494 | 352 | + | + | 35 | | | - | - |
| 3b | F | 13 | 731 | 629 | + | + | - | <2% | = | = | = | = | = | = | = | | = | = |
| 4 | F | 10 | 485 | 428 | + | + | - | 15% | 36 | 318 | 223 | - | - | 35 | 345 | 271 | + | - |
| 5 | M | 10 | 500 | 424 | + | + | - | <2% | - | 300 | - | - | - | - | 400 | - | - | - |
| 6 | F | 12 | 800 | 708 | + | + | - | - | 42 | 390 | - | + | - | - | 390 | - | - | - |
| 7 | M | 13 | 585 | 526 | + | + | - | <2% | 39 | 350 | - | - | - | 36 | 280 | - | - | - |
| 8 | M | 16 | 635 | - | + | + | + | - | - | 410 | - | + | - | - | 370 | - | + | - |
| 9 | F | 17 | 515 | 475 | + | + | + | 5% | 51 | 280 | 210 | - | - | 48 | 370 | - | + | - |
| 10 | F | 21 | 670 | 616 | + | + | + | <2% | 50 | 400 | - | - | + | 46 | 315 | 253 | - | - |
| 11 | F | 16 | 540 | - | + | + | - | - | 38 | 310 | - | + | - | 38 | 355 | - | + | - |
| Mean | | | 641 +142 | 562 +150 | | | | | | 362 +70 | 244 +60 | | | | 354 +35 | 232 +39 | | |

TC = Total Cholesterol
LDL C = LDL cholesterol
CX = cutaneous xanthomas
TX = tendinous xanthomas
CV = cardiovascular ischemic disease

## TABLE II    Group II

| | | | PROPOSITUS | | | | | | FATHER | | | | | MOTHER | | | | |
|---|---|---|---|---|---|---|---|---|---|---|---|---|---|---|---|---|---|---|
| Family | Sex | Age Years | TC | LDL C | CX | TX | CV | LDL receptor | Age | TC | LDL C | TX | CV | Age | TC | LDL C | TX | CV |
| 1a | F | 14 | 635 | 585 | + | + | - | 35% | 42 | 285 | | - | - | 38 | 200 | 169 | - | - |
| 1b | F | 15 | 570 | 484 | + | + | + | 35% | = | | 210 | = | - | = | | | = | - |
| 2 | F | 15 | 655 | - | + | + | - | | 47 | 325 | - | - | - | 44 | 235 | - | - | - |
| 3a | M | 10 | 575 | - | + | + | - | - | 51 | 273 | - | - | - | 47 | 183 | - | - | - |
| 3b | F | 8 | 630 | - | + | + | - | - | = | | | = | = | = | | | = | |
| 3c | F | 6 | 685 | - | + | + | - | - | = | | | = | = | = | | | = | |
| 4 | M | 16 | 335 | 249 | + | + | - | 20% | 42 | 330 | 197 | + | - | 40 | 220 | 127 | - | - |
| 5 | M | 8 | 665 | 552 | + | + | - | 15% | ? | ? | ? | ? | ? | 29 | 220 | 180 | - | - |
| 6 | F | 10,5 | 760 | 510 | + | + | + | <2% | 33 | 403 | 233 | - | + | 29 | 273 | 185 | - | - |
| Mean | | | 612 +119 | 476 +133 | | | | | | 323 +51 | 213 +18 | | | | 222 +31 | 165 +26 | | |

## Table III    Group III

| | | | PROPOSITUS | | | | | | FATHER | | | | | MOTHER | | | | |
|---|---|---|---|---|---|---|---|---|---|---|---|---|---|---|---|---|---|---|
| Family | Sex | Age Years | TC | LDL C | CX | TX | CV | LDL receptor | Age | TC | LDL C | TX | CV | Age | TC | LDL C | TX | CV |
| 1a | F | 7 | 670 | 520 | + | + | - | 100% | 42 | 235 | 142 | - | + | 39 | 180 | 92 | - | - |
| 1b | F | 1 | 585 | - | - | - | - | - | = | | | - | = | = | | | = | = |
| 2 | F | 9 | 565 | 465 | + | + | - | 40% | 45 | 275 | 175 | - | - | 43 | 250 | 165 | - | - |
| 3 | F | 5 | 660 | 600 | + | + | - | - | 37 | 215 | 136 | - | - | 38 | 215 | 164 | - | - |
| Mean | | | 620 +53 | 528 +68 | | | | | | 242 +31 | 151 +21 | | | | 215 +35 | 140 +42 | | |

# The Impact of Analbuminemia on Lipid Transport and Lipoproteins

R. Fellin, G. Baldo, E. Manzato, M. R. Baiocchi, C. Lista, G. Baggio, F. Fabiani, S. Pauluzzi, and G. Crepaldi

## A. Introduction

Analbuminemia or better hypoalbuminemia is a rare disease, first described in 1954 by Bennhold et al.(1), and is characterized by the almost total absence of albumin. This disease is inherited and is probably transmitted by a recessive autosomal gene (2,3). The defect is not complete. The albumin traces present in circulation on immunoelectrophoresis show the same mobility as normal albumin (4) and no antigenic differences between normal albumin and that in subjects with analbuminemia have been detected (5). In this desease an increased catabolism or loss of this protein may also be ruled out: perfusion of albumin labelled with radioactive iodine has in fact shown a remarkable increase in the half-life of albumin (6,7).

A constant feature in analbuminemic patients is hyperlipidemia characterized by a rise in cholesterol and phospholipids with usually normal triglyceride levels (7).

The aim of this study was to examine the distribution and the composition of plasma lipoproteins in 2 subjects (brother and sister) with analbuminemia and in 3 of their first-degree relatives.

## B. Patients and Methods

Two patients with analbuminemia, R.U. and his sister R.R., 51 and 44 years old respectively, were studied. Their father (R.P.) and mother (D.A.) were first-degree cousins. The parents of the patients and the only healthy sister, R.M., were also studied. Another sister, R.S., died perinatally (cause of death unknown).

Objectively R.U. presented a mild hepatomegaly and the outcome of a peripheral paralysis of the right facial nerve. R.R. showed a moderate hepatomegaly. Neither patients had cutaneous or tendinous xanthomas nor clinical signs of atherosclerosis. Pretibial edema was absent and no signs of edema were referred. Despide their age, the parents were in good health, as was the sister R.M..

The lipoprotein fractions (VLDL,LDL and HDL) were separated by sequential preparative ultracentrifugation. HDL$_2$ and HDL$_3$ levels were determined according to Gidez et al.(8).

Apoproteins A-I and B were determined according to a modification of the Laurell immunoelectrophoretic method, using monospecific antibodies raised in our laboratory.

Apoproteins in the VLDL and HDL lipoprotein fractions were evaluated by polyacrylamide gel electrophoresis (PAGE), according to Kane.

## C. Results

Both patients had very high cholesterol levels (Table I) with normal esterified fraction. Phospholipids were elevated, while triglycerides were 73 mg/dl in R.U. and 220 mg/dl in R.R.

Table I. Total serum cholesterol (TC)(mg/dl), free (FC) and esterified (EC%) cholesterol, triglycerides (TG), phospholipids (PL), total protein (TP)(g/dl) and albumin
(mg/dl) in 2 analbuminemic patients and in 3 first-degree relatives

| Patients | | Age(yrs) | TC | FC | EC | TG | PL | TP | Albumin |
|---|---|---|---|---|---|---|---|---|---|
| R.U. | brother | 51 | 407 | 101 | 75% | 73 | 308 | 5.8 | 11 |
| R.R. | sister | 44 | 639 | 165 | 74% | 220 | 424 | 6.0 | 7 |
| Relatives | | | | | | | | | |
| R.P. | father | 81 | 254 | 70 | 72% | 112 | 234 | 6.9 | 4928 |
| D.A. | mother | 81 | 341 | 90 | 74% | 178 | 278 | 6.8 | 4610 |
| R.M. | sister | 48 | 265 | 67 | 75% | 167 | 222 | 6.3 | 4658 |

Lipoprotein electrophoresis in the whole serum (Fig.1) showed a remarkable increase
in the α and β bands in both patients. The pre-β band is almost absent in R.U.; in
R.R. it is barely visible and not well separated from the β band. The overall pattern
does not correspond to any of the phenotypes in Fredrickson's classification. After
heparin injection the changes in lipoprotein electrophoresis pattern suggest a normal
lipoprotein lipase activity; in R.R., an intensity reduction in the β-band with trail-
ing up to pre-β position is present.

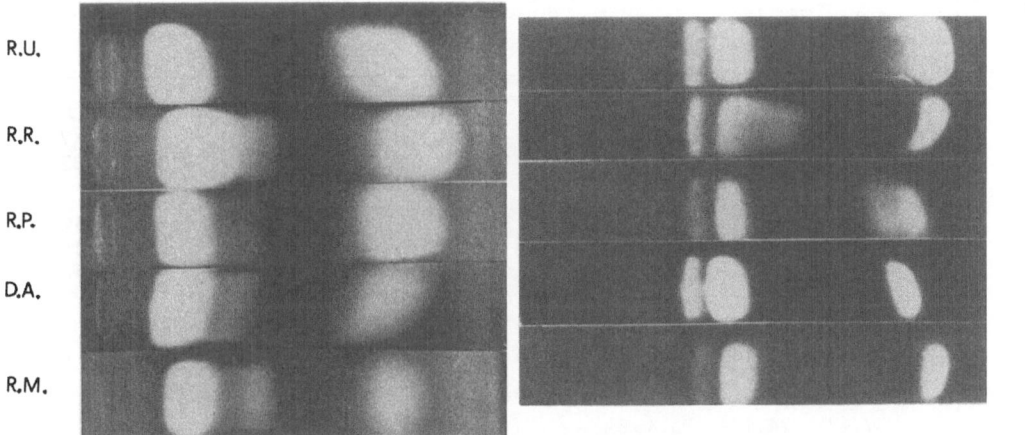

Fig. 1. Lipoprotein electrophoresis of whole serum (left) and of plasma 10 min. after
heparin injection (60U/kg)(right) of 2 analbuminemic patients and of 3 first-degree
relatives

Plasma VLDL concentration (Table II) is sharply reduced in R.U., normal in R.R. and
in the 3 family members. LDL concentration is distinctly increased in R.U. and in
R.R.; it is also high in D.A. and R.M. and is within upper normal limits in R.P..
HDL levels are sharply increased in the patients, slightly augmented in R.P., within
upper normal limits in D.A. and normal in R.M.. Compared to reference values, significant differences in the lipid-protein composition were not observed in the patients
or their family members (Table II).

108

Table II. Serum VLDL, LDL, HDL total mass (mg/dl) and protein-lipid composition (% of total mass) in 2 analbuminemic patients and in 3 first-degree relatives

| Patients | mass mg/dl | VLDL CT | TG | PL | PR | mass mg/dl | LDL CT | TG | PL | PR | mass mg/dl | HDL CT | TG | PL | PR |
|---|---|---|---|---|---|---|---|---|---|---|---|---|---|---|---|
| R.U. | 27 | 15 | 48 | 25 | 12 | 570 | 48 | 8 | 21 | 23 | 696 | 16 | 2 | 28 | 54 |
| R.R. | 90 | 13 | 56 | 18 | 13 | 1158 | 43 | 12 | 19 | 26 | 530 | 14 | 2 | 30 | 54 |
| Relatives | | | | | | | | | | | | | | | |
| R.P. | 70 | 10 | 56 | 18 | 16 | 391 | 41 | 15 | 21 | 23 | 442 | 16 | 2 | 30 | 52 |
| D.A. | 122 | 13 | 64 | 13 | 10 | 558 | 46 | 13 | 25 | 16 | 415 | 13 | 3 | 25 | 59 |
| R.M. | 139 | 14 | 63 | 11 | 12 | 468 | 42 | 14 | 23 | 21 | 349 | 12 | 3 | 28 | 57 |
| Normal | 63–137 | 19 | 55 | 18 | 8 | 229–371 | 45 | 12 | 22 | 21 | 233–361 | 18 | 4 | 24 | 55 |

Total HDL and HDL$_3$-cholesterol was increased in both patients (Table III). HDL$_2$-cholesterol was increased in R.U. and slightly reduced in R.R..The HDL$_2$/HDL$_3$ cholesterol ratio was normal in R.U., very reduced in R.R.. R.P. also showed an increase in HDL-cholesterol with a high HDL$_2$-cholesterol and HDL$_2$/HDL$_3$ cholesterol ratio. In D.A. cholesterol distribution in the HDL fractions was normal while R.M. showed a low HDL-cholesterol with a very reduced HDL$_2$-cholesterol.

Table III. Plasma concentration of total HDL,HDL$_2$,HDL$_3$-cholesterol (mg/dl) and of Apo A-I in whole serum (WS) and HDL and Apo B in WS,VLDL and LDL (mg/dl) in 2 analbuminemic patients and in 3 first-degree relatives

| Patients | HDL | HDL$_2$ | HDL$_3$ | Apo A-I WS | HDL | Apo B WS | VLDL | LDL |
|---|---|---|---|---|---|---|---|---|
| R.U. | 99 | 34 | 65 | 261 | 250 | 202 | / | 177 |
| R.R. | 72 | 18 | 54 | 161 | 137 | 372 | 10 | 358 |
| Relatives | | | | | | | | |
| R.P. | 62 | 30 | 32 | 215 | 187 | 143 | 8 | 121 |
| D.A. | 49 | 20 | 29 | 137 | 132 | 190 | 12 | 151 |
| R.M. | 34 | 7 | 27 | 137 | 125 | 187 | 16 | 145 |
| *Normal | M 47.25±1.37 | 16.30±1.14 | 31.07±0.83 | M+F 157.3±13.9 | | 81±21.3 | | |
| | F 57.47±1.37 | 24.12±1.24 | 33.45±0.79 | | | | | |

*Data from our laboratory (m±S.E.)

In patient R.U. and his father R.P., apo A-I is increased both in total serum and in the HDL fraction (Table III). In patient R.R., total serum apo A-I is within upper normal limits. Apo B is sharply increased in both patients in the total serum as well as in the LDL fraction. A slight increase in apo B levels was also seen in all the 3 family members, particularly D.A..

Due to the low concentration of the VLDL fraction, in patient R.U. it was not possible to visualize the apoproteins normally detectable with polyacrylamide gel electrophoresis. In patient R.R. the VLDL pattern appears normal. In the HDL fraction of R.U., an intensification of the group C peptide bands was seen, particularly the apo C-III band; in addition, a double band in the C-II position was observed.

FFA basal levels in R.R. were very low (0.10 mEq/l), and slightly reduced in the other family members. The FFA/Alb. molar ratio in R.R. was extremely high (104.6).

## D. Discussion

As in other reported cases, the hyperlipidemia of our patients consisted essentially of a hypercholesterolemia. The plasma cholesterol level of the patient R.R. is the highest described (9). In both cases the hypercholesterolemia is due to a selective increase in the LDL and HDL concentrations. With regard to the latter, the literature data are conflicting; in one case they are low (5), in another high (10). In patient R.U., who presents HDL levels which are compatible with a diagnosis of "hyperalphali poproteinemia", there is an increase of both $HDL_2$ and $HDL_3$ subfractions; in R.R. only $HDL_3$ are increased. Esterified cholesterol fractions were normal and this agrees with Fröhlich et al.(10), who reported normal LCAT activity in a child with analbuminemia. However, it must be considered that the mother (D.A.) showed a sharp increase in LDL, while the father showed an HDL increase.

The increased LDL and HDL concentrations explain the rise in plasma phospholipids which is also a typical finding in patients with analbuminemia. Our patients showed another lipoprotein abnormality: R.U., whose triglyceride values are within the lower normal limit, showed a marked decrease in the pre-β band on electrophoresis and in VLDL fraction following centrifugation. R.R. had slightly increase triglyceride levels with a normal VLDL fraction concentration. Nonetheless on lipoprotein electrophoresis there was poor separation of the pre-β band, probably due to the remarkable increase in β lipoproteins. This finding might explain also the rise in plasma triglyceride in this patient. Conflicting reports are present in the literature regarding this point; in most cases normal triglyceride levels are recorded (7,10), in others triglyceride levels are high with a type IIb electrophoretic pattern (5).

It is interesting to note that despite the marked alterations in the lipoprotein concentration, its composition is normal in both the patients and their family members. The only qualitative abnormality found in this study is the presence of an intermediate band between C-II and $C-III_1$ on PAGE analysis of the HDL apoproteins in patient R.U.. Further studies are in course to define this finding more precisely.

The change in the lipoprotein electrophoretic pattern following heparin that were observed in the patients and their family members indirectly suggest the presence of good lipoprotein lipase activity. Basal FFA concentration in R.R. was very low; in 2 other reported cases (2,11) it was elevated, in one case normal (9).

Generally hyperlipidemia in analbuminemia is considered "secondary" to the severe albumin reduction, but the mechanisms by which the albumin reduction determines an increase in plasma cholesterol are unknown. This hypothesis is supported by the reduction (7) or the normalization (9,11) of cholesterol and phospholipids levels following albumin transfusion and the gradual increase in these parameters is parallel with the progressive decrease in transfused albumin. In our 2 patients, however, we cannot exclude a genetic component for the hypercholesterolemia. Their mother, in fact, presents a sharp LDL increase and their sister also shows high LDL values. The high HDL-cholesterol level found in the father only added to the problem of interpreting the hypercholesterolemia in our 2 cases.

Clinical signs of precocious atherosclerosis were absent in our patients, but they have been decribed in this disease. It may not be excluded that the high HDL levels found in our patients might have exerted a protective effect againt atherosclerotic complications.

References

1. Benhold H, Peters H, Roth E (1954) Über einer Fall von kompletter Analbuminaemie ohne wesentliche klinische krankheintszeichen. Verhandl. Deutsch. Gesellsch. Inn. Med. 60, 630

2. Goullé JP, Laine G, Sauger F, Maitrot B, Bouillerot A, Gray H, Blondet P, Dieryck B (1976) Etude biochimique du premier cas d'analbuminémie en France. Ann. Biol. Clin. 34, 403

3. Gitlin D, Gitlin JD (1975) Genetic alterations in the plasma proteins of man. In: "The plasma proteins",Putnam FW ed., p.321, Vol.II, Academic Press, New York

4. Irunberry J, Abbadi M, Khati B, Benabadji M, Rocha E (1971) Trois cas d'analbu minemie dans une fratrie. Rev. Europ. Etudes Clin. et Biol. 16, 372

5. Boman H, Hermodson M, Hommond CA, Motulsky AG (1976) Analbuminemia in an American Indian Girl. Clin. Genet. 9, 513

6. Bennhold H., Kallee E (1959) Comparative studies on the half-life of $I^{131}$-labelled albumins and non-radioactive human serum albumin in a case of analbuminemia. J. Clin. Invest. 38, 863

7. Waldmann AT, Gordon RS, Rosse W (1964) Studies on the metabolism of the serum pro teins and lipids in a patient with analbuminemia. Am. J. Med. 37, 960

8. Gidez LI, Miller GJ, Burstein M, Eder HA (1979) Analyses of plasma high density lipoprotein subclasses by a precipitation procedure: correlation with preparative and analytical ultracentrifugation . In: "Reported of the high density lipoprotein methodology workshop, Lippel K (ed) Public Health Service National Institute of Health, San Francisco California p 328

9. Cormode EJ, Lyster DM, Israels S (1975) Analbuminemia in a neonate. J. Pediat. 86, 862

10. Frohlich J, Pudek MR, Cormode EJ, Sellers EM, Abel JG (1981) Further studies on plasma proteins, lipids, and dye-and drug-binding in a child with analbuminemia. Clin. Chem. 27,1213

11. Weinstock JV, Kawanishi H, Sisson J (1979) Morphologic biochemical and physiologic alterations in a case of idiopathic hypoalbuminemia (analbuminemia). Am. J. Med. 67, 132

# Familial Hypertriglyceridemia: Incidence, Genetics and Possible Defect in Cellular Metabolism

D. K. Henze and N. Zöllner

Among the inherited disorders of lipoprotein metabolism, familial hypertriglyceridemia (FHT) is one of the least well understood. In FHT all affected relatives have elevated serum triglyceride levels only, while in familial combined hyperlipidemia, serum triglyceride, cholesterol or both may be elevated in affected family members (1). Genetic studies have suggested an autosomal dominant trait (1), but up to now no clinical or biochemical genetic marker are known which can distinguish patients with FHT from individuals who suffer from other forms of hypertriglyceridemia. The diagnosis of familial hypertriglyceridemia can only be made with certainty if the patient has a sufficiently large family to allow family studies. The gene seems to have a low penetrance. Thus, full expression of the gene appears to occur only after the age of 25 to 30. Serum triglyceride levels can therefore not be used in children, adolescents and young adults for genetic screening.

The little knowledge about the defect in cellular metabolism in this disease is rather surprising, because FHT is possibly one of the most frequent inherited disorders of lipid metabolism. Among unselected survivors of myocardial infarction below the age of 60 studied in Seattle, about 5,2 percent were found to have FHT as defined by the presence in the family of at least one relative with hypertriglyceridemia (2). Among the general population in the same city the frequency of familial hypertriglyceridemia has been estimated to be around 0.2-0.3 percent (2).

However most of the studies relating to the pathogenesis of hypertriglyceridemia were done on patients with endogenous hypertriglyceridemia. Endogenous hypertriglyceridemia describes a heterogenous group of primary familial and sporadic hypertriglyceridemia. In 1976 J.D. Brunzell and E.L. Bierman investigated the relation insulin-triglyceride plasma levels in patients with well defined FHT (5). As described by other authors there was a correlation between plasma triglyceride and insulin concentrations in the group of affected family members as well as in the control group. However for the same plasma insulin concentration the hypertriglyceridemic relatives had higher triglyceride levels as compared to the normotriglyceridemic relatives. These data suggested that a higher cellular sensitivity to insulin might play a role in the pathogenesis of FHT.

A. Chait and coworkers recently observed an increase VLDL-apoprotein B turnover rate in patients with FHT as well as in patients with familial combined hyperlipidemia suggesting that hypertriglyceridemia seen in both genetic disorders was due to very low density lipoprotein overproduction (6). The turnover rate of very low density lipoprotein apoprotein B was however greater in familial combined hyperlipidemia than in FHT, while plasma triglyceride turnover rate was higher in FHT. The disparity in the turnover rates of apoprotein B and triglycerides between these disorders was accompanied by a higher VLDL triglyceride / apoprotein B ratio in FHT as compared to familial combined hyperlipidemia or to controls. The authors concluded that the hypertriglyceridemia of combined hyperlipidemia is due to an overproduction of very low density lipoprotein of normal composition, while that of FHT is due to oversecretion of triglyceride enriched VLDL.

Our group at the Poliklinik der Universität München has investigated the lipogenic capacity of cultured diploid fibroblasts from patients with FHT from sufficiently large families as described previously (7). The basal and insulin stimulated activities of acetyl-CoA carboxylase, the rate limiting enzyme of fatty acid synthesis, did not differ in fibroblasts of patients with FHT as compared to controls (8). However incorporation of $^{14}$-C-acetate into triglyceride fatty acids was slightly increased in cells derived from patients with FHT. Addition of triiodothyronine to the cell layers produced a significant increase in $^{14}$-acetate incorporation into fatty acids in the cells derived from patients with FHT (fig).1.In normal cell lines used as controls this hormone did not stimulate fatty acid synthesis. The stimulatory effect of triiodothyronine was dose dependent with a maximum at a concentration of 5 ng/ml. Insulin increased acetate incorporation in both cell types, but without significant differences. In agreement with these results the activity of acetyl-CoA-carboxylase was increased by triiodothyronine in FHT-cells but not in controls. The magnitude of the stimulatory effect of triiodothyronine in the FHT-Cells is however quite different from one cell line to another ranging from 140 to 250 %. The reason for these differences are presently under investigation. In cells derived from unaffected family members and normal controls the stimulatory effect of triiodothyronine could not be shown.

Our results indicate a higher lipogenic capacity of the cultured fibroblasts from patients with FHT. They are in agreement with studies of Chait (6) who demonstrated an excess production and turnover of triglyceride enriched VLDL-particles in FHT.

The higher lipogenic capacity of cultured fibroblasts from patients under FHT might be an important basis in the search for a genetic marker of this disorder.

This project was supported by Deutsche Forschungsgemeinschaft Dr.C.Lemmen took care of the cell culture and most of the analytical work.

References
1. Fredrickson D.S., Goldstein J.L, Brown M.S.: The familial hyperlipoproteinemias. In: The Metabolic Basis of Inherited Disease (Ed.J.B.Stanbury, J.B.Wyngaarden and D.S.Fredrickson, Mc Graw Hill Book Company New York 1980, 605-655.
2. Goldstein J.L., Hazzard W.R., Schrott H.G.,Bierman E.L. and A.G. Motulsky: Hyperlipidemia in Coronary Artery Disease. J.Clin. Invest. 52, 1533-1568, 1973.
3. Nikkilä E.A.: Metabolism of plasma triglycerides in endogenous hypertriglyceridemia. Horm. Metab. Res. Suppl. 4, 34-38, 1974.
4. Havel R.J., Jane J.P., Balasse E.O., Segel N. and L.V. Basso: Splanchnic metabolism of free fatty acids and production of triglycerides of VLDL in normotriglyceridemic and hypertriglyceridemic humans J.Clin. Invest. 49, 2017-2035, 1970.
5. Brunzell J.D., Biermann E.L.: Plasma triglyceride and nsulin levels in familial hypertriglyceridemia. Ann. Int. Med. 87, 198-199, 1977.
6. Chait A., Albers J.J. and J.D.Brunzell: Very low density lipoprotein overproduction in genetic forms of hypertriglyceridemia. Eur. J. Clin.Invest. 10, 17-22, 1980
7. Henze K., Wallmüller A., Barth C.A., Wolfram C and N. Zöllner: Untersuchungen zur Genetik der primären Hypertriglyceridämie. Vhdlg. Dtsch. Ges. Inn. Med. 83, 395-298, 1977
8. Lemmen C., Wolfram G., Barth C. and N. Zöllner: Hormonal regulation of lipogenesis in human dipoloid fibroblasts from normal subjects and from patients with familial hypertriglyceridemia (submitted for publication 1982).

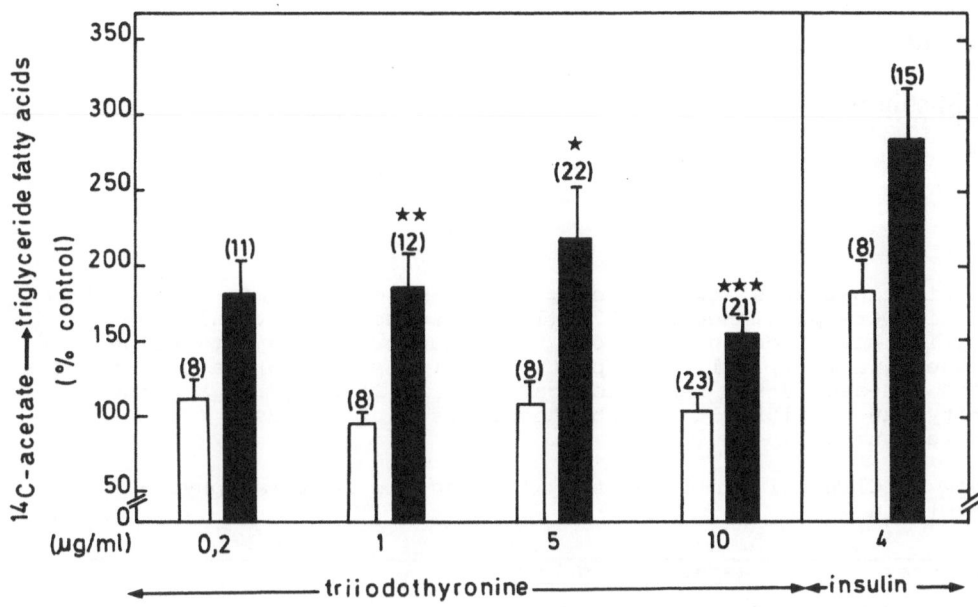

Fig. 1.

Confluent cell monolayers were kept for 72 hoursin incubation medium
containing triodothyronine and insulin as indicated. Control dishes
received no hormone. Values are expressed as mean $\pm$ S.E.M. with the
number of experiments in brackets.
Open bars.
Controls Closed bars: FHT cells.
(P-values for FHT versus controls are:

```
+        = p < 0,05;
++       = p < 0,01;
+++      = p < 0,001.
```

# Phytosterolemia

T. A. Miettinen

The first patients, two sisters, with β-sitosterolemia and xanthomatosis were published in 1974 (1). Subsequently several other
families have been found (2-6), total number of subjects being
sixteen (Table 1). Clinical picture includes also premature coronary
heart disease (7-9), hematological abnormalities (7,9) and the
entity can coexist with cerebrotendinous xanthomatosis
(cholestanosis).

Table 1. Clinical and laboratory findings in familial phytosterolemia

| Parameter | Reference number | | | | | |
|---|---|---|---|---|---|---|
| | 2 | 8 | 7 | 6 | 9 | 3-5 |
| No. of cases | 3 | 5 | 1 | 1 | 1 | 5 |
| Age, years | 20-31 | 28 | 27 | 20 | 42 | 4-19 |
| Males, no. | 0 | 2 | 1 | ND | 1 | 2 |
| Cholesterol | NL | High | NL | High | Low | NL |
| ApoB | High | High | ND | High | ND | ND |
| Cholestanol | - | - | - | + | + | + |
| Campesterol | + | + | + | + | + | + |
| Stigmasterol | Tr | Tr | + | + | Tr | ND |
| β-sitosterol | + | + | + | + | + | + |
| Avenasterol | - | - | + | (+) | - | - |
| Sitostanols | ND | ND | - | ND | ND | ND |
| Bile acids | NL | ND | NL | ND | AL | AL |
| Xanthomas | 3/3 | 5/5 | 1 | 1 | 1 | 3/5 |
| CHD | - | 3/5 | + | ND | + | ND |

ND = not determined or mentioned; NL = normal; AL = abnormal; Tr =
traces; CHD = coronary heart disease

β-sitosterol, campesterol and stigmasterol are the major components
of phytosterols found in different plant materials. These plant
sterols differ structurally from cholesterol in that the side chain
may contain substituents, e.g. methyl group (campesterol = methyl
cholesterol), ethyl group (β-sitosterol = methyl cholesterol) or
double bonds. The corresponding 5α-series is also detectable (e.g.,
methyl cholestanol and ethylcholestanol). It is owing to
differences in the side chain that plant sterols, especially the 5α-
series, are poorly absorbed. Absorption of campesterol appears to be
higher than that of β-sitosterol, indicating that the less polar the
side chain the lower the absorption. This has been demonstrated for
shellfish sterols (10).

Analogously to cholesterol, unabsorbed plant sterols are converted
to secondary products (coprostanol and coprostanone derivatives) by
colonic bacterias (11). Under normal dietary conditions dietary
plant sterols are quite quantitatively recovered in feces, a finding
signifying poor absorbability. However, in formula fed human
subjects relatively large portion of β-sitosterol is degraded to

undetectable products (12). Since this degradation is similar to
that of cholesterol β-sitosterol has been widely used in sterol
balance studies as an internal marker for correction of cholesterol
losses possibly taking place during the intestinal transit.

Normally less than five percent of dietary β-sitosterol is absorbed
(13). This would result in a marked β-sitosterolemia, especially on
high intake, e.g. during treatment of hypercholesterolemia, unless
elimination were effective. In fact, only small amounts of plant
sterols, usually <2 mg/100 ml, are normally found in plasma lipoproteins, campesterol frequently predominating. The distribution of
β-sitosterol in plasma lipoproteins resembles that of cholesterol
(13, Table 2) but the ester fraction tends to be lower. Elimination
of plasma plant sterols is faster than that of cholesterol.
Fractional conversion to bile acids appears to be similar but
biliary secretion of plant sterols is two-three times that of
cholesterol (13, Table 3). One third of absorbed β-sitosterol may
be eliminated via the skin (cf. 2).

Table 2. Sterols in maternal milk, and in maternal and infant
(2 months old) plasma lipoproteins  (Mean±SE; n = 6)

| Fraction | Cholesterol | Desmosterol | Lathosterol | Campesterol | β-sitosterol |
|---|---|---|---|---|---|
| | | *Maternal milk* | | | |
| Total[*] | 0.44±0.07 | 1447±217 | 64±12 | 25±6 | 19±4 |
| | | *Maternal plasma* | | | |
| Total[*] | 5.94±0.54 | 355±108 | 271±76 | 391±60 | 283±42 |
| VLDL[x] | 1.5 (56) | 1.0 (46) | 3.0 (59) | 1.2 (53) | 3.4 (59) |
| LDL[x] | 73.3 (71) | 78.6 (84) | 76.9 (57) | 73.6 (66) | 66.5 (61) |
| HDL[x] | 25.2 (80) | 20.4 (85) | 20.1 (68) | 25.2 (77) | 30.1 (74) |
| | | *Infant plasma* | | | |
| Total[*] | 3.55±0.20 | 273±37 | 149±13 | 32±4 | 87±45 |
| VLDL[x] | 7.3 (54) | 8.6 (51) | 120 (52) | 4.7 (53) | 17.1 (68) |
| LDL[x] | 63.4 (66) | 57.2 (73) | 57.0 (45) | 78.1 (69) | 45.8 (61) |
| HDL[x] | 29.3 (79) | 34.3 (83) | 31.0 (64) | 17.2 (51) | 37.0 (49) |

[*]Cholesterol = mmol/l, other sterols = µg/dl; [x]percent of total,
ester percent in parenthesis. Analysis performed with gas chromatography on SE-30 capillary column.

Table 3. Plasma and biliary campesterol and cholestanol in patients
with familial hypercholesterolemia without and with ileal bypass
and in a case (7) with phytosterolemia; (µg/100 mg cholesterol)

| Group | Plasma, free | | Plasma, esters | | Bile, total | |
|---|---|---|---|---|---|---|
| | Campe-sterol | Chole-stanol | Campe-sterol | Chole-stanol | Campe-sterol | Chole-stanol |
| Control | 291±79[*] | 129±9 | 248±64[*] | 141±8 | 671±219[*] | 756±41 |
| Bypass | 418±46 | 129±12 | 344±37 | 114±10 | 966±117 | 765±52 |
| Case(7) | 12160±1116 | .. | 7425±197 | .. | 11293±1471 | .. |

[*]p<0.05 from control on log scale; total plasma plant sterol
concentration exceeded 1.5 mg/dl in 2 out of 8 controls and in 7
out of 8 bypassed patients.

Lactating women and infants appear to develop phytosterolemia (14,
15). On a low cholesterol, phytosterol-rich diet plant sterols of
maternal and infant plasma, and maternal milk reach quite high
values. Thus, the plasma phytosterol levels increase up to 10-20
mg/dl, the values seen only in patients with familial phytosterolemia.

116

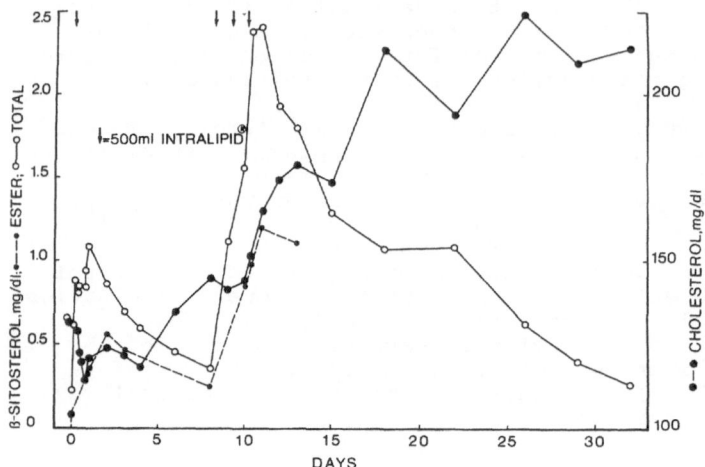

<u>Fig. 1.</u> β-sitosterol concentration in plasma of a patient on
parenteral nutrition. Each 500 ml of Intralipid[R] contained 75-130 mg
of β-sitosterol (other plant sterols are not included) and 101-192
mg of cholesterol. Increase of cholesterol is due to improvement of
patient's condition.

Our results have revealed lower values (Table 2) and less consistent
association with dietary phytosterols. Another transient phytosterolemia is caused by intravenous infusion of plant sterol-
containing fat emulsions during parenteral nutrition (Fig. 1). A
phytosterol peak occurs one day after the infusion followed by a
rapid equilibration with the exchangeable sterol pools in tissues
and elimination out from the body. We have found a third form of
secondary mild phytosterolemia in patients with familial hypercholesterolemia and ileal bypass (Table 3). In these patients the biliary
elimination of plant sterols appears to be effective, and plasma and
biliary cholestanol is normal.

The original two sisters with β-sitosterolemia and xanthomatosis
were characterized by tendon and tuberous xanthomata since young
age, by the absence of hypercholesterolemia or other significant
physical or routine laboratory findings, but by the presence of
plant sterols, β-sitosterol, campesterol and some stigmasterol, in
exchangeable sterol pool (1,2). Plant sterols comprised 11-16% of
the plasma total sterols (normally <1%), were transported mainly in
LDL and HDL, negligibly in VLDL, and were esterified normally. The
major abnormality was a greatly increased intestinal absorption of
β-sitosterol, 18-35% vs. <5% normally. Our case (7) showed, in
addition to other plant sterols, avenasterol in plasma and bile
(Fig. 2), low biliary cholesterol secretion, relative impairment in
biliary plant sterol output (cf. Table 3; plasma and biliary plant
sterol/cholesterol ratios are similar in phytosterolemia, while in
hypercholesterolemia the ratio is twice higher in the bile than in
the plasma), very low molar percentage of biliary sterols, especially
during cholestyramine treatment, and a high plant sterol absorption.
A quite high cholesterol absorption and low biliary secretion explained the low elimination of cholesterol as fecal neutral sterols,
while basal bile acid production was normal and cholesterol synthesis
was low. Cholestyramine decreased serum cholesterol and plant sterols

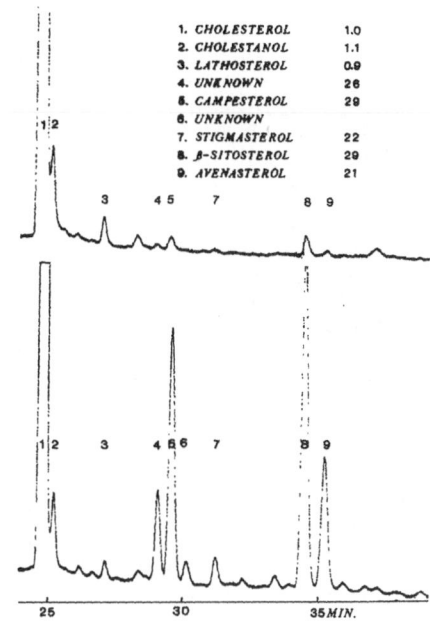

| | |
|---|---|
| 1. CHOLESTEROL | 1.0 |
| 2. CHOLESTANOL | 1.1 |
| 3. LATHOSTEROL | 0.9 |
| 4. UNKNOWN | 26 |
| 5. CAMPESTEROL | 29 |
| 6. UNKNOWN | |
| 7. STIGMASTEROL | 22 |
| 8. β-SITOSTEROL | 29 |
| 9. AVENASTEROL | 21 |

**Fig. 2.** Gas chromatography of biliary sterols on SE-30 capillary column. Retention time in minutes. Upper run from a normal subject, the lower one from a patient with phytosterolemia (7). Value after each sterol is the patient/normal ratio when the ratio for cholesterol is 1.0. The peaks 4 and 6 are unknown but include apparently 24-methylenecholesterol (7). No plant stanols are detectable.

similarly and increased bile acid and cholesterol synthesis moderately. Severe coronary atheromatosis and hypersplenism (requiring splenectomy) were major clinical findings, in addition to xanthomatosis.

Familial phytosterolemia appears to be a heterogenous entity inherited as an autosomal recessive trait. Limited data available suggests that two or three different subsets can be separated. The patients in references 2 and 8 of Table 1 seem to have the original β-sitosterolemia with xanthomatosis. Some of them have premature coronary heart disease and hyperapobetalipoproteinemia occurs in some family members even without phytosterolemia. Low stigmasterol, and absence of other plant sterols and of excessive 5α-sterols may be characteristic. The two patients in references 6 and 7 resemble each other in that stigmasterol and other side chain-unsaturated plant sterols (Fig. 2), including avenasterol, are clearly observable. Coprostanol derivatives of plant sterols are not detectable (Fig. 2). The older patient had severe premature coronary heart disease, normal bile acids and cholesterol but no 5α-plant sterols, while the younger one developed cholestanolosis especially when off cholestyramine. The patients in references 3-5 and 9 have coexisting cerebrotendinous xanthomatosis and phytosterolemia. They have high cholestanol and plant sterol levels in blood and tissues, and defective synthesis of chenodeoxycholic acid associated with increased tetra- and pentahydroxy bile acid precursors in bile and feces. Coronary heart disease and hematological abnormalities can be found.

118

References

1. Bhattacharyya AK, Connor WE (1974) J Clin Invest 53: 1033
2. Bhattacharyya AK, Connor WE (1978) In: Stanbury JB, Wyngaarden JB, Fredrickson DS (eds) The Metabolic Basis of Inherited Disease. McGraw-Hill Book Co, New York, Chapt. 31
3. Khachadurian AK, Clancy KF (1978) Clin Res 26: 329 (Abstract)
4. Khachadurian AK, Salen G (1978) Clin Res 26: 297 (Abstract)
5. Dayal B, Tint GS, Verga D, Salen G (1980) Fed Proc 39: 1904 (Abstract)
6. Whitington GL, Ragland JB, Sabesin SM, Kuiken LB (1979) Circulation 60: Part II: II-33 (Abstract)
7. Miettinen TA (1980) Eur J Clin Invest 10: 27
8. Kwiterovich PO, Bachorik PS, Smith HH, McKusick VA, Connor WE, Teng B, Sniderman AD (1981) Lancet i: 466
9. Wang C, Lin HJ, Chan T-K, Salen G, Chan W-C, Tse T-F (1981) Am J Med 71: 313
10. Connor WE, Lin DS (1981) Gastroenterology 81: 276
11. Miettinen TA, Grundy SM, Ahrens EH Jr (1965) J Lipid Res 6: 411
12. Grundy SM, Ahrens EH Jr, Salen G (1968) J Lipid Res 9: 374
13. Salen G, Ahrens EH Jr, Grundy SM (1974) J Clin Invest 49: 952
14. Mellies M, Glueck CJ, Sweeney C, Fallat RW, Tsang RC (1976) Ishikawa Pediatrics 57: 60
15. Mellies MJ, Ishikawa TT, Gartside P, Burton K, MacGee J, Allen K, Steiner PM, Brayd D, Glueck CJ (1978) Am J Clin Nutr 31: 1347

# Familial Chylomicronaemia Due to a Circulating Inhibitor of Lipoprotein Lipase

N. E. Miller, P. Alaupovic, J. Brunzell, C. Cortese, J. St. Hilaire, B. Lewis, and C. S. Wang

## Introduction

The currently recognised causes of familial chylomicronaemia are absence or deficiency of lipoprotein lipase (LPL), and absence of the cofactor for LPL, apoprotein (apo) CII, each of which is recessively inherited. This report concerns a family in which chylomicronaemia was inherited through three generations in an autosomal dominant manner, and was due to a circulating inhibitor of LPL.

## Clinical description of proband

The proband (F1) was a 47 y old Caucasian female who was found to have massive hypertriglyceridaemia after developing eruptive xanthomas on the outer aspects of both feet. There were no other xanthomas or xanthelasma. She gave a history of recurrent undiagnosed abdominal pain since the age of 16 y. Alcohol intake was minimal, and she was not taking any hormone preparations. On examination the spleen was palpable, but there was no hepatomegaly. She was not obese. There was no clinical evidence of atherosclerotic disease. Oral glucose tolerance was normal. Conventional biochemical indices of renal, thyroid and hepatic function were also normal. There was no paraproteinaemia. On an unrestricted diet, lipoprotein fractionation by serial preparative ultracentrifugation gave the following results (mmol/l): chylomicron triglyceride, 20.5; VLDL triglyceride, 6.8; VLDL cholesterol, 1.9; LDL triglyceride, 1.8; LDL cholesterol, 0.81; HDL triglyceride, 0.34; HDL cholesterol, 0.36. Reduction of dietary fat intake to 5 g/d reduced chylomicron triglyceride by 80% after 48 h. Nicotinic acid therapy had no lipid-lowering effect.

## Family members

The proband's father died at age 39 y after surgery for acute abdominal pain. Screening of other family members demonstrated normal lipid levels in the proband's mother, sister, brother and husband. However, her only child (F2) also had marked hypertriglyceridaemia. He had no xanthomas or hepatosplenomegaly, and was asymptomatic. Severe hypertriglyceridaemia was also found in the proband's grandson (F3)(Table 1).

Table 1. Clinical details of affected subjects

| Subject | Age | Sex | Plasma trigly-ceride (mmol/l) | Plasma cholesterol (mmol/l) |
|---------|-----------|-----|------|------|
| F1 | 47 y | F | 43.7 | 11.7 |
| F2 | 21 y | M | 40.6 | 7.5 |
| F3 | 4 months | M | 28.1 | 6.4 |

## Post-heparin plasma lipolytic activity

Post-heparin plasma LPL and hepatic lipase (HL) activities were measured in F1 and F2 during a heparin infusion of 4 h duration after an overnight fast. A bolus of heparin was injected (2280 u/m$^2$ body surface area; approximately 60 u/kg), followed by an infusion of 2000 u/m$^2$/h. Post-heparin plasma was incubated with and without rat antiserum to human HL, and then assayed for triglyceride hydrolase activity, as previously described[1]. The lipolytic activity in the presence of antiserum and apo CII was regarded as LPL activity.

One hour after starting the infusion post-heparin plasma LPL activity in both patients was less than 25% of (and more than two SD below) the mean value in 6 normal subjects. After 4 h of infusion, the activity in both was approximately 30% of mean normal.

## Adipose tissue LPL activity

Needle biopsies of gluteal adipose tissue were collected from F1 and F2 in the fasted state, and assayed for heparin-elutable LPL activity, as previously described[2], using pooled normal human serum as the source of apo CII. The enzyme activity was very high in F1 and moderately high in F2, relative to results from normal controls (173 and 9.2 nmol FFA/min/g versus 5.6±5.4(SD), n=12).

## Demonstration of an inhibitor of LPL in serum

There was no measurable LPL activity when serum from F1 or F2 was used to activate LPL eluted from normal human adipose tissue with heparin. Nor was there any LPL activity when a 1:1 (v:v) mixture of pooled normal human serum and serum from F1 or F2 was used as activator.

In other experiments the d>1.25 g/ml infranatants of serum from F1 and F2 were found to inhibit the lipolytic activity of normal post-heparin plasma by 80%. In contrast, the d>1.25 g/ml fraction of serum from two normal subjects produced less than 10% inhibition.

Chylomicron-free serum from F1 and F2 also inhibited the lipolytic activity in heparin eluates of rat epididymal adipose tissue, assayed in the presence of normal human serum as activator (Table 2).

Table 2. Effect of chylomicron-free serum from F1 and F2 on LPL activity eluted with heparin from rat epididymal adipose tissue

| Serum included in incubation mixture | LPL activity (nmol FFA/min/g) |
|---|---|
| 2 vols normal human serum | 47.0 |
| 1 vol normal plus 1 vol F1 serum | 0.6 |
| 1 vol normal plus 1 vol F2 serum | 0.1 |

The inhibitor in the d>1.25 g/ml fraction was non-dialyzable and was stable when serum was heated to 55$^{\circ}$C for 2 h. It was unstable, however, to freezing and thawing (x3).

## Apoprotein assays

The concentrations of apoproteins in plasma from F1 and F2 were measured by electroimmunoassay[3],[4]. The results for apo CII and apo CIII are compared in Table 3 with those obtained from patients with untreated chylomicronaemia due to familial LPL absence or familial apo CII absence[5].

Table 3. Apoprotein concentrations (mg/dl)

|  | F1 | F2 | LPL absence | CII absence | Controls* |
|---|---|---|---|---|---|
| CII | 21 | 8 | 11 | 0 | 4±1 |
| CIII | 54 | 24 | 15 | 39 | 8±2 |

* 25 normolipidaemic subjects aged 20-39 y

Thus, all 4 patients had elevated concentrations of apo CIII, and F1, F2 and the patient with LPL absence had very high apo CII levels.

Isoelectric focussing of VLDL apoproteins of subject F1 demonstrated an additional band on the cathodic side of apo $CIII_0$ which was not seen in VLDL from fifty normal subjects and 6 subjects with hypertriglyceridaemia.

## Discussion

The results of these studies demonstrate vertical transmission of chylomicronaemia through three generations. The mother and husband of the proband had normal triglyceride levels. Thus, the data are compatible with autosomal dominant inheritance. It seems possible that the acute abdominal emergency suffered by the proband's father was acute pancreatitis, and hence that a fourth generation was affected by the disorder.

The low post-heparin LPL activity in plasma associated with the hypertriglyceridaemia was shown not to be due to apo CII deficiency or adipose tissue LPL deficiency. Although the concentration of apo CIII, which inhibits LPL in vitro[6], was elevated, this was commensurate with the degree of hypertriglyceridaemia, high apo CIII concentrations being found also in patients with chylomicronaemia due to absence of LPL or apo CII.

The presence of an inhibitor of LPL was demonstrated in both the proband and her son using three different assay systems (normal post-heparin plasma, LPL eluted from normal adipose tissue, and LPL eluted from rat adipose tissue). The inhibitor was heat-stable and was present in the d>1.25 g/ml fraction of plasma.

In the light of these findings, a familial LPL inhibitor should be considered in any patient with chylomicronaemia and low post-heparin lipolytic activity. This is particularly so when there is clinical or laboratory evidence of chylomicronaemia in a parent or child, since unlike deficiencies of LPL and apo CII this condition appears to be dominantly inherited.

The very high adipose tissue LPL activity in F1 was similar to that previously observed in a patient with familial apo CII deficiency[5]. This raises the possibility that the tissue content of LPL increases in an adaptive manner when the enzyme is in a non-functional state in the capillary endothelium.

## Acknowledgement

We thank Drs. J. Huttunen, E. Nikkila and C.Enholm for providing the rat antiserum to human post-heparin hepatic lipase. Part of this work was supported by NIH grants AM 02456, HL 18687 and HL 23705 (Dr. J. Brunzell).

## References

1. Brunzell JD, Chait A, Nikkila EA, Ehnholm C, Huttunen JK, Steiner G (1980) Heterogeneity of primary lipoprotein lipase deficiency. Metabolism 29:624-629

2. Schwartz RS, Brunzell JD (1981) Increase of adipose tissue lipoprotein lipase activity with weight loss. J Clin Invest 67:1425-1430

3. Curry MD, McConathy WJ, Fesmire JD, Alaupovic P (1981) Quantitative determination of apolipoproteins C-I and C-II in human plasma by separate electroimmunoassays. Clin Chem 27:543-548

4. Curry MD, McConathy WJ, Fesmire JD,Alaupovic P (1980) Quantitative determination of human apolipoprotein C-III by electroimmunoassay. Biochim Biophys Acta 617:503-513

5. Miller NE, Rao SN, Alaupovic P, Noble N, Slack J, Brunzell JD, Lewis B (1981) Familial apolipoprotein CII deficiency: plasma lipoproteins and apolipoproteins in heterozygous and homozygous subjects and the effects of plasma infusion. Eur J Clin Invest 11:69-76

6. Brown WV, Baginsky ML (1972) Inhibition of lipoprotein lipase by an apoprotein of human very low density lipoprotein. Biochem Biophys Res Commun 46:375-82

# 1.3 Animal Models of Atherosclerosis

# Experimental Nonhuman Primate Atherosclerosis

R. N. Chakravarti

Research on experimental animals has provided valuable information regarding the pathogenesis and therapy of atherosclerosis. Earlier studies were done mostly on small laboratory animals, rabbits, rats and chicken. For the last 2-3 decades the emphasis has fallen on larger animals like dogs, pigs and subhuman primates because of obvious advantages. Various species of nonhuman primates including the old and new world monkeys have been employed for creation of an experimental model of atherosclerosis bearing close resemblance to the human disease and different methods of therapeutic control have been evaluated. At our center in Chandigarh, India we have been studying this problem in rhesus monkeys ($\underline{M}$. $\underline{mulatta}$) for the lasttwenty years. In this species we have observed athero-arteriosclerotic lesions occurring spontaneously in the wild state and found these macaques very suitable for producing human type of atherosclerotic disease by experimental procedures.

## Spontaneously occurring athero-arteriosclerosis and thrombosis in wild monkeys

Apes, baboons and monkeys develop atherosclerotic lesions in the aorta, and much less frequently in the coronary and cerebral arteries, in their wild habitat or when kept under captivity for long periods (1-6). Studies on rhesus monkeys have been done extensively in our Institute also(7,8).Three consecutive studies on a total number of 329 recently captured wild rhesus macaques have revealed that fatty streaks, atheroma and fibrous plaques in aorta are not infrequent, but these lesions are less commonly seen in coronary and cerebral arteries (8-10). In the latest study (10) 27 percent of 124 monkeys were found to have in their aorta fatty streak/atheromatous lesion, 13 percent fibrous plaques and 22 percent intimal fibrosis without lipid. Mural thrombi adherent to subjacent arterio/atherosclerotic plaques were seen in 3 animals. Coronary arteries showed atherosclerosis, particularly in the epicardial segment in 10 percent of the animals. In the cerebral arteries fibrous plaques with little lipid were seen in 5 out of 20 monkeys and complicated atherosclerosis in one animal (11).

## Experimental atherosclerosis in new and old world monkeys

About two decades back Taylor and his colleagues in USA produced experimental atherosclerosis in rhesus monkeys by feeding a diet rich in animal fat mixed with cholesterol (12). When this diet was fed over a period of several years typical atherosclerotic lesions in the aorta, coronary arteries, renal and peripheral arteries were produced. A couple of such monkeys developed myocardial infarction and gangrene of the limbs (13). The results obtained by him on this species prompted other workers to use nonhuman primates for atherosclerosis research. Thus McGill and Strong at New Orleans, Wissler and colleagues at Chicago, Clarkson and his co-workers at Bowman Gray School of Medicine, Winston-Salem and several other groups carried out extensive research on both new and old world monkeys as well as baboons. They could produce various grades of atherosclerosis involving the aorta

Department of Experimental Medicine, Postgraduate Institute of Medical Education and Research, Chandigarh, India.

and coronary arteries of monkeys by feeding high fat and high cholesterol diet alone or by combining it with renal hypertension (14-16).

## Catecholamine induced aggravation of aortic and coronary atherosclerosis in rhesus monkeys

It is known that stressful situations promote endogenous liberation of catecholamines which produce acute haemodynamic disturbances as well as cause endothelial damage by direct toxic action. In view of this atherogenic diet fed rhesus monkeys were given daily intravenous injection of adrenaline in a dose of 250 ug/animal for a period of seven months. There was a marked rise of systolic and diastolic blood pressure following adrenaline injection which returned to the normal level within an hour. Significant hypercholesterolemia was produced in animals which were fed atherogenic diet alone (Gr.I) or when atherogenic diet was combined with adrenaline injections (Gr.II). In the former group the mean serum cholesterol was 286.4 $\pm$ 25.57 mg/100 ml while in the latter it was 295.16 $\pm$ 17.34 mg/100 ml. There was a significant increase of aortic cholesterol in monkeys of group II, mean value in groups I and II being 2.76 $\pm$ 0.42 and 6.44 $\pm$ 1.63 mg/g (P $\angle$ 0.05). Phospholipids, TG, hydroxyproline and collagen content of aorta in monkeys of these two groups did not show significant variation. Again, extent of aortic sudanophilia was greater in group I animals, the mean value being 35.66 $\pm$ 6.84 against the value of 17.56 $\pm$ 4.29 in group II monkeys (P $>$ 0.05). Microscopic assessment of height of the largest aortic plaque did not show significant variation between the two groups, the mean value in group I being 388.0 $\pm$ 66.83 um and in group II 356.62 $\pm$ 65.2 um. The frequency of involvement with atherosclerotic plaques (fatty or fibrous) at different sites in the aorta was 25 percent in group I and 23 percent in group II.

The coronary atherosclerosis index in monkeys of groups I and II were 10.92 $\pm$ 1.25 and 10.43 $\pm$ 1.49, the difference being insignificant. The largest plaque in coronary arteries of these two groups of monkeys showed a mean height of 61.25 $\pm$ 11.64 um in group I as against 63.08 $\pm$ 17.29 um in group II (P $>$ 0.05).

## Morphology of experimental atherosclerosis

Three types of atherosclerotic lesions were detected in aorta and coronary arteries of groups I and II monkeys. These were fatty streak, atheromatous plaque and fibrous plaque. The greatest incidence of aortic fibrous plaques was in group II, 5 out of 6 monkeys (83.5 percent) as against 50 percent in group I monkeys. Calcification of the plaques was not detected. In aorta mural thrombosis was noted in 2 monkeys of group I and one monkey of group II while coronary artery showed this lesion in one animal of group II only.

## Reversibility of experimentally induced atherosclerosis in monkeys

One of the important aspects of atherosclerosis research is the evaluation of various diets, drugs and other intervention in the prevention or regression of atherosclerotic lesions. At the present time lot of emphasis is being given on the primary prevention of atherosclerosis, particularly in human population groups exposed to the risk of ischaemic heart disease and stroke. Since primary prevention starts quite early in life and is spread over several decades to cover the major portion of one's life span it is a cumbersome and difficult procedure to follow. Even then certain studies carried out in USA have definitely shown beneficial effects of primary prevention and incidence of deaths from acute myocardial infarction/stroke has been reduced to some extent. Since atherosclerotic lesions cause marked narrowing of the arterial lumen and cause significant reduction in blood supply to tissue they produce ischemic lesions or frank necrosis. Attempts to widen the already narrowed arteries and bring about increased blood flow to the ischemic tissue is being elucidated these days. Based on the observations both on human subjects as well as in experimental animals various dietary regimens, drugs and other interventions are being evaluated for effecting regression of already existing atherosclerotic plaques(15,17-20).

Table. Mean ($\pm$ SE) values of cholesterol and TG in serum (mg/100 ml) and aorta (mg/g wet wt) in control atherosclerotic (CA) and treated (T)monkeys

| Group | Serum | | | | Aorta | | | |
|---|---|---|---|---|---|---|---|---|
| | Cholesterol | | TG | | Cholesterol | | TG | |
| | CA | T | CA | T | CA | T | CA | T |
| Mustard oil (a) | 261.68 $\pm$ 24.29 | 144.16* $\pm$ 14.88 | 94.20 $\pm$ 7.10 | 32.42** $\pm$ 8.10 | 6.44 $\pm$ 1.63 | 2.48* $\pm$ 0.39 | 2.77 $\pm$ 0.27 | 6.61** $\pm$ 1.06 |
| Peanut oil (b) | 252.86 $\pm$ 18.24 | 154.96* $\pm$ 11.95 | 94.4 $\pm$ 7.67 | 66.54 $\pm$ 8.95 | " | 1.50* $\pm$ 0.18 | " | 4.91 $\pm$ 1.51 |
| Clofibrate (c) | 231.12 $\pm$ 10.68 | 162.46** $\pm$ 7.79 | 83.8 $\pm$ 1.90 | 39.48*** $\pm$ 3.75 | " | 4.12 $\pm$ 1.36 | " | 8.46*** $\pm$ 0.64 |
| Propranolol (d) | 236.92 $\pm$ 10.98 | 159.16** $\pm$ 12.19 | 85.0 $\pm$ 1.67 | 50.04** $\pm$ 4.22 | " | 1.86* $\pm$ 0.60 | " | 5.61* $\pm$ 0.86 |
| Stock diet (e) | 252.05 $\pm$ 14.85 | 138.83** $\pm$ 14.69 | 81.25 $\pm$ 2.15 | 55.96** $\pm$ 9.11 | " | 1.41* $\pm$ 0.42 | " | 7.72 $\pm$ 3.16 |

P $<$ 0.05 (*); $<$ 0.01 (**); $<$ 0.001 (***)
Intra group comparisons after therapy

Serum cholesterol – N.S.     Aorta cholesterol – a vs b *
Serum TG – a vs b *          Aorta TG – c vs d *
           c vs e *

In this laboratory work is being continued for the last many years on the production of experimentally induced advanced atherosclerosis in rhesus monkeys (21) and methods for its control by feeding a low fat low calorie diet or diet rich in polyunsaturated fatty acids, safflower oil (19). Several other dietary agents viz. mustard and peanut oil and low fat diet as well as drugs like clofibrate and propranolol have been tested on this model to elucidate their reversibility potential. It has been observed that these therapeutic diets and drugs bring about a marked reversal of the elevated levels of serum cholesterol and TG towards normal levels within a period of 7 months (Table). The aortic lipids also showed a decline in cholesterol content but increase in TG following the administration of the therapeutic diets(Table). Aortic hydroxyproline and collagen content, however, did not show significant change from the untreated atherogenic diet fed control (Kukreja, 1982).

The extent of aortic sudanophilia did not show significant variation in the treated animals as compared to baseline control values. Intra group comparisons after therapy showed significantly less aortic sudanophilia in mustard oil fed monkeys as compared to clofibrate administered animals 14.8 $\pm$ 3.21 vs 31.25 $\pm$ 4.42 (P $<$ 0.05). The frequency incidence of aortic atheromatous or fibrous plaques showed almost similar values in treated animals except those given mustard oil where the value was relatively high. As regards plaque size there was significant reduction in all the treated groups as compared to the baseline control value. However, coronary atherosclerotic plaque size did not show significant reduction. As far as coronary atherosclerosis index was concerned there was no significant variation from the value of baseline control.

In summary it can be said that the monkey model of atherosclerosis provides a suitable experimental situation having close similarity to the human disease. Further, that established lesions of atherosclerosis in this species can be partially reversed has been amply demonstrated following the use of various diets and drugs.

## References

1.  Fox, H (1933) Arteriosclerosis in lower mammals and birds. its relation to the disease in man. Arteriosclerosis E.V. Cowdry, Ed. (Macmillan Co., New York) p 617.

2.  Ratcliffe HL and Cronin MTI (1958) Changing frequency of arteriosclerosis in mammals and birds at the Philadelphia Zoological garden. Circulation 18: 41.

3.  McGill, HC, Strong JP, Holman RL, Werthessen NT (1960) Arterial lesion in the Kenya baboons. Circ. Res 8: 670.

4.  Lapin BA, Yakovleva LA (1963) Comparative pathology of monkeys. Charles C Thomas Publ USA.

5.  Malinow MR, Maruffo CA (1965) Aortic atherosclerosis in free ranging howler monkeys. Nature 206: 948

6.  Middleton CC, Rosal J, Clarkson TB, Newman WP III, McGill HC Jr(1967) Arterial lesions in squirrel monkeys. Arch Pathol 83: 352.

7.  Chakravarti RN, Chawla KK (1966) Spontaneously occurring mural throm bi in arteries of macaca mulatta. J. Atheroscler Res 6: 455.

8.  Chawla KK, Murthy CDS, Chakravarti RN, Chhuttani PN (1967) Arteriosclerosis and thrombosis in wild rhesus monkeys. Am Heart J 73: 85

9.  Chakravarti RN, Mohan AP, Komal HS (1976) Atherosclerosis in macaca mulatta - Histopathological, morphometric and histochemical studies in aorta and coronary arteries of spontaneous and induced atherosclero sis. Exp Mol Pathol 25: 390.

10. Chakravarti RN, Kukreja RS (1981) Naturally occurring athero-arterio sclerosis in rhesus monkeys. Indian J Med Res 73: 603

11. Bharadwaj JR (1982) Experimental study of cerebral atherosclerosis in rhesus monkeys. Ph.D. thesis PGI Chandigarh, India

12. Taylor CB, Cox, GE, Manalo Estrella P, Southworth, J, Patton, DE Cathcart C (1962) Atherosclerosis in rhesus monkeys - Arterial lesion associated with hypercholesterolemia induced by dietary fat and cholesterol. Arch Path 74: 16.

13. Taylor CB, Patton DE, Cox GE (1963) Atherosclerosis in rhesus monkeys VI Fatal myocardial infarction in a monkey fed fat and cholesterol Arch Path 76: 404

14. McGill HC, Frank MH, Geer JC (1961) Aortic lesions in hypertensive monkeys. Arch Path 71: 96.

15. Strong JP (1976) Atherosclerosis in primates. Prim Med 9: 1.

16. Bond MG, Bullock BC, Bellinger DA, Hamm TE (1980) Myocardial infarction in a large colony of nonhuman primates with coronary artery atherosclerosis. Am J Path 101: 675.

17. Armstrong ML, Warner ED, Connor WE (1970) Regression of coronary atheromatosis in rhesus monkeys 57: 59.

18. Vesselinovitch D, Wissler RW, Hughes R, Borensztajn J (1976) Reversal of advanced atherosclerosis in rhesus monkeys. Atherosclerosis 23: 155.

19. Chakravarti RN, Sasikumar B, Nair CR, Kumar M (1977) Reversibility of cholesterol adrenaline induced atherosclerosis in rhesus monkeys : Evaluation of safflower oil and low fat low calorie diet. Atherosclerosis 28: 405.

20. Wagner WD, St.Clair RW, Clarkson TB (1980) A study of atherosclerosis regression in macaca mulatta : Chemical changes in arteries from animals with atherosclerosis induced for 19 months then regressed for 24 months at plasma cholesterol concentrations of 300 or 200 mg/dl. Exptl Mol Path 32: 162.

21. Kukreja RS, Datta BN, Chakravarti RN (1981) Catecholamine induced aggravation of aortic and coronary atherosclerosis in monkeys. Atherosclerosis 40: 291.

22. Kukreja RS (1982) Role of diet and drugs on the reversibility of experimentally induced atherosclerosis in rhesus monkeys. Ph.D.thesis PGI Chandigarh, India.

# Platelets and Atherogenesis in Normal and von Willebrand Disease Pigs

V. Fuster

## Introduction

There is increasing evidence that platelet-arterial wall interaction is an important step in the genesis of arteriosclerotic lesions (1). The genesis of these lesions may involve the following factors (2): (a) continued endothelial injury; (b) adherence and aggregation of platelets to damaged endothelial cells or to exposed subendothelial tissue; (c) local release of platelet constituents, including a mitogenic protein (platelet-derived growth factor) that stimulates growth of cultured smooth muscle cells, and passage of such platelet constituents into the underlying arterial wall; (d) migration of smooth muscle cells through the internal elastic lamina into the intima and platelet-mediated intimal proliferation of smooth muscle cells; (e) formation of a connective tissue matrix by the smooth muscle cells through synthesis and secretion of collagen, elastic fiber proteins, and glycosaminoglycans; and (f) accumulation of intracellular and extracellular lipids.

For several years, we have maintained a breeding colony of pigs with von Willebrand's disease (3). These animals have the observed impairment of primary hemostasis and the other hemostatic abnormalities noted in the severe form of the disease in humans (3,4): a serious autosomally transmitted bleeding tendency, a long bleeding time, reduced retention of platelets in a column filled with glass beads, reduced levels of factor VIII coagulant activity (VIII:C), very low levels of factor VIII-related antigen (VIII R:AG), and a lack of ristocetin cofactor (Willebrand factor VIII:RWF) in the plasma (3,5). This ristocetin cofactor is closely allied with, or identical to, the factor VIII-related antigen.

If indeed platelet-arterial wall interaction is a step in the genesis of atherosclerosis (1), we thought that a good deal of information might be obtained by investigating whether pigs with an affected platelet function in the form of von Willebrand's disease are resistant to the development of arteriosclerosis. Thus far our approach has been: 1) to evaluate whether there is a resistance to aortic arteriosclerosis in von Willebrand pigs under a controlled high fat-high cholesterol diet, and under a controlled low fat-low cholesterol diet--such an approach might be a first step in testing the concept of the possible importance of platelets in the genesis of arteriosclerosis; 2) to evaluate, by aortic transplantation, whether the donor normal pig aorta becomes resistant to the development of arteriosclerosis when it is transplanted into the host von Willebrand pig--such an approach might provide information on the possible contribution of the arterial wall or the circulating blood in the development of arteriosclerosis in the pig; and 3) to evaluate, after a superficial injury of the endothelium of the carotid artery, whether platelet deposition over the injured surface is decreased in pigs with von Willebrand's disease when compared with normal pigs--such an approach might provide "in vivo" evidence that the platelet-arterial wall interaction is impaired in von Willebrand's disease.

## 1. Aortic Arteriosclerosis Studies

Pigs with von Willebrand's disease have a severe bleeding diathesis and bleed to death periodically from exsanguinating gastrointestinal haemorrhage and severe epistaxis. For unknown reasons, the epistaxis always starts in the posterior nose, and because porcine turbinates are convoluted, the bleeding site cannot be visualized. At post-mortem, it was observed that there was negligible aortic arterio-sclerosis. This observation was interesting and unexpected because pigs have an arterial system closely resembling that of man (6), and they usually develop arteriosclerotic lesions early in life (7). Following the post-mortem observations, a retrospective study of spontaneous arteriosclerosis was started in 1974. The incidence of spontaneous aortic arteriosclerosis in 11 von Willebrand pigs was compared with the incidence in 11 normal pigs obtained from the slaughterhouse. The normal pigs were of the same breed as the von Willebrand pigs—a cross between Poland-China and Yorkshire-Hampshire. The aortas of the 11 normal pigs were examined, and 6 were found to have multiple raised fatty or fibrous atherosclerotic plaques (8). None of the aortas of the 11 von Willebrand pigs had multiple plaques, four had single plaques, but only one was more than 2 mm in diameter.

The first retrospective study, therefore, showed that there was a striking difference between the normal pig and pigs with von Willebrand's disease in the incidence and extent of arteriosclerotic lesions in the aorta. However, the study had a number of shortcomings: it was retrospective, the body mass of the controls was higher than that of the pigs with von Willebrand's disease, and we did not have exact information about the diets of the normal pigs. We, therefore, decided in the following year to initiate a prospective study in which the pigs were matched for breed, age and sex and the diet was strictly controlled (8). Eighteen newborn pigs were fed with maternal milk supplemented with cows' milk until 3 months of age at which time they received an atherogenic high fat-high cholesterol diet (approximately 500 g/40 kg body mass, containing 2% cholesterol) for a period of 6 months. Seven pigs had homozygous von Willebrand's disease and there were 11 normal control pigs. The 11 control pigs all developed raised fatty or fibrous arteriosclerotic plaques on the aorta; thus, an average of 18% of the aortic surface below the renal arteries was involved by arteriosclerosis. In the von Willebrand pigs there was a striking contrast: only an average of 3% of the aortic surface below the renal arteries was involved by arteriosclerosis (Table 1).

Table 1. Porcine Arteriosclerosis

| Type of study | Type of pig | Arteriosclerosis (% aortic surface) | P value |
|---|---|---|---|
| High cholesterol diet (6 mo) | Normal (11) Homozygous vWd (7) | 18 3 | 0.01 |
| Normal diet (4 yr) | Normal (5) Homozygous vWd (5) | 27 7 | 0.01 |

Dietary-induced arteriosclerosis may, of course, be different from the spontaneously occurring variety, so a prospective study of spontaneous arteriosclerosis was also undertaken (9). Ten newborn

pigs were fed with maternal milk supplemented with cows' milk until
3 months of age, at which time they received a low fat-low cholesterol
diet for a period up to 4 years.  Five pigs had homozygous von
Willebrand's disease and five were normal control pigs.  Of the normal
pigs, an average of 27% of the aortic surface below the renal arteries
was involved by arteriosclerosis.  In contrast, of the von Willebrand
pigs, only an average of 7% of the aortic surface below the renal
arteries was involved by arteriosclerosis (Table 1).

These three studies, therefore, are evidence that pigs with von
Willebrand's disease are resistant to the development of arteriosclerosis.  There are a number of possible explanations for these
findings, and one of them may lie in the abnormal platelet--blood
vessel interaction seen in von Willebrand's disease (10).  In such
case, these studies would support the concept of the importance of
platelets and of a normal platelet-blood vessel interaction in the
genesis of arteriosclerosis in the pig model.

## 2.   Aortic Transplantation Studies

Aortic segments of 5 cm length and proximal to the trifurcation of
the aorta from four normal control pigs were transplanted into four
host von Willebrand pigs.  The appropriate control operations between
normal pigs were also done, and we have actually performed 18 such
procedures.  The von Willebrand pigs were infused with 60 ml of normal
pig cryoprecipitate about three hours before the procedure, to improve
haemostasis.  Ten days after operation, at which time the effect of
cryoprecipitate had disappeared, the pigs began to receive an
atherogenic high fat-high cholesterol diet.  The diet was continued
for 6 months, the pigs were killed, and the aortas were removed,
examined and measured for gross arteriosclerotic plaques.  It was
found that the aortic segments from control pigs that were transplanted
into von Willebrand pigs had a significant decreased capability of
developing arteriosclerosis when compared with the control study (9);
in addition, it was shown by immunofluorescence that they lost their
Willebrand factor, which normally is present in the aortas of the
control pigs (11).

For complete interpretation of the data of these transplantation
studies, we need to know whether the donor aortic segments are totally
or partially replaced by the host aortas.  We can say, however, that
the resistance to arteriosclerosis correlated with the absence of
von Willebrand factor.  Thus, the results obtained are compatible with
the hypothesis that in pigs with homozygous von Willebrand's disease,
the absence of Willebrand factor may be responsible for an impairment
of platelet-arterial wall interaction and the resistance to arteriosclerosis in these animals.

## 3.   Carotid Artery Injury Studies

As indicated above, there are several lines of evidence indicating
that platelet-vessel wall interaction is impaired in von Willebrand's
disease.  However, good "in vivo" evidence of this phenomenon has not
yet been fully established.  Accordingly, we evaluated, after a
superficial injury of the endothelium of the carotid artery, whether
platelet deposition over the injured surface is decreased in pigs
with von Willebrand's disease when compared with normal pigs (12).
Selective endothelial injury was produced in a 4 cm segment of carotid

artery by drying for 3 minutes in a stream of air which entered one end (100 ml/min) and exited through a small hole in the other end. This procedure was performed in 5 normal and 3 von Willebrand pigs 24 hours after the intravenous infusion of [111]Indium-labeled platelets. Carotid blood flow was re-established and the pigs were sacrificed 24 hours later. The ratio of radioactivity (cpm/g) of injured/ noninjured carotid arteries was decreased in the von Willebrand pigs. Electron microscopy confirmed endothelial damage in all injured segments and the platelets attached to the vessel wall appeared less activated in the von Willebrand pigs than in the normal pigs.

This "in vivo" evidence of impaired platelet-vessel wall interaction in von Willebrand's disease is now leading us to pursue in the carotid model the following objectives: 1) to determine whether in the normal pig, neutralization of Willebrand factor results in impairment of platelet adhesion and intimal proliferation; and 2) to determine whether in the von Willebrand pig, transfusion of purified Willebrand factor leads to platelet adhesion and intimal proliferation.


## Conclusion

The study of von Willebrand's disease is giving us and other groups important new information about the physiology of haemostasis as well as a new avenue for investigation of arteriosclerosis (8,9,13). Von Willebrand's disease in pigs is an excellent example of how an animal model can lead to important advances in our understanding of human disease.


## References

1. Ross R, Glomset JA (1976) The pathogenesis of atherosclerosis. N Engl J Med 295:369-377; 420-425
2. Fuster V (1981) Role of platelets in the development of atherosclerotic disease and possible interference with platelet inhibitor drugs. Scand J Haematol 27(Suppl. 38):1
3. Bowie EJW, Owen CA Jr, Zollman PE, Thompson JH Jr, Fass DN (1973) Tests of hemostasis in swine: normal values and values in pigs with von Willebrand's disease. Am J Vet Res 34:1405-1407
4. Mannucci PM, Pareti FI, Holmberg L, Nilsson IM, Ruggeri ZM (1976) Studies on the prolonged bleeding time in von Willebrand's disease. J Lab Clin Med 88:662-671
5. Fass DN, Brockway WJ, Owen CA Jr, Bowie EJW (1976) Factor VIII (Willebrand) antigen and ristocetin-Willebrand factor in pigs with von Willebrand's disease. Thromb Res 8:319-327
6. French JE, Jennings MA, Florey HW (1965) Morphological studies on atherosclerosis in swine. Ann NY Acad Sci 127:780-799
7. Getty R (1965) The gross and microscopic occurrence and distribution of spontaneous atherosclerosis in the arteries of swine. In Comparative Atherosclerosis: The Morphology of Spontaneous and Induced Atherosclerotic Lesions in Animals and Its Relation to Human Disease. J. C. Roberts, Jr., and R. Straus, editors. Harper & Row Publishers, Inc., New York, 11-20
8. Fuster V, Bowie EJW, Lewis JC, Fass DN, Owen CA Jr (1978) Resistance to arteriosclerosis in pigs with von Willebrand's disease. Spontaneous and high cholesterol diet-induced arteriosclerosis. J Clin Invest 61:722-730
9. Fuster V, Fass DN, Kaye MP, Josa M, Zinsmeister AR, Bowie EJW (in press) Arteriosclerosis in normal and von Willebrand pigs: Long-term prospective study and aortic transplantation study. Circ Res

134

10. Booyse FM, Quarfoot AJ, Bell S, Fass DN, Lewis JC, Mann KG,
    Bowie EJW (1977) Cultured aortic endothelial cells from pig with
    von Willebrand's disease: _in vitro_ model for studying the
    molecular defect(s) of the disease.  Proc Nat'l Acad Sci USA
    74:5702-5706
11. Fuster V, Bowie EJW, Josa M, Kaye MP, Fass DN (1979) Athero-
    sclerosis in normal and von Willebrand pigs:  cross-aortic
    transplantation study (abstr) Thromb and Haemost 42(1):425
12. Fuster V, Dewanjee MK, Kaye MP, Fass DN, Bowie EJW (1980)
    Evaluation of platelet deposition following selective endothelial
    injury of the carotid artery in normal and von Willebrand pigs
    (abstr) Circulation 62(Suppl. 3):98
13. Griggs TR, Reddick RL, Sultzer D, Brinkhous KM (1981) Susceptibil-
    ity to atherosclerosis in aortas and coronary arteries of swine
    with von Willebrand's disease.  Am J Pathol 102:137-145

# Lipid Accumulation in the Rabbit Aortic Wall in Response to Injury

S. Moore

## Introduction

Lipid-rich lesions can be induced in the arterial wall of rabbits fed a normal diet by repeated or continuous mechanical injury (1) or by repeated immunological injury (2). These lesions develop rapidly and accumulate large amounts of lipid (3). When the injury stimulus is no longer present the lesions regress rapidly, becoming smaller, depleted of lipid and calcium and eventually evolving to intimal plaques composed of smooth muscle cells and interstitial connective tissue (4,5). This type of injury is characterized by the formation of abundant platelet-fibrin thrombus and consumption of platelets (6). When the injury is removed the thrombus rapidly disappears, presumably by the process of organization. The development of the lesions can be inhibited or prevented by the induction of severe thrombocytopenia, employing an antiserum raised in goats to rabbit platelets (7).

Lesions, which are lipid-rich, can also be induced by a different kind of injury, induced by removal of the endothelial layer by a Fogarty balloon catheter (8). These lesions do not require repeated injury for the accumulation of lipid to occur. Moreover, the lesions persist and progress over time, the amount of lipid increasing, together with the thickness of the lesions (9). These lipid containing lesions occur in the areas of the aortic wall that have been covered by regenerated endothelium. Areas remaining uncovered by regenerated endothelium, although showing proliferation of SMC to form a neo-intima, have very little lipid as shown by histochemical staining and chemical analysis of the lipid content of the tissue.

These two forms of injury, although both are associated with plaque formation and lipid accumulation, differ markedly in terms of the interaction of formed elements of the blood with the vessel wall, the persistence of lipid in the lesions, and the tendency of one type of lesion to regress and for the other type to progress. Although both can be inhibited by severe thrombocytopenia induced by antiplatelet serum (10), indicating that platelet interaction with the vessel wall plays a significant part in their development, the character and extent of the interaction of formed elements of the blood with the vessel wall is also very different in the two types of lesion (6).

## Two Types of Injury Induced Lesions

For convenience, the type of lesion resulting from continuous and repeated mechanical damage to the intima or repeated immunological injury is designated the Type 1 lesion. The lesion resulting from removal of the endothelium is referred to as the Type 2 lesion.

In the last ten years we have become familiar with the concept of
atherosclerosis induced experimentally in normal fed animals.  In
most of these experiments repeated or continuous injury has been
required for the formation of lipid-rich lesions as in the Type 1
lesion (11).  However, it is now clear that a single injury, in
which only the endothelial layer is removed from the vessel wall is
associated with a progressing lesion in which lipid accumulation
persists and two years following de-endothelialization with a
Fogarty balloon catheter contains large amounts of lipid (9).  Cholesteryl ester is a significant component of the lesion lipid.  In
this (Type 2) lesion lipid accumulates preferentially or exclusively
in the neointima which has been covered by regenerated endothelium
(8,9).

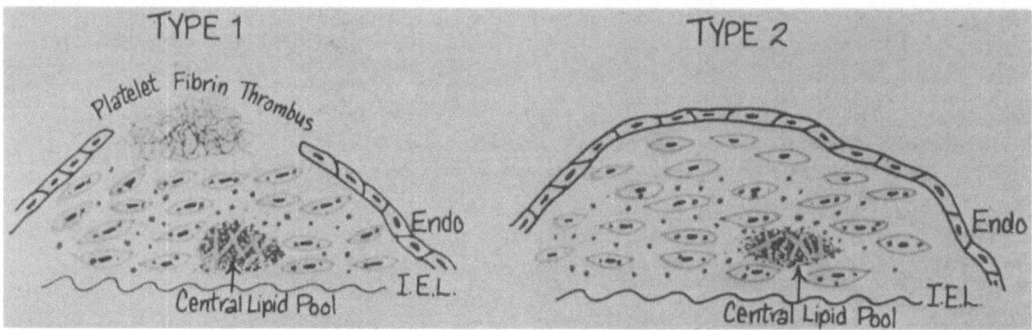

Fig. 1

Recently we have examined the lipid content of intima-media samples
of rabbit aortic wall from areas covered by regenerated endothelium,
areas not so covered and undamaged areas (12).  Free cholesterol was
48% higher in areas not covered by endothelium, compared to undamaged
areas, at six months following one balloon catheter removal of the
endothelium and remained at the same level at 12 and 24 months.  In
areas covered by regenerated endothelium free cholesterol was 1.6,
1.8 and 2.0 times higher than control at 6, 12 and 24 months respectively.  The changes in cholesteryl ester were more pronounced; in the
endothelium covered tissue being 40-68 times higher than control;
whereas there was only a slight elevation in the areas remaining
uncovered by endothelium.  These findings confirm the morphological
estimate of lipid accumulation observed previously in oil red-0
stained frozen sections of rabbit aorta.  These showed an increase-
ing amount of lipid over time following one balloon removal of the
endothelium.  The amounts were similar at comparable intervals after
one balloon removal of the endothelium to those seen after the first
of six balloon removals.

## Mechanisms of Lipid Accumulation

The mechanisms by which lipid accumulates in the endothelium covered neointima following one balloon removal of the endothelium in normal fed rabbits are of current interest. Some of the mechanisms which might be involved are new synthesis of lipid (3), alteration of enzyme metabolism particularly a relative decrease in cholesteryl ester hydrolase (13) or trapping of lipids by proteoglycans or the glycosaminoglycan (GAG) components of the proteoglycan complex (6). Support for a "trapping" mechanism comes from histochemical evidence (14), the isolation of GAG-lipoproteins complexes from lesion tissue (15), chemical analysis of tissue (16) and studies of the in-vitro interaction of GAG and plasma lipoproteins (17). Taking advantage of the ability of ruthenium red to stain proteoglycans we have recently demonstrated, in tissues viewed by transmission electron microscopy, an increased concentration of large particles in the endothelium covered neointima with a decrease in the areas lacking endothelial cover. Enzymes which break down sulphated GAGs of the condroitin sulphate or dermatan sulphate type remove these particles from the tissue. Small granules, considered to be heparan sulphate are very much reduced in concentration in the areas remaining uncovered by endothelium (18). Normally these granules occur in greatest quantity, just beneath the endothelium and are considered to regulate permeability (19).

The kinetics of $^{125}I$-LDL uptake comparing areas of endothelial regrowth with areas of neointima lacking endothelium and with uninjured arterial wall support a trapping mechanism. Although LDL uptake is initially higher in endothelium denuded areas the label does not persist for long. In contrast the uptake into endothelium covered areas is initially less than into the denuded areas though much more than into the undamaged wall, but persists for longer. This is accompanied by a sharp decay in the $^{125}I$-labelled-LDL in the plasma, indicating that the LDL which enters the endothelium covered neointima is retained (20). Thus, the accumulation of LDL in the endothelium covered neointima is associated with apparent increase in sulphated GAGs in the tissue.

More recently the relationship of lipid accumulation to GAG content has been examined in the Type 1 lesion, induced by the placement of an indwelling aortic catheter and followed during the period of regression of lesions after removal of the catheter. This study was also a morphometric evaluation of the proteoglycan content of lesions. Two observations support the mechanism of trapping of LDL by GAG, in this experimental setting (21). First, early lipid accumulation related to the occurrence of lipid vacuoles in macrophages in the superficial portion of raised lesions, characterized by abundant thrombus deposition, showed no increase in ruthenium red positive granules.

Secondly, deeper in the raised lesions around smooth muscle cells containing lipid vacuoles, there was an increased concentration of the particles. The same finding occurred in intimal plaques containing lipid in the smooth muscle cells, whereas areas of intimal thickening without lipid showed a decrease in the number of interstitial ruthenium-red-positive granules. Later, the concentration of sulphated GAG particles decreased when lipid disappeared from the lesions.

Thus in both Type 1 and Type 2 lesions the presence of lipid in lesions appears to be associated with an increased concentration of the sulphated GAG moieties of proteoglycans.

138

It is not clear why in Type 1 lesions, regression occurs when the
injury stimulus is removed, following induction of an apparently
more severe injury than the Type 2 lesion, which persists and apparently progresses over time following an apparently lesser injury. In
both an initial interaction of platelets with the vessel wall is
needed to stimulate the proliferative response which forms the substrate for lipid accumulation. Also, in both lesions an increased
synthesis of proteoglycans appears to play an important part in the
process of lipid accumulation.

These lesions, which are similar to human atheromatous plaques, represent two different responses of the arterial wall to injury. The
Type 1 lesion, which is capable of undergoing marked regression,
resembles the complicated human lesion with mural thrombus formation.
The Type 2 lesion, which is progressive, resembles the human fibro-
fatty plaque. A better understanding of the biology of these reactions may provide some insight into mechanisms of progression and
regression of human atheromatous lesions.


<u>References</u>

1.  Moore S, (1973) Thromboatherosclerosis in normolipemic rabbits:
    A result of continued endothelial damage.  Lab Invest 29: 478-
    487
2.  Friedman R, Moore S, Singal DP (1975) Repeated endothelial
    injury and induction of atherosclerosis in normolipemic rabbits.
    Lab Invest 30: 404-415
3.  Day AJ, Bell FP, Moore S, Friedman RJ (1974) Lipid composition
    and metabolism of thrombo-atherosclerotic lesions produced by
    continued endothelial damage in normal-fed rabbits.  Circ Res
    34: 467-476
4.  Friedman RJ, Moore S, Singal DP, Gent M (1976) Regression of
    injury-induced atheromatous lesions in rabbits.  Arch Pathol
    Lab Med 100: 185-196
5.  Moore S, Friedman RJ, Gent M (1977) Resolution of lipid-contain-
    ing atherosclerotic lesions induced by injury.  Blood Vessels
    14:  193-203
6.  Moore S (1981) Responses of the arterial wall to injury: Diabetes
    Suppl 30: 8-13
7.  Moore S, Friedman RJ, Singal DP, Gauldie J, Blajchman MA, Roberts
    RJ (1976) Inhibition of injury-induced thromboatherosclerotic
    lesions by antiplatelet serum in rabbits.  Thrombos Haemostas
    35: 70-81
8.  Moore S, Ihnatowicz IO (1978) Vessel injury and atherosclerosis.
    In Thrombosis: Animal and clinical models edited by H James Day,
    Basil A molong, Edward E Nishigawa, Ronald H Rynbrant. Plenum
    Publishing Corporation, New York
9.  Moore S, Belbeck LW, Richardson M, Taylor W (1982) Lipid accumulation in
    the neointima found in normal-fed rabbits in response to one or
    six removals of the aortic endothelium.  In Press Lab Invest
10. Friedman RJ, Stemerman MB, Wenz B, Moore S, Gauldie J, Gent M,
    Tiell ML, Spaet TH (1977) The effect of thrombocytopenia on exper
    imental arteriosclerotic lesion formation in rabbits 1. Smooth
    muscle cell proliferations and re-endothelialization. J  Clin
    Invest 60: 1191-1201
11. Ross R (1981) Atherosclerosis: A problem of the biology of arter-
    ial wall cells and their interaction with blood components.
    Arteriosclerosis 1: 293-311

12. Alavi M, Moore S (1982) The lipid composition in the neointima of rabbit aortic wall following the removal of the endothelium by a balloon catheter. Submitted for publication

13. Hajjar DP, Falcone DJ, Fowler S, Minick CR (1981) Endothelium modifies the metabolism of the injured aortic wall. Am J Pathol 102: 28-39

14. Moon HD, Reinhart JF (1952) Histogenesis of arteriosclerosis. Circulation 6: 481-488

15. Srinivasan SR, Dolan P, Radakrishnamurthy B, Pargaonkar PS, Berenson GS (1975) Lipoprotein-acid mucopolysaccharide complexes of human atherosclerotic lesions. Biochim Biophys ACTA 388: 58-70

16. Nakashima Y, Nakamura M, Kikuchi Y (1981) Cerebral atherosclerosis in Japanese Part 6: The interactions of plasma lipoproteins with glycosaminoglycans isolated from the cerebral arteries and aortas. Artery 9: 151-165

17. Bihari-Varga M, Vegh M (1967) Quantitative studies on the complexes formed between aortic mucopolysaccharides and serum lipoproteins. Biochim Biophys ACTA 144: 202-210

18. Richardson M, Ihnatowycz IO, Moore S (1980) Glycosaminoglycan distribution in rabbit aortic wall following balloon catheter de-endothelialization: An ultrastructural study. Lab Invest 43: 509-516

19. Kanwar YS, Farqhar MG (1979) Isolation of glycosaminoglycans (heparan sulphate) from glomerular basement membranes. Proc Natl Acad Sci USA 76: 4493-4497

20. Alavi M, Moore S (1982) Kinetics of low density lipoprotein interactions with rabbit aortic wall following balloon catheter de-endothelialization. Submitted for publication

21. Moore S, Richardson M (1981) Glycosaminoglycan (GAG) distribution in catheter induced lesions in rabbit aortae in relation to Lipid accumulation. Thrombos Haemostas 478: 221 Abstr

# WHHL Rabbit. A Heritable Animal Model of Familial Hypercholesterolemia

Y. Watanabe, Y. Tsujita, and A. Izumi

## Introduction

WHHL rabbit is short for the Watanabe Heritable Hyperlipidemic rabbit. This strain has been inherited by inbreeding a mutant of hyperlipidemic rabbit found in Japanese white rabbits (Oryctolagus cuniculus Var. domesticus).

The characteristics of this strain are as follows: 1) Abnormally high levels of serum cholesterol, triglyceride and phospholipid from new born (1). 2) LDL receptor deficiency in cells from skin, liver and adrenal gland (2,3,4,5). 3) The occurrence of spontaneous atherscle- rosis in aorta and coronary artery in premature stage (1,7).

## 1) Serum lipid and Lipoprotein Concentration

Serum cholesterol, triglyceride and phospholipid levels in WHHL rabbit are about 10 times high as compared with those in normal rabbits (Table 1). Although the serum cholesterol of normal rabbit was mainly present in HDL, most of elevated cholesterol in WHHL rabbit was local- ized in LDL (Table 2).

Electrophoretic patterns of serum lipoproteins in WHHL rabbit were characterized by deeply stained bands for pre-beta and beta-lipopro- teins and faintly stained band for alpha-lipoprotein, indicating in- creases in VLDL and LDL, and decrease in HDL.

Table 1. Serum Lipid Levels of WHHL rabbit

| Month of age | | 1 | 6 | 12 | 24 |
|---|---|---|---|---|---|
| Cholesterol (mg/dl) | WHHL | 595+143 | 510+ 90 | 385+ 90 | 352+96 |
| | Normal | 65+ 27 | 41+ 10 | 46+ 16 | 43+10 |
| Triglyceride (mg/dl) | WHHL | 535+145 | 354+ 88 | 304+115 | 330+55 |
| | Normal | 55+ 20 | 34+ 19 | 49+ 30 | 68+22 |
| Phospholipid (mg/dl) | WHHL | 402+ 58 | 545+125 | 370+44 | |
| | Normal | 120+ 18 | 89+ 17 | 94+ 19 | 69+24 |

Table 2. Serum Lipoprotein Concentration

| | Lipoprotein Cholesterol (mg/dl serum) | | | | | FC/TC |
|---|---|---|---|---|---|---|
| | VLDL | IDL | LDL | HDL | Total | |
| WHHL | 39.7+17 | 43.3+25 | 846+287 | 3.0+0.6 | 932+256 | 0.267 |
| Normal | 1.4+ 0.7 | n.d. | 6.2+1.0 | 16.0+0.7 | 23.6+1.6 | 0.254 |

n.d.: not detected

## 2) Deficiency of LDL receptor

The time courses of binding and degradation of $^{125}$I-LDL by intact skin fibroblast from a normal rabbit are shown in Fig. 1a. The amount of $^{125}$I-LDL bound to the cells reached a maximum 2 hour and remained constant thereafter, whereas, the degradation of $^{125}$I-LDL proceeded almost linearly. However, neither binding nor degradation of $^{125}$I-LDL took place in the cells from WHHL rabbit (Fig. 1b).

When the normal and WHHL rabbit cells were incubated in lipoprotein deficient medium, the activity of HMG CoA reductase, the rate limiting enzyme in cholesterol synthesis was very high in the both cells. However, LDL was added to medium, the reductase activity was markedly suppressed in the normal cells but not in the WHHL cells (Fig. 2).

The average LDL receptor activities in WHHL cells were 1/16 in binding, 1/18 in internalization and 1/24 in degradation, compared with those in normal cells (2,3).

The cholesterol esterification activity in WHHL cells was 1/14 of that in normal cells, whereas, the cholesterol synthetic activity in WHHL cells was 5.2-fold higher than in normal cells (2,3).

These observations indicate that LDL pathway does not function in the fibroblasts from WHHL rabbit.

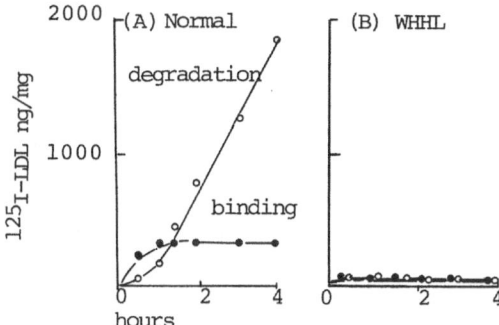

Fig.1 Activities of LDL binding and degradation in fibroblast from a normal(A) and a WHHL rabbit(B)

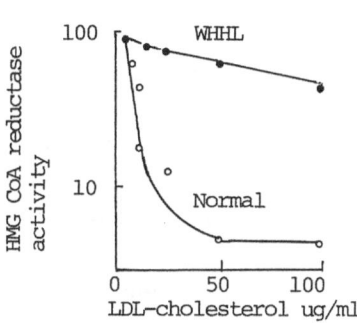

Fig.2 HMG CoA reductase activity in fibroblast from a normal and a WHHL rabbit

## 3) Spontaneous Lesion

### Aorta

Aortic atherosclerosis started to develop from three months of age and the lesion was found in all cases at the 5 months of age in premature stage (Table 3). The microscopic features of the lesions in the aorta was a marked fibrous thickening of the intima accompanied with accumulation of form cells.

## Coronary artery

Coronary atherosclerosis was first observed at 5 months of age (Table 3). The coronary branch narrowed more than 50% was found in 17% of young stage (5-12 months of age), 33% of middle aged stage (13-24 months of age) and 53% of advance stage (25-36 months of age). In spite of the narrowing in the coronary artery, the myocardiac degeneration was not observed.

The narrowed lesion occurred in the origin of left coronary (46%), in the circumflex branch (25%), in the right coronary (13%) and in the anterio descending branch (11%).

## Xanthoma

The Xanthoma on digital joints developed at 5 months of age, and the incidence after 5 months of age was about 70% (Table 3).

## Fat Necrosis of Osteocytes

The fat necrosis of osteocytes of femoral head occurred about 70% after 12 months of age. The bone trabeculae are thickened and the marrow spaces are filled with fatty tissue (6).

Table 3. Incidence of spontaneous atherosclerosis and xanthoma in WHHL rabbit

| Months of age | Atherosclerosis | | Xanthoma |
|---|---|---|---|
| | Aorta | Coronary artery | |
| 1 - 4 | 55% ( 6/11) | 0% ( 0/11) | 0% ( 0/ 6) |
| 5 - 15 | 100% (78/78) | 37% (25/68) | 67% (41/61) |
| 16 - 24 | 100% (19/19) | 47% ( 8/17) | 61% (11/17) |
| 25 - 36 | 100% (15/15) | 69% ( 9/13) | 87% (13/15) |

## 4) Process of Development of the Strain

A hyperlipidemic mutant gene was introduced into 10 normal Japanese white rabbits, and the mutant gene were inherited by five sister-brother mating lines and five back crossing lines.

Seven lines died out by 3rd generation due to low reproductive ability, high sensitivity to infectious diseases and appearance of malformation (Mandiblar prograthism and splay leg).

The survived three lines were inherited by intercross mating among these lines after 5th generation. Since then the WHHL rabbit strain has been kept as a closed colony.

## 5) Inheritance Mode

The first generation derived from the mating between a normal and a WHHL rabbit showed normal serum lipid levels in all cases. At the 2nd generation, the ratio of segregation of hyperlipidemia in the back crossing and sister-brother mating is one to one and three to one, respectively. The mating between two hyperlipidemic rabbits produced all hyperlipidemic rabbits.

According to the law of dominance and segregation, the hyperlipidemia in the WHHL rabbit is inherited by a recessive single gene.

## 6) Weak Points of the Strain

The weak points of the WHHL rabbit strain are low ability of reproduction and high sensibility to pasteurellosis (Pastrella matlocida) which is the most common naturally occurring disease of rabbits. Whether it's sensitive to other infectious diseases is not clear because other infectious diseases except pasteurellosis are not common in Japan.

These weaknesses are probably attributed to the hyperlipidemia with atherosclerosis in premature stage and to the high coefficient of inbreeding (about 60% at 5th generation).

In conclusion, the WHHL rabbit is a suitable animal for human familial hypercholesterolemia.

Acknowledgments  I am indebted to Drs. M. Kuroda, K. Tanzawa, Y. Shimada, M. Arai, K. Kawai and Mr. T. Ito for collaborating in part of the experiments.

## References

1. Watanabe Y (1980) Serial inbreeding of rabbit with hereditary hyperpipidemia (WHHL) - Incidence and development of atherosclerosis and xanthoma. Atherosclerosis 36 (2): 261-268
2. Tanzawa K, Shimada Y., Kuroda M., Tsujita Y., Arai M, Watanabe Y (1980) WHHL rabbit, a low density lipiprotein receptor-deficient animal model for familial hypercholesterolemia. FEBS Let 118 (1): 81-84
3. Shimada Y., Tanzawa K., Kuroda M., Tsujita Y., Arai M, Watanabe Y (1981) Biochemical characterization of skin fibroblast derived from WHHL rabbit, a notable animal model for familial hypercholesterolemia. Eur J Biochem 118: 557-564
4. Kita T, Brown MS, Watanabe Y, Goldstein JL (1981) Deficiency of LDL receptor in liver and adrenal gland of the WHHL rabbit, An animal model of familial hypercholesterolemia. Proc Natl Acad Sci USA 78 (4) 2268-2272
5. Attie AC, Pittman RC, Watanabe Y, Steinberg D (1981) Low density lipoprotein receptor deficiency in cultured hepatocytes of the WHHL rabbit. J Biol Chem 256 (19): 9789-9792
6. Kawai K, Maruno H, Watanabe Y, Hirohata K (1980) Fat necrosis of osteocytes as a causative factor in idiopathic osteonecrosis in hyperpipidemic ra-bits. Clin Orthopaedics 153: 273-282
7. Ito T, Watanabe Y, Shiomi M (1982) Spontaneous coronary atherosclerosis in immature stage of WHHL rabbit. J Jap coll Angiol 22 (4): 229-232

# Hypertensive Rat Models of Atherosclerosis

Y. Yamori, R. Horie, Y. Nara, M. Kihara, H. Wang, and K. Ikeda

## Introduction

The development of hypertensive rat models for atherogenesis and myocardial lesions by a selective inbreeding from spontaneously hypertensive rats (SHR) (1) has added new experimental approach to the pathogenesis, regression and prevention of these very common cardiovascular diseases in man. In this paper the development of various rat models for cardiovascular diseases is reviewed with a special reference to basic vascular lesions noted in hypertension, and then our models for atherogenesis and thrombogenesis, and also a new model for myocardial infarction which is caused by the combination of both thrombosis and atherosclerosis are reported together with our recent findings on the regression of atherosclerosis.

## I. Development of Various Rat Models for Cardiovascular Diseases

Various models for cardiovascular diseases have been developed at our laboratory. In addition to the well-known SHR, stroke-prone and -resistant substrains (SHRSP, SHRSR) (2) were established by selecting the offspring from the SHR which died of stroke. We further developed rats with spontaneous thrombogenesis (STR) (3) which died mainly of cerebral thrombosis, and arteriolipidosis-prone rats (ALR) (4) which developed wide-spread arterial fat deposits when fed high-fat-cholesterol (HFC) diets. Finally, we have developed a new rat model, myocardial ischemic rats (MIR) (5), with a high prevalence of ischemic heart disease which occurs spontaneously but is worsened when HFC diets are ingested.

## II. Basic Vascular Lesions in Hypertensive Models

SHRSP develop severe hypertension over 200 mmHg at the age of 10 to 15 weeks and die of typical cerebral hemorrhage or infarction. The basic pathological changes causing these cerebrovascular lesions are *arterionecrosis* of small intracerebral arteries which results in cerebral hemorrhage with rupture as well as in cerebral infarction with thrombosis. And pathogenic mechanism of stroke in this model is summarized as follows: Severe hypertension with cerebral circulatory disturbance increases vascular permeability and induces arterionecrosis. When microaneurysms formed at the necrotic arterial wall rupture, hemorrhage occurs. On the other hand, thrombosis occurs often at the necrotic arterial wall or within microaneurysms and causes infarction. Therefore, stroke in this model is *arterionecrothrombogenic stroke* caused by hypertension (6) but not *atherothrombotic stroke* caused by atherosclerosis.

However, basic vascular alteration in hypertension is initially functional reversible vasoconstriction which increases peripheral vascular resistance but hypertension itself as well as increased vasomotor tone accelerate collagen and noncollagen protein synthesis of arterial walls and quickly induce hypertrophy or hyperplasia of the medial smooth muscle cells (7): Incorporation of labelled amino acid into the collagen and noncollagen of the aorta and mesenteric arteries or prolyl hydroxylase activity in the aorta are increased in SHRSP and SHRSR even at the age of 4 or 5 weeks without a significant stable increase in blood pressure compared with Wistar-Kyoto normotensive rats (WKY).

In order to rule out the effect of mild hypertension on the vascular protein synthesis, smooth muscle cells from the aorta were cultured by an explant method. Even under tissue culture condition free from blood pressure, smooth muscle cells from SHR and SHRSP grew faster than those from WKY. This was also biochemically confirmed by increased incorporation of tritiated thymidine or $^{14}$C-leucine into DNA or protein, of cultured vascular smooth muscle cells from hypertensive rats (8). Ornithine decarboxylase activity, which is the rate limiting step of polyamine biosynthesis, therefore, regarded as a good biochemical indicator of cellular hypertrophy or hyperplasia, is also increased in cultured vascular smooth muscle cells from hypertensive rats. Therefore, we can conclude that vascular smooth muscle cells in genetic hypertension are more vulnerable to hyperplasia in response to hypertension. Their predisposition to proliferation is considered as the basic vascular lesions in hypertension, and they may contribute to atherogenesis and thrombogenesis when superimposed with lipidemia or with disorders of fibrinolysis or prostacycline system.

In summary, basic vascular lesions in hypertension are initially functional and then fibromuscular hyperplasia with active protein synthesis, that is, generally called *arteriosclerosis*, but severe hypertension induces *arterionecrosis* in certain organs such as the brain. However, if lipidemia is added to hypertension, atherosclerotic process is accelerated as shown in the following section.

## III. Hypertensive Rat Models for Atherogenesis and Thrombogenesis

Models for atherosclerosis have been established by selecting rats for greater reactive hypercholesterolemia from SHR. In the 3rd generation and thereafter, serum cholesterol levels became elevated up to 500 and 800 mg/dl in males and females, respectively even after one week of HFC diet feeding. Since they developed not only hypercholesterolemia but also fat deposits in small arteries such as mesenteric arteries within a few weeks when fed HFC diets, they were named *arteriolipidosis-prone rats* (ALR) (4).

Microscopically, fat deposits are noted in the intima and media of small arteries and vascular lumen is sometime narrowed with localized fat deposits. Although rats are generally regarded as being resistant to fat deposition in arteries, especially in cerebral arteries, ALR develop ring-like fat deposits in cerebral arteries which are easily detectable by Sudan staining. Since such segmental fat deposits are noted in human cerebral arteries, ALR would be considered a good model for cerebrovascular sclerosis.

Pathogenesis of atherogenesis in ALR is hypertension and lipidemia. The importance of hypertension in the development of arterial fat deposition was shown by delay and reduction of arterial fat deposition in ALR treated with antihypertensive agents in comparison with non-treated ALR. Without HFC diet feeding, serum cholesterol level is not high but HDL level is significantly decreased, therefore, atherogenic index, the ratio of LDL to HDL is increased compared with WKY. Abnormal lipid metabolism in ALR disclosed up to the present are increased intestinal absorption of cholesterol, decreased catabolism of cholesterol into bile acids and decreased HDL level, and they appear to be biochemical bases for acute arterial fat deposition and reactive hypercholesterolemia (9).

On the other hand, since SHRSP developed cerebral hemorrhage and infarction at various ratios, we started a selective breeding from among SHRSP to develop a model for thrombosis, and established 2 substrains; one developed severe hypertension quickly and frequently died of cerebral hemorrhage, while the other strain developed severe hypertension more slowly and died of thrombosis nearly in 100%. Therefore, the latter was named *spontaneous thrombogenic rats* (STR) (3).

Moreover, one of the mechanisms of thrombosis was proven to be the impairment of fibrinolytic system; plasminogen activator in the blood was decreased in STR compared with the age-matched WKY, while anti-plasmine was increased in younger age (3). Since these results were suggestive of endothelial cell-dysfunction in SHRSP, we further measured the metabolites of prostacycline in the blood. The plasma level of 6-keto $PGF_{1\alpha}$, the stable metabolite of prostacycline, was decreased in SHRSP at the age of 3 months, especially when they were fed on HFC diet. On the other hand, plasma level of $TXB_2$ from $TXA_2$ was significantly increased in them, indicating the imbalance between prostacycline-thromboxane $A_2$ system was the basis for high incidence of thrombosis in these models.

## IV. Development of a New Rat Model for Myocardial Infarction

Since the combination of atherosclerosis and thrombosis in hypertrophic or hyperplastic coronary arteries in hypertension is the basic vascular lesion causing myocardial infarction, we have selectively bred from the relevant SHR substrains a new substrain which develops ischemic heart disease spontaneously in a high incidence (5).

Rats of this substrain show typical symptoms of congestive heart failure and die with extensive ischemic lesions scattered in the myocardium. Correspondingly to such symptoms of heart failure, vectorcardiograms show obvious abnormalities indicating myocardial lesions in comparison with the control vectrocardiographic pattern of SHRSP; they are deformity and inverse rotation of QRS loop, markedly prolonged QRS duration, P-Q interval prolongation, etc. The incidence of cardiac death in this substrain within one year after birth was 75% when they were fed HFC diets, but no cardiac death was observed in SHRSP under the same condition.

At autopsy, atherosclerotic vascular lesions with intimal proliferation were frequently noted within a relatively short period when they were fed HFC diets. Sudan staining demonstrated marked fat deposition in the thickened intima which caused typical narrowing of coro-

nary arteries. Thrombosis was frequently noted at the small branches
of coronary arteries. Since such atheromatous lesions with thrombosis resulted in scattered fibrosis, ischemic myocardial lesions
similar to myocardial infarction, they were named *myocardial-ischemic
rats* (MIR) (5).

The pathogenesis of severe atherosclerotic lesions in MIR may be
ascribed to low HDL level. Especially when they are fed HFC diets,
not only serum cholesterol level but also atherogenic index, that is,
the ratio of LDL to HDL, is elevated markedly because of the greater
lowering of HDL level under HFC diet feeding in comparison with WKY
on the same diet.

In summary, hypertensive rat models for thrombogenesis and atherogenesis were established from among the substrains of SHR. We are
further developing a new rat model for ischemic myocardial diseases
which are predisposed to both atherosclerosis and thrombosis. Genetic factors and environmental influence, especially diets affect hypertension, lipidemia and thrombosis in each model, and the combination
of all three factors results in myocardial infarction in this new
model. That is, hypertension causes basic myointimal thickening of
coronary arteries and superimposed lipidemia accelerates fat deposits
and intimal proliferation. Additional impairments of fibrinolytic
and prostacycline systems induce thrombosis and finally atherothrombotic process results in myocardial infarction.


## V. Application for Experimental Regression of Atherosclerosis


Since MIR, ALR and SHRSP on HFC diets quickly develop arterial fat
deposits within a short period, these models can be applied for
studies on prevention and regression of atherosclerotic arterial
lesions. Dietary effect on the regression of atherosclerosis was
observed as follows: After 1-month-feeding of HFC diet feeding (20%
of suet, 5% cholesterol and 2% bile acid), diets were changed into
low (10%), normal (23%), high (46%) soy bean protein diets and the
normal protein diet containing 3% of taurine, and one month after
dietary changes, these animals were sacrificed to check cholesterol
and triglycerides in the serum and the liver. Serum cholesterol and
triglycerides were significantly lower in the group on high soy bean
protein diet (61 ± 3, 27 ± 4 mg/dl, respectively) than those on low
protein diet (103 ± 7, 41 ± 8 mg/dl). Similarly, triglyceride level
in the liver was also significantly decreased in the high protein
diet-fed group (20 ± 1 mg/g) compared with the low protein diet-fed
group (54 ± 3 mg/g). Dietary effect on lipoprotein profiles was also
observed, because in comparison with the profiles in rats fed normal
protein diet, HFC diets increased and broadened LDL fraction and
decreased one of 3 HDL fractions demonstrated by polyacrylamide gel
electrophoresis. Fish protein diet and the diet rich in taurine,
that is, sulfur amino acids abundantly contained in the fish protein,
accelerated the recovery of one of HDL fractions after the dietary
changes from HFC diet feeding. These experiments suggest dietary
maneuvers affect lipoprotein profiles and accelerate the recovery
from hypercholesterolemia, and may stimulate the regression of
atherosclerosis.

## Conclusion

1) Hypertensive rat models for stroke (SHRSP), thrombosis (STR), atherosclerosis (ALR) and myocardial infarction (MIR) have been established by selective breeding from SHR.
2) Basic vascular lesions in hypertension are fibromuscular sclerosis and arterionecrosis in SHR and SHRSP.
3) With impaired lipid metabolism and hypertension, ALR quickly develop arterial fat deposition.
4) MIR develop myocardial infarction due to atherosclerotic and thrombotic coronary lesions.
5) Protein-rich diets accelerate the regression of atherosclerosis in these animal models.

These new models will hopefully contribute to the further progress in research on atherosclerosis and myocardial infarction which are the most preponderant cardiovascular diseases in man.

## Acknowledgement

This study was supported by grants from the Science and Technology Agency of the Japanese Government, the Ministry of Education, the Ministry of Health and Welfare, and the Japanese Heart Foundation.

## References

1. Okamoto K, Aoki K (1963) Development of a strain of spontaneously hypertensive rats. Jpn Circ J 27: 282-293
2. Yamori Y, Nagaoka A, Okamoto K (1974) Importance of genetic factors in hypertensive cerebrovascular lesions: An evidence obtained by successive selective breeding of stroke-prone and resistant SHR. Jpn Circ J 38: 1095-1100
3. Yamori Y, Ohta K, Horie R, Ohtaka M, Nara Y, Ooshima A (1979) A new model for cerebral thrombosis and its pathogenesis. Jpn Heart J 20 (Suppl 1): 343-345
4. Yamori Y (1977) Selection of arteriolipidosis-prone rats (ALR). Jpn Heart J 18: 602-603
5. Yamori Y, Kihara M, Nara Y, Horie R (1982) Myocardial-ischemic rats (MIR), coronary vascular alteration induced by a lipid-rich diet. Atherosclerosis 42: 15-20
6. Yamori Y, Horie R, Akiguchi I, Nara Y, Ohtaka M, Fukase M (1977) Pathogenic mechanisms and prevention of stroke in stroke-prone SHR. In: De Jong W, Provoost AP, Shapiro APA (eds) Progress in Brain Research, Elsevier, Amsterdam, p 219-234
7. Yamori Y (1976) Neural and non-neural mechanisms in spontaneous hypertension. Clin Sci Mol Med 51: 431s-434s
8. Yamori Y, Igawa T, Kanbe T, Kihara M, Nara Y, Horie R (1981) Mechanisms of structural vascular changes in genetic hypertension: Analyses on cultured vascular smooth muscle cells from spontaneously hypertensive rats. Clin Sci 61 (Suppl 7): 121s-123s
9. Yamori Y, Iritani N, Nara Y, Fukuda E, Kitamura Y (1979) Cholesterol metabolism of arteriolipidosis-prone rats (ALR). Jpn Heart J 20 (Suppl 1): 349-351

# Seeking for More Similarity Between Animal Models and Human Atherosclerosis

G. N. Chaldakov

A cell quartet represented by arterial endothelial cell and smooth muscle cell (SMC), platelet and monocyte-derived macrophage is recently recognized as cellular machinary which makes up the atherosclerotic plaques. Although more than 200 risk factors for atherosclerosis were recently reported, the hypercholesterolemia and platelet hyperaggregability are considered to be primarily involved in the initiation and development of atherosclerotic plaques. Respectively, the receptor-mediated endocytosis of low density lipoprotein (LDL) by endothelial cells and SMC (1), and the prostacyclin-thromboxan equilibrium are considered as main molecular triggers in the atherogenesis. The SMC proliferation and its sequelae, an increased secretion of extracellular matrix components, are the end, but reversible, issue of the plaque story both in animal and human atherosclerosis.

A searching for heritable animal atherosclerosis models with disturbances in LDL receptor-mediated pathway and/or platelet-derived growth factor receptor-mediated internalization by arterial SMC (2), and in prostacyclin-thromboxan system may bring more similarity between the animal models and human atherosclerosis. In this respect, the recent data of GOLDSTEIN, ANDERSON, BROWN (1979) have demonstrated three genetically determined LDL receptor-mediated endocytosis disturbances ( $R\ b^o$, $R\ b^-$, $R\ b^+, i^o$ ) which are closely related to human familial hypercholesterolemia are very promisful for profilaxis and therapy of atherosclerosis. We have described coated pits and coated vesicles in rabbit aorta and pulmonary trunk SMC (3), and recently receptosomes (2) both in arterial endothelial cells and SMC ( CHALDAKOV, GHENEV, PETROV, MORENO, 1982). It should seem interesting to pursue how the receptor-mediated endocytosis of LDL operates in WHHL rabbit, a heritable animal model of familial hypercholesterolemia.

Acknowledgments    I am very much indebted to Drs. P. Ghenev, S. Stoev, B. Balev, S. Slavov, K. Dikranian, Z. Angelov and to my students, Ch. Petrov, W. Moreno Barrero and J. Etta, and S. Dandanov for cooperation and discussions.

References

1. Goldstein, JL, Anderson M, Brown MS, (1979) Coated pits, coated vesicles, and receptor-mediated endocytosis. Nature 279: 679-685
2. Pastan IH, Willingham MC, (1981) Journey to the centrum of the cell: role of receptosome. Science 214: 504-509
3. Chaldakov G, Nikolov S (1975) Adv exp Med Biol 57: 14-20
4. Chaldakov GN, Ghenev PI, Petrov ChD, Moreno WB (1982) Fine morphological aspects of the receptor-mediated endocytosis in arterial smooth muscle cells. I. Coated pits, coated vesicles and receptosomes. ( submitted in abstract form in 3rd Internat Symp Physiol Pharmacol Smooth Muscle, September 1982, Varna )

# Lipoproteins, Blood Cells and Endothelial Integrity in Atherosclerosis: What Role for Eicosanoids?

L. Larrue

Experimental animal models of atherosclerosis not only support and extend some aspects of the disease process relative to human atherosclerosis but, before all, provide opportunities to explore the mechanisms leading to atherosclerosis. Animal models can be particularly useful in the formation of testable questions that interelate the biology of each of the cells of the artery wall and of the blood and their interactions with one another and with plasma components. One of the most impressive progress concerns the ability to utilize a number of genetically selected strains exhibiting essential risk factors such as hypertension, hypercholesterolemia or diabetes together with selective injury (endothelial trauma ...) or altered nutritional balance leading to new concepts concerning some of the most important questions in the atherosclerotic development and regression processes.

The observations presented in this session raise several questions focused on the aspect of interactions between blood cells, lipoprotein metabolism and endothelial integrity. Among them, the following points appear important to discuss :

    - Is endothelial cell regeneration modified by hypercholesterolemia ? Is this process depending or not on the extend of injury ? Does LDL interact with endothelial cell migration or proliferation or both in vivo ?

    - Do intimal smooth muscle cells play a role in the endothelial cells regeneration ?

    - Do eicosanoids formed by stimulated blood and arterial cells influence cell migration and/or proliferation and how do lipoproteins modify the capacity of the cells to metabolize arachidonic acid ?

Much remains to be learnt concerning the role of eicosanoids, but it is of interest that proliferative intimal smooth muscle cells synthesize high levels of prostacyclin (1, 2), that hydroxyeicosatetraenoic acids (HETE) stimulate smooth muscle cell migration (3) and that arachidonic acid metabolism may be modified by lipoproteins (4).

The ability to utilize the tools of animal models to probe these problems promise to generate useful information which may promote new approches of atherosclerosis and its complications.

References

1. Eldor A, Falcone D J, Hajjar D P, Minick C R, Wexsler B B (1981). Recovery of prostacyclin production by deendothelialized rabbit aorta. J. Clin. Invest., 67, 735-741
2. Larrue J, Bricaud H (1982) Prostacyclin synthesis by proliferative smooth muscle cells. Vasa (in the press).
3. Nakao J, Ooyama T, Chang W.C, Murota S, Orimo H (1982) 12 HETE stimulates aortic smooth muscle cell migration in vitro (this volume)
4. Szczeklik A, Gryglewski R J, Domagala B, Zmuda A, Hartwich J, Wozny E, Grzywacz M, Mady J, Gryglewska T (1981) Serum lipoproteins, lipid peroxydes and prostacyclin synthesis in patients with coronary heart disease. Prostaglandins, 22 : 795-807

# 1.4 Measurement and Identification of Atherosclerosis

# Chairman's Comments on the Discussion at the Workshop on Measurement of Atherosclerosis

C. W. M. Adams

It is widely held that atherosclerotic lesion must be more accurately measured, both as regards their size and their contents. Too often one sees quite crude non-validated visual assessments or descriptions of lesion as "WHO Grade II +++". Even though one was one-self guilty of some of these errors 20 years ago, there is now a clear need for much greater precision.

The papers presented by Drs NEWMAN and VESSELINOVITCH outlined the well-known point-counting and graticule methods for the surface measurement of atherosclerotic lesions. In addition, Dr Newman told us about graded illustrative cards for rapid use as "standards" with human autopsy material. These illustrations have been validated for observer error and against quantitative assessments of surface involvement and cholesterol content.

A simplified method for surface measurement has been introduced by Dr HATA from Tokyo. The opened artery is placed within a polythene bag and then it is xerographed in a standard commercial Xerox machine. The Xerox copy can be read with a graticule placed over it; considerable image intensification can be obtained with this method. We have previously described the preparation of a graticule by the simple manoeuvre of photographing squared paper of the required size directly onto photographic glass plate. Clearly, there is considerable scope for preparing cheap, clean and simple measurement systems. An important limitation of non-computerized systems is eye fatigue!

It was emphasized by Dr DAOUD and others that these surface methods only measure two dimensions and that the third dimension of depth is required to establish the real magnitude and volume of the lesion, i. e. depth should be measured at many points throughout the lesion. Dr VESSELINOVITCH described measurements of the sectional areas of lesions by computerized planimetry. All agreed that pressure-perfusion fixation at mean blood-pressure is required with sectional of lumenal measurements to stretch the internal elastic membrane and tunica media to the size that they were in vivo. Clearly, without such pressure perfusion, the lumen would be too small, and the wall and lesion distorted inwards. It is a common fallacy at autopsy to regard a coronary artery with a pinhole lumen as necessarily thus representing the situation obtained in vivo.

Dr VESSELINOVITCH said that the computerized planimetric apparatus for measurement of the sectional area of lesions can also be used to measure accumulated lipid deposits. The chairman presented some illustrative data on measurements obtainable with the Vickers M 85 microdensitometer. This apparatus allows spectrophotometric estimations within defined areas (plugs) in the tissue section with a scanning technique over some 10,000 points in the plug during the 9 - 5 seconds taken for measurement. This method is applicable to stained lipid, elastic collagen and smooth muscle in sections of the aterial wall.

A simple manual planimetric method has been in use for many years. The optical image is projected onto paper, the outlines are traced with pencil, the relevant areas of paper are cut out and then weighed to establish size. The method may be adapted to photography by weighing the cut-out samples, or by estimating the silver in them. This procedure can be used to good effect with relatively small numbers of tissues and, for example, we have previously measured the dilatation of coronary arteries with advancing age in this way.

Dr DAOUD discussed the measurement of regression in induced atherosclerotic lesions in swine. Apart from the mechanical aspects of area and volume quantification, he presented data about changes in lipids, glycosaminoglycans and collagen. A difficulty here is the reference point for the expression of biochemical data. Reference to DNA and non-collagen protein may avoid some of the pitfalls associated with a growing or regressing lesion. However, any change in cell population may affect the use of DNA as a reference point. Reference to net weight or dry weight is invalidated by changes in weight of the growing or regressing lesion. Even lipid-free dry weight is not truly representative when much scarring has occurred, with its attendant increase in collagen content. The problem could be overcome by chemical analysis of the whole aorta, but this is rarely practical. A compromise solution is to use a suitable size of cork-borer to remove circles of tissue of constant surface area.

Dr K. T. LEE discussed the measurement of glucose-6-phosphate dehydrogenase isomers in arterial wall cells as evidence of monotypic change. The material was obtained from normal and atherosclerotic aortas from heterozygous black women and hybrid hares. Other studies showed that cultured skin fibroblasts from both the black women and hybrid hares either undergo monotypic change or show a predominance of one isomer or the other. The monotypic change is increased by exposure to a cytotoxic compound, such as 25-hydroxycholesterol. These results, together with previous publications, suggest that the frequent presence of monotypic or "monoclonal" atherosclerotic lesions is an example of cellular adaptation, in that one or other allele provides a survival advantage under certain conditions.

Dr ELSPETH SMITH discussed the gelatinous lesion or elevation described first by VIRCHOW in the last century. This is an oedematous lesion which cannot readily be recognized in fixed tissue and, thus, is often missed. Although there is an increased lipoprotein content in the fluid of the lesion, this is not an established atherosclerotic process, even though it may be a precursor. Perhaps it should be regarded as a focal example of markedly increased permeability (insudation or plasmatic vasculosis). One even wonders whether vasoactive inflammatory compounds may play a part in its genesis.

A workshop on the measurement of atherosclerosis had previously been held at Silver Springs, Maryland, USA in February, 1982. Drs BOND and INSULL were the chairmen and they kindly offered to discuss the importance of the various pathological methods of measurement at autopsy described above, particularly the need for pressure perfusion-fixation. They also discussed the various types of non-invasive clinical (antemortem) methods for estimating the extent of atherosclerosis. These included Doppler probe, computerized radiology and B-mode ultrasound. All these techniques have yet to be fully evaluated (see Dr BLANKENHORN in Plenary Session No 1). B-mode ultrasound seems to be most promising; but it has the limitation that the frequency to obtain good definitive (8 - 10 mHz) allows penetration of only 3,6 cms. Thus, this apparatus is of most use with the more superficial arteries, such as the carotids.

# Measurement of Regression in Atherosclerosis

A. S. Daoud, K. E. Fritz, J. Jarmolych, and B. Wiener

During the last few decades, a large body of morphologic, biochemical and clinical measurements indicated that diet-induced atherosclerotic lesions in many species of animals regressed after withdrawal of the dietary stimulus.

## A. Morphologic Measurements

These encompass a spectrum of techniques ranging from gross evaluation to light microscopic and scanning and transmission electron microscopic measurements. The gross evaluation has included the surface area affected with lesions. Characteristics which have been measured on light microscopic sections include lesion area, lesion thickness, lumen area, area enclosed within the external and internal elastic membranes, area of media, percent lumen stenosis, cross-sectional area of fibro-muscular caps, area of necrosis and area of mineralization. Measurement has been made by micrometers or grids mounted in the eyepiece of a microscope or by point counting. More recently, hand-activated digitizers, as well as automated scanners are being used. By these instruments data not only can be generated more rapidly and easily, but more accurately and reproducibly, than by older methods. Light microscopic sections have also been used for enumeration of cells in the lesion and media; and, by the use of $H_3$ thymidine pulse labeling, the degree of cell proliferation has been evaluated. Transmission and scanning electron microscopy have been used mainly for qualitative studies. The work of Armstrong et al (1), Daoud et al (2) and Wissler and co-workers (3) are examples of the role of morphologic evaluation of regression. As an example of the type of information which can be obtained from morphological studies, in a sequential study of the regression of coronary atherosclerosis in swine, we have found that there were no significant differences in the morphometric measurements between the reference and 6 weeks regression, or between the 5 and 14 mos regression lesions. But in the combined 5 and 14 mos regression groups, as compared with the combined reference and 6 weeks regression, there was a significant decrease in size of the lesion, in necrosis and in percent of luminal stenosis. There was no significant change in calcification (Table 1.). We also found that the overall size of the artery decreased during regression. Unexpectedly, in spite of the decrease in the percent luminal occlusion observed during regression, the actual size of the lumen did not increase. Comparison of size of the lesion with either the size of the artery or the size of the lumen showed a positive correlation at a highly significant level (p<0.0005).

However, the morphologic techniques are not without limitations, some of which are: 1) Morphologic measurements of components, such as lipids, connective tissue and GAG, can detect only qualitative or very large quantitative differences. Even with the addition of the most sophisticated techniques they suffer from the problems of staining specificity and uniformity. 2) Detecting quantitative differences in lesion cellularity requires tedious cell counts and careful sampling to avoid du-

156

Table 1

|  | Early Reference + 6 Wks Mean ± S.E.M.** | Late 5 & 14 Mos Regr. Mean ± S.E.M.** |
|---|---|---|
| Total Lesion Area (mm$^2$) | 1.6* ± 0.39 | 0.61 ± 0.15 |
| Total Necrosis Area (mm$^2$) | 0.78*± 0.24 | 0.15 ± 0.07 |
| Total Calcified Area (mm$^2$) | 0.10 ± 0.03 | 0.08 ± 0.01 |
| % Lumen Occlusion | 24.5* ± 3.2 | 15.2 ± 4.8 |

* Sig. > Late Lesion by Duncan's Multiple Range or Student's "T" Tests
** S.E.M. = Standard Error of the Mean

plicate counts of the same cell or to achieve a count which is truly representative of a heterogeneous lesion. 3) Since the morphometric measurements are carried out on postmortem specimens which are subjected to various procedures such as sampling, fixation and staining, their relationship to the in vivo situation is not clear.

B.  Biochemical Measurement

Exclusively biochemical studies can be divided into those in which whole arteries are analyzed and those in which lesions are dissected from non-lesion areas and both types of tissue analyzed separately. As examples of the former, Armstrong et al (4) and St. Clair et al (5) analyzed entire aortas or pools of entire aortas, while Meeker and Jobling (6) reported free and esterified cholesterol concentrations of dissected aortic lesions vs normal areas.  The use of whole or pooled vessels is obviously required when available aortic tissue is severely limited, but does result in a "dilution" of lesion values by the non-lesion contribution.

The advantages of the biochemical measurements are that they are specific and that they allow quantitative assessment.  Their disadvantages are, first, total lack of localization of the constituent under study, and secondly, their requirement of larger amounts of tissue, even for ultramicroanalyses, than that needed for sections.

C.  Clinical Measurements

The major clinical techniques used in the evaluation of atherosclerosis are contrast arteriography, venous arteriography, Doppler ultrasound, B-scan real-time imaging and A-mode imaging.  Probably the most promising evidence that human atherosclerosis may regress was obtained recently by studying changes in the size of the lesion as it appeared in arteriograms.  A group of investigators at the University of Minnesota School of Medicine showed, by sequential coronary arteriograms, that some individuals whose serum cholesterol had been reduced by partial ileal bypass, exhibited a decrease in plaque size (Knight et al, 1972) (7).  Using computer controlled image dissection, Barndt et al, 1977 (8) from the University of S. California, Los Angeles, studied changes in early atherosclerosis as they appeared in the angiograms of femoral arteries of twelve patients with type IV hyperlipoproteinemia and thirteen with type II hyperlipoproteinemia.  Elevated blood lipids and blood pressure were treated with medication and diet.  After an interval of thirteen months on the regimen, repeat angiograms showed regression of atherosclerosis in nine patients, no changes in three and progression in thirteen. The clinical methods have the advantages of allowing measurement of the disease in vivo and of permitting serial examination of the lesions to assess prevention or therapy. However, the extent and/or composition of the lesion can not be studied by these methods; the only parameter susceptible to definitive characterization by these methods is lumen stenosis. In addition, the data generated from most of these methods can be altered by such variables as vasospasm, vasodilation and arterial pulsation effects.

## D. Combined Methods

In recent years, more investigators have turned to the correlation of morphologic with biochemical studies. In some studies, chemical analysis has been made on one arterial bed, the morphologic studies on others. Another approach is to use one of paired arteries for biochemical and the other for morphologic examination. Alternately, both morphologic and biochemical approaches can be applied to defined areas, such as lesion or non-lesion tissue.

While the combined approach provides the opportunity for the study of correlation among various vessel features, it does pose some problems. For instance, how will the available tissue be allotted to the various aspects of the study? At the time of sacrifice how is the experiment organized so that the tissue destined for each type of analysis receives optimal processing? Since formalin or glutaraldehyde fixation is, in most cases, not compatible with biochemical analysis (certainly not with synthesis studies!), should perfusion be avoided, with the attendant problems in interpretation of some features, such as lumen area? Is there enough skilled manpower available to make the tedious ultramicrochemical assays needed for combined studies feasible?

Even considering the problems cited above, the potential results of combined studies are so attractive, especially when monitoring changes resulting from continuing regimens, that, in many cases, they are worth the effort. One of our recent experiments (9,10) may serve as an example of perhaps the most extensive study feasible. We chose the swine, based on the similarity of type and distribution of aortic lesions to those of man, and because the swine aorta is large enough to make feasible the analysis of lesions separated from non-lesion tissue. For distribution of available lesions we divided the abdominal aorta in half longitudinally. The left half was dedicated to morphologic examination, including percent of the surface area involved in sudanophilic lesion, and extensive morphometric studies of the entire half of the aorta sectioned at 2mm intervals longitudinally. After stripping and discarding the adventitia, examples of three types of lesion from the right half were used for autoradiography, lipid staining and enzyme histochemistry at both the light and electron microscopic levels. Similar lesions were analyzed for the concentrations of DNA, total cholesterol, triglyceride and phospholipid and for rates of synthesis of DNA and total protein. Remaining lesions were pooled, as were the non-lesion areas, and analyzed for the concentrations of free and esterified cholesterol, collagen and GAG, and the synthesis of 5 lipid classes, collagen and GAG. Alternatively, the above tissue could have been analyzed for various hydrolytic enzyme activities or for the phagocytic activity of lesion cells.

Table 2. presents some of the data from this sequential study of the fate of very severe lesions for comparison with the same features from a previous study of moderately severe lesions. In both studies, there was a change in cholesteryl ester and DNA concentrations and in the rate of DNA synthesis towards normal values. However, while there was a significant decrease in the size of the moderately severe lesion, the very severe lesions did not become smaller. In the latter, a marked increase in calcium concentration was noted, suggesting a possible cause and effect relationship between increasing amounts of calcium and a lack of regression.

Table 2

|  | Mod. Severe Lesions | | Very Severe Lesions (Sequential Study) | | | |
|---|---|---|---|---|---|---|
|  | Ref.[t] | Regr.[tt] | Ref.[t] | Regr.[tt] (6wks) | Regr.[tt] (5 mos) | Regr.[tt] (14 mos) |
| Cholesterol (µg/mg dry wt) | | | | | | |
| Total | 15.0 | 3.8* | 107.8 | 63.5 | 53.0 | 55.8 |
| Esterified | 11.2 | 0.4* | 74.5 | 50.0 | 26.1* | 27.6 |
| DNA (µg/mg dry wt) | 6.6 | 4.2* | 3.3 | 3.6 | 2.7 | 2.4* |
| Synthesis (dpm $^3$H-Thymidine/µg DNA) | 846 | 201* | 2,302 | 3,776 | 1,108 | 290* |
| Calcium a) No. of calcified areas or b) µg/mg dry wt | (a) 28 | (a) 48 | (b) 9.1 | (b) 55.5 | (b) 87.2* | (b) 128.6* |
| Lesion Thickness / Media Thickness | 0.65 | 0.29* | 1.27 | 1.27 | 0.88 | 1.22 |

[t] Reference    [tt] Regression    * Sig. diff. from Ref. value

Combined angiographic and morphologic technics have been used to measure coronary atherosclerosis in man. We recently compared in vivo angiographic vs postmortem morphometric measurements of coronary atherosclerosis in swine. Preliminary results indicate that 1) the lumen, as it appears in angiograms, was consistently larger than that measured on the histologic sections, 2) extensive diffuse atherosclerosis was not detectable by angiography and 3) under favorable conditions, lesions shown by morphometry to cause a 20% narrowing of the lumen, could be detected, but not lesions obstructing less than 20% of the lumen.

E. Summary

Many morphometric, biochemical and clinical methods have been used in assessing the regression of atherosclerosis in man and experimental animals. The wealth of data generated to the present indicate that most of the features of the plaque will regress, at least under favorable conditions.

Recent advances in morphometric measurements, which involve the use of digitizers, have improved the accuracy and reproducibility of these measurements. The introduction of ultramicrochemical analyses has allowed investigators to carry out extensive chemical analyses on carefully dissected lesions and non-lesion tissue. The use of computer controlled image dissection in measuring angiographic images may improve the in vivo measurements of lesion features. However, all of these various techniques still have their limitations and pitfalls and their usefulness depends on the state of the material available and on the question to be answered. The use of combined approaches decreases the scope of these limitations, thus allowing a broader view of the regression process.

Acknowledgments   The authors gratefully acknowledge the expert technical support of Patricia Condella and Amy Voorhees.

This work was supported by the Veterans Administration and by NIH Grant #HL 20993.

## References

1.  Armstrong ML, Warner ED, Connor WE (1970) Regression of coronary atheromatosis in rhesus monkeys after regression diets. Circ Res 27:59-67
2.  Daoud AS, Jarmolych J, Augustyn JM, Fritz KE, Singh JK, Lee KT (1976) Regression of advanced atherosclerosis in swine. Arch Path Lab Med 100:372-379
3.  Vesselinovitch D, Wissler RW, Hughes R, Borensztajn J (1976) Reversal of advanced atherosclerosis in rhesus monkeys. Atherosclerosis 23:155-176
4.  Armstrong ML, Connor WE, Warner ED (1969) Tissue cholesterol concentration in the hypercholesterolemic rhesus monkey. Arch Path 87:87-92
5.  St. Clair RW, Clarkson TB, Lofland HB (1972) Effects of regression of atherosclerotic lesions on the content and esterification of cholesterol by cell-free preparation of pigeon aorta. Circ Res XXXI:664-671
6.  Meeker DR, Jobling JW (1934) A chemical study of the arteriosclerotic lesions in the human aorta. Arch Path 18:252-257
7.  Knight L, Scheibel R, Amplatz K, Varco RL, Buchwald L (1972) Radiographic appraisal of the Minnesota partial ileal bypass study. Surg Forum 23:141-142
8.  Barndt R, Blankenhorn DH, Crawford DW, Brooks SH (1977) Regression and progression of early femoral atherosclerosis in treated hyperlipoproteinemic patients. Ann Int Med 86:139-146
9.  Daoud AS, Jarmolych J, Augustyn JM, Fritz KE (1981) Sequential morphologic studies of regression of advanced atherosclerosis. Arch Path Lab Med 105:233-239
10. Fritz KE, Augustyn JM, Jarmolych J, Daoud AS (1981) Sequential study of biochemical changes during regression of swine aortic atherosclerotic lesions. Arch Path Lab Med 105:240-246

# Measurement of Monotypism in Atherosclerosis

K. T. Lee, W. A. Thomas, C. D. Murray, and K. Janakidevi

In 1973, Dr. Earl Benditt and his associate reported extremely interesting and provocative findings in regard to the origin of atherosclerotic lesions (1). These investigators have been studying atherosclerotic lesions in autopsy specimens from black women who were heterozygous for glucose-6-phosphate dehydrogenase (G-6-PD), using techniques
that had been developed for investigating the origin of neoplasms.
They found many advanced atherosclerotic lesions are monotypic or at
least have monotypic foci. With these findings they concluded that
each atherosclerotic lesion probably arose from a single, genetically
transformed cell and thus constituted a single clone (monoclonal origin). This had been shown to be the case for leiomyomas and for certain other neoplasms. The obvious inference to be drawn was that
atherosclerotic lesions were in fact neoplasms. Since then many observations have been made on this phenomenon in a number of laboratories
including ours. We have studied similar atherosclerotic lesions with
monotypic foci and have concluded, from similar data to those reported
by Dr. Benditt and his associate that the observed monotypism has
causes other than monoclonism and hence it does not indicate monoclonal origin of the lesions (2).

Basis for these studies in black women who are heterozygous for G-6-PD
as well as hybrid hares that are also heterozygous for G-6-PD, is
Lyon's hypothesis (3). According to Lyon's hypothesis, one or the
other of the two X-chromosomes in females is inactivated on a random
basis early in embryonic life. If the individual is heterozygous for
any genes on the X-chromosome, the body will henceforth consist of a
mixture of cells of the two phenotypes, since the cells have been shown
to breed true. In the mature organism the mixture of cells is not
homogeneous, but instead, cells of one or the other phenotype are found
in small patches (mosaicism).

In order to detect the presence of cells of two different phenotypes,
a marker is needed. The most readily available marker at present is
G-6-PD. The two most common types of G-6-PD are referred to as A and
B. G-6-PD's from those two different phenotypes can readily be separated by electrophoresis, and the relative activity of each can be
estimated by a densitometric method.

G-6-PD mosaicism for A and B is common among black females in the
United States, with approximately one-third being G-6-PD heterozygotes.
If a neoplasm arose from a single cell, such a tumor is by definition
monoclonal in origin. In a heterozygote, the tumor will of necessity
have only one type of G-6-PD (monotypism), while the normal tissue will
have two types (ditypism).

However, monoclonal origin is not the only possible cause of monotypism. Cells with one X-chromosome may have survival or growth characteristics not shared by the other (because of differences involving any
or all genes on the X-chromosome) and may overgrow and eventually replace the other type, especially under adverse conditions and when the
cells are undergoing frequent divisions. A probable example of this

phenomenon has been reported recently for skin fibroblasts from G-6-PD heterozygotes grown in tissue culture (4). Cultures of fibroblasts from 19 black female heterozygotes started as a mixture of A and B phenotypes; but after multiple passages, one or the other phenotype completely disappeared. Hence, cultures originally ditypic became monotypic.

Our data on monotypism in atherosclerotic lesions and in normal media of G-6-PD heterozygous black women can be summarized as follows. From each lesion or media up to 25 samples were taken for G-6-PD analysis for both human and experimental animal studies.

Monotypism is infrequent in thin lesions and it becomes progressively more frequent as lesions get thicker. In thin lesions of either fatty streak or non-fatty streak type of 200μ or less, monotypism is found in less than 7% of the lesions examined. It becomes progressively more frequent as the lesions get thicker and in thick fibrous plaque of over 600μ in thickness monotypism is found in approximately 60% of the lesions examined.

Nearly all thick lesions with monotypic foci also have many ditypic foci; and monotypic foci in a given lesion are nearly always of the same phenotype. When multiple samples are taken from thick fibrous plaque-type lesions, monotypism is found in multiple foci of one type, either A or B. These data strongly suggest that lesions do not orig- inate from a single cell and monotypism is a secondary phenomenon.

Approximately 84% of monotypic foci found in all lesions are of the phenotype predominant in the media of the aorta. This observed bias of monotypism toward the phenotype predominant in the media is signifi- cantly greater than expected by chance, at the P value of 0.005 level. Furthermore in 14 out of 24 aortas with monotypic foci, the monotypism was exclusively of the same phenotype in a given aorta.

We can conclude from these observations that one phenotype has a selec- tive advantage over the other in the abnormal microenvironment of atherosclerotic lesions. We suspect that the above accounts for most of the monotypism observed, but not all, since 16% of the lesions showed the phenotype that is not predominant in the media of the aorta. The exact cause of this phenomenon is not known at this time.

During the course of our studies on heterozygous black women, it be- came obvious to us that it·would be useful to have available an animal model with similar characteristics as black women, and which would permit experimental procedures in time series. We found such a model described by Ohno et al. in 1965 (5), a female hybrid hare obtained from cross between two species of wild hare, Lepus timidus and Lepus europaeus. They are heterozygous for G-6-PD and the allozymes of G-6-PD are distinct from the human A and B, and are designated by us as T and E representing the parent species names. These allozymes can be separated by electrophoresis and quantitated by densitometer as in the case of A and B in black women. The following are some character- istics we have observed in these hybrid hares (6, 7, 8).

The G-6-PD T:E ratio in the normal aorta was approximately 65:35 on the average (or expressed as 65% T ± 3). There is relatively little varia- tion among animals, and cholesterol feeding does not appear to change appreciably the T:E ratios in the normal media.

Sixteen of the heterozygous hybrid hares fed cholesterol 6-17 months before sacrifice showed extensive atherosclerotic lesions in the aorta.

In seven hares, T:E ratios in multiple samples from lesions showed significant shift from the T:E ratios in their media; of the seven, three shifted toward E and four toward T (Table I). No monotypic foci were found in any of these lesions; hence these lesions are not monoclonal in origin. However, it is important to note that there were significant shifts in T:E ratios and the direction of the shift was always the same in a given aorta, regardless of the number of lesions examined.

Table I. % T(G-6-PD) in samples of aortic lesions showing significant shift in seven hybrid hares fed HL diet

| Hare # | Duration of Diet, Mo. | % T in Normal Media* | % T in Lesion* | Significance | Direction of shift |
|--------|------|-------|--------|--------|--------|
| 7 | 6 | 68 ± 2 (15) | 53 ± 2 (27) | P <.001 | → E |
| | | | 56 ± 3 (15) | P <.001 | → E |
| | | | 54 ± 2 (24) | P <.001 | → E |
| 133 | 11 | 68 ± 1 (23) | 63 ± 3 (20) | P <.03 | → E |
| 126 | 11 | 69 ± 2 (12) | 76 ± 2 (12) | P <.01 | → T |
| 11 | 12 | 61 ± 3 (16) | 73 ± 1 (14) | P <.001 | → T |
| | | | 72 ± 1 (16) | P <.001 | → T |
| | | | 72 ± 2 (13) | P <.003 | → T |
| 5 | 12 | 63 ± 3 (17) | 56 ± 2 (15) | P <.01 | → E |
| | | | 50 ± 3 (10) | P <.003 | → E |
| | | | 53 ± 2 (19) | P <.003 | → E |
| 36 | 16 | 69 ± 2 (12) | 73 ± 1 (18) | P <.01 | → T |
| 41 | 17 | 56 ± 6 (3) | 67 ± 2 (10) | P <.01 | → T |
| | | | 62 ± 1 (20) | P <.03 | → T |
| | | | 63 ± 1 (14) | P <.01 | → T |

*Mean ± SEM. Numbers in parentheses are the number of samples taken from each media or lesion.

Four of the hares that were given a mixture of 25-hydroxycholesterol (an autoxidation product of cholesterol) and cholesterol for 6-8 months were found to have similarly advanced atheroscerotic lesions. Two of the four hares showed monotypic foci in lesions as well as in non-lesion areas in the aorta. These results suggest that the appearance of monotypic foci may be due to acquisition of resistance to 25-hydroxycholesterol. This is further substantiated by the work of Sinensky (9) who has isolated a mutant of mammalian cells resistant to 25-hydroxycholesterol.

We have also carried out tissue culture experiments using fibroblasts grown from skin punches of these heterozygous hybrid hares. Cells from primary cultures were used for subsequent serial passages. Before every passage cells were analyzed for G-6-PD phenotype. Skin fibroblasts from 39 hybrid hares were cultured through multiple passages. A total of 21 cultures became monotypic, that is 100% T, after 1-12 passages. Only two cultures became 100% E after the 4th passage. The remaining 16 cultures did not become monotypic (Table II) but 12 showed shifts toward one or the other phenotype. Thus, the majority of cultures either changed systematically in the ratios of G-6-PD variants, or exhibited, at some transfer one type only. Changes occurred in both directions; toward higher T:E ratios or toward lower T:E ratios. These results are similar to those found in skin fibroblast cultures of heterozygous black female G-6-PD mosaics (4), and suggest the presence of factors, in one or the other of the X-chromosomes, that confer a selective advantage on the cells of the corresponding type.

Table II. Skin fibroblast cultures from 39 hares heterozygous for G-6-PD carried through multiple passages

| | | No. of Passages | | |
|---|---|---|---|---|
| | 1 | 2-5 | 6-12 | Total |
| 1. No. of cultures exhibiting 100% T at passage indicated | 8 | 6 | 7 | 21 |
| 2. No. of cultures exhibiting 100% E at passage indicated | 0 | 2 | 0 | 2 |

Remaining 16 cultures did not become monotypic but 12 showed a shift toward either T (3) or E (9).

Skin fibroblast cultures from 11 hares were exposed to 25-hydroxychol-esterol in six different concentrations ranging from 0-50 µg/ml of medi-um. Eight cultures showed a significant shift in T:E ratios toward E with increasing concentration of 25-hydroxycholesterol in the media. Three of the eight showed monotypic cultures, and they were all E-type. None showed a significant shift toward T. The change of T:E ratios toward E appears to occur because the 25-hydroxycholesterol is more toxic for the T-type cells (8).

In another study we are making use of the mosaic model to determine if the direction of phenotypic shift in tissue culture correlates with the in vivo shift in atherosclerotic lesions. For this purpose in vivo and in vitro studies were carried out in the same animal. Skin biopsies were taken before animals were put on a hyperlipidemic diet. Thirteen hares have been examined thus far for this study. Changes to monotyp-ism were observed in skin fibroblast cultures in nine hares and a sig-nificant shift in T:E ratios in two hares. Six of these 11 hares also showed a significant shift in T:E ratios in atherosclerotic lesions in vivo (Table III). It is interesting to note that in all six hares the

Table III. Correlation of significant changes in T:E ratios in culture with that in vivo

| Hare # | 11 | 36 | 7 | 126 | 133 | 41 | 13 | 14 | 69 | 129 | 22 | 31 | 30 |
|---|---|---|---|---|---|---|---|---|---|---|---|---|---|
| Monotypic or pre-dominant phenotype in culture (in vitro) | T | T | E | T | E | T | T | T | T | T | E | NS | NS |
| Direction of signif. phenotypic shift in lesion (in vivo) | T | T | E | T | E | T | NS | NS | NS | NS | NS | NS | NS |
| Duration of diet, mos. | 12 | 16 | 6 | 11 | 11 | 17 | 12 | 12 | 9 | 11 | 11 | 15 | 14 |

predominant phenotype is the same. These data suggest that the changes in T:E ratios in fibroblast culture would be an in vitro indicator of the changes that take place in vivo of T:E ratios in lesions. Furthermore, these data suggest that the phenotype that has a selective advantage in the tissue culture environment also has a selective advantage in the abnormal microenvironment of atherosclerotic lesions.

In summary, our in vivo and in vitro observations do not support a monoclonal origin of atherosclerotic lesions but instead indicate that observed monotypism is due to a possible existence of factors that confer a selective advantage on one phenotype.

Acknowledgement    This work is supported by USPHS grant HL 20993.

References

1.  Benditt EP, Benditt JM (1973) Evidence for a monoclonal origin of human atherosclerosis plaques. Proc. Nat. Acad. Sci. USA 70: 1753-1756
2.  Thomas WA, Reiner JM, Janakidevi K, Florentin RA and Lee KT (1979) Population dynamics of arterial cells during atherogenesis. X. Study of monotypism in atherosclerotic lesions of black women heterozygous for glucose-6-phosphate dehydrogenase. Exp. Mol. Path. 31: 367-386
3.  Lyon MF (1962) Sex chromatin and gene action in the mammalian X-chromosome. Amer. J. Hum. Genet. 14: 135-148
4.  Zavala C, Herner G, and Fialkow PJ (1978) Evidence for selection in cultured diploid fibroblast strains. Exp. Cell Res. 117: 137-144
5.  Ohno S, Poole J, and Gustavsson I (1965) Sex-linkage of erythrocyte glucose-6-phosphate dehydrogenase in two species of wild hares. Science 150: 1737-1738
6.  Lee KT, Thomas WA, Janakidevi K, Kroms M, Reiner JM, and Borg KY (1981) Mosaicism in female hybrid hares heterozygous for glucose-6-phosphate dehydrogenase. I. General properties of a hybrid hare model with special reference to atherogenesis. Exp. Mol. Path. 34: 191-201
7.  Janakidevi K, Lee KT, Thomas, WA, Reiner JM, and Murray CD (1981) Mosaicism in female hybrid hares heterozygous for glucose-6-phosphate dehydrogenase. II. Changes in the ratios of G-6-PD types in skin fibroblast cultures carried through multiple passages. Exp. Mol. Path. 34: 202-208
8.  Murray CD, Lee KT, Thomas WA, Reiner JM, and Janakidevi K (1981) Mosaicism in female hybrid hares heterozygous for glucose-6-phosphate dehydrogenase. III. Chnages in the ratios of G-6-PD types in skin fibroblast cultures exposed to 25-hydroxycholesterol. Exp. Mol. Path. 34: 209-215
9.  Sinensky M (1977) Isolation of a mammalian cell mutant resistant to 25-hydroxycholesterol. Biochem. Biophys. Res. Comm. 78: 863-867

# Measurement of Human Atherosclerosis

W. P. Newman III, G. T. Malcom, L. H. McMahan, and R. E. Tracy

The need for accurate assessment of atherosclerosis has long been recognized. Lesions of some degree have been found in almost all individuals in populations systematically surveyed. The quantitation of atherosclerosis is essential for meaningful comparisons among populations and for a better understanding of the disease.

## MEASUREMENT METHODS

Several methods with various modifications have been and are being used to grade atherosclerosis both for extent and type of lesion involvement. Pathologists at autopsy have for years either cross sectioned arteries or opened them longitudinally and estimated the amount of atherosclerosis, frequently quantitating the disease using terms like severe, marked, moderate, or minimal, and percent stenosis as an estimate of the reduction in lumen diameter. As interest in the disease increased, methods were developed that allowed for some degree of lesion measurement "standardization."

Visual estimation of surface area involvement with different types of atherosclerotic lesions after Sudan staining has been used in many population studies at our institution and in collaboration with other investigators (1). The procedure is simple, yet large interobserver bias is a problem without training and testing. EGGEN, STRONG, and McGILL performed optical electronic analyses of photographs of opened stained vessels. The precision is better than with visual estimation, but instrumentation is complex and costly (2). Planimetric procedures with grid overlays or tracing paper are more reproducible than visual estimation; however, the procedure is slower and more tedious (3,4,5). Calipers have been used to estimate wall thickness on limited samples of the arterial wall with good reproducibility (6).

Postmortem angiography was pioneered by SCHLESINGER in 1938 (7) and has been used in some studies to evaluate the status of the coronary arteries (8,9). Angiography postmortem most often underestimates the disease when compared to examination of the vessels, whether opened longitudinally or in cross section; lack of agreement between methods varies from report to report. Because of projection on a plane, overlapping vessels, and inadequate filling, some lesions may be missed. In a study designed to evaluate postmortem angiograms for lumen stenosis and/or occlusion, we found we could not determine stenosis and occlusion with confidence from the angiogram alone, but evaluation of the postmortem angiogram in conjunction with evaluation of the opened coronary arteries aided in grading stenosis and occlusion (unpublished data).

Morphometric studies, both light and electron microscopic, have furnished important information and are being addressed in detail by other participants in this Symposium.

Interest in pressure perfusion fixation discussed at the Workshop on Quantitative Evaluation of Atherosclerosis, Silver Springs, Maryland, February 22-23, 1982, by S. GLAGOV and C. ZARINS has suggested the need for increased cooperation between the clinician and the morphologist in assessment of arterial disease including the carotid system, accessible to ultrasound imaging.

## VISUAL GRADING

The reproducibility of our visual estimates of lesion involvement undergoes continual scrutiny. For example, in investigating whether atherosclerosis has decreased in New Orleans (10), we have used our cardiovascular pathology archive containing specimens collected over two time periods. Specimens are blindly coded in such a way that those collected between 1960 and 1964 are indistinguishable from those collected from 1969 through 1978. Specimens then are arranged in random order and graded independently by three pathologists. In addition, "standard sets" of specimens are graded repeatedly, and selected specimens are routinely re-graded (without the graders' knowledge that they have been graded previously).

The contribution of various sources of error in the grading process can be derived from estimates of components of variance computed for three pathologists' evaluations of specimens in a standard set. Square roots of estimated components and their contributions to total variability (percentage of the sum of components) are presented in Table 1.

It is apparent from the data that the proportion of variability attributable to pathologists (graders) is small compared to that for specimens. The variability of lesion involvement among the specimens accounts for the vast majority of the total variability: 78.5% for lesions in the thoracic aorta, and 87.2% for lesions in the abdominal aorta. For coronary arteries, the largest proportion of the total variability is also in the specimens--84.1% to 88.3%.

## CORONARY ARTERY CALCIFICATION

Percentage surface area involved with calcified lesions was estimated independently by four pathologists using the visual grading procedure of the opened coronary arteries and x-rays of the arteries in a 10-year study of atherosclerosis in 25-44 year old men. If the average grading for the four pathologists was greater than zero, the gross specimen was classified as having calcification present. The radiographic image was also inspected for areas of calcification. Calcification was classified as present by both methods in 208 of 952 sets of coronary arteries (Table 2); calcification was recorded as absent by both methods in 600 specimens. Thus, agreement between methods was about 85% (808/952).

There were 46/952, or slightly less than 5%, in which calcification was detected on x-ray but was not noted on visual inspection of the gross specimen. In only 2 of these 46 specimens was the percentage surface involvement as determined by evaluation of the x-ray greater than 1%. In about 10% of the specimens, pathologists thought calcification was present in fibrous plaques, but it was not detected on the x-ray.

Table 1. Square root of estimates of three variance components and the contribution of the component to the total variability in raised lesions in arterial segments

| Arterial segment | Square root of estimated component of variance | | | % of sum of estimated components | | |
|---|---|---|---|---|---|---|
| | Pathologist | Specimen | Residual | Pathologist | Specimen | Residual |
| Thoracic aorta | 2.6 | 14.5 | 7.1 | 2.5 | 78.5 | 19.0 |
| Abdominal aorta | 5.0 | 22.7 | 7.1 | 4.2 | 87.2 | 8.6 |
| Right coronary | 0.8 | 16.8 | 7.2 | 0.2 | 84.1 | 15.6 |
| Left circumflex coronary | 1.9 | 10.6 | 3.4 | 2.7 | 88.3 | 8.9 |
| Left anterior descending coronary | 2.7 | 16.1 | 5.3 | 2.4 | 88.2 | 9.4 |

Table 2.  Presence or absence of calcification in coronary arteries, by visual classification of gross specimen and radiographic image

| Radiographic image | Gross specimen | | Total |
| --- | --- | --- | --- |
| | $Ca^{++}$ absent | $Ca^{++}$ present | |
| $Ca^{++}$ absent | 600 | 98 | 698 |
| $Ca^{++}$ present | 46 | 208 | 254 |
| Total | 646 | 306 | 952 |

## CHEMICAL AND VISUAL GRADING COMPARISONS

Visual estimates of the extent of grossly assessed raised lesions in one half of the abdominal aorta have been compared with chemical analysis of dry defatted weight and total lipid (chemical lipid) extracted from the intima.  This study included 76 men dying in New Orleans, Louisiana, USA, and 77 men dying in Guatemala (11,12). The extent of grossly evaluated raised lesions was highly correlated with dry defatted weight in specimens from New Orleans (0.899) and Guatemala (0.860)--Table 3.  High correlations also were found between chemical lipid and dry defatted weight (0.847 and 0.908) suggesting that lipid and nonlipid components are proportional to each other.  The correlation between raised lesions and chemical lipid was not as good in the Guatemalan specimens (0.670) as in the New Orleans specimens (0.800).

Table 3. Correlation coefficients for selected measures of arterial condition, New Orleans and Guatemalan men aged 15-54 years

| Measure | RL | DDW | CL |
| --- | --- | --- | --- |
| RL | | 0.899 | 0.800 |
| DDW | 0.860 | | 0.847 |
| CL | 0.670 | 0.908 | |

New Orleans, n = 76
Guatemala, n = 77

   RL = gross raised lesions; DDW = dry defatted weight; and CL = chemical lipid.

## SUMMARY

Many methods have been used to evaluate and estimate the extent and severity of human atherosclerosis, both clinically and at autopsy. With increasing sophistication in clinical measurement including arteriography and ultrasound imaging, correlation with pathologists' autopsy findings will be needed.  Improved techniques, pressure

perfusion fixation and measurement methods including the use of digitizers for more reproducible measurement, will be important in these
correlations. There still exists a need for information for the
understanding of the underlying processes. Voids in our knowledge
about the basic processes underlying atherosclerosis may be answered
in part by continued surveillance of arterial disease as it exists in
populations. Methods that are best for measuring fatty streaks,
fibrous plaques, and calcified lesions may not be the most suitable
for measuring stenosis and occlusion. Methods for assessing "severity"
may not be suited for evaluating the extent of individual types of
lesions. Methods designed to investigate basic mechanisms of atherosclerosis may not be best for evaluating lesions detected clinically.

The type of measurement--whether gross, microscopic, ultrastructural,
or chemical--will depend on the level of precision and accuracy
needed to answer the questions formulated.

*Acknowledgments* This research was supported in part by funds from the
National Heart, Lung, and Blood Institute, National Institutes of
Health, Grant Number HL-08974 and Contract Number N01-HV 12911.

REFERENCES

1. Strong JP, McGill HC Jr (1962) The natural history of coronary
   atherosclerosis. Am J Pathol 40:37-49
2. Eggen DA, Strong JP, McGill HC Jr (1962) An objective method for
   grading atherosclerotic lesions. Lab Invest 11:732-742
3. Mitchell JRA, Schwartz CJ (1962) Relationship between arterial
   disease in different sites: A study of the aorta and coronary,
   carotid, and iliac arteries. Br Med J 1:1293-1301
4. Cranston WI, Mitchell JRA, Russell RWR, Schwartz CJ (1964) The
   assessment of aortic disease. J Atheroscler Res 4:29-39
5. Mitchell JRA, Cranston WI (1965) A simple method for the quantitative assessment of aortic disease. J Atheroscler Res 5:135-144
6. Daoud AS, Goodale F, Florentin R, Beadenkopf WG (1962) Chemico-
   anatomic studies in geographic pathology: A practical method
   for the quantitation of coronary atherosclerosis. Arch Pathol
   73:74-81
7. Schlesinger MJ (1938) An injection plus dissection study of
   coronary artery occlusions and anastomoses. Am Heart J 15:528-568
8. Eusterman JH, Achor RWP, Kincaid OW, Brown AL (1962) Atherosclerotic disease of the coronary arteries. A pathologic-
   radiologic correlative study. Circulation 26:1288-1295
9. Hutchins GM, Bulkley BH, Ridolfi RL, Griffith LSC, Lohr FT,
   Piasio MA (1977) Correlation of coronary arteriograms and left
   ventriculograms with postmortem studies. Circulation 56:32-37
10. Strong JP, Guzman MA (1980) Decrease in coronary atherosclerosis
    in New Orleans. Lab Invest 43:297-301
11. Malcom GT (1978) Extent of atherosclerosis and lipid composition
    of abdominal aorta in Guatemala and New Orleans. PhD disserta-
    tion, Department of Pathology, Louisiana State University Medical
    Center
12. Restrepo C, Tracy RE, Malcom GT, Strong JP, Toca VT (1982)
    Microscopic morphometry of abdominal aorta from males in New
    Orleans and Guatemala. Arteriosclerosis 2

# Identification of the Gelatinous Lesion

## B. Smith

In 1856, Virchow published a detailed description of gelatinous lesions: "Im ersten Anfange der Veranderungen sieht man gewohnlich leichte Anschwellungen der inneren Arterienhaut, ..... Diese Anschwellungen treten entweder fleckweise, oder auch wohl in mehr diffuser Form auf, so dass die ganze Gefassoberflache weicher, gequollen, uneben erscheint. Im Anfange sind die geschwollenen Theile wohl immer saftreicher und sie erreichen nicht selten einen so grossen Gehalt an wasserigen Theilen, dass sie vollstandig gallertartig aussehen. Diess sind die gallertartigen oder albuminosen Exsudationen." (1). As a biochemist, I failed to read Virchow, but noticed these lesions about 1964 and thought, from their gelatinous appearance, that they might contain large amounts of glycosaminoglycans (GAG). However, compared with adjacent normal intima GAG were increased in only one of seven samples, and decreased in five (2).

In the post-war period of rapidly expanding atherosclerosis research these lesions were overlooked or ignored by a majority of British and American pathologists, but in Canada their morphology and histochemistry were extensively studied by Haust, More and coworkers who showed that the lesions contained large amounts of insudated plasma macromolecules (reviewed by Haust, reference 3).

Using quantitative immunoassay techniques, we have shown that, on the basis of tissue dry weight, the concentration of low density lipoprotein is increased 2-3-fold compared with adjacent normal intima, with parallel increases in $\alpha_2$-macroglobulin, HDL, albumin and $\alpha_1$-antitrypsin, and a greater increase in fibrinogen (4,5). Haust (3) suggests that organization of the insudate leads to local increase of connective tissue, and I feel no doubt that gelatinous lesions are the principal precursors of fibrous plaques.

## Recognition of Gelatinous Lesions on Macroscopic Inspection of Fresh Arteries

Failure to see gelatinous lesions on routine inspection is probably the main reason for their neglect. Most lesions are translucent, and neutral in colour; smaller lesions are difficult to detect with the naked eye but are clearly seen at 2-2.5x magnification under a lens surrounded by a circular fluorescent tube light. Oblique lighting helps to confirm focal thickening, as seen in Fig. 2a. Even abruptly raised large lesions (Fig. 1a) are inconspicuous although the central area may become slightly greyish or opaque. Some lesions are yellow, and characterized by finely dispersed perifibrous lipid along the collagen strands; others are pinkish, and contain traces of haemoglobin. Gelatinous areas are frequently found surrounding white fibrous plaques; in the most usual distribution there is a narrow gelatinous border - 1-2mm in width - at the proximal edge and sides of the white fibrous cap, and a large gelatinous tail that may extend for a centimetre in length and be 1000-2000μm thick at its thickest point.

Texture is a useful aid to recognition of gelatinous lesions. If gently palpated with the back of curved forceps the lesions feel soft, and if gentle pressure is applied and the forceps moved from side to side the lesions wobble. In normal areas of adult coronary arteries the diffusely thickened intima is slightly translucent and has a soft texture, which makes recognition of gelatinous lesions more difficult than in aorta.

## Distribution of Gelatinous Lesions in Aorta

Gelatinous lesions occur in all parts of the aorta and their distribution is dependent on age and severity of atherosclerosis. In the second decade there may be quite extensive areas of flat, translucent thickening in the lower abdominal segment. Sometimes these are edged with a narrow band of fat-filled cells, and occasionally fat-filled cells are scattered through all or part of the thickening, giving a mixed gelatinous-fatty streak lesions. In older age groups these seem to be replaced by white, fibrous thickenings and lipid-rich lesions. In the descending thoracic and upper abdominal segments small translucent thickenings may occur in any position in the second decade and increase in size and number with age. Translucent gelatinous lesions which may have greyish centres are frequently found round the orifices of the intercostal branches in the third and fourth decades. Elongated, strap-like gelatinous lesions in the mid-anterior sector of the proximal thoracic aorta may extend for up to 6cm in length (Fig. 2a) and are particularly characteristic of the fourth and fifth decades. In older age groups gelatinous areas are seen as surrounds and tails of plaques with white fibrous centres, as flattish translucent thickenings between two plaques, and as large, translucent lesions with visible fat in the deep layers.

## Histological and Biochemical Characteristics

As emphasized by Virchow (1), a striking characteristic of the lesions is their high fluid content. Fluid may flow out of the lesion on incision (5), and histological examination suggests increased extracellular space (Figs. 1b and 2c) and swelling of the collagen fibres (3,6). These impressions are confirmed by analysis; in a comparison of gelatinous lesions with adjacent normal intima (11 pairs) the water content, expressed as mg water/100mg dry tissue, was approximately doubled. From the concentrations of plasma proteins in the isolated interstitial fluid (7) and in the intact tissue (4,5) it can be calculated that the interstitial fluid compartment and the "bound plus intracellular water" compartments increased to about the same extent. Analysis also confirms the low lipid content of most gelatinous lesions; total cholesterol concentration was $6.6 \pm 1.2$ (SEM) mg/100mg dry tissue compared with $7.5 \pm 1.1$mg in the normal intima. Both chemical and histochemical analysis indicate reduced concentration of GAG (2,3,6). Cellularity is variable: there may be very numerous large smooth muscle cells throughout the lesion, as in Figs. 1 and 2; loss of cells in the deepest part of the lesion, presumably as a result of hypoxia; occasionally, cells seem to have disappeared throughout the lesion (3,6). Loss of cells, particularly in the deep layers of the lesion, may be accompanied by changes in the morphology of the collagen in which the linear architecture is replaced by a network and the thick collagen bundles are attenuated. Presumably this is an indication of necrosis. However, in diffuse cell loss the collagen bundles may appear unchanged.

## Measurement of Gelatinous Lesions

Most studies on the incidence and extent of arterial lesions have been made on formalin-fixed sudan-stained arteries (8,9). On formalin fixation the gelatinous lesions lose their characteristic translucency and softness. Large lesions become indistinguishable from fibrous plaques and small diffuse thickenings may be graded as normal intima, thus they are not only missed, but may be a major source of inaccuracy in measurement of fibrous plaques and normal intima. The difference between macroscopic and microscopic classifications in coronary arteries have been examined by Velican and Velican (10). The identity of gelatinous lesions in their terminology is not clear, but they probably correspond with "mucoid", and "necrotic/early atheroma" lesions, and macroscopically these were classified either as fibrous plaques or normal intima. In the 21-30 age group only 53% of macroscopically normal areas were normal on microscopic examination, and 35% were probably gelatinous lesions. Measurement of gelatinous lesions could only be

172

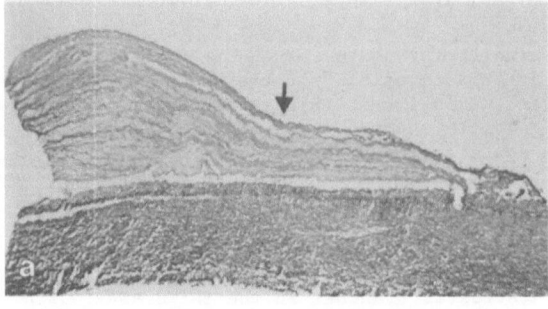

A

FIG. 1. Gelatinous plaque from woman aged 60; maximum thickness 1600μm. A. Low power view of half the lesion (12.5x). B. Higher power view through whole intima at ↓ . Graphite grains (arrows) mark strip planes for interstitial fluid and tissue analysis (85x; Fettrot/Mayer's haemalum).

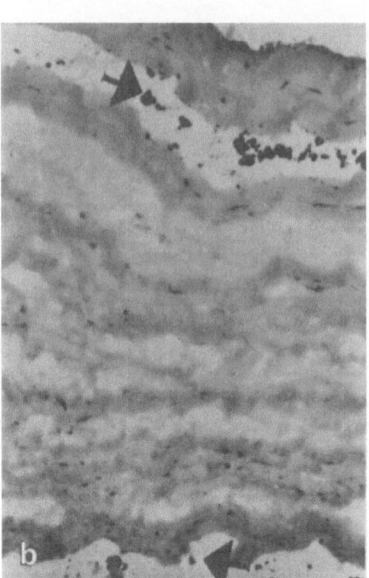

B

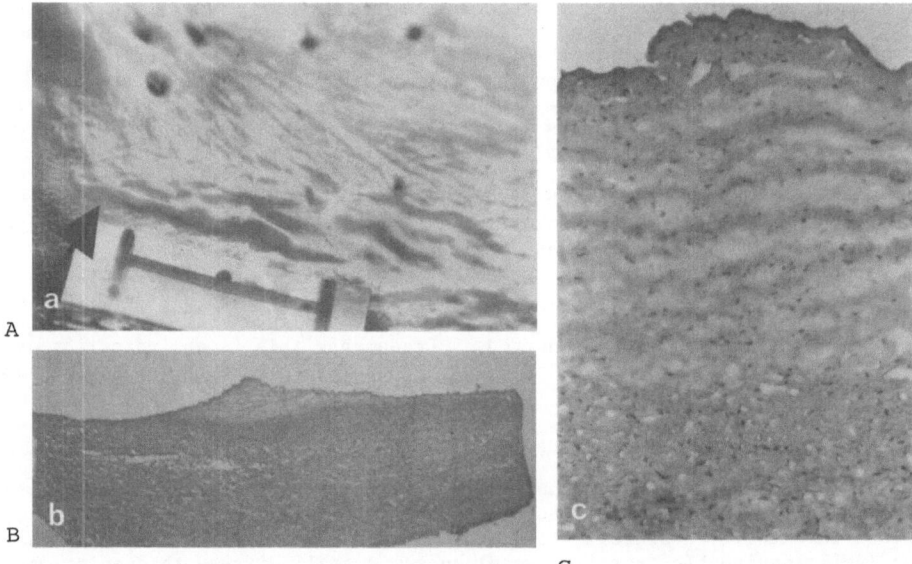

A

B

C

FIG. 2. Elongated gelatinous lesion, extending from intercostal branches 1-6, in mid-anterior quadrant of aorta from man aged 42. A. Macroscopic appearance of proximal part, viewed with oblique lighting; 2cm marker. B and C. Section across leading edge of lesion (arrow). B. Magnification 10x; C. Magnification 85x showing typical separated collagen bundles with variable numbers of smooth muscle cells; maximum thickness 550μm (Fettrot/Mayer's haemalum).

accomplished in fresh arteries, and this presents difficulties with respect to preservation of the anonymity of the case  so that it is truly assessed blind, and exchange of specimens for cross standardization of grading between pathologists. Cross-standardization is of particular importance because classification of the slightly opaque centre of a lesion as "grey gelatinous" or "white fibrous", or the point from which the gelatinous surround of a lesion should be measured are highly subjective judgments.   Thus although the gelatinous lesions are probably the most significant early lesions, their measurement on an epidemiological scale present serious difficulties.

Acknowledgements    The author's work was supported by grants from the Medical Research Council and the British Heart Foundation.

References

1.    Virchow R (1856) Gesammelte Abhandlungen zur Wissenschaftlichen Medicin. Meidinger Sohn & Co, Frankfurt AM, 496-497.
2.    Smith EB (1965) The influence of age and atherosclerosis on the chemistry of aortic intima:  Part 2 - Collagen and mucopolysaccharides.  J Atheroscler Res. 5: 241-248.
3.    ·Haust MD (1971) The morphogenesis and fate of potential and early athero-sclerotic lesions in man.   Human Pathol 2:1-29.
4.    Smith EB, Slater RS (1973) Lipids and low density lipoproteins in intima in relation to its morphological characteristics.   In: Atherogenesis: Initiating Factors.   Ciba Foundation Symposium 12 (new series).   Associated Scientific Publishers, Amsterdam, p39-52.
5.    Smith EB, Staples EM (1982) Intimal and medial plasma protein concentrations and endothelial function.   Atherosclerosis 41: 295-308.
6.    Movat HZ, Haust MD, More RH (1959) The morphologic elements in the early lesions of arteriosclerosis. Amer J Path 35: 93-97.
7.    Smith EB, Staples EM (1982) Collection of interstitial fluid from human aortas and measurement of its plasma protein content.  J Physiol 324: 48P.
8.    McGill HC (1968) The geographic pathology of atherosclerosis.  Lab Invest 18: 463 et seq.
9.    World Health Organization (1976) Atherosclerosis of the aorta and coronary arteries in five towns.    Bull WHO 53: 485-645.
10.  Velican C, Velican D (1982) Discrepancies between data on atherosclerotic involvement of human coronary arteries furnished by gross inspection and by light microscopy.   Atherosclerosis 43: 39-49.

# Quantitation of Certain Qualitative Differences in the Atherosclerotic Process*

D. Vesselinovitch and R. W. Wissler

To obtain quantitative information regarding the status of atherosclerotic disease and its consequences, the process is measured
through functional effects and visually either *in vivo* or postmortem.
Due to rapid developments in instrumentation, it is now becoming more
feasible to correlate antemortem to postmortem findings. Moreover,
quantitative evaluation of atherosclerosis in tissue, including the
utilization of biochemical and immunohistochemical methods, may soon
make it possible to relate visual information to functional process.

In spite of these achievements some difficulties and requirements remain. A common difficulty in quantitating atherosclerosis is the lack
of methods which are precise, replicable and relatively simple. A
number of visual or morphometric approaches with both advantages and
limitations have been described which permit lesion quantitation at
the macroscopic and microscopic level (1-8).

The study of atherosclerosis for comparative and correlative purposes
depends on careful evaluation of lesion extent, severity, composition
and the relationship to other micro-architecture. The following requirements should be fulfilled: a) approximate antemortem configuration in postmortem tissue by controlled pressure-perfusion fixation;
b) delineation of vessel wall and the lesion; c) standardization of
sampling sites; d) uniformity of fixation, orientation and staining;
and e) selection of measurable parameters and standardization of
methods for measurement. Careful histological preparations taking
into consideration all of these parameters should avoid some of the
difficulties which arise when an attempt is made to correlate angiographic findings with histological measurements (10,11). Variability
in methodology and technical complications such as angulation, motion,
overlapping during *in vivo* measurements, as well as shrinkage, dis-
tortion and staining differences during the preparations of microscopic specimens, should be considered when correlations between
antemortem and postmortem findings are made. Moreover, observer
variability in interpretation of the results is important.

Furthermore, different sets of criteria need to be applied to elastic
arteries (aorta, common carotid) and muscular arteries (coronary, femoral), dictated by their size and functional role. The conductive
nature of elastic arteries and their need to withstand the rapid
changes in pulse pressure make them vulnerable to any changes affecting components of their wall. Thus equal evaluation of intimal and
medial involvement is of utmost importance, with special attention

*The studies reported here which were performed in this laboratory
were supported partially by NIH grants No. HL 15062 and HL 17648 and
by the University of Chicago's Cardiovascular Research Founcation.

given to fibrous cap formation, calcification, necrosis, and existence of any form of aneurysms. Muscular arteries, on the other hand,
control blood distribution by contraction, thus features to be carefully evaluated are the size of the artery, the size of the lumen and
lesions, the position of the lesions as well as lesion components.

Volume and mass of plaque may be less important than is the composition of the lesion (12). Moreover, concentric or eccentric plaques,
as well as transmural or largely intimal and inner medial lesions,
should be identified (13). These latter features have an apparent
role in the further fate of the lesion and the functional abilities
of the artery. When examining coronary arteries in two macaque
species, we have found that concentric lesions were seen in 46% of
lesions in cynomolgus monkeys as opposed to 10% in rhesus monkeys.

To measure atherosclerotic lesions we had previously used "point-
counting" methods (4,6,9,14). Recently we have been using the Neo-
Palmer projecting microscope (Leitz) combined with a digitizer-
computer listed as "Hewlett Packard System 45" (10,15). Diagrams of
an aortic and a coronary artery section, as produced by this system,
are shown in figures 1a and b. On the left (a) is aortic lesion and
on the right (b) is coronary artery lesion in a cynomolgus monkey fed
peanut oil-cholesterol diet for a period of 12 months.

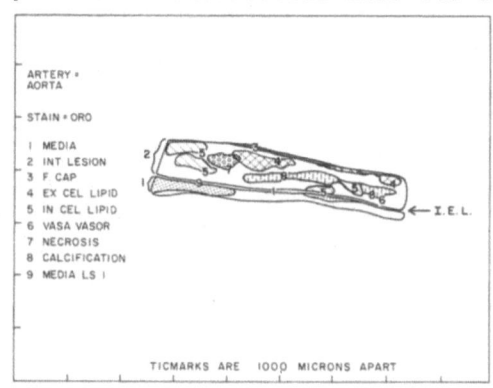 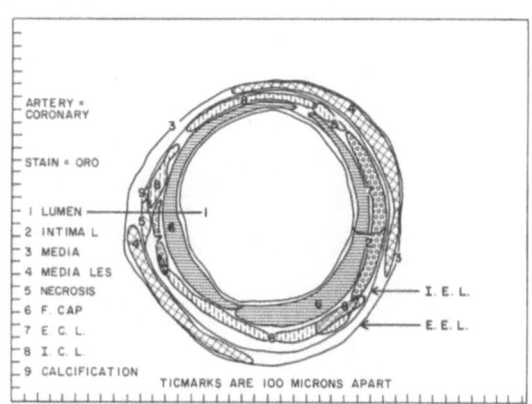

Fig. 1a,b

Contours of lesions, and the lumen, the whole artery and the media,
as well as lesion components, are traced in order to evaluate lesion
size, shape and the area occupied by intra and extracellular lipid,
fibrous caps, necrotic areas, calcification, fibrosis, vasa vasorum,
etc. Special programs have been developed to allow recording and
analysis of lines, points and contours resulting in a hard copy of
total tracing with accompanying pertinent calculations. This method
is highly reproducible, accurate and time conserving. It convincingly documents the qualitative and quantitative changes which
occur during induction and regression of atherosclerosis (16).

Lesions in the coronary arteries of two rhesus monkeys fed two different atherogenic diets for a 12-month period are shown in figure
2a and b. The lesion on the left (a) was induced by a peanut oil-
cholesterol enriched diet and the one on the right (b) by coconut oil-
butter fat cholesterol diet. Differences in lesion size and components are evident and can be measured.

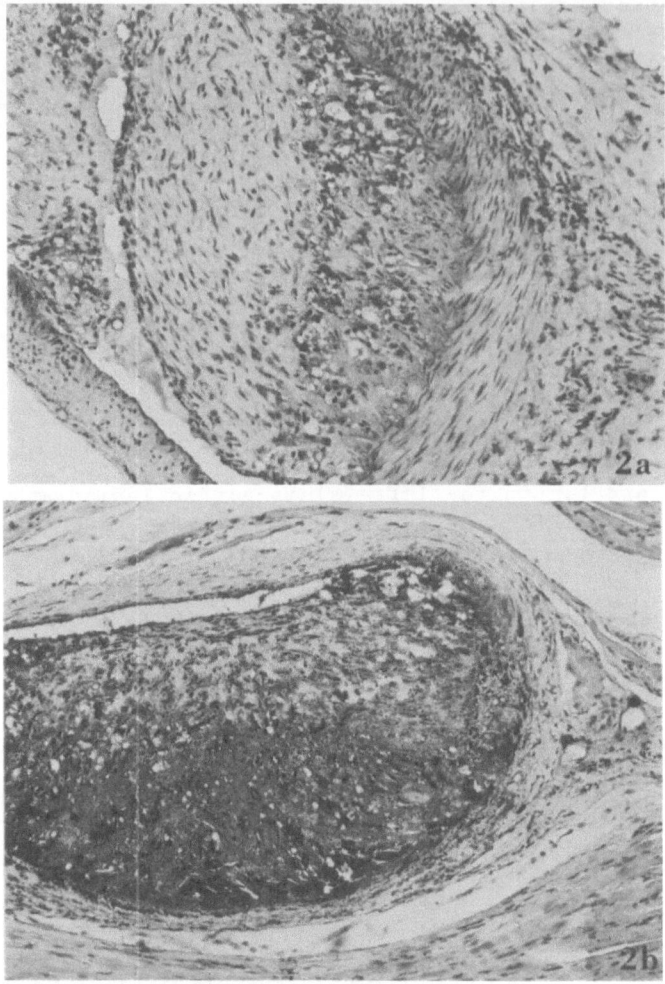

Fig. 2a,b

Lesions size and components in the aortas of two macaque species fed
the same atherogenic diets for 12 months were measured by this system
and the results are summarized in Table 1.

Table 1. Plaque components in the aortic lesions in Macaques
fed atherogenic diets for 12 months

| Lesion Components | Peanut Oil and Cholesterol | | Coconut Oil-Butterfat Cholesterol | |
|---|---|---|---|---|
| | Rhesus (12 mos.) | Cynomolgus (12 mos.) | Rhesus (12 & 14 mos.) | Cynomolgus (12 mos.) |
| Area of lesion | 40 ($\mu m^2$) | 98 ($\mu m^2$) | 84 ($\mu m^2$) | 87 ($\mu m^2$) |
| Lesion thickness | 190 $\mu$ | 403 $\mu$ | 300 $\mu$ | 360 $\mu$ |
| Medial lesion vs. total medial (%) | 5 | 17 | 13 | 47 |
| Necrosis (%) | 1 | 3 | 2 | Not done |
| Total lipids (%) | 41 | 43 | 35 | Not done |
| Intracellular (%) | 15 | 30 | 22 | 21 |
| Extracellular (%) | 26 | 13 | 13 | Not done |

Evidently lesion thickness and the degree of intimal and medial involvement, as well as the extent of necrosis and lipid depositions,
are influenced both by the type of dietary fats and the species
studied. Lesion area and thickness, as well as medial involvement,
are generally greater in cynomolgus than in rhesus monkeys regardless
of the diet fed. When two atherogenic diets were compared, it became
apparent that the lesions were bigger in rhesus monkeys fed the
coconut oil-butterfat cholesterol diet, while peanut oil-cholesterol
enriched rations resulted in larger lesions in the cynomolgus monkeys.
Table 2 compares the data from left coronary artery on area of intimal lesion and artery size in both species of macaque fed peanut oil-
cholesterol diet, as well as the effect of two atherogenic diets in
rhesus monkeys. A significant correlation exists between area of
lesion and artery size for all three parts of the left coronary artery.

Table 2. Area of coronary artery size and lesions in two Macaque
species fed atherogenic diets for 12 months

| Left Coronary Arteries | Coconut Oil-Butterfat and Cholesterol | | | | Peanut Oil and Cholesterol | |
|---|---|---|---|---|---|---|
| | Rhesus[b] | | Cynomolgus[c] | | Rhesus[d] | |
| | Area of Intimal Lesion ($\mu m^2$) | Size of Artery[a] | Area of Intimal Lesion ($\mu m^2$) | Size of Artery[a] | Area of Intimal Lesion ($\mu m^2$) | Size of Artery[a] |
| Main | 37 | 109 | 86 | 218 | 107 | 282 |
| Anterior descending | 44 | 118 | 65 | 189 | 102 | 266 |
| Circumflex | 46 | 122 | 107 | 280 | 81 | 192 |

[a]Area of artery as measured by outer limit of medial.

[b]Area of intimal lesion
   to size of artery      R = 0.94
[c]  "          "        "     R = 0.84   } n = 47 for each artery segment
[d]  "          "        "     R = 0.97

Similar observations using slightly different correlation were reported by Bond et al. (17). Although still quite preliminary, this
type of investigation should prove fruitful in elucidating the effects of lesion size, type and shape on the general function of the
circulatory system.

Although some difficulties remain, attempts are underway to resolve
them. Exciting new methods, which should provide superior morphometric data, are being developed rapidly and should soon yield substantial advances in our ability to make quantitative measurements
on the atherosclerotic plaque, both *in vivo* and at autopsy. They
should also help us to interpret qualitative changes in the diseased
artery wall in the living human subject--an advance which should improve choice of therapy, evaluation of therapeutic results and prognosis.

References

1.  McGill HC Jr, Brown BW, Gore I, McMillam GC, Paterson JD,
    Pollak OJ, Roberts JC Jr, Wissler RW (1968) Grading human
    atherosclerotic lesions using a panel of photographs. Report
    of Committee on Grading Lesions, Council on Atherosclerosis.
    Circulation 37:455-459.

2.  Al-Hashimi AS, Williams G (1971) A morphometric method for
    assessment of atherosclerotic lesions. Atherosclerosis 14:
    401-409.

3.  Morgan RS, Adams CWM (1974) A graticule for measuring athero-
    sclerosis. Atherosclerosis 19:347-388.

4.  Howard CF Jr (1979) Aortic atherosclerosis in normal and
    spontaneously diabetic *Macaca nigra*. Atherosclerosis 33:479-
    493.

5.  Cornhill JF, Roach MR (1974) Quantitative method for the evalu-
    ation of atherosclerotic lesions. Atherosclerosis 20:131-136.

6.  Vesselinovitch D, Wissler RW, Schaffner TJ (1982) Quantitation
    of lesions during progression and regression of atherosclerosis
    in rhesus monkeys. In: Nutrition and Heart Disease, Chapter 9,
    SP Medical and Scientific Books, New York.

7.  Blankenhorn DH (1975) Diagnostic methods for the study of
    human atherosclerosis. In: Sirtori C, Ricci C, Gorini S (eds),
    Diet and Atherosclerosis. Plenum, New York, pp. 119-124.

8.  Clarkson TB, Bond MG, Marzetta CA, Bullock BC  (1980)  Approaches
    to the study of atherosclerosis regression in rhesus monkeys:
    Interpretation of morphometric measurements of coronary arteries.
    In:  Grotto AM Jr, Smith LC, Allen B (eds), Atherosclerosis V.
    Springer-Verlag, New York, pp. 739-748.

9.  Vesselinovitch D, Fischer-Dzoga K  (1981)  Techniques in pathology
    in atherosclerosis research.  Advances in Lipid Research 18:
    1-63.

10. Glagov S, Grande J, Vesselinovitch D, Zarins CK  (1981)  Quanti-
    tation of cells and fibers in histologic sections of arterial
    walls:  Advantages of contour tracing on a digitizer plate.  In:
    McDonald TF, Chandler AB (eds), Connective Tissues in Arterial
    and Pulmonary Disease.  Springer-Verlag, New York, pp. 57-93.

11. Zarins CK, Zatina MA, Glagov S  (1982)  Correlation of postmortem
    angiography and pathologic anatomy:  Quantitation of athero-
    sclerotic lesions.  Workshop on Quantitative Evaluation of
    Atherosclerosis, February 22, Silver Spring, Md (in press).

12. Roberts WC  (1977)  Coronary heart disease.  A review of ab-
    normalities observed in the coronary arteries.  Cardiovasc Med.
    2:29-49.

13. Wissler RW, Vesselinovitch D  (1982)  Atherosclerosis--Relation-
    ship to coronary blood flow.  Am J Cardiol (in press).

14. Vesselinovitch D, Wissler RW, Schaffner TJ, Borensztajn J
    (1980)  The effect of various diets on atherogenesis in rhesus
    monkeys.  Atherosclerosis 35:189-207.

15. Wissler RW, Vesselinovitch D, Schaffner TJ, Glagov S  (1980)
    Quantitating rhesus monkey atherosclerosis progression and re-
    gression with time.  In:  Gotto AM, Smith LC, Allen B (eds),
    Atherosclerosis V.  Springer-Verlag, New York, pp. 757-761.

16. Vesselinovitch D, Wissler RW  (1981)  Correlation of types of
    induced lesions with regression of coronary atherosclerosis in
    two species of monkeys.  In:  Noseda G, Fragiacomo C, Fuma-
    galli R, Paoletti R (eds), Lipoproteins and Coronary Athero-
    sclerosis.  Elsevier Biomedical, pp. 401-424.

17. Bond MG, Adams MR, Bullock BC  (1981)  Complicating factors in
    evaluating coronary artery atherosclerosis.  Artery 9:21-29.

Acknowledgments

The authors are grateful for the assistance they have received in
preparing this manuscript from Joan King, Myrtle Tuzar, and Gertrud
Friedman.  They also acknowledge the excellent technical assistance
of Timothy Bridenstine, Laura Harris, and other members of the SCOR
Atherosclerosis staff.

# 1.5 Regression

# Chairman's Introduction to Workshop on Regression

R. W. Wissler

Regression of advanced atherosclerosis has now been well documented in experimental animals and humans (1 - 4). Regression, like the pathological state to which it is applied, is a multifactorial process which seems to take place at varying rates depending on the methods of measurement and/or the plaque components being evaluated (5). The most prominent beneficial aspects of regression of the established atherosclerotic plaque which have been well documented now in the "best" (most human-like) animal models* utilized to study this process are as follows:

1. Smaller overall size of the plaque.
2. Necrotic center decreases or disappears.
3. Intracellular and non fiber-bound extracellular lipid are diminished greatly.
4. Cell proliferation is greatly retarded and number of cells in lesion decrease.
5. Endothelial injury heals.
6. Collagen and elastin become more condensed and decrease relative to anatomical units.
7. Calcium sometimes becomes less prominent.

These changes have been illustrated diagramatically recently (6) and this diagram is reproduced here (Figure 1).

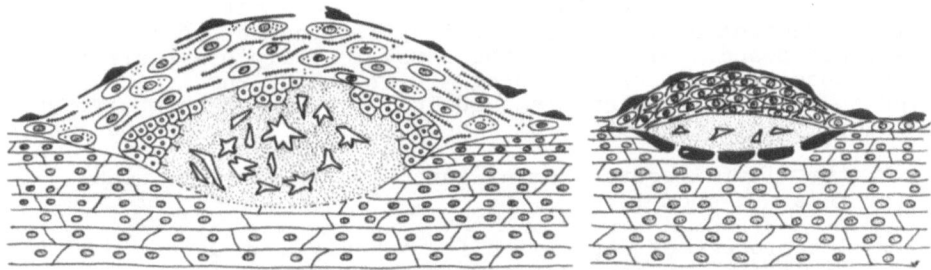

Fig. 1

The rates of these various changes can now be established by sequential studies of regression. We are currently engaged in completing four separate experiments in which all of these parameters and several others besides (most of them biochemical analyses) will be quantitated at four month intervals during both progression and regression. Selected changes with time from one of these experiments, in which both progression and regression were studied, are shown graphically in Figure 2.

---

* rhesus monkey and Yorkshire swine.

184

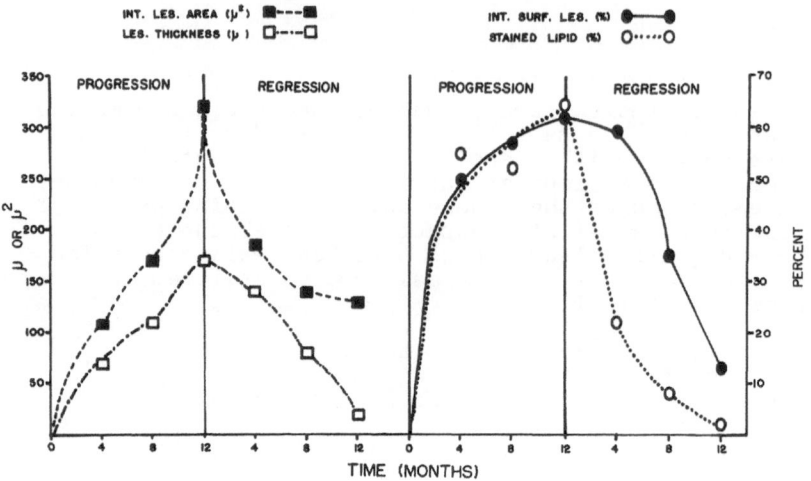

PROGRESSION AND REGRESSION OF AORTIC ATHEROSCLEROSIS
IN RHESUS MONKEYS WITH TIME

Fig. 2

It is evident from the data depicted in this figure that the
various lesion measurements plotted have substantially different
rates of progression and regression as compared to others. Perhaps
the most promising result is the relatively rapid decrease of 50%
of total intimal lesion area in 4 - 5 months. At that time over
80% in the reduction of lesion size which is going to occur in one
year has taken place. Similarly, the removal of lipid appears to
occur much more rapidly than expected. Over 50% of the lipid
deposited in one year has been removed in 3 months and this will go
on to virtually total depletion of excess visible lipid in one year.

Therefore, the first important point which should serve as background for this workshop is:

    ·1.  The process of regression is probably much more
         rapid than we have previously appreciated.
The second important point which should be made by way of introduction is that:

    2.   Concentric, transmural lesions are resistant to
         effective regression (7 - 9) as compared to eccen-
         tric, largely intimal plaques (10).

Fortunately the latter is the common type of advanced lesion observed in human muscular arteries (11, 12). Comparative pathological experiments conducted in this laboratory by Davis,
Vesselinovitch and myself indicate that this resistance to regression in the cynomolgus (M. fascicularis) monkeys is probably
associated with circulating immune complexes*. The resulting athero-
arteritis (10) which others have associated with these kinds of

*Performed in the WHO Reference Laboratories directed by
Dr. Peter Lambert in Geneva, Switzerland.

Table 1.

CONTRAST OF RHESUS AND CYNOMOLGUS RESPONSE INDUCED
BY CONSTANT DIET FED FOR SAME LENGTH OF TIME

| Response | Rhesus | Cynomolgus |
|---|---|---|
| Serum Cholesterol & LDL Elevation | + + + | + + + + |
| Circulating Immune Complex Elevation | ± | + + + |
| Circulating Lipophages | + | + + |
| Monocyte Derived Macrophages in Arterial Lesions | + | + + + + |
| Concentric Pattern of Atheromatous Lesions | + | + + + |
| Transmural Atheromatous Lesions | + | + + + + |
| Arterial Medial Destruction and Inflammation | + | + + + + |
| Arterial Dilatation as Lesion Progresses | + | + + + |
| Arterial Adventitial Foam Cells | ± | + + + |
| Regression of Arterial Atherosclerosis | + + + | + |
| Lumen Increase Following Lipid-Lowering Therapy | + + + | 0 |
| Lumen Decrease Following Lipid-Lowering Therapy | 0 | + to + + |

lesions in lupus, heart transplantation, serum sickness in rabbits, and in other pathological states (13 - 15) is associated with accelerated atherogenesis and very severe lesions in muscular arteries. These types of lesions appear to produce constriction and scarring of the media and narrowing of the lumen when the animals are placed on a serum lipid-lowering diet (7 - 9) - a paradoxical effect compared to most results published relative to the response of the non-human primate plaque to this type of therapy (12).

This workshop is designed to offer maximum opportunity to explore the many unanswered questions about factors which may affect the rate and effectiveness of the regression process, and to survey the current status of regression in human atherosclerotic disease not only as it affects the endothelium and the lumen of the arteries, but also the changes in disease components of the wall of the artery relative to the types of reactions I have just introduced.

References

1.    Armstrong ML (1976) Regression of atherosclerosis, In: Paoletti R, Gotto AM, Jr (eds) Atherosclerosis Reviews, Vol. 1, New York, Raven Press: 137-155

2.    Wissler RW (1978) Current status of regression studies, In: Paoletti R, Gotto AM, Jr (eds) Athero- sclerosis Reviews, Vol. 3, New York, Raven Press: 213 - 245

3.    Malinow MR (1980) Atherosclerosis: Regression in non-human primates, Circ Res 46: 311 - 320

4.      Blankenhorn DH, Sanmarco ME (1979) Angiography for
        study of lipid-lowering therapy, Circ 59: 212 - 214

5.      Vesselinovitch D, Wissler RW (1982) Quantitation of certain
        qualitative differences in atherosclerotic lesions,
        Atherosclerosis VI Procedings (in this same
        volume: Workshop w-5 on June 15, 82)

6.      Wissler RW (1980) Principles of the pathogenesis of
        atherosclerosis  In:  Braunwald E (ed) A Textbook of
        cardiovascular medicine, Philadelphia, WB Saunders Co: 1221
        - 1245

7.      Armstrong ML, Megan MB (1974) Responses of two macaque
        species to atherogenic diet and its withdrawal,  In:
        Schettler G, Weizel A (eds) Atherosclerosis III, New York,
        Springer Verlag: 336 - 338,

8.      Hollander W, Kirkpatrick B, Paddock B, Colombo J, Nagraj M,
        Prusty S (1979) Studies on the progression
        and regression of coronary and peripheral atheroscler-
        osis in the cynomolgus monkey, Exp Mol Pathol 30: 55-73

9.      Vesselinovitch D, Wissler RW (1982) Correlation of
        types of induced lesions with regression of coronary
        atherosclerosis in two species of monkeys, In: Noseda G,
        Fragiacomo C, Formagalli R, Paoletti R (eds) The
        lipoproteins in atherosclerosis, Amsterdam, Elsevier,  401 -
        405
10.     Wissler RW, Vesselinovitch D (1982) Atherosclerosis
        relationship to coronary blood flow, in press In:
        "Proceedings of Sixth Triennial Australian National Heart
        Foundation Conference on Physiology and Pathology of
        Coronary Heart Disease", Supplement of Am J Cardiol

11.     Roberts WC (1975) The coronary arteries in coronary heart
        disease, morphologic observations, Pathobiol Ann 5: 249 -
        282

12.     Roberts WC (1977) Review of abnormalities observed in the
        coronary arteries, Cardiovasc Med 2: 29 - 49

13.     Tsakraklides VG, Blieden LC, Edwards JE (1973) Coronary
        atherosclerosis and myocardial infarction associated with
        systemic lupus erythematosis, Am Heart J 87: 637 - 650

14.     Minick CR, Murphy GE (1973) Experimental induction of
        atheroarteriosclerosis by the synergy of allergic injury to
        arteries and lipid rich diet. II Effect of repeatedly
        injected foreign protein in rabbits fed a lipid-rich, choles-
        terol-poor diet, Am J Pathol 73: 265 - 300

15.     Alonso DR, Starek PK, Minick CR (1977) Studies on the
        pathogenesis of atheroarteriosclerosis induced in rabbit
        cardiac allografts by the synergy of graft rejection and
        hypercholesterolemia, Am J Pathol 87: 415 - 442

# Preliminary Report on Coronary Lesions and Serum Lipids Before and After 2 Years Dietary Intervention in 22 Patients

A. C. Arntzenius[1], J. D. Barth[2], A. V. G. Bruschke[3], B. Buis[1], C. M. van Gent[4], U. M. T. Houtsmuller[5], N. Kempen-Voogd[6], D. Kromhout[7], J. H. C. Reiber[2], S. Strikwerda[1], E. A. van der Velde[8], and L. A. van Wezel[6]

## Introduction

It is of importance to examine if certain interventional procedures can possibly influence the rate of progress of coronary sclerosis in man. In femoral atherosclerosis, Blankenhorn has already shown that computer estimate of atherosclerosis percent change was significantly correlated with triglyceride and cholesterol level (1). Recently Blankenhorn has also shown that coronary atherosclerosis regression studies can be done with computer processed angiograms and, that comparison between human and computer measures on diameter stenosis can be satisfactory (2). The importance of the influence of the diet on coronary atherosclerosis has recently once more been underscored in an impressive way by the study of Hjermann et al, where it was shown in middle-aged men at high risk of CHD that advice to change eating habits and to stop smoking significantly reduced the incidence of the first event of myocardial infarction and sudden death (3).

The aim of the study on which we here report and which was originally triggered off by the publication of Barndt et al (4), was to examine the possible influence of dietary intervention on coronary sclerotic narrowing in patients with known angina who were for some reason not going to be operated upon. Ideally for such intervention study one would try and make use of a control group of patients. Practically this proved to be impossible as outlined in the paragraph on patient selection. It was therefore felt that comparison first and second coronary angiograms should perhaps be made as reliable as possible by having two techniques of "reading" cineangio. One was done by human eye: two independent cardiologists not involved in the study and not knowing sequence of films, both of the Dept. of Cardiology, St. Antonius Hospital Utrecht (chief Dr. A.V.G. Bruschke) and the second by the computer-based Coronary Angiography Analysis System, developed by J.H.C. Reiber Ph.D. at Thorax Center (chief Prof. P.G. Hugenholtz), Erasmus University, Rotterdam.

## Patient selection

We studied 53 patients who in 1977/1978 had been examined clinically because of angina of effort. Their coronary angiograms showed at least symptoms of 50% narrowing in at least one vessel. Coronary by-pass surgery had not been recommended to them, either because coronary arteries were technically not suitable, or because of poor left ventricular contraction patterns, or because of patients having one vessel disease only.

1. Dept. of Cardiology, Leiden University, Leiden
2. Thorax Center, Erasmus University, Rotterdam
3. St. Antonius Hospital, Utrecht
4. Gaubius TNO Research Laboratory, Leiden
5. Unilever Research Laboratory, Vlaardingen
6. Dietician
7. Dept. Social Medicine, Leiden University, Leiden
8. Dept. of Medical Statistics, Leiden University, Leiden

On two mornings with fortnight in between, patients had been given
information about purpose of study, dietary intervention and blood
sampling, as well as the need to have a repeat angiogram after two
years of dieting. The 53 patients gave their consent for the study.
On the two mornings each time blood samples (S.cholesterol, HDL cholesterol and fatty acid pattern of cholesterol esters), body weight,
physical examination, blood pressure and 12-lead ECG were taken for
baseline reading.
All 53 patients were seen regularly at the out patient clinic: every
4 weeks in first half a year, and in following 18 month period bi-
monthly. Blood samples in first half a year were taken every two
month, later every 4 month. After two years of dietary intervention
patients were admitted to the hospital where repeat coronary angiograms were carried out and final blood samples were taken. Drug
treatment was as usual and individually tailored. Patients were adviced to refrain from smoking but ceasing to smoke was no prerequisite for the study.
We tried to set up a control group but met with problems. First and
foremost it was unfair to expect some 50 patients of a possible control group to come for regular visits and then not counsel them on
diet etc. We therefore chose to find matched patients for age, sex
and symptoms in whom two years earlier angina symptoms had prompted
coronary angiography, showing at least 50% narrowing. Patients, in
whom no bypass surgery was to be carried out. When the matched controls were asked consent for repeat coronary angio the response was
poor (50%) and blood examination of those who came revealed that they,
like the intervention group had high levels of linoleic acid content
of cholesterol esters: they had been dieting to much the same degree.

## Methods

### Diet

Diet was vegetarian with 30 to 40 energy % fat content, half of
which consisted of linoleic acid. Cholesterol was limited to less
then 100 mg/day and great care was taken by two dieticians, who in-
terviewed and adviced patients at each out patients visit, that diet
contained sufficient proteins and vitamins. We hope later to publish
on the relation of diet and lipoproteins and fatty acids content of
cholesterol esters of patients examined.

### Laboratory tests on lipid variables

Measurements of S.lipids and lipoprotein were carried out at Gaubius
TNO Research Institute, Leiden. Serum HDL - cholesterol was determined after precipitation of other lipoproteins with magnesium-phos-
photungstate and determination of cholesterol in the supernatant.
The method results were within recommended ranges of Lipids Research Centers of Prague and Atlanta. S. triglycerides were not determined because patients coming from far could not be expected to
to arrive in a fasting state. Fatty acid pattern of cholesterol esters was determined at Unilever Research Laboratory, Vlaardingen,
using thin layer chromatography and gaschromatography.

### Non-lipid variables

Age, sex, relative body weight, blood pressure, smoking and ECG. On
the latter both the Minnesota code and the Cardiac Injury Score were
applied on the 9 ECG's taken of each participant prior and during
the 2 year intervention period.

## Coronary angiography

Clinical left ventricular and coronary cineangiogram were obtained in routine fashion, using the Judkins technique via percutaneous transfemoral catheterisation. Angiograms were recorded on 35 mm film using the 6-inch field of a Philips image intensifier. In addition to right and left anterior oblique projection, craniocaudal projections were used in all cases. Great care was taken to ensure no appreciable differences with regard to angles of projections used.

## Human reading of coronary projector angiograms (St.Antonius Hospital Utrecht)

Independently two cardiologists not involved in the study and not knowing sequence of films, compared both angiograms (viewed on a Tago Arno projector) of each patient. Obstructions were estimated and recorded in percent narrowing of luminal diameter on a 5% step scale. In the Utrecht coding system the coronary tree is divided into 32 segments (5). Collateral pathways also were noted down but narrowings in them were not quantified.

## Leiden scoring system applied to human reading of percentage narrowing of luminal diameter.

Blankenhorn has pointed out that scoring coronary narrowing by lump estimates of the degree of the stenosis into groups such as 0 - 25 percent, 25 - 50 percent, etc. is not satisfactory for the study of lesion change (2). Our scoring system therefore was based on the 5% step values of the maximally 32 segments present, as noted down by the human readers in Utrecht.

A scoring system was developed by which in each of the 3 main vessels the patency percentage is calculated for each abnormal site. Whenever (which frequently is the case) two obstructions are seen one behind the other, the two patency percentages are multiplied with one another so as to arrive at a score for each succeeding segment. An example of calculating the score for 3 obstructions in one right coronary artery is given underneath fig.1.

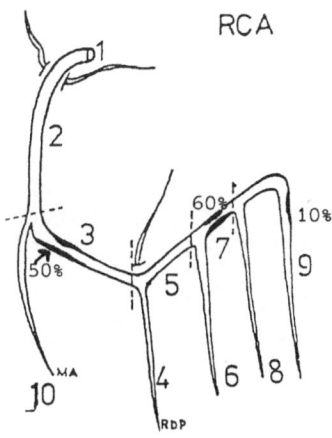

Example of calculating Leiden scoring system applied to Right Coronary Artery (RCA) with 50% narrowing of segment 3, 60% of segment 7 and 10% of segment 9. Patency through to sector 4 will be 0.5, to sector 6 also 0.5. Sector 8 will get blood through 0.5 x 0.4 = 0.2 patency, sector 9 will have 0.5 x 0.4 x 0.9 = 0.18 and sector 10 will have 1.0.
RCA score will thus be

$$1 - \frac{0.5+0.5+0.2+0.18+1}{5} \quad \text{or } 52\%$$

Fig. 1

Computer-based Coronary Angiography Analysis System (Thorax Center, Erasmus University, Rotterdam)

Coronary cineangiograms were analyzed quantitatively with the computer-based Coronary Angiography Analysis System (6). Selected cine-
frames are converted into video format with a video camera and selected regions of interest can be digitized and stored in the PDP 11/44
computer for subsequent processing. User-interaction consists of indicating a number of centerline positions within a arterial segment
to be analyzed; the contours of the segment are then detected auto-
matically. From these contour positions the diameter function of the
segment is computed. The diameter values are given in absolute
values (mm), since the contrast catheter is used as a scaling device.
The severity of an obstruction is expressed as a percentage diameter
reduction with respect to a user-defined reference position and by
means of the absolute value of the minimal obstruction diameter
(Fig. 2.) For arterial segments without any obstruction the mean
diameter value is computed.

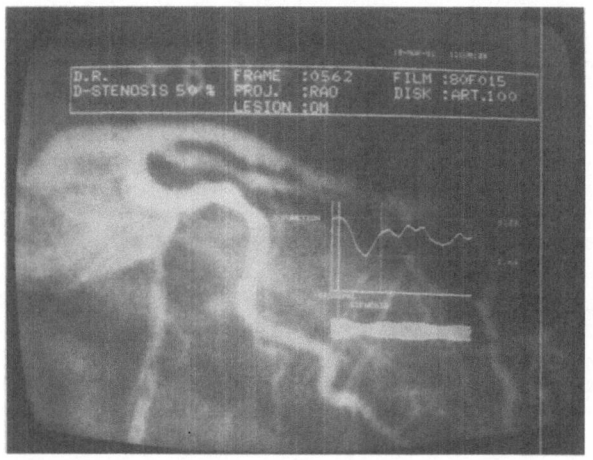

Fig. 2

Example of selected cineframe of the left coronary artery in the RAO
30 projection with computer output of the analyzed lesion in the
obtuse   marginal branch. The diameter narrowing is 50%.

Rotterdam scoring system

The large coronary arteries are divided into a total of 9 coronary
segments and for each coronary segment the severity of an obstruction
is computed, if present, as well as one or more mean diameter values.
From all the data two scores are derived, a percentage coronary score
and an absolute coronary score. The percentage score is determined
as follows: for each obstruction the percentage area stenosis is computed from the percentage diameter stenosis assessed from two projections, assuming elliptical cross sections, and multiplied with a
flow dependent weighting factor specific for that particular coronary segment (7). The total percentage coronary score is obtained by
adding these weighted area stenosis values for all the obstructions
in the large coronary arteries.
The absolute coronary score is determined as follows: for each of
the large coronary arteries (RCA, Main, LAD, Cx) the mean obstruction diameter in mm is computed. If there is no obstruction present

in the artery the mean value of the computed average diameter
measurements for the different segments of this artery is substituted. Adding these 4 mean diameter values results in the absolute
coronary score.
The changes in the percentage and absolute coronary scores over the
two year diet period are simply determined as the differences in the
pre- and post- diet coronary scores.

## Results

53 patients with angina and coronary obstructions of at least 50% in
one vessel entered the study. In 2 yrs of study period 4 patients
died (3 during acute myocardial infarction, 1 suddenly). Seven
patients underwent bypass-surgical procedures, because of increasing
symptoms of angina pectoris not responding satisfactorily to drug
treatment. In 3 patients no second coronary angiogram was carried
out: two patients developed a malignancy, the third refused a second
cine angio to be made.
Data on 22 of 39 remaining patients are now available and some results are presented in this preliminary report. Serum lipids and lipoprotein were measured twice with two weeks interval prior to intervention, the mean of which is called initial value.  The mean
of the 8 values obtained during 2 years of dietary intervention period are given as mean 2 years.

|  | Initial value | mean 2 yrs | P | |
|---|---|---|---|---|
| S. cholesterol (mmol/l) | 6.96 | 6.05 | <0.001 | (fig. 3) |
| HDL cholesterol(mmol/l) | 1.02 | 0.99 | ns | |
| $\frac{\text{S. cholesterol}}{\text{HDL cholesterol}}$ | 7.05 | 6.24 | <0.01 | (fig. 4) |
| Linoleic acid content of chol.esters | 52.17% | 60.69% | <0.001 | (fig. 5) |

## Changes in coronary obstructions

Preliminary results of comparison of stenotic lesions between first
coronary angiogram, prior to intervention and second angiogram after
two years of dietary intervention. With human reading of 32 segments
of coronary tree by St. Antonius Hospital Utrecht, to which the
Leiden scoring system is applied, initial value is 50.98 and after
2 years final value amounts to 58.15 which implies a significant
rate of progression of the mean of the coronary changes with P=0.002.
With complete reading of 9 coronary segments of the first and last
coronary angiograms the mean change of the absolute value of the
coronary diameter score proved to be -0.58 mm, which is a not significant decrease in diameters.
And when the percentage score is applied, again on computer aided
reading, the values are 4.3% and 4.6% respectively (P=0.12).
Variability of rate of atherosclerosis change from one person to the
next was great. Whatever reading or scoring system was used: in
quite a few patients the coronary narrowing progressed considerably
and in some there was slight regression seen, or at least no lesion
growth. It was also sometimes noted that in one patient one segment
would show progress of sclerosis and another would show slight regression.
With human reading and scoring in 8/22 patients no lesion growth
was noted and with computer aided  percentage as well as absolute
measurements 7/22 patients showed no lesion growth.

## Correlations

Comparison of human and computer measures:
Of the initial angiograms there proved to be a correlation between
the scores of the human reading and the computer system (percentage
narrowing) with r = 0.73 (P = 0.002), see fig. 6.

Relation between changes in angiograms and mean 2 years levels of
blood lipids:
Changes in human scores between first and second coronary angiograms
proved to be correlated to mean 2 year value of S .cholesterol/HDL-
cholesterol with r = 0.57 (P = 0.001), see fig. 7.

No significant correlation was found so far between changes in computer scores of coronary narrowing and mean 2 year value of
S. cholesterol/HDL-cholesterol.

## Discussion

### Preliminary results only

With the data as presented here of a diet intervention study on 53
anginal patients one should keep in mind that results are only available on 22 of the 39 patients who finished the study without surgical intervention. The rate of progression of atheromatous lesions in
general will show great individual variations and may also vary in
the same individual at different times and at different vascular
regions as Nikkilä has pointed out (8). Great care should therefore
be taken not to overinterpret results. The individual responses to
diet in our study also varied a great deal: some patients developing
slight signs of regression of atherosclerosis or at least suppression of atherosclerotic lesion growth and on the other hand around
66% of the patients showing either moderate or sometimes severe progression of obstruction.
Authors feel that the great individual variation in the rate of
progression can perhaps be "understood" to a certain degree when one
accepts that coronary obstruction is influenced on the one hand by a
very slow process called atheroma which will take between 20 and 30
years to reach significant obstruction of the coronary vessel and on
the other hand by fast processes such as spasm, platelet aggregation,
bleeding in vessel wall or in atheroma and thrombosis: fast processes, which in the course of days or even hours may increase the
degree of obstruction by 50 or more %. Until we are able not only to
measure coronary diameters but as well to gain information on the bulk,
consistency or exact 3-dimensional configuration of lesions, it will not
easily be possible to differentiate the fast from the slow process.
Also, quite clearly, once non-invasive methods are developed to
measure the atherosclerotic lesion at an early stage, much insight
into understanding of growth as well as treatment of atheroma will
be gained.

With the results of a weak correlation between computerised measurements and human eye reading of coronary angiograms it is well to remember that the computer reading is carried out on 9 segments whereas in Utrecht, Dr. Bruschke and co-workers looked at and coded all
lesions in a total of 32 segments, which takes the small branches as
well into account.

There appears to be a weak but significant association between changes of coronary narrowing (as read by the human eye) and mean 2 year
S. cholesterol/HDL cholesterol values. If this keeps up when the
data on the 39 patients are vailable, firm ground is gained for diet-

coronary relationship and hopefully it may next inspire further clinical studies to be set up on the same topic.
There is no doubt that the 22 patients (as did the total group of 53) kept to the diet in an exemplary fashion. The data on changes of linoleic acid content in cholesterol esters warrant this statement.

Authors want to thank the patients of the Leiden intervention study who made it all possible.

Acknowledgements. Authors want to thank for their help C. Groen, J. Hillers, J. Kraal, A. Kramp, J.H.M. Moorrees, L. de Pagter, H.L. Roeters van Lennep, R. van Schie, H. v.d. Voort.

## References

1. Blankenhorn DH, Brooks SH, Selzer RH, Barndt R (1978) The rate of atherosclerosis change during treatment of hyperlipoproteinemia. Circulation vol 57 no 2: 355-361.
2. Blankenhorn DH, Cashin WL, Selzer RH, Brooks SH (1982) Human coronary atherosclerosis regression studies with computer processed angiograms. In: Lipoproteins and Coronary Atherosclerosis. Editors: G Noseda, C Fragiacomo, R Fumagalli, R Paoletti. Elsevier Biomedical.
3. Hjermann I, Holme I, Velve Byre K, Leren P (1981) Effect on diet and smoking intervention on the incidence of coronary heart disease. The Lancet, 12 Dec: 1303-1310.
4. Barndt R, Blankenhorn DH, Crawford DW, Brooks SH (1977) Regression and progression of early femoral atherosclerosis in treated hyperlipoproteinemic patients. Ann. of Internal Medicine 86: 139-146.
5. Bruschke AVG, Wijers TS, Kolsters W, Landman J (1981) The anatomic evolution of coronary artery disease demonstrated by coronary arteriography in 256 nonoperated patients. Circulation vol 63 no 3: 527-536.
6. Reiber JHC, Gerbrands JJ, Booman F, Troost GJ, Den Boer A, Slager CJ, Schuurbiers JCH (1982) Objective characterization of coronary obstruction from monoplane cineangiograms and three dimensional reconstruction of an arterial segment from two orthogonal views. In: Applications of computers in Medicine. Edited by MD Schwartz. IEEE. Cathalogue nr: TH0095-0. pages 93-100.
7. Leman DM, Brower RW, Meester GT, Serruys P, van den Brand M (1981) Coronary artery atherosclerosis: severity of the disease, severity of angina pectoris and compromised left ventricular funktion. Circulation vol 63 no 2: 285-292.
8. Nikkilä EA (1981) Is human atherosclerosis reversible? In: Lipoproteins, Atherosclerosis and Coronary Heart Disease. Editors: N.E. Miller and B. Lewis. Elsevier/North Holland Biomedical Press Amsterdam: 155-164.

194

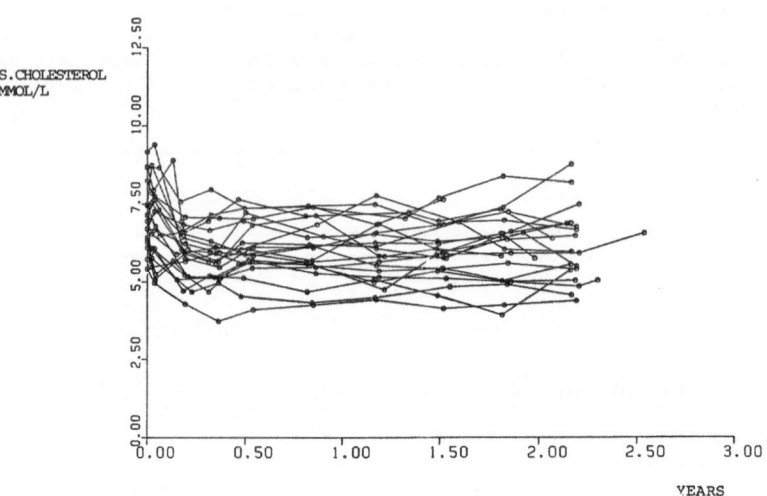

Fig. 3

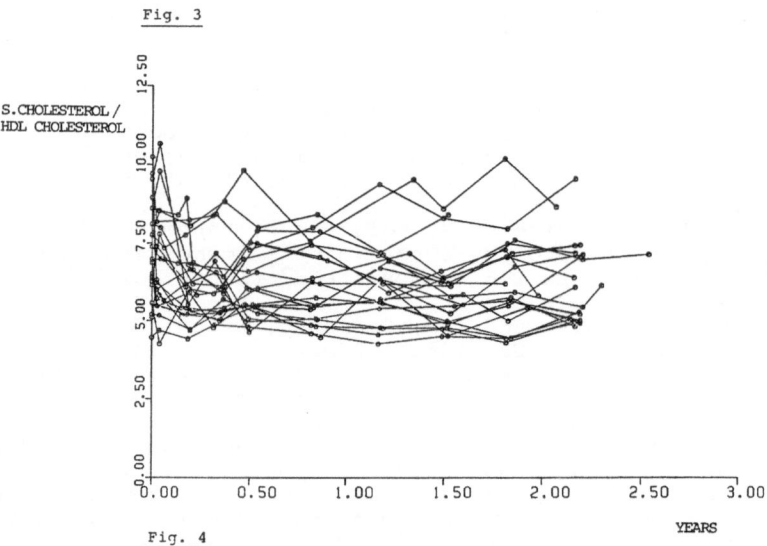

Fig. 4

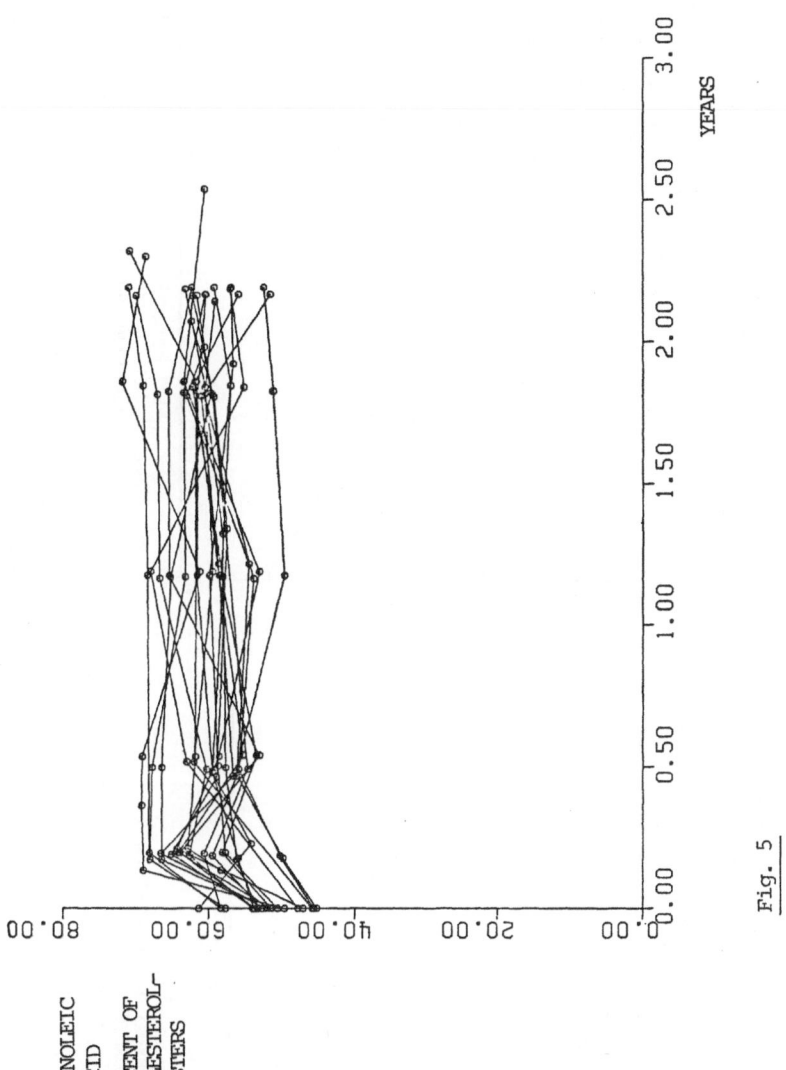

Fig. 5

196

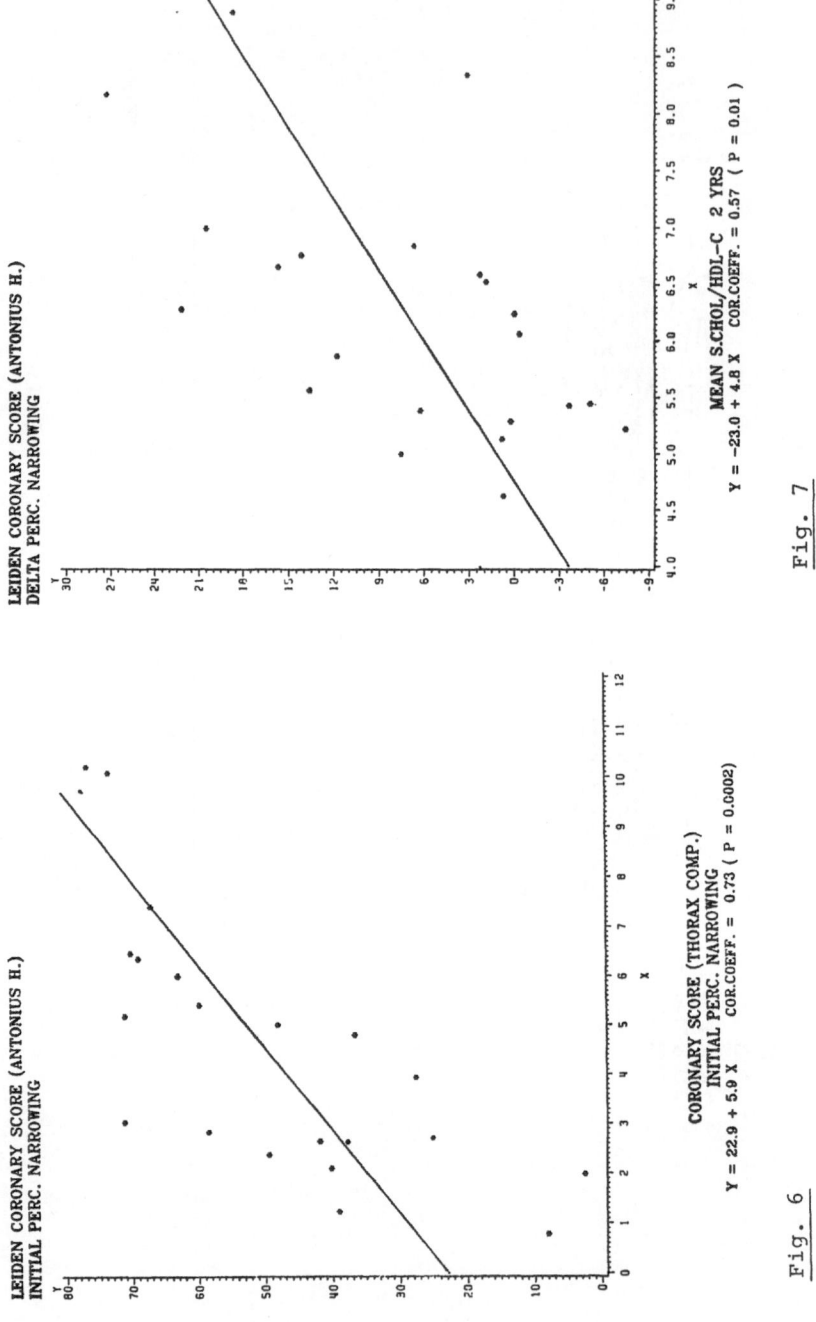

LEIDEN CORONARY SCORE (ANTONIUS H.)
DELTA PERC. NARROWING

X
MEAN S.CHOL/HDL-C  2 YRS
Y = -23.0 + 4.8 X    COR.COEFF. = 0.57  ( P = 0.01 )

Fig. 7

LEIDEN CORONARY SCORE (ANTONIUS H.)
INITIAL PERC. NARROWING

X
CORONARY SCORE (THORAX COMP.)
INITIAL PERC. NARROWING
Y = 22.9 + 5.9 X    COR.COEFF. = 0.73  ( P = 0.0002)

Fig. 6

# Measurement of Atherosclerosis by Arteriography and Microdensitometry: Model and Clinical Investigations

U. Erikson, G. Helmius, A. Hemmingsson, G. Ruhn, and A. G. Olsson

## Introduction

In recent years it has become clear that the use of clinical end
points such as myocardial infarcts as a measure of the effect of
serum lipid lowering carry considerable drawbacks, although it is
the final goal of the preventive treatment. To get a more direct
estimate of the effect of the treatment on the target - the atheroma
- methods have been developed to quantitate small atheroma present
in vivo in human beings (1). The present ongoing study uses as end
point sequential computer estimated femoral atherosclerosis derived
from arteriography. Asymptomatic men with massive hyperlipidaemia
have been treated vigorously with potent serum lipid lowering drugs.
Here we describe the angiographic and densitometric procedure and
report the effect on atheroma development in the first eight consecutive cases treated with diet and drugs.

## Material and methods

### Subjects

The eight men are the first in a series of sixty asymptomatic men
in the age of 40 to 60 years presenting hyperlipidaemia at a health
control. Men who at repeated serum lipid analysis have fasting
serum cholesterol above 9.00 mmol/l and/or serum triglycerides (TG)
above 3.5 mmol/l are admitted to the metabolic ward for further
examination. No subjects are hypertensive or diabetic.

### Design of study

The study has a single blind design. After the first angiogram all
subjects are treated with a moderate serum lipid lowering diet (2)
for six months when a second angiogram is performed. Half of the
patients are then randomly allocated either to active treatment
with a combination of fenofibrate 200 mg x 2 and nicotinic acid in
the starting dose of 1 g 4 times daily (3) or to placebo treatment.
In case of insufficient lipid lowering effect the nicotinic acid
dose may be increased. Angiograms are then performed after 6, 12
and 24 months on drug treatment.

### Chemical methods

Serum lipids and lipoproteins were determined according to routine
procedures of the laboratory (4). Typing of hyperlipidaemia was performed according to WHO (5).

### Arteriography

Femoral arteriography followed the routine at the Department with
the following specifications: The focal spot was 0.1 x 0.1 mm,
focus film distance 87 cm and leg-film distance 48 cm; enlargement

2.2. An AOT film changer 24 x 30 cm with a coal fiber top (Siemens, Stockholm) was used. In most cases the settings were 90 kV, 32 mA and 0.64 s and 1 film/s during 7 s. The screens were Lanex fine (Kodak), the film Orto G (Kodak) and no grid was used.

By an automatic contrast injector (Medrad, Pittsburg, USA) 20 ml of Urografin 45% (220 mg I/ml) was injected by a speed of 10 ml/s. In addition an intraarterial injection of prostaglandin $E_1$ was performed, with a dose rate of 0.005 mg/ml (conc. 0.005 mg/ml) during about 3 min., immediately followed by an additional arteriography (6).

## Densitometric procedures

Scan procedure:
The region of interest, i.e. the femoral artery in the adductor channel, was outlined on the angiogram. The area was 50-80 x 30 mm, corresponding to an actual area of 23-36 x 14 mm due to the optical enlargement 2.2x. The optical densities in the region of interest were analysed by means of a drumscanner. Photoscan System P-1000 (Optronix International Inc, Chelmsford, Massachusetts, USA). Every individual measuring area was 200 x 200 μm on the angiogram, corresponding to a real area of 90 x 90 μm. The scans were placed 200 μm apart. The density values were stored on a floppy-disc (Norsk Data, Oslo, Norway).

Computer analysis:
From the floppy-disc every scan was displayed as a density profile on a graphic display unit Tektronix 4006-1 (Tektronix, Beaverton, Oregon, USA). The inflexion points from the density profile were defined as edges of the artery. These points and the background densities were entered into the computer to calculate the chord lengths of the artery (1).

The cross sectional area for each scan was calculated from a formula according to Crawford et al. (1). From all cross sectional areas the longitudinal lumen of the vessel was determined as a curve. A line was drawn between parts of the curve which had the largest cross sectional areas. These cross sectional areas were defined as normal vessel. The amount of atherosclerosis was defined as the enclosed area between this line and the longitudinal curve, as measured with planimetry.

This enclosed area is a relative value of the amount of atherosclerosis (atherosclerosis estimation, AE) and is given in radiological units (RU) k x $mm^3$. Investigations were performed correlating the AE with real lumen decrease in phantoms and the correlation coefficient obtained was 0.99 (7).

The atherosclerosis quantitation procedure was performed in randomized order without knowledge of at what stage of the study each angiogram had been made.

To improve the visualization of the artery changes the density-profiles are superposed to a three-dimensional picture (Fig. 1).

## Results

Of the eight men one was typed as having a type II A, six as type II B and one as type IV hyperlipoproteinaemia. The mean serum lipo-

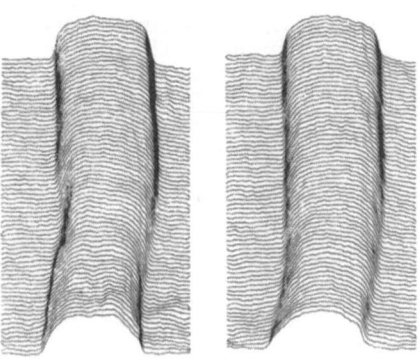

Figure 1. Visualization by computer of atheromatous femoral artery in one of the eight patients. In the left panel the artery before drug treatment on Sept. 20, 1979, shows irregularities suggesting early atherosclerosis. On Oct. 30, 1980, after one year of pronounced lipid lowering irregularities have disappeared suggesting regression (right panel).

protein concentrations before, during dietary treatment and during the combined treatment with diet, fenofibrate and nicotinic acid is given in Table 1. The mean body weight decreased significantly by about 2 kg during the dietary treatment and remained at a lower level during the drug treatment. Small decreases in total cholesterol and triglycerides were noted on diet alone. The only lipoprotein changing significantly during diet was very low density lipoprotein (VLDL) triglycerides.

Table 1. Mean serum lipid (TG = triglycerides, Chol = cholesterol) and lipoprotein concentrations (+SEM) before the study, during six months of dietary treatment and during one year of treatment with fenofibrate and nicotinic acid in 8 asymptomatic men.

| | Total | | VLDL | LDL | HDL |
|---|---|---|---|---|---|
| | TG | Chol | TG | Chol | Chol |
| Before | 3.26+0.93 | 10.10+0.16 | 2.93+0.64 | 7.15+0.37 | 1.47+0.11 |
| Diet | 2.74+0.58 | 9.49+0.32 | $1.57+0.42^{xx}$ | 6.92+0.48 | 1.60+0.08 |
| Drugs | $1.18+0.14^{x}$ | $6.17+0.29^{xxx}$ | $0.53+0.11^{xxx}$ | $3.93+0.23^{xxx}$ | $1.93+0.17^{xxx}$ |

Drug treatment induced dramatic changes in serum lipids and lipoproteins, serum total triglycerides and cholesterol decreasing by 64 and 39 percent respectively. VLDL triglycerides and low density lipoprotein (LDL) cholesterol decreased by 82 and 45 percent respectively, while high density lipoprotein (HDL) cholesterol increased by 31 percent.

Mean times between angiograms during dietary and dietary + drug treatment were 7 (range 6 to 8) and 12.5 (7 to 18) months respectively. Although asymptomatic all subjects had varying amounts of atherosclerosis in the femoral arteries. Mean monthly change in AE during diet alone was 0.05+0.05 (SEM) k x $mm^3$ (n=3, n.s.) and during drug treatment -0.12+0.05 k x $mm^3$ which was significantly different from 0 on the 5 percent level. The individual changes in AE is given in Figure 2. During drug treatment AE decreased in 6 of the 8 cases. The serum lipoprotein concentrations and concentration

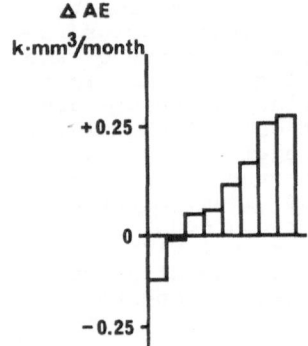

Figure 2. Individual changes in AE/month in the eight patients (positive sign = decrease in AE, negative sign = increase in AE).

changes during drug treatment were correlated to changes in AE. The r-values for VLDL triglycerides and LDL cholesterol decreases and AE decreases were 0.07 and 0.41 respectively and between HDL cholesterol increase and AE decrease 0.10. The r-values for VLDL triglyceride and LDL and HDL cholesterol concentrations during treatment and AE decreases were -0.20, -0.50 and 0.29 respectively. No correlation was so far significant but tendencies showed that decreases of elevated LDL cholesterol levels and low LDL cholesterol concentrations seem to be of greatest importance to achieve regression of early femoral atherosclerosis.

## Comment

Little is known at present regarding the natural course of atheroma development in femoral (and coronary) atherosclerosis. The present finding of significant decrease of AE over one year's pronounced serum lipid lowering in asymptomatic hyperlipidaemic men needs to be put in relation what happens in the same category of patients whose serum lipids are not affected. This will be made possible with the use of control group in this study. More subjects must be studied to see whether significant correlations exist between serum lipoprotein changes and changes in atheroma development.

*Acknowledgements.* The work was supported by grants from Cilag Chemie Stiftung, Swedish Medical Research Council (19X-204), Tore Nilson's Fund for Medical Research, Swedish National Association against Heart and Lung Diseases, Albert and Gerda Svensson's Fund, Loo and Hans Osterman's Fund, Nordisk Insulinfond and Åke Wibergs Stiftelse.

## References

1. Crawford DW, Brooks SH, Selzer RH, Barndt Jr R, Beckenbach ES, Blankenhorn DH (1977) Computer densitometry for angiographic assessment of arterial cholesterol content and gross pathology in human atherosclerosis. J Lab clin Med 89: 378-392.
2. Fredrickson DS, Levy RI, Jones E, Bonnell M, Ernst N (1971) Dietary management of hyperlipoproteinemia. NHLBI Bethesda, Maryland.

3. Rössner S, Olsson·AG (1980) Effects of combined procetofene -
   nicotinic acid thearpy in treatment of hypertriglyceridaemia.
   Atherosclerosis 35: 413-417
4. Carlson K (1973) Lipoprotein fractionation. J clin Path, 26,
   suppl (Ass Clin Path) 5: 32-37
5. Beaumont JL, Carlson LA, Cooper GR, Fejfar Z, Fredrickson DS,
   Strasser T (1970) Classification of hyperlipidaemias and hyperlipoproteinaemias. Bull Wld Hlth Org 43: 891-915
6. Carlson LA, Ericsson M, Erikson U (1973) Prostaglandin $E_1$
   ($PGE_1$) in peripheral arteriographies. Acta Radiol 14: 583-587
7. Ruhn G, Erikson U, Helmius G, Hemmingsson A (1982) Computerized
   quantitation of atherosclerosis by arteriography and micro-
   densitometry - A model study. Acta Radiol, in press

# Role of Macrophages in Regression of Swine Atherosclerosis

K. E. Fritz, A. S. Daoud, and J. Jarmolych

## A. Presence of Macrophages in Lesions during Regression

Over the years numerous investigators have noted the presence of macrophages or "macrophage-like cells" in arterial lesions in various species in both the progression and regression phases of atherogenesis.
Using various combinations of enzyme histochemistry and immune adherence tests on light and/or electron microscopic levels, some information as to the prevalence of cells with at least some of the characteristics of macrophages in regressing lesions has been obtained. Ultrastructurally, Stary (1) documented in rhesus monkeys a rapid decrease in the number of "macrophage-derived foam cells" within four to
six months after imposition of a regression diet. These findings are
similar to those of Tucker et al (2), who also showed electron microscopically a dramatic decrease in the number of "lipid laden monocytes"
in aortic intimal lesions of rhesus monkeys after a four month regression regimen. Daoud et al (3) showed, in a sequential study of the
changes in swine aortic lesions resulting from withdrawal of an atherogenic diet after a six month induction period, that macrophages, numerous in the baseline lesions, first increased in number in the initial
six weeks of the regression regimen, then decreased after five and fourteen months of regression until they were rare in the latter period.
They were intimately associated with necrosis, and their decrease paralleled the nearly complete disappearance of necrosis by the termination
of the experiment. Histochemical demonstration of non-specific esterase
on the light microscopic level paralleled these findings (4), showing
intensely reactive cells, often near necrotic and/or calcified areas, to
be prevalent in the reference and six week regression lesions, more limited at five months and relatively few at fourteen months of regression,
when no reaction product-containing macrophages were present in the limited samples available for electron microscopy.

## B. Possible Effects of Lesion Macrophages on Regression

These findings raise the important question of what effect(s) the macrophages may be having on the resolution of lesions, since the documented
functions of these cells are so many, varied and wide ranging. For example, they are "professional phagocytes" and, as such, are actively
involved in the resolution of inflammation and/or bacterial infection
(5); they will even phagocytize mineralized calcium (6). Under varying
circumstances they have been shown to synthesize collagen and glycosaminoglycans (GAG) (7), as well as proteinases which will degrade the major extracellular components of the artery wall (8). They secrete an
impressive array of other substances: complement components and acid
hydrolases (9); and peroxidase, superoxide dismutase, enzyme inhibitors
and chemotactic factors (10). Of special interest as regards their role
in atherosclerosis is their secretion of a growth factor which stimulates proliferation of both SMC and endothelial cells (11,12), and of
fibronectin (13), a protein involved in cell adhesion and in non-immune
opsonization of particles for phagocytosis.

These functions suggest that the presence of macrophages may be a "two-edged sword"--beneficial on the one hand, contributing to the resolution of lesions, or, on the other hand, detrimental and exacerbating development of the lesion. As a beneficial function, perhaps primary might be their phagocytic capacity. They may be acting as scavengers of particulate matter--partially degraded cells or extracellular constituents. This function may be enhanced by the macrophage's own production of fibronectin, which, with its affinity sites for collagen, fibrin, GAG and cell membranes, serves as an effective "non-specific" opsonin (14,15). Their extensive potential complement of hydrolytic enzymes may also aid in the resolution of necrosis by degradation of cell- and extracellular substance-derived debris to soluble, and thus diffusible, components. But this same hydrolytic capacity, if directed towards normal arterial wall components, might equally plausibly contribute to the disorganization and degradation typical of lesion development.

The overall effect of the production of collagen and GAG may be debatable. The accumulation of collagen is viewed by some as an unfortunate sequela of atherogenesis, but by others as part of a healing process. Likewise, the secretion of GAG may help restore normal arterial composition. On the other hand, depending on the type and quantity of GAG produced, this may enhance retention of low density lipoprotein in the lesion through the documented affinity of this lipoprotein for several species of GAG (16).

So far we have dealt only with direct functions of macrophages, but their effects via interactions with the other major cell type, SMC, may also be important. The SMC mitogen produced by macrophages may be a major cause of the demonstrated high level of DNA synthesis by lesion cells (17), reflecting a localized high concentration of the mitogen in proximity to the target cells. Experiments in which macrophages secreted a factor which enhanced the production of collagenase by fibroblasts (18) suggest other possible avenues of macrophage influence on lesion cells which have yet to be documented.

Thus far the possible effects of the macrophage in its role as an effector cell in the immune response have not been considered. Yet it is well established that active immunization, as with BCG, will result in nonspecific enhancement of many of the previously mentioned functions of macrophages. This can occur on a systemic basis, or in localized areas of antigen accumulation. The degree of such enhancement or "activation" of lesion macrophages is not known. Yet they may, indeed, reflect the immune status of the host. The possibility of manipulating the overall immune reactivity of an individual as a means of modulating the activity of lesion macrophages is intriguing.

On a more localized level, an activation of lesion macrophages could result from the presence of immune complexes. The demonstration in experimental lesions of the components of a circulating immune complex resulting from a single episode of serum sickness (19) raises the possibility of macrophage activation via binding of the Fc fragment of the immunoglobulin, perhaps through the involvement of C3 derived either from the plasma or secreted by the lesion macrophages, themselves. Perhaps an even more likely source of an immune complex within a lesion would be an altered arterial wall component to which a plasma-derived autoantibody had bound. The presence of autoantibodies which bound selectively to aortic lesions, but not to adjacent normal aortic tissue, has been reported (20). Such insoluble complexes, with C3, might prove chemotactic for, as well as activate macrophages.

Results of the sequential study of regression in swine (3,17) suggest that overall the contribution of the macrophages to the regression process was positive. They were present in large numbers concomitantly with a biochemically defined decrease in cholesterol concentration a decrease in the number of foam cells. Their prominence when necrosis was most marked and their proximity to necrotic areas, combined with the parallel decrease in obvious macrophage involvement and extent of necrosis suggests a role for them in the resolution of necrosis. The documented elevated levels of such hydrolytic enzymatic activities as -glucuronidase and cholesteryl ester hydrolase, in florid progression lesions similar to those seen in early phases of the swine sequential study (3,21), may reflect, in part, the production of these enzymes by lesion macrophages, whether activated or not. The fact that the macrophage population was greatly depleted in the later stages of the regression regimen, even though the lesion size had not decreased, suggests that their greatest importance may lie in the early phases of regression of advanced atheromata, but these conclusions are largely speculative.

## C.  Aspects of Macrophage Involvement which Need to be Addressed

Of prime importance is the problem of identifying, localizing and quantitating the relative numbers of macrophages and/or cells of macrophage origin in lesions. So far, positive identification has been restricted to electron microscopic identification of typical macrophages, and even this approach is not suitable for quantitative study because of the severely limited size and numbers of samples feasible, and the extreme heterogeneity of lesion composition. In situ demonstration of cells of macrophage origin is one obvious goal, since the procedures involved, at least in swine, in releasing cells from lesions cannot be expected to yield representative proportionate data, and may, in fact, alter the surface and/or functional properties on which identification is based. As yet, no absolutely characteristic histochemically definable feature is available. The most desirable approach would be the use of a specific antibody in immunohistochemical and/or cytochemical staining procedures on tissue sections. Indeed, efforts in this direction are under way in several laboratories, most involving the production of monoclonal antibodies using hybridoma techniques. One problem with this approach lies in the fact that most such antibodies are against cell surface antigens, and must be exhaustively tested to document their macrophage specificity. However, it is also entirely possible, in analogy to other cell types, that macrophages express different cell surface antigens at different stages of maturation or under different environmental conditions, so that a given antibody might be useful in identifying only a certain group of macrophage-derived cells. This possibility adds to the complexities and technical problems associated with this admittedly promising approach.

The definition of the state of activation of lesion macrophages is a major question which should be addressed. It is feasible to use Schaffner's technique (22) of releasing cells from lesions by mincing for quantitating the number of cells releasable under standard conditions and their mean phagocytic activity. Enzyme histochemical study of these cells can also give a qualitative assessment of the complement of some enzymes. But the number of such released cells is too small to allow for quantitative biochemical analysis of enzyme activity. An alternative approach, the relevance of which to the activity of lesion macrophages has yet to be demonstrated, is to monitor the enzyme activities of peritoneal or alveolar macrophages. Sufficient macrophages to study several functions can be harvested repeatedly from an individual animal.

Similarly, plasma fibronectin levels can be monitored at various phases of regression.

The immune status of an animal is of importance because of its effect(s) on macrophage activation. One aspect of this is susceptible to assessment, on a systemic basis, by monitoring the serum for the presence of autoantibodies directed against arterial components. Likewise, efforts to modulate the immune response, as by active immunization with BCG, are feasible, and the effect, if any, of such an intervention on the actual regression of atherosclerosis in the experimental animal should be determined. It should be noted that a similar intervention has been reported to be effective in prolonging survival times of patients with early lung cancer (23).

These admittedly indirect approaches to assessing changes in macrophage function, and thus in their contribution to lesion changes during a regression regimen, should provide useful information on the dynamics of the regression process. But investigators should be ever alert to potential new approaches which would allow more direct assessment of lesion macrophage activities.

Acknowledgements   We thank Elsie Collier, Judi Ciani, and John Safarik for expert technical contribution to these studies.

This work was supported by the Veterans Administration and by NIH Grant #HL 20993.

## References

1.  Stary HC, Strong JP, Eggen DA (1980) Differences in the degradation rate of intracellular lipid droplets in the intimal smooth muscle cells and macrophages of regressing atherosclerotic lesions of primates. In: Gotto AM, Smith LC, Allen B (eds) Atherosclerosis V, Springer-Verlag, Berlin-Heidelberg-New York, pp 753-756
2.  Tucker CF, Catsulis C, Strong JP, Eggen DA (1971) Regression of early cholesterol-induced aortic lesions in rhesus monkeys. Amer J Path 65:493-502
3.  Daoud AS, Jarmolych J, Augustyn JM, Fritz KE (1981) Sequential morphologic studies of regression of advanced atherosclerosis. Arch Path Lab Med 105:233-239
4.  Fritz KE, Daoud AS, Jarmolych J (1980) Non-specific esterase activity during regression of swine aortic atherosclerosis. Artery 7: 352-366
5.  Steinman RM, Cohn ZA (1974) The metabolism and physiology of the mononuclear phagocytes. In: Zweifach BW, Grant L, McClusky RT (eds) The Inflammatory Process, Academic Press, New York, San Francisco, London, pp 449-510
6.  Rifkin BR, Baker RL, Somerman MJ, Pointon SE, Coleman SJ, Au WYW (1980) Osteoid resorption by mononuclear cells in vitro. Cell Tiss Res 210:493-500
7.  Kulonen E, Potila M (1980) Macrophages and the synthesis of connective tissue components. Acta Path Microbiol Scand Sect C:7-13
8.  Werb Z, Band MJ, Jones PA (1980) Degradation of connective tissue matrices by macrophages. I. Proteolysis of elastin, glycoproteins and collagen by proteinases isolated from macrophages. J Exp Med 152:1340-1357
9.  Unanue ER (1976) Secretory function of mononuclear phagocytes. Am

J Path 83:396-417

10. Ross R (1981) Atherosclerosis: a problem of the biology of arterial wall cells and their interactions with blood components. Arteriosclerosis 1:293-311

11. Martin BM, Gimbrone MA, Jr, Unanue ER, Cotran RS (1981) Stimulation of nonlymphoid mesenchymal cell proliferation by a macrophage-derived growth factor. J Immuno 126:1510-1515

12. Glenn KC, Ross R (1981) Human monocyte-derived growth factor(s) for mesenchymal cells: activation of secretion by endotoxin and concanavalin A (CON A). Cell 25:603-615

13. Alitalo K, Hovi T, Vaheri A (1980) Fibronectin is produced by human macrophages. J Exp Med 151:602-613

14. Pearlstein E, Gold LI, Garcia-Pardo A (1980) Fibronectin: a review of its structure and biological activity. Mol Cell Biochem 29:103-128

15. Yamada KM, Kennedy DW, Kimata K, Pratt RM (1980) Characterization of fibronectin interactions with glycosaminoglycans and identification of active proteolytic fragments. J Biol Chem 255:6055-6063

16. Bihari-Varga M (1965) Precipitation of complexes formed from mucopolysaccharides and serum $\beta$-lipoprotein with the introduction of metal ions. Acta Clin Acad Sci Hung 45:219-229

17. Fritz KE, Augustyn JM, Jarmolych J, Daoud AS (1981) Sequential study of biochemical changes during regression of swine aortic atherosclerotic lesions. Arch Path Lab Med 105:240-246

18. Huybrechts-Godin G, Hauser P, Vaes G (1979) Macrophage-fibroblast interactions in collagenase production and cartilage degradation. Bioch J 184:643-650

19. Lamberson HV, Jr, Fritz KE (1974) Localization of antigen, antibody and permeability changes in immunologically enhanced rabbit atherosclerosis. Fed Proc 33:235

20. Harper GR, Fritz KE (1974) Demonstration of autoimmunity in experimental atherosclerosis. Circulation 50, Suppl III, 264

21. Fritz KE, Daoud AS, Jarmolych J (1981) Cholesteryl ester hydrolase and $\beta$-glucuronidase activities in swine aortic lesions. Fed Proc 40:351

22. Schaffner T, Taylor K, Bartucci EJ, Fischer-Dzoga K, Beeson JH, Glagov S, Wissler RW (1980) Arterial foam cells with distinctive immunomorphologic and histochemical features of macrophages. Amer J Path 100:57-73

23. McKneally MF, Maver C, Kausel HW, Alley RD (1976) Regional immunotherapy with intrapleural BCG for lung cancer. Surgical considerations. J Thor Cardiovasc Surg 72:335-338

# Potential for Atherosclerosis Regression in Perspective

M. R. Malinow

In closing this part of the workshop, I will contrast atherosclerosis regression in animals and in humans. For this purpose, I
will use, as an illustration of the numerous animal experiments
reported in the last decades, a recent experiment of mine involving
*Macaca fascicularis* (1). For 6 months, 51 monkeys ingested semipuri-
fied food containing about 42% of the calories as fat (mainly
saturated) and 1.2 mg of cholesterol/Cal. At the end of this
induction period, 17 monkeys (group I) were killed for baseline
data. The remaining monkeys were assigned randomly to two groups
(II and III) of 17 animals each. The cholesterol content of the
diet was reduced to 0.3 ml/Cal to bring cholesterolemia to the
300-400 mg/dl level in the positive control group (II). In the
intervention group (III), the same diet also contained 1.2% of an
extract of alfalfa hay--operationally termed *alfalfa saponins* (2).
The monkeys were observed for the next 18 months, and the extent
of atherosclerosis was determined. Table 1 indicates the extents

Table 1. Aortic and coronary atherosclerosis[a] in *Macaca fascicularis*[b]

| Group | | Number of animals | Aortic atherosclerosis (+ to 5+)[c] | Coronary atherosclerosis (maximum % lumen encroachment)[d] |
|---|---|---|---|---|
| I | induction | 17 | $3.7 \pm 0.2$ | $24.7 \pm 4.3$ |
| II | intervention (controls) | 17 | $3.1 \pm 0.3$ | $19.5 \pm 4.3$ |
| III | intervention (saponins) | 17 | $2.4 \pm 0.2$ | $11.1 \pm 2.7$ |

[a]Data given as means $\pm$ SE

[b]Taken from Malinow et al. (in press) (1)

[c]Kruskal-Wallis test: the three groups are significantly different.
$P$ (Wilcoxon-Mann-Whitney statistics): I versus II, not significant; I versus III and II versus III, $< 0.05$

[d]$P$ (Student's $t$ test): I versus II and II versus III, nonsignificant; I versus III, $< 0.01$

of aortic and coronary atherosclerosis in the three groups. Figure
1 shows the extent of sudanophilia in the aortas of monkeys from
groups I and III. Figure 2 shows sections of coronary arteries
that are representative for the same groups. These results demonstrate that aortic and coronary atherosclerosis regressed in the
monkeys receiving alfalfa saponins. Extensive hematologic,

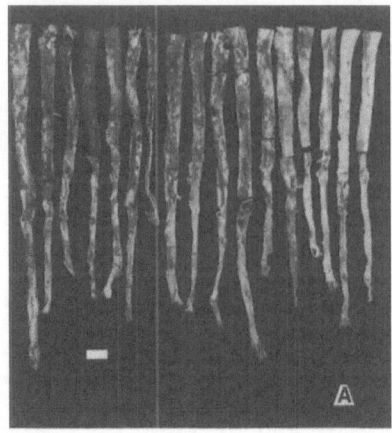
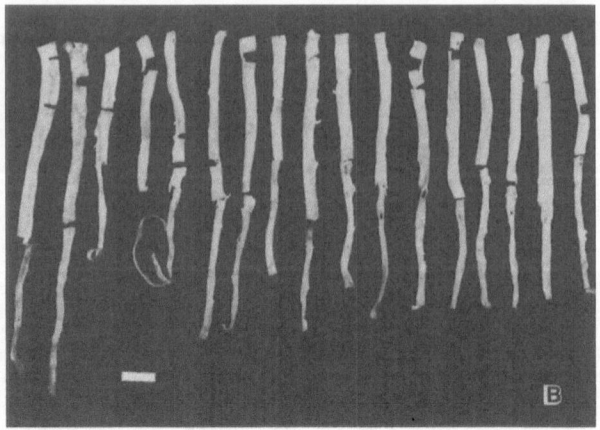

Fig. 1. Aortas of monkeys from group I (A) and group III (B).
The aortas have been split longitudinally and stained with Sudan
IV. The intimal surfaces of one half of the aortas are shown.
Group III monkeys have much less sudanophilia than group I monkeys,
probably associated with regression of atherosclerosis. Scale:
horizontal bar = 1 cm

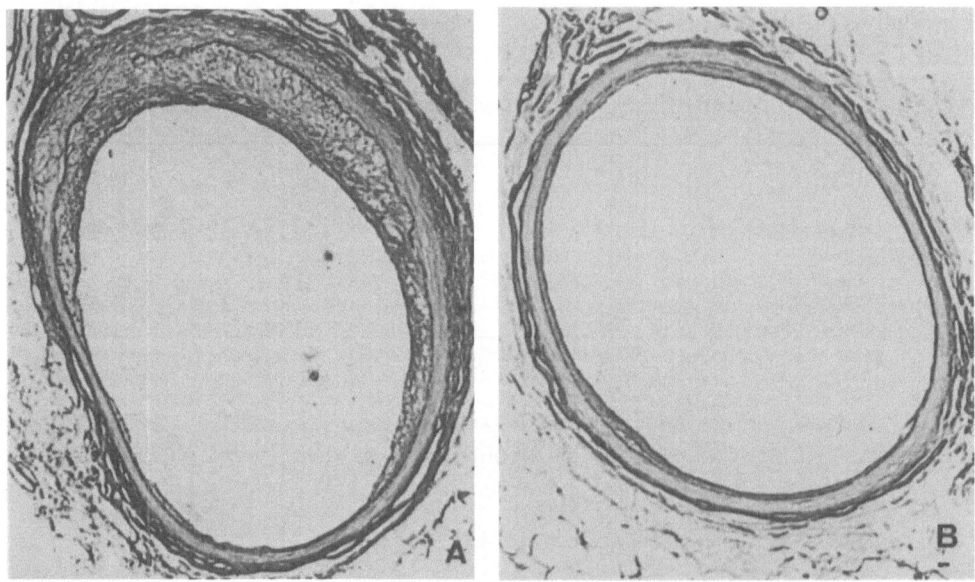

Fig. 2. Sections of representative coronary arteries from groups I
(A) and III (B). The obstructions of the lumen secondary to
intimal thickenings (A = 32%; B = 7%) demonstrate regression of
atherosclerosis induced by alfalfa saponins. Orcein elastic
stain; A 85 x; B 140 x

biochemical, immunologic, and anatomical analyses revealed no toxic effects associated with the ingestion of alfalfa saponins (3); therefore, the saponins induced regression of atherosclerosis without toxicity.  The mechanisms through which alfalfa saponins reduce atherosclerosis may include:  decreases in cholesterolemia without changes in levels of high-density cholesterol, impairment of cholesterol absorption, and increases in fecal excretion of neutral steroids and of bile acids (1, 4).

Let us turn our attention to the regression of atherosclerosis in humans.  The evidence of regression in humans was gathered in studies involving serial contrast angiography.  Table 2 shows data

Table 2.  Angiographically documented regression of human athero-sclerosis in patients with various treatments (5)[a]

| Number of insti-tutions | Number of patients | Arterial bed | X-ray interval (years) | Therapy | Patients with regression |
|---|---|---|---|---|---|
| 8 | 110 | femoral coronary, renal, aorta | 0.3 to 3.5 | "mild" to "vigorous" | 26 |

[a]Patients from references 29 and 33 (5) have been deleted.

on 110 patients reported by 8 groups of investigators:  regression was demonstrated in 26 cases, usually after dietary modification, exercise, avoidance of cigarette smoking, reduction of blood pressure when appropriate, and the administration of various drugs (5).  In certain of these studies, regression was associated with a reduction in cholesterolemia.  In three additional series, 16 of 477 patients requiring coronary angiography because of clinical indications showed signs of regression (Table 3); the treatment in these series was not reported.

Table 3.  Angiographically documented regression of human athero-sclerosis in patients without specific treatment

| Reference | Number of patients | Arterial bed | X-ray interval (years) | Patients with regression |
|---|---|---|---|---|
| 6 | 174 | coronary | 1 to 4 | 4 |
| 7 | 256 | coronary | 1 to 7 | 11 |
| 8 | 47 | coronary | 1.5 | 1 |
| Totals | 477 | | | 16 |

In one series, Bruschke et al. (7) studied the evolution of athero-sclerosis in four main coronary arteries; in 11 patients they found decreases in the degree of stenosis in one artery with simultaneous increases or no change in the stenosis of other coronary arteries. This simultaneous progression and regression emphasizes the importance of local vascular factors in these processes.

Since angiographic data are by necessity limited to artery lumina, an apparent decrease in the degree of stenosis could also be due to release of spasm; growth or ectasia of the arteries; thinning of the media with outward bulging of the plaques; or recanalization and lysis of thrombi. It is unlikely that all cases of human regression are due to these mechanisms, but it still needs to be demonstrated that an angiographically observed decrease in the degree of stenosis is in fact associated with the arterial wall changes described as regression in animals. This evidence will be hard or impossible to obtain until we have noninvasive means of differentiating vascular wall thickening from superimposed thrombi. Nevertheless, apparent shrinking of lesions with associated functional improvement has been noted in many patients by different investigators (5), an indication that functional regression occurs in humans. Atherosclerosis regression--already demonstrated over many decades in animals (9-11)--constitutes an exciting new concept in human pathology.

*Acknowledgments*   This is Publication No. 1208 of the Oregon Regional Primate Research Center, supported in part by Grants RR-00163 and HL-16587 from the National Institutes of Health.

References

1. Malinow MR, McLaughlin P, Stafford C, Livingston AL, Senner JW (in press) Effects of alfalfa saponins on regression of atherosclerosis in monkeys. In: Hauss WH (ed) Clinical Implications of Recent Research Results in Arteriosclerosis, Westdeutscher Verlag, Opladen, West Germany
2. Malinow MR (in press) Triterpenoid saponins in mammals: Effects on cholesterol metabolism and atherosclerosis. In: Ness SW, Fuller G, Tsai LS (eds) Proceedings of Symposium on Regulation and Function of Isopentenoids in Plants, Marcel Dekker, New York
3. Malinow MR, McLaughlin P, McNulty WP, Houghton DC, Kessler S, Stenzel P, Goodnight SH Jr, Bardana EJ Jr, and Palotay JL (in press) Lack of toxicity of alfalfa saponins in monkeys. J Med Primatol
4. Malinow MR, Connor WE, McLaughlin P, Stafford C, Lin DS, Livingston AL, Kohler GO, McNulty WP (1981) Cholesterol and bile acid balance in *Macaca fascicularis*: Effects of alfalfa saponins. J Clin Invest 67: 156-162
5. Malinow MR (1981) Regression of atherosclerosis in humans: Fact or myth? Circulation 64: 1-3
6. Gensini GF, Esente P, Kelly A (1974) Natural history of coronary disease in patients with and without coronary bypass graft surgery. Circulation 49 & 50 (Suppl II): II-98-II-102
7. Bruschke AVG, Wijers TS, Kolsters W, Landmann J (1981) The anatomic evolution of coronary artery disease demonstrated by coronary arteriography in 256 nonoperated patients. Circulation 63: 527-536
8. Brown BG, Bolson EL, Dodge HT (1982) Arteriographic assessment of coronary atherosclerosis. Review of current methods, their limitations, and clinical applications. Arteriosclerosis 2: 2-15

9.  Wissler RW, Vesselinovitch D (1977) Regression of atheroscle-
    rosis in experimental animals and man.  Mod Concepts Cardio-
    vasc Dis 46:  27-32
10. Malinow MR (1980) Atherosclerosis:  Regression in nonhuman
    primates (review).  Circ Res 46:  311-320
11. Malinow MR (1980) Regression of atherosclerosis in nonhuman
    primates.  An overview.  In: Kalter SS (ed) Use of Nonhuman
    Primates in Cardiovascular Diseases, University of Texas
    Press, Austin and London, pp 181-220

# The Biochemical Basis for Anatomical Regression of Atherosclerosis

W. St. Clair

Although several, early studies suggested the potential for regression of atherosclerosis, it was largely due to a report by Armstrong and coworkers (1) in 1970,
showing conclusive evidence for regression of coronary artery atherosclerosis in
nonhuman primates, that interest in further studies on regression of atherosclerosis was renewed. Since that time, numerous studies have confirmed and extended
Armstrong's observations such that we now have a much more comprehensive understanding of the variety of biochemical and metabolic changes that occur in regression of atherosclerosis.

The purpose of this paper will be to summarize the biochemical changes that have
been shown to accompany the regression of atherosclerotic lesions and to indicate
how these biochemical changes relate to the anatomic and morphologic changes seen
in the regressed plaque.

Regression is a complicated process in which a variety of components of the atherosclerotic lesion change (either increasing or decreasing). The temporal sequence of change is not the same for all components and can be markedly affected by
the initial severity and characteristics of the lesions and the conditions under
which regression occurs. Upon regression, there are changes that occur in the
lipids, connective tissue, mineral, and cellular elements of the lesion.

A considerable body of data using a variety of animal models and experimental conditions has shown a consistent decrease in both the free (FC) and esterified cholesterol (EC) components of the atherosclerotic plaque during regression (2-7). As
shown in Fig. 1, the decrease in lesion cholesterol content can be detected after
less than two months of regression and reaches maximum depletion by eight months in
pigeons with severe aortic atherosclerosis. A similar time course for cholesterol
depletion has been reported for swine (6). In fatty streaks (8) as well as in
moderately severe, raised lesions (9,10), the FC and EC contents return to near

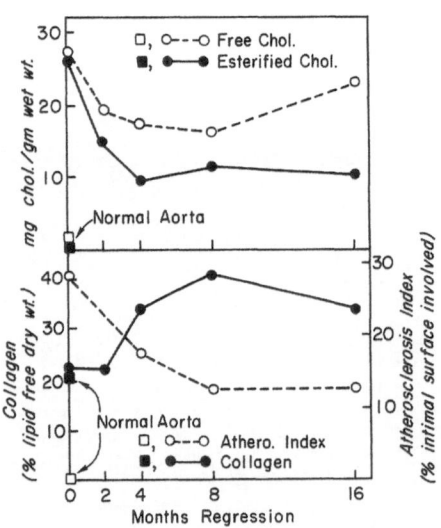

Fig. 1. Plaque cholesterol and collagen
content and extent of atherosclerosis in
White Carneau pigeons fed cholesterol for 1
year, followed by regression for up to 16
months. Adapted from (2) with permission
of authors

normal levels, given a sufficient duration of regression. The rate of depletion of EC appears to be more rapid than that of FC, however (Fig. 1). Whether the lesion cholesterol content returns to normal or plateaus at a concentration above normal (as in Fig. 1) depends on the initial severity of the lesions. In these more severe lesions, even with regression periods of nearly 4 years, cholesterol concentrations do not return to normal (4,11). The failure to mobilize some of the pool of atheroma cholesterol appears to be closely correlated with the physical form of the cholesterol in the lesion. Extracellular cholesterol crystals, for example, appear to regress slowly (2,12) as indeed they would be expected to do on a physical chemical basis (13). Intracellular ECs, on the other hand, are rapidly cleared from the lesions and this clearance is closely correlated with the disappearance of foam cells (2,14). Extracellular CEs, however, are also mobilized from the lesion but in severe lesions this mobilization is not complete (Fig. 1). The mechanisms responsible for clearance of both intra- and extracellular cholesterol are largely unknown. A number of mechanisms have been suggested for the loss of foam cells with regression, including cell death (8), foam cell migration from the lesion (15), and cellular EC hydrolysis with excretion of FC from the cell in the presence of a suitable acceptor. The depletion of extracellular cholesterol has been hypothesized to occur in part by phagocytosis by macrophages (14).

The effect of initial lesion severity and of plasma cholesterol concentrations on depletion of arterial cholesterol during regression is shown in Table 1. In this experiment, rhesus monkeys were fed an atherogenic diet for either 19 or 38 months to produce atherosclerotic lesions with different degrees of severity (16). The animals were then exposed to a regression period of 24 or 48 months at a plasma cholesterol concentration of either 200 or 300 mg/dl. Regression at 200 mg/dl caused significantly greater depletion of arterial FC and EC than at 300 mg/dl. In addition, the more severely diseased aortas from animals fed the atherogenic diet for 38 months showed less cholesterol depletion.

The magnitude of the accumulation of other lipids, such as triglycerides and phospholipids, is much less in the atheroma than is the accumulation of cholesterol. Regression results in a depletion of some or all of these lipids as well (4,9).

Table 1. Effect of initial lesion severity on cholesterol content of the abdominal aorta of rhesus monkeys after regression for 24 or 48 months at plasma cholesterol concentrations of 200 or 300 mg/dl

| Group (mo. regression) | N | Plasma cholesterol mg/dl | Cholesterol (mg/g wt wt.) | | |
|---|---|---|---|---|---|
| | | | Total | Free $\bar{x}$ ± SEM | Esterified |
| Control | 4 | 201 | 1.35 ± 0.19 | 1.06 ± 0.08 | 0.29 ± 0.13 |
| 19 mo. induction (regression) | 12 | 785 | 10.3 ± 1.22 | 5.33 ± 0.51 | 4.95 ± 0.72 |
| 24 mo. | 16 | 300 | 5.27 ± 0.82 | 3.42 ± 0.45 | 1.86 ± 0.40 |
| 24 mo. | 18 | 200 | 1.97 ± 0.15 | 1.46 ± 0.07 | 0.49 ± 0.08 |
| 48 mo. | 18 | 300 | 5.14 ± 0.70 | 3.14 ± 0.36 | 2.00 ± 0.36 |
| 48 mo. | 18 | 200 | 2.17 ± 0.18 | 1.57 ± 0.09 | 0.60 ± 0.09 |
| 38 mo. induction (regression) | 19 | 629 | 12.1 ± 1.13 | 6.12 ± 0.58 | 5.98 ± 0.68 |
| 24 mo. | 19 | 300 | 5.70 ± 0.61 | 3.51 ± 0.35 | 2.19 ± 0.28 |
| 24 mo. | 18 | 200 | 4.61 ± 0.54 | 2.99 ± 0.34 | 1.63 ± 0.22 |
| 48 mo. | 19 | 300 | 8.96 ± 0.94 | 4.14 ± 0.42 | 4.82 ± 0.61 |
| 48 mo. | 20 | 200 | 5.18 ± 0.12 | 2.14 ± 0.33 | 2.15 ± 0.23 |

The design of this experiment has been described in detail elsewhere (16)

There have been only a relatively few studies conducted to show metabolic changes with regression. The synthesis of phospholipids, triglycerides and CEs are marked-ly decreased with regression as is total protein synthesis (6,17). Cholesterol esterification is decreased to near normal levels even in arteries that continue to contain large amounts of excess cholesterol. This suggests that it is the plasma lipoprotein cholesterol that elevates the rate of lesion cholesterol esterification and not the atheroma cholesterol (17).

The development of atherosclerotic plaques (but generally not fatty streaks) is associated with an increased collagen content (16,18). During regression virtually all studies report a further increase in the collagen component of the lesion as observed morphologically (1,2,7,19). Results have not been as consistent, however, when based on the content of collagen measured chemically. There are reports of decreases, increases, or no change in the collagen content of the arterial wall during regression (3,4,7,9,18). These differences between the morphological and chemical results are probably related to differences in the initial severity of the lesions in some studies as well as the distribution of collagen in the athero-sclerotic arterial wall. Microscopic evidence indicates that the collagen change with regression occurs almost exclusively in the plaque, and even though this change may be substantial, the amount of plaque collagen relative to the total arterial wall collagen is small and, as a result, changes in plaque collagen content may be diluted by the mass of collagen in the remainder of the arterial wall. Most studies now indicate that in more complicated lesions the collagen content does indeed increase during regression, and that this can be detected chemically (2,4,6,7). In pigeon atherosclerotic lesions this increase in collagen lags behind the drop in lesion cholesterol content (Fig. 1). The accumulation of fibrous connective tissue can be so extensive that it can largely replace the space previously occupied by foam cells, resulting in the maintenance of considerable intimal thickening (2,7,20), and in severe cases prevent any substantial decrease in intimal area with regression. This is illustrated in Fig. 2 for the individual animals that compose the groups of rhesus monkeys described in Table 1. Fig. 2A shows that with regression at plasma cholesterol concentrations of 200 mg/dl for 48 months there is greater depletion of cholesterol than at 300 mg/dl. This was associated with a slight increase in the intimal area involved with atherosclerosis with regression at both 200 and 300 mg/dl (Fig. 2B). Part of this failure to observe a decrease in intimal area following regression can be attributed to re-placement of the space previously occupied by foam cells with collagen (Fig. 2C). This is particularly evident for the animals in the upper 25% of the distribution.

Elastin content also increases in the atherosclerotic artery (4,7,18), and although many studies report a return of elastin concentrations to normal with regression (4,18) others have reported further increases in elastin with regression (17).

Calcium content has consistently been shown to increase in the arterial wall with regression (4,6,7,14). This is particularly true early in the regression process (14).

Total glycosaminoglycan (GAG) concentrations do not show major changes with either induction or regression of atherosclerosis. There are changes in individual GAGs with regression, with an increase in hyaluronic acid and heparan sulfate, while dermatan sulfate and chondroitin 6-sulfate decrease (20).

## Correlation of biochemical and morphologic features

The major space-occupying components of the atherosclerotic lesion are cells (such as foam cells that arise either from proliferation of arterial smooth muscle cells or from influx of monocytes from the blood), connective tissue, and extracellular material including necrotic debris and lipid. During regression all of these com-ponents can change to a greater or lesser extent. Cell proliferation decreases with regression (22,23) which reduces the input of new cells into the lesion. In addition, foam cells are rapidly lost from the lesion, which correlates closely with the loss of cholesteryl esters and a decline in the rate of production of new cholesteryl esters (17).. The actual mechanisms involved in the loss of foam cells are not known. Not only can the cellular lipids be mobilized during regression but extracellular lipids and debris can also be cleared, but here again the extent of mobilization of these extracellular components is probably limited by the initial severity of the lesions. All of these changes are associated with considerable remodeling of the plaque as is evidenced by the increases in connective tissue components, particularly collagen. The magnitude of fibrosis may actually determine to a large extent the degree of reduction in lesion area that is achieved during regression.

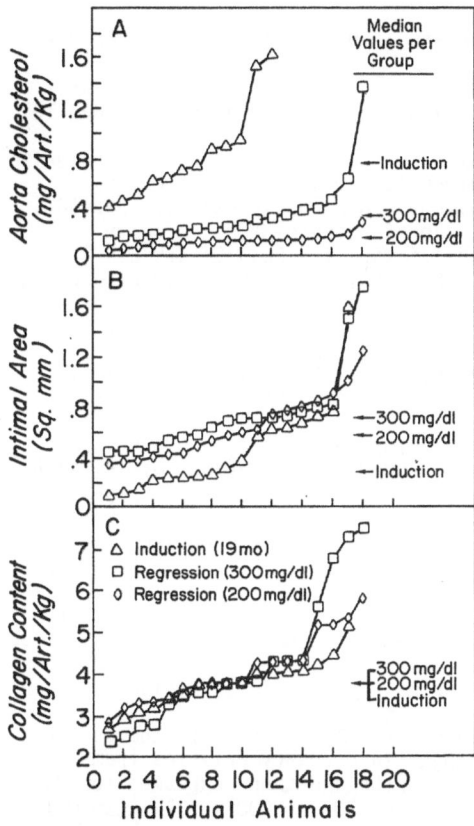

Fig. 2. Changes in abdominal aorta total cholesterol content, intimal area involved with atherosclerosis and collagen content in rhesus monkeys fed an atherogenic diet for 19 months (induction) followed by regression for 48 months at plasma cholesterol concentrations of 200 or 300 mg/dl. The distribution for all animals is shown along with the median values for each group. Results have been taken from previously published studies in which only mean values were presented (4,19).

References

1. Armstrong ML, Warner ED, Connor WE. (1970) Regression of coronary atheromatosis in rhesus monkeys. Circ Res 27: 59-67.
2. Clarkson TB, King JS Jr, Lofland HB, Feldner MA, Bullock BC. (1973) Pathologic characteristics and composition of diet-aggravated atherosclerotic plaques during "regression". Exp Mol Pathol 19: 267-283.
3. Vesselinovitch D, Wissler RW, Hughes R, Borensztajn J. (1976) Reversal of advanced atherosclerosis in rhesus monkeys. Part 1. Light-microscopic studies. Atherosclerosis 23: 155-176.
4. Wagner WD, St Clair RW, Clarkson TB, Connor JR. (1980) A study of atherosclerosis regression in Macaca mulatta. III. Chemical changes in arteries from animals with atherosclerosis induced for 19 months and regressed for 48 months

216

at plasma cholesterol concentrations of 300 or 200 mg/dl. Am J Pathol 100: 633-650.

5. Kokatnur MG, Malcom GT, Eggen DA, Strong JP. (1975) Depletion of aortic free and ester cholesterol by dietary means in rhesus monkeys with fatty streaks. Atherosclerosis 21: 195-203.

6. Fritz KE, Augustyn JM, Jarmolych J, Daoud AS. (1981) Sequential study of biochemical changes during regression of swine aortic atherosclerotic lesions. Arch Path Lab Med 105: 240-246.

7. Hollander W, Kirkpatrick B, Paddock J, Colombo M, Nagraj S, Prusty S. (1979) Studies on the progression and regression of coronary and peripheral atherosclerosis in the cynomolgus monkey. 1. Effects of dipyridamole and aspirin. Exp Mol Pathol 30: 55-73.

8. Stary HC. (1979) Regression of atherosclerosis in primates. Virchows Archiv 383: 117-134.

9. Fritz KE, Augustyn JM, Jarmolych J, Daoud AS, Lee KT. (1976) Regression of advanced atherosclerosis in swine. Chemical studies. Arch Pathol Lab Med 100: 380-385.

10. Srinivasan SR, Patton D, Radhkrishnamurthy B, Boster TA, Malinow MR, McLaughlin P, Berenson GS. (1980) Lipid changes in atherosclerotic aortas of Macaca fascicularis after various regression regimens. Atherosclerosis 37: 591-601.

11. Armstrong ML, Megan MB. (1972) Lipid depletion in atheromatous coronary arteries in rhesus monkeys after regression diets. Circ Res 30: 675-680.

12. Wagner WD, Clarkson TB. (1973) Slowly miscible cholesterol pools in progressing and regressing atherosclerotic aortas. Proc Soc Exp Biol Med 143: 804-809.

13. Katz SS, Small DM. (1980) Isolation and partial characterization of the lipid phases of human atherosclerotic plaques. J Biol Chem 255: 9753-9759.

14. Daoud AS, Jarmolych J, Augustyn JM, Fritz KE. (1981) Sequential morphologic studies of regression of advanced atherosclerosis. Arch Path Lab Med 105: 233-239.

15. Gerrity RG. (1979) The movement of foam cells through arterial endothelium overlying atherosclerotic lesions. In: Bailey GW (ed) Proceedings of the 37th Annual Meeting of the Electron Microscopy Society of America, Baton Rouge, LA. Clavitors Publications, pp 88-89.

16. Clarkson TB, Lehner NDM, Wagner WD, St Clair RW, Bond MG, Bullock BC. (1979) A study of atherosclerosis regression in Macaca mulatta. I. Design of experiment and lesion induction. Exp Mol Pathol 30: 360-385.

17. St Clair RW, Clarkson TB, Lofland HB. (1972) Effects of regression of athero-sclerotic lesions on the content and esterification of cholesterol by cell-free preparations of pigeon aorta. Circ Res 31: 664-671.

18. Armstrong ML, Megan MB. (1975) Arterial fibrous proteins in cynomolgus monkeys after atherogenic and regression diets. Circ Res 36: 256-261.

19. Clarkson TB, Bond MG, Bullock BC, Marzetta CA. (1981) A study of atherosclero-sis regression in Macaca mulatta. IV. Changes in coronary arteries from animals with atherosclerosis induced for 19 months and then regressed for 24 or 48 months at plasma cholesterol concentrations of 300 or 200 mg/dl. Exp Mol Pathol 34: 345-368.

20. Pick R, Prabhu R, Glick G. (1978) Diet-induced atherosclerosis and experimental hypertension in stumptail macaques (Macaque arctoides). Effects of antihyper-tensive drugs and a non-atherogenic diet in the evolution of lesions. Atherosclerosis 29: 405-429.

21. Radhakrishnamurthy B, Ruiz HA, Dalferes ER Jr, Vesselinovitch D, Wissler RW, Berenson GS. (1979) The effect of various dietary regimens and cholestyramine on aortic glycosaminoglycans during regression of atherosclerotic lesions in rhesus monkeys. Atherosclerosis 33: 17-28.

22. Stary HC. (1974) Proliferation of arterial cells in atherosclerosis. Adv Exp Med Biol 43: 59-81.

23. Thomas WA, Scott RF, Florentin RA, Reiner JM, Lee KT. (1981) Population dynamics of arterial cells during atherogenesis. XI. Slowdown in multipli-cation and death rates of lesion smooth muscle cells in swine during the period 105-165 days after balloon endothelial cell denudation followed by a hyper-lipidemic diet. Exp Mol Pathol 35: 153-162.

# The Endothelial Changes During Regression of Atherosclerotic Lesions in Animal Models

G. Weber

An extremely important role is attributed to endothelium in the main tenance of the arterial wall integrity. To endothelial injury, what- ever its kind, great relevance is given as to the initial event in atherosclerosis. "Denuding and non-denuding": the problem has been well focused by Schwartz et al. (1); "dysfunction" (2) or "subtle functional derangements" (3) being the terms which may help us to fur ther understand what is expected to happen in the arterial wall when the endothelial layer is somehow "supplanted".

We know well how the intimal surface looks like at scanning electron microscopy, in a normal aorta, for instance of a New Zealand rabbit: the regularly disposed endothelial cells are flow-oriented and look well joined, in a continuous layer.

If the continuity of the endothelial layer is lost already after a short-term hypercholesterolic diet is still an open and debated que- stion. Quite recent observations of ours (4) have confirmed, by means of morphometric mesurements of denuded areas (on pressure-perfusion- fixed, silver-stained aortas) that, the continuity of the endothelial layer is lost (after 7 days) in about 8% of the whole measured areas, chosen far from the origin of the collateral branches. In control rab bits only single endothelial cells, sparsely disseminated, are lost, possibly due to silver-staining. Over the largely denuded areas of rabbits on hypercholesterolic diet, after 15 days, red blood cells, platelets and fibrin-like deposition are found, clearly showing that endothelial injury has taken place during life. Similar observations had been collected by us also in rabbits after immunologic injury (5, 6).

When advanced atherosclerotic lesions are developed, the continuity of the endothelial layer over them may result more or less largely lost both in aortas of Rhesus monkeys and of New Zealand rabbits on atherogenic diets (7,8).

It is generally accepted that in Rhesus monkeys, under the effect of regression diets and/or drugs, the arterial plaques loose lipid, cells and matrix and are largely remodeled, their dimensions being gradual= ly reduced together with the lumen stenosis (cfr. Wissler, 9).

At scanning electron microscopy, the regressing plaques have the sur= face completely covered by endothelial cells, when the lipemia levels have returned to normal values. Most of the endothelial cells look well distended and appear flow-oriented. These features of the re= generated endothelial cells have been observed after 12-18 months of regression diet. More recently Wissler and Jones (cfr. Wissler, 10) have shown that the repair of the endothelial layer is going on already four months after the beginning of a regression diet, sup= plemented or not with cholestyramine.

In atherosclerotic New Zealand rabbits, submitted to partial ileal by-pass (11), we have observed regression of atherosclerotic lesions with features, at light and transmission electron microscopy observa

tion, similar to the ones observed in Rhesus monkeys. The hyperchole=
sterolemia levels, which during atherosclerosis induction (2 months -
1% chol. diet)  could overpass the 1000mg/dl were dramatically redu=
ced after surgery to 100mg/dl or less; a substantial reduction, up to
disappearance, of gross aortic lesions (mean intimal surface area in=
volved from 85% to 12,43%) together with histologically relevant loss
of lipid and foam cells reduction from the residual lesions (from a
73,04 to a 39,21 percentage of foam cells). At scanning electron mi=
croscopy examination, the aortic lesions (which after the 60 days a=
therogenic diet are very bulging and large, with discontinuities of
the endothelial layer due to loss of cells and of groups of cells) ap
pear now regressed, almost flat, with the surface of the residual le=
sions almost completely covered by flattened endothelium. This endo=
thelium may still present, however, some irregularities both in the
shape and the orientation of the cells. In some areas, the juxta-po=
sed cells of this "neo-endothelial" layer are rather square, not yet
"flow-oriented" and appear very loosely joined to each other. In other
areas, the regeneration of the endothelial cells appears very intense,
with many small, "plump", crowding cells. Also upon transmission elec
tron microscopy examination, over the regressing aortic lesions, the
endothelial cells appear frequently cuboidal and small, with inter-en
dothelial junctions rather loose and almost straight, and only few
plasmalemmal vesicles at the luminal surface of the cell membrane.

While studying these features, we have been impressed by another fin=
ding, quite unusual, consisting in the presence of a Con A reactive
layer well evident not only at the luminal surface, where it is expec
ted to be (12,13) but also at the abluminal surface of regenerating
endothelial cells. We know, from Wight and Ross (14), that the ablu=
minal surface of the endothelial cells doesn't usually stain with
Ruthenium red, nor was ever observed by us any staining at this surfa
ce making use of the Bernhard and Avrameas Con-A reaction (15) in nor
mal rabbits.

On role and function of regenerating endothelial cells, see also re=
cent data reported by Hansson (16), Fisher and Betz (17), Bylock (18),
Schwartz et al. (1).

I shall only remind here that regenerating endothelial cells may be
functionally altered both in endocytosis and in proteoglycan produc=
tion (19,20,21,22) and may show large amount of basement membrane ma
terial in the sub-endothelial layer (23,24); the surface of the re=
gressing lesions results not yet perfectly organised (see 25,26,27,
28,29,30); increased arterial permeability has been found wherever
regenerated endothelial cells overlap the myo-intima (3). Loss of junc
tions between regenerating arterial endothelial cells has been obser=
ved by means of freeze-etching technique by Spagnoli et al. (31), thus
confirming data by Schwartz et al. (23). In cultured bovine aortic en
dothelial cells, after confluence, it has been evidenced by us, making
use of the freeze-etching technique (32), a diminished number of pino
cytotic vesicles.

Both from literature data and from our observations it seems possible
to assume that many regenerating endothelial cells observed by us du=
ring regression of atherosclerotic aortic lesions of rabbits, submit=
ted to partial ileal by-pass, look in the whole as simplified in their
plasma-membrane, some of the areas at the surface of the regressing
lesions appearing moreover "not yet perfectly organised", as sugge=
sted also by the positive Con-A reaction found at the abluminal cell
surface. Such regenerating endothelial cells of rabbits could so be

interpreted as "dysfunctioning" endothelial cells (see Gimbrone, 2; Stemerman, 3).

We wonder if and when these "dysfunctioning" endothelial cells of our rabbits will ever acquire the features of a well functioning endothe= lial layer: a topic on which much work indeed has still to be done.

# References

1.  Schwartz SM, Gajdusek CM, Selden SC (1981) Vascular wall growth control: the role of the endothelium. Arteriosclerosis 1: 107-126.
2.  Gimbrone MA (1981) Endothelial dysfunction and the pathogenesis of atherosclerosis. In: Gotto AM, Smith LC, Allen B (eds) Athero sclerosis V, Springer Verlag, New York Heidelberg Berlin, pp 415-425.
3.  Stemerman MB (1981) Effect of moderate hypercholesterolemia on rabbit endothelium. Arteriosclerosis 1: 25-33.
4.  Weber G, Toti P (1981) Osservazioni morfometriche in microscopia elettronica a scansione sul distacco di cellule endoteliali della aorta di coniglio a dieta ipercolesterolica di breve durata. Boll. Soc. It. Biol. Sper. 57: 2170-2175.
5.  Weber G (1980) Ultrastructural aspects of experimental atheroge= nesis. Degenerative lesions in the early stages of experimental cholesterol and immunological atherogenesis in rabbits. In: Con= stantinides P, Pratesi F, Cavallero C, Di Perri T (eds) Immunity and atherosclerosis, Academic Press, London New York Toronto Sid ney San Francisco, pp 109-110.
6.  Weber G, Orazioli D, Fabbrini P, Resi L (1980) Lesioni degenera= tive precoci dellaparete arteriosa in conigli sottoposti ad inie zioni di omogenato eterologo di aorta. Giorn. Arteriosclerosi 5: 105-111.
7.  Weber G, Fabbrini P, Resi L, Jones R, Vesselinovitch D, Wissler RW (1977) Regression of arteriosclerotic lesions in Rhesus mon= key aortas after regression diet. Atherosclerosis 26: 535-547.
8.  Weber G, Fabbrini P, Resi L (1979) Arterial intimal changes in early phases of experimental atherogenesis. Ather. Rev. 4: 97-117.
9.  Wissler RW (1978) Progression and regression of atherosclerotic lesions. In: Chandler AB, Eurenius K, McMillan GC, Nelson CB, Schwartz CJ, Wessler S (eds) The thrombotic process in atheroge= nesis, Plenum Press, New York London, pp 77-109.
10. Wissler RW (1981) Neueste Studien über die Pathogenese und Rück-bildung der Atherosklerose. Therapie Woche, pp 1-7.
11. Weber G, Fabbrini P, Papi F, Pescatori GF, Resi L, Sforza V, Tan ganelli P (1981) Regression of aortic lesions in rabbits withdrawn from a hypercholesterolic diet and subjected to partial ileal by-pass: SEM and TEM observations. Exp. Molec. Path. 34: 244-252.
12. Weber G, Fabbrini P, Barbaro A, Resi L (1972) Reattività alla Con canavalina A sull'endotelio aortico di coniglio nella norma e nel le prime fasi dell'aterogensi colesterolica sperimentale. (Osser-vazioni preliminari in microscopia elettronica a trasmissione). Boll. Soc. It. Biol. Sper. 48: 1009-1010.
13. Weber G, Fabbrini P, Resi L (1973) On the presence of a Concana= valin A reactive coat over the endothelial aortic surface and its modifications during early experimental cholesterol atherogenesis in rabbits. Virchows Arch. Anat. Path. A 359: 299-307.
14. Wight TN, Ross R (1975) Proteoglycans in primate arteries I Ultra structural localization and distribution in the intima. J. Cell Biol. 67: 670-674.

15. Bernhard W, Avrameas S (1971) Ultrastructural visualization of cellular carbohydrate components by means of Concanavalin A. Exp. Cell Res. 64: 232-236.
16. Hansson GK (1980) Endothelial injury and monocyte adhesion in a= therogenesis. Experimental studies in the rabbit. Göteborg, pp 1-20.
17. Fisher H, Betz E (1981) Das Gafässendothel. Wissenschaftliche Ver lagsgesellschaft mbH, Stuttgart, pp 1-144.
18. Bylock A (1981) The arterial surface ultrastructure. Effects of cholesterol feeding and mechanical injury. Göteborg, pp 1-53.
19. Davies PF, Ross R (1978) Mediation of pinocytosis in cultured smooth muscle and endothelial cells by platelet-derived growth factor. J. Cell Biol. 79: 663-671.
20. Vlodavsky I, Fielding PE, Fielding CJ, Gospodarovictz D (1978) Ro le of contact inhibition in the regulation of receptor-mediated uptake of low density lipoprotein in cultured vascular endothelial cells. Proc. Nat. Acad. Sci. USA 73: 356-360.
21. Davies PF, Selden SC, Schwartz SM (1980) Enhanced rates of fluid pinocytosis during exponential growth and monolayer regeneration by cultured arterial endothelial cells. J. Cell Phys. 102: 119-128.
22. Wight TN, Curwen K, Homan W (1979) Effect of regenerated endothe= lium on glycosaminoglycan accumulation in the arterial wall. Fed. Proc. 38: 1075.
23. Schwartz SM, Stemerman MB, Benditt EP (1975) The aortic intima. II Repair of the aortic lining after mechanical denudation. Am. J. Pathol. 81: 15-42.
24. Stemerman MB, Ross R (1972) Experimental atherosclerosis. I: Fi= brous plaque formation in primates. An electron microscopy study. J. Exp. Med. 136: 769-789.
25. Buck RC (1979) Contact guidance in the subendothelial space. Re pair of rat aorta in vitro. Exp. Mol. Pathol. 31: 275-283.
26. Buck RC (1979) The longitudinal orientation of structures in the subendothelial space of rat aorta. Am. J. Anat. 156: 1-14.
27. Christensen BC, Chemnitz J, Tkocz I, Kim CM (1979) Repair in arte rial tissue. I Endothelial regrowth, subendothelial tissue chan= ges and permeability in the healing rabbit thoracic aorta. Acta Path. Microbiol. Scand. Sect. A 87: 265-273.
28. Christensen BC, Chemnitz J, Tkocz I, Kim CM (1979) Repair in ar= terial tissue. II Connective tissue changes following an embolec tomy catheter lesion. The importance of the endothelial cells to repair and regeneration. Acta Path. Microbiol. Scand. Sect. A 87: 275-283.
29. Weber G, Fabbrini P, Resi L, Sforza V, Tanganelli P (1980) "Lesio ni" e "disfunzione" delle cellule endoteliali nella aterogenesi sperimentale e nell'ateroregressione. Arch. De Vecchi 64: 175-182.
30. Reidy MA, Schwartz SM (1981) Endothelial regeneration. III Time course of intimal changes after small defined injury to rat aor= tic endothelium. Lab. Invest. 144: 301-308.
31. Spagnoli LG, Pietra GG, Villaschi S, Johns LW (1982) Morphometric analysis of gap junctions in regenerating arterial endothelium. Lab. Invest. 46: 139-148.
32. Weber G, Bianciardi G, Giacchi M, Toti P, Vatti R, Weber E (1981) Ultrastructural features of BAEC, studied by freeze-etching tech= nique. 2nd Italian Austrian Atherosclerosis Meeting Igls April 30 May 2, 34.

# 1.6 Diet

# Diet and Carcinogenesis[1]

## K. K. Carroll[2]

## A. Introduction

It is well-recognized that the level of serum cholesterol can be lowered significantly in human subjects by substituting polyunsaturated fat for saturated fat in their diet (1-3). Since a high level of serum cholesterol is considered to be a major risk factor for cardiovascular disease, individuals with elevated serum cholesterol are often advised to decrease their intake of saturated fat and to eat more polyunsaturated fat. A change in this direction was also recommended for the population of the United States as a whole in the Dietary Guidelines prepared by a Select Committee of the United States Senate. These Guidelines suggested that dietary fat intake be reduced to 30% of calories and that the proportions be altered so as to provide approximately equal amounts of polyunsaturated, monounsaturated, and saturated fat (4).

## B. Possible Impact of Dietary Recommendations on Carcinogenesis

These recommendations are focussed primarily on reducing the risk of cardiovascular disease, and it is worth considering whether they may at the same time alter the risk of other major diseases such as cancer. Interest in this possibility was stimulated by results of clinical trials with diets high in polyunsaturated fat, since these provided some indication that such diets might increase the risk of death from cancer. Although the evidence is at best suggestive, the possibility of adverse effects from diets high in polyunsaturated fat remains a matter of continuing concern (5).

In studies on dietary fat in relation to mammary cancer in rats, it was found that polyunsaturated fats promoted mammary tumor development more effectively that saturated fats (6). Similar results have recently been reported for pancreatic cancer in rats (7). Dietary fat also promotes the development of intestinal tumors in rats, but in this case, the type of fat appears to be relatively unimportant (8).

In our experiments on mammary cancer, it was found that saturated fats were as effective as polyunsaturated fats in promoting carcinogenesis when they were fed in combination with a small amount of polyunsaturated fat, which by itself was ineffective (9). It appeared from our results that the polyunsaturated fat was providing essential fatty acids which, in addition to a high-fat diet, were necessary for promotion of mammary carcinogenesis (10). Further experiments indicated that the amount of polyunsaturated fat required increased as the total amount of fat in the diet decreased (Fig. 1) suggesting that the two requirements may be interrelated (11).

[1] Supported by the National Cancer Institute of Canada.
[2] Career Investigator of the Medical Research Council of Canada.

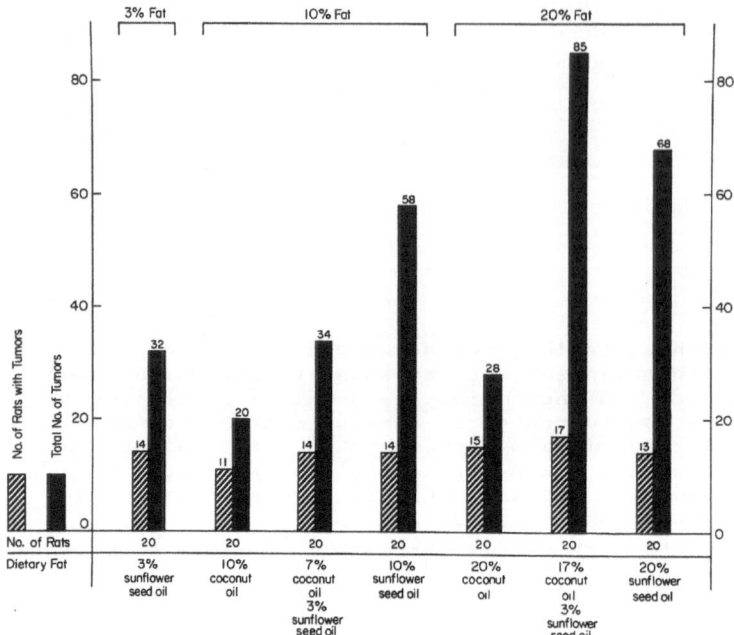

Fig. 1. Effects of different levels and types of dietary fat on incidence and yield of mammary tumors induced in female Sprague-Dawley rats by 7,12-dimethylbenz(a)anthracene (see Ref. 11)

Analysis of epidemiological data has shown strong positive correlations between the amount of fat available for consumption in different countries and mortality from cancer at a number of different sites, including breast, colon, prostate and rectum (12). Similar correlations are obtained for dietary animal fat, but the correlations with vegetal fat are much weaker or absent (Table 1).

These observations may seem to be in disagreement with the results of experiments with animals described above, since fats derived from plants tend to be more unsaturated than those derived from animals. However, the evidence from epidemiological data and experimental studies can be rationalized as follows: At high levels of fat intake only small amounts of polyunsaturated fatty acids are required for promotion of mammary carcinogenesis in rats, and such small amounts would probably be supplied by the national food supplies of most countries. Although the experiments with rats indicate that a higher proportion of polyunsaturated fat is required for cancer promotion at lower levels of fat intake, it is still reasonable to expect that cancer mortality should show a better correlation with total dietary fat than with degree of unsaturation. This conclusion is even more logical in the case of colon cancer, where the type of dietary fat seems to make little difference in animal experiments.

Overall, the evidence suggests that at high levels of fat intake (40% of total calories) substitution of polyunsaturated fat for saturated fat in the diet poses no additional risk for cancer, and may help to reduce risk of cardiovascular disease. At lower levels of fat intake (e.g. 20% of total calories) the results of experiments with animals indicate that a higher proportion of polyunsaturated fat is associated with more effective promotion of mammary cancer and possibly other types of cancer as well.

Table 1. Correlation coefficients between per caput availability of dietary fat in different countries and age-adjusted mortality in those countries from malignant neoplasms at different sites[1]

| Site | Sex | Correlation coefficients | | |
|------|-----|--------------------------|---|---|
|      |     | Total fat | Animal fat | Vegetal fat |
| Breast | F | +0.865 | +0.837 | +0.297 |
| Intestine (except rectum) | M | +0.850 | +0.861 | +0.162 |
| Intestine (except rectum) | F | +0.807 | +0.830 | +0.143 |
| Prostate | M | +0.766 | +0.749 | +0.231 |
| Rectum | M | +0.727 | +0.771 | +0.042 |
| Rectum | F | +0.666 | +0.729 | -0.017 |

[1]The correlation coefficients were calculated from age-adjusted mortality for 1975 compiled by Segi et al (13) and values for dietary fat over the 15-year period prior to and including 1975 (14). Only data for countries with populations greater than 2 million in 1975 were used.

## C. Cholesterol and Carcinogenesis

The possibility of a relationship between cholesterol and carcinogenesis has been considered with respect to intake of dietary cholesterol, fecal excretion of cholesterol and bile acids, and the level of cholesterol in blood.

Evidence from both epidemiological data and experiments with animals has led to the suggestion that dietary cholesterol is co-carcinogenic for colon cancer (15, 16). It is possible that dietary cholesterol (15) and dietary fat (8, 17) may both influence intestinal cancer by increasing fecal excretion of cholesterol and/or bile acids. Nigro and his associates found that colon carcinogenesis in rats was enhanced either by feeding cholestyramine or by diverting bile to the distal part of the small intestine (18). They also reported (19) that the yield of intestinal tumors in rats was increased by the polyene macrolide, candicidin, which appears to inhibit cholesterol absorption from the intestine. The animals excreted much larger amounts of neutral sterols, mainly as coprostanol, but there was little effect on bile acid excretion.

Rats treated with cholestyramine developed significantly more tumors in the large intestine, whereas those fed candicidin had more tumors in the distal small intestine. This suggests that bile acids may have a greater promoting effect in the large intestine, whereas the effect of neutral sterols may be greater in the distal small intestine (19).

Reddy and Watanabe (20) found that cholesterol administered intrarectally did not promote colon carcinogenesis in rats, although bile acids were effective when given by this route. Any effect of dietary cholesterol on colon cancer is thus more likely to be mediated by increased excretion of bile acids rather than neutral sterols. It

is thus of interest that dietary cholesterol has been shown to increase bile acid production in rats, dogs and monkeys, but generally
not in humans (21-23).

Although addition of cholesterol to the diet of rats has been reported to increase their susceptibility to colon cancer (15,17), from
other experiments it appears that vegetable oils, which contain no
cholesterol, promote colon cancer in rats as least as effectively
as animal fats (8). Polyunsaturated vegetable oils were actually
found to be more effective than animal fats in promoting mammary
tumors in rats (6).

Another recent cause for concern has been the indication from a number of epidemiological studies of an inverse correlation between
serum cholesterol levels and cancer incidence (5,24-26). It is known
that people living in non-industrialized countries tend to have low
serum cholesterol levels and also to be at low risk from cancer,
but it is still possible that individuals with low serum cholesterol
levels in countries where the average level is high may have some
special characteristics that make them more susceptible to cancer
(27).

Although an inverse relationship between cancer mortality and level
of serum cholesterol has been reported in a number of studies, it
is not apparent in others (5,24-26,28) and more work is required
to assess the significance of these observations. This topic will
be discussed in detail at the workshop on Hypocholesterolemia and
Cancer.

## References

1.  Kinsell LW (1963) Relationship of dietary fats to atherosclero-
    sis. Progr Chem Fats & Other Lipids 6: 137-170
2.  McGandy RB, Hegsted DM (1975) Quantitative effects of dietary
    fat and cholesterol on serum cholesterol in man. In: Vergroe-
    sen AJ (ed) The Role of Fats in Human Nutrition, Acad Press,
    NY. pp 211-230
3.  Grundy SM (1975) Effects of polyunsaturated fats on lipid meta-
    bolism in patients with hypertriglyceridemia. J Clin Invest 55:
    269-282
4.  Select Committee on Nutrition and Human Needs, United States
    Senate (1977) Dietary Goals for the United States, Second Edi-
    tion, U.S. Government Printing Office, Washington, DC
5.  Oliver MF (1981) Serum cholesterol - The knave of hearts and
    the joker. Lancet 2: 1090-1095
6.  Carroll KK, Khor HT (1971) Effects of level and type of dietary
    fat on incidence of mammary tumors induced in female Sprague-Daw-
    ley rats by 7,12-dimethylbenz(α)anthracene. Lipids 6: 415-420
7.  Roebuck BD, Yager JD, Jr, Longnecker DS, Wilpone SA (1981) Pro-
    motion by unsaturated fat of azaserine-induced pancreatic carci-
    nogenesis in the rat. Cancer Res 41: 3961-3966
8.  Reddy BS, Cohen LA, McCoy GD, Hill P, Weisburger JH, Wynder EL
    (1980) Nutrition and its relationship to cancer. Adv Cancer Res
    32: 237-345
9.  Carroll KK, Hopkins GJ (1979) Dietary polyunsaturated fat versus
    saturated fat in relation to mammary carcinogenesis. Lipids 14:
    155-158
10. Carroll KK, Hopkins GJ, Kennedy TG, Davidson MB (1981) Essential

fatty acids in relation to mammary carcinogenesis. Progr Lipid Res 20: 685-690

11. Carroll KK, Davidson MB (1982) The role of lipids in tumorigenesis. In: Arnott MS, van Eys J, Wang Y-M (eds) Molecular Interrelations of Nutrition and Cancer, Raven Press, NY, pp 237-245

12. Carroll KK, Khor HT (1975) Dietary fat in relation to tumorigenesis. Progr Biochem Pharmacol 10: 308-353

13. Segi M, Hattori H, Segi R (1980) Age-adjusted death rates for cancer for selected sites (A-classification) in 46 countries in 1975. Segi Institute of Cancer Epidemiology, Nagoya, Japan

14. Food Balance Sheets - 1975-77 Average and Per Caput Food Supplies - 1961-65 Average, 1967 to 1977 (1980) Food and Agriculture Organization of the United Nations, Rome

15. Cruse P, Lewin M, Clark CG (1979) Dietary cholesterol is co-carcinogenic for human colon cancer. Lancet 1: 752-755

16. Liu K, Moss D, Persky V, Stamler J, Garside D, Soltero I (1979) Dietary cholesterol, fat, and fibre, and colon-cancer mortality. Lancet 2: 782-785

17. Reddy, BS (1981) Dietary fat and its relationship to large bowel cancer. Cancer Res 41: 3700-3705

18. Nigro, ND (1981) Animal studies implicating fat and fecal steroids in intestinal cancer. Cancer Res 41: 3769-3770

19. Nigro ND, Campbell RL, Gantt JS, Lin YN, Singh DV (1977) A comparison of the effects of the hypocholesteremic agents, cholestyramine and candicidin, on the induction of intestinal tumors in rats by azoxymethane. Cancer Res 37: 3198-3203

20. Reddy BS, Watanabe K (1979) Effect of cholesterol metabolites and promoting effect of lithocholic acid in colon carcinogenesis in germ-free and conventional F344 rats. Cancer Res 39: 1521-1524

21. Quintão E, Grundy SM, Ahrens EH Jr. (1971) Effects of dietary cholesterol on the regulation of total body cholesterol in man. J Lipid Res 12: 233-247

22. Myant NB (1981) The biology of cholesterol and related steroids. William Heinemann Medical Books Ltd. London. pp. 481-484

23. Lin DS, Connor WE (1980) The long term effects of dietary cholesterol upon the plasma lipids, lipoproteins, cholesterol absorption and the sterol balance in man: the demonstration of feedback inhibition of cholesterol biosynthesis and increased bile acid excretion. J Lipid Res 21: 1042-1052

24. Lilienfeld AM (1981) The Humean fog: Cancer and cholesterol. Am J Epidemiol 114: 1-4

25. Feinleib M (1981) On a possible inverse relationship between serum cholesterol and cancer mortality. Am J Epidemiol 114: 5-10

26. Heller RF (1981) Coronary heart disease, cancer, lipoproteins, and the effects of clofibrate: Is enzyme induction a common link and are lipoproteins red herrings? Lancet 2: 1258-1260

27. Broitman SA (1981) Cholesterol excretion and colon cancer. Cancer Res 41: 3738-3740

28. Dyer AR, Stamler J, Paul O, Shekelle RB, Schoenberger JA, Berkson DM, Lepper M, Collette P, Shekelle S, Lindberg HA (1981) Serum cholesterol and risk of death from cancer and other causes in three Chicago epidemiological studies. J Chron Dis 34: 249-260

# Effects of Dietary Cholesterol and Saturated Fat on the Appearance of HDLc in Peripheral and Cardic Lymph

P. Julien and A. Angel

## A.  Introduction

Several studies on the kinetics of plasma LDL clearance and turnover indicate that up to 30 to 40% of LDL and HDL distribute in extravascular pools (1,2).  Apoproteins known to be associated with VLDL, LDL and HDL have been detected in human peripheral (pedal) lymph by Reichl et al (3).  In previous work, we have demonstrated that cholesterol-rich lipoproteins, LDL and HDL, are present in cardiac lymph of pigs and dogs at concentrations 36 to 59% that of plasma and that cardiac lymph contained VLDL-like particles (4).  Dietary effects on lipoproteins in peripheral lymph were observed by Courtice et al (5) who cannulated lymphatic vessels in hind limbs of hyperlipoproteinemic rabbits.  Presumably lipoproteins in the interstitial space can undergo metabolic transformations because of the presence of lipid metabolizing enzymes (6) and because of proximity to lipoprotein binding sites on various parenchymal and mesenchymal cells.

Mahley et al (7) showed significant changes in plasma lipoproteins in dogs fed diets rich in cholesterol and containing the antithyroid drug propylthiouracil.  Feeding of cholesterol-rich diets to hypothyroid dogs increased plasma VLDL, $\beta$VLDL and LDL and induced the appearance of Apo E rich $HDL_c$ (7).  In the present study, we examined the effect of a cholesterol and saturated fat supplemented diet on peripheral and cardiac lymph lipoproteins.  Euthyroid animals were employed to avoid the confounding effects of hypothyroidism on lipoprotein metabolism (8,9) and on interstitial fluid volume and composition (10).  Cholesterol and saturated fat feeding produced a marked increase in peripheral and cardiac lymph $HDL_c$ cholesterol indicating wide interstitial distribution of this unique lipoprotein.

## B. Methods

Healthy dogs weighing 20-25 kg were fed a diet containing 1% cholesterol, 30% saturated-fat (lard) and 69% Purina dog chow for 3 weeks.  After an overnight fast, blood and lymph samples were obtained during general anesthesia (1.5% fluothane in $NO_2:O_2$ 2:1).  Cardiac lymph vessels were cannulated as previously described (11) and peripheral lymph was obtained by cannulating a hindleg superficial lymph vessel distal to the popliteal lymph node.  Lymph flow was maintained by passive ankle flexion.  Microhematocrit centrifugation of lymph confirmed the absence of red blood cells, as no visible sedimentation occurred.

Plasma and lymph lipoproteins were analysed by ultracentrifugation at density 1.006 (VLDL), 1.006-1.063 (LDL, $HDL_1$, $HDL_2$), 1.063-1.087 ($HDL_1$, $HDL_c$, $HDL_2$) and 1.087-1.21 ($HDL_2$) according to previously described methods (4).  LDL, $HDL_1$ and $HDL_c$ obtained at density 1.006-1.063 were separated by Pevikon electrophoresis (11) and then eluted from the gel with 0.15M NaCl.  Lipids were extracted from total plasma, lymph and lipoprotein fractions by the method of Folch et al (12).

Total cholesterol and triglycerides were measured by Technicon Auto-
analyser and phospholipids using Bartlett's method (13).

Purified plasma HDLc, was radioiodinated (14) and 120 µCi of $^{125}I$-HDL$_c$
was administered i.v. to 4 anesthetized dogs.  Peripheral lymph and
plasma samples were collected at frequent intervals over 3 hours.
Plasma or lymph HDL$_c$ radioactivity was determined by measuring the
TCA (10%) precipitable activity (4).


## C. Results

The plasma and lymph lipid composition in normal and cholesterol fed
dogs is presented in table 1.  Normal peripheral lymph cholesterol was
17% that of plasma and normal cardiac lymph contained twice the cholesterol of peripheral lymph.  Cholesterol feeding increased total
plasma cholesterol by 72% with a doubling in peripheral and cardiac
lymph cholesterol.  With respect to phospholipids, the peripheral lymph
was again 17% that of plasma and the normal cardiac lymph phospholipid
was twice that of peripheral lymph.  Cholesterol feeding increased
plasma phospholipid by 41% and increased peripheral lymph phospholipid
but had little effect on cardiac lymph.  With respect of triglyceride,
control cardiac lymph was more than twice that of peripheral lymph and
cholesterol feeding had no apparent effect on plasma and lymph.


Table 1. Plasma and lymph lipids in dogs fed diets rich in cholesterol and saturated fat

|  |  | n | Cholesterol | Phospholipid | Triglyceride |
|---|---|---|---|---|---|
| Plasma | Control | 5 | 142.9 ± 7.5 | 261.0 ± 16.4 | 30.2 ± 3.2 |
|  | Diet | 5 | 246.3 ± 19.5 | 368.9 ± 36.5 | 36.6 ± 6.3 |
| Lymph peripheral | Control | 2 | 23.7 ± 5.9* | 45.3 ± 0.8* | 4.1 ± 0.9* |
|  | Diet | 3 | 54.0 ± 13.2 | 79.1 ± 28.7 | 7.2 ± 0.9 |
| cardiac | Control | 5 | 52.1 ± 7.2 | 108.7 ± 14.1 | 11.5 ± 6.6 |
|  | Diet | 3 | 98.8 ± 15.3 | 116.1 ± 20.8 | 8.3 ± 4.8 |

*Results are expressed as mg/100 ml (mean ± range) of values, all
others : mean ± SEM
Diet: cholesterol (1%), lard (30%), dog chow (69%), 3 weeks


The cholesterol distribution among plasma lipoprotein fractions is
shown in Table 2.  HDL$_2$ (d 1.087-1.21) was the major plasma cholesterol
carrier in control dogs.  In cholesterol fed dogs, HDL$_2$ was still the
principal cholesterol carrier but 4-6 fold increases in fractions
containing HDL$_c$ (1.006-1.063 and 1.063-1.087) occured.  Three out of
4 dogs showed a decrease in HDL$_2$ concentration but the variation pre-
cluded statistical significance to the reduction in mean values.

Plasma and lymph lipoproteins in density 1.006-1.063 were separated
by Pevikon electrophoresis into LDL, HDL$_1$ and HDL$_c$ fractions (Table 3).
Only the HDL$_1$ fraction is present in normal plasma and lymph.  HDL$_1$
and HDL$_c$ comigrate in preparative electrophoresis, therefore the relative amounts of HDL$_1$ and HDL$_c$ present in plasma and lymph of cho-

Table 2. Plasma lipoprotein cholesterol distribution in dogs fed diets rich in cholesterol and saturated fat

| Fraction | Control | Diet | Δ | P |
|----------|---------|------|---|---|
| d <1.006 | 2.5 ± 0.3* | 2.6 ± 1.4 | 0.2 ± 1.3 | N.S. |
| 1.006-1.063 | 13.3 ± 1.6 | 88.4 ± 21.1 | 75.2 ± 21.1 | <0.025 |
| 1.063-1.087 | 5.8 ± 1.2 | 26.4 ± 6.1 | 20.7 ± 5.0 | <0.025 |
| 1.087-1.21 | 121.3 ± 6.6 | 103.9 ± 11.1 | -17.6 ± 15.0 | N.S. |

*Results are expressed as mg/100 ml (mean ± SEM, n=4)
N.S. = not significant
Diet: cholesterol (1%), lard (30%), dog chow (69%), 3 weeks

Table 3. Effect of cholesterol rich diets on LDL and HDL subfractions purified from dog plasma and lymph, d 1.006-1.063

| | | Control | Diet |
|---|---|---------|------|
| | | cholesterol, mg/100 ml | |
| Plasma | | | |
| | LDL | 5.9 ± 2.9 | 33.3 ± 6.2 |
| | $HDL_1 + HDL_c$ | 7.3 ± 3.5 | 49.6 ± 22.3 |
| | $HDL_2$ | 82.3 ± 6.6 | 112.1 ± 1.4 |
| Lymph | | | |
| peripheral* | | | |
| | LDL | 3.5 ± 2.3 | 3.7 ± 2.3 |
| | $HDL_1 + HDL_c$ | 1.5 ± 0.3 | 5.3 ± 3.2 |
| | $HDL_2$ | 15.2 ± 5.1 | 32.5 ± 14.2 |
| cardiac | | | |
| | LDL | 5.0 ± 3.1 | 5.5 ± 1.7 |
| | $HDL_1 + HDL_c$ | 4.5 ± 1.4 | 9.4 ± 1.3 |
| | $HDL_2$ | 34.8 ± 3.4 | 51.7 ± 9.9 |

*Results: mean ± range of duplicate, all others, mean ± SEM, n=3
Diet: cholesterol (1%), lard (30%), dog chow (69%), 3 weeks

Table 4. Plasma and peripheral lymph $^{125}I$-$HDL_c$ radioactivity following i.v. injection of 120 μCi $^{125}I$-$HDL_c$ in a dog

| Time after injection (min) | Plasma (μCi/ml) | Peripheral lymph (μCi/ml) | $\frac{lymph}{plasma}$ x 100 |
|---|---|---|---|
| 15 | 181,348 | 180 | 0.1 |
| 30 | 180,600 | 1,630 | 0.9 |
| 60 | 178,186 | 16,308 | 9.2 |
| 120 | 171,000 | 14,713 | 8.6 |
| 180 | 170,620 | 13,589 | 8.0 |

lesterol-fed animals could not be distinguished. During cholesterol feeding plasma LDL increased from 5.9 to 33.3 mg/100 ml and $HDL_c$ appeared in the amount of 49.6 mg/100 ml. A similar increase also occured in lymph $HDL_c$. No significant increase in lymph LDL occured during cholesterol feeding but the $HDL_2$ concentration doubled in peripheral and cardiac lymph.

To test whether the $HDL_c$ in lymph originated from plasma, the appearance of $^{125}I-HDL_c$ was measured in peripheral lymph after i.v. injection of $^{125}I-HDL_c$. The $HDL_c$ radioactivity appeared during the first 15 minutes, increased rapidly and plateaued in less than one hour. Table 4 shows the appearance of labelled $HDL_c$ in peripheral lymph. At plateau, the lymph:plasma ratio ranged between 8.0 and 9.2%. Similar experiments in 3 dogs confirmed these findings.


## D. Discussion

The present study shows that feeding diets rich in cholesterol and saturated fat to euthyroid dogs produced an increase in plasma cholesterol (72%) and phospholipid (41%) with no change in triglyceride. Parallel increases in cholesterol also occured in peripheral lymph and cardiac lymph (table 1). Most of the plasma cholesterol increase was in the density fraction 1.006-1.063 which contains a mixture of LDL, $HDL_1$ and $HDL_c$ , the apo E rich lipoprotein typically induced by cholesterol feeding. The increase in plasma $HDL_c$ was associated with the appearance of $HDL_c$ in peripheral and cardiac lymph. Cholesterol feeding resulted in an increase in plasma LDL which is similar to the response in man fed cholesterol and saturated fat diets (15). There is no explanation for the lack of increase in LDL cholesterol in lymph from cholesterol fed animals.

It is noteworthy that no increase in plasma VLDL occured with cholesterol feeding (table 1). As our experiments were performed in euthyroid animals, it is likely that the increases in VLDL observed in cholesterol-fed dogs (7) and rats (9) is due to the associated hypothyroidism.

The study with $^{125}I-HDL_c$ (table 4) demonstrates that lymph $HDL_c$ originates by direct entry of plasma $HDL_c$ into the extravascular pool. Thus, $HDL_c$ like LDL, $HDL_1$ and $HDL_2$ distributes widely in the interstitial space. A question worth considering is whether $HDL_c$ in peripheral interstitial compartments has any metabolic function. While the liver is thought to be the major site of metabolic clearance (16) evidence has appeared to suggest that peripheral tissues may be involved (17). Recent work from this laboratory (17), has shown that dog adipocytes specifically bind $HDL_c$ with high capacity. This may explain the mechanism whereby cholesterol feeding results in expansion of adipose tissue cholesterol stores (18).

The concentration of total cholesterol, LDL and $HDL_c$ in cardiac lymph was consistantly higher than that of peripheral lymph. The pathophysiological significance of this observation is not established but if the atherogenic effects of high cholesterol diets proves to be a function of interstitial lipoprotein levels, the predilection for the coronary bed may be partly explained.


Acknowledgements  Dr. Pierre Julien was a Scholar of the Canadian Heart Foundation and this work was supported by grants from the Ontario Heart Foundation. The authors acknowledge the expert technical assistance of Ms. Laura Sheu and Ms. Erica Klazynski. We thank the Lipid Research Clinic, University of Toronto, for measurements of cholesterol and triglycerides.

# References

1.  Sniderman AD, Carew TE, Steinberg D (1975) Turnover and tissue distribution of $^{125}$I-labelled low density lipoprotein in swine and dogs. J Lipid Res 16: 293–299
2.  Shepherd J, Packard CJ, Patsch JR, Gotto AM and Taunton OD (1978) 61:1582–1592
3.  Reichl D, Postiglione A, Myant NB, Pflug JJ Press M (1975) Observation on the passage of apoproteins from plasma lipoproteins into peripheral lymph in two men. Clin Sci Mol Med 49: 419–426
4.  Julien P, Angel A (1981) Composition and metabolism of very low density lipoproteins in dog cardiac lymph. Can J Biochem 59: 709–714
5.  Courtice FC, Munoz-Marcus M, Garlick DG (1964) The permeability of the blood capillaries of the leg to the lipoproteins in various hyperlipaemic states in the rabbit. Q J Exp Physiol 49: 441–456
6.  Julien P, Angel A (1981) Lipoprotein metabolizing enzymes in cardiac lymph. Arteriosclerosis 1: 381A–382A
7.  Mahley RW, Weisgraber KH, Innerarity T (1974) Canine lipoproteins and atherosclerosis. II Characterization of the plasma lipoproteins associated with atherogenic hyperlipodemia. Circ Res 35: 722–733
8.  Sykes M, Cnoop-Koopmans WM, Julien P, Angel A (1981) The effects of hypothyroidism, age and nutrition on LDL catabolism in the rat. Metabolism 30: 733–738
9.  DeLamatre JG, Roheim PS (1981) Effect of cholesterol feeding on apo B and apo E concentrations and distributions in euthyroid and hypothyroid rats. J Lipid Res 22: 290–306
10. Parving HH, Hansen JM, Steen LN (1979) Mechanism of edema formation in myxedema – Increased protein extravasation and relatively slow lymphatic drainage. N Engl J Med 301:460–465
11. Julien P, Downar E, Angel A (1981) Lipoprotein composition and transport in the pig and dog cardiac lymphatic system. Circ Res 49: 248–254
12. Folch J, Lees M, Sloane Stanley GH (1957) A simple method for the isolation of purification of total lipids from animal tissues. J Biol Chem 226: 497–509
13. Bartlett GR (1959) Phosphorus assay in colum chromatography. J Biol Chem 234: 466–468
14. Angel A, D'Costa MA, Yuen R (1979) Low density lipoprotein binding, internalization, and degradation in human adipose cells. Can J Biochem 57: 578–587
15. Schonfeld G, Patsch W, Rudel LL, Nelson C, Epstein M, Olson RE (1982) Effects of dietary cholesterol and fatty acids on plasma lipoproteins. J Clin Invest 69: 1072–1080
16. Mahley RW, Hui DY, Innerarity TL, Weisgraber KH (1981) Two independent lipoprotein receptors on hepatic membranes of dog, swine and man. Apo-B,E and apo-E receptors. J Clin Invest 68: 1197–1206
17. Fong B, Rodrigues P, Julien P, Angel A (1982) Lipoprotein receptors in adult human adipocyte plasma membranes. Clin Res 30: 523A
18. Angel A, Farkas J (1974) Regulation of cholesterol storage in adipose tissue. J Lipid Res 15: 491–499

# Dietary Fibres for Prevention of CVD

M. Mancini, A. Rivellese, G. Riccardi, and A. Postiglione

## Introduction

Many epidemiological studies have clearly demonstrated that dietary habits are strongly related to the incidence of Cardiovascular Diseases (CVD) in different countries (1,2). The diet commonly used by people living in South Europe is generally considered protective against CVD. Such diet is not only poor in saturated fat and cholesterol, but also rich in dietary fibre. Therefore potential benefits on cardiovascular risk factors from a high-fibre diet, composed exclusively by natural foods and adequate in calories, need to be evaluated.

So far fibre added to foods in form of guar or pectin or bran have proved to be effective in reducing blood glucose levels in diabetic patients. Moreover the soluble type of dietary fibre has been reported to reduce serum cholesterol by about 10% in hyperlipidemic subjects (3,4).

However fibre supplements in form of guar or pectin are not well tolerated because of their poor taste and hence not suitable for long term treatments as needed for diabetic and hyperlipidemic patients.

Therefore the aim of this study was to evaluate the influence of a diet composed of naturally fibre rich foods on two major cardiovascular risk factors like hyperlipoproteinemia and hyperglicemia.

## Subjects and Methods

Three different dietary experiments have been performed with three different groups of patients:

Experiment 1). 5 patients with type II hyperlipoproteinemia (two with type II A and three with type II B) underwent two isocaloric diets identical in the distribution of nutrients (CH 53%, Fat 30%, Proteins 17%) and relatively high in saturated fats (40g/die). The only difference between the two diets was the amount of dietary fibre (15g/die vs 62g/die).

Experiment 2). 6 patients with type II hyperlipoproteinemia (three with type II A and three with type II B) performed an identical dietary experiment as the previous group with two diets different only in the amount of dietary fibre (15g/die vs 62g/die) but, in this case, the two

diets were low in saturated fat (17g/die).
Experiment 3). 5 patients with diabetes mellitus and type II hyperlipoproteinemia (3 with type II A and 2 with type II B) underwent the
same dietary experiment as group 2.

All the experiments were performed in a metabolic ward for consecutive
periods of 10 days each. Patients were allocated at random on the high
or low fibre diet and then continued with the other diet.

All diets were composed by natural food-stuffs available at the usual
shops.

At the end of each dietary period a fasting serum specimen was analysed
by preparative ultracentrifugation and both cholesterol and triglycerides were measured on each major lipoprotein class.

## Results

No significant weight change was recorded between the two dietary
periods for each of the three groups of patients.

Experiment 1) (table 1).

During the high fibre diet there was a significant reduction in both
total cholesterol (16%, $p < .025$) and LDL cholesterol (13%, $p < .025$)
without any significant change in other lipoproteins. However there
was a trend towards a reduction in VLDL cholesterol and an increase
in HDL cholesterol. Total and VLDL triglycerides were practically not
modified by dietary fibre.

Table 1. Lipoprotein composition (M+SD) at the end of each dietary
period in patients with type II hyperlipoproteinemia (n=5)

| Diets: | LFHS | HFHS |
|---|---|---|
| Cholesterol (mmol/l) | | |
| Tot. | 8.68+1.53 | 7.23+ .98°° |
| VLDL | 1.74+2.56 | 0.98+1.06 |
| LDL | 5.88+1.40 | 5.08+1.01°° |
| HDL | 1.04+ .36 | 1.19+ .39 |
| Triglyceride (mmol/l) | | |
| Tot. | 5.39+5.70 | 5.67+5.92 |
| VLDL | 4.88+5.02 | 4.74+4.52 |

Abbreviations: LFHS= Low fibre-high saturated fats
               HFHS= High fibre-high saturated fats

°°$p < .025$

Experiment 2) (table 2).

The only significant modification on serum lipoproteins induced by the
high fibre diet in this experimental condition (diets low in saturated

fat) was a 10% reduction in LDL cholesterol (p<.05). The other lipoprotein classes remained practically unchanged during the two different
diets.

Table 2. Lipoprotein composition (M+SD) at the end of each dietary
period in patients with type II hyperlipoproteinemia (n=6)

| Diets: | LFLS | HFLS |
|---|---|---|
| Cholesterol (mmol/l) | | |
| Tot. | 7.59+1.24 | 7.23+1.35 |
| VLDL | .78+ .54 | .91+ .78 |
| LDL | 5.80+1.45 | 5.21+1.27° |
| HDL | 1.04+ .23 | 1.09+ .18 |
| Triglyceride (mmol/l) | | |
| Tot. | 1.84+ .78 | 2.27+1.08 |
| VLDL | 1.29+ .84 | 1.29+ .80 |

Abbreviations: LFLS= Low fibre-low saturated fats
                HFLS= High fibre-low saturated fats

°p < .05

Experiment 3) (table 3).

Despite the fact that the two diets utilized for this group of patients with diabetes were identical to the previous experiment, this
time the influence of the high fibre diet on serum lipoproteins was
much more remarkable. Both total and LDL cholesterol were dramatically
reduced by this diet (30%, p< .005 and, respectively, 34%, p<.02)
and this reduction was significantly higher (p<.01) than that obtained
in experiment 2. However a significant reduction was recorded also for
HDL cholesterol (15%; p<.02). VLDL-TG were only slightly reduced by
the high fibre diet and the ratio LDL-chol+VLDL-TG/HDL-chol. was reduced by roughly 19%. For this group of patients dietary fibre were also
able to improve blood glucose control: during the high fibre diet postprandial blood glucose significantly decreased by 27% (p<.05).

236

Table 3. Lipoprotein composition (M+SD) at the end of each dietary period in diabetic patients with type II hyperlipoproteinemia (n=5)

| Diets: | LFLS | HFLS |
|---|---|---|
| **Cholesterol (mmol/l)** | | |
| Tot. | 7.10+ .96 | 4.97+ .34°° |
| VLDL | .65+ .32 | .48+ .17 |
| LDL | 4.93+ .88 | 3.25+ .31°° |
| HDL | 1.50+ .36 | 1.27+ .44° |
| **Triglyceride (mmol/l** | | |
| Tot. | 1.57+ .34 | 1.47+ .27 |
| VLDL | 1.06+ .30 | .87+ .18 |

Abbreviations: LFLS= Low fibre-low saturated fats
              HFLS= High fibre-low saturated fats

°p <.02; °°p <.005

Discussion and conclusion

Our study demonstrates that a high fibre diet composed of naturally high fibre foodstuffs has a significant hypocholesterolemic and hypoglicemic effect.

As this type of diet is safe and well tolerated by the patients, it can be adequately used for dietetic treatment of diabetes (5,6) and type II hyperlipoproteinemia. This diet can be expecially useful for the treatment of diabetic patients with type II hyperlipoproteinemia as in these patients it can reduce to a large extent deranged values of both blood glucose and LDL cholesterol.

The high fibre diet reduces LDL cholesterol also when the dietary amount of saturated fat is low and therefore it is possible to hypothisize that a reduction in dietary saturated fat and an increase in dietary fibre have a synergistic effect on lowering LDL cholesterol in hypercholesterolemic patients.

In conclusion the diet commonly used by people living in South Europe may be protective against CVD not only for its low content of saturated fats, but also because it is rich in foods containing a high amount of dietary fibre.

References

1. Kawate R., Yamokido M., Nishimoto Y., Bennett P.A., Hammon R.F. and Knowler W.C. (1979) Diabetes Mellitus and its vascular complications in Japanese Migrants on the Island of Hawaii. Diabetes Care 2: 161.
2. Trowell H. and Burkitt H.D. (1977) Dietary fibre and cardiovascular disease. Artery 3: 107-19.

3. Jenkins D.J.A., Leeds A.R., Slavin B., Mann J., Jepson E.M. (1979) Dietary fibre and blood lipids: reduction of serum cholesterol in type II hyperlipidemia by guar gum. Am.J.Clin.Nutr. 32: 16-18.
4. Jenkins D.J.A., Reynolds D., Slavin B., Leeds A.R., Jenkins A.L. and Jepson E.M. (1980) Dietary fibre and blood lipids: treatment of hypercholesterolemia with guar crispbread. Am.J.Clin.Nutr. 33: 575-581.
5. Riccardi G., Rivellese A., Patti L., Pacioni D., Genovese S., and Mancini M. (1981) A high fibre diet as a possible mean to treat hyperglycemia and hyperlipoproteinemia. Proceedings of European Atherosclerosis Group. Spring Meeting 1981, Padova, in press.
6. Rivellese A., Riccardi G., Giacco A., Pacioni D., Genovese S., Mattioli P.L., Mancini M. (1980) Effect of dietary fibre on glucose control and serum lipoproteins in diabetic patients. Lancet 2: 447-450.

# Dietary Cholesterol and Plasma Lipoproteins

J.Nestel and T.Billington

Although dietary cholesterol undoubtedly affects the plasma cholesterol level, the magnitude of this effect depends on several factors:
1. the amount of cholesterol ingested; 2. the amount of dietary
fat; 3. the type of dietary fat; 4. the efficiency of metabolic
compensatory mechanisms; 5. interactions with other dietary factors.
Some of these are not sufficiently well recognized and account for
considerable confusion. For instance, studies in which the addition
of a single egg (250mg cholesterol) to a daily diet already rich in
cholesterol, carried out in outpatients in whom other dietary constituents are surmised but not established, cannot be interpreted.
The apparent absence of a clear relationship between dietary cholesterol and coronary disease within a single affluent society (in contrast to studies between populations) is similarly clouded, although
such a relationship has recently been shown in the Chicago Western
Electric Study (1).

The purpose of this paper is to summarize the several dietary and
metabolic factors that influence the effect of dietary cholesterol
on the serum cholesterol, and to present new data showing in man an
increase in intermediate density lipoprotein production when cholesterol is eaten. This may be relevant to the formation of atherosclerosis because the particle that is formed is rich in cholesterol
and apoprotein E.

## Dietary cholesterol, amount and type of fat

When cholesterol is incorporated into a controlled diet and compared
strictly with a similar diet almost devoid of cholesterol there is on
average a rise in serum cholesterol. This has been established in
many studies and summarized recently (2). Equally impressive is the
direct correlation between dietary cholesterol and serum cholesterol
in the Tarahumara Indians who eat less than 300 mg cholesterol daily
(3). The type of dietary fat is also important; when 500 mg cholesterol is added to a diet rich in polyunsaturated fatty acids, the
rise in serum cholesterol is only half that seen when the fat is rich
in saturated fatty acids (4,5).

The amount of fat eaten with the cholesterol can be critical; the
serum cholesterol is much lower with a low than an average fat intake
(6).

## Metabolic compensatory mechanisms

Another reason for individual variability in the response to dietary
cholesterol lies in the subject's capacity to suppress synthesis or
stimulate excretion of cholesterol. We have shown this to apply
equally in normal subjects and in those with familial hypercholesterolaemia (7,8). Mistry et al. (9) have shown a direct inhibition of
HMGCoA reductase in blood mononuclear cells of subjects eating
cholesterol.

## Increased production of IDL

When massive hypercholesterolaemia is induced in animals fed
cholesterol, a prominent circulating lipoprotein is a cholesteryl
ester, apo-E rich particle, termed β- very low density lipoprotein,
which is held responsible for the severe atherosclerosis. We have
sought changes within VLDL of humans eating diets high in cholesterol
(10). When 1700 mg cholesterol was eaten daily, distinct changes
occurred in plasma lipoproteins, even when the plasma cholesterol
concentration changed little. Within VLDL, the proportion of apoprotein E rose, the ratio of cholesteryl ester : triglyceride rose,
and there was an increase in particles that bound to heparin, on
heparin-Sepharose columns, (Figure 1). In later studies we have
established that heparin-bound VLDL metabolically resemble IDL or
partly catabolized VLDL. Since VLDL transport was not increased we
postulated that this increase in heparin-bindable particles represented enhanced formation of IDL, required to transport the additional
cholesterol, either from the gut or more probably from the liver.

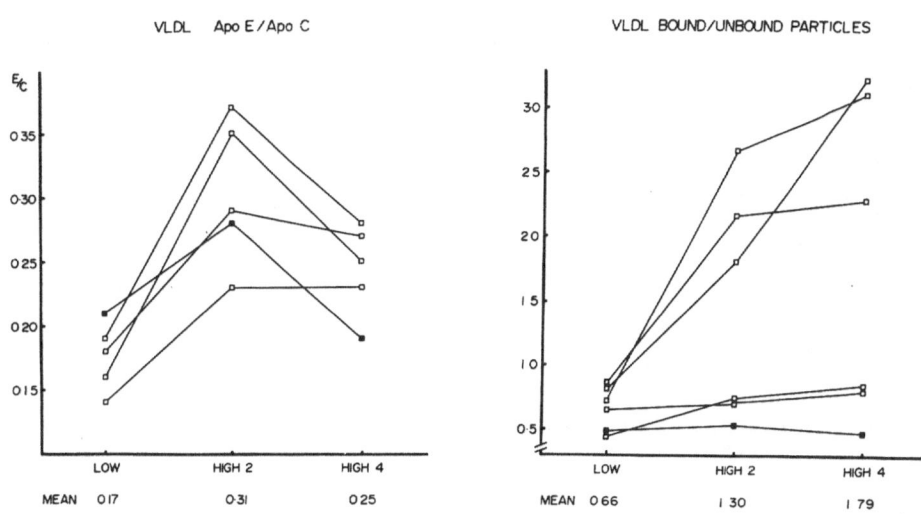

Fig.1. Apoprotein E:C ratios in VLDL, derived from scanning SDS-
polyacrylamide gels (left). Ratios of bound:unbound particles in
VLDL, derived from proportions of protein retained and not retained
on heparin-sepharose columns (right). Measurements were made at end
of low cholesterol intake (LOW) and at the end of two (HIGH 2) and
four (HIGH 4) weeks of cholesterol loading: each value is the mean
of two samples. Difference between LOW and HIGH 2 significant at
<0.5%; difference between LOW and HIGH 4 significant at <0.5%

We have confirmed this in further studies of 8 subjects in whom IDL
(Sf 12-20 or Sf 12-60) transport was compared at cholesterol intakes
of 200 mg and 1700 mg per day. Lipoproteins were labelled with
$^{125}$I, reinjected and reisolated from plasma obtained over 48 hr.
Transport (mg/kg/day) was calculated for IDL apoprotein B by 2-pool

kinetics.    Figure 2 summarizes the findings: in 7 of 8 subjects transport rose so that there was on average a highly significant increase in production with cholesterol loading.    In fact the increase in production correlated directly with the rise in serum cholesterol.    These studies demonstrate for the first time that dietary cholesterol stimulates the formation of a specific lipoprotein which appears to be responsible for the rise in total plasma cholesterol.    Since the latter reflects mainly an increase in low density lipoprotein, as well as of IDL, (present studies and ref. 9), it is highly likely that the LDL are derived from the IDL, although additional independent input of LDL is possible.

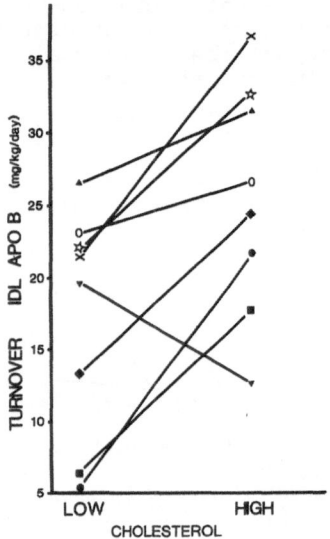

Fig.2.    Transport of IDL apoprotein B with low and high cholesterol diets

References

1. Shekelle RB, Shryock AM, Oglesby P, Lepper M, Stamler J, Liu S, and Raynor WJ  (1981)  Diet, serum cholesterol, and death from coronary heart disease.  The Western Electric Study.  New Engl. J Med. 304: 65-70
2. Roberts SL, McMurry MP and Connor WE  (1981)  Does egg feeding (i.e. dietary cholesterol) affect plasma cholesterol levels in humans?  The results of a double-blind study.  Am J Clin Nutr 34: 2092-2099
3. Connor WE, Cerqueira MT, Wallace RW, Malinow RB, and Casdorph HE (1978)  The plasma lipids, lipoproteins and diet of the Tarahumara Indians of Mexico.  Am J Clin Nutr 31:  1131-1142
4. Nestel PJ (1977)  Practical considerations of changing dietary cholesterol.  In:  Schettler G, Goto Y, Hata Y, Klose G (eds) Atherosclerosis IV, Springer-Verlag, Berlin, NY, p 442-444
5. Bronsgeest-Schoute DC, Hautvast GAJ and Hermus JJ  (1979) Dependence of the effects of dietary cholesterol and experimental conditions on serum lipids in man.  1.  Effects of dietary cholesterol in a linoleic acid-rich diet  Am J Clin Nutr 32: 2183-2187
6. Schaefer EJ, Levy RI, Ernst ND, Van Sant FD and Brewer HB (1981)  The effects of low cholesterol, high polyunsaturated fat, and low fat diets on plasma lipid and lipoprotein cholesterol levels in normal and hypercholesterolemic subjects. Am J Clin Nutr 34: 1758-1763
7. Nestel PJ and Poyser A (1976)  Changes in cholesterol synthesis and excretion when cholesterol intake is increased  Metabolism 25: 1591-1599
8. Martin GM and Nestel P  (1979)  Changes in cholesterol metabolism with dietary cholesterol in children with familial hypercholesterolaemia  Clin Sci 56:  377-380
9. Mistry P, Miller NE, Laker M, Hazzard WR and Lewis B  (1981) Individual variation in the effects of dietary cholesterol on plasma lipoproteins and cellular cholesterol homeostasis in man J Clin Invest 67:  493-502
10. Nestel P, Tada N, Billington T, Huff M and Fidge N  (1982) Changes in very low density lipoproteins with cholesterol loading in man  Metabolism (in press)

# Experience with Soybean Protein Diets in Treating Hypercholesterolemias

C. R. Sirtori and G. C. Descovich

## A. Introduction

The soybean diet treatment for hypercholesterolemia has gained increasing popularity, particularly in countries, e.g., Italy, West Germany, Switzerland, where preparations suitable for human use have been made available (1-3). Some conclusions about the efficacy and scope of clinical applications have become quite clear in the past few years:

a) type II patients, similarly to hypercholesterolemic animals, are definitely more responsive than normolipidemic subjects;

b) textured products (TVPs) seem to be more efficacious than soybean isolates for human treatment; isolates have been, however, shown to be active in some studies (4); a high percentage of calories from TVP (not less than 18% of total calories) also appears to be a requisite for maximal hypocholesterolemic activity;

c) the mode of action in humans may differ from that described in animals (5), i.e. a clear cholesterol mobilization is not noted (6).

These conclusions, at present, allow perhaps to explain some of the reported failures with this dietary treatment. In the negative studies, patients were normolipidemic or with a minimal degree of hypercholesterolemia; the administered diets, moreover, were in the form of isolates and provided a low intake of vegetable proteins (7). In this report, a brief outline of long-term studies in type II patients, treated initially with total, then with partial substitution of animal proteins with TVP, will be presented. Moreover, the results of some clinical studies, pertaining to the evaluation of cholesterol balance in treated patients and to changes in plasma free aminoacid levels will also be analyzed.

## I. Long-term evaluation of the soybean protein diet

In most of the published studies by our groups (1,8) only data collected during Metabolic Ward or relatively short-term outpatient studies were presented. More recently, we tried to maintain the cholesterol lowering effect of the diet for more prolonged periods of time, generally by administering six meals per week with complete substitution of the animal proteins with TVP.

We have now complete data on 27 patients (13 males, 14 females, age range 20-60 y.o.), who have been followed, while on this regimen, for over 2 years. After 2 months of total substitution of dietary proteins, the patients were instructed to take at least six meals per week of TVP (Cholsoy[R]). No significant side effects were encountered and the results are clearly consistent with the maintenance of the hypocholesterolemic activity, up to 2 years and longer. A small, progressive rise of HDL cholesterol levels was also noted. These patients have been monitored for changes in xanthoma size and for cardiovascular changes. Significant improvements in xanthomata and in angina symptoms were observed in some.

## II. Studies on the mechanism of the soybean protein diet

1. Sterol biosynthesis and excretion in humans following different dietary proteins

A limited number of studies have described changes in sterol biosynthesis and excretion in humans following dietary protein changes. Potter and Nestel (9), in infants, described a significant increase of neutral sterol excretion, upon shifting from standard milk to soybean milk. More recently, the same Authors (10) reported a reduced LDL biosynthesis in vegetarians, together with a low excretion of neutral sterols and bile acids. These findings are at variance with the expected sterol excretory changes in the presence of a high dietary fiber intake and are consistent with a mode of action unrelated to non-absorbable dietary components. Animal studies (5,11,12) have consistently shown an increased excretion of neutral sterols and bile acids in animals (rabbits, mini-pigs) administered high fat diets with soybean protein, compared to the same diets with casein.

In recently completed studies on the steroid excretory pattern of type II hyperlipoproteinemic subjects, treated with TVP, we failed to note any significant change in the pattern of fecal steroid excretion (6). When the in- and out-movements of sterols from plasma and tissues after injection of [14]C-cholesterol were monitored, no changes in the slope of the plasma specific activity decay curve could be detected (Fig. 1). The mechanism of the soybean protein diet is thus different from that of drugs increasing steroid excretion into the gut lumen (e.g., clofibrate) and of drugs interfering with bile acid reabsorption (e.g., cholestyramine).

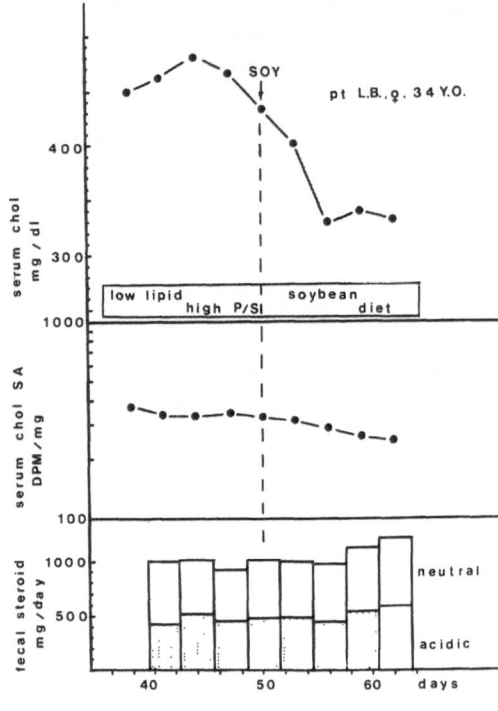

Fig. 1. Plasma total cholesterol,
[14]C-cholesterol specific activity
and fecal steroid excretion in a
type II female patient after
switching from a standard low lipid,
to the soybean diet. Changes in both
specific activity decay curve and
fecal steroid excretion are
negligible (6)

2. Changes in hormonal secretion and plasma free aminoacid pattern

The relative arginine richness of soy proteins has been suggested as being possibly responsible for the observed changes in plasma cholesterol levels. Arginine (A) might, in fact, directly activate liver lipoprotein receptors (13), resulting in the described changes of liver cholesterol metabolism in treated rodents (14). It may also stimulate hormonal release, e.g., of glucagon, and finally it may regulate the secretion of specific lipoproteins in cholesterol-fed animals.

Hormonal changes in treated humans were described by Noseda et al. (15): the release of glucagon during A stimulation increases after one week of soybean diet treatment in normal volunteers and type II patients. More recent data by the same Authors show, however, similar findings after a diet rich in casein (16). It is likely that these changes may be related to the protein richness of both diets, since total aminoacid intake, rather than specific aminoacids, may directly stimulate glucagon secretion (17). Subjects treated with the soybean diet show, on the other hand, an increased plasma content of small molecular weight glucagon, apparently most active on metabolic regulation (15).

The relative arginine richness of soy protein, and particularly the reduced lysine/arginine ratio (L/A), could be also responsible for changes in lipoprotein secretion. L inhibits liver arginase (18), thus possibly increasing the production of arginine rich protein (apo E) in cholesterol fed animals. The atherogenicity of different proteins may, therefore, be related to their L/A ratio, as recently shown (19). On the other hand, trypsin hydrolysates of soy protein are definitely more effective in lowering cholesterol than aminoacid mixtures corresponding to the same protein, and different aminoacid substitutions within a casein diet fail to modify its cholesterol raising properties (20).

The issue of A richness of soy protein and of the low L/A ratio being still controversial, it is of interest to note that humans treated with this regimen show, at the end of two months of treatment, a 25.8% increase of free A in plasma, with a -5.1% reduction of free L (Fig. 2). The L/A ratio is reduced 22.8% (p <0.01).

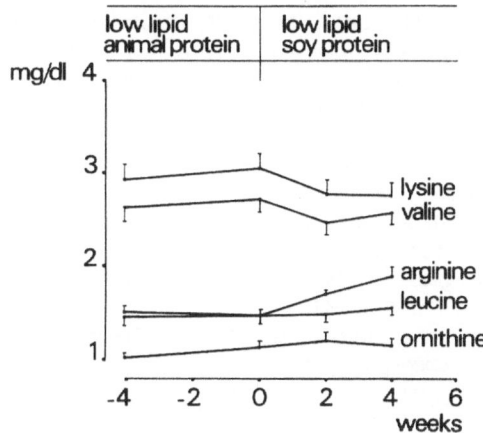

Fig. 2.  Changes in free aminoacid levels in plasma during and after the soybean diet treatment. The increase in free arginine, with decreased lysine and consequent increased L/A ratio are noteworthy

## B. Conclusions

The soybean diet treatment for hypercholesterolemia has a well established efficacy in type II patients. Its mechanism, however, is still unclear. The lack of an increase in fecal steroid excretion during the diet is noteworthy, and may indicate some kind of "hormonal effect", regulating both synthesis and excretion (9). The relative arginine richness of the diet has been suggested by many Authors as the basic mechanism. Experimental results are controversial. Human studies indicate, on the other hand, a marked reduction of the lysine/arginine ratio after diet treatment.

References

1. Sirtori CR, Agradi E, Conti F, Gatti E, Mantero O (1977) Soybean protein diet in the treatment of type II hypercholesterolemia. Lancet 1: 275-277
2. Noseda G, Fragiacomo C, Bosia C, Ramelli F, Sirtori CR (1979) Behandlung der Hyperlipidämia Typ II mit Sojabohnen. Schweiz Med Wschr 109: 1852-1853
3. Schwandt P, Richter WO, Weisweiler P (1981) Soybean protein and serum cholesterol. Atherosclerosis 40: 371-372
4. Wolfe BM, Giovannetti PM, Cheng DCH, Roberts OCK, Carroll KK (1981) Hypolipidemic effect of substituting soybean protein isolate for all meat and dairy protein in the diets of hypercholesterolemic men. Nutr Rep Int 24: 1187-1198
5. Kim DN, Lee KT, Reiner JM, Thomas WA (1980) Increased steroid excretion in swine fed high-fat, high cholesterol diets with soy protein. Exp Mol Pathol 33: 25-35
6. Fumagalli R, Soleri L, Farina R, et al (1982) Fecal cholesterol excretion studies in type II hypercholesterolemic patients treated with the soybean diet. Atherosclerosis, in press
7. Van Raaij JMA, Katan M, Hautvast JGAJ, Hermus RJJ (1981) Effects of casein versus soy protein diets on serum cholesterol and lipoproteins in young healthy volunteers. Am J Clin Nutr 34: 1261-1271
8. Descovich GC, Ceredi C, Gaddi A, et al (1981) Multicenter study of soybean protein diet for outpatient hypercholesterolaemic patients. Lancet 2: 709-711
9. Potter JM, Nestel PJ (1976) Greater bile acid excretion with soybean than with cow milk in infants. Am J Clin Nutr 32: 1645-1653
10. Nestel PJ, Billington T, Smith B (1981) Low density and high density lipoprotein kinetics and sterol balance in vegetarians. Metabolism 30: 941-945
11. Fumagalli R, Paoletti R, Howard AN (1978) Hypocholesterolaemic effect of soya. Life Sci 22: 947-952
12. Huff M, Carroll KK (1980) Effects of dietary protein on turnover, oxidation and absorption of cholesterol, and on steroid excretion in rabbits. J Lipid Res 21: 546-558
13. Gotto AM (1982) Literature review on the effects of protein on lipid metabolism. Atheroscler Rev, to be published
14. Bosisio E, Ghiselli GC, Galli Kienle M, Galli G, Sirtori CR (1981) Effects of dietary soy protein on liver catabolism and plasma transport of cholesterol in hypercholesterolemic rats. J Steroid Biochem 14: 1201-1207
15. Noseda G, Fragiacomo C, Descovich GC, Fumagalli R, Bernini F, Sirtori CR (1980) Clinical studies on the mechanism of the soybean protein diet. In: Fumagalli R et al. (Eds) Drug Affecting Lipid Metabolism, Elsevier, Amsterdam, p 355
16. Noseda G, Fragiacomo C, Gatti E, Descovich GC, Sirtori CR (1982) Glucagon release following experimental diets in man: effects of soybean and casein enriched diets. Pharmacol Res Comm, submitted for publication
17. Eisenstein AB, Strack I, Gallo-Torres H, Georgiadis A, Neal Miller (1979) Increased glucagon secretion in protein fed rats: lack of relationship to plasma aminoacids. Am J Physiol 5: E20-E27
18. Cittadini D, Pietropaolo C, De Cristoforo D, D'Ayjello-Caracciolo M (1964) In vivo effect of l-lysine on rat liver arginase. Nature 203: 643-644
19. Kritchevsky DL, Tepper SA, Czarnecki SK, Klurfeld DM (1982) Atherogenicity of animal and vegetable protein. Atherosclerosis 41: 429-431
20. Huff MW, Carroll KK (1980) Effects of dietary proteins and aminoacid mixtures on plasma cholesterol levels in rabbits. J Nutr 110: 1676-1685

# Dietary Fatty Acids as Prostaglandin Precursors

A. J. Vergroesen

In the course of the past ten years it has become increasingly accepted that the prostaglandin system, together with the steroids, biogenic amines and polypeptides, belongs to the endogenic compounds which have an important physiological regulating function.

The prostaglandin (PG) system comprises substances synthesised by means of cyclo-oxygenase (prostaglandins E, D, $F_\alpha$, I and thromboxanes (TXA)). In addition a large series of compounds are now known (various monohydroxy and dihydroxy fatty acids, such as 5-HETE and 5,12,-diHETE, and the leucotrienes $LTA_4$, $B_4$, $C_4$ and $D_4$) which are produced from the common substrates dihomo-$\gamma$-linolenic acid (20:3 n-6,9,12), arachidonic acid (20:4 n-6,9,12,15) and eicosapentaenoic acid (20:5 n-3,6,9,12,15) under the influence of lipoxygenase.
None of these substrates can be produced by animals themselves. This means that for an adequate PG-biosynthesis we depend on the presence of these fatty acids or their precursors linoleic acid (18:2 n-6,9) and $\alpha$-linolenic acid (18:3 n-3,6,9) in the diet.
The role of the dietary $\alpha$-linolenic acid and eicosapentaenoic acid in respect of PG biosynthesis in vivo has been reviewed recently by Willis (1). He concluded that it has not yet been convincingly concluded that the biosynthesis of the n-3 series of PG's and TXA's can have a major physiological function since 20:5 n-3 is a poor substrate for cyclo-oxygenase (see also: 2,3,4).
On the other hand 20:5 n-3 (and 22:6 n-3) are incorporated very efficiently in cellular membranes at the expense of mainly linoleic and arachidonic acid as has been observed also in men consuming diets high in marine fish oil (5,6). This change in membrane composition will change membrane fluidity which is thought to influence various receptor sites on the cellular membrane and the biochemical events following stimulation of a receptor. Although 20:5 n-3 is a poor substrate for the cyclo-oxygenase it is very well accepted by lipoxygenase leading to the biosynthesis of various mono- en dihydroxy derivatives of 20:5 n-3 which on further study may show to have pathophysiological significance (7).

The pharmacological effects of the various PG's on blood circulation have been studied fairly extensively.

Increase in capillary permeability: $LTC_4$ and $D_4$
Aggregation of blood platelets    : $TXA_2$
Disaggregation of blood platelets : $PGE_1$, $D_2$, $I_2$, $I_3$
Sodium and water diuresis         : $PGE_1$, $E_2$ and $I_2$ (promoting effect)
                                  : $PGF_{2\alpha}$ (inhibitory effect)
Vasodilation and lowering of
blood pressure                    : $PGE_1$, $E_2$, $I_2$
Vasoconstriction                  : $TXA_2$, $PGF_{1\alpha}$ and $PGF_{2\alpha}$

$LTC_4$ and $D_4$ are also vasoconstrictive, yet, when injected intravenously, they lower the blood pressure.

This incomplete list shows that a large number of highly active substances which are capable of interaction are produced in vivo from two of the three possible substrates. It is also known that the various tissues differ in respect of the type of prosta-glandins that are made on stimulation and that there exist significant differences between various animal species.
The best known example is the antagonism between $PGI_2$ from the vascular endothelium and $TXA_2$ from blood platelets, which forms the basis of the hypothesis of Moncada et al. (8) that the ratio of $TXA_2$ to $PGI_2$ is the most important factor determining

arterial thrombosis tendency and eventually the risk of developing atherosclerosis. Other investigators, such as Willis and Smith (9) are of the opinion that the TXA/PGI are only of minor importance as adhesion-stimulated platelet aggregation (a process not dependent on PG) is probably the most important factor in arterial thrombosis.

Another complicating factor is the biphasic reaction of the arachidonic acid concentrations in cell membranes to changes in the linoleic acid concentration in the diet. An increase in the linoleic acid concentration in the diet from 0 to 3 en% results in an increase in the arachidonic acid concentration in the tissue at the cost of eisosatrienoic acid (20:3 n-9,12,15). A further increase of the linoleic acid concentration in the diet does not, however, result in a further increase in the arachidonic acid concentration; on the contrary, it even induces a slight drop in the arachidonic acid concentration (10). Yet, the excretion of one of the most important PG metabolites via the urine shows an increase, which points to an increase instead of the expected decrease in PG biosynthesis (11,12).

Apparently, analytical data on the fatty acid composition of cellular membranes are of little value in predicting the amount of total PG-biosynthesis and they indicate even less about the types of products formed.
Another complicating factor is the fact that PG-biosynthesis is mainly determined by the degree (and type?) of tissue stimulation. For example, Ten Hoor et al. (13) have shown that differences in dietary linoleic acid intake will result only in a different $PGI_2$ biosynthesis in pulsatingly perfused arterial tissue, but not in unstimulated isolated perfused aortae. This observation indicates that differences in substrate availability might only manifest themselves if the tissues studied are sufficiently and/or properly stimulated. Blood platelets are frequently used in this type of studies and one should realize that the normal procedures by which they are concentrated from blood always involve a severe degree of stimulation. This may influence the response of platelets to the next trigger to an unknown degree.
Furthermore, Ten Hoor et al. (13) have demonstrated an antagonistic effect of dietary saturated fatty acids and of eicosapentaenoic acid. The latter is especially effective in inhibiting both endothelial $PGI_2$ production and $TXA_2$ synthesis by collagen-stimulated rat platelets, so it seems that on feeding eicosapentaenoic acid the ratio of $PGI_2$ to $TXA_2$ does not change to an important extent, although both $PGI_2$ production are decreased significantly. The pathologically increased bleeding times observed in fish oil fed rats and men (5,6) can be explained by the low $TXA_2$ production preventing, to a great extent, platelet-plug formation in the damaged vessel wall. Other potentially harmful effects of eicosapentaenoic acid are also too frequently neglected and I should like to draw attention to e.g. Gudbjarnasson's studies (14,15) on the role of eicosapentaenoic and docosahexaenoic acids in the development of cardiac necrosis and an increased sensitivity to catecholamine stress.
Finally, I would like to stress that the conversion of linoleic acid via dihomo-$\gamma$-linoleic and arachidonic acid into PG, TXA, LT and HETE is irreversible and contributes to the EFA requirements of men and animals. Depending on the duration and degree of stimulation occurring in an individual the EFA-requirement can be significantly increased to above the generally accepted basal requirement of 1-3 en% of EFA. As the EFA are also required for tissue growth and regeneration it is the combination of these two factors which determines actual EFA requirements. Standard laboratory chow for mice, rats and rabbits rarely exceeds 3 en% of EFA as is also the case with most human food compositions. One example where this seems to play an important role can be found in a series of experiments to determine EFA requirements in the prevention and therapy of $Na^+$-induced hypertension (16,17). In these studies an excess of $Na^+$ caused an increased requirement of linoleic acid in order to maintain basal blood pressure and to prevent hypertension - in the absence of excess $Na^+$ various levels of dietary linoleic acid did not influence blood pressure.

These data - and many others which could not be reviewed within the limitations of this overview - indicate that the manifold and frequently opposite physiological effects of the minute amounts of PG, TXA, LT and HETE synthesised from the fatty acid precursors strongly suggest a regulating role in a great range of cellular functions but that the variety of factors which determine their synthesis are not yet sufficiently understood to allow predictions to be made on the basis of analytical data on the prevalence of the substrates in the various tissues.

The numerous nutritional and clinical studies published up till now, however, clearly indicate that increased dietary linoleic concentrations do result in:
- increased coronary perfusion rate and myocardial contractility in perfused isolated rat hearts (18,19).
- reduced aggregation tendency of blood platelets in vivo (rat (20); rabbit (21); man (22,23,24).
- lowering of blood pressure in the case of sodium-sensitive hypertension both in rats (16,17) and man (25,26,27,28,29).
- prevention of retinal microangiopathy and coronary heart disease in insulin-independent diabetes mellitus patients (30).

This remarkable combination of favourable effects of increased consumption of linoleic acid can be explained, at least in part, by a beneficial change of PG biosynthesis as in many cases the effects of dietary modification can be counteracted by drugs which inhibit the conversion of the substrates into the various PG's.
The exact biochemical explanation of how these effects are produced, however, cannot yet be given.

## References

1. Willis AL (1981) Nutritional and pharmacological factors in eicosanoid biology. Nutrition Reviews 39: 289-301
2. Lands WEM, Le Tellier PR, Rome LH, Vanderhoek JY (1973) Inhibition of prostaglandin biosynthesis. Adv Biosci. 9: 15-28
3. Needleman P, Raz A, Minkes MS, Ferrendelli JA, Sprecher H (1979) Triene prostaglandins: Prostacyclin and thromboxane biosynthesis and unique biological properties. Proc Natl Acad Sci USA 76: 444-948
4. Struyk CB, Beerthuis RK, Pabon HJJ, Van Dorp DA (1966) Specificity in enzymic conversion of polyunsaturated fatty acids into prostaglandins. Recl Trav Chem Pays Bas 85: 1233-1250
5. Dyerberg J, Bang HO, Stoffersen E, Moncada S, Vane JR (1978) Eicosapentaenoic acid and prevention of thrombosis and atherosclerosis. Lancet ii: 117-119
6. Siess W, Scherer B, Böhlig B, Roth P, Kurzman J, Weber PC (1980) Platelet membrane fatty acids, platelet aggregation, and thromboxane formation during a mackerel diet. Lancet i: 441-444
7. Vergroesen AJ, Ten Hoor F, Hornstra G (1981) Effects of dietary essential fatty acids on prostaglandin synthesis. In Beers Jr RF, Bassett EG (eds) Nutritional factors: Modulating effects on metabolic processes. Raven Press, New York p 539-549
8. Moncada S, Gryglevski RJ, Bunting S, Vane JR (1976) An enzyme isolated from arteries transforms prostaglandin endoperoxides to an unstable substance that inhibits platelet aggregation. Nature 263: 663-665
9. Willis AL, Smith JB (1981) Some perspectives on platelets and prostaglandins. Progress in Lipid Research 20: 387-406
10. Holman RT (1970) Biological activities of and requirements for polyunsaturated acids. In: Holman RT (ed) Progress in the Chemistry of Fats and other Lipids, Vol 9, Polyunsaturated Acids Part 5. Pergamon Press Oxford, p 611-682
11. Nugteren DH, Evert WC, Soeting WJ, Spuy JH (1980) Effect of different amounts of linoleic acid in the diet on the excretion of urinary prostaglandin and metabolites in the rat. In: Samuelsson B; Ramwell PW, Paoletti R (eds) Advances in Prostaglandin and Thromboxane Research, Vol 8. Raven Press New York, p 1793-1796
12. Zöllner N, Adam O, Wolfram G (1979) The influence of linoleic acid intake on the excretion of urinary prostaglandin metabolites. Res Exp Med (Berl) 175: 149-153
13. Ten Hoor F, De Deckere EAM, Haddeman E, Hornstra G, Quadt F (1980) Dietary manipulation of prostaglandin and thromboxane synthesis in heart, aorta and blood platelets of the rat. In: Samuelsson B, Ramwell PW, Paoletti R (eds) Advances in Prostaglandin and Thromboxane Research, Vol 8. Raven Press, New York, p 1771-1781

14. Gudbjarnasson S, Hallgrimsson J (1976) The role of myocardial membrane lipids in the development of cardiac necrosis. Acta Med Suppl 587: 17:27
15. Gudbjarnasson S (1980) Pathophysiology of long-chain polyene fatty acids in heart muscle. Nutr Metab 24 (Suppl 1): 142-146
16. Triebe G, Block HU, Förster W (1976) Ueber das Blutdruckverhalten kochsalz-belasteter Ratten bei unterschiedlichem Linolsäuregehalt des Futters. Acta Biol Med Germ 35: 1223-1224
17. Ten Hoor F, Van de Graaf HM (1978) The influence of a linoleic acid-rich diet and acetyl salicylic acid on NaCl-induced hypertension, $Na^+$ and $H_2O$-balance, and urinary prostaglandin excretion in rats. Acta Biol Med Germ 37: 875-877
18. Ten Hoor F (1980) Cardiovascular effects of dietary linoleic acid. Nutr Metab 24 (Suppl 1): 162-180
19. Hoffmann P, Förster W (1981) Zur Bedeutung einer an polyungesättigten Fetten reichen Ernährung für die Prävention und Therapie von Herz-Kreislauf-Krankheiten. Dt Gesundh.-Wesen 35: 2001-2012 and Dt Gesundh.-Wesen 36: 145-152
20. Hornstra G (1974) Dietary fats and arterial thrombosis. Haemostasis 2: 21-52
21. Galli C, Agradi E, Petroni A, Tremoli E (1981) Differential effects of dietary fatty acids on the accumulation of arachidonic acid and its metabolic conversion through the cyclooxygenase and lipooxygenase in platelets and vascular tissue. Lipids 16: 165-172
22. Hornstra G, Lewis B, Chait A, Turpeinen O, Karvonen MJ, Vergroesen AJ (1973) Influence of dietary fat on platelet function in men. Lancet i: 1155-1157
23. Renaud S, Dumont E, Godsey F, Morazain R, Thevenen C, Ortchanian E (1980) Dietary fats and platelet function in French and Scottish farmers. Nutr Metab 24 (Suppl 1): 90-104
24. Fleischman AI, Justice D, Bierenbaum ML, Stier A, Sullivan A (1975) Benificial effect of increased dietary linoleate upon in vivo platelet function in man. J of Nutr 105: 1286-1290
25. Iacono JM, Judd JT, Marschall MW, Canary JJ, Dougherty RM, Mackin JF, Weinland BT (1981) The role of dietary essential fatty acids and prostaglandins in reducing blood pressure. Progress in Lipid Research 20: 349-364
26. Vergroesen AJ, Fleischman AI, Comberg HU, Heyden S, Hames CG (1978) The influence of increased dietary linoleate on essential hypertension in man. Acta Biol Med Germ 37: 879-883
27. Stern B, Heyden S, Miller D, Latham G, Klimas A, Pilkington K (1980) Intervention Study in high school students with elevated blood pressures: Dietary experiment with polyunsaturated fatty acids. Nutr Metab 24: 137-147
28. Rao Harsha R, Rao Brahmaji U and Srikantia SG (1981) Effect of polyunsaturate-rich vegetable oils on blood pressure in essential hypertension. Clin Exp Hypertension 3: 27-38
29. Oster P, Arab L, Schellenberg B, Henck CC, Mordasini R, Schlierf G (1980) Linolsäure in der Diätbehandlung der Hypertonie. Ernährungs-Umschau 27: 143-144
30. Houtsmuller AJ, Van Hal-Ferwerda J, Zahn KJ, Henkes HE (1981) Favorable influences of linoleic acid on the progression of diabetic micro- and macroangiopathy in adult onset diabetes mellitus. Progress in Lipid Research 20: 377-386

# Effects of Dietary Treatment on Lipoplitic Activities and Lipids and Apolipoproteins in Patiens with Uremia

T. Yasugi

## I. Introduction

Lipid metabolism and effects of diet on lipid metabolism in Patients with uremia under hemodialysis(H.D.) has been investigated since the hyperlipidemia and high incidence of coronary heart disease had been reported in such patients.

## II. Methods

Separation and determination of serum lipoproteins: ultracentrifugation. Apolipoproteins: PAG electrophresis. PHLA: method of Carlson. LCAT: method of Akanuma and Glomset. TC and TG: enzymatic method. TG: acetylacetone method.

## III. Results

### 1. Serum lipids and Lipoproteins

In 191 cases of H.D. patients, 60% showed hypertriglyceridemia, 20% combined hyperlipidemia and remained 20% within normal lipid levels (Fig. 1.).

Fig.1. Serum TC and TG in H.D.

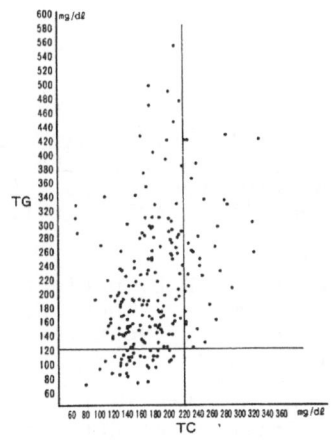

In the lipoprotein levels, LDL increased and $HDL_2$ and $HDL_3$ decreased. In the LDL subfractions, Sf12-20 increased significantly, but Sf0-12

did not increase(Table 1.).

Table 1.  Serum Lipoprotein Levels in H.D.

|          | n  | VLDL   | LDL    | HDL    | HDL$_2$ | HDL$_3$ |
|----------|----|--------|--------|--------|---------|---------|
| controls | 36 | 127±11 | 252±13 | 244±12 | 84±4    | 158±10  |
| H.D.     | 20 | 131±18 | 311±22 | 145±21 | 40±7    | 105±15  |

mean±SE, mg/dl

In the lipid components of various lipoproteins, it was remarkable
that TG content in LDL and HDL increased significanyly, and TC
content in LDL and HDL decreased.  Aminoacid components in apo-LDL
and apo-HDL were almost similar between H.D. and controls.

## 2.  PHLA and LCAT Activities, and Apolipoproteins

PHLA and LCAT activities significantly decreased in the H.D. patients.
Apo-C/B ratio of VLDL and apo-AI/AII ratio of HDL also decreased
significantly(Table 2.)

Table 2.  PHLA and LCAT Activities, and Apoproteins in H.D.

|                        | control       | H.D.          |
|------------------------|---------------|---------------|
| PHLA (mEq/l)           | 0.493±0.082 n=5 | 0.262±0.058 n=6 |
| apθ-C/apo-B (VLDL)     | 1 n=10        | 0.64 n=5      |
| LCAT (n mol/ml/hr)     | 89±2 n=6      | 40±6 n=8      |
| apo-AI/apo-AII (HDL)   | 1 n=10        | 0.7 n=6       |

apoprotein ratio: shown control value as 1, mean±SE

## 3. Effect of Diet

Our regular diet for H.D. patients(40 cal/Kg/day, protein 15%, carbo-
hydrate 55%, fat 30%, P/S=0.7) was changed by the following two ways;
Diet P/S=1.5: P/S ratio was changed from 0.7 to 1.5 and Diet P/S=1.5,
F: carbohydrate was changed from 55% to 40%, fat from 30% to 45% and
P/S ratio from 0.7 to 1.5.

The regular diet in which 13 cases of H.D. patients were maintained
was changed to Diet P/S=1.5 for 4 weeks.  Then, after the 4 weeks of
interval on regular diet, the 4 cases of volunteering patients were
given again Diet P/S=1.5,F for 2 weeks.

Results are listed in Table 3.,4.·,and 5.  In the Diet P/S=1.5,
decreases of VLDL and LDL, and increase of HDL were observed.  In the
Diet P/S=1.5,F, although LDL decreased, VLDL increased and HDL decreased significantly.  In the both diet groups, tendencies of increases of PHLA and LCAT were observed but, these did not recover to
the control values.  In the apo-AI/AII ratio of HDL, recover to the

control value(1.5 to 2.0) was observed under the Diet P/S=1.5. However, apo-AI/AII ratio of HDL rather decreased (1.5 to 1.1) under the Diet P/S=1.5,F.  Subunits of HDL apo-C were not affected by the both diet.

Table 3.  Effects of Diet on Serum Lipids and Lipoproteins

Diet P/S=1.5

|        | TC       | TG      | PL      |
|--------|----------|---------|---------|
| before | 187±13   | 158± 9  | 212± 6  |
| after  | 163±13   | 128±12  | 196±10  |

|        | VLDL   | LDL     | HDL     | $HDL_2$ | $HDL_3$  | $HDL_2/HDL_3$ |
|--------|--------|---------|---------|---------|----------|---------------|
| before | 99±10  | 365±30  | 153±17  | 50±8    | 103±13   | 0.36±0.06     |
| after  | 73±10  | 301±30  | 194±14  | 54±7    | 140±12   | 0.63±0.09     |

Diet P/S=1.5,F                                   n=13,   mg/dl

|        | TC       | TG      | PL      |
|--------|----------|---------|---------|
| before | 199±25   | 158±19  | 212±13  |
| after  | 191±16   | 175±31  | 203± 9  |

|        | VLDL   | LDL      | HDL     | $HDL_2$ | $HDL_3$  | $HDL_2/HDL_3$ |
|--------|--------|----------|---------|---------|----------|---------------|
| before | 64±21  | 411±62   | 193±23  | 60±11   | 134±19   | 0.45±0.12     |
| after  | 102±12 | 310±109  | 163±17  | 46±15   | 117±10   | 0.51±0.12     |

                                                  n=4,    mg/dl

Table 4.  Effects of Diet on PHLA and LCAT Activities and Apo-AI/AII Ratio of HDL

|              | PHLA          | LCAT      | AI/AII  |
|--------------|---------------|-----------|---------|
| control      | 0.493±0.082   | 89 ±2.0   | 2.0±0.2 |
| Diet P/S=1.5 |               |           |         |
| before       | 0.245±0.048   | 48.2±5.0  | 1.5±0.1 |
| after        | 0.381±0.056   | 54.0±4.3  | 2.0±0.2 |
| Diet P/S=1.5,F |             |           |         |
| before       | 0.213±0.060   | 42.9±3.3  | 1.5±0.1 |
| after        | 0.237±0.036   | 49.9±6.8  | 1.1±0.1 |

         PHLA:mEq/l,   LCAT:nmol/ml/hr,   mean±SE

IV.  Discussions

Increases of TG content in LDL and HDL should be noticed in the H.D. patients.  These phenomena may induce the higher incidence of hyper triglyceridemia than that of hypercholesterolemia.  The evidences that PHLA and LCAT activities significantly decreased in the H.D. patients, might be one of the causative factors to disturb the meta-

254

bolism of triglycerides.  Several reports on the enzyme activities in uremia show similar tendencies(1-4).  In this study, we found that apo-C in the VLDL and apo-AI in the HDL decreased in the H.D. patients. These may partially play a rol in the decreases of enzyme activities.

Table 5.  Effects of Diet P/S=1.5 on HDL Apo-C

|          | before   | after    |
|----------|----------|----------|
| C-I      | 3.4±0.4  | 3.1±0.3  |
| C-II     | 6.0±0.6  | 5.1±0.3  |
| C-III    | 9.8±0.4  | 9.1±1.2  |
| C-II/C-III | 0.6±0.1 | 0.5±o.1 |

Concerning the effectiveness of diet on the hyperlipidemia in uremia, Cattran et al reported the following results.  Namely, low carbohydrat diet reduced serum triglyceride level and high carbohydrate diet elevated the level.  Furthermore, serum cholesterol level maintained constant value during the each diet period(5).  In this study, slight decrease of carbohydrate(from 55% to 50%) and the increase of P/S ratio(from 0.7 to 1.5) decreased both TC and TG levels.  Serum LDL and VLDL levels also decreased and HDL increased.  Furthermore, this diet(Diet P/S=1.5) recovered HDL apo-AI/AII ratio to the normal value. These results suggest that the increase of P/S ratio to 1.5 gives favorite effects on the lipid metabolism in H.D. patients.  Even though above mentioned favorite effects, Diet P/S=1.5 could not re-cover the enzyme activities and also did not affect the HDL apo-C sub-units.  On the other hand, the decrease of carbohydrate intake(from 55% to 40%), the increase of fat intake(from 30% to 45%) and the in-crease of P/S ratio to 1.5 did not give any convenient effects in respect of serum lipid levels, the enzyme activities and the apolipo-proteins.  These evidences that the diet does not improve the re-duction of enzyme activities and the status of apolipoproteins might indicate that the hyperlipidemia in H.D. patients is not caused by the dietary factors only.

Concerning the atherogenesis in H.D. patients, the change to HDL lipid component to be rich in triglycerides and reduction of LCAT activity might be noticed since the both phenomena are pointed out to impare the removal of cholesterol from cell membrane.

V. Conclusions

Incidence of hypertriglycridemia is dominant than that of hyper-cholesterolemia in H.D. patients.  This triglyceridemia seems to be caused by the reductions of lipolitic enzyme and LCAT activities. And it seems to be difficult improve the hyperlipidemia by the dietary treatment since the apolipoproteins and the enzyms may stand against to improve the hyperlipidemia effectively.  However, the dietary treatment which increases the P/S ratio to 1.5 may still be recomended to H.D. patients in order to improve the hyperlipidemia.

Acknowledgment  The author is grateful to doctors T. Shimizu, T. Konno, H. Izumida, T. Tochihara, G. Mizuno, K. Kishi, T. Fujioka and U. Hara for their cooperations.

## References

Bagdade JD, Porte DJ, Bierman EI (1968) Hypertriglyceridemia, a metabolic consequence of chronic renal failure. New England J Med. 279: 181-186

Huttunen J, Ehnholm C, Kinnunen P, Nikkila EA (1975) An immunochemical method for the selective measurement of two triglyceride lipase in human postheparin plasma. Clinica Chimica Acta. 63:335-347

Applebaum-Bowden D, Goldberg AP, Hazzard WR, Sherrard DJ, Brunzell JD, Huttunen J, Nikkila EA, Ehnholm C (1979) Postheparin plasma triglyceride lipase in chronic hemodialysis. Metabolism. 28:917-924

Guarnieri GF, Moracchiello M, Campanacci L, Ursini F, Ferri L, Marina V, Gregolin C (1978) Lecithin-cholesterol acyltransferase(LCAT) activity in chronic uremia. Kidney International. 13:Suppl.8, S26-S30

Cattran DC, Steiner G, Fenton SSA, Ampil M (1980) Dialysis hyperlipidemia: response to dietary manipulations. Clinical Nephrology. 13: 177-182

# 1.7 Exercise

# Introduction

P. D. Wood

It is my privilege to introduce this workshop on Exercise.
I believe that this marks the first occasion on which exercise, and
its relation to atherosclerosis, has been accorded a major subsection
of the proceedings of this International Symposium. For many years
exercise occupied the neglected end of the energy input - energy output continuum, a Cinderella subject, overshadowed by her sisters,
diet and drugs. I am sure I speak for all the participants here
today in thanking the organizers of this Symposium for recognizing
exercise as a research area whose time has come, and indeed, for
increasing the general emphasis on the scientific study of prevention of atherosclerosis at this meeting.

I should like to clarify the term "exercise" as we shall use
it this afternoon. We are referring to the rather more vigorous or
aerobic forms of physical activity: stair climbing, brisk walking,
running, cross-country skiing, cycling, swimming and the like. Lei-
surely golf, American Football and bowling do not qualify. One may
question the relevance of these aerobic sports and occupations; and,
indeed, the infrequent practice of aerobic activities, particularly
by the middle-aged, has perhaps justified the meager attention paid
to exercise in relation to atherosclerosis in the past. In many
countries (but not all) this is now changing, and increased physical
activity in leisure time has become a prominent feature of modern
life in North America. Some 30 million joggers are believed to fre-

quent American parks and streets. The annual San Francisco "Bay-to-Breakers" race over 8 miles, which had a field of 110 in 1963, attracted 50,000 runners in 1982.

It seems, therefore, that large-scale participation in exercise can quite rapidly become part of a national lifestyle, and so its study is now clearly relevant. The great majority of people of all ages and both sexes can take part in some type of aerobic exercise. Exercise tends to be addictive, its practice is reinforcing since it produces desirable results quite rapidly in many people, it is readily modelled to the inactive by its exponents, and it has a certain vitality that is refreshing.

Regular exercise produces countless physiological and psychological changes in the sedentary person, many of which we shall hear about this afternoon, since they relate in one way or another to atherosclerosis. The exerciser, compared to the sedentary individual, is usually lean; in spite of this he frequently eats more than the sedentary person, which has several interesting consequences. Exercisers tend not to smoke. They have serum lipoprotein patterns that appear to be associated with lowered risk of cardiovascular disease. Exercise modifies many enzyme systems, with changed activity levels for respiratory chain, lipoprotein lipase and hepatic lipase enzymes, among others. The processes of clotting and fibrinolysis in blood are modified. Exercise appears to change the concentrations of prostaglandins and endorphins in blood. And there are strong indications from epidemiological studies in man, and from animal studies in sub-human primates, that long-term exercise has a role in the prevention, and perhaps regression, of atherosclerosis.

Most of these numerous characteristic effects of exercise are generally interpreted as advantageous from the point of view of preventing heart disease. We might expect, therefore, that the

growing habit of exercising regularly will be followed in due course
by a clear decrease in death and disability from heart disease.  I
believe there is reason for considerable optimism in this regard;
but it is important for us to ensure that the study of exercise is
not the sole province of zealots and enthusiasts.  Solid, scientific
study of all aspects of the influence of increased exercise on the
atherosclerotic  process is vital, given the clear movement towards
more physically active populations.  The study of possibly deleterious
effects of exercise must also receive due attention.

Mark Twain was of the opinion that he obtained all the exercise he needed by helping to carry the coffin at the funerals of his
more active friends.  I suspect we shall prove him wrong; but we must
do so with well designed studies, hard facts and an unbiased approach.
The speakers here this afternoon represent the vanguard of distinguished scientists who will dedicate themselves to this task.

# Therapeutical Effects of Endurance Training in Primary Hyperlipoproteinemia

M. Hanefeld, W. Leonhardt, S. Fischer, U. Julius, E. Schubert, A. Trübsbach, and H. Haller

Physical inactivity plays an important role in the pathogenesis of hyperlipoproteinemia (HLP) and associated coronary risk factors. A study with 444 first degree relatives of index cases with primary HLP proved that relatives without regular physical training (PT) are more prone to elevated blood lipids than those exercising during leisure (Hanefeld et al. 1982).
Considerable evidence has accumulated indicating that vigorous PT substantially reduces serum triglycerides (TG). The efficacy on total cholesterol (TC) is less impressive. However, more detailed analysis revealed an increase in HDL-C and decrease in LDL-C induced by PT (Wood et al. 1976).
Recently published reviews showed a significant reduction of hypertriglyceridemia (HTG) and hyperinsulinemia in type IV HLP. So far, little information exists about the therapeutical effect of mild to moderate PT in middle-aged sedentary patients with HLP under the conditions of sustained lipid lowering diet. We therefore investigated the efficacy of a moderate PT regimen on lipid and lipoprotein fractions in patients with HLP.

## Material and Methods

Since 1974 more than 160 patients with primary HLP, e.g. TG levels before treatment $> 250$ mg/dl and/or TC $> 300$ mg/dl were trained 4 weeks at a health resort. The patients were at least 4 weeks before and during the training program on a standardized lipid lowering diet (p/s ratio $\sim 1.0$, cholesterol intakte p.d.

300 mg, recommendations for restriction of refined carbohydrates and alcohol resp.). The exercise program involved jogging, terrain training, gymnastics and volleyball. The prescribed daily load was 45 minutes at pulse rates of 130 - 180/M.
This paper deals with:

I       65 patients with HTG (59 M, 6 F, aged 41.9 $\pm$ 10.2 yrs.) excess weight $<$ + 15 kg. Additional 21 had calorie restrictions (food supply 1000 - 2000 cal. p.d.)

II      16 M with familial type V treated in the same way

III     36 M (27 HTG, 9 familial hypercholesterolemia) with isocaloric diet-supply who additionally trained twice daily 10 M on a bicycle ergometer with 80% $VO_2$ max.

Serum lipids and lipoproteins were determined with routine methods. The intravenous fat tolerance test was performed with Lipofundin (Braun-Melsungen) according to the procedure described by Rössner (1974) to calculate the fractional removal rate (p). The exercise capacity (Watt) was measured by bicycle ergometry.

Effect on Serum Lipids: Relation to Weight Loss and Starting Level

In study I diurnal TG conc. decreased by about 35% after 9 days PT (Fig. 1).

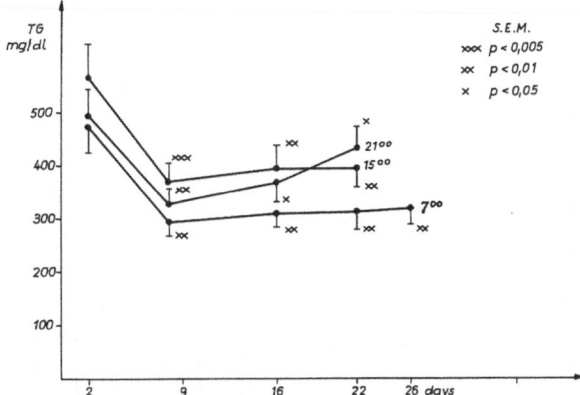

Fig. 1 Effect of PT on diurnal TG conc. in primary HTG (n=65)

The TG-minimum at this time was followed by a small increase despite a continuing loss of weight (Fig.2). Obviously, this rebound is more expressed in the postprandial state which could be confirmed in the below mentioned study with obese HTG patients. Since this phenomenon could not be observed with weight-stable subjects (Fig.4) one could speculate that elevated levels of FFA may contribute to an enhanced hepatic VLDL synthesis in weight-losing patients at this time

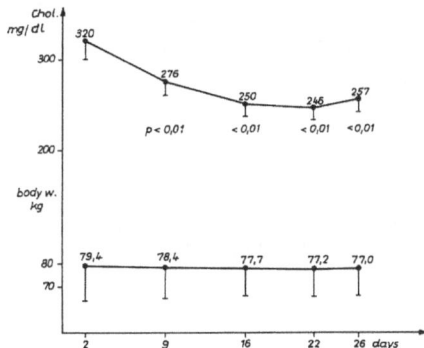

Fig. 2 Effect of PT on TC conc. and body weight in primary HTG (n=65)

TC react slowlier to PT reaching its lowest level after 22 days PT. The decrease in blood lipids was mainly due to the superimposed weight-loss. The TG-fall (starting TG conc.-TG conc. at the 22nd day) signi-ficantly correlated to weight-loss (r=0.25, p < 0.05). Another impor-tant factor influencing the response to PT was the lipid level before the training program (Fig.3)

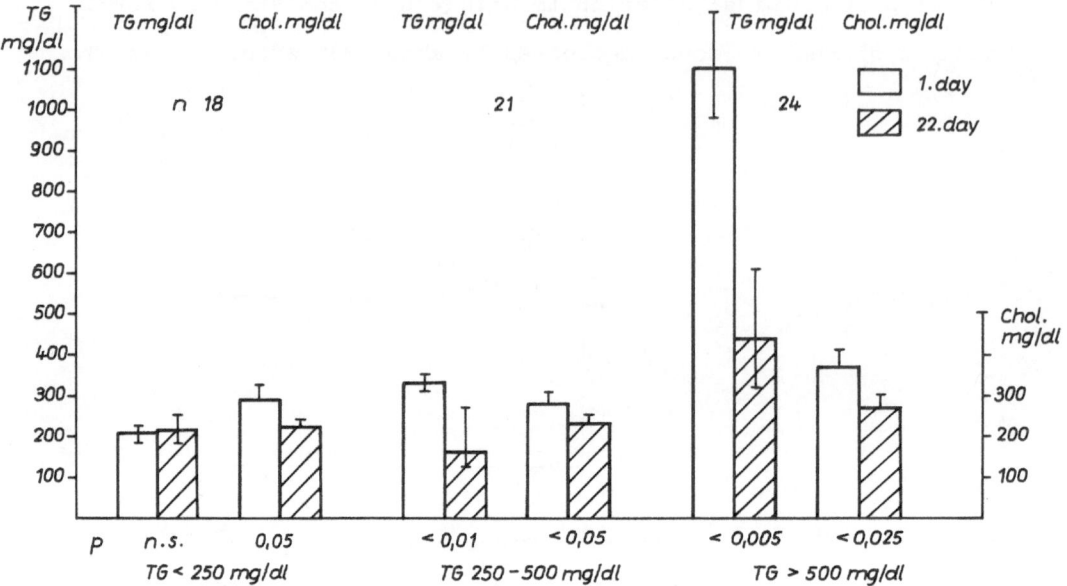

Fig. 3 Effect of PT on blood lipids in relation to TG starting level

The best therapeutical results were obtained in the category with
initial TG levels above 500 mg/dl. These data confirm a previously
published study (Hanefeld et al. 1981) with 41 obese HTG patients
where a highly significant correlation of TG and TC levels at
entry to lipid lowering efficacy of PT could be domonstrated. There
seem to be at least two exceptions from this rule: familial type V
and familial hypercholesterolemia


Relation between Lipoprotein Fractions, Intravenous Fat Tolerance
Test and Working Capacity

The effect on lipoprotein fractions in weight-stable patients
(study III) with HTG is demonstrated in Fig. 4

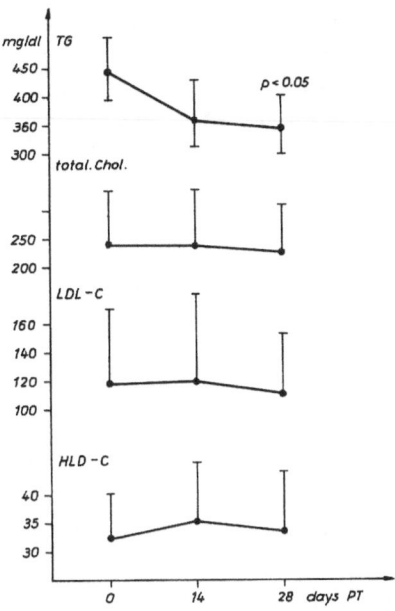

Fig. 4 Effect of PT on blood lipids in 26 middle-aged male patients with HTG (BWI before PT 1.15, after 1.13, working capacity before PT 125 Watt, after PT 147 Watt)

Despite a substantial decrease in TG conc. no significant influence on cholesterol fractions could be obtained. Contrary to findings with long-lasting heavy exercise we observed no significant changes in HDL-C. This confirms previously reported results (Hanefeld et al. 1981) with 18 patients with HTG who underwent the same program as group I. Recently, Farrel and Barboriak (1980) described a biphasic course of HDL-C changes in subjects undergoing a moderate training program: a slight drop in the first 4 weeks was followed by a significant rise after 8 weeks.

The changes in TG level ($\Delta$ TG) were significantly correlated to improved intravenous fat tolerance test ($\Delta$ P Lipofundin) as indicated in Tab. 1. Furthermore, there was a positive correlation between enhanced working capacity ($\Delta$ Watt) and fractional removal rate.

Tab. 1 Correlations between changes in working capacity, lipid conc. and lipid removal (P Lipofundin) induced by PT in HTG with stable body weight ($\Delta$ =value before-value after 28 days PT)

| | lg TG (before) | HDL-C (before) | $\Delta$ lg TG | $\Delta$ HDL-C | $\Delta$ lg P Lipofund. |
|---|---|---|---|---|---|
| lg TG(before) | – | | | | |
| HDL-C(before) | -0.48[a] | – | | | |
| $\Delta$ lg TG | 0.40[b] | -0.23 | – | | |
| $\Delta$ HDL-C | 0.20 | 0.26 | -0.23 | – | |
| $\Delta$ lg P Lipof. | 0.09 | 0.01 | -0.50[a] | -0.07 | – |
| $\Delta$ Watt | 0.01 | -0.07 | -0.27 | 0.03 | 0.38[b] |

a) $p < 0.01$         b) $p < 0.05$

This could be caused by an elevated lipoprotein lipase activity in trained subjects. This supports the assumption that accelerated catabolism of TG-rich lipoproteins could be a major mechanism by which PT lowers TG and TC in HLP. More studies are needed to show whether PT also influences hepatic secretion of VLDL.
We have studied in 5 patients with HTG the relationship of Apo CIII/CII ratio to TG concentrations before and during the training at the health resort and found a highly significant correlation between Ap CIII/CII and lg VLDL-TG (Tab.2).

Tab. 2 Correlations between apoprotein and lipoprotein fractions before and during 26 days PT (6 values per patient)

| Variables | CIII/CII (VLDL) | lgTG | lgVLDL-TG | lgVLDL-C | AI (HDL) | AII (HDL) | HDL-TG |
|---|---|---|---|---|---|---|---|
| CIII/CII | - | +0.72$^a$ | +0.68$^a$ | +0.55$^b$ | - | - | - |
| AI | - | - | - | - | - | -0.75$^a$ | -0.57$^c$ |
| AII | - | - | - | - | - | - | +0.53$^d$ |

a) $p < 0.001$,    b) $p < 0.005$    c) $p < 0.01$    d) $p < 0.05$

These data suggest that besides a direct effect of PT on VLDL removal via enhanced adipose tissue and muscle lipoprotein lipase activity changes in Apo C and Apo A pattern must be considered. Obviously manouvres to lower blood lipids by exercise affect both removal and lipoprotein production.


Effect of PT in Familial HLP

Investigations published on exercise effects mainly concern inhomogeneous groups of patients with HTG differing in genetics and pathogenesis. Scarce information exists on exercise treatment of familial HLP whose lipid abnormality does not so much depend on environmental factors. A study with familial type V patients (Tab.3) reveals less impressive lowering of blood lipids.

Tab. 3 Effect of physical training on blood lipids (X + SEM, mg/dl) in Type V hyperlipoproteinemia (n=16)

| Parameter | O | 22 days | decrease(%) | p |
|---|---|---|---|---|
| TG | 2109+1575 | 1447+1126 | 31 | n.s. |
| Cholesterol | 486+ 270 | 373+ 183 | 23 | n.s. |

In some cases even an increase could be observed. The same applies for familial hypercholesterolemia (Fig.5) which is rather resistent to PT.

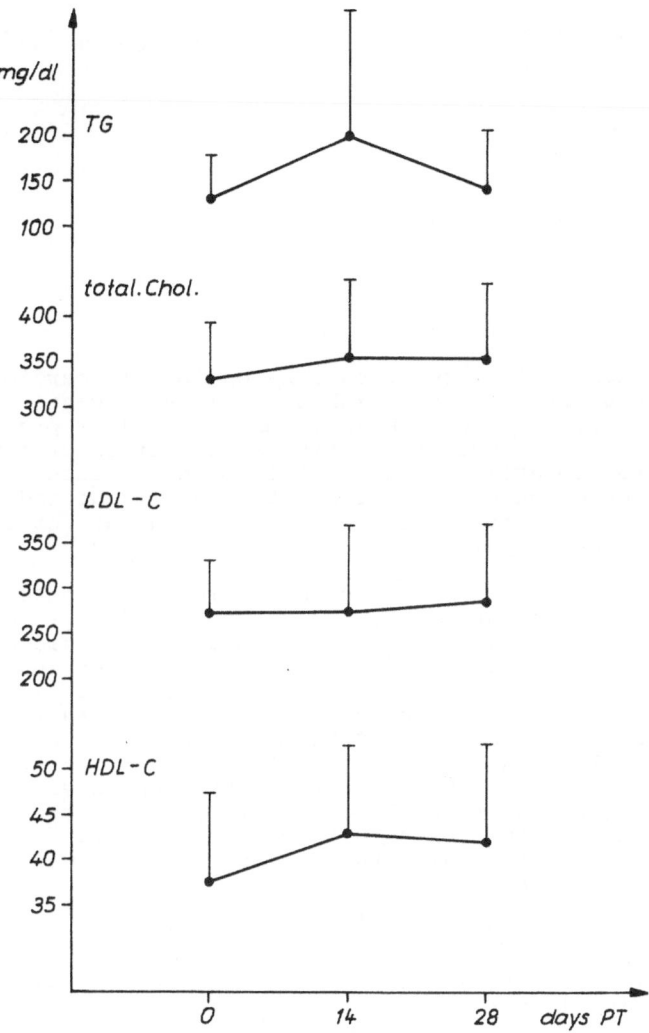

<u>Fig. 5</u> Effect of PT on blood lipids in familial hypercholesterolemia (n=9) (BWI before 1.10, after 1.08, working capacity before 121 Watt, after 147 Watt)

Further investigations are needed to define the types of HLP which preferentially should be treated with exercise. The same applies for optimal techniques and intensity to use PT as a powerful tool in the prevention of HLP and vascular complications.

# Atherosclerotic Disease in Non-Human Primates: Its Prevention and Regression by Moderate Conditioning Exercise

D. M. Kramsch, A. J. Aspen, and R. L. Spicer

The precise influence of exercise on atherosclerotic cardiovascular disease in man has not been established (1-2). As recently reviewed (4), pertinent studies in lower mammals and birds have produced contradictory results, some even suggesting acceleration of atherosclerosis by exercise. To gain more insight into the effects of physical training on the cardiovascular system with and without induced atherosclerosis, chronic moderate exercise conditioning was tested for the first time in non-human primates.

Five groups of 8 or 9 adult male Macaca fascicularis monkeys each were studies for 42 months or 36 months, respectively. Two groups were first exercise conditioned for 18 months while on a control diet, after which time 1 group was given an atherogenic diet (10% butter and 0.1% cholesterol by weight) with both groups continuing chronic exercise for 24 months. Two other groups were not chronically exercised throughout the study and designated "sedentary". Both of these groups were given the control diet for 12 months, after which time 1 group received the atherogenic diet for 24 months while the other continued the control diet. The fifth group was first kept sedentary and on the atherogenic diet for 24 months and then exposed to a gradually increasing exercise program for 18 more months while the atherogenic diet was continued. Chronic conditioning exercise consisted of running on a treadmill for 1 hour three times a week at an average speed of 3.5 km/h (a good jogging pace for monkeys of 4 - 5 kg body weight). All animals were subjected periodically to short test exercise (10 minutes) or extensive exercise tests (up to 1 hour) while the electrocardiogram was monitored by radiotelemetry.

The heart rates of exercising monkeys at rest and test exercise decreased drastically after conditioning regardless of diet and of time sequence in which the exercise program was introduced (Fig. 1, left). In contrast, all monkeys which remained sedentary (Fig. 1, right) retained the same high heart rates at rest and test exercise. The mean serum content of total cholesterol rose markedly from values of 102 mg/dl in sedentary or exercising normal controls to about 620 mg/dl in the sedentary or exercise-conditioned groups on the atherogenic diet. These increases in cholesterol were mainly due to large increases in LDL + VLDL-cholesterol in all cholesterol-fed animals. However, in both exercise-conditioned groups receiving the atherogenic diet, there was also a small but significant (p < 0.01) increase in HDL-cholesterol content as compared with the sedentary group on the same diet, but not with the sedentary normal controls.

In sedentary monkeys receiving the atherogenic diet for 24 months, the cholesterol feeding induced striking grossly visible atherosclerosis of the coronary and other major arteries (Fig. 2). In contrast, the arteries of monkeys that were exercise-conditioned before and during the feeding of the high cholesterol diet revealed remarkably less in-

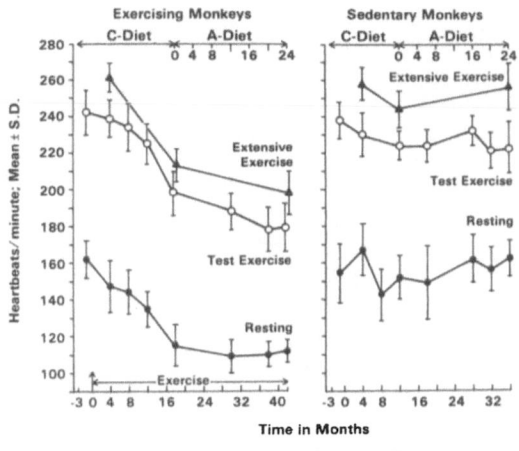

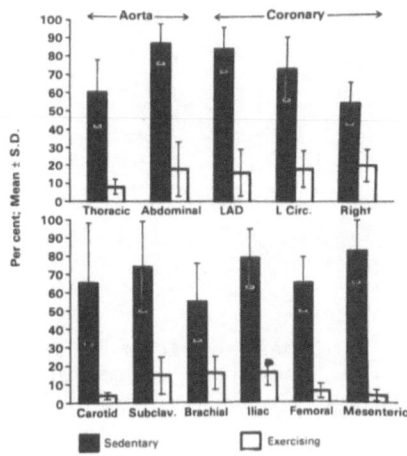

Fig. 1. Heart rates of exercising (left) and sedentary (right) monkeys on atherogenic diet for 24 months

Fig. 2. Intimal surface involved with lesions in sedentary and exercising monkeys on atherogenic diet for 24 months

timal lesions. Similar marked reductions in gross lesion involvement were obtained when exercise-conditioning was introduced after the animals had been on the atherogenic diet and sedentary for 24 months. No lesions were observed in sedentary or exercising animals on the control diet.

The hearts of exercise-conditioned monkeys, whether on control or atherogenic diets (Fig. 3), were considerably larger than those of sedentary animals on the atherogenic diet or sedentary normal controls. The heart weights of conditioned monkeys also were much greater than those of either sedentary group. The increases in heart size and weight were mainly due to significant (p < 0.01) increases in left ventricular mass. Although lesions were present in the coronary artery segments from predetermined sites in all groups on the atherogenic diet, the disease

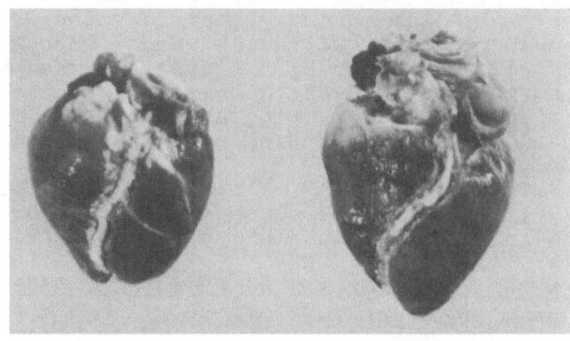

Fig. 3. Hearts of monkeys on atherogenic diet for 24 months: left = sedentary; right = exercise-contioned

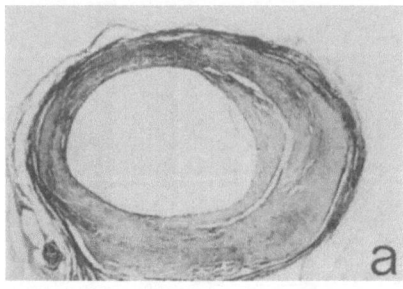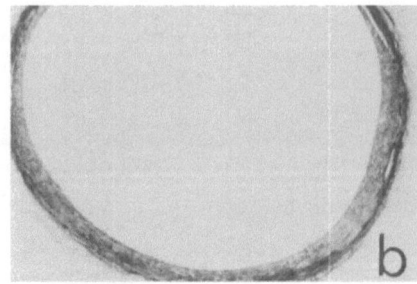

**Fig. 4.** Cross sections of left cirumflex coronary arteries, atherogenic diet: a. Sedentary 24 months; b. Sedentary 24 months then exercised 18 months

was markedly different in exercise-conditioned monkeys. Conditioning resulted in lesions of less than half the intimal thickness found in lesions of sedentary animals, regardless of whether the exercise was introduced <u>before</u> or <u>after</u> starting the atherogenic diet. Furthermore, there was a significant ($p < 0.01$) increase in the size of the coronary-artery lumina outlined by the internal elastica (IEL-lumina) in all conditioned monkeys as compared with the IEL-lumina of sedentary animals on the atherogenic diet (Fig. 4) and those of sedentary normal controls. It is of interest to note that the IEL-lumina of coronary arteries in exercise-conditioned normal controls also were significantly ($p < 0.01$) larger than those of either sedentary group.

Thus, in exercise-conditioned monkeys, an increase in vessel caliber and a decrease in lesion size seemed to act in concert to reduce the substantial coronary-artery narrowing induced in sedentary monkeys by the atherogenic diet to "clinically" inapparent levels. Our studies provide direct evidence that long-term regular exercise, even at moderate levels, may be capable of retarding and/or reversing generalized atherosclerosis and atherosclerotic coronary heart disease in primates.

Supported by a grant (HL 18060) from the US Public Health Service.

## References

1. Milvy P, Sieger AJ (1981) Physical activity levels and altered mortality from coronary heart disease with an emphasis on marathon running: a critical review. Cardiovasc Rev Rp 2: 233-236
2. Froehlicher VF (1978) Exercise and the prevention of coronary atherosclerotic heart disease. Cardiovasc Clin 9 (3): 13-23
3. Paffenbarger RS Jr, Wing AL, Hyde RT (1978) Physical activity as an index of heart attack risk in college alumni. Am J Epidemiol 108: 161-175
4. Kramsch DM, Aspen AJ, Abramowitz BM, Kreimendahl T, Hood WB Jr (1981) Reduction of coronary atherosclerosis by moderate conditioning exercise in monkeys on an atherogenic diet. N Engl J Med 305: 1482-1489

# The Effect of Different Types of Exercise on Serum Lipids

A. Lehtonen

With respect to evidence suggestive of the fact that reduced HDL-cholesterol and elevated LDL-cholesterol may predispose to athero-sclerosis it seems logical that alteration of their levels should be beneficial in reducing the incidence of coronary heart disease. Therefore, it has been much interest to determine lipoprotein changes produced by increased physical activity.

## Physical Activity During Leisure

Carlsson and Mossfeldt (1) found decreased levels of very low density lipoprotein (VLDL) and high levels of HDL-cholesterol in skiiers participating in a 90 km skiracing. Measurements of VLDL cholesterol in male and female long distance runners have confirmed that triglyceride-rich VLDL is indeed at a very low level in these very active individuals (2). Plasma triglyceride concentration and age are positively correlated in sedentary subjects but not in athletes (3). Wood et al. (4) determined plasma lipoproteins in very active men (running > 25 km/wk for the previous year, mean age 47 years) and in a comparison group of men. The runners had significantly decreased plasma LDL cholesterol concentrations and a higher mean level of HDL cholesterol than the comparison group. We have determined the serum lipids of 23 regularly training men, over 30 year old, who trained more than 25 km/week, running or skiing (5). The exercise increased serum HDL cholesterol concentration and the ratio of HDL cholesterol to total cholesterol and decreased serum triglyceride levels. There was a positive correlation between the amount of weekly exercise in km and plasma HDL cholesterol level. Hartung et al. (6) investigated the effect of diet on HDL cholesterol in marathon runners, joggers (running at least 3.2 km three times per week) and inactive men. Their results suggest that HDL differences among the three groups were primarily the result of distance run, not dietary factors. Distance run was also the best predictor of the HDL: total cholesterol ratio and of total cholesterol ( a negative correlation ).

Chronic heavy endurance exercise alters serum lipoproteins, but it also has been shown changes in serum lipids after a single exposure to exercise (7,8). HDL cholesterol increased by 12 % of the pre-race level immediately after the 70 km cross country ski race and was still elevated 4 days after the race (7). LDL and VLDL chole-sterol showed a tendency to decrease immediately after the race and were reduced on the following two days (7). Serum total cholesterol and triglyceride concentration decreased after a 42-km footrace but only small increase in HDL cholesterol levels were noted after exercise (8).

A change in HDL cholesterol may reflect only a change in the propor-tion of cholesterol in relation to the other lipoprotein components i.e. the apoproteins, A-I, and A-II and phospholipids. As physical activity seems to cause higher HDL cholesterol levels it is of

interest to know whether this increase could also be demonstrated
for the apoproteins A-I and A-II or whether is is a result of increased cholesterol protein ratio. Athletes running as an average
at least 25 km per week had significantly higher apolipoprotein A-I
concentrations than the inactive controls (9). No significant
difference was noted in apoprotein A-II concentration between the
groups. In about half of the athletes apoprotein A-I concentrations
were above the upper limit of the controls. Kraus et al. (10) have
found the significantly higher $HDL_2$ concentrations in serum of long
distance runners than in sedentary persons, $HDL_3$ was not different.

## Work Activity

There are only few reports about the effect of vigorous physical
activity at work on serum lipids. Lehtonen and Viikari (11) have
compared the serum lipid concentrations of full-time lumberjacks
(13 men) whose occupational physical activity is most vigorous with
those of a group of ordinary electricians. HDL cholesterol levels
of lumberjacks were significantly higher than those of electricians,
but there were no differences in VLDL + LDL cholesterol values.
Three lumberjacks with overweight had lower HDL cholesterol values
than other lumberjacks, whose HDL levels were clearly higher than
normal. The study of Kuusela et al. (12) also shows that the
effect of vigorous work activity on serum HDL cholesterol and on
triglycerides is similar to that of exercise in leisure.

## The Quality of Exercise

The metabolism during endurance exercise is most aerobic. There
are many popular kinds of sports, where the anaerobic part of metabolism is more prominent. When soccer players and ice-hockey
players were compared in model matches, it was found that the energy
expenditure in soccer players was 0.18 kcal/min/kg whereas the
respective figure of ice-hockey players was 0.43 kcal/min/kg (13).
The anaerobic part of the metabolism of ice-hockey players is
approximately two-thirds of the total energy expenditure. Lehtonen
and Viikari (14) determined serum lipids of top-class football and
ice-hockey players during different training programs. The serum
levels of total cholesterol, HDL cholesterol and the ratio of HDL
cholesterol to total cholesterol were increased in those football
players having more aerobic exercise in their training program. This
aerobic part consisted of running at a speed of 4-5 min/km which
induced a pulse level of about 140 beats/min. The concentrations
of HDL cholesterol and the HDL cholesterol to total cholesterol
ratio were lowest in the ice-hockey players whose training is most
anaerobic. The training program of ice-hockey players had been
planned to maintain the pulse rate mostly above the level of 180
beats per min. Each of the actions lasted 30-90 min. The ice-
hockey team trained 7 times per week (about 10 hrs per week).
According to the results of this study the differences of serum
lipids seem to be in connection with the kinds of sport that differ
in their energy metabolism requirements. However, the age of
athletes may be of importance. The mean age of football players
was about 23 years and of ice-hockey players about 25 years. When
the serum lipids of young men (16-20 years old) were investigated,
there were no significant differences in HDL cholesterol levels of
top-class endurance runners, sprinters and controls with ordinary
physical activity (15). The serum LDL cholesterol concentration

was lowest in sprinters, who had also some endurance training. The lipid profile of young men is relatively advantageous and although the high amount of exercise seems to cause a tendency to higher HDL cholesterol and lower LDL cholesterol levels the changes are small. The importance of the quality of exercise has also been shown in the study of Nikkilä et al. (16). The serum lipids of sprinters, whose chief training consisted most of athletic exercises of short duration did not differ significantly from those of controls. The long distance runners had higher mean levels of HDL cholesterol than respective controls. Tennis is also a very popular sport in many countries. Vodak et al.(17) have evaluated plasma lipoprotein concentration in middle-aged male (mean age 42 years) and female (mean age 32 years) tennis players. During the time of investigation the men played an average 6.7 hr/wk; the women played an average 5.4 hr/wk. When compared to a sedentary group matched for age, sex and education, the tennis players exhibited similar plasma total cholesterol and LDL cholesterol concentrations and lower triglyceride levels. Plasma HDL cholesterol was significantly higher in the tennis players. The strength exercise like weight lifting does not effect favourable on serum lipids (18).

## The Quantity of Exercise

As seen previously cross-sectional studies report that dedicated runners and skiers have relatively high concentration of HDL cholesterol as compared to predominantly inactive controls matched for age. The quantity of exercise in the groups investigated is very high. Active long distance runners, joggers and skiers have usually trained regularly several years, several times per week. In most of these studies the persons investigated are middle-age (about 40 years old) men. Lehtonen and Viikari (5) found a positive correlation between the number of km run per week and the plasma HDL cholesterol concentration. Although there was a tendency to a higher than average HDL cholesterol concentration in the whole group of runners the concentrations were clearly higher than normal when the amount of running exceeded 70 km/week. Prospective studies on sedentary subjects who increase their physical activity are important to establish the effects of exercise on lipids. Several studies of this nature have been done (19,20,21,22,23) some report decreases in lipids and the others report no changes. Vigorous regular walking of obese men resulted in an increase of plasma HDL cholesterol (21). Men and women can have different lipid patterns in response to exercise, despite equivalent increases in maximal oxygen uptake (23). Men showed an increase in HDL cholesterol and in the HDL/LDL ratio, but women showed a small decrease in HDL cholesterol and no significant change in the HDL/LDL ratio (23). Because of the amount of physical exercise needed to cause prominent changes in plasma lipoproteins seems to be relatively great the contradictory results of training programs (19,29) are understandable.

References

1. Carlson LA, Mossfeldt F (1964)  Acute effects of prolonged,
   heavy exercise on the concentration of plasma lipids and lipoproteins in man.  Acta Physiol Scand 62: 51-59
2. Wood BD, Haskell WL, Stern MP, Lewis S, Perry C (1977) Plasma
   lipoprotein distributions in male and female runners.  The
   Marathon: Physiological, Medical, Epidemiological and Psychological Studies.  N Y Acad Sci 301: 748-761
3. Hurter R, Peyman MA, Schwale J, Barnett CWH (1972)  Some
   immediate and long-term effects of exercise on the plasma lipids.
   Lancet 2: 671-675
4. Wood PO, Haskell W, Klein H, Lewis I, Stern MP, Farguhar JW
   (1976)  The distribution of plasma lipoproteins in middle-aged
   male runners.  Metabolism 25: 1249-1257
5. Lehtonen A, Viikari J (1978)  Serum triglycerides and cholesterol
   and serum high-density lipoprotein cholesterol in highly physically active men.  Acta Med Scand 204: 111-114
6. Hartung GH, Foreyt JP, Mitchell RE, Vlasek J, Gotto AM (1980)
   Relation marathon runners, joggers and inactive men.  New Engl
   J Med 302: 357-361
7. Enger SC, Strömme SB, Refsum HE (1980)  High density lipoprotein
   cholesterol, total cholesterol and triglycerides in serum after
   a single exposure to prolonged heavy exercise.  Scan  J Clin Lab
   Invest 40: 341-345
8. Thompson PD, Cullinane E, Henderson LO, Herbert PN (1980)  Acute
   ffects of prolonged exercise on serum lipids.  Metabolism 29:
   662-665
9. Lehtonen A, Viikari J, Ehnholm C (1979)  The effect of exercise
   on high density (HDL) lipoprotein apoproteins.  Acta Physiol
   Scand 106: 487-488
10. Krauss RM, Lindgren FT, Wood PO, Haskell WL, Albers JJ, Cheung
    MC (1977)  Differential increases in plasma high density lipo-
    protein subfractions and apolipoproteins (Apo-LP) in runners.
    Circulation 56: 4
11. Lehtonen A, Viikari J (1978)  The effect of physical activity
    at work on serum lipids with a special reference to serum high-
    density lipoprotein cholesterol.  Acta Physiol Scand 104: 117-
    121
12. Kuusela P, Voutilainen E, Kukkonen K, Rauramaa R (1980)  Lipo-
    protein pattern in lumberjacks.  Scand J Sport Sci 2: 13-16
13. Seliger V (1968)  Energy metabolism in selected physical exer-
    cise.  Int Z Angew Physiol 25: 104-120
14. Lehtonen A, Viikari J (1980)  Serum lipids in soccer and ice-
    hockey players.  Metabolism 29: 36-39
15. Rönnemaa T, Lehtonen A, Järveläinen H, Vihersaari T, Viikari J
    (1980)  Serum lipids and lipoproteins on young male athletes
    and the effect of their sera on cultured human aortic smooth
    muscle cells.  Scand J Sport Sci 2: 33-38
16. Nikkilä EA, Taskinen M-R, Rehunen S, Härkönen M (1978)  Lipo-
    protein lipase activity in adipose tissue and skeletal muscle of
    runners: Relation to serum lipoproteins.  Metabolism 27: 1661-
    1671
17. Vodak PA, Wood PD, Haskell WL, Williams PT (1980)  HDL-
    cholesterol and other plasma lipid and lipoprotein concentra-
    tions in middle-aged male and female tennis players. Metabolism
    29: 745-752

18. Farrell PA, Maksud MG, Pollock ML, Foster C, Anholm J, Hare J,
    Leon AS (1982) A comparison of plasma cholesterol, triglyceri-
    des and high density lipoprotein-cholesterol in speed skaters,
    weight-lifters and non-athletes. Eur J Appl Physiol 48: 77-82
19. Huttunen JK, Länsimies E, Voutilainen E, Ehnholm C, Hietanen E,
    Penttilä J, Siitonen O, Rauramaa R (1979) Effect of moderate
    physical exercise on serum lipoproteins. A controlled clinical
    trial with special reference to serum high-density lipoproteins.
    Circulation 60: 1220-1229
20. Shephard RJ, Youldon PE, Cox M, West C (1980) Effects of
    6-month industrial fitness programme on serum lipid concentra-
    tions. Atherosclerosis 35: 277-286
21. Leon AS, Conrad J, Hunninghake DB, Serfass R (1979) Effects of
    vigorous walking program on body composition and carbohydrate
    and lipid metabolism of obese young men. Am J Clin Nutr 32:
    1776-1787
22. Streja D, Mymin D (1979) Moderate exercise and high-density
    lipoprotein-cholesterol: observation during a cardiac rehabilita-
    tion program. JAMA 242: 2190-2192
23. Brownell KD, Bachorik PS, Ayerle RS (1982) Changes in plasma
    lipid and lipoprotein levels in men and women after a program
    of moderate exercise. Circulation 65: 477-484

# Physical Exercise as Protection Against Heart Attack

R. S. Paffenbarger, Jr.

Exercise makes an important contribution to health and sense of well-being through improvements in many body systems. There is a strong inverse association between exercise and the incidence of heart attack, and evidence accumulates that this relationship largely represents protection (that is, a cause of reduced heart attack incidence) rather than selection (an effect of heart attack symptoms).

In 1953 Professor J.N. Morris observed in pioneering studies that London bus conductors who continually scrambled about the double-decker buses had lower heart attack rates than bus drivers who merely worked sitting at the wheel. Morris concluded that this difference in exercise was an independent contributor to risk chiefly responsible for the difference in heart attack rates (1). Twenty years later Morris reached similar conclusions when he reviewed the leisure-time exercise patterns of British civil servants and found that men engaged in vigorous exercise were at lower risk of heart attack than their less active counterparts (2). Further studies of work- or leisure-time physical activity and heart attack rates have concerned letter carriers and postal clerks (3), rural and urban residents (4), Israeli kibbutzim workers in various jobs (5), railroad workmen and clerks (6), residents of Framingham, Massachusetts, and of 2 counties of Eastern Finland with various lifestyles (7, 8), San Francisco cargo handlers and dockworkers (9), college alumni in various activities (10), and a number of others. While these studies showed lower heart attack rates with higher activity levels, they did not address all questions of diet, cigarette smoking, blood pressure level, heredity, stress, and other potentially confounding factors. Relative risks of heart attack for contrasting levels of physical activity within some of these populations are given in Table 1.

Table 1. Relative risks of heart attack, by sedentary lifestyles (selected studies)

| Study | Work- or leisure-time activity | High risk group or activity level | Prevalence of high risk group % | Relative risk of heart attack |
|---|---|---|---|---|
| London Transport [1] | Work | Bus drivers | 50 | 1.8 |
| San Francisco Long-shoremen [9] | Work | <8500 Kcal/wk | 69 | 1.8 |
| British Civil Service [2] | Leisure | No vigorous exercise | 88 | 2.2 |
| Harvard Alumni [10] | Leisure | <2000 Kcal/wk | 60 | 1.6 |
| Harvard Alumni [10] | Leisure | No vigorous sports | 60 | 1.4 |
| Framingham Men [7] | Combined | Low-moderate activity | ∿70 | ∿2.0 |
| Framingham Women [7] | Combined | Low-moderate activity | ∿85 | ∿1.5 |
| East Finland Men [8] | Work | Low activity | 22 | 1.6-1.5* |
| East Finland Men [8] | Leisure | Low activity | 33 | 1.4-1.2* |
| East Finland Women [8] | Work | Low activity | 25 | 2.7-2.4* |
| East Finland Women [8] | Leisure | Low activity | 27 | 1.7-1.5* |

*Relative risks of acute myocardial infarction by low physical activity levels: first figure, age-adjusted; second figure, "risk-factor adjusted"

Not all studies have shown differences in heart attack rates by levels of energy expenditure within job assignments or by leisure-time life-styles, perhaps because physical activity on the job was insufficient or because other influences were not taken into account. Special difficulties arise in defining or assessing exercise levels on a global scale.

Data on the habitual leisure-time activity patterns and health status of some college alumni have helped to distinguish between a protective and selective effect of exercise on heart attack risk. Study of 16,936 Harvard alumni who entered college from 1916 through 1950 provided information on leisure-time exercise habits in the 1960's and on 10-year follow-up patterns of fatal and nonfatal heart attack. Between the ages of 35-74 a total of 572 alumni experienced heart attacks, 215 fatal and 357 nonfatal. Age-adjusted rates and relative risks of first heart attack were computed according to differences in physical exercise. The one-third of alumni who reported climbing fewer than 50 stairs per day were at 25 percent increased risk of heart attack over those who climbed more. There was a similar increased risk for the one-quarter of alumni who walked fewer than five blocks daily as compared with those who walked more. The one-quarter of alumni who played no sports were at similar risk as compared with those who played only light sports. But the 60 percent who played no vigorous sports were at 38 percent greater risk than those who did. These measures of exercise are not mutually exclusive; they are indices rather than absolute expressions of the relation between physical activity and heart attack risk (10).

A composite physical activity index constructed from the energy equivalents required to ascend stairs, walk, and play at specific sports showed that 60 percent of the alumni expended less than 2000 kilocalories weekly and were at 64 percent greater risk of heart attack than their classmates who were more active. Age-specific heart attack rates declined consistently with an increase in energy expenditure by each activity-- climbing, walking, sports play, and the composite physical activity index. These trends were similar for both fatal and nonfatal events. Fig. 1 shows age-specific rates of first heart attack by the physical activity index. Rates for an index of less than 500 kilocalories per week were increased 176, 32, 147, and 131 percent over an index of 2000 or more in successive 10-year age classes 35-44 through 65-74.

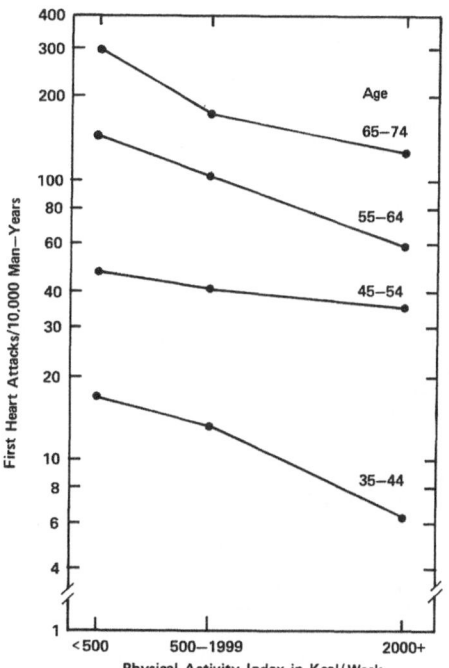

Fig. 1. Age-specific first heart attack rates among Harvard alumni in a 10-year follow-up, by physical activity index

Persistence of these findings was demonstrated by comparing relative risks of heart attack by physical activity index over successive intervals of time, 1-3 years and 4-6 years of follow-up from exercise

278

assessment. During these intervals, the risk with an index of less than 2000 kilocalories energy expenditure per week was, respectively, 66 percent and 80 percent higher, than the risk for more active alumni. In addition, data on a number of personal characteristics known to influence heart attack risk were obtained from student records and alumni questionnaires. These included cigarette habits; blool pressure levels; stature and weight-for-height ratios; and history of hypertension, diabetes, stroke, and parental heart attack and hypertension. Both in the presence and in the absence of each of these student and alumni characteristics, a physical activity index of less than 2000 kilocalories per week was accompanied by a higher heart attack risk than an index of 2000 or more. Relative risks attached to the lower index ranged from a high of nearly 300 percent for alumni with a history of diabetes to a low of 33 percent for alumni who were one-quarter or more overweight for their height.

Rates and relative risks of heart attack were computed by physical activity index at the 2000 kilocalorie breakpoint and the clinical type of heart attack. For the less active alumni, risk of angina pectoris alone was nearly doubled, risk of nonfatal myocardial infarction was increased by one-third, and risk of fatal heart attack was more than doubled as compared with more active alumni.

The college alumni study addressed the question of whether a physically active lifestyle in adult life was independent of activity in youth as a predictor of lower heart attack risk. Table 2 shows age-adjusted rates of first heart attack by cross tabulation of Harvard student and alumni activity levels. College activity was considered as varsity or intramural sports participation, and alumni activity as kilocalories expended weekly in climbing, walking, and sports play expressed at three levels: less than 500, 500-1999, and 2000 or more. Thus, heart attack rates are given for men less active as students but more active as alumni, or vice versa, or for men who showed little change in activity level from youth to adulthood. The findings indicate that student athleticism per se was unrelated to heart attack risk later in life. Student athletes and non-athletes alike experienced low heart attack risks only if they had a high physical activity index as alumni.

Table 2. Age-adjusted rates* of first heart attack among Harvard alumni in a 10-year follow-up, by student and alumnus activity patterns

| Student activity | Alumnus physical activity index in kilocalories per week | | | | | |
| | <500 | | 500-1999 | | 2000+ | |
| | %M-Y[†] | Rate | %M-Y | Rate | %M-Y | Rate |
|---|---|---|---|---|---|---|
| Varsity athlete | | | | | | |
| No | 15.9 | 70.7 | 46.3 | 53.3 | 37.8 | 35.3 |
| Yes | 9.3 | 92.7 | 34.7 | 45.2 | 56.0 | 35.2 |
| Sports play in hours per week[‡] | | | | | | |
| <5 | 17.6 | 85.6 | 49.9 | 54.9 | 32.5 | 33.3 |
| 5+ | 14.3 | 61.2 | 43.8 | 49.4 | 41.9 | 28.4 |

*No. with heart attack per 10,000 man-years of observation. [†]Percent man-years of observation. [‡]Excludes varsity athletes.

The college alumni study also permitted examination of the relative importance of strenuous vs. more casual energy expenditures as they affected heart attack risk. Fig. 2 presents a multiple logistic regression analysis of the reduction in heart attack risk for vigorous sports or other activities expressed as habitual and leisure exercise in the physical activity index. Using a reference level of less than 100 kilo-

calories expended weekly, each
curve represents a reduction in
heart attack risk as energy expenditure is increased for one
type of exercise with the effect
from the other type of exercise
being held constant. The data
are adjusted for differences in
age and follow-up interval. A
reduced risk of heart attack is
seen with increasing energy output from each type of activity,
but at any given level, the risk
is significantly lower for vigorous sports play than for casual
activities. When adjustment is
made for the unfavorable influences of cigarette habit, hypertension, and obesity, the reduction in heart attack risk remains
strongly related to vigorous activities but is reduced somewhat for more
casual activities.

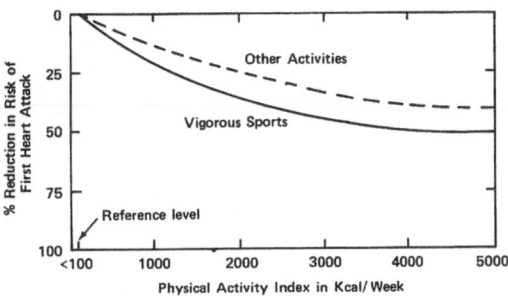

Fig. 2. Percent reduction in risk of
first heart attack among Harvard
alumni in a 10-year follow-up, by
physical activity index for vigorous
sports and other activities

It is possible to set aside the effects of age, follow-up interval,
cigarette smoking, hypertension, obesity, and history of parental heart
attack so as to delineate the role of energy output in establishing
heart attack risk. Table 3 presents the results of a multiple logistic
regression analysis showing relative and attributable risks attached to
each of these characteristics. (Attributable risks are estimates of the
potential reduction in heart attack rates that would have been achieved
if the characteristics had been changed from high to low risk levels.)

Table 3. Relative and attributable risks* of first heart attack among
Harvard alumni in a 10-year follow-up study, by selected characteristics

| Characteristic | Prevalence % | Relative Risk $\overline{m} \pm$ 1SE | P | Attributable Risk % Clinical | Community |
|---|---|---|---|---|---|
| Sedentary lifestyle[†] | 61.2 | 1.49 ± 0.18 | <.001 | 33.1 | 23.1 |
| Cigarette smoking[‡] | 51.7 | 1.30 ± 0.14 | .016 | 23.2 | 13.4 |
| Hypertension[§] | 8.7 | 2.34 ± 0.31 | <.001 | 57.4 | 10.4 |
| Obesity[‖] | 37.6 | 1.32 ± 0.14 | .010 | 24.5 | 10.7 |
| Parental heart attack[¶] | 38.6 | 1.28 ± 0.14 | .024 | 21.8 | 9.8 |

*Adjusted for age, follow-up interval, and each of other characteristics
listed. [†]Energy expenditure of less than 2000 kilocalories per week in
walking, climbing stairs, and sports. [‡]Any amount. [§]Physician diagnosed. [‖]About 20 percent or more over ideal weight-for-height. [¶]Ei-
ther father or mother.

For example, the relative risk of heart attack among sedentary men was
49 percent higher than the risk in more active men, and this inactive
lifestyle might have accounted for 33 percent of heart attacks in sedentary men and 23 percent in the total population of men. Also, the
relative risk of heart attack was 134 percent higher in hypertensive
than normotensive men; 57 percent of the added risk in hypertensive men
might have been due to hypertension; and 10 percent of the added risk
in the total population might have resulted from this cause. Review of
the findings of Table 3 shows that each of these five characteristics
made a contribution to heart attack risk that was independent of age
and the other four characteristics. Hypertension would seem to have

made the strongest contribution to risk in a clinical sense, but because of its high prevalence, as defined, a sedentary lifestyle might have made a more potent contribution in a community sense. In the wider scope, it is promising that physical activity would tend to reduce the influence of hereditary, familial, and other circumstances.

Report No. XXIV in a series on chronic disease in former college students.

Acknowledgments  This work was supported by the U.S. Public Health Service research grant HL 24133 from the National Heart, Lung and Blood Institute, the Marathon Oil Foundation, Inc., the Mobil Foundation, and the Phillips Petroleum Foundation, Inc.

## References

1. Morris JN, Kagan A, Pattison DC, Gardner MJ, Raffle PAB (1966) Incidence and prediction of ischaemic heart-disease in London busmen. Lancet 2: 553–559
2. Morris JN, Everitt MG, Pollard R, Chave SPW, Semmence AM (1980) Vigorous exercise in leisure-time: protection against coronary heart disease. Lancet 2: 1207–1210
3. Kahn HA (1963) The relationship of reported coronary heart disease mortality to physical activity of work. Am J Public Health 53: 1058–1067
4. Zukel WJ, Lewis RH, Enterline PE, Painter RC, Ralston LS, Fawcett RM, Meredith AP, Peterson B (1959) A short-term community study of the epidemiology of coronary heart disease: a preliminary report on the North Dakota study. Am J Public Health 49: 1630–1639
5. Brunner D, Manelis G, Modan M, Levin S (1974) Physical activity at work and the incidence of myocardial infarction, angina pectoris and death due to ischemic heart disease: an epidemiological study in Israeli collective settlements (Kibbutzim). J Chronic Dis 27: 217–233
6. Taylor HL, Klepetar E, Keys A, Parlin MS, Blackburn H, Puchner T (1962) Death rates among physically active and sedentary employees of the railroad industry. Am J Public Health 52: 1697–1707
7. Dawber TR (1980) The Framingham Study. The Epidemiology of Atherosclerotic Disease. Harvard University Press, Cambridge, Massachusetts. Chapter 10, pp. 157–171
8. Salonen JT, Puska P, Tuomilehto J (1982) Physical activity and risk of myocardial infarction, cerebral stroke and death: a longitudinal study in Eastern Finland. Am J Epidemiol 115: 526–537
9. Paffenbarger RS, Hale WE (1975) Work activity and coronary heart mortality. N Engl J Med 292: 545–550
10. Paffenbarger RS, Wing AL, Hyde RT (1978) Physical activity as an index of heart attack risk in college alumni. Am J Epidemiol 108: 161–175

# Exercise and Fibrinolysis

R. S. Williams

## A. Introduction

Epidemiologic studies have demonstrated a consistent inverse relationship between habitual levels of vigorous physical activity and the incidence of death due to cardiovascular disease (1). However, the biologic sequelae of regular exercise that account for this apparent protective effect have not been completely defined. Profound alterations in lipoprotein constituents of plasma (2), and in the neural control of the circulation (3) clearly occur in individuals who exercise regularly, and can be plausibly hypothesized to retard the atherosclerotic process or to limit the propensity to sudden cardiac death in individuals with established atherosclerosis. However, the prominent role of humoral and platelet mediated coagulation processes in current theories of both the pathogenesis of atherosclerosis (4) and in the precipitation of clinical events such as myocardial infarction, stroke, and venous thromboembolism (5) has led several investigators to examine the effects of exercise upon hemostasis, seeking further insight into the apparent protective effects of regular exercise on cardiovascular risk. Since the overall propensity to intravascular thrombus formation is determined by the balance between humoral and platelet mediated mechanisms that produce clot formation, and the fibrinolytic mechanisms that produce clot dissolution, specific attention has been directed to the relationship between exercise and fibrinolysis.

Fibrinolytic activity in human plasma derives from the conversion of plasminogen, an inactive circulating plasma protein, to its active form, plasmin, by the action of one of several types of plasminogen activators. Plasmin is a trypsin-like non-specific protease, but its directed action in the proteolysis of fibrin is related to the presence of plasma inhibitors, notably $\alpha_2$ anti-plasmin, that limit its activity except at sites of clot formation, where the higher affinity of plasmin for fibrin leads to its absorbance into the clot where it is less susceptible to inhibition by $\alpha_2$ anti-plasmin (6).

Plasminogen can be activated to plasmin by exogenously administered compounds (urokinase), by tumor-derived factors, by a Hageman Factor dependent pathway, by factors derived from activation of the alternate complement pathway, by circulating activators that are probably of hepatic origin and by a newly described plasma compound termed Protein C (6-9). However, current interest has focused upon plasminogen activator derived from vascular endothelium (10), since, in contrast to the circulating activators, the release of this vascular tissue activator appears to undergo dynamic regulation by factors such as exercise or venous stasis (11,12). Furthermore, except for rare cases of inherited deficiencies of plasminogen or of Protein C (13), defective release of endothelial-cell-derived plasminogen activator appears to be more strongly associated with vascular disease states (coronary artery disease, stroke, venous thromboembolism, diabetic retinopathy) than abnormalities of resting fibrinolysis that primarily assess the effects of circulating activators (14 - 17). Vascular plasminogen activator purified from tissue culture or from human cadaveric perfusates is a 60,000 dalton peptide (10). Extensive investigations are exploring the use of purified vascular plasminogen activators as therapeutic agents for acute thrombotic disorders.

## B.  Enhancement of fibrinolysis by acute exercise

A number of interventions have been shown to enhance fibrinolytic capacity of
plasma including administration of epinephrine or nicotinic acid, venous stasis,
and exercise (11,12,19).  Fibrinolysis also undergoes diurnal variation in normal
adults (18).  Whereas many studies of activation of fibrinolysis by drugs or physical stimuli antedated current knowledge of the various sources of plasminogen
activators, it is likely that these factors that exert dynamic control over fibrinolysis do so by regulation of the release of vascular plasminogen activators from
vascular endothelium.

Although there is universal agreement that acute exercise enhances fibrinolytic
activity, the intensity of exercise required for release of vascular plasminogen
activators has not been entirely defined.  In healthy young subjects HEYERS et al
reported no significant enhancement of fibrinolysis during 5 min of treadmill exercise at 1/3 of maximum oxygen consumption ($VO_2$ max), slight enhancement at 2/3 of $VO_2$
max, and marked enhancement at peak exercise ($\angle 0$), whereas MENON et al (21) demonstrated markedly enhanced fibrinolysis after only 1.5 min on a step test that
elevated mean heart rate by only 27 bpm above resting levels, but no further increase
in fibrinolysis with more strenuous (though submaximal) exercise.  The enhanced
fibrinolysis produced by acute exercise persists for up to 90 min following cessation
of exercise, and this persistence appears to be independent of either the intensity
or the duration of exercise (11,20), though these factors have not been systemically
studied in the same study population.  In addition, in contrast to the effects of
acute exercise on Factor VIII procoagulant activity, enhanced fibrinolysis produced
by acute exercise is not inhibited by beta-adrenergic blockade (22).

## C.  Physical conditioning and fibrinolysis

Resting fibrinolytic capacity, which primarily assesses the activity of circulating
plasminogen activators, has been observed to decline following short-term (4-10 wks)
moderate physical conditioning in two longitudinal studies of healthy adults (23,24).
However, other investigators observed that a longer duration (6 mo) of training
produced enhanced resting fibrinolysis in their subjects (25).  No effect on resting
fibrinolysis was observed in a small group of coronary patients who trained for 6
weeks (26).  Two cross-sectional studies observed enhanced resting fibrinolysis
among athletes who were compared to sedentary controls (21,27), although a third
report found no correlation between leisure or occupational physical activity
quantitated by questionnaire and resting fibrinolysis (28).  Thus, although resting
fibrinolytic activity declines with short-term exercise training, it appears that
different effects may be observed with longer durations of training.

On the other hand, both cross-sectional and longitudinal data from our own laboratory,
as well as from other investigators, indicate that moderate exercise training
enhances the release of endothelial plasminogen activators in response to venous
occlusion or to acute exercise.  In a group of 69 healthy middle-aged adults
(Table I) we found the enhancement of fibrinolysis produced by 5 min of venous
occlusion (reflecting release of vascular plasminogen activators) to be significantly correlated with aerobic fitness assessed by symptom-limited treadmill
performance (24).  Furthermore, we found 10 weeks of a moderate conditioning program
(30-45 min of walk/jog at 60-75% $VO_2$ max, 3X weekly) to significantly enhance
(52% increase) plasminogen activator release in response to venous occlusion.  This
effect of exercise training was most marked in individuals with the lowest level
of exercise capacity prior to the conditioning program.  It was more prominent in
women than in men, but did not appear to be related to age or to change in body
weight.

Table 1. Fibrinolytic activity stimulated by venous occlusion (SFA) in healthy middle-aged adults: Response to 10 weeks of exercise-training (adapted from WILLIAMS et al (24))

| Subpopulation | Number of Subjects | Pre-training SFA* | Post-training SFA | P-value† |
|---|---|---|---|---|
| Entire group (unstratified) | 69 | 21.7 | 33.8 | 0.0037 |
| Fitness before training§ | | | | |
| Lowest third | 22 | 13.5 | 29.4 | 0.0315 |
| Middle third | 27 | 23.9 | 35.9 | 0.0686 |
| Highest third | 19 | 28.8 | 37.2 | 0.2495 |

*Fibrinolytic activity measured by radioenzymatic casein hydrolysis assay and expressed in arbitrary units
†Student's t-test for paired samples (two-tailed)
§Assessed by maximal graded treadmill exercise

KEBER et al (25) observed a similar increase (+75%) in vascular plasminogen activator release stimulated by acute exercise in response to a 6 month conditioning program in 10 male alpinists aged 25-51 years. In a separate study, fibrinolytic response to acute exercise was increased in two of six patients with coronary disease after 6 weeks of training, but the change in the group mean was not significant (26).

KEBER et al (25) also studied 9 of 10 of their subjects who had completed a six month conditioning program following a subsequent six-week climbing expedition to the Andes. In contrast to the enhanced plasminogen activator release noted in these subjects with a moderate conditioning program (1 hr, 3X weekly), plasminogen activator release in response to acute exercise fell markedly following their climbing expedition. Although the subjects underwent extreme physical exertion over this six-week period, it is difficult to ascribe their subsequent results to exercise alone, since the subjects also were exposed to extremes of cold and altitude. These authors hypothesized that repeated, prolonged bouts of strenuous exertion may lead to depletion of endothelial stores of plasminogen activator, and therefore limit release of activators in response to provocative stimuli. Techniques to quantitate plasminogen activator stores in human vein biopsy specimens have been reported (29), but have not been applied to studies of exercise to test this hypothesis.

D. Summary

Acute bouts of exercise stimulate fibrinolytic activity, probably by promoting the release of endothelial cell-derived plasminogen activator. Moderate physical conditioning enhances the stimulation of fibrinolytic activity produced either by acute exercise, or by venous occlusion, presumably by increasing the amount of vascular plasminogen activator released in response to these acute stimuli. The effect of physical conditioning upon endothelial stores of plasminogen activator is not known. This effect of physical conditioning can be plausibly hypothesized to reduce the likelihood of intravascular thrombus formation, particularly in the venous circulation, but conceivably in the arterial circulation as well. However, with the exception of rare kindreds with profound deficiencies of components of the fibrinolytic system, the role of subnormal fibrinolysis as a causative factor in venous thromboembolism or in atherosclerotic vascular disease remains conjectural. Likewise, clinical benefits as a result of enhanced endothelial plasminogen activator release produced by physical conditioning must be regarded as speculative.

## References

1. Paffenbarger RS, Hale WE (1975) Work activity and coronary heart mortality. N Engl J Med 292: 545-550
2. Wood PD, Haskell W, Klein H, Lewis S, Stern MP, Farquhar JW (1976) The distribution of plasma lipoproteins in middle-aged runners. Metabolism 24: 1249-1257
3. Scheuer J, Tipton CM (1977) Cardiovascular adaptations to physical training. Ann Rev Physiol 39: 222-251
4. Ross R, Glomset JA (1976) The pathogenesis of atherosclerosis. N Engl J Med 295: 369-377, and 420-425
5. Oliva PB (1981) Pathophysiology of acute myocardial infarction. Ann Int Med 94: 236-244
6. Wiman B, Collen D (1978) Molecular mechanism of physiologic fibrinolysis. Nature 272: 549-550
7. Kaplan AP, Castellino FJ, Collen D, Wiman B, Taylor FB (1978) Molecular mechanisms of fibrinolysis in man. Thrombos Haemostas 39: 263-283
8. Comp PC, Esmon CT (1981) Generation of fibrinolytic activity by infusion of activated Protein C into dogs. J Clin Invest 68: 1221-1228
9. Astrup T (1978) Fibrinolysis: An overview. Prog Chem Fibrinol Thrombol 3: 1-57
10. Binder BR, Spragg J, Austen KF (1979) Purification and characterization of human vascular plasminogen activator derived from blood vessel perfusates. J Biol Chem 254: 1988-2003
11. March N, Gaffney P (180) Some observations on the release of extrinsic and intrinsic plasminogen activators during exercise in man. Haemostasis 9: 238-247
12. Walker ID, Davidson JF, Hutton I (1976) Fibrinolytic potential: The response to a 5 minute venous occlusion test. Thromb Res 8: 629-638
13. Griffin JH, Evatt B, Zimmerman TS, Kleiss AJ, Wideman C (1981) Deficiency of Protein C in congenital thrombotic disease. J Clin Invest 68: 1370-1373
14. Walker ID, Davidson JF, Hutton I, Laurie TDV (1977) Disordered fibrinolytic potential in coronary heart disease. Thromb Res 10: 509-520
15. Pizzo SV, Lewis JG, Campbell EE, Dreyer NA (1981) Fibrinolytic response of oral contraceptive-associated thromboembolism. Contraception 23: 181-186
16. Mettinger KL, Nyman D, Kjellin KG, Siden A, Soderstrom CE (1979) Factor VIII related antigen, antithrombin III, spontaneous platelet aggregation and plasminogen activator in ischemic cerebrovascular disease. J Neurol Sci 41: 31-38
17. Clayton JK, Anderson JA, McNicol GP (1976) Preoperative prediction of post-operative deep vein thrombosis. Br Med J 2: 910-912
18. Rosing DR, Redwood DR, Brakman P, Astrup T, Epstein SE (1973) Impairment of the diurnal fibrinolytic response in man. Circ Res 32: 752-758
19. Cash JD, Woodfield DE (1968) Fibrinolytic response to moderate exercise in 50 healthy middle-aged adults. J Appl Physiol 40: 287-292
20. Heyers TM, Martin BJ, Pratt DS, Dreisin RB, Franks JJ (1980) Enhanced thrombin and plasmin activity with exercise in man. J Appl Physiol 48: 821-825
21. Menon S, Burke F, Dewar HA (1967) Effects of strenuous and graded exercise on fibrinolytic activity. Lancet 1: 699-702
22. Rosing DR, Redwood DR, Brakman P, Astrup T, Epstein SE (1978) The fibrinolytic response of man to vasoactive drugs measured in arterial blood. Thromb Res 13: 419-428
23. Ferguson EW, Guest MM (1974) Exercise, physical conditioning, blood coagulation and fibrinolysis. Thromb Diath Haemorrh 34: 63-71
24. Williams RS, Logue EE, Lewis JL, Barton T, Stead NW, Wallace AG, Pizzo SV (1980) Physical conditioning augments the fibrinolytic response to venous occlusion in healthy adults. N Engl J Med 302: 987-991

25. Keber D, Stegnar M, Keber I, Acetto B (1979) Influence of moderate and strenuous daily physical activity on fibrinolytic activity of blood: Possibility of plasminogen activator stores depletion. Thrombos Haemostas 41: 745-755

26. Redwood DR, Rosing DR, Epstein SE (1972) Circulatory and sympatomatic effects of physical training in patients with coronary artery disease and angina pectoris. N Engl J Med 286: 959-965

27. Moxley RT, Brakman P, Astrup T (1970) Resting levels of fibrinolysis in blood in inactive and exercising men. J Appl Physiol 28: 549-552

28. Korsan-Bergsten K, Wilhelmsen L, Tibblin G (1973) Blood coagulation and fibrinolysis in relations to degree of physical activity during work and leisure time: A study based on a random sample of 54 year old men. Acta Med Scand 193: 73-77

29. Pandolfi M, Nilsson IM, Robertson B, Isacsom S (1967) Fibrinolytic activity of human veins. Lancet 2: 127-137

# Regulation of Serum Triglycerides in Trained Subjects

A. Wirth

## Serum triglyceride concentration

Cross-sectional and longitudinal studies have demonstrated that serum triglycerides (TG) can be lowered by physical activity (19). As
shown in epidemiological studies, TG levels are lower in active subjects at work and leisure-time (11). Therefore, the type of exercise
seems to be of minor importance provided that dynamic exercise includes large muscle groups. On the contrary, power athletes with a
static type of exercise exhibit elevated concentrations of TG (4).

Training programs in hypertriglyceridemic patients markedly reduce
serum TG concentrations of up to 45 % (6). Since similar decreases
in serum concentrations have been reported in comparative studies,
the question whether or not the training-induced reduction depends
on the initial serum TG concentration is still open.

Differences in food intake in physically active and inactive people
are probably of minor importance with regard to differences in serum
TG. Kiens et al (9) found similar changes in serum TG when food intake was switched from a fat-rich to a fat-poor diet. Gyntelberg et
al (6) noticed the same reduction in TG concentration when the increased caloric expenditure was compensated for by increased food intake. Similar results could be obtained during extreme endurance
exercise. We noticed that despite the higher calorie consumption
serum TG fell by 43 % (17). These results indicate that the serum
concentration of TG decreases with exercise-training per se.

## Catabolism of triglyceride rich lipoproteins

The effect of physical training on the removal of endogenous TG has
not been determined directly in man. The disappearance of TG from
the blood after a fat-loading meal was enhanced following exercise-
training (1). A similar training effect could be shown recently in
hypertriglyceridemic patients who were given exogenous fat intravenously (18).

Lipoprotein lipase (LPL) is considered an important factor in the
regulation of serum TG. As shown first in animals, LPL activity is
increased after physical conditioning in both muscle and adipose
tissue (2). These results were confirmed later in man in cross-
sectional and longitudinal studies (13). Therefore, by increasing
LPL activity, physical training might accelerate the removal of TG
at this metabolic site. Since this enzyme is primarily located on
the capillary endothelium and the capillary density is increased
by physical training the enhanced activity might derive from an endothelial proliferation rather than an induction.

## Triglyceride synthesis and mobilization in fat stores

Following hydrolysis of triglyceride-rich lipoproteins free fatty acids are liberated and incorporated into various tissues. A training-induced, stimulated oxidation of free fatty acids has been proven in skeletal muscle (7). As far as the esterification of free fatty acids is concerned the situation is less clear. Whereas Askew et al (3) found changes in enzyme activities indicating an enhanced lipogenesis in rat adipose tissue others noticed opposite effects (10). By measuring the incorporation and esterification of fatty acids in humans we also noticed a reduced lipogenesis in adipose tissue (18).

In several studies a reduced basal and enhanced stimulated lipolysis was shown in both rats and humans (5). Catecholamine-stimulated lipolysis is increased and it seems that not only maximal response but also sensitivity are enhanced (5). The mechanisms by which training induces the accelerated breakdown of TG are not well understood. Binding of dihydroalprenolol seems to be unaffected by training, and adenylate cyclase activity is rather reduced than stimulated (5, 8, 14). Since lipolysis is also increased by drugs bypassing the adenylate cyclase complex such as theophylline and dibutyryl cyclic AMP an alteration at a metabolic step distal to stimulus recognition by adrenoreceptors is postulated (5).

## Triglyceride secretion

Data on training-induced changes in TG secretion in man are not available. Using the Triton method Simonelli and Eaton (15) found an appreciable reduction in TG secretion by 52 % in trained hyperlipemic, obese Zucker rats and 78 % in their normolipemic thin littermates. Similar results were obtained by Zavaroni et al (20), who applied the liver perfusion technique. In their study the carbohydrate-induced hypertriglyceridemia could be prevented by exercise training. The basis for this diminished increase in VLDL-TG secretion rate may be seen either in lower hepatic insulin concentration or in an improved disposal of glucose (20).

## Conclusion

Serum TG can be markedly lowered by endurance exercise as shown in both cross sectional and longitudinal studies. Dietary habits seem to be of minor importance (fig. 1). The precise mechanisms, whereby serum concentrations are decreased by physical activity, are currently not known. There is some evidence that lipoprotein lipase activity is increased in postheparin plasma as well as in muscle, heart, and adipose tissue. This adaptation is in line with a stimulated uptake and oxidation of fatty acids into muscle tissue. The uptake and esterification of fatty acids into adipose tissue, however, seem to be reduced. The hormone-stimulated mobilization of depot TGs is clearly increased in the training state, leading to a reduction in adipose tissue mass. In animals an appreciable reduction in TG secretion has been demonstrated following training.

Figure 1

## REGULATION OF SERUM TRIGLYCERIDES IN THE TRAINING STATE

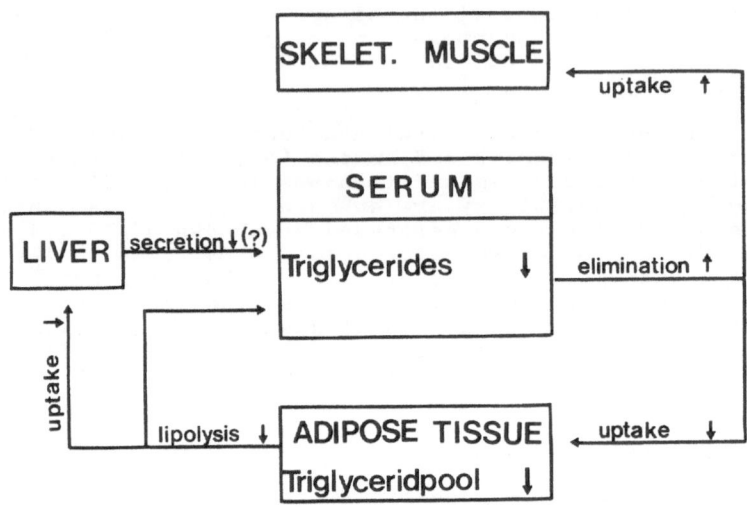

Regulation of serum triglycerides in trained subjects in the
basal state

## References

1. Altekruse EB, Wilmore JH (1973) Changes in blood chemistries
   following a controlled exercise program. J. Occ. Med. 15:110–113
2. Askew EW, Dohm GL, Huston RL, Sneed TW, Dowdy RP (1972) Response
   of rat tissue lipases to physical training and exercise. Proc.
   Soc. Exptl. Biol. Med. 141:123–127
3. Askew EW, Huston RL, Dohm GL (1973) Effect of physical training
   on esterification of glycerol-3-phosphate by homogenates of
   liver, skeletal muscle, heart, and adipose tissue of rats.
   Metabolism 22:473–480
4. Berg A, Ringwald G, Keul J (1980) Lipoprotein-cholesterol in
   well-trained athletes. A preliminary communication: reduced HDL-
   cholesterol in power athletes. Int. J. Sports Med. 1:137–138
5. Bukowiecki L, Lupien J, Follea N, Paradis A, Richard D, LeBlanc J
   (1980) Mechanism of enhanced lipolysis in adipose tissue of exercise trained rats. Am. J. Physiol. 239:E422–E429
6. Gyntelberg F, Brennan R, Holloszy J.O, Schonfeld G, Rennie MJ,
   Weidman SW (1977) Plasma triglyceride lowering by exercise
   despite increased food intake in patients with type IV hyperlipoproteinemia. Am J. Clin. Nutr. 30:716–720
7. Holloszy J (1967) Biochemical adaptations in muscle. Effects of
   exercise on mitochondrial oxygen uptake and respiratory enzyme
   activity in skeletal muscle. J. Biol. Chem. 242:2278–2282

8. Holm G, Jacobson B, Toss L, Smith U, Björntorp P (1980) The effect of physical exercise on the regulation of beta adrenergic receptors and adenylate cyclase in rat adipocytes. 3rd International Congress on Obesity, Rome

9. Kiens B, Jörgensen I, Lewis S, Jensen G, Lithell H, Vessby B, Hoe S, Schnohr P (1980) Increased plasma HDL-cholesterol and apo A-1 in sedentary middle-aged men after physical conditioning Eur. J. Clin. Invest 10:203-209

10. Lopez-S A, René A, Bell L, Herbert JA (1975) Metabolic effects of exercise. I. Effect of exercise on serum lipids and lipogenesis in rats. Proc. Soc. Experim. Biol. and Medicine 148:640-645

11. Morris JN, Everitt MG, Pollard R, Chave SPW, Semmence AM (1980) Vigorous exercise in leisure time: protection against coronary heart disease. Lancet II:1207-1210

12. Nikkilä EA, Taskinen M-R, Rehunen S, Härkönen M (1978) Lipoprotein lipase activity in adipose tissue and skeletal muscle of runners: relation to serum lipoproteins. Metabolism 27:1661-1671

13. Peltonen P, Marniemi J, Hietanen E, Vuori I, Ehnholm Ch (1981) Changes in serum lipids, lipoproteins, and heparin releasable lipolytic enzymes during moderate physical training in man: a longitudinal study. Metabolism 30:518-526

14. Shepherd RE, Noble EG, Klug GA, Gollnick PhD (1981) Lipolysis and cAMP accumulation in adipocytes in response to physical training. J. Appl. Physiol. 50:143-148

15. Simonelli C, Eaton RP (1978) Reduced triglyceride secretion: a metabolic consequence of chronic exercise. Am. J. Physiol. 234: E221-E227

16. Wirth A, Holm G, Lindstedt G, Lundberg P-A, Björntorp P (1981) Thyroid hormones and lipolysis in physically trained rats. Metabolism 30:237-241

17. Wirth A, Diehm C, Kohlmeier M, Heuck CC, Vogel I (1982) Effect of long-lasting intermittent exercise on serum lipids and lipoproteins. Submitted for publication

18. Wirth A, Welte J, Hanel W, Schlierf G (in preparation) Mechanisms of reduced serum triglycerides in hypertriglyceridemia after physical training

19. Wood PD, Haskell WL, Stern MP, Lewis S, Perry Ch (1977) Plasma lipoprotein distributions in male and female runners. Ann. N.Y. Acad. Sci.

20. Zavaroni I, Chen YI, Mondon CE, Reaven GM (1981) Ability of exercise to inhibit carbohydrate-induced hypertriglyceridemia in rats. Metabolism 30:476-480

# Exercise and Arachidonic Acid Metabolites: Effect of Adrenergic Beta Blockade

K. Laustiola, E. Seppälä, T. Nikkari, and H. Vapaatalo

Few reports on the relationships between prostaglandins (PGs) and exercise have been published, although PGs may participate in many physiological events during and after physical stress. Adrenergic beta blocking drugs also affect the prostaglandin system, and patients treated with these drugs are often exposed to stress. We describe the effect of submaximal physical exercise on PGs, and the ability of different types of beta blocking drugs to modify these responses.

Six healthy male students (19-23 years) volunteered in a randomized, cross-over, single blind trial. A submaximal ergometer test was arranged every second week. The work load was individually adjusted to reach a steady-state heart rate of 130/min. The subjects were given i.v. either placebo or equipotent increasing doses of atenolol (total 0.19 mg/kg), practolol (0.64 mg/kg) or propranolol (0.19 mg/kg) at 5 min intervals. Blood samples were drawn immediately before the exercise, at exhaustion, and after 30 min of recovery. Plasma free AA was measured with GLC. RIA was used for the quantification of AA metabolites in plasma, and the assay of spontaneous formation of $TxB_2$ during clotting.

The results are presented in Table 1. During submaximal exercise (E) there was an increase of plasma AA, 6-keto-$PGF_{1\alpha}$, $TxB_2$, as well as of the formation of $TxB_2$ by platelets. They remained elevated, or increased even further during the recovery period (R); also $PGE_2$ was increased. The effects of atenolol did not markedly differ from those of placebo, while practolol and propranolol reduced exercise induced changes.

Table 1. Concentrations of AA, $PGE_2$, 6-keto-$PGF_{1\alpha}$ and $TxB_2$ in plasma, as well as $TxB_2$ formation by platelets during and after submaximal exercise, and the effects of beta adenergic blocking drugs on them

| | AA | | $PGE_2$ | | 6-keto-$PGF_{1\alpha}$ | | $TxB_2$ | | $TxB_2$ formation | |
|---|---|---|---|---|---|---|---|---|---|---|
| Control level | 3.6 | | 177 | | 347 | | 138 | | 32 | |
| | E | R | E | R | E | R | E | R | E | R |
| Placebo | 5.9*** | 5.5*** | 162 | 281 | 481* | 380 | 265** | 273** | 47 | 121** |
| Atenolol | 4.2* | 4.6** | 145 | 270 | 352 | 346 | 228 | 442*** | 46 | 168*** |
| Practolol | 3.9 | 4.8*** | 145 | 150 | 347 | 339 | 188 | 214 | 18 | 32 |
| Propranolol | 3.2* | 4.8*** | 138 | 107 | 402 | 381 | 154 | 252* | 42 | 77* |

The values are means of determinations; AA nmol/ml, $PGE_2$, 6-keto-$PGF_{1\alpha}$, $TxB_2$ pg/ml, $TxB_2$ formation ng/ml. *$p<0.05$, **$p<0.01$, ***$p<0.001$ compared to the control level.

We conclude that submaximal physical exercise induces marked increase in the plasma concentrations of AA and its various metabolites. Adrenergic beta blockade can reduce these changes. There are, however, differences between various types of adrenergic beta blocking drugs.

Acknowledgements   The study was supported by ICI-Pharma, Finland, and the Academy of Finland.

# Effect of Physical Training on Blood Pressure and Serum Lipoproteins in Middle-Aged Men with Borderline Hypertension

R. Rauramaa, J. T. Salonen, K. Kukkonen, E. Voutilainen, and E. Länsimies

Hypertension and dyslipoproteinemias are established risk factors for coronary heart disease. Since prospective studies have revealed that even mild hypertension contributes to an increased risk for coronary heart disease, its drug treatment seems to be indicated. Because of the adverse effects of drugs, various nonpharmacological methods have also been attempted. Physical training studies have suggested a blood pressure lowering effect of exercise on mildly hypertensive persons. Furthermore, regular physical training of mild to moderate intensity has a favourable effect on plasma lipoproteins. We carried out a randomized controlled trial on the effects of physical training on blood pressure and serum lipoproteins in middle-aged men.

Thirty-four normotensive and 25 borderline hypertensive men (aged 35-50 years) were randomized into a training or sedentary group. The mean pretraining blood pressure was 133/86 mmHg in the normotensive training group, 129/85 in the normotensive sedentary group, 143/99 in the borderline training group and 139/98 in the borderline sedentary group. The ratio of HDL to LDL cholesterol was 0.26, 0.31, 0.29 and 0.28, respectively. The training programme consisted of first bicycle ergometer training for two months and then walking-jogging for two months. The training intensity was moderate, the frequency three times a week and the duration of the sessions 50 to 60 minutes.

Except for the systolic blood pressure in the borderline hypertensive sedentary subjects, systolic (SBP) and diastolic (DBP) blood pressure decreased in both trained and sedentary groups during the four-month training period (Table 1). The HDL/LDL cholesterol ratio increased slightly in all groups (Table 1). However, the difference in the change of SBP between the training and sedentary group was greater in the borderline hypertensives than in the normotensives ($p < 0.05$, two-way ANCOVA). There was also a similar nonsignificant trend in DBP.

Table 1. Age-adjusted changes in the resting SBP and DBP (mmHg) and in the HDL/LDL-cholesterol ratio (HDL/LDL) in the normotensive and borderline hypertensive men during physical training

| Group | SBP | DBP | HDL/LDL |
|---|---|---|---|
| Normotensive | | | |
| Training | -5.8 | -6.7 | +0.06 |
| Sedentary | -6.0 | -10.2 | +0.04 |
| | | | |
| Borderline | | | |
| Training | -9.1 | -11.9 | +0.001 |
| Sedentary | +2.1 | -7.8 | +0.02 |

We conclude that physical training programme used in this study does not seem to have any notable influence on resting blood pressure either in the normotensive or in the borderline hypertensive middle-aged men. Physical training programmes of longer duration are needed to study the possibilities to modify blood pressure and serum lipoproteins, the two major risk factors for coronary heart disease.

Acknowledgements The support from Juho Vainio Foundation and from Ministry for Social Affairs and Health is gratefully appreciated.

# 1.8 Drug Therapy of Hyperlipoproteinemias

# The Treatment of Hyperlipaemia by Gemfibrozil: A Comparison with Clofibrate

A.N.Howard and J.Marks

## A. Pharmacology in the rat

Gemfibrozil is structurally related to clofibrate and was investigated because of its greater hypotriglyceridaemic activity in the rat. In this species there are some major differences in pharmacological response between the two compounds. In contrast to clofibrate, gemfibrozil has no effect on total plasma cholesterol or fibrogen, but does increase HDL-cholesterol (1).

The latter effect is particularly pronounced in cholesterol – cholic acid fed rats (2). As shown in Table 1, clofibrate has no effect in this model and lipantyl is only moderately active.

Whilst clofibrate increased rat liver $\alpha$ -glycerophosphate dehydrogenase, carnitine acyl transferase, and fatty oxidation, gemfibrozil has no effect. Clofibrate increases cholesterol biosynthesis and HMG Co-A reductase, but gemfibrozil effects a decrease (3).

Table 1.  Elevation of rat HDL-cholesterol: comparative effects of gemfibrozil, clofibrate, lipantyl and U-41792

| Drug | Dose (mg/kg) | Elevation % |
|------|------|------|
| Gemfibrozil | 50 | 334 |
|  | 100 | 406 |
| Clofibrate | 50 | 0 |
|  | 100 | 0 |
| Lipantyl | 50 | 26 (N.S.) |
|  | 100 | 50 |
| U-41792 | 50 | 434 |
|  | 100 | 700 |

Control HDL-C was $6.5 \pm 0.7$ mg/dl
Diet:   1.5% cholesterol
        0.1% cholic acid
U-41792 is used as a positive control

B.    Clinical pharmacology in hyperlipaemia

1.    Efficacy

In man, the hyperlipoproteinaemias most likely to be affected are types IIb, III, IV and V and many trials in the United Kingdom and Scandinavia have confirmed this (Table 2). Serum triglycerides are reduced 30-40% and cholesterol 10-20% ( 1 ).

Table 2.    Effect of gemfibrozil on serum lipids
            Summary of multicentre trials

| HLP Type | No. of Trials | No. of Patients | Mean % decrease in Cholesterol | Triglyceride |
|---|---|---|---|---|
| IIa | 13 | 80 | 14.4 | 32.5 |
| IIb | 16 | 100 | 18.0 | 42.3 |
| III | 4 | 16 | 20.2 | 37.6 |
| IV | 17 | 122 | 14.4 | 37.2 |
| V | 3 | 4 | 13.4 | 34.4 |

Gemfibrozil has a potentially beneficial effect on serum lipoproteins (Table 3).

In type IIa, LDL-cholesterol is decreased by 25%; in type IIb, VLDL-triglyceride decreased by 60% and LDL-cholesterol by 18%.  In type IV, VLDL is normalized, but there is no effect on LDL-cholesterol (4).

Table 3.    Effect of gemfibrozil on serum lipoproteins

| Serum lipid | Lipoprotein fraction | No. of trials | No. of patients | % change in mean |
|---|---|---|---|---|
| Cholesterol | CHYLO | 4 | 18 | − 58.1 |
|  | VLDL | 14 | 135 | − 46.9 |
|  | LDL | 13 | 115 | − 6.1 |
|  | HDL | 17 | 135 | + 14.5 |
| Triglycerides | CHYLO | 1 | 3 | − 79.0 |
|  | VLDL | 9 | 105 | − 43.0 |
|  | LDL | 8 | 102 | − 25.8 |
|  | HDL | 10 | 82 | − 23.2 |

An important effect is an elevation of HDL-cholesterol of 10-30% in all the above-mentioned hyperlipaemias.  For example, in 12 patients treated with 1.2g/day, MANNINEN et al (1982) obtained an increase of 26% in total HDL-cholesterol, consisting of increases in both $HDL_2$ and $HDL_3$ (5).

## 2. Comparison with clofibrate

In several cross–over studies (Table 4) gemfibrozil (0.8–1.2g/day) has proved more effective than clofibrate (1.5–2g/day) in lowering serum triglycerides, whilst having the same activity in lowering cholesterol (4).

Table 4.       Comparison of effects of gemfibrozil and clofibrate in type IIb/IV

Serum cholesterol and triglycerides

| Author | No. | Drug | Dose g/day | Serum Cholesterol Decrease % | Triglyceride |
|--------|-----|------|------------|-------------|--------------|
| Eisalo | 16 | Clofibrate | 1.5 | 15 | 49 |
|        |    | Gemfibrozil | 0.8 | 15 | 60 |
| Nikkila | 11 | Clofibrate | 2.0 | 10 | 27 |
|        |    | Gemfibrozil | 0.8 | 9 | 50 |
| Howard | 11 | Clofibrate | 2.0 | 8 | 21 |
|        |    | Gemfibrozil | 1.2 | 12 | 42 |

For example, in eleven type IIb/IV patients, treated randomly with both drugs (Fig. 1) gemfibrozil was twice as potent as clofibrate in lowering LDL-cholesterol and triglycerides (6). Whilst clofibrate had no significant effect on HDL-cholesterol, gemfibrozil caused a 30% increase. This latter difference has also been reported by two other groups using 0.8g/day gemfibrozil ( 1).

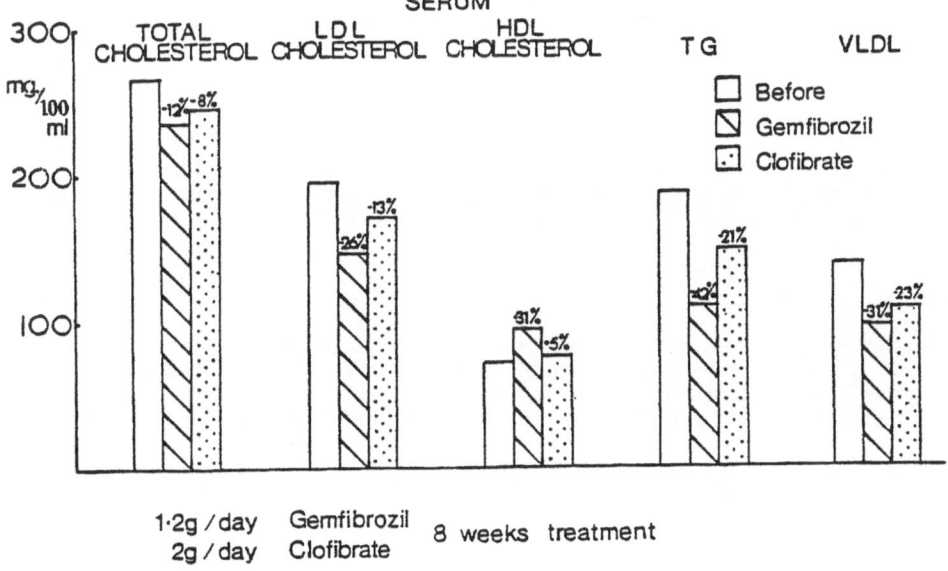

Fig. 1    Effect of gemfibrozil compared with clofibrate in same eleven patients

Table 5.    Comparison of gemfibrozil and clofibrate in 16 diabetics

| Drug | | Serum cholesterol | Serum HDL cholesterol mg/100ml | Triglycerides |
|------|---|-------------------|--------------------------------|---------------|
| Gemfibrozil | Before | 235 | 106 | 267 |
| (1.2g/day) | After | 220 | 130 | 158 |
| | % change | -6 | +23 | -41 |
| Clofibrate | Before | 228 | 95 | 197 |
| | After | 224 | 96 | 190 |
| | % change | 0 | +1 | -4 |

A potentially beneficial property of clofibrate is its effect in decreasing plasma fibrinogen; this is not seen with gemfibrozil (4).

The difference in efficacy is even more evident in diabetics in which hypertriglyceridaemia occurs in high incidence (40-50%). In a double blind cross-over trial, 16 mature onset diabetics, controlled by diet alone or with clorpropamide, and with type IV or IIb hyperlipoproteinaemia, were treated with 1.2g/day gemfibrozil and 2.0g/day clofibrate for eight weeks (7). With gemfibrozil, triglycerides were decreased by 41% and HDL-cholesterol raised by 23%. Clofibrate had no effect. With neither drug was there any important changes in the diabetic status of the patients or an ADP-induced platelet aggregation. Clofibrate increased SGPT and decreased serum alkaline phosphatase, whereas gemfibrozil had no significant effect.

## 3.    Safety

Clofibrate has the disadvantage of increasing the lithogenic index of bile and the incidence of gallstones. In a study of normolipaemic volunteers, gemfibrozil, in contrast to clofibrate, did not significantly increase the lithogenic index, and the number of volunteers having saturated bile was less (8). Whether this difference is seen in hyperlipaemic patients has yet to be determined.

Gemfibrozil has a much shorter half life (1.5 hr.) compared with clofibrate (12 hr.); this may explain why it is tolerated to a much greater extent in hyperlipaemic patients with uremia or nehprotic syndrome. Thus MANNINEN et al reported that gemfibrozil, in contrast to clofibrate, was able to combat effectively dyslipidaemia in these conditions safely without side-effects and deterioration in renal function (9).

## 4.    Conclusions

Gemfibrozil is structurally related to clofibrate but has some important pharmacological differences. It is a much more potent hypotriglyceridaemic agent, and consistently elevates serum HDL-cholesterol where this is abnormally low. It has proved superior in the treatment of hyperlipaemia in diabetes, and safer in uremia and nephrotic syndrome.

## References

1. Hodges RM (1976)  Gemfibrozil: A new lipid lowering agent.  Proc. Roy. Soc. Med. 69: 1-113
2. Maxwell RE (1981)  Personal communication
3. Maxwell RE, Nawrocki JW, Uhlendorf PD (1982)  Some differences in effects of clofibrate, bezafibrate, cholestyramine and ML-236B on lipid metabolism in rats  Res. & Clin. Forum 4: (2)  In Press
4. Gorringe J (1982)  Personal communication
5. Manninen V, Malkonen M, Nikkila EA (1982)  Effect of gemfibrozil on blood levels of high density lipoprotein subfractions $HDL_2$ and $HDL_3$.  Res. & Clin. Forum 4: (2)  In Press
6. Howard AN (1982)  Unpublished
7. Marks J, Howard AN (1982)  A comparative study of gemfibrozil and clofibrate in the treatment of hyperlipidaemia in patients with maturity-onset diabetes.  Res. & Clin. Forum 4: (2)  In Press
8. Hall MJ, Nelson LM, Russell RI, Howard AN (1981)  Gemfibrozil - The effect on biliary cholesterol saturation of a new lipid lowering agent and its comparison with clofibrate.  Atherosclerosis 39: 511-516
9. Manninen V, Malkonen M, Eisalo A (1982)  Gemfibrozil treatment of dyslipidaemias in renal failure with uremia or in nephrotic syndrome.  Res. & Clin. Forum 4: (2) In Press

# Lipid-Lowering Agents and Apolipoproteins B, A-I and A-II – A Long-term Study

R. Mordasini and W. Riesen

Lipid Research Laboratory of the Institute for Clinical Protein
Research (Tiefenauspital) of the University of Berne/Switzerland

LIPID-LOWERING AGENTS AND APOLIPOPROTEINS B, A-I AND A-II –
A LONGTERM STUDY

R. Mordasini and W. Riesen

## Summary

Changes in serum lipids, the individual lipoprotein fractions after
ultracentrifugation and the apoproteins B, A-I and A-II were studied
in 66 patients with primary hypercholesterolaemia under treatment
with different lipid-lowering agents. After three months with dietary
treatment alone and a four-week placebo period, the patients were
given bezafibrate (3 x 200 mg daily), colestipol (2 x 10 g per day)
or probucol (2 x 500 mg daily) for 12 months, followed by another
four-week placebo period at the end of the study.

Colestipol showed the best lipid-lowering effect (total- and LDL-Cholesterol were decreased by 20 % and 23 % respectively) but satisfactory total- and LDL-cholesterol lowering results were also obtained
with the other substances. However, the changes in HDL differed widely among the three substances: bezafibrate increased HDL-cholesterol
and the HDL-apoproteins A-I and A-II significantly, colestipol did
not alter these parameters, while probucol treatment was followed
by a significant decrease in both HDL-cholesterol and the apoproteins A-I and A-II.

## Introduction

Raised levels of the low-density lipoproteins (LDL), which transport
the majority of plasma cholesterol, are considered to be highly atherogenic. On the other hand, the high-density lipoproteins (HDL) appear to have a protective effect against the manifestation of atherosclerotic vascular complications (3,4,9).

The atherogenicity of a disturbance of lipid metabolism may be characterized best today by measurement of some apoproteins, the carrier
proteins of the serum lipids (1,13): The atherogenic LDL possess
only one apoprotein, apoprotein B; the apoproteins A-I and A-II constitute the majority of the HDL apoproteins (2,11).

The aim of the present study was the analysis of different standard
substances of the lipid-lowering drug treatment with regard to their
influence on the major LDL- and HDL-apoproteins. There was special
interest in the behavior of HDL. The clofibrate derivative bezafibrate, the anion exchange resin colestipol and the synthetic antioxidant probucol were tested.

## Patients and methods

### Patients

66 male patients were included in the study. The average age was
44.1 years (29 to 58 years). In 36 patients, there was a primary
pure hypercholesterolemia, in 30 cases there was a type II b- pattern.

The body weight of the patients increased during the duration of
the study by an average of 1.1 kg.

### Methods

Cholesterol and triglycerides were measured in whole serum and in
the isolated lipoprotein fractions after ultracentrifugation (6).
The chemical lipid determinations were performed with enzymatic methods in a Technicon AA-II autoanalyzer. Apolipoprotein B (apo B)
was measured by radial immunodiffusion on commercially available
immunoplates (Behringwerke Marburg, 7). The apolipoproteins A-I
and A-II (apo A-I and A-II) were determined with an electroimmuno-
diffusion test developed in our own laboratory (10).

### Study design

All patients received a fat-reduced and fat-modified diet for three
months prior of the beginning of the study. Then the patients were
divided into 3 groups and received after administration of a placebo
for four weeks A) bezafibrate (3 x 200 mg per day), B) colestipol
(2 x 10 g per day) and C) probucol (2 x 500 mg per day). 22 patient
records could be evaluated in group A, 24 patient records in group
B and 20 patient records in group C. The duration of treatment was
12 months. At the end of the study, the patients again received a
placebo for one month. During the entire duration of the trial, clinical and laboratory checks were performed in 4 to eight week intervals.

### Results

Colestipol showed the best reduction of the total and LDL-cholesterol after the whole treatment period lasting 12 months (average reduction: 20 % and 23 % respectively). With a decrease of 13 % in
total cholesterol and 17 % in the LDL-cholesterol fraction, probucol
followed in second place. 13 % reduction of total cholesterol in the
mean resulted under the administration of Bezafibrate (Table 1).

Apo B also was reduced to the greatest extent by the anion exchange
resin with an average of 16.5 %, form the initial placebo period.
The effect of Probucol was very similar with 16 % in the mean, whereas a 9 % decrease of apo B resulted under Bezafibrate.

The analysis of the HDL revealed a significant increase both for
HDL-cholesterol and the HDL apoproteins A-I and A-II (Table 1).
These parameters were not significantly altered by the anion exchange

Table 1. Lipids, lipoprotein fractions and apoproteins during treatment with a) Bezafibrate, b) Colestipol and c) Probucol

|  | Preperiod | Placebo | 4 months | 8 months | 12 months | Placebo |
|---|---|---|---|---|---|---|
| **A. Bezafibrate** | | | | | | |
| Cholesterol | 298 ± 15 | 292 ± 11 | 253 ± 16** | 258 ± 17** | 253 ± 12** | 304 ± 14 |
| Triglycerides | 166 ± 21 | 154 ± 18 | 99 ± 12 | 109 ± 14 | 103 ± 16 | 122 ± 18 |
| LDL-Cholesterol | 181 ± 9 | 178 ± 7 | 152 ± 6** | 156 ± 9** | 156 ± 7** | 185 ± 10 |
| HDL-Cholesterol | 39 ± 4 | 41 ± 6 | 49 ± 3** | 50 ± 6** | 53 ± 4** | 44 ± 6 |
| Apo B | 134 ± 10 | 134 ± 6 | 118 ± 9** | 120 ± 7** | 122 ± 5** | 140 ± 11 |
| Apo A-I | 119 ± 6 | 123 ± 9 | 131 ± 7* | 128 ± 3* | 130 ± 5* | 126 ± 7 |
| Apo A-II | 38 ± 4 | 40 ± 3 | 46 ± 6* | 44 ± 6** | 44 ± 4** | 39 ± 5 |
| **B. Colestipol** | | | | | | |
| Cholesterol | 296 ± 14 | 289 ± 11 | 234 ± 7** | 241 ± 14** | 231 ± 8** | 284 ± 16 |
| Triglycerides | 176 ± 24 | 169 ± 17 | 194 ± 29 | 186 ± 22 | 174 ± 14 | 170 ± 29 |
| LDL-Cholesterol | 181 ± 10 | 176 ± 9 | 144 ± 7** | 140 ± 9** | 136 ± 11** | 172 ± 11 |
| HDL-Cholesterol | 41 ± 6 | 42 ± 4 | 36 ± 4** | 39 ± 7 | 43 ± 3 | 42 ± 6 |
| Apo B | 131 ± 11 | 125 ± 8 | 114 ± 2** | 106 ± 9 | 104 ± 7** | 126 ± 9 |
| Apo A-I | 116 ± 7 | 119 ± 9 | 115 ± 11 | 112 ± 4 | 111 ± 9* | 110 ± 11 |
| Apo A-II | 34 ± 4 | 32 ± 7 | 33 ± 3 | 36 ± 5 | 34 ± 5 | 34 ± 4 |
| **C. Probucol** | | | | | | |
| Cholesterol | 336 ± 24 | 322 ± 19 | 287 ± 14** | 279 ± 21** | 278 ± 12** | 329 ± 29 |
| Triglycerides | 187 ± 35 | 166 ± 41 | 156 ± 31 | 160 ± 28 | 174 ± 49 | 178 ± 34 |
| LDL-Cholesterol | 234 ± 18 | 227 ± 11 | 184 ± 9** | 187 ± 17** | 189 ± 17** | 216 ± 11 |
| HDL-Cholesterol | 39 ± 9 | 42 ± 7 | 35 ± 8* | 35 ± 5* | 33 ± 9* | 40 ± 10 |
| Apo B | 146 ± 27 | 140 ± 21 | 121 ± 19* | 124 ± 26* | 117 ± 28* | 142 ± 36 |
| Apo A-I | 103 ± 14 | 106 ± 11 | 89 ± 7** | 84 ± 9** | 82 ± 11** | 100 ± 13 |
| Apo A-II | 34 ± 9 | 37 ± 7 | 31 ± 4** | 26 ± 5** | 27 ± 8** | 35 ± 7 |

$*p < 0.01$;  $**p < 0.001$

resin therapy, whereas probucol significantly lowered both HDL-cholesterol and the HDL apoproteins A-I and A-II.

The best lipid-lowering effect was already obtained after two months
of treatment with all three substances investigated. It remained almost unchanged during the whole duration of the study. On the other
hand, the greatest effects on HDL were only observed in the control
after 12 months of treatment.

Serious undesired side effects were not observed in the patients
treated with probucol. Slight epigastric pain was noted in four cases, but did not necessitate cessation of therapy. With bezafibrate,
we had to discontinue treatment in one patient due to the occurrence
of muscle pain with marked increase in CPK (this is an undesired
side effect which is well-known under clofibrate, 5). Three patients
complained of nausea and feeling of pressure in the upper abdomen
which largely declined with time on continuation of therapy. In the
colestipol group, the treatment of four patients was discontinued
because of constipation, feeling of fullness and other problems in
taking the preparation; four further patients complained of in some
cases severe constipation and feeling of fullness despite administration of the substance in two daily doses and the recommendation that
it be taken in fruit juice.

Discussion

All three substances tested led to a significant decrease of total-
and LDL-cholesterol. The best effect was obtained with colestipol.
However, bezafibrate and probucol were only slightly inferior to this
result. Apo B, the carrier protein of the atherogenic LDL, was accordingly also reduced to the greatest extent in patients treated with
the anion exchange resin.

However, analysis of the probably "antiatherogenic" HDL showed that
the tested substances had very different effects on the HDL: there
was a significant increase of both HDL-cholesterol and apo A-I and
A-II under bezafibrate, whereas there were no major alterations of
these parameters with colestipol. Probucol even caused a significant
reduction of the plasma HDL level. This result was found consistently both in the measurement of HDL-cholesterol and in the determination of the main HDL-apoproteins A-I and A-II. The decrease in the
HDL with probucol treatment was present at any control during the
whole duration of the study.

The aim of lipid-lowering drug treatment is primarily to lower the
levels of atherogenic lipoproteins, above all of the LDL. It has not
been proved yet whether an increase of HDL (as would be assumed for
theoretical reasons) entails an additional antiatherogenic effect
(11).

It is therefore also difficult to assess the significance of the reduction of HDL under treatment with probucol. This finding is a confirmation of previously published results (8,12). On the basis of
theoretical considerations, it may be observed that caution in the
application of a lipid-lowering substance which significantly reduces the HDL appears to be justified at present. However, on the

other hand, in our opinion the rise of HDL under bezafibrate is not a sufficient argument in order to prefer this substance to the anion exchange resin which leaves the HDL essentially unchanged.

It can be stated out in conclusion that the three lipid-lowering drugs tested alter the HDL in a very different way with comparable total- and LDL-cholesterol-lowering efficacy: The clofibrate derivative bezafibrate increases the HDL significantly, the anion exchange resin colestipol leaves them almost unchanged, and the synthetic antioxidant probucol leads to a significant reduction of HDL. Even if it is too early to accord this different influence on the HDL decisive importance in the choice of a lipid-lowering agent, this observation nevertheless deserves increasing attention. On the basis of what we know about HDL today, caution in the administration of substances which lower HDL appears to be justified at present.

# R e f e r e n c e s

1. Avogaro P., Bon G., Cazzolato G., Quinci G., Sanson A.,
   Sparla M., Zagetti G., Caturelli G.:
   Variations in apolipoproteins B and A-I during the
   course of myocardial infarction.
   Eur. J. clin. Invest. 8, 121 (1978).

2. Blum C., Levy R., Eisenberg S., Hall H., Goebel R.,
   Berman M.:
   High density lipoprotein metabolism in man.
   J. clin. Invest. 60, 795 (1977).

3. Carew T., Hayes S., Kochinsky T., Steinberg D.:
   A mechanism by which high density lipoproteins may slow
   the atherogenic process.
   Lancet 1976/1, 1315.

4. Castelli W., Doyle J., Gordon T., Hames C., Hjortland M.,
   Hulley S., Kagan A., Zukel W.:
   HDL-cholesterol and other lipids in coronary heart disease.
   Circulations 55, 767 (1977).

5. Langer T., Levy R.:
   Acute muscular syndrome associated with administration of
   clofibrate.
   New. Engl. J. Med. 279, 856 (1968).

6. Lipid Research Clinic Program:
   In: Manual of Laboratory Operations.
   Vol. I. U.S. Government Printing Office, Washington DC
   (1974).

7. Mancini G., Carbonara A., Heremans J.:
   Immunochemical quantitation of antigens by single radial
   immunodiffusion.
   Immunochemistry 2, 2 (1955).

8. Miettinen T., Huttunen J., Kumlin T., Naukkarinen V.,
   Matila S., Enholm C.:
   High density lipoprotein cholesterol and apolipoproteins A-I and A-II during longterm treatment with clofibrate and probucol.
   Annual Meeting Europ. Atherosclerosis Group, Lugano
   (1979).

9. Miller G., Miller N.:
   Plasma high-density lipoprotein concentration and de-
   velopment of ischaemic heart disease.
   Lancet 1975/1, 16.

10. Mordasini R., Riesen W.:
    Electroimmunoassay and radioimmunoassay for the quantitation
    of high density apolipoproteins A-I and A-II.
    J. clin. Chem. clin. Biochem. 18, 917 (1980).

11. Mordasini R., Riesen W., Oster P.:
    HDL - die Unbekannte mit dem grossen Gewicht.
    Schweiz. med. Wschr. 111, 309-314 (1981).

12. Riesen W., Keller M., Mordasini R.:
    Probucol in hypercholesterolemia. A double blind study.
    Atherosclerosis 36, 201-207 (1980).

13. Riesen W., Mordasini R., Salzmann C., Theler A., Gurtner H.P.:
    Apoproteins and lipids as discriminators of severity of
    coronary heart disease.
    Atherosclerosis 37, 157 (1980).

# Compliance and Cholestorol-Lowering in Clinical Trials: Efficacy of Diet

B. M. Rifkind, R. Goor, and B. Schucker

Cholesterol lowering by dietary or pharmacological means to reduce coronary heart disease (CHD) incidence has been the object of much effort over the past few decades. Prospective studies show that the higher the cholesterol level, the greater the risk of CHD. Cholesterol-lowering therapy is prescribed on the assumption that reduction of cholesterol will be accompanied by decreased CHD risk. The greater the reduction in cholesterol, the greater will be the likely reduction in the risk. Accordingly, there has been a search for agents that would consistently produce a considerable reduction in cholesterol. Since hypercholesterolemia is common and the rationale for cholesterol lowering requires that it be lifelong, cholesterol-lowering regimens are widely used.

In assessing the efficacy of cholesterol-lowering regimens, the impact of compliance on efficacy has received insufficient attention. Compliance to a regimen is clearly important in determining its capabilities. While it is a truism that failure to take a powerful cholesterol-lowering agent makes it worthless, there is probably insufficient recognition of the serious impact that various compliance problems have on a regimen's effectiveness.

Achieving good compliance is by no means easy. Treating patients with medication requires considerable cooperation on the part of the patient. It is especially troublesome when it involves long-term therapy in asymptomatic subjects, and is sometimes associated with side effects.

The evaluation of promising cholesterol-lowering agents, after their initial development and study in animals, is largely based on small-scale clinical studies. This intensive scrutiny is important to obtain a detailed picture of the drug's potency as well as other information. It is generally required that several such studies be performed to obtain an overall, hopefully accurate picture of the drug's capabilities.

Although a critical stage in the development of cholesterol-lowering agents, the shortcomings of such small-scale clinical studies in describing the efficacy of a drug may be insufficiently recognized. They tend to be of relatively short duration, usually several weeks or months, whereas the actual prescription of the cholesterol-lowering drugs would cover years, and perhaps the lifetime of the individual. By the time a subject has entered into a typical short-term study, many selection biases are likely to have operated, some overt and others less obvious. Often the patients, who have various forms of hyperlipidemia often accompanied by vascular disease, are well-motivated towards reducing their high cholesterol levels. By necessity, the number of subjects studied is usually few, often between 20–50. Such studies are usually performed in a specialized clinical setting and involve frequent clinic visits. Leaving aside the impact of these shortcomings in assessing the potential long-term toxicity of cholesterol-lowering agents, such study design features may seriously impair the assessment of cholesterol-lowering by providing insufficient information on long-term compliance. In general, many of these features can be expected to result in overstating the degree of cholesterol-lowering that would occur in routine clinical practice, involving very large numbers of asymptomatic, less motivated subjects and less frequent clinic visits in less specialized settings.

Large-scale clinical trials of CHD prevention through cholesterol lowering, on the other hand, provide a more realistic assessment of the cholesterol-lowering capabilities of drugs and other regimens. They usually involve much larger numbers of subjects who are more representative of the population eligible for treatment, are of several years' duration, and have less frequent clinic visits. Thus the large-scale trial often more closely approximates the conventional clinical care situation than the initial small-scale studies, and provides a more realistic assessment of the efficacy of the drug in clinical practice, especially as it relates to compliance with the therapeutic recommendations. It has to be pointed out, however, that even the large-scale trial may have features that make it significantly different from conventional clinical practice.

A large number of clinical trials of the efficacy of cholesterol-lowering in preventing CHD have been reported. These comprise primary or secondary prevention studies, employing diet and/or drugs designed to obtain cholesterol lowering in predominantly middle-aged males with different degrees of hypercholesterolemia.

We have summarized the cholesterol-lowering reported in many such studies employing drugs (Table 1) and diet (Tables 2 and 3). It should be noted it is not clear from some reports how the cholesterol reduction was calculated. Some of the trials of hypolipidemic agents for the prevention of CHD actually fail to report the degree of cholesterol-lowering or to make a clear statement regarding it. In some reports, subjects who withdrew from the study, or from whom data was not available because of missed clinic visits, may have been omitted from calculation. This would have the effect of producing an average cholesterol reduction greater than that actually achieved in all subjects initially entered into the treatment group. Account is not always taken of the duration of the study which can vary considerably; the longer the study, the more likely that decreased compliance will occur. Often the cholesterol lowering is not calculated and averaged for the total duration of the study. Allowance is not always made for the possibility of regression of the original entry cholesterol values to the mean so that, again, cholesterol lowering may be overstated. Adjustment for any changes in the control group is not always made. To what extent, in dietary studies, such adjustments should be made is not clear since trends in a control group may reflect coincident changes in their dietary intake.

## Drug Trials

The W.H.O. Clofibrate Study (1) is the major primary prevention trial that used a drug to lower cholesterol. In the three participating centers, the blinded use of clofibrate resulted in a 8.2-9.7% reduction in cholesterol over seven years, varying from 7% in Budapest to 11% in Edinburgh. Small-scale studies suggest that clofibrate is capable of lowering cholesterol by about 10-15%.

Table 1. Cholesterol-lowering in large-scale drug studies

| Study | Drug | Primary or Secondary | Double-Blind | Duration (Yrs.) | % Cholesterol Reduction |
|---|---|---|---|---|---|
| V.A. Drug-Lipid[8] Coop. Study | Aluminum Nicotinate | S | + | 5 | 12.6 |
| | DT4 | S | + | 5 | 6.5 |
| Coronary Drug Proj.[5,7] | Clofibrate | S | + | 6 | 6.5 |
| | Nicotinic Acid | S | + | 6 | 9.9 |
| | DT4 | S | + | 3 | 12.0 |
| Newcastle[3] | Clofibrate | S | + | 5 | M 11 / F 15 } at 6 mos. |
| Scotland[4] | Clofibrate | S | + | 6 | 16 |
| United Airlines[2] | Clofibrate | P&S | - | 2-5 | 15 |
| Upjohn[9] | Colestipol | P&S | - | 1-3 | 10 |
| W.H.O.[1] | Clofibrate | P | + | 8 | 8.2 - 9.7 |

Most of the secondary prevention studies have also employed clofibrate. Average cholesterol falls of 15% were reported (2) for the United Airlines Study (mixed primary and secondary), 11% in males and 15% for females in Newcastle, England (3), and 16% in the last two years of a study in Scotland (4). The largest secondary prevention study was the Coronary Drug Project (CDP). The group receiving clofibrate obtained only a 6.5% reduction (over five years) when allowance was made for changes in the placebo group (5). The group receiving nicotinic acid obtained a corresponding fall of 9.9% (5). The CDP also evaluated 2.5 mg of conjugated estrogen which produced a slight reduction in serum cholesterol (6), 5 mg/day of conjugated estrogen for which the cholesterol-lowering was not reported (7), and dextrothyroxine which produced a 12% fall over the 3 years of its use (7).

The earlier V.A. Drug-Lipid Cooperative Study also evaluated several cholesterol-lowering agents (8). Estrogen (1.25 mg/day) had no appreciable effect on the cholesterol level. Over the five years of the study, dextrothyroxine and aluminum nicotinate respectively produced average falls of 6.5% and 12.6% after adjustment for trends in the control group.

The only large-scale study of a biliary sequestrant is actually an aggregate of several studies of primary or secondary prevention using colestipol (9). After three years, a 10% reduction was achieved. In contrast, falls of 15-25% in cholesterol have been reported in short-term, small-scale studies of sequestrants such as colestipol or cholestyramine.

Recently attention has been focussed on regimens that combine two lipid-lowering agents in an attempt to produce better cholesterol-lowering, though the enhanced potency of two agents might be expected to be offset by greater problems in compliance. An interim report on myocardial infarction survivors in Stockholm found that a combined regimen of nicotinic acid and clofibrate produced an average fall of 14% in serum cholesterol, though this result was influenced by omitting data on subjects who dropped out of the study (10).


Diet Trials


Diet studies generally aim to decrease the dietary cholesterol and saturated fat intake while increasing that of polyunsaturated fat. Many of the diet studies, especially the more recent ones, are of primary prevention, reflecting the interest in primary prevention of CHD, the reluctance to use drugs for this purpose, and the assumption that cholesterol-lowering diets are less likely to be toxic.

Table 2. Cholesterol-lowering in large-scale diet studies

| Study | Primary or Secondary Intervention | Double-Blind | Duration (Yrs.) | % Cholesterol Reduction | Comments |
|---|---|---|---|---|---|
| Diet-Heart [21] | P | + | 1 | 8 | Free-living |
| | | – | 1 | 11 | Free-living |
| L.A. V.A. [17] | P & S | + | 8 | 13 | Institutional |
| Finnish Mental Hospital [15] | P | – | 6 | 15 | Institutional |
| N.Y. Anti-Coronary Club [18] | P | – | 14 | 8.7 in first yr. 13.5 in fourth yr. | Free-living |
| Minnesota [19] | P | + | 4.5 | 13 | Institutional |
| Oslo [16] | P | – | 5 | 23.5 | Free-living |
| MRFIT [20] | P | – | 4 | 6-7% active intervention group | Free-living |

Table 3.  Cholesterol-lowering in large-scale diet studies (Derived from Mann & Marr, 1981) [22]

| Study | Primary or Secondary Intervention | Duration (Yrs.) | % Cholesterol Reduction |
|-------|-----------------------------------|-----------------|-------------------------|
| Morrison [14] | S | 8 | 29 |
| Rose [12] | S | 2 | 20 |
| Leren [13] | S | 11 | 18 |
| M.R.C. [11] | S | 2-6 | 17 at 3 yrs. |

In contrast to the drug studies, many of the diet studies achieved cholesterol reductions of 15% or more, for example, those of the M.R.C. (11), Rose (12), Leren (13), Morrison (14), and most recently, the Finnish Mental Hospital Study (15) and the Oslo Study (16).  Studies which resulted in falls of 10-15% include the Los Angeles-VA Study (17), the New York Anti-Coronary Club (18), and that of Frantz (19) in Minnesota.  The MRFIT study reported a 7.4% reduction in cholesterol after 4 years.  This more modest fall may reflect the impact of coincident interventions to control blood pressure and smoking, which might be expected to aggravate compliance problems.  Mention must also be made of the Diet-Heart Feasibility Study, which obtained an overall reduction of 11% in free-living urban men (21).

## Concluding Remarks

Our review has important implications.  The results of the drug studies are generally disappointing, though some may have been adversely influenced by blinding.  It is likely that knowing the response of one's cholesterol level to treatment encourages compliance.  So far as drugs are concerned, none has established itself as a consistently effective, powerful and safe cholesterol-lowering agent.  Although some of the clofibrate studies have found falls of about 15%, others, including the two largest, have reported less impressive falls, and found it to be toxic.  The single biliary sequestrant study gave an average reduction far below its capability as reflected by small-scale studies; it is likely that compliance problems relating to side-effects, bulk and taste account for this discrepancy.  Other drugs, apart from dextrothyroxine, which is toxic, achieved a fall of less than 10%.  Although wider use of nicotinic acid has been advocated, its side-effects have seriously interfered with its widespread adoption.  Combined therapy with nicotinic acid and sequestrants has reportedly produced impressive reductions in cholesterol but has not yet been assessed in large clinical trials. At present, no single drug can be regarded as qualified to obtain considerable cholesterol reduction in large numbers of free-living hypercholesterolemic subjects over long periods of time.  Of course, considerable reductions can often be achieved by drugs, in combination with diet, in many subjects who are able to comply with, and are responsive to the regimen.

In contrast to the drug studies, however, the results of the dietary studies are encouraging in demonstrating that long-term compliance is feasible.  They indicate that 10-20% average reductions in cholesterol can be achieved in large, diverse, free-living populations.  These observations may not only apply to subjects with hypercholesterolemia, but have implications for cholesterol reduction in the general population.  They confirm that dietary change in the general population is attainable and can produce cholesterol changes of a magnitude that, on the basis of the cholesterol/CHD relationship seen in prospective epidemiological studies, might result in considerable reductions in CHD incidence.  That diet change is effective is also encouraging since it is likely to be free of the toxicity associated with long-term drug use.

References

1.  Committee of Principal Investigators (1978) A co-operative trial in the primary prevention of ischemic heart disease using clofibrate. Brit Heart J 40: 1069–1118

2.  Krasno LR, Kidera GJ (1972) Clofibrate in coronary heart disease. Effect on morbidity and mortality. JAMA 219: 845–851

3.  Physicians of the Newcastle Upon Tyne Region (1971) Trial of clofibrate in the treatment of ischaemic heart disease. Brit Med J 4: 767–775

4.  Scottish Society of Physicians Research Committee (1971) Ischaemic heart disease: A secondary prevention trial using clofibrate. Brit Med J 4: 775–784

5.  The Coronary Drug Project Research Group (1975) Clofibrate and niacin in coronary heart disease. JAMA 231: 360–381

6.  The Coronary Drug Project Research Group (1973) The Coronary Drug Project. Findings leading to discontinuation of the 2.5 mg/day estrogen group. JAMA 226: 652–657

7.  The Coronary Drug Project Research Group (1970) The Coronary Drug Project. Initial findings leading to modifications of its research protocol. JAMA 214: 1303–1313

8.  Detre KM, Shaw L. (1974) Long-term changes of serum cholesterol with cholesterol-altering drugs in patients with coronary heart disease. Veterans Administration Drug-Lipid Cooperative Study. Circulation 50: 998–1005

9.  Dorr AE, Gunderson K, Schneider JC, Spencer TW, Martin WB (1978) Colestipol hydrochloride in hypercholesterolemic patients – Effect on serum cholesterol and mortality. J Chron Dis 31: 5–14

10. Rosenhamer G, Carlson LA (1980) Effect of combined clofibrate-nicotinic acid treatment in ischemic heart disease. Atherosclerosis 37: 129–138

11. Research Committee to the Medical Research Council (1968) Controlled trial of soya bean oil in myocardial infarction. Lancet ii: 693–700

12. Rose GA, Thomson WB, Williams RT (1965) Corn oil in treatment of ischaemic heart disease. Brit Med J 1: 1531–1533

13. Leren P (1970) Oslo Diet-Heart Study. 11-year report. Circulation 42: 935–942

14. Morrison IM (1955) A nutritional program for prolongation of life in coronary atherosclerosis. JAMA 159: 1425–1428

15. Turpeinen O (1979) Effect of cholesterol-lowering diet on mortality from coronary heart disease and other causes. Circulation 59: 1–7

16. Hjermann I, Holme I, Velvebyre K, Leren P (1981) Effect of diet and smoking intervention on the incidence of coronary heart disease. Lancet 2: 1303–1310

17. Dayton S, Pearce, ML, Hashimoto S, Dixon WJ, Tomiyasu U (1969) A controlled clinical trial of diet high in unsaturated fat in preventing complications of atherosclerosis. Circulation 39 & 40 (Suppl. II)

18. Christakis G, Rinzler SH, Archer M, Kraus A (1966) Effect of the Anti-Coronary Club Program on coronary heart disease risk factor status. JAMA 198: 129–136

19. Frantz ID, Dawson EA, Kuba K (1975) The Minnesota Coronary Survey: Effect of diet on cardiovascular events and deaths. Circulation 51–52 (Suppl. II–4)

20. Caggiula AW, Christakis G, Farrand M, Hulley SB, Johnson R, Lasser NL, Stamler J, Widdowson G (1981) The Multiple Risk Factor Intervention Trial (MRFIT) IV. Intervention on blood lipids. Prev Med 10: 443–475

21. Brown HB (1968) The National Diet-Heart Study – Implications for dietitians and nutritionists. J Amer Diet Assn 52: 279–287

22. Mann JI and Marr JW (1981) Coronary heart disease prevention – Trials of diets to control hyperlipidaemia. In: (Miller NE and Lewis B, eds.) Metabolic Aspects of Cardiovascular Disease. I. Lipoproteins, Atherosclerosis and Coronary Heart Disease. Amsterdam: Elsevier/North Holland Biomedical Press, pp 197–210

# Long-term Treatment of Hypercholesterolaemia with Guar Gum: Comparison with Probucol

L. A. Simons and S. Balasubramaniam

## Introduction

The potential for long-term side effects is a cause for concern when treating patients with absorbable lipid-lowering drugs. This underlies the current interest in non-absorbable plant fibres as clinical cholesterol-lowering agents. Guar gum is one of the few members of a heterogeneous group of substances having confirmed cholesterol-lowering action (1). A new formulation of Guar gum having improved palatability was recently developed. We now present the results of one year's treatment with Guar gum in patients with primary hypercholesterolaemia. The findings are compared with those in a companion group of patients who received the partially-absorbed drug Probucol.

## Methods

Nineteen patients with hypercholesterolaemia ($>6.5$mmol/l) who were already stabilised on a standard cholesterol-lowering diet were enrolled for treatment with Guar gum. The clinical details are presented in Table 1.

Table 1. Summary of clinical details

| | | |
|---|---|---|
| Patients | : | 9 male, 10 female |
| Ages | : | 35 - 75 years |
| Placebo plasma cholesterol | : | 6.7 - 9.6mmol/l |
| Placebo plasma triglycerides | : | 1.3 - 4.8mmol/l |
| Lipid phenotypes | : | 18 Type IIb, 1 Type IIa |

The trial was conducted single-blind, each patient acting as his own control. During an initial 4 week period patients consumed a matching placebo t.d.s. with meals and provided two fasting blood samples. Active Guar formulation was then commenced in a dose of 6g t.d.s. with meals and this was continued for up to 12 months. Fasting blood samples were obtained monthly for the first three months of treatment and thereafter three monthly up to twelve months. Lipid and lipo-protein measurements were performed according to previously described methods (2).

The flavoured Guar formulation was developed by Wellcome Australia Limited and was presented as 6g of active principle packaged in a foil-lined sachet. The dose was shaken vigorously with 170ml of water and remained in a palatable and completely fluid state. Upon reaching the acid pH of the stomach, the Guar reverted to its natural state, absorbed water and became a highly viscous gel.

## Results and Discussion

Ten patients immediately manifested gastro-intestinal side effects, such as abdominal bloating or loose stools. In 8 patients these symptoms resolved spontaneously within 7 to 10 days, but two patients did withdraw within 2 weeks of entry because of severe diarrhoea. Seventeen patients completed three months of Guar treatment and 13 patients completed 12 months.

The cholesterol and triglyceride results from 17 patients completing three months of Guar treatment are presented in Fig. 1.

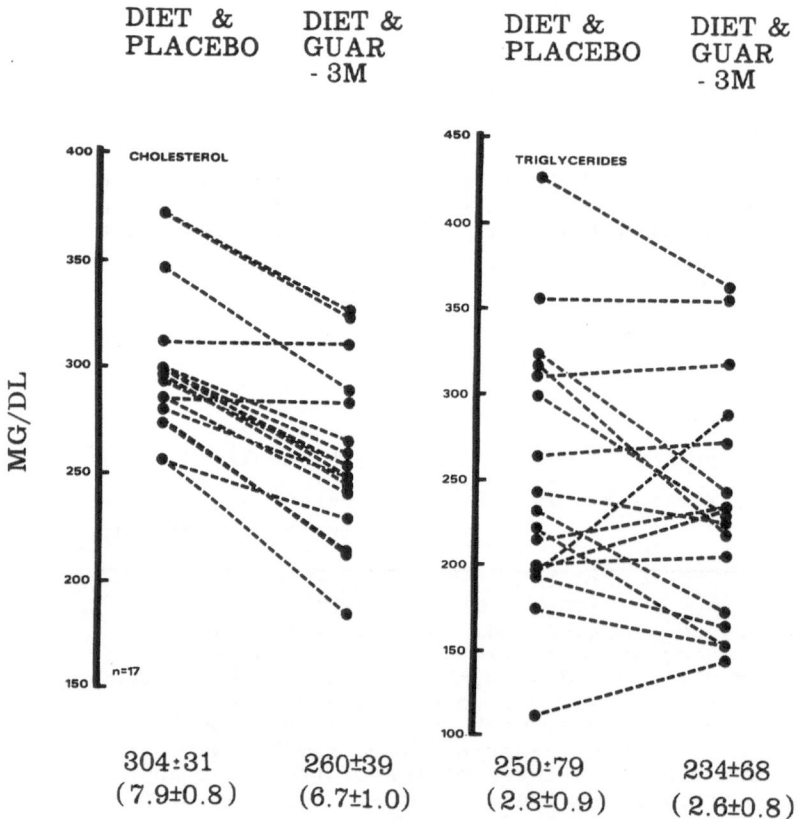

**Fig. 1.** Changes in plasma cholesterol and triglyceride levels in 17 patients completing 3 months treatment with Guar gum

There was a significant 15% fall in mean plasma cholesterol level, but no significant change in plasma triglycerides. In 13 patients continuing for one year, the plasma cholesterol remained significantly lower for the whole period.

The changes in lipoprotein cholesterol concentration over 12 months are presented in Fig. 2.

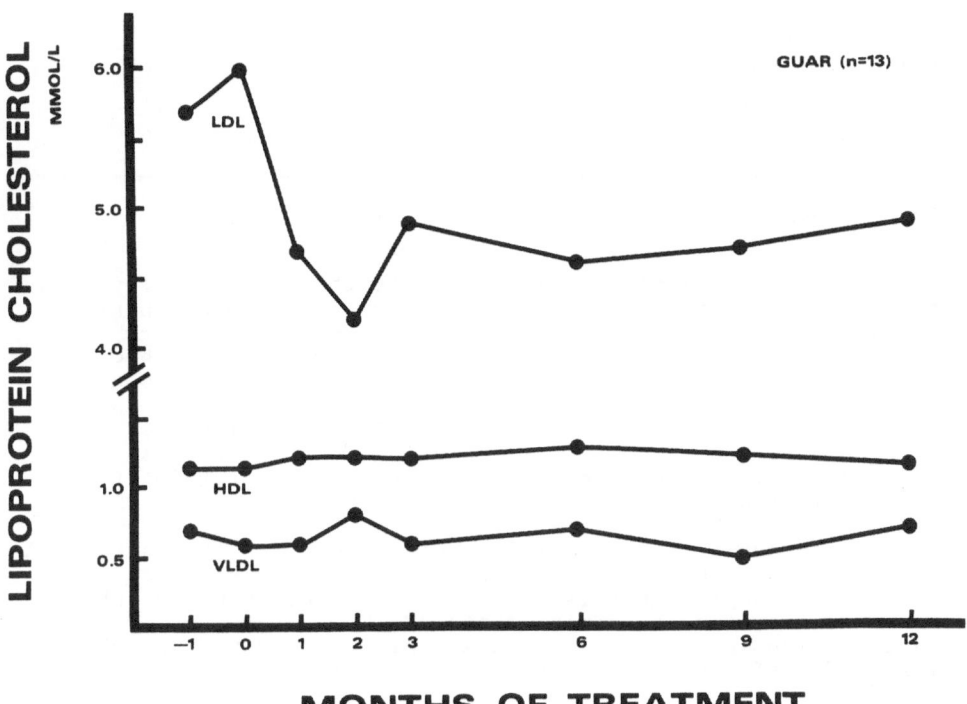

**MONTHS OF TREATMENT**

Fig. 2. Changes in lipoprotein cholesterol levels in 13 patients completing 12 months treatment with Guar gum

The sustained fall in plasma cholesterol was associated with a mean 20% fall in LDL cholesterol, but with no significant change in the level of VLDL or HDL cholesterol.

The results in patients taking Guar gum have been compared with previously published findings in a separate but comparable group of patients treated with Probucol (500mg b.d.) in our clinic (2) (see Table 2). Probucol was clinically tolerated to a better extent than Guar gum, while the plasma cholesterol-lowering efficacy was quite similar for both agents. However, the plasma cholesterol decrement induced by Probucol was due to significant falls in LDL and HDL cholesterol levels. With Guar gum the decrement was solely due to a fall in LDL cholesterol. The ratio of total to HDL cholesterol fell with guar gum but increased with Probucol treatment.

314

Table 2. Comparison of results in patients treated with Guar gum or Probucol

|  | GUAR GUM* | PROBUCOL** |
|---|---|---|
| Duration | 12 months | 6 months |
| Numbers | 13 | 16 |
| Control plasma cholesterol (mmol/l) | 7.7 ± 0.6 | 8.4 ± 1.4 |
| Plasma cholesterol change | −15% | −16% |
| LDL cholesterol change | −20% | −14% |
| HDL cholesterol change | + 4% | −41% |
| TC/HDL cholesterol change | −17% | +40% |

\* Present study                    \*\* See Reference 2

Although current epidemiologic data suggests that LDL is a positive risk factor and HDL is a negative risk factor for coronary heart disease, we have no information available as to the long-term effects, if any, of an induced fall in HDL cholesterol which occurs in parallel with a fall in LDL cholesterol, as seen with Probucol treatment. The use of Probucol remains appropriate in the management of patients with significant degrees of hypercholesterolaemia. However, the observed changes in lipoproteins with Guar treatment could theoretically be beneficial in preventing or retarding the progression of atherosclerosis.

Before Guar gum can be more generally recommended for the management of hypercholesterolaemia, a number of questions remain to be answered. For example, what is the minimum effective dose? What is the necessary frequency of administration? What is the optimum mode of administration in relation to meals? Are there any more subtle long-term side effects asssociated with its use?

References

1.  Jenkins DJA (1979) Dietary fibre, diabetes and hyper-
    lipidaemia. Progress and prospects. Lancet 2:1287−1290
2.  Simons LA, Balasubramaniam S, Beins DM (1981) Metabolic
    studies with Probucol in hypercholesterolaemia.
    Atherosclerosis 40:299−308

## 1.9 Flow Restituting, Nonsurgical Intervention in Cardiovascular Disease

# Gross Endothelial Layer Blistering and Vascular Injury

P. L. Blackshear, Jr., G. L. Blackshear, M. K. Newell, P. F. Emerson, and S. J. Kayser

## A.   Introduction

In 1856 Virchow proposed that injury to the vascular endothelium was the pre-
cipitating event which lead to the formation of an atherosclerotic plaque (1) .
Recently Ross and Harker (2) and others have demonstrated plaque like lesions
in experimental animals following intentional endothelial layer desquamation.
The siting of atherosclerotic lesions in humans has led investigators familiar
with the laws of fluid mechanics to suspect that factors related to fluid flow
influence the patterns and that through a careful study of arterial fluid mechanics a mechanism of arterial endothelial injury could be dicovered (3) .
Many mechanisms have been proposed:  1. Concentration polarization of macromolecules or platelets may occur due to ultra filtration across the artery
wall; this would lead to injury at sites of low fluid shear rate.  2. Fluid
shearing stress causes the endothelium to become more permeable to macromolecules; this would lead to injury at sites of high or fluctuating fluid shear
rate (4) .  3. Regions of low fluid hydrostatic pressure cause subendothelial
fluid to accumulate at these sites; injury should be focused at local pressure
minima (5) .  The agreement between observed frequency of plaque siting and
the estimated site of a local pressure minimum is good  (5) .

This paper describes research into the movement of water across the artery wall
at steady pressure and following a step change in mean systemic pressure.  It
leads to the suggestion of a mechanism whereby a rapid change in the hydrostatic
(or colloid osmotic) pressure will predispose the arterial endothelium, in particular at the local pressure minima, to desquamation by fluid shear forces.
The consequences of sudden postural chhanges similar to those occurring in daily
life are considered in the light of the processes examined.  It appears that the
fluid movement may play a role in the pathogenesis of abdominal aortic atherosclerosis and peripheral vascular disease.

## I.   Water Movement in Response to a Constant Pressure Differential

Segments of rabbit and dog thoracic aortas are inflated and superfused with
Krebs Ringers containing 1% albumin.  The change of weight is recorded with and
without the endothelium present (after ballooning) and from this information
the hydraulic conductivity, $L_p = 8 \cdot 10^{-7}$ m/s bar, for the endothelial layer
and the permeability of the arterial media were found (6) .  This value of
$L_p$ of the endothelial layer is in close agreement with measurements of heart
and muscle capillary $L_p$'s.  The permeability, $k = 1.6 \cdot 10^{-18}$ $m^2$, agrees

well with estimates in porcine and rabbit arterial tissue in the literature.
All of these values determined in vivo are somewhat higher than the estimates
derived from dye penetration studies in the rabbit aorta in vivo (7) .

## II.  Water Movement in Response to a Step Change in Pressure Differential

Air inflated dog aortas are superfused internally with a thin fluid film, enclosed in a fluid filled chamber and subjected to a step change in pressure differential.  The resulting weight transient provides the transient fluid movement across the inner wall if the artery is without an intact endothelium. A transient hydraulic conductivity $L_p' \equiv v'/ p'$ where $v'$ is the transient

velocity, positive in the radial direction and $p'$ the imposed pressure step. $v' < o$ when $p' < o$ and vice versa so $L_p' > o$.  The values of $L_p'$ vs time for 11

dog thoracic aortic segments are given in Ref. (8) .  This data has been compared to the predictions of Kenyon (9)
for the consolidation of an isotropic
porous tube.  Here it is expected that
the interstitial fluid pressure, $p_t'$,

will undergo a perturbation, $p_t' = - 5 p'$,

where the quantity 5 is related to the
ratio of media thickness to artery radius.
In brief, the consolidation process represents a relaxation of $p_t'$ at the inner and

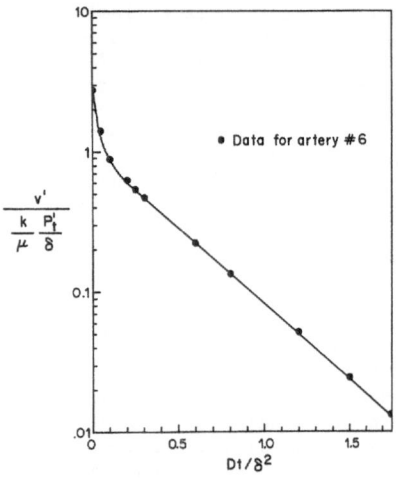

outer surfaces of the artery according
to the diffusion equation.  Then with
the fluid movement obeying Darcy's law
for flow in a porous media, the response
should be as shown by the solid line in
Fig. 1 (10) (data from a single artery).
The parameters derived from a best fit
to the model of all the data are D =
$1.95 \cdot 10^{-10}$ m$^2$/s, $p_t' = - 5.12 p'$,
for $\delta = 2 \cdot 10^{-4}$.  In Fig. 1, $v'$
is interstitial fluid viscosity and $\delta$ is
half thickness of the unvascularized media.

A useful measure of the change in volume
of a slice of tissue in consequence of a
change in tissue pressure is tissue compliance.  This quanitity was calculated:
$\int_0^\infty v' dt/\delta p_t' = 0.8$ bar$^{-1}$.  When compared with
the compliance of other tissues, arterial
media was found to be more compliant than
cartilage but less than skeletal muscle.

Fig 1.  Transient interfacial
velocity $v'$ in response to a
luminal pressure change $p'$.
Tissue pressure, $p_t' = -5.12$ $p'$,
$k/\mu\delta = 8 \cdot 10^{-7}$ m/s bar, $\delta^2/D = 205$ s

## III.  The Effect of a Negative $v'$ at the Intimal Surface Predisposing the Endothelial Layer to Desquamation

Micrographs of an edematous intima show the endothelial cells to be tethered
to the internal elastic lamina, IEL, at intervals of approximately 1 μm and
capable of displacements from the IEL of the same magnitude before the tethers break (11) .  It is not known at what hydrostatic pressure the tethers will
part; shear stress thresholds for desquamation suggest the pressure elevation
over the luminal pressure to be approximately $4 \cdot 10^{-3}$ bars (12) .  Thus fluid
leaving the media in response to an arterial pressure fall will first displace
the endothelium uniformly until the tethers are forced to part.  The behavior
expected for this type of localized subendothelial edema is expected to be very
like blister formation in elastomeric paints and lacquers (13) .  We have fixed
the endothelium of a rabbit thoracic aorta 5 minutes after a fall in pressure
and obtained the blisters thus shown in Fig. 2.  Fluid filling the blister is

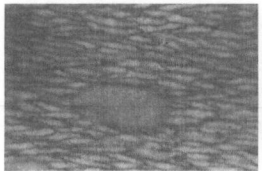 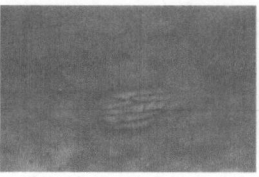 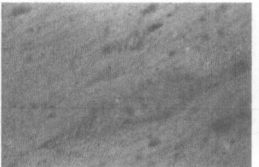 

Fig 2. Blisters in a rabbit endothelium caused by a sudden drop in pressure
L to R. Low flow: focus at base of blister; focus at crest of blister; high
flow, blisters removed before staining: high magnification; low magnification

drawn from the surrounding subendothelium relieving the pressure there. If
the pressure in the subendothelium is uniform prior to blister formation, the
largest driving force for blister development should be at the local pressure
minimum dictated by the flowing blood. Once the blister is formed the elevated
endothelium is now more vulnerable to local shear stress, $\tau$. If the blister
achieves a length , $\ell$, and the endothelium tears at a tension, $\sigma$, then desquamation should occur when $\sigma = \ell\tau$. Fry has shown in a partially blocked artery
with an assumed nonblistered endothelium $\tau$ must be in excess of 40.0 $N/m^2$ (much
greater than values for normal arteries found in vivo) in order to cause desquamation (12) . Fig. 2 also shows blisters that underwent desquamation at
0.4 $N/m^2$. From these results we estimate $\sigma$ to be of order $10^{-4}$ N/m.

IV. Predisposition to Vascular Injury Caused by Postural Change

To learn if there is a reason for concern in postural change we applied the consolidation theory with values taken from (10) to a model vascular tree employing
arterial dimensions for a 1.8 m man.
The perturbation pressure p′ was
assumed to be equal to the change in
head of water from the carotid sinus
to the artery of interest. This is
the reduction in arterial pressure
perturbation felt upon lying down.
The calculation produced the total
fluid displacement that would occur
before the sign of fluid movement
reversed at the positions shown in
Fig. 3 (10) . Here it can be seen
that if the $L_p$ were zero for the en-

dothelial layer, the average displacement throughout would exceed the
1 μm for the onset of blisters, and parts
of the entire aorta would be at elevated
risk each time we lay down. For comparison the graded severity of atherosclerotic
lesions from 70 year olds (who died of
other than cardiovascular causes) is also
given in Fig. 3 (14) . The jump at the
thoraco-abdominal boundary is worthy of
note. The reason for the jump in the
model calculations is that at this point
the medial vasa vasorum disappear and an
increased thickness of unvascularized
media (and thus the interstitial fluid

GRADED SCORE OF SEVERITY OF
ARTHEROSCLEROTIC LESIONS REF 10

1 2 3 4

THORACIC
ABDOMINAL

0 20 40 60 80 μm

▪ D_PMET, FOLLOWING POSTURAL
PRESSURE FALL

Fig 3. The risk of lying down

that must exit at the intima) of the abdominal aorta is nearly double the unvascularized media in the adjacent thoracic aorta.

## V.    Methods for Avoiding the Risk Introduced by Rapid Pressure Change

Our results suggest that to avoid rapid pressure change, one should lie down slowly.  Rates taken from the dog artery suggest that the artery relaxes in 5 to 10 minutes (10) .  The entire plasma volume shift from extra to intra vascular space of 7 to 20% that occurs when we lie down is virtually complete in 20 minutes.  Thus lying down in 2 - 3 stages of 5 minutes each might significantly reduce the  rate at which fluid is introduced to the subendothelial space from the media.

## B.    Concluding Remarks

There is ample evidence that blisters can form in the vascular endothelium.  We have presented evidence that when blisters are present the fluid shear stress required to cause endothelial layer dequamation can be reduced to the shear stress range normally found in arteries, if the blisters are sufficiently large. In examining the transient velocity when an excised dog artery is exposed to a sudden pronounced drop in pressure, nearly 10% of the interstitial water was seen to leave the artery.  We infer less water movement in arteries in situ in living rabbits.  Perhaps lowering the pressure in a human artery in vivo produces less fluid movement than shown in Fig. 3.; the actual amount is unknown. It is reasonable to suppose that intramural fluid movement would increase with increased edema and be dependent upon local arterial anatomy.  In addition, the thicker intima in human arteries may offer protection against blistering.  But the prediction of consolidation theory (9) and the findings reported in (10) and here suggest that a pronounced sudden pressure fall can under some circumstances produce sufficient fluid movement to inflate vulnerable blisters in the endothelium.

Experiments have shown that repeated endothelial damage can give rise to atherosclerotic plaque-like lesions in experimental animals without the need for a high cholesterol diet.  We propose that lying down suddenly could represent a form of minimal, but repeated endothelial damage that influences the growth of lesions; the effect could be intensified by the additional effect of other risk factors in the lower aorta and peripheral arteries; there is a possibility that without such repeated injury the lesions would subside.  Such a cessation of injury could be achieved by having the individual lie down slowly.

In addition to the hydrostatic pressure gradient, a gradient in macromolecule concentration across the endothelial layer can cause associated water movement and blister formation.  Thus an artery where slow moving blood produces a subendothelium equilibrated at a relatively high colloid osmotic pressure because of concentration polarization could, when demand increases its blood flow (4) , present the endothelium with a suddenly lower colloid osmotic pressure and a consequent driving force for blister formation and its sequellae.  Disorders that produce drastic swings in osmolarity (e.g., diabetes, chronic uremia with dialysis) would be likely prospects for osmotic blister producing episodes.

Acknowledgements   We thank C. Vargas, J. Pribyl, and Prof. F. Vargas for their work on developing the artery weighing technique.

This work was supported by NIH Grant No. 5 R01 H121188-05

References

1.  Virchow R (1856) Aus dem pathologisch--anatomischen Curse.  Wien, med. Wschr. 6:  809
2.  Ross R, Harker L (1976) Hyperlipidemia and atherosclerosis.  Science, 193:  1094
3.  Nerem RM, Cornhill JF (1980) The role of fluid mechanics in athero-genesis, J of Biochem Eng 102:  181-189
4.  Lutz RJ, et al (1979) Shear stress patterns in a model canine artery: their relationship to atherosclerosis.  In:  Hwang NHC (ed) Quantitative Cardiovascular Studies, University Park Press, Baltimore, pp. 233-237
5.  Texon M (1979) The hemodynamics basis of atherosclerosis, Hemisphere Pub Co, Washington, DC
6.  Vargas CB, et al (1979) Hydraulic conductivity of the endothelial and outer layers of the rabbit aorta, Am J Physiol 236:  H53-H60
7.  Colton CK, et al (1980) Labeled albumin transport into the normal and de-endothelialized rabbit thoracic aorta in vivo.  In:  Nerem R (ed) Hemo-dynamics and the Arterial Wall, Proceedings of a Specialists Meeting Sponsored by NSF
8.  Blackshear PL Jr, et al (1981) Artery wall water movement related to atherogenesis Part I: Experimental method and results.  submitted to J of Biomech Eng
9.  Kenyon DE (1979) A mathematical model for water flux through aortic tissue.  Bull of Math Biol, Vol 41, pp 79-90
10. Blackshear PL Jr, et al (1981) Artery wall water movement related to atherogenesis Part II:  The application of pseudo consolidation theory to experimental results.  submitted to J of Biomech Eng
11. Tsao C and Glagov S (1970) Basal endothelial attachment tenacity at cyto-plasmic dense zones in the rabbit aorta.  Lab Inv 23:  510
12. Fry DL (1976) Certain histological and chemical responses of the vascular interface to acutely induced mechanical stress in the aorta of the dog. Circ Res 24:  363-367
13. van der Meer-Lerk LA and Heertjes PM (1975) Blistering of varnish films on substrates induced by salts.  J Oil Col Chem Assoc 58:  79-84
14. Roberts JD Jr, et al (1959) Autopsy studies in atherosclerosis in patients dying without morphologic evidence of atherosclerotic catastrophe.  Circ 20:  522

# Haemodynamic Influences on Platelets in Haemostasis and Thrombosis

G. V. R. Born

When blood vessels are injured so that they bleed, circulating platelets adhere to the damaged vessel walls and aggregate, so diminishing
or arresting the haemorrhage. This interaction between platelets and
vessel walls therefore has an easily demonstrable physiological function. There is much clinical and experimental evidence that a deficiency
or defect in circulating platelets is associated with "spontaneous"
haemorrhages from small vessels. This suggests that platelets are somehow essential for the functional integrity of these vessels, but no
mechanism has yet been established.

Claims are made that agents released from platelets are able to damage
vessel walls, either acutely (Mustard et al., 1977b) or by contributing
to atherogenesis (Ross & Glomset, 1973). The evidence for these propositions is indirect and circumstantial and no such effects have been
incontrovertibly established (see Walton, 1975). On the other hand,
there is conclusive evidence that occlusive thrombi in arteries damaged
by atherosclerosis contain platelets as a major, if not the main, component (Davies & Thomas, 1981). The formation of platelet thrombi appears so similar to that of haemostatis plugs of platelets that analysis of the mechanism of the latter is likely to provide an understanding of the former. This introduction poses questions about how
the plugging mechanism depends on the haemodynamic environment in which
platelets aggregate on vessel walls.

Both the gross and the histological appearance of arterial thrombi
establish that the central mass consists mainly of aggregated platelets. What, therefore, is the mechanism responsible for rapid and extensive platelet aggregation in an artery as an apparently random event
in time (see Born 1979)? Close serial sectioning of obstructed coronary
arteries established some time ago that the platelet thrombus responsible
is invariably associated with recent haemorrhage into an underlying
atherosclerotic plaque (Friedman, 1970; Constantinides, 1966). The
haemorrhages occur through fissures or fractures in the plaque; and the
sudden appearance of such a fissure or fracture may well be the random,
individually unpredictable event affecting coronary arteries that has
to be assumed to occur to account for the clinical onset of acute coronary thrombosis (Born, 1979).

How does haemorrhage into a ruptured plaque start off platelet thrombogenesis? This can be regarded as part of the general question of how
platelets are caused to aggregate through haemorrhage, and most effectively through haemorrhage from arteries. Until recently this question
was commonly answered by assuming that the process depends on the adhesion of platelets to collagen which is exposed where damaged vessel
walls are denuded of endothelium. Adhering platelets then release other
agents, including thromboxane $A_2$ and ADP, which in turn are responsible
for the adhesion of more platelets as growing aggregates. This explana
tion is unlikely to be correct, for the following reasons. First, haemo-

static and thrombotic aggregates of platelets grow without delay and very rapidly. For example, when an arteriole 200 µm in diameter is cut into laterally, the rate of accession of platelets to the haemostatic plug is of the order of $10^4$/s (Born & Richardson, 1979). In contrast, although the adhesion of platelets to collagen itself is almost instantaneous, the subsequent aggregation of platelets, even under optimal conditions for their reactivity, begins only after a delay or lag period of at least 15 to 30 s (Wilner et al., 1969). Secondly, platelets tend to aggregate as mural thrombi when anti-coagulated blood flows through the plastic vessels of artificial organs such as oxygenators or dialysers (Richardson et al., 1976) that contain no collagen or anything else capable of activating platelets similarly. This implies that there are conditions under which platelets are activated in the blood by something other than collagen or other constituents of the walls of living vessels.

The plaque on which a thrombus grows has usually narrowed the arterial lumen. At constant blood pressure the flow of blood is faster through the constriction than elsewhere in the artery. Therefore, high flow and wall shear rates are no hindrance to the aggregation of platelets as thrombi (Born, 1977). Indeed, the question arises of whether the activation of platelets which precedes their aggregation depends in some way on such abnormal haemodynamic conditions.

The effectiveness of platelet aggregation in plugging a leak is at least as effective in arterioles as in venules. As the haemodynamic situation should be more unfavourable to the formation of aggregates in arterioles than in venules, an explanation of arteriolar haemostasis is likely to account in principle also for that in venules. For that reason, the following considerations are limited to arterioles.

When an arteriole is cut, platelets are seen to adhere with great rapidity to the damaged vessel wall, while the red cells continue to rush by. This high flow velocity in relation to the small size of the vessels implies the presence in the fluid of strong mechanical forces acting normally and tangentially on and near the vessel walls. The cut causes peripheral resistance to the flow to diminish suddenly; and if the inflow pressure remains constant the mean flow velocity increases. Thus the fluid-mechanical forces on platelets adhering and aggregating on the vessel wall become greater still. With increasing size the platelet aggregates tend to constrict the cut, causing a further, although usually temporary, increase in flow velocity.

In spite of wall shear stresses of $10^5$ to $10^6$ µN/cm$^2$ which are one or two orders of magnitude greater than anywhere in the normal circulation, platelets succeed into haemostatically effective plugs. The blood-flow velocities that would be experienced by platelets closest to the vessel wall and therefore with the highest probability of colliding with the sites of damage can be calculated (Schmid-Schönbein et al., 1976). Human platelets have a major diameter of about 1.5 µm. In an arteriole of medium size the flow velocity of plasma and of any cells in it at a distance of 1 µm from the wall is of the order of 10-100 µm/ms. Therefore, a platelet flowing within a distance no greater than its own diameter would pass an injury site 100 µm long in at most 10 ms. In the absence of other influences, this would seem to be the time available for such a platelet to adhere to the damaged wall.

The time just calculated as available to circulating platelets "at risk" for adhering to a wall lesion has to be compared with what is known about the time required for platelets to be activated into a condition in which their collision with such a lesion would very probably result in adhesion. That a process of activation is an essential prerequisite for adhesion and aggregation is inferred from the non-reactivity of normal circulating platelets.

As activation is indicated by adhesiveness, the change must involve one or more constituents of the outer surface of platelets. There is evidence that the essence is the exposure of surface receptors for fibrinogen, which has long been known to be an essential and specific plasma co-factor for platelet aggregation (Born & Cross, 1964; Corss, 1964). The activation time of platelets may then be defined as the interval between the encounter of platelets with an activating agent such as ADP and their ability to react with plasma fibrinogen.

That circulating platelets can be activated to adhere in much less time than that required by their gross changes in shape (Born, 1970) is indicated by direct experimental observations. An arteriole can be irradiated by a laser in such a way that damage is limited to a few square micrometers of endothelium (Arfors et al., 1976). The site of damage is covered almost immediately with platelets that must have been activated in small fractions of a second.

Very similar events follow the application of the activating agent ADP by micro-iontophoresis to the outside of an arteriole or venule under conditions in which appropriate controls indicate that there is no evidence at all of damage to the endothelial layer (Begent & Born, 1970). Platelet aggregates grow in the vessel exactly opposite the tip of the micropipette, while the blood continues to flow rapidly and without noticeable disturbance over the site. This is explained most simply by assuming that sufficient ADP diffuses between the endothelial cells into the blood to reach platelets passing close to the wall and that this ADP activates them in a few seconds.

An extension of this technique has provided a basis for calculating an average activation time for circulating platelets. It was found that the size of platelet aggregates produced by the iontophoretic application of ADP increases exponentially. The rate constant of this increase depended on the mean blood flow velocity, determined in the same vessels at the same time (Begent & Born, 1970). The shape of the experimentally determined curve was simulated closely by a theoretical curve (Richardson, 1973), which was derived on the single assumption that platelets require an activation time of about 100 ms to 200 ms. This time is still one order of magnitude greater than that indicated by the earlier theoretical considerations, so either this experimental derivation overestimates the true activation time or the earlier considerations failed to take something into account that would allow flowing platelets more than a few milliseconds for activation. More time would, for example, be available if the blood flow near the vessel wall were non-laminar, so that platelets caught up in vortices, however small, might be exposed to localized activating conditions for longer than they would otherwise be. When branching vessels of the microcirculation are observed microscopically, platelets can often be seen trapped in vortices for variable times of up to several seconds. Such delays may occur in the immediate vicinity of major vessel wall lesions, whether caused by disease such as the sudden rupture of an atheromatous plaque (Friedman & Van den Bovenkamp, 1966; Davies & Thomas, 1981) or by traumatic injury such as a puncture or transection. However, there is no evidence of even the smallest disturbances in the flow of blood in a normal vessel in which platelets are caused to adhere by iontophoretically applied ADP. Moreover, it seems most unlikely that any endothelial unevenness produced by laser injury would give rise to flow disturbances large enough to delay the passage of platelets.

The old thrombogenic hypothesis of atherosclerosis (von Rokitansky, 1841; Duguid, 1949) has recently reappeared in modern costume as claims that *platelets* contribute to atherogenesis in three ways: first, through damaging arterial endothelial cells by releasing injurious agents, presumably where circulating platelets adhere (Mustard et al., 1977a); secondly, through the release in such situations of a factor responsible for smooth muscle proliferation in the arterial wall (Ross & Glomset, 1973); and thirdly through the formation of persistent mural thrombi which are organized into intimal thickenings. Such evidence as there is for these propositions fails to establish any of them as relevant to atherosclerosis in animals or human beings (see Walton, 1975). Underlying all three claims is the assumption that some normal circulating platelets settle on arterial walls for long enough to release some of their contents. There is no observational basis for this assumption in normal arteries. Therefore it is assumed further that arterial endothelium is continuously subject to "damage" or "injury" of some kind as a precondition for the adherence of platelets. There is no convincing evidence for this generalization, especially not in human beings. The only finding that could conceivably apply to human arteries is that guinea pig aorta has a higher replacement rate of endothelium around the openings of branches than elsewhere (Payling-Wright & Born, 1971). This is most simply explained by assuming that endothelial turnover depends, *inter alia*, on haemodynamic effects due to non-laminar blood flow over such areas. But this should be thought of more correctly as a quasi-physioligical effect and, even there, platelets are rarely if ever seen adhering to the walls. The turnover rate of endothelium is increased in experimental hypertension (Payling-Wright, 1972). This is compatible with hypertension as a "risk factor" for coronary heart disease. It seems most likely that this is due to an accelerating effect of interendothelial gaps on plasma lipoprotein accumulation (Stehbens, 1965; Caro, 1977) than to an increase in the indiscriminate or even selective deposition of platelets on arterial walls.

This Session is therefore concerned inter alia with questions, most of them unanswered, about the effects of haemodynamics on the interactions of cellular and other constituents of the circulating blood with the walld of the vessels, particularly with those of arteries.

## References

Arfors KE, Cockburn JS & Gross JF, 1976. Measurement of growth rat of laser-induced intravascular platelet aggregation, and the influence of blood flow celocity. Microvasc Res 11: 79-87

Begent NA & Born GVR 1970. Growth rate in vivo of platelet thrombi produced by iontophoresis of ADP, as a function of mean blood flow velocity. Nature (Lond) 227: 926-930

Born GVR 1970. Observations on the change in shape of blood platelets brought about by adenosine diphosphate. J Physiol 209: 487-511

Born GVR 1977. Fluid-mechanical and biochemical interactions in haemostasis. Br Med Bull 33: 193-197

Born GVR 1979. Arterial thrombosis and its prevention (Proc VIII World Congr Cardiol, Tokyo 1978) Excerpta Medica, Amsterdam, ICS 470, p 81-91

Born GVR & Cross MR 1964. Effects of inorganic ions and of plasma proteins on the aggregation of blood platelets by adenosine diphosphate. J Physiol (Lond) 170: 394-414

Born GVR & Richardson PD 1979. Activation time of blood platelets. Proc R Soc Lond B Biol Sci (submitted)

Caro CG 1977. Mechanical factors in atherogenesis. In: Cardiovascular flow dynamics and measurement. University Park Press, Baltimore

Constantinides P 1966. Plaque fissures in human coronary thrombosis. J Atheroscler Res 6: 1-17

Cross MJ 1964. Effect of fibrinogen on the aggregation of platelets by adenosine diphosphate. Thromb Diath Haemorrh 12: 524-527

Davies MJ & Thomas T 1981. The pathological basis and microanatomy of occlusive thrombus formation in human coronary arteries. Phil Trans R Soc Lond B 294: 225-229

Duguid JB 1949. Pathogenesis of atherosclerosis. Lancet 2: 925

Friedman H 1970. Pathogenesis of coronary thrombosis, intramural and intralumunal haemorrhage. In: Halonen LA (ed) Thrombosis and coronary heart disease. Karger, Basel, vol 4: 3

Friedman M & Van den Bovenkamp GJ 1966. The pathogenesis of a coronary thrombosis. Am J Pathol 48: 19-44

Mustard JF, Moore S, Packham MA, Kinlough Rathbone RL 1977a. Platelets, thrombosis and atherosclerosis. Proc Biochem Pharmacol 13: 312-325

Mustard JF, Packham MA, Kinlough Rathbone RL 1977b. Platelets, thrombosis and atherosclerosis. Adv Exp Med Biol 104: 127-144

Payling-Wright, HP 1972. Mitosis patterns in aortic endothelium. Atherosclerosis 15: 93-95

Payling-Wright, HP, Born, GVR 1971. Possible effect of blood flow on the turnover rate of vascular endothelial cells. In: Hartert HH, Copley AL (eds) Theoretical and clinical hemorheology. Springer Berlin, p 220-226

Richardson PD 1973. Effect of blood flow velocity on growth rate of platelet thrombi. Nature (Lond) 245: 103-104

Richardson PD, Galetti P, Born GVR 1976. Regional administration of drugs to control thrombosis in artificial organs. Trans Am Soc Artif Intern Organs 22: 22-29

Ross R, Glomset JA 1973. Atherosclerosis and the arterial smooth muscle cell. Proliferation of smooth muscle is a key event in the genesis of the lesions of atherosclerosis. Science (Wash DC) 180: 1332-1339

Schmid-Schönbein H, Rieger H, Fischer T 1976. Blood vessels: problems arising at the borders of natural and artificial blood vessels. In: Effert S, Meyer-Erkelenz J (eds) Springer Berlin p 57-63

Stehbens WE 1965. Endothelial cell mitosis and permeability. J Exp Physiol (Cogn Med Sci) 50: 90-92

von Rokitansky (1841-46) Handbuch der pathologischen Anatomie. Braumüller & Seidel, Vienna

Walton KW 1975. Pathogenetic mechanisms in atherosclerosis. Am J Cardiol 35: 542-558

Wilner GD, Nossel HL, LeRoy EC 1969. Aggregation of platelets by collagen. J Clin Invest 47: 2616-2621

# Effect of Stresses on the Uptake of Material by the Arterial Wall

C.G.Caro, M.J.Lever, A.Baldwin, and A.Tedgui

Theories involving mechanical stresses and mass transport have been
proposed to account for the localisation of atheromatous lesions
both within the arterial tree (1, 2) and through the thickness of
the arterial wall (3, 4, 5, 6, 7). In attempt to clarify these problems,we have examined the uptake of relatively inert extracellular
tracers by excised arteries under various conditions (8, 9, 10, 11).

## Methods

Most of the experimental procedures have been described (7). 4-7
month old New Zealand white rabbits, fed a normal diet were
anaesthetised with sodium pentobarbitone and heparinised. The common
carotid arteries or aorta were exposed and excised. Experiments
were conducted with the vessels incubated at $38 \pm 1^{\circ}C$ when (i) at
relaxed length and zero transmural pressure (non-pressurized) (ii)
at in vivo length and pressurized to 70 mmHg with air (air-pressurized)
(iii) at in vivo length and pressurized to 70 mmHg with liquid
(liquid pressurized).

The non-pressurized vessels were cut into segments about 0.5cm in
length and immersed in Tyrodes solution containing 4% bovine serum
albumin together with tracer. Bubbling 5% $CO_2$ in air through the
incubating solution did not affect tracer uptake. The air-pressurized
vessels were cannulated in situ, excised and incubated without being
allowed to shorten, to lessen the likelihood of endothelial damage.
The downstream cannula was clamped to prevent air flow along the
vessels. The external solution was Tyrodes solution containing tracer
and 2% albumin. The liquid-pressurized vessels were similarly
prevented from shortening. They were pressurized with Tyrodes
solution containing 4% albumin and tracer, the downstream cannula again
being clamped. The external incubating solution was Tyrodes solution
containing 2% albumin and tracer at the same concentration as in the
lumen. Smooth muscle tone was varied in some experiments with the
use of noradrenaline (NA), sodium nitrite ($NaNO_2$) or the long-acting
vasodilator isosorbide dinitrate (ISDN). In some studies all
segments, including the controls, were incubated with $10^{-7}M$ NA, in
order to induce additional tone in the excised vessels. In other
studies, the endothelium was removed by passing a rubber tube along
the lumen.

Following incubation, the vessels were opened axially, frozen and
subjected to sequential frozen sectioning parallel to the intima at
20 µm intervals. The tissue/solution tracer concentration ratio, $C_T/C_P$
(cpm $cm^{-3}$ tissue/cpm $cm^{-3}$ incubating solution) was determined and
concentration profiles were constructed. In order to allow for variation of wall thickness, medial thickness was non-dimensionalised being
made equal to 100 units.To avoid the transition region between the media
and adventitia, mean medial and adventitial values were calculated by

averaging values for sections lying between 0-80 and 120-180 units
from the lumen respectively.  It was presumed, in view of the long
times required to reach steady values, that no significant change
occurred of wall tracer distribution in the few minutes required
to prepare segments for freezing.

## Results

### Carotid arteries

**Non-pressurized vessels**    The mean medial $C_T/C_P$ for $^{125}I$ albumin
became steady by 90 min with $10^{-7}NA$, $10^{-7}M$ NA + $10^{-3}M$ NaNO$_2$ and
$10^{-7}M$ NA + $10^{-3}M$ ISDN.   The respective values were 0.048 SD 0.008
(n = 12), 0.058 SD 0.009 (n = 12) and 0.066 SD 0.010 (n = 12). The
NA value was significantly lower than the NA + Na NO$_2$ (p < 0.02)
and NA + ISDN (p < 0.001) values.   We have previously reported that
in segments incubated without a vasoactive agent, a gradual increase
of mean medial albumin uptake occurs after 90 min and that NA at a
concentration exceeding $10^{-9}M$ decreases and NaNO$_2$ at a concentration
exceeding $10^{-4}M$ increases the value above that of the controls (11).

**Air-pressurized vessels**    The 90 min mean medial values for albumin
for vessels incubated with no vasoactive agent, $10^{-5}M$ NA and $10^{-4}M$
NaNO$_2$ were respectively 0.035 SEM 0.007 (n = 9), 0.027 SEM 0.003
(n = 6) and 0.051 SEM 0.008 (n = 6).   The NA values are significantly
lower than the controls and the NaNO$_2$ values are significantly higher.

**Liquid-pressurized vessels** The 90 min mean medial values for albumin
for segments incubated with $10^{-7}M$ NA, $10^{-7}M$ NA + $10^{-3}M$ NaNO$_2$ and
$10^{-7}M$ NA + $10^{-3}M$ ISDN were respectively 0.062 SD 0.011 (n = 17),
0.046 SD 0.011 (n = 11) and 0.045 SD 0.007 (n = 9).   The NA values
are significantly higher than those obtained with NA plus either
vasodilator (p < 0.05 and p < 0.001 respectively).

### Aorta

**Liquid-pressurized** vessels   The 90 min mean medial value for albumin
was 0.15 SD 0.03 (n = 4) in de-endothelialised vessels and 0.056 SD
0.003 (n = 5) in intact vessels.   The steady mean medial value for
$^{14}C$-sucrose was 0.443 SD 0.029 (n = 7) for de-endothelialised vessels
and 0.418 SD 0.015 (n = 11) for intact vessels (p < 0.05).

## Discussion

Tracer uptake was studied in these experiments when convection across
the wall was absent, approximately normal or increased.  It could be
expected that convection would be absent when transmural pressure
was zero or when vessels were pressurized with air and interfacial
forces would prevent fluid inflow to the wall.   Since the wall is
compressible, convection could occur transiently following relaxation of, or air-pressurization of, a vessel.   It was expected,
however, to have become small at the longer incubation times, which

probably exceeded consolidation times (6). Convection was
believed to be approximately normal in the liquid-pressurized
intact vessels and was enhanced in the de-endothelialised vessels.
The labelled albumin is thought to have been distributed principally in the interstitium and changes in tracer uptake are believed
to represent mainly changes in interstitial properties, since the
steady uptake of the smaller species $^{51}$Cr EDTA was always within
the normal range.

A steady-state concentration can be achieved in the interstitium
both in the absence of and in the presence of convection. It need
not, however, take the same value in the two conditions, even when,
as in these studies, the bulk concentration of tracer was the same
in the luminal and external incubating solutions. A feature of
the studies was the increase of the steady mean medial uptake of
albumin with increase of convection; the value was lower in the
absence of convection (non-pressurized and air-pressurized vessels)
than in the presence of convection (liquid-pressurized vessels) and
was substantially elevated, when convection was enhanced
(de-endothelialised vessels). A small increase was also seen in
these last vessels of the steady mean medial uptake of $^{14}$C-sucrose.

The mechanisms underlying these changes are not clearly established.
However, it can be expected that the steady distribution of an
inert extracellular tracer will depend on interaction of the tracer
with the solvent, for example solvent drag, interaction of the
tracer with the wall, and interaction of the solvent with the wall.
The geometry of the wall will depend in addition on its mechanical
properties, including the contribution from smooth muscle.

We have given preliminary consideration to crude macroscopic
schemes which might shed light on solvent/wall interactions and on
these results. In the absence of convection through the wall, it
might be expected that pressure within the interstitium would fall
towards lymphatic pressure and that some compaction would occur of
the interstitium. An increase of convection, as in the case of
removal of the endothelium, might in contrast elevate interstitial
pressure and expand the interstitium.

It is of interest to see whether this scheme might also aid understanding of the other responses of the arterial wall. Reduction
of the diameter of arteries by NA in the absence of convection was
associated with reduction of the steady medial uptake of labelled
albumin. An increase of the tone of the medial smooth muscle
might be expected to compress the interstitium and dilatation of
the vessel might have the opposite effect.

The effects of the vasoactive agents in liquid pressurized vessels
are unexpected and less readily explained. A possible mechanism
which might account for the effects is that NA enhanced permeability
of the endothelium (12) and, hence, convection through the wall.
Consistent with that idea, we observed in vessels treated with NA,
but not in vessels treated with NA plus a vasodilator, patchy staining of the intima with Trypan blue and marked convolution of the
plasmalemma of a small fraction of the endothelial cells.

## Acknowledgements

We acknowledge helpful discussions with Dr. K. H. Parker. Support for the work derived from the Medical Research Council, National Heart Research Fund and Sanol Schwarz Pharmaceuticals Ltd., UK. The ISDN was kindly provided by Pharma Schwarz, Monheim, Germany.

## References

1. Fry DL (1969) Certain chemorheologic considerations regarding the blood vascular interface with particular reference to coronary artery disease. Circulation 39 and 40: Suppl 4: 38-57
2. Caro CG, Fitz-Gerald JM, Schroter RC (1971) Atheroma and arterial wall shear: Observation correlation and proposal of a shear dependent mass transfer mechanism for atherogenesis. Proc Roy Soc Lond B 177: 109-159
3. Jellinek H, Veress B, Balint A, Nagy Z (1970) Lymph vessels of rat aorta and their changes in experimental atherosclerosis: an electronmicrosopic study. Exp Mol Path 13: 370
4. Adams CWM (1973) Tissue changes and lipid entry in developing atheroma. In: Porter R, Knight J (eds) Atherogenesis Initiating Factors, Ciba Foundation Symposium No 12 (New Series), Elsevier, Amsterdam, pp 5-37
5. Walton KW (1975) Pathogenetic mechanism in atherosclerosis. Amer J Cardiol 15: 542
6. Blackshear PL Jr, Vargas FF, Emerson, PF, Newell, MJ, Vargas CB, Blackshear GL (1980) Water and ion flux through the artery wall in: Haemodynamics and the Arterial Wall, Proceedings from a Specialists Meeting, Nerem RM and Guyton JR (Eds) University of Houston, Texas
7. Caro CG, Lever MJ, Laver-Rudich Z, Meyer F, Liron N, Ebel W, Parker KH, Winlove CP (1980a) Net albumin transport across the wall of the rabbit common carotid artery perfused in situ. Atherosclerosis 37: 497-511.
8. Lever MJ, Tedgui A (1981) Oedema and albumin space in the rabbit aorta following intimal damage. J. Physiol 319: 37-38
9. Caro CG, Lever MJ (1980) Effect of vasoactive agents on the albumin space of the arterial wall. J. Physiol 305: 112
10. Baldwin A, Lever MJ, Caro CG (1982) Effect of vasoactive drugs on distribution volume for $^{125}I$ albumin in rabbit carotid artery Fed Proc 41 (4): 5626
11. Caro CG, Lever MJ, Tedgui A (1980b) Effect of active and passive stresses on distribution volume in the arterial wall in: Hemodynamics and the Arterial Wall, Proceedings from a Specialists Meeting, Nerem RM and Guyton JR (Eds) University of Houston, Texas
12. Robertson AL, Khairallah PA (1972) Effects of angiotensin II and some analogues on vascular permeability in the rabbit. Circulation Res 31: 923-931

# Percutaneous Transluminal Angioplasty in the Treatment of Peripheral Vascular Disease

G. Hudon, Y. Hébert, L. Lemarbre, and C. Goulet

Percutaneous transluminal angioplasty (PTA) is a therapeutic application of angiography and a method to increase regional blood flow to either an ischemic organ or vascular bed (1). This procedure may be performed to dilate a vascular stenosis (fig. 1) or to recanalize an obstructed artery (fig. 2) (2).

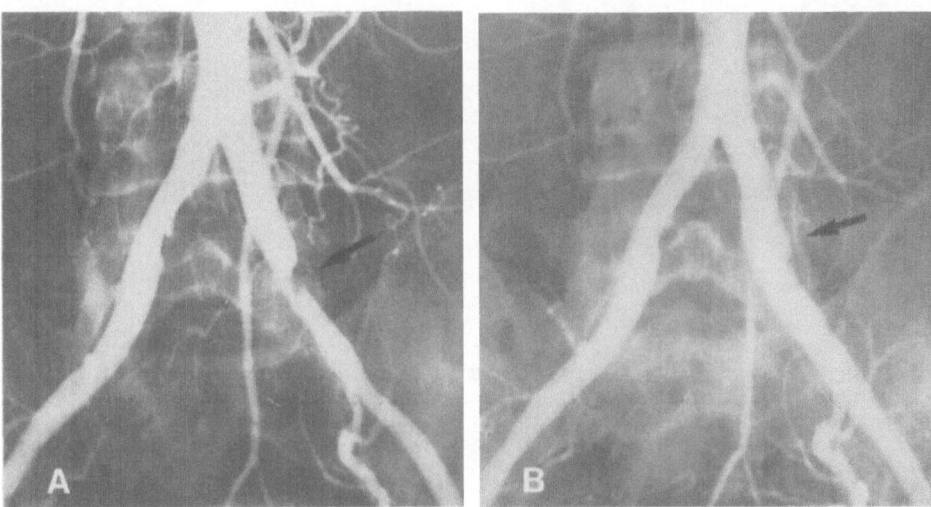

<u>Fig. 1.</u> A: Left common iliac artery with significant stenosis before PTA
B: Widely patent artery 15 months after PTA

## History

The suggestion that arterial stenoses could be permanently dilated was first presented by DOTTER and JUDKINS in 1964 (3). Unfortunately, DOTTER's original system of coaxial telescopic catheters had many disadvantages (4) and its procedure met a great deal of resistance in his own country (5). In 1974, GRÜNTZIG and HOFF (5) refined DOTTER's concept and developed a non-elastomeric balloon of relatively fixed volume that was placed on a double-lumen catheter body (fig. 3). The availability of this new dilating catheter then expanded areas of application, improved success rates and reduced complications associated with dilatation procedures (5).

## Pathophysiology

Since the introduction of the angioplasty, DOTTER postulated that atheromatous lesions are dilated by circumferential compression and longitudinal redistribution of the atheroma along the arterial wall, and by "squeezing-out" some of the lipids from the atheroma. He thought that the outer diameter of the vessel would not be changed (3).

However, CASTANEDA-ZUNIGA (6) et al, using cadaver and animal models, recently pointed out that compression or redistribution of atherosclerotic material could not be demonstrated histologically following angioplasty. They postulated that a predominant mechanism for the increased caliber of arteries following a dilatation procedure is the permanent overstretching of the media, causing a permanent histological derangement of both elastic fibers and smooth

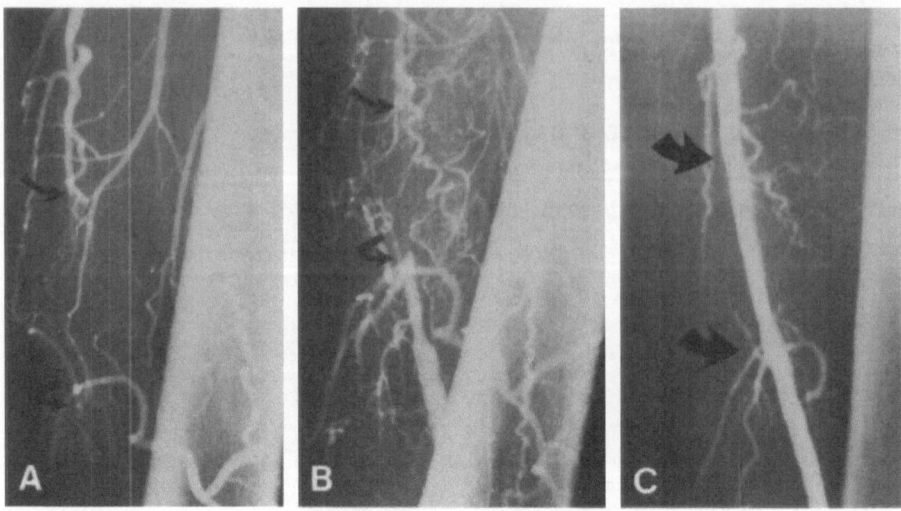

Fig. 2 A and B. Completely occluded superficial femoral artery (between arrows). C: Patent artery immediately after angioplasty

muscle. Cracking of the intima (7) and separation of this layer from the media were also demonstrated. After dilatation, the media would distend, carrying with it intima and atheromatous material, resulting in an increase of both internal and external arterial caliber. Healing of the disrupted arterial layers is by formation of a neointima and scar tissue similar to that which is formed following endarterectomy.

## Patient selection

At the present time, all patients for whom PTA is considered should conform to surgical indications for revascularization, having either limb-threatening resting ischemia or ischemia with exercise which severely limits ability to work or perform everyday activities (8). Probably in the future, these indications will be altered or expanded, especially in superficial artery disease resulting in intermittent claudication which only midly or moderately hampers patient's activity (1). Consultation between the patient's referring physician, a vascular surgeon and a vascular radiologist should be encouraged to optimize the choice of therapy for each patient (2, 4). The presence of a lesion on arteriography is not per se an indication for PTA.

## Evaluation of the lesion

In peripheral vascular disease, it appears that PTA is well suited for the treatment of short-segment focal disease (1 cm, 2-5 cm stenoses (9)) involving the iliac, femoral and popliteal arteries. In patients with multiple-segment or long-segment involvement (stenosis longer than 5 cm in iliac and femoral arteries or occlusion longer than 10 cm in superficial femoral and popliteal arteries (4)), the results are less favorable (10).

## Technique

PTA is ideally done under fluoroscopic control in the angiography room of the radiology department (2). The procedure is done following local anesthesia in a patient under mild sedation. PTA equipment is shown in figure 3 (11).

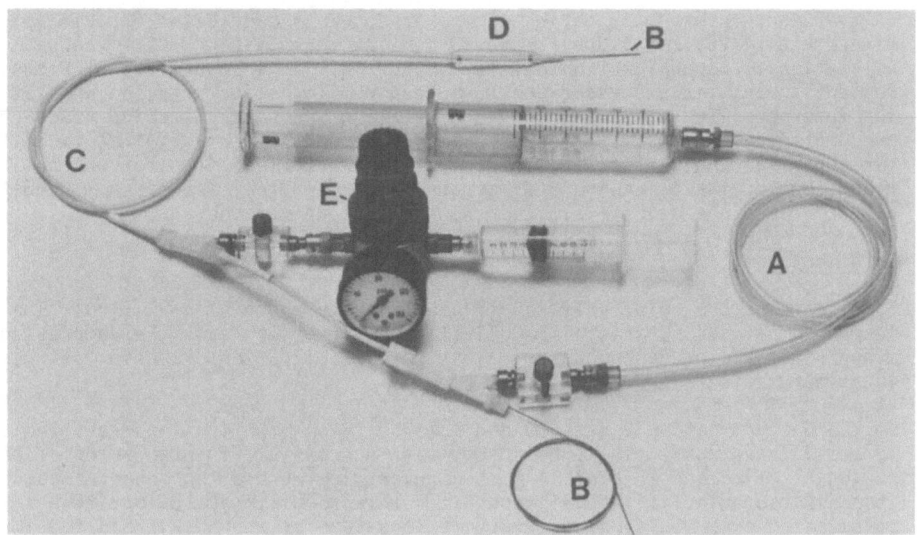

Fig. 3. Equipment for PTA. A: Flexible tube to flush catheter and to connect to pressure monitor. B: Guide wire. C: Double-lumen Grüntzig balloon catheter. D: Expanded balloon. E: Pressure gauge to monitor balloon pressure during dilatation (11) (with permission, Union Méd. du Canada)

## Results

In order to evaluate both preliminary and long-term results of this thera-peutic procedure in our institution, a clinical research protocol was estab-lished where data collection has taken place for two years and patients follow-up will last for an additional two years. Informed consent was obtained in all patients. Each selected patient had a symptomatic peripheral vascular disease, documented with Doppler ultrasonography. Clinical evaluation was made by a vascular surgeon regarding the advisability of a treatment. The extent, site and morphology of the lesion(s) had been documented by arterio-graphy. Research protocol included:

A.: At time of PTA:
    Before procedure:   Doppler ultrasonography; antiplatelet therapy for 24 h
                              (ASA and dipyridamole)
    During procedure:   Heparin 5000 I.U.
    After procedure :   Doppler ultrasonography; antiplatelet therapy for 3
                              weeks
    Patient is urged to stop cigarette smoking.

B.: Long-term follow-up:
    Six (6) months        : Doppler ultrasonography
    Twelve (12) months    : Doppler ultrasonography; control arteriography
    Twenty-four (24) months : Doppler ultrasonography

C.: Criteria of successful PTA:
    Angiographic : ↓ > 50% of stenosis or occlusion
                   e.g. 80% stenosis → 40% residual stenosis
    Hemodynamic   : ↓ > 50% of pressure gradient
    Doppler ultrasonography : improved or normal velocity curve
    Clinical improvement

In a 23 month period, 82 patients were accepted as candidates for PTA (63 males: age 34-76, $\overline{M}$ 54.1 years and 19 females: age 34-67, $\overline{M}$ 52.2 years). Dilatation or recanalization were attempted in 134 iliac or femoral arterial segments. Initial success rates have been 86% for iliac arteries and 72% for femoropopliteal arteries. When dilatation and recanalization procedures are considered separately, success rates are much better for dilatation: (95% for the iliac and 81% for the femoropopliteal arteries) than for recanalization (44% for the iliac and 56% for the femoropopliteal arteries). Long-term patency rates are under evaluation with objective methods.

## Complications

Complications are relatively few (1), within the range of 5-7% (13). The most feared complication, distal embolization of fragments from the compressed atherosclerotic plaque, occurs in less than 5% of patients and in most cases is asymptomatic (1).

We had 6 complications, 5 minor and 1 major. Two embolizations resulted in a successful and uneventful embolectomy with successful PTA; two arterial perforation (1 iliac and 1 femoral) with a guide wire were of no consequence; one stenosis (superficial femoral) converted to a complete occlusion. One failure at dilating a common femoral artery (contra-lateral approach) resulted in acute severe limb-threatening ischemia for which surgical revascularization was successfully performed but eventually resulted in patient's death.

## Conclusion

Any new procedure must be compared with existing modes of treatment, in this case, surgical revascularization, which has been in use for thirty years (8). PTA must be examined and compared in terms of acute hemodynamic effectiveness, mortality and morbidity, specific indications, long-term results and consequences of long-term failure. At present time, there is no question that the incidence of successful dilatation and patient improvement is quite high in competent hands (8), and that complication rates are acceptably low (4, 12). Patients are ambulatory the day following PTA and typical hospitalization time is about 48 hours: advantages in both patient discomfort and hospitalization costs compared with reconstructive surgery are obvious (5). PTA can be used as a replacement for surgery or as an adjunct to surgery (to increase either inflow or outflow in a subsequent bypass graft) (7). PTA can be used as a palliative measure in a large group of patients who are no longer surgical candidates because of poor run-off or other associate conditions (13).

The PTA procedure seems to be an effective mean of treating certain types of occlusive vascular disease. Its preliminary results compare favorably with bypass surgery when all aspects are considered (9, 10).

## References

1. Athanasoulis CA (1980) Therapeutic applications of angiography. N Engl J Med 302: 1174-1178
2. Athanasoulis CA (1980) Percutaneous transluminal angioplasty: general principles. Amer J Roent 135: 893-900
3. Dotter CT, Judkins MP (1964) Transluminal treatment of arteriosclerotic obstruction. Circulation 30: 654-670
4. Sos TA, Sniderman KW (1981) Percutaneous transluminal angioplasty. Seminars in Roentgenology 16: 26-41

5. Grüntzig A, Kumpe DA (1979) Technique of percutaneous transluminal angioplasty with the "Grüntzig balloon catheter". Amer J Roent 132: 547-552
6. Castaneda-Zuniga WR, Formanek A, Tadavarthy M, Vlodaver Z, Edwards JE,
   Zollikofer C, Amplatz K (1980) The mechanism of balloon angioplasty.
   Radiology 135: 565-571
7. Block PC, Fallon JT, Elmer D (1980) Experimental angioplasty: lessons
   from the laboratory. Amer J Roent 135: 907-912
8. Abbott WM (1980) Percutaneous transluminal angioplasty: surgeon's view.
   Amer J Roent 135: 917-920
9. Spence RK, Freiman DB, Gatenby R et al (1981) Long-term results of transluminal angioplasty of the iliac and femoral arteries. Arch Surg 116:
   1377-1386
10. Neiman HL, Brandt TD, Greenberg M (1981) Percutaneous transluminal angio-
    plasty. An angiographer's viewpoint. Arch Surg 116: 821-828
11. Hudon G, Goulet C (1980) Angioplastie transluminale percutanée: principes
    et revue de la littérature. Union Méd Canada 111: 8-21, 76-77
12. Zeitler E (1978) Complications in and after percutaneous transluminal re-
    canalization. In: Zeitler E, Grüntzig A, Schoof W, eds. Percutaneous vas-
    cular recanalization. Berlin, Springer-Verlag 123
13. Motarjeme A, Keifer JW, Zuska AJ (1980) Percutaneous transluminal angio-
    plasty and case selection. Radiology 135: 573-586

# Metabolic and Haemodynamic Effects of Plasma-Exchange in Familial Hypercholesterolemia

A. Postiglione, P. Rubba, N. Scarpato, G. Marotta, S. Montefusco, and M. Mancini

## Introduction

Plasma-exchange (PE) is a procedure whereby blood is removed continuously from the patients and cells separated and returned to the donor
after resuspension in plasma protein fraction.This procedure was at
first performed in patients with immunological diseases,with circulating exogenous toxins or with very high concentrations of some plasma
costituents (1-3).Thompson et al. first reported the periodical use
of PE in the treatment of patients with homozygous Familial Hypercho-
lesterolemia(FH)(4) and thereafter other authors have confirmed the
effectiveness of this procedure (5,6).In fact long term PE,when performed every two weeks and associated to drug therapy,reduces the rate of progression of atheroma in patients with homozygous FH and possibly induces regression in the heterozygotes (7).More recently important developments of this technique  have been suggested for the treat
ment of FH by Stoffel et al. with selective removal of LDL from plasma
by affinity chromatography (8,9).Thompson has proposed moreover the
infusion of HDL or its analogous into circulation at the end of PE
in order to promote efflux of cholesterol from the extravascular
pool (10).

We have shown recently a marked increase of arterial blood flow to the
lower limbs (11) and to the cerebral district (12) lasting at least
 for seven days after PE.It has been suggested that this effect,pos-
sibly related to a reduction of plasma and whole blood viscosity,might
be useful in FH.In the present paper both metabolic and haemodinamic
effects of PE are evaluated for two weeks.

## Patients and methods

Four patients with FH periodically performed PE in our department.Three
of them were homozygous for FH gene(s),while the fourth had the heterozygous form.All of them had diffuse xanthomatas with pathological
bruits over the aortic root and several arteries.No patient smoked for
two days before and throughout the study.Before and during the whole
period of investigation the patients were under lipid lowering diet
and drug therapy (cholestyramine 20g/day and nicotinic acid 2.4 g/day
or fenofibrate 300 mg/day).

PE was performed using a Transfer 90 Bell Co centrifuge.Anticoagulation
was mantained with A.C.D. (Citric Acid-Sodium Citrate-Dextrose) in a
1:8 ratio to total blood.Plasma removed was exchanged with isotonic

saline containing 5% human albumin.

Arterial blood flow to the lower limbs was determined at baseline and at day 1,4,7,8,11,14 after PE by using a venous occlusion plethysmo-graph (Periflow,Janssen,Beerse,Belgium).A cuff was placed on the pro-ximal portion of the limb to be evaluated.The cuff pressure was higher than the venous pressure,but lower than the diastolic arterial pressure. After a well defined  inflow time,the arterial flow was derived from the increase in circumference of the limb.Triggering of the venous occlusion intervals by means of ECG allowed semicontinuous measurements of flow.Each study was performed at 22 C after at least 20 minutes of supine rest in the room at that temperature.After ten minutes of rhyt-mic venous occlusion blood flow registration was performed for two mi-nutes.Results were expressed in ml/min/dl of leg volume.In two experi-ments reactive hyperemia test was performed in order  to evaluate ma-ximal flow over the calf.A three minute arterial occlusion was perfor-med by inflating the same cuff used for venous occlusion at a supra-systolic pressure.After the release of arterial occlusion reactive hy-peremia occurred and postischemic peak flow could be determined.

Plasma cholesterol and triglyceride concentration was determined by enzymatic method  (13) at the time of each arterial flow study.Plasma apolipoprotein B and plasma fibrinogen concentrations were assayed by radial immunodiffusion technique.

Results

Percent of plasma exchanged was on average 43% and more than 5 g of cholesterol was withdrawn by a single PE.Table 1 shows mean plasma concentration of cholesterol,triglyceride,apolipoprotein B,haemato-crit and fibrinogen during the first (day 1,4,7) and the second (day 8,11,14) week in our FH patients.Plasma cholesterol was significantly reduced by 24% during the first week of treatment and by 15% during the second one (n.s.).Similar variations occurred for apoprotein B during the first week,while no significant difference from baseline could be detected during the second period of observation.

Table 1. Plasma lipids,apoprotein B,fibrinogen and packed cell volume before and during 2 weeks after plasma-exchange in 4 patients with FH

| After P.E. (weeks) | Cholesterol | Triglyceride (mg/dl) | apoprotein-B | PCV (%) | Fibrinogen (mg/dl) |
|---|---|---|---|---|---|
| 0 | 761±132 | 178±70 | 340±25 | 41±7 | 311±30 |
| 1 | 580±108* | 160±64 | 265±24* | 41±7 | 289±28 |
| 2 | 646±83 | 154±70 | 335±34 | 41±7 | 311±40 |

*$p < 0.05$                                                        (M±SE)

Fibrinogen was only slightly reduced (less than 10%) during the first week and rose to pretreatment value thereafter.Haematocrit did not change in any patient after the procedure,while plasma triglyceride concentration returned to baseline together with plasma globulin within few days.

Fig.1 shows the results of nine experiments measuring blood flow over the calf in our four patients.In all experiments resting flow over the calf was increased during the first week after PE (p< 0.01,Wilcoxon); resting flow during the second week was found to be markedly increased in four out of six experiments (n.s.).Increase in peak flow could be demonstrated during the first and the second week in the two patients performing reactive hyperemia test.

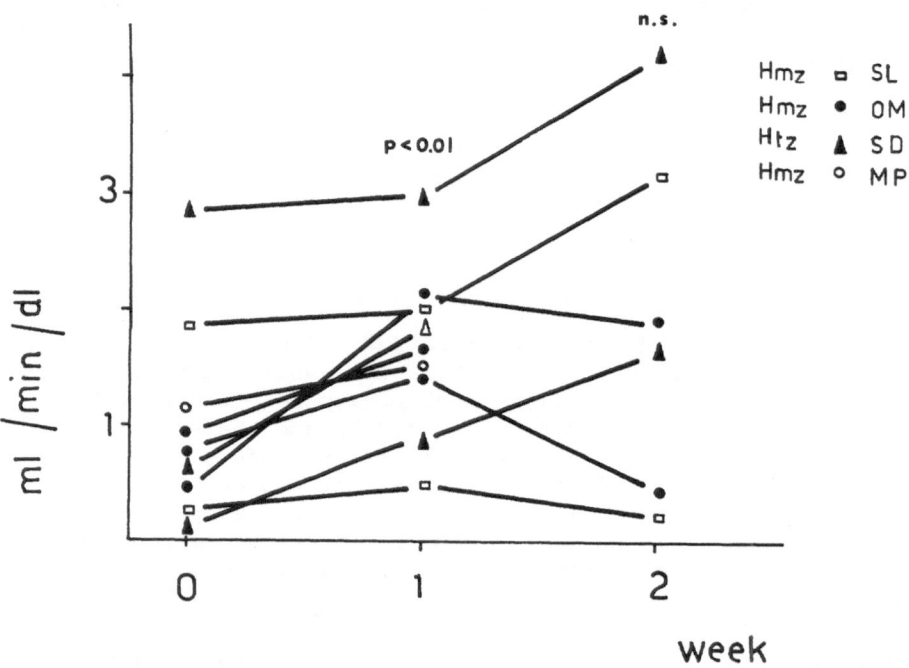

Fig. 1.Effect of plasma-exchange on resting blood flow over the calf in Familial Hypercholesterolemia

## Discussion

The present observations confirm the useful metabolic and haemodinamic effects of PE in patients with FH.The reduction of plasma cholesterol and of apoprotein B concentrations are expected to produce slower progression of the atherosclerotic process.Removal of atherogenic particles (LDL) from the circulation will interfere with lipid deposition

in the arterial wall and possibly will also promote transfer of cholesterol from the extra- to the intravascular space.There are in fact
several observations suggesting that plasma cholesterol after PE is
at least in part derived from the extravascular pool,including the arterial wall (10,14).An additional effect of PE is related to the function  of circulating platelets,which are known to be hypersensitive
to aggregating substances in hypercholesterolemic patients.When observed by electron microscopy they show increased amount of cell wall irregularities as compared to normocholesterolemic subjects.After PE
the amount of cell wall abnormalities is markedly reduced (15).The arterial  blood flow improvement after PE is probably a rheological effect of the procedure associated with a reduction of whole blood viscosity at low shear rate by 20-83% together with a decrease of plasma
viscosity (16).An additional modification probably contributing to the
increased arterial blood flow in these patients is the enhanced eri-
throcyte filtration rate (17).Furthermore changes in the arterial wall
resulting from removal of cholesterol from atherosclerotic plaque can
not be excluded especially after a prolonged period of treatment.

## References

1. Verrier Jones,J ,Cummings,R H ,Bucknall, RC.,Asplin,C M,Fraser,ID,
   Bothamley,J,Davis,P,Hamblin,TJ (1976)Plasmapheresis in the management of acute systemic lupus erythematosus.Lancet 1:709-711
2. Buckner,CD,Clirr,RA,Thomas,LD (1975)Plasma-exchange with the continuous flow centrifuge.In: Goldman JM & Lowenthal RM (eds)Leukocytes:
   Separation,collection,transfusion,Academic Press,p 578-580
3. Editorial (1977)Plasmapheresis in macroglobulinaemia.Lancet 2:807-
   808
4. Thompson,GR,Lowenthal,R,Myant,NB (1975)Plasma exchange in the management of homozygous familial hypercholesterolemia. Lancet 1:1208-
   1211
5. Berger,GMB,Miller,JL,Bonnici,F,Joffe,HS,Dubovsky,DW (1978) Continuous flow plasma exchange in the treatment of homozygous familial
   hypercholesterolemia.Am. J. Med. 65:243-251
6. Simons,LA,Gibson,JC,Isbister,JP,Biggs,JC (1978) The effects of plasma exchange on cholesterol metabolism. Atherosclerosis 31:195-204
7. Thompson,GR,Myant,NB,Kilpatrick,D,Oakley,CM,Raphael,MJ,Steiner,RE
   (1980) Assessment of long term plasma-exchange for Familial Hypercholesterolemia. Br. Heart J. 43:680- 690
8. Stoffel,W,Demant,T (1981) Selective removal of apolipoprotein B-containing serum lipoproteins from blood plasma.Proc. Nat. Acad. Sci.
   78:611-615
9. Stoffel,W,Borberg,H,Greve,V (1981) Application of Specific Extracorporeal Removal of low density lipoprotein in Familial Hypercholeste-
   rolemia.Lancet 2: 1005-1007
10.Thompson,GR (1981) Plasma exchange for hypercholesterolemia.Lancet
   1: 1246-1247
11.Postiglione,A,Rubba,P,Scarpato,N,Iannuzzi,A,Mancini,M (1982) Increased arterial blood flow to lower limbs in patients with Familial
   Hypercholesterolemia after plasma-exchange.Atherosclerosis 41:412-416

12. Postiglione,A,Soricelli,A,Scarpato,N,Lamenza,F,Mancini,M (1982)
    Increased cerebral blood flow after plasma-exchange in patients
    with Familial Hypercholesterolemia.Clinical Haemorheology (in press)
13. Oriente,P,Di Marino,L,Mastranzo,P,Iovine,C,Patti,L (1979)Simultane-
    ous determination of cholesterol and triglycerides in serum and lipo-
    protein fractions by enzymatic authomated methods.In:Burlina A &
    Galzigna L (eds) Clin.Enzym. Symposium,Piccin,p 387-402
14. Scarpato,N,Postiglione,A,Gnasso,A (1982) Passaggio di colesterolo
    dal compartimento extravascolare a quello intravascolare dopo plas-
    ma exchange in pazienti con Ipercolesterolemia Familiare.La Trasfu-
    sione del sangue (in press)
15. Weber,G,Bianciardi,Toti,P,Scarpato,N,Postiglione,A,Mancini,M.Ultra-
    structural features of circulating platelets from hypercholestero-
    lemic (typeIIa) patients submitted to plasma exchange.A freeze-et-
    ching study (in press)
16. Kilpatrick,D,Fleming,J,Clyne,C,Thompson,GR,(1979) Reduction of blo-
    od viscosity following plasma-exchange.Atherosclerosis 32:301-306
17. Postiglione,A,Soricelli,Lamenza,Scarpato,N,Montefusco,S.Plasma-
    exchange for the treatment of cerebrovascular occlusive disease in
    Familial Hypercholesterolemia  (in press)

# 2 Arterial Wall and Plasma Components

# Role of Endothelial Dysfunction In Vivo in Smooth Muscle Proliferation

S. M. Schwartz, A. Reidy, and G. Hansson

Göran Hansson

## Introduction

Our concept of the endothelium as a semipermeable tube able to contain blood changed with the advent of culture systems able to propagate endothelial cells. The resulting biochemical characterization of endothelial cell functions has led to new concepts for possible roles of the endothelial cell in atherosclerosis. From the point of view of this review, suggestions that endothelial injury plays a central role in the pathogenesis of smooth muscle proliferation are of particular interest. Until recently, this has taken the form of the hypothesis that endothelial denudation leads to platelet thrombosis and release of the platelet-derived growth factor that stimulates smooth muscle proliferation. As we will discuss, however, the evidence for endothelial denudation *in vivo* is limited. In contrast, cytochemical studies suggest that other forms of endothelial injury do occur *in vivo*. We will suggest that these changes represent an important direction for future study.

Our principal interest is in the etiology of abnormal cell growth. For the endothelium, we are concerned with growth as a repair process that is necessary to replace endothelial cells lost through normal turnover. We want to know the initial resting state of these two cell types and what are the stimuli that initiate their growth and permit the maintenance of continuity. The growth control issues for the other vascular wall cells is quite different. Both *in vivo* and *in vitro* endothelial cells rest in a diploid state and do not respond to conventional polypeptide mitogens (1). In contrast, smooth muscle cells at rest *in vivo* and *in vitro* show a large number of tetraploid cells. The nature of these cells is not known (2, 3). Smooth muscle cell growth, at least *in vitro*, depends on exogenous growth factors (4). While *in vivo* data are limited, there is also evidence that growth of smooth muscle in response to hypertension requires sympathetic innervation (5). Furthermore, it appears that factors made by endothelial cells are able to either stimulate or inhibit smooth muscle growth *in vitro* (1, 6, 7, 8, 9).

These data on ploidy or a growth requirement in culture do not tell us how abnormal smooth muscle growth occurs *in vivo*. Ross and his colleagues (4) have suggested that the smooth muscle cells in lesions are stimulated to grow by exposure to abnormal quantities of growth factors---analogous to the studies of action of growth factors on other cell types (10). In contrast, two other groups have suggested that the mechanism is "intrinsic," resulting from neoplastic growth (11) or from abnormal development of the smooth muscle cells (12). From the viewpoint of endothelial biology, the distinctive feature of the Ross hypothesis, release of platelet-derived growth factor, is loss of endothelial integrity (4). In contrast, the intrinsic hypotheses do not require endothelial injury as a critical initiating event (12, 13). In any case, there is no doubt that endothelial injury and thrombosis occur as lesions progress. This should promote lesion progression. Thus, the concept of endothelial integrity is central to our concept of the interrelationships between endothelial and smooth muscle cell growth control.

## Endothelial Integrity

Most morphological and physiological studies have treated the endothelium as a simple sheet of neutral material pierced by holes. This is no longer valid. We know that the endothelium contains high affinity receptors for plasma molecules including LDL, acetyl LDL, thrombin, alpha-macroglobulin and insulin, as well as complex patterns of surface change. For review see Ross and Schwartz, 1982 (14).

A more important fault with this simple model of the endothelium is that it neglects cell turnover. Rheologic data predicts higher shear forces at sites known to have a predilection for lesion formation. Vessel walls are subject to wear and tear. The conclusions of studies of endothelial cell turnover are remarkably consistent: cell turnover in the aortic endothelium is low ($10^{-3}$ cell/day) except in focal areas including regions of high shear (15, 16, 17, 18, 19). The presence of these focal areas of turnover raises the possibility that spontaneously denuded areas might occur. This, however, does not appear to be the case. Studies of similar areas of scanning electron microscopy (SEM) and transmission electron microscopy (TEM) have not as yet demonstrated such discontinuities in normal animals. There is no compelling evidence, moreover, that during the early phases (1-2 months) of hypercholesterolemia, that endothelium is actually denuded in these studies. In contrast, Ross and Harker observed endothelial denudation in the aorta of monkeys fed a hypercholesterolemic diet for two years (4). Thus, denudation is likely to be more important to lesion progression than it is to initiation of lesions.

## Initial Growth State of Smooth Muscle Cells

As noted above, smooth muscle cells *in vivo* rest in two growth states: diploid and tetraploid. In hypertension, even higher ploidy states may be reached. The wall also contains multinucleated smooth muscle cells. The frequency of hyperploidy is greatly increased in animals with elevated pressure (2, 3). These data may have significance for atherosclerosis aside from the relevance to hypertension. From our studies, we know that tetraploid smooth muscle cells do not represent cycling cells, since the frequency of cells in S, as measured by $^3$HTdR autoradiography of dispersed cells, was approximately $10^{-3}$ or less (2). Since this cell type is able to endoreplicate as well as undergo true cell division, present concepts of muscle cell growth may be simplistic. For example, thymidine index data can no longer be considered a satisfactory measure of changes in smooth muscle cell number (20). We should also consider the possibility that subpopulations of cells in quite different states of growth arrest may proliferate differently. Very little is known about the properties of tetraploid cells in any system. Pero and his colleagues (21) reported an abnormal rate of unscheduled DNA synthesis, i.e., "repair," in the nuclei of lymphocytes from hypertensive patients. It is interesting to speculate about the possible effects of instabilities of the genome of tetrapliod cells on their ability to proliferate. This could be the basis for the monoclonal nature of smooth muscle cells in atherosclerotic plaques (11).

## Initial Growth State of Endothelial Cells

Wound models have been quite important in studies of the endothelium both *in vivo* and *in vitro*. Endothelial regeneration *in vitro* is, at least formally, comparable to regeneration following a wound *in vivo*. In both cases the apparent stimulus is loss of a portion of the cell layer. Also in both cases, growth occurs without addition of exogenous growth factors to the overlying medium during growth stimulation (1, 22). These *in vitro* wound healing studies may resolve some of the confusion over the growth requirements of endothelial cells. Conflicting claims on growth requirements of sparsely plated cells (1) may result from the fact that endothelial cells are able to condition their own medium and to synthesize a matrix that may obviate the requirement for exogenous growth factors (6, 7, 23). As might be expected, however, the requirement for conditioned medium disappears as cell density increases. Thus, it is not surprising that our studies have failed to find a growth factor requirement for endothelial cells plated at densi-

ties approaching those seen *in vivo*, or for regeneration of these cells at a wound
edge (1, 22).

The *in vitro* model has also been very important to our attempts to define the
changes in a wound layer required to permit regeneration. For example, endothelial cells appear to be required to move before they can initiate cell replication. Cytochalasins selectively inhibit DNA synthesis at the wound edge. The
kinetics of entry into S after arrest with cytochalasin D suggest that the event
affected by this drug must be quite close to the time of wounding itself (24, 25).
In contrast, if the wound is small enough so that cells move together in less than
eight hours, no replication occurs (26). A relationship of endothelial replication to cell movement is also suggested by our observation that growth is
stimulated by the application of vinblastine or by overlaying cells with
polymerized collagen (13, 25). The effective doses cause a marked change in cell
shape with partial retraction of each cell from the other.

## Interrelationships of Endothelial and Smooth Muscle Growth States

At this point we can return to the hypothesis that endothelial injury is the
initial event in atherosclerosis (4). This hypothesis rests on the fact that
denudation of the endothelium leads to adhesion of platelets with release of the
platelet-derived growth factor. Surprisingly little is known about actual loss of
the endothelium either spontaneously or in response to atherosclerosis risk
factors. As noted above, there are focal areas with high rates of cell turnover.
Endothelial replication is increased ion response to acute hypertension (27) or
hyperlipemia (20). The effects of hypertension, however, are limited to its
acute, early stages (28). Evidence for spontaneous denudation is lacking, either
in normal animals or in animals exposed to hypertension or hyperlipemia (29).
This lack of convincing evidence for spontaneous denudation does not prove that
the subendothelium cannot be exposed for brief repeated episodes. It is possible
to estimate the duration of exposure of the thrombogenic subendothelium, and the
interval of denudation required for stimulation of smooth muscle proliferation.
Our studies, as well as work by Hirsch and his co-workers (1, 18, 26, 30, 31),
have examined the response of the aorta of rats and rabbits to denudation. Total
denudation by the balloon technique leads to intimal accumulation of smooth muscle
cells. Smooth muscle lesions, however, are formed only in those areas requiring
several days for endothelial regeneration. This suggests that there is a "critical lesion size;" i.e., brief exposures to platelet releasate are not sufficient
to stimulate smooth muscle proliferation. The importance of this critical interval is further illustrated by studies of platelet adhesion. Again, most of the
platelet adhesion and release of granules occurs in the first few hours following
experimental denudation (32, 33). It is interesting to speculate whether the
initial platelet interactions play a special role in the stimulation of smooth
muscle cell proliferation.

In contrast to these data, studies of endothelial regeneration imply that the
surface is unlikely to remain denuded; in fact, endothelial desquamation may
normally occur without denudation. Areas of denudation two cells wide are
re-covered within eight hours (26). Recent work from our laboratory has studied
the loss of single cells. Although we can detect a five-fold increase in
endothelial cell replication in response to endotoxin, there is no evidence of
denudation (34). These data imply that the endothelium may be able to regenerate
rapidly enough to obviate any exposure of the subendothelium. This would explain
the paradox of cell replication studies which show focal areas of high cell
turnover while scanning electron microscopy studies continue to show a continuous
endothelium (18).

## Nondenuding Injuries In Vivo

If endothelial denudation *per se* is not an early event in atherosclerosis, we need
to consider the role of other possible forms of endothelial response. Unfortunately, the data here are very incomplete. Despite extensive data on endothelial

346

cell function *in vitro*, there are as yet no obvious ways to determine the role of these functions in an intact animal. Morphologic studies, with two exceptions, have led to very subjective concepts of "injury." The first exception is the accumulating evidence that monocytes accumulate in or on the endothelium during hyperlipemia (1). This is clear evidence for "injury" affecting one or both of these cell types. It is interesting to speculate about the possible role of macrophage-derived growth factor in atherosclerosis (14).

The second form of morphologic data comes from recent studies begun by Hansson in Goteborg, and continued in our laboratory. Earlier work by Bjorkerud provided evidence that some endothelial cells were permeable to trypan blue (35). Since permeability of cultured cells to trypan blue is an indicator of cell death and breakdown of the plasma membrane, Hansson reasoned, the cytoplasm of these cells should contain serum proteins and the cells should be dead. We find that about 3% of the aortic endothelial cells in a rat show cytoplasmic IgG. These same cells bind chlortetracycline, implying extensive calcification of the cell, presumably of the level of the mitochondria. These observations strongly imply that we are detecting dead cells in the aortic endothelium *in vivo*. *In vitro*, the IgG binding appears to be attributable to a specific binding site. Cultured cells with these properties undergo two- or three-day agonal periods, gradually breaking apart and falling off the monolayer. The surrounding cells, as suggested by our *in vivo* studies, undermine the dying cell, thus maintaining continuity (29).

The significance of this phenomenon of "death *in vivo*" remains to be determined. We might speculate, however, about the probable effects of the products of cell death on surrounding cells and about the alterations in endothelial cell function at sites having large numbers of such cells. Two speculations are of interest to us. First, cell death is known to be associated with activation of phospholipase A2 (36). This should lead to release of fatty acids, many of which are likely to have important biologic activities. Second, recent studies from our laboratory demonstrate the release of mitogenic cells from dying endothelial cells (7). It is intriguing to speculate on the effects that these poorly defined materials might have on surrounding or underlying cells *in vivo*.

## Summary

As of now, we do not know a great deal about the interrelationships of growth in these two cell types. *In vitro* , endothelial cells produce mediators able to stimulate or inhibit smooth muscle proliferation. Whether these mediators exist or play a role *in vivo* is difficult to determine. Moreover, when large amounts of the endothelium are removed mechanically, smooth muscle cell proliferation results. The problem here is that proliferation does not occur when the extent of the wound is very small, and there is no good evidence for denudation as an early event in atherogenesis. Central issues would appear to be the presence or absence of endothelial denudation at various time points of lesion formation, the definition of more subtle forms of endothelial injury, and the design of experiments able to measure the effects of growth factors in the whole animal. In contrast, our new data suggest that spontaneous endothelial cell death does occur in the intact animal. The function of these dead cells remains to be determined.

## References

1. Schwartz, S.M., Gajdusek, C.M. and Selden, S.C., III: Vascular wall growth control: The role of the endothelium. Arteriosclerosis 1:107-161, 1981.

2. Owens, G.K., Rabinovitch, P.S. and Schwartz, S.M: Smooth muscle cell hypertrophy versus hyperplasia in hypertension (polyploidy/spontaneously hypertensive rat/cell cycle). Proc Natl Acad Sci USA 78:7759-7763, 1981.

3. Grünwald, J., Robenek, H., Mey, J., Hauss, W.H: *In vivo* and *in vitro* cellular changes in experimental hypertension: Electromicroscopic and

morphometric studies of aortic smooth muscle cells. Exp. Mol. Pathol. 36:164-176, 1982.

4.  Ross, R. and Harker, L: Hyperlipidemia and atherosclerosis. Chronic hyper-lipidemia initiates and maintains lesions by endothelial cell desquamation and lipid accumulation. Science 193:1094-1100, 1976.

5.  Bevan, R.D., Tsuru, H: Functional and structural changes in the rabbit ear artery after sympathetic denervation. Circ. Res. 49:478-485, 1981.

6.  Gajdusek, C.M. and Schwartz, S.M: Self stimulation by endothelial cell con-ditioned medium. J. Cell Biol. 87:X2619, 1980. (abst).

7.  Gajdusek, C.M. and Schwartz, S.M: Ability of endothelial cells to condi-tion culture medium. J. Cell. Physiol. 110:35-42, 1982.

8.  Harris-Hooker, S.A., Gajdusek, C.M., Schwartz, S.M. and Wight, T: Role of endothelial cell products in vascular growth responses and neovasculariza-tion. J. Cell. Physiol. (in press) 1982.

9.  Castellot, J., Addonizio, M., Rosenberg, R. and Karnovsky, M: Cultured endothelial cells produce a heparin-like inhibitor of smooth muscle cell growth. J. Cell Biol. 90:372-379, 1981.

10. Herschman, H.R: Nerve growth factor and epidermal growth factor. In: *Growth Factors* . Moderator D.W. Golde. Ann. Intern. Med. 92:650-662, 1980.

11. Benditt, E.P. and Gown, A.M: Atheroma: The artery wall and the environment. Int. Rev. Exp. Pathol. 21:55-118, 1980.

12. Velican, C. and Velican D: Study on the onset of atherosclerotic lesions in human coronary arteries. Rev. Roum. Med-Med. Int. 17:131-149, 1979.

13. Delvos, U., Gajdusek, C., Sage, H., Harker, L.A. and Schwartz, S.M: Inter-actions of vascular wall cells with extracellular matrix. Lab. Invest. 1982 (in press).

14. Ross, R. and Schwartz, S.M: Platelet-endothelial interactions. In: *Handbook of Physiology* . Editor A.B. Fisher. University of Pennsylvania, Philadelphia. (in press).

15. Schwartz, C.J., Gerrity, R.G. and Lewis, L.J: Arterial endothelial structure and function with particular reference to permeability. Atherosclerosis Reviews. 3:109-124, 1978.

16. Schwartz, S.M. and Benditt, E.P: Clustering of replicating cells in aortic endothelium. Proc. Nat. Acad. Sci. USA 73:651-653, 1976.

17. Schwartz, S.M: Role of endothelial integrity in atherosclerosis. Artery 8:305-314, 1980.

18. Schwartz, S.M., Gajdusek, C.M., Reidy, M.A., Selden, S.C., III and Haudens-child, C.C: Maintenance of integrity in aortic endothelium. Fed. Proc. 39:2618-2625, 1980.

19. Kunz, J., Schrejter, B., Schubert, B., Voss, K., Krieg, K: Experimentelle Untersuchungen über die Regeneration der Aortenendothelzellen. Automatische und visuelle Auswertung von Autoradiogrammen. Acta. Histochem. 61:53-63, 1978.

348

20. Florentin, R.A., Nam, S.C., Lee, K.T. and Thomas, W.A: Increased $^3$H-thymidine incorporation into endothelial cells of swine fed cholesterol for 3 days. Exp. Mol. Path. 10:250-255, 1969.

21. Pero, R.W., Bryngelsson, C., Mitelman, F., Thalin, T. and Norden, A: High blood pressure related to carcinogen induced unscheduled DNA synthesis, DNA carcinogen binding and chromosonal aberration in human lymphocytes. Proc. Natl. Acad. Sci. 73:2496-2500, 1976.

22. Schwartz, S.M., Selden, S.C., III and Bowman, P: Growth control in aortic endothelium at wound edges. In: *Hormones and Cell Culture*, *Vol*. 6. Editors R. Ross and G. Sato. Cold Spring Harbor 3rd Conference on Cell Proliferation. Cold Spring Harbor, New York. pp. 593-611, 1979.

23. Gospodarowicz, D. and Ill, C: Extracellular matrix and control of proliferation of vascular endothelial cells. J. Clin. Invest. 65:1351-1364, 1980.

24. Selden, S.C., III and Schwartz, S.M: Cytochalasin B inhibition of endothelial proliferation at wound edges *in vitro*. J. Cell Biol. 81:348-354, 1979.

25. Selden, S.C., III, Rabinovitch, P.S. and Schwartz, S.M: Effects of cytoskeletal disrupting agents on replication of bovine endothelium. J. Cell. Physiol. 108:195-211, 1981.

26. Reidy, M.A. and Schwartz, S.M: Endothelial regeneration III. Time course of intimal changes after small defined injury to rat aortic endothelium. Lab. Invest. 44:301-308, 1981.

27. Schwartz, S.M. and Benditt, E.P: Aortic endothelial cell replication. I. Effects of age and hypertension in the rat. Circ. Res. 41:248-255, 1977.

28. Schwartz, S.M. and Standaert, D.M: Effect of chronic hypertension and antihypertensive therapy on endothelial cell replication in the spontaneously hypertensive rat. Lab. Invest. (in press).

29. Hansson, G.K. and Schwartz, S.M: Endothelial dysfunction without cell loss. In: *Biochemical Interactions at the Endothelium* Editor A. Cryer. Elsevier/North Holland Biomedical Press, London (in press).

30. Haudenschild, C.C. and Schwartz, S.M: Endothelial regeneration II. Restitution of endothelial continuity. Lab. Invest. 41:407-418, 1979.

31. Hirsch, E.Z. and Robertson, A.L: Selective acute arterial endothelial injury and repair. I. methodology and surface characteristics. Atherosclerosis 28:271-287, 1977.

32. Goldberg, I.D., Stemerman, M.B. and Handin, R.I: Vascular permeation of platelet factor IV after endothelial injury. Science 209:610-612, 1980.

33. Groves, H.M., Kinlough-Rathbone, R.L., Richardson, M., Moore, S. and Mustard, J.F: Platelet interaction with damaged rabbit aorta. Lab. Invest. 40:194-200, 1979.

34. Reidy, M.A. and Schwartz, S.M: Mechanisms of endothelial repair after injury. Fed. Proc. 39:1109, 1980.

35. Björkerud, S., Bondjers, G: Endothelial integrity and viability in the aorta of the normal rabbit and rat as evaluated with dye exclusion tests and interference contrast microscopy. Atherosclerosis 15:285-300, 1972.

36. Farber, J.L., Chien, K.R., Mittnacht, S. The pathogenesis of irreversible cell injury in ischemia. Am. J. Pathol. 102:271-281, 1981.

# Derivation and Progression of Atherosclerotic Plaques

M.D.Haust[1]

## A. Introduction

The incidence of clinical disease and mortality from atherosclerosis increased alarmingly in advanced industrialized societies following World War II. Some elements of modern life appeared to aggravate and accelerate this disease with the coronary circulation being particularly affected. In the mid-sixties atherosclerotic heart disease assumed almost epidemic proportions and over half of all deaths in the United States of America were in some way associated with atherosclerosis (1). In several European countries with traditionally low mortality rates from coronary heart disease the involvement with atherosclerosis gradually approached that in the U.S.A. (2).

Around 1968 a remarkable change became apparent in the U.S.A. as death rates from atherosclerotic disease began to fall noticeably, the decline ranging in various studies from 6.2% to 30% (3,4) for different population groups. This encouraging trend continues, is - to say the least - intriguing, but remains to be explained (5,6). Whereas it is true that better public awareness of the risk factors of the atherosclerotic disease (hypertension, cigarette smoking, hyperlipidemia, and other) and intensified measures to reduce these may have contributed to this decline, this trend cannot be explained entirely on that basis. Moreover, it cannot be predicted, given our present status of knowledge, whether the favourable course might reverse itself again! Are we at the mercy of trends of atherosclerosis that behave at will? As long as we are unable to unravel totally the etiology and pathogenesis of the early lesions and the factors of progression that culminate in the clinically important atherosclerotic plaques, we may remain unable to influence in a rational way the natural course of this disease.

## B. Atherosclerotic Plaques (Advanced Atherosclerotic Lesions)

"Atherosclerotic plaques" is a generic term used often interchangeably with "advanced lesions" either in a collective sense or in reference to one of the two generally acknowledged forms; one form consists almost exclusively of fibrous tissue (white or pearly-white fibrous plaque), and the second contains in addition a baso-central atheroma (atheromatous plaque).

These lesions have been the acknowledged hallmark of atherosclerosis and are the least controversial lesions with respect to their appear-

---

[1]Department of Pathology, The University of Western Ontario, London, Ontario, Canada.

ance, nature and significance (7-16); their derivation (17,18) however, still remains contentious in some scientific "quarters" (see below). Whereas the term relates to lesions that on gross inspection have a characteristic appearance, in reality the lesion may not only represent two distinct forms, but in addition "embraces" various stages in the development of the plaque and the morphological counterparts of recurring episodes of the atherosclerotic process. Analysis of the nature of these recurrent processes not only was important from the point of view of learning how a given atherosclerotic plaque enlarges progressively, but in addition was instrumental in recognizing also that similar and related tissue reactions underlie the earliest forms of atherosclerotic lesions, i.e., the lesions of inception (12-15, 17, 18).

## I.   White or Pearly-White Plaques

The characterization of this lesion is based on external features and those on cross-cut sectioning. Light microscopic examination often is required for the confirmation of the gross appearance.

The lesion on gross examination may vary from a white-opaque to a pearly-white plaque, and the size may range from a few millimeters to over one centimeter. The plaques are usually elongated in the longitudinal axis of the artery such as the aorta. On cross-sectioning the lesion consists exclusively of a focal fibrous connective tissue accumulation that merges imperceptibly on each side with the adjacent normal intima. The plaques begin to appear in the human aorta at the end of the second or early third decade, and their distribution resembles that of fatty dots and streaks of early life (14,17,18). However, once they develop in the abdominal aorta, they become here more numerous, prominent and larger than the plaques in the thoracic aorta. The plaques appear first on the posterior wall, but some may develop at the same time elsewhere. The new fibrous plaques develop usually in the ventral direction and the same applies to the extensions of the existing lesions on the posterior wall. In middle and old age the fibrous plaques occupy a considerably larger surface and are more prominent in the abdominal than in the thoracic aorta. These prominent lesions may encroach on the orifices of and impede the blood supply to the aortic branches.

Light microscopic examination of fibrous plaques may show a wide range of tissue changes. At one hand of the scale a plaque may consist of connective tissue which is in the same stage of maturation. This tissue is composed of collagen and fine elastic fibers intermingled with smooth muscle cells (SMCs), all arranged parallel to each other and to the longitudinal axis of the aorta. They are embedded in ground substance which is aboundant in glycosaminoglycans (GAGs)(19-23). The arrangement of the connective tissue components resembles closely that of normal intima and no capillaries are present in the typical uncomplicated fibrous plaque. With age and maturation of the plaque the amount of ground substance, particularly its GAGs-component, decreases. Similarly, the collagen fibers and the elastic components vary considerably from lesion to lesion depending upon its maturation and aging as well as the simplicity or complexity of the fibrous plaque (see below). In a young lesion the SMCs are free of intracellular lipids, but lipid droplets may be present in SMCs in the old lesions. Moreover, in the latter the SMCs may show various stages of atrophy and

the collagen and elastic tissue fibers may be in part or completely
hyalinized. At the other end of the range, the fibrous plaque may
consist of several layers of connective tissues, all displaying the
characteristic features of arrangement and composition as described
above; the effect of "layering" is best demonstrated by special connective tissue stains. Each layer is believed to represent an episode
in the evolution of the plaque, the oldest being present at the base
and the most recent at the immediately subendothelial region. The
most superficial layer of the plaque may show features of insudation,
and albumin, fibrin, and high-, and low-density lipoproteins may all
be identified by special techniques in those layers (see: 13-15,19).
The features of insudation are identical to those observed in the grey
gelatinous elevations, one of the three forms of early atherosclerotic
lesions. The amount of albumin and fibrin varies inversely with the
maturity of the connective tissues of the fibrous plaque.

Other fibrous plaques may show on microscopic examination the presence
of a superimposed mural thrombus. Fibrinous remnants may be also observed either in the deep or superficial layers of the fibrous plaque.
In still other instances several layers of mural thrombi may be superimposed upon each other. Usually in such instances, the thrombi are
in different stages of organization, merging with each other and with
the connective tissues of the underlying fibrous plaque. Occasionally,
a white fibrous plaque with a grey hue on gross inspection proves to
be composed almost entirely of numerous layers of thrombi in various
stages of organization (14,15,24-26).

The cells present in the fibrous plaques are smooth muscle cells (SMCs).
These cells are responsible for the elaboration of all connective tissue elements (11-15,19-26), and show a propensity for proliferation.
This is particularly evident at the ultrastructural level, as many immature forms are often present. These forms are endowed with cytoplasmic organelles concerned with secretion; the cells are capable of forming all the connective tissue components: GAGs-containing ground substance, microfibrils of the extracellular space (27), collagen fibrils
and elastic tissue elements (28). The SMCs elaborate their own basal
lamina which corresponds to the closely enveloping, PAS-positive layer
previously observed around the SMCs by light microscopy (22). By electron microscopy (21) it proved to be a basement membrane (BM) resembling those associated with epithelial and endothelial cells. Morphologically, this BM appears to be a single structure consisting of a
lamina lucida (adjacent immediately to the cytoplasmic membrane) and
an outer lamina densa. It is quite remarkable how complex this BM-
structure proved to be (29,30). It is known to-day that the lamina
lucida consists of a large molecular glycoprotein, laminin (31-34).
The lamina densa on the other hand consists of type IV non-fibrillar
collagen that is characteristically localized to the BM (35-38). Most
recent studies indicate that the collagen in the BM is arranged in a
honey-comb-like lattice, thus representing a unique network of collagenous molecules which impart upon the underlying cells or tissue layers, both tensile strength and elasticity (39). The lamina lucida and
the lamina densa are "cemented" to each other by a narrow layer of a
heparan sulphate-proteoglycan (BM$_1$-Proteoglycan)(38-40). A similar
layer is interposed between the external surface of the lamina densa
and the surrounding interstitial tissue, or fibronectin (39). The previously identified anionic sites in the BM have been localized to the
heparan sulphate-PG. Some studies suggest that the heparan sulphate
forms an ionic shield over the BM which blocks the passage of negatively charged macromolecules (see: 39). Whereas the above information
regarding the BM of different cell types has not all been confirmed
yet for the SMC-related BM, some data on that subject have been forth-

coming recently (34,35).

In atherosclerotic plaques the BMs often are thick and appear to proliferate in a "reticular" pattern (12,15,28) reminiscent of that observed in hypertension. In a recently developed model of atherosclerosis the BM-proliferation of the intimal SMCs was a particularly striking feature (41).

It is also of considerable interest that the arterial SMCs synthesize
and secrete at least four forms of collagen: type I, type III, type IV
and type V (35,42). Whether they may be also secreting the so-called
"linkage", i.e., type VI collagen (35) has not been determined to-date.

In normal arteries collagen does not appear to have antigenic properties and its affinity for lipids is apparently moderate (43). It accounts for approximately 5% of all arterial protein synthesis, the rate
of which is for collagen approximately 97 ng/g/4h (44). In atherosclerotic arteries the synthesis of collagen reportedly increases to 14%
of all proteins, as does also the affinity of lipids for binding to
insoluble collagen (44). The collagen in the lesions exhibited antigenic properties and a small amount of collagen-bound IgG appeared to
be synthesized locally (45). Moreover, it was reported (44,46) that
the ratio of synthesis of type I and type III collagens was reversed,
i.e., in atherosclerotic plaques 65% of collagen was of type I and 35%
of type III. However, data published most recently (47) indicate that
the composition of normal aortae and that of atherosclerotic plaques
does not differ significantly with respect to the content of collagens
type I and type III, as there was only a small shift in favour of type
I in the atherosclerotic plaques. These recent data do not support
the previously proposed concept (46) that atherosclerosis involves a
"transformation" of SMCs to fibroblast-like cells, whereby a major
switch in the synthesis occurs from largely type III to type I collagen in the atherosclerotic plaques. In the above quoted most recent
study (47), type V collagen was also tested and found to be increased
in the plaques relative to the interstitial collagens.


II.  Atheromatous Plaques

The appearance of these lesions on gross examination is indistinguishable from that of the white or pearly-white fibrous plaques (see above).
However, the cross-section discloses that the lesion consists of a
baso-central yellow softening, i.e., the atheroma, and the overlying
fibrous cap. This is the typical and universally accepted atheromatous plaque as originally defined by Marchand (see: 15). This form of
atherosclerotic plaque is more common than is the purely white fibrous
variety.

Microscopic examination shows that the baso-central atheroma consists
of a pool of amorphous proteinaceous and fatty substances intermingled
with cellular debris and cholesterol crystals. In addition, various
amounts of fibrin or fibrinoid, GAGs and a deeply basophilic, finely
dispersed or crystalloid substance, interpreted as calcium complexes,
may be present (15). The atheroma usually merges gradually with the
overlying fibrous cap. All the components of connective tissues and
the cells of this fibrous cap resemble those of the white and pearly-
white fibrous plaques with respect to the basic components and their
arrangement, but there are subtle differences. The SMCs in the fibrous
cap, particularly those in the vicinity of the atheroma, contain a

variable number of large, cytoplasmic droplets, even in the presence of normal, i.e., non-hyalinized connective tissues. In the interstitium of the connective tissue, similar droplets may be present and presumably originate from the disintegrating fat-containing SMCs. An increased amount of the finely dispersed extracellular fat-variety is present between the various connective tissue fibers. In the region between the atheroma and the base of the fibrous cap foam cells, surrounding remnants of unorganized fibrin or fibrinoid, may be present. This association is similar to that observed around unorganized fibrin remnants in the deep layers of mural thrombi and in sero-fibrinous insudate in some gelatinous lesions (see below; 13,17).

Electron microscopic examination confirms largely the above observations. At times it is possible to identify the foam cells in the fibrous cap and those surrounding the unorganized fibrinous remnants as myogenic foam cells (17,48). The accumulation of cytoplasmic fat varies considerably from one cell to another, and it appears to be related inversely to the distance from the atheroma. In the immediate vincinity of the atheroma myogenic foam cells are in various stages of disintegration. The ultrastructural characteristics of connective tissue components of the fibrous cap do not differ appreciably from those observed in the purely fibrous plaques. The atheromatous core itself contains granular lipoid substances, identical to those observed in the extracellular space of fatty streaks and in the interstitium of the fibrous cap. The electron-dense granular material is intermingled with electron-dense crystals (probably representing calcium or its complexes) and with less electron-dense substances. In addition, electron-lucent clefts, i.e., empty spaces formerly occupied by cholesterol crystals lost in the course of tissue-preparation, may be seen in the atheroma. The ratio of the width of the fibrous cap to the size of the atheroma varies from one atheromatous plaque to another. When the overlying fibrous cap becomes extremely thin the lesion may appear yellow rather than white on gross inspection, and in such instances the advanced (atheromatous) plaque, is on its way to become a complicated lesion.

## C. Derivation of Plaques

It has been generally accepted that atherosclerotic plaques may be derived from three different precursor lesions: fatty dots or streaks, grey gelatinous elevations, and microthrombi (12-15,17-19). These so-called early lesions of atherosclerosis are defined on the basis of combined gross, and light and electron microscopic examination, but most of the microthrombi are detected only on microscopic examination.

*The Fatty Dots and Streaks* appear as yellow, usually well circumscribed, flat or slightly elevated small lesions and reflect largely the accumulation of fat-droplets in the intimal SMCs. The number of fat-droplets in the individual SMCs as well as the number of the cells involved determine the size of the lesion. It is assumed that as long as the fat-droplets are confined to the SMCs, the lesion is reversible. However, once the number of fat-droplets accumulating in the cytoplasm surpasses the ability of these cells to metabolize this fat, cellular necrosis ensues. Necrotizing SMCs release the fat into the extracellular space and induce changes that ultimately culminate in the formation of an atherosclerotic plaque. Necrosis of SMCs stimulates local SMC-mitosis. Connective tissues damaged by the released fat-droplets are also replaced by proliferation of collagen and elastic fibers.

Macrophages, stimulated by cellular and extracellular tissue damage migrate into the area to phagocytize the debris. They may only perform that function in the superficial layers, as they do not survive under anaerobic conditions prevailing deep in the lesions (see: 15). All the above new local conditions may change the integrity of the overlying endothelium and thus result in an influx of blood constituents into the intima and/or deposition of a mural thrombus. These new complex tissue reactions continue to induce repeated episodes of similar changes that ultimately, over two or three decades, culminate in the formation of an atherosclerotic plaque (17). As is evident from the surface distribution of fatty dots and streaks and of atherosclerotic plaques, not all of the former are converted to the latter lesions.

*The Grey Gelatinous Elevation (Insudative Lesion)* represents the second form of early atherosclerotic lesions and reflects a focal intimal insudate containing blood constituents. Probably, the underlying cause for the intimal accumulation of the insudate is the damage to either endothelium or to the intimal connective tissues. When the damage is not severe, the resulting lesion may represent a serous edema, containing only a small amount of albumin. This may be absorbed into the circulation relatively promptly, with a complete restitution to normal of the area involved. However, if the edema is massive or alternatively, the damage to the endothelium so severe that large molecules enter the intima, the resultant sero-fibrinous insudate may not be effectively and promptly absorbed. Fibrinogen that precipitates in tissues to fibrin cannot be absorbed by diffusion and would have to be phagocytized. Unabsorbed insudate (= edema fluid) may be organized by forces of repair provided that the intimal SMCs remain unaffected. The organization results in local connective tissue accumulation. This tissue is extremely well adapted structurally and perhaps functionally to the local conditions. The organizing forces do not always suffice to "act" swiftly and efficiently; the stagnated insudate may in time change the metabolic conditions of the local SMCs resulting in their fatty metamorphosis and ultimate necrosis (see above). The massive edema may also fragment and distort the local connective tissue fibrils providing a stimulus for replacement by proliferating connective tissues. The process is further complicated if the large molecules of prebeta- and beta lipoproteins are contained in the insudate. Even the completely organized insudative lesion represents a focus of altered metabolism and the likely site for further pathological changes, i.e., fatty metamorphosis of the local SMCs, thrombus deposition, and recurrent insudation. Thus, (a chain of)events may be initiated that are indistinguishable from those beginning as fatty dots and streaks, and ultimately culminate in the formation of a fibrous atherosclerotic plaque.

*Microthrombi.* Tiny mural thrombi occurring in the arteries of animals and man (see: 15,17,49) also represent an early form of atherosclerotic lesions. There is evidence that in an intact circulation of man and animals fibrin forms and is being removed constantly by fibrinolysins. The delicate balance between formation and lysis of these deposits may be disturbed by many factors that either promote coagulation or inhibit fibrinolytic activity. The endothelium itself also possesses fibrinolytic properties. The formation of microthrombi is intimately associated with the dynamics and status of platelets in the circulation. In addition to having a role in thrombosis, platelets may relate to the formation of atherosclerotic plaques by releasing various substances capable of increasing vascular permeability (intermediates of arachidonate metabolism, nucleotides, prostaglandins, serotonin, and a cationic protein)(49), form and release an elastase (49) and a collagenase that is capable of digesting collagen (50). Moreover, when present in the microthrombus they may release mitogens that stimulate

the proliferation of SMCs in the focally affected area (for review
see: 23). When the microthrombus is not lysed but remains and becomes
organized to connective tissues it represents again a nidus upon which
repeated precipitation of mural thrombi may occur. In addition, the
persisting microthrombus may become secondarily altered or induce changes in the underlying intima. Whether organized or not, it may "permit" a considerable influx of plasma proteins into its substance. An
organized microthrombus that is incorporated into the intima may influence a nutritional state and the metabolism of SMCs in the subjacent
area with consequent fatty metamorphosis of these cells. In such instances it is not possible to determine whether the microthrombus was
deposited upon a pre-existing small fatty streak, or alternatively, if
the appearance of lipids in the intimal SMCs followed the deposition
of a microthrombus (15,17). Thus, even a small microthrombus may induce several tissue changes that progress, become complex and their
interactions culminate in the formation of a typical atherosclerotic
plaque in a fashion indistinguishable from that induced by the two
other lesions of inception (see above).


D.  Progression of Plaques


Once established, an atherosclerotic plaque may progress into a large
size-lesion by two basic processes that are followed by a cellular
proliferative reaction. These two processes were discussed in the
section on derivation of the advanced lesions, and involve recurrent
deposition of mural thrombi and/or insudation from the lumen into the
substance of the established atherosclerotic plaque. Following either
of the two processes, SMCs of the existing plaque migrate into the
areas of the lesion affected by the deposition of the proteinaceous
substances derived from the blood, multiply, and organize the proteinaceous substances derived from the blood to connective tissues. It
follows therefore that any atherosclerotic plaque that is advanced and
of large size results from sequential recurring episodes of either
thrombus deposition or insudation into the pre-existing fibrous tissue
of the originally small atherosclerotic plaque. Whenever the forces
of organization by SMCs do not suffice and fibrin-containing substances
remain unorganized within the lesions, these remnants degenerate and
give rise to a nidus of atheroma. It is therefore understandable that
by special stains it is possible to demonstrate in some, e.g., the coronary arteries, that an eccentric atherosclerotic lesion in reality
consists of numerous alternating layers of a connective tissue cap and
an atheroma (12,15). This alternating pattern of many layers of fibrous cap and atheroma is less frequently observed in the aorta, perhaps because in this large artery the organizational forces by SMCs
are of greater magnitude than they exist in smaller calibre arteries.

Paraphrasing the process of "progression", one could state that ultimately the atherosclerotic plaques "progress" further to the formation
of complicated lesions. However, the complicated lesions characterized
by several degenerative changes, constitute a separate category. Clinical manifestations of atherosclerosis reflect usually events that are
caused as a consequence of the complicated lesions. Nevertheless, a
prominent uncomplicated atherosclerotic plaque may also precipitate a
grave clinical manifestation by a mural thrombus occluding the arterial lumen narrowed by the prominent plaque.

## E.  Closing Comments

Despite the presently continued favourable trend with respect to the morbidity and mortality from atherosclerosis, it remains of paramount importance to continue the search for factors initiating the early lesions as well as those that are responsible for the progression from the innocuous early lesions to the atherosclerotic plaques.  It is evident that no matter which of the three different forms of early lesions is the initiating change, it may in turn induce the two other basic tissue reactions and in each instance the process may finally culminate in the formation of the complex, typical and clinically important atherosclerotic plaque.

Various factors relating to the peculiar nature of the arterial wall, the existing hemodynamic conditions, and the status of the circulating blood constituents may be injurious either to the endothelium or to the elements of the underlying intima (51,52).  Injury to the endothelium may be followed by an influx (insudation) of plasma constituents into the intima,  by the deposition of a microthrombus, or both. Both processes may induce fatty metamorphosis of the SMCs in the underlying intima and in addition the insudation may cause mechanical damage to the intimal connective tissues.  The failure to organize or remove the insudate or the thrombus may furnish substances that induce further lipid accumulation and provide a stimulus for tissue reactions (53) - including SMCs-proliferation.  The latter phenomenon may be enhanced in part by platelet factors, and by the nature of lipoproteins and other blood-derived substances contained in the insudate itself (for recent review see: 23).

It would appear that at present we are unable to prevent the development of the early lesions (of inception) of atherosclerosis and that some or all of these three forms are present in all men.  However, the clinical manifestations of the disease are produced by advanced stages in the evolution of the lesions that take place over at least two to three decades.  It is therefore logical that attention is being directed of late towards the early life in the hope of retarding the conversion of the earliest lesions to the advanced fibrous and clinically important atherosclerotic plaques. Identification of the factors involved in the conversion of the former to the latter became particularly important in the attempts at retarding this conversion and thus furthering the present trend of decreasing the morbidity and mortality from atherosclerosis.

*Acknowledgements*  This work was supported by a grant-in-aid of research T.3-11 from the Ontario Heart Foundation, Toronto, Ontario, Canada. The author wishes to thank Ms. Irena Wojewodzka for her efficient assistance with the library work, and Mrs. Lya Motesharei for her competent typing of the manuscript and loyalty.

## References

1. Atherosclerosis. A Report by the National Heart and Lung Institute Task Force on Arteriosclerosis, Vol II (1971) DHEW Publication No (NIH), US Government Printing Office, Washington, DC

2. Rose G (1970) Current developments in Europe. In: Jones RJ (ed) Atherosclerosis, Proceedings of the Second International Symposium, Springer-Verlag, New York-Heidelberg-Berlin, p 310
3. Gordon T, Thom T (1975) The recent decrease in CHD mortality. Prev Med 4: 115-125
4. McMillan GC (1979) Atherosclerotic disease and the vessel wall. Exp Mol Pathol 31: 163-168
5. Walker WJ (1977) Changing United States lifestyle and declining vascular mortality: cause or coincidence? N Engl J Med 297: 163-165
6. Fourth Report of the Director of the National Heart, Lung, and Blood Institute (1977) DHEW Publication No (NIH) 77-170, US Government Printing Office, Washington, DC
7. Benditt EP, Gown AM (1980) Atheroma: the artery wall and the environment. Int Rev Exp Pathol 21: 55-118
8. French JE (1966) Atherosclerosis in relation to the structure and function of the arterial intima, with special reference to the endothelium. Int Rev Exp Pathol 5: 253-353
9. Geer JC, McGill HC Jr, Strong JP (1961) The fine structure of human atherosclerotic lesions. Am J Pathol 38: 263-287
10. Ghidoni JJ, O'Neil RM (1967) Recent advances in molecular pathology: a review. Ultrastructure of human atheroma. Exp Mol Pathol 7: 378-400
11. Haust MD, More RH, Movat HZ (1959) The mechanism of fibrosis in arteriosclerosis. Am J Pathol 35: 265-273
12. Haust MD (1978) Light and electron microscopy of human atherosclerotic lesions. Adv Exp Med Biol 104: 33-59
13. Haust MD (1978) Zur Morphologie der Arteriosklerose. Internist (Berlin) 19: 621-626
14. Haust MD (1981) The natural history of atherosclerotic lesions. In: Moore S (ed) Vascular Injury and Atherosclerosis, Marcel Dekker Inc, New York, p 1
15. Haust MD (1982) Atherosclerosis; - lesions and sequelae. In: Silver MD (ed) Cardiovascular Pathology, Churchill-Livingstone, New York, In Press
16. Marshall JR, Adams JG, O'Neal RM, DeBakey ME (1966) The ultrastructure of uncomplicated human atheroma in surgically resected aortas. J Atheroscler Res 6: 120-131
17. Haust MD (1971) The morphogenesis and fate of potential and early atherosclerotic lesions in man. Human Pathol 2: 1-29
18. Haust MD (1978) Atherosclerosis in childhood. In: Rosenberg HS, Bolande RP (eds) Perspectives in Pediatric Pathology, Vol 4, Year Book Medical Publishers Inc, Chicago, Illinois, p 155
19. Geer JC, Haust MD (1972) Smooth Muscle Cells in Atherosclerosis. In: Pollak OJ, Simms HS, Kirk JE (eds) Monographs on Atherosclerosis, Vol 2, S Karger, Basel-London-New York
20. Haust MD, More RH (1958) New functional aspects of smooth muscle cells. Fed Proc 17: 440
21. Haust MD, More RH (1963) Significance of the smooth muscle cell in atherogenesis. In: Jones RJ (ed) Evolution of the Atherosclerotic Plaque, University of Chicago Press, Chicago, p 51
22. Haust MD, More RH, Movat HZ (1960) The role of smooth muscle cells in the fibrogenesis of arteriosclerosis. Am J Pathol 37: 377-389
23. Haust MD (1982) Atherosclerosis and smooth muscle cells. In: Stephens NL (ed) Biochemistry of Smooth Muscle, CRC Press Inc Number 6575, Boca Raton, Florida, In Press
24. Haust MD, More RH (1960) The thrombotic basis of arteriosclerosis. Heart Bull 9: 90-92
25. Haust MD (1977) Thrombosis in the inception and progression of coronary atherosclerotic lesions. In: Schettler G, Horsch A, Mörl H, Orth H, Weizel A (eds) Der Herzinfarkt, FK Schattauer Verlag, Stuttgart-New York, p 120

26. More RH, Movat HZ, Haust MD (1957) Role of mural fibrin thrombi of the aorta in genesis of arteriosclerotic plaque. AMA Arch Pathol 63: 612-620

27. Haust MD (1965) Fine fibrils of extracellular space (microfibrils). Their structure and role in connective tissue organization. Am J Pathol 47: 1113-1137

28. Haust MD, More RH (1966) Mechanism of fibrosis in white atherosclerotic plaque of human aorta: an electron microscopic study. Circulation 34(III): 14

29. Kefalides NA (1973) Structure and biosynthesis of basement membranes. Int Rev Conn Tiss Res 6: 63-104

30. Kefalides NA, Alper R, Clark CC (1979) Biochemistry and metabolism of basement membranes. Int Rev Cytol 61: 167-228

31. Foidart JM, Bere EW Jr, Yaar M, Rennard SI, Gullino M, Martin GR, Katz SI (1980) Distribution and immunoelectron microscopic localization of laminin, a noncollagenous basement membrane glycoprotein. Lab Invest 42: 336-342

32. Rohde H, Wick G, Timpl R (1979) Immunochemical characterization of the basement membrane glycoprotein laminin. Eur J Biochem 102: 195-201

33. Timpl R, Rohde H, Robey PG, Rennard SI, Foidart JM, Martin GR (1979) Laminin--a glycoprotein from basement membranes. J Biol Chem 254: 9933-9937

34. Voss B, Rauterberg J, Jander R, Timpl R (1982) Localization of different collagen types, fibronectin and laminin in blood vessel walls. Abstract (Poster Session P18) No 649, Program, 6th International Symposium on Atherosclerosis, Berlin, June 13-17, p 36

35. Gay S (1982) Immunology of collagens. In: Wagner BM, Fleischmajer R (eds) Connective Tissue and Diseases of Connective Tissue, Williams & Wilkins Co, Baltimore, In Press

36. Hahn E, Wick G, Pencev D, Timpl R (1980) Distribution of basement membrane proteins in normal and fibrotic human liver; collagen type IV, laminin, and fibronectin. Gut 21:63-71

37. Miller EJ, Gay S (1982) The multiple types and forms of collagen - an overview. In: Cunningham LW, Fredrickson DW (eds) Methods in Enzymology, Academic Press, New York

38. Thesleff I, Barrach HJ, Foidart JM, Vaheri A, Pratt RM, Martin GR (1981) Changes in the distribution of type IV collagen, laminin, proteoglycan, and fibronectin during mouse tooth development. Develop Biol 81: 182-192

39. Martin GR, Robey PG, Hassell JR, Liotta LA (1982) Structure and function of basement membranes. In: Wagner BM, Fleischmajer R (eds) Connective Tissue and Diseases of Connective Tissue, Williams & Wilkins Co, Baltimore, In Press

40. Kjellen L, Oldberg A, Höök M (1980) Cell-surface heparan sulfate. Mechanisms of proteoglycan-cell association. J Biol Chem 255: 10407-10413

41. Jellinek H, Harsing J, Füzesi Sz (1982) A new model for arteriosclerosis. An electron-microscopic study of the lesions induced by i.v. administered fat. Atherosclerosis 43: 7-18

42. Leushner JRA, Haust MD (1982) The isolation and characterization of type V collagen from bovine aortae. Abstract (Poster Session P12) No 439, Program, 6th International Symposium on Atherosclerosis, Berlin, June 13-17, p 32

43. Nikkari T, Heikkinen E (1968) The lipids of collagen preparations. Acta Chem Scand 22: 3047-3052

44. McCullagh KG, Ehrhart LA (1974) Increased arterial collagen synthesis in experimental canine atherosclerosis. Atherosclerosis 19: 13-28

45. Hollander W, Colombo MA, Kramsch DM, Kirkpatrick B (1974) Immunological aspects of atherosclerosis. Adv Cardiol 13: 192-207

46. McCullagh KA, Balian G (1975) Collagen characterization and cell transformation in human atherosclerosis. Nature 258: 73-75
47. Morton LF, Barnes MJ (1982) Collagen polymorphism in the normal and diseased blood vessel wall. Investigation of collagens types I, III and V. Atherosclerosis 42: 41-51
48. Balis JU, Haust MD, More RH (1964) Electron-microscopic studies in human atherosclerosis. Cellular elements in aortic fatty streaks. Exp Mol Pathol 3: 511-525
49. Mustard JF (1975) Function of blood platelets and their role in thrombosis. Trans Am Clin Climatol Ass 87: 104-127
50. Chesney C Mcl, Harper E, Colman RW (1974) Human platelet collagenase. J Clin Invest 53: 1647-1654
51. Haust MD (1970) Injury and repair in the pathogenesis of atherosclerotic lesions. In: Jones RJ (ed) Atherosclerosis, Proceedings of the Second International Symposium, Springer-Verlag, New York-Heidelberg-Berlin, p 12
52. Haust MD, More RH (1972) Development of modern theories on the pathogenesis of atherosclerosis. In: Wissler RW, Geer JC (eds) The Pathogenesis of Atherosclerosis, Williams & Wilkins Co, Baltimore, p 1
53. Haust MD (1974) Reaction patterns of intimal mesenchyme to injury, and repair in atherosclerosis. Adv Exp Med Biol 43: 35-57

# Hemodynamics as a Factor in Lesion Localization

R. Nerem and M. J. Levesque

## A. Introduction

In this discussion of hemodynamics as a factor in the localization of atherosclerotic lesions, it is the evidence for a hemodynamic involvement which first will be briefly reviewed. This evidence includes both the pattern of the disease as well as hypertension being a risk factor. As indirect as this evidence is, it has provided the primary motivation for the resurgence of interest in the study of blood flow through large arteries which has taken place over the last 15 years.

The detailed characteristics of arterial flows will be considered next. Blood flow in the major mammalian arteries presents a number of interesting and challenging problems. Such flows are pulsatile and pass through vessels which are complex both in geometry and in their elastic nature. It is the former which is of particular interest with regard to atherosclerosis. It now appears that it is this geometric complexity, as represented by vessel branching and the general tortuosity of the vasculature, which may be all important, not only in determining the detailed characteristics of arterial flows, but also the spatial nature of any hemodynamic involvement in the disease process.

The possible mechanisms through which any such hemodynamic involvement might manifest itself have also been the subject of extensive study. As the interface between the arterial wall and the flowing blood, it is the vascular endothelium which has been focused on in terms of hemodynamics as a factor in atherogenesis. In this there has been a primary interest in the role of mechanical forces, as imposed by the flow of blood, on endothelial morphology and function, and it is this which will be reviewed here.

Finally, these preceding elements will be used to discuss the role of hemodynamics in the disease process. Severe atherosclerosis produces changes in the geometry of some of the larger arteries, and in doing so alters and interferes with blood flow. This is particularly important for the heart and the brain, with the result being myocardial or cerebral ischemia or even a myocardial infarction or stroke. However, even in the early stages of the disease process, i.e. during atherogenesis, it is believed that there is an important relationship between the disease and the characteristics of the blood flowing through the arteries. This is not because the disease in any way has altered the blood flow properties, but rather it is because of the possibility that there may be blood flow or hemodynamic related factors involved in the initiation and early development of the disease. In these early stages of the disease, the vascular geometry is unaltered from its normal state, although this normal geometry may vary considerably from individual to individual. Thus, if there is a role of hemodynamics or arterial fluid dynamics in the early development of atherosclerosis, it is the fluid dynamics of the normal cardiovascular system which is of interest.

Furthermore, considering the characteristic time of this disease, the role of hemodynamics is quite possibly an extremely subtle one. This

suggests that it is the rather detailed hemodynamic characteristics
that may be important, and it is the evidence for such a subtle involvement, the detailed flow characteristics themselves, and the mechanisms
that may be participatory that are discussed here and used to speculate
on the role of hemodynamics in lesion localization.

## B. Evidence for a Hemodynamic Involvement

Although the possible importance of hemodynamics in atherogenesis has
provided a requirement for a more detailed knowledge of the properties
of arterial blood flow, there is some question as to what is the evidence for the involvement of fluid dynamics in the atherosclerotic
process?  The answer here centers primarily on the pattern of the disease (1-3).  Not only is it the aorta as well as the iliac, femoral,
coronary, and cerebral arteries which are most commonly affected, but
to be more specific, it appears that it is often regions of arterial
branching and sharp curvature which have the greatest predilection
for the development of atherosclerosis.  These are also regions where
the flow will assume unusual characteristics or at least deviate from
what otherwise might be considered a well-behaved arterial flow.  It
is the indictment provided by this indirect evidence, particularly
as it relates to the bifurcations and geometrical contortions of the
arterial vasculature, which motivates much of the present interest in
arterial fluid dynamics.

Unfortunately, in terms of understanding the hemodynamic factors in
the atherosclerotic process it is not enough to identify the general
regions of branching and sharp curvature.  This is because such general regions may include locations of flow separation, localized positions of accentuated secondary motion, areas where the wall shear
stress will be high and others where it will be low, and portions of
the wall itself where the stresses within will be intensified and
others where stress levels may be lessened.  The net result is that
any indictment of hemodynamics as a disease factor which is based on
the pattern of the disease only raises questions relative to the details.

Fortunately, there is some information available on the specifics of
the pattern of the disease in man and animals.  These results seem
to divide into two groups.  In human fetuses, neonates and infants
(4) and in experimental diet-induced animal studies (5), the pattern
of the disease appears to favor the occurence of lesions in regions
which, as we will see in the next section, are believed to be high
shear.  However, in adult human disease (3,6,7) and in the White Carneau pigeon (8) where spontaneous atherosclerosis occurs, the disease
pattern appears to favor low shear regions.  This difference in spatial
location between lesions raises important questions, both with regard
to the possible importance of hemodynamics in atherogenèsis and also
in terms of differences in the development of experimental as opposed
to spontaneous disease.

In addition to the pattern of the disease, there is another piece of
evidence with potential hemodynamic implications.  This is that hypertension is a risk factor in coronary artery disease.  A basic question,
the answer to which has considerable implication for hemodynamics, is
whether it is a systolic, diastolic or mean pressure effect or whether
it is a pulse pressure effect.  Unfortunately, the answer to this question is not all clear.  This is because individuals with an elevated
mean arterial pressure in general also have an elevated pulse pressure.

Another logical question is what is the role of blood pressure? At one time it was thought that blood-arterial wall lipid transport was due to a pressure driven, bulk flow process. However, data now available tends to refute any major importance of such a pressure effect (9). There of course still could be a major effect of pressure on the endothelium. Furthermore, if it is mean blood pressure that is important in terms of a hypertension effect, then it may be due to its effect on arterial geometry or on wall metabolism. The former would affect local flow details, while the latter would represent a hemodynamic effect of a very indirect type. Furthermore, if it is an elevated pulse pressure that is important in hypertension being a risk factor, then there is another possibility which presents itself. This is that, associated with an increased pulsed pressure, there would be an altered velocity waveform, an increased peak velocity, and an increased level of wall shear stress (10).

With regard to a pressure effect on arterial geometry, it has been reported that gross elevation of aortic pressure distorts the geometry of the aortic tree to the point where angles of branching are markedly changed (11). This could have the effect of changing a relatively streamlined flow system into one considerably more tortuous which would tend to accentuate the type of complicated fluid dynamic phenomena already discussed. There are also data showing an accelerated occurrence of atherosclerosis in subjects with a human coronary geometry deviating from that normally found (12). Furthermore, aortic coarctation, which represents a major change in vessel geometry, results in a significant alteration in the uptake of Evans Blue dye (13), and our own recent studies have demonstrated a similar effect on endothelial geometry and orientation. In considering the various factors involved in atherogenesis, the one that clearly and most directly would be influenced by arterial geometry would be the detailed hemodynamic characteristics. This suggests that vasculature geometry and the way it influences the local detailed flow properties may be a primary determinant of a hemodynamic effect on atherosclerosis, and this will be explored further in the next few sections.

## C. Detailed characteristics of Arterial Flows

Until recently little information existed about the detailed nature of viscous flow phenomena in the arterial system. This is at first surprising since the subject of viscous flow has been of continuing interest and importance in a wide range of engineering contexts. In general, however, the problem in the arterial system has been uniquely difficult, not only because of the unsteady nature of the basic flow, but also because of limitations on instrumentation and access.

Partly as a result of the motivation provided by a possible role for hemodynamics in atherogenesis, there has been a great deal learned about arterial flows in the last 15 years. A major achievement was the development of the ability to make point-velocity measurements within blood vessels. Such measurements have become possible with the hot-film constant temperature anemometer and the pulsed ultrasonic Doppler systems. These techniques have provided for the first time insight into the temporal and spatial velocity variations present locally in the vascular system. In vivo studies using such point velocity measurement systems have been carried out in a variety of animals and in humans (14-18). Furthermore, laser Doppler anemometry has been used in physical model studies (7). From this combination of approaches a much clearer picture of arterial fluid dynamics has emerged.

The classical problem used to explain the detailed characteristics of flowing blood is that of Poiseuille flow. In this the flow is likened to that in a long, rigid, circular pipe with a constant flow rate. The velocity pattern or velocity profile, i.e., the variation in velocity as one moves radially across the lumen of the vessel from one wall to the other, is characterized as being parabolic. However, we now know that flow in the circulation system in general is not Poiseuillian in nature, i.e. it is not a fully developed viscous flow characterized by a parabolic profile.

There are many reasons for this. Primary among these is the unsteady nature of the flow in large arteries--the concept of Poiseuille flow strictly speaking only applies under steady state flow conditions. There is also the possibility of transition to turbulence (16) at least in the aorta. In the context of our interests here, however, one of the very major complexities of blood flow is that the vessels involved are often curved, and they branch repeatedly. This asymmetric geometry quite naturally produces asymmetries in the velocity patterns, complicated secondary motions, entry phenomena and even flow separation, all of which are far more difficult to analyze than the simple problem of steady state, fully developed Poiseuille flow (10).

The entrance effect, or the existence of an entry length, is a well-known problem in fluid dynamics (19). In general, when a flow passes from a large diameter vessel into a smaller one, the velocity distribution at the entrance to the smaller vessel is found to be rather blunt. A wall boundary layer, initially very thin at the entrance of the vessel, increases in thickness as the flow proceeds distally. At a distance from the entrance called the entry length, the boundary layer closes in on itself, and at this point the frictional effect of a viscous fluid passing through the vessel has spread across the entire lumen of the vessel. If one calculates the entry lenth for flow in the human aorta (10), the result is a length of at least 150 cm which is far greater than the length of the aorta. The flow in the aorta thus cannot be characterized as fully developed, and this has been shown experimentally (14-16). In fact, all the larger arteries of the circulatory system, including the epicardial coronary vessels, are subject to entrance effects.

An additional complexity of the arterial system is that its asymmetric geometry, including vessel branching and curvature, quite naturally produces asymmetries in the velocity patterns. For example, at a bifurcation the flow in the upstream parent vessel divides into the two daughter vessels so as to bring relative high velocity blood at the center of the parent vessel in close proximity to the wall of the flow divider and this has been demonstrated both for aortic (14,15) and coronary flows (17). Skewing of the velocity profile also occurs in a curved vessel. The nature of this skewing depends on whether the flow is largely inviscid or fully viscous. By largely inviscid is meant a flow such as present in the ascending aorta which is an entrance region where viscous effects are confined to a thin wall boundary layer (15). In the fully viscous case, on the other hand, the flow is skewed towards the outer wall. An example of this is the flow in the left common coronary artery (17). Furthermore, the bifurcation of the left common into the LAD and the left circumflex coronary arteries represents a case where there is skewing both due to branching and curvature. Our own studies demonstrate that the skewing produced by the curving of these vessels over the heart in many cases dominates that associated with the bifurcation process, depending of course on the exact geometry.

Associated with the flow in a bifurcation or a curved vessel is the

secondary motion induced by the curved path the fluid must follow.
Secondary flows are characterized by a swirling, helical component
superimposed on  the main streamwise velocity along the tube axis.
The most familiar example is that of steady flow in a pipe (19) a
relevant example, since the arch of the aorta is in effect a pipe
bend.   Secondary motions are also produced by branchings, where, just
as in a curved pipe, the curvature associated with the change in flow
direction is accompanied by a centrifugal pressure gradient.   Although
there have been numerous fluid dynamic studies of secondary flow phenomena (10), instrumentation limitations have prevented any in vivo observations.

An additional complication introduced by the geometry of the arterial
system is that the flow may actually separate from the wall giving
rise to a recirculating, dead-water region which can be slow moving,
almost stagnant fluid.   For example, for steady flow in a bifurcation the flow may separate because of the adverse pressure gradient
associated with the deceleration of the fluid as it passes from the
parent vessel into daughter vessels whose combined cross-sectional area
exceeds that of the parent vessel.   Downstream of the bifurcation the
flow will reattach to the wall.   The bubble or recirculation region
located between the points of separation and reattachment contains
recirculating fluid.   Needless to say, the occurrence of flow separation in pulsatile flows is an extremely complex phenomena.   In a
pulsatile flow, the recirculation region is itself unsteady in nature
and flow separation and reattachment points, if present, can change
location or even disappear and then reappear as the flow pulses.   Flow
patterns for oscillatory flows obviously will be more complicated than
for steady flows, and very little is yet known about the details of
many of the phenomena discussed here for arterial blood flow conditions.

Associated with the local velocity pattern, there will be a mechanical, hemodynamic force exerted by the flowing blood on the arterial
wall.   The effect of this force has been of particular interest in
terms of any hemodynamic-endothelium interaction.   The force per unit
wall area is denoted as a stress, and the total stress imposed on the
artery wall by the flow of blood is manifested through both a normal
and a tangential component.   The normal component of the stress is
essentially equal to the blood pressure.   The tangential component is
a frictional force per unit area and is termed the wall shear stress.
The wall shear stress is equal to the product of the fluid viscosity
and the shear rate, S, evaluated at the wall.   The latter is by defi-
niton equal to rate of change in the streamwise velocity component as
one moves away from the wall, across the lumen of the vessel.

Whereas a blood pressure of 100 mm Hg represents a normal force in
excess of $10^5$ dynes/cm$^2$, wall shear stresses are believed to be several
order of magnitudes lower.   Limited experimental data (some of which
is suspect) as well as theoretical determinations indicate peak shear
stresses at the level of 100-200 dynes/cm$^2$ (10).   Although the shear
stress levels are obviously much smaller than the stress due to normal
pressure, it may well be that the arterial wall is designed to take a
much higher normal stess.

It is through our understanding of arterial blood flow, as summarized
here, that we believe we can characterize vascular regions as high
shear or low shear as done in the previous section.   For example, in
a region of branching in general we would expect the flow divider to
experience higher shear, while immediately proximal to the branch, the
shear should be relatively lower.   However, there is a certain element

of risk in doing this for in complicated flow regions the shear stress
can vary considerably over a very short distance. For example, in the
region of the iliac bifurcation one might speculate that the shear
would be low on the outer walls. However, there is now data suggesting
that as the flow passes into the daughter vessels, there is a significant increase in the shear stress level (20). Thus, depending exactly
on where you are located on the outer wall, it may be a region of low
shear stress on one of high shear stress.

## D. Mechanical Influences on the Endothelium

Early studies of a possible influence of hemodynamic events on the
endothelium focused on transendothelial transport. Fry's results
(21) suggest that the wall shear stress influences the rate of transport of macromolecules between blood and the arterial wall, and the
results of Caro and Nerem (22) using $^{14}C$-4-cholesterol have shown
that it is not an effect of wall shear on diffusion boundary layer
transport, but one considerably more subtle in the terms of an effect
of shear stress on the properties of the arterial wall. Similar steady
flow results have been obtained using $^{131}I$-albumin, and data from both
radioactively labelled albumin and cholesterol experiments indicating
that is is not only the mean component of arterial pressure and flow,
but also the oscillatory nature of the phenomena which has an important influence on the blood-arterial wall transport of macromolecules
(23-24). These results suggest that, at a shear stress level greater
than 50 dynes/cm$^2$, there is a much stronger dependence of the transport rate on shear stress (9). The more recent results of Thibault
et al. (25) confirm this, but raise the question as to whether excised
vessels at such stress levels have an intact endothelium.

The interest in shear-dependent macromolecule transport stems from it
being the link between luminal hemodynamic events and biochemical
processes within the arterial wall. However, there are at least two
other mechanisms which lend themselves to a shear-dependent hypothesis. The first of these is hemodynamics being a controlling factor
in determining the availability of oxygen to the intima (10,26). There
have been a number of observations correlating hypoxic conditions and
the incidence of atherosclerosis, and assuming that the diffusion
boundary layer is rate-limiting oxygen transport, then it is low shear
regions of the wall which would have the greater predilection for
tissue hypoxia. The other way in which hemodynamic considerations
would favor a low shear hypothesis is if shear does in fact determine
platelet deposition. As inferred earlier, there may be many ways in
which endothelial injury can occur, possibly on a continuing and random basis. Such injury might then be followed by platelet deposition, release reactions, and smooth muscle cell proliferation -- in
some cases leading to repair of the wall and in some cases leading to
atherogenesis. If platelet deposition is enhanced in low shear regions (27), then a disease pattern would emerge which would be consistent with a low shear hypothesis.

There is also a body of accumulating data which indicates that endothelial cell geometry and orientation is determined by hemodynamic
forces. If the functioning of a cell is influenced by its shape, then
this could be a means whereby a hemodynamic effect becomes manifest.
Whether this would support a high shear or low shear interpretation
of the pattern of the disease would of course depend on the exact
nature of any relationship between cell function and cell shape. Of
particular interest in our studies of arterial endothelium has been
the influence of hemodynamic forces, i.e. the effect or pressure and
of wall shear stress. Using the vascular casting technique, endo-

thelial cell patterns in the region of intercostal ostia, as determined
from casts of rabbit aortae, have been shown to be very much suggestive
of the complicated flow patterns that one might expect to be present
(28). Recently in vitro studies of the endothelial cellular dynamics
have been initiated using cultured populations of vascular cells. Dewey
et al. (29) have reported the use of a rotating cone-plate viscometer to
study cultured bovine aortic endothelial cells under conditions of a
uniform fluid shear stress. In our own laboratory we are using a parallel plate, channel flow device for similar studies. Our initial studies
also have involved the use of cultured bovine aortic endothelial cells
(second and third passage), on either a polystyrene or glass substrate,
and exposed to a constant shear stress in the range of 8-16 dynes/cm$^2$
for a time period of anywhere from one to five hours. Although only
preliminary results are available at this time, there has been a clear
indication of the presence of a shear stress effect. For example, using
a glass substrate with only a one hour exposure to a shear stress of
9 dynes/cm$^2$, there is almost a total orientation of the cells with the
direction of flow. Although the orientation of the cells was initially
random, within the one hour period 60 per cent of the cells had achieved
an angle of orientation of within 10$^0$ to the direction of flow, another
32 per cent of the cells had an angle between 10$^0$ and 20$^0$, and only 8
per cent of the cells had an angle of orientation greater than 20$^0$. This
is to be contrasted with a similar population of endothelial cells on a
polystyrene substrate exposed to a shear stress of 16 dynes/cm$^2$ and where,
although here also there was a tendency to orient the cells in the direction of the flow, even after five hours 60 per cent of the cells still
had an angle of orientation greater than 20$^0$. Furthermore, whereas the
cells on a glass substrate showed a strong correlation between shape and
angle of orientation after one hour, the cells on a polystyrene substrate showed no such correlation, even after five hours. The preliminary data obtained thus suggest that there is a definite shear stress
effect on endothelial morphology, but one which is highly dependent on
substrate attachment. If cell function is in some manner related to cell
shape, then it would not be surprising if, for example, endothelial cell
turnover rate was influenced by hemodynamic events. Certainly, in vivo
data (30) suggest that endothelial cell turnover rate may be different
in regions which are believed to be different in shear.

E. Concluding discussion

All of the evidence for a hemodynamic involvement presented here are in
fact geometry related. This thus suggests that vascular geometry, and
the way it influences the local detailed flow properties, may be the primary determinant of a hemodynamic effect on atherosclerosis. Under such
a hypothesis whatever affects vascular geometry would alter the local,
detailed flow characteristics and correspondingly influence endothelial
morphology and function. For an individual subject, that geometry might
be inherited, i.e. a family history or genetic effect, and as such one's
geometry may in and of itself be a risk factor. Alternatively, a subject's vascular geometry may have been significantly altered by a risk
factor such as hypertension. However, whatever the effect, the primary
determinant of the pattern of atherogenesis would be vascular geometry,
and whether or not an individual has an abnormal predilection for the
disease would depend not only on biochemically related factors, but also
on the exact nature of the geometry, e.g. branching pattern and degree of
curvature and/or tortuosity, and the resulting detailed hemodynamic
characteristics.

A few years ago the prevailing view was that if one could produce a sta-

tistically significant picture of the pattern of the disease and a correspondingly statistically significant picture of the flow pattern,
then one could draw conclusions on the relationship of hemodynamics to
atherogenesis.  However, it now appears that it is not the normal
pattern of disease (in the sense of mean data representing the statistically normal situation) nor the normal flow pattern which are of
interest.  Rather, it is *deviations* from the *normal* which are important, and it is in this context that *vascular geometry* may be a *risk
factor*.  From this point of view, vascular geometry, whether inherited
or as altered by the influence of a factor like elevated blood pressure, would determine the local, detailed hemodynamics and the resulting influence on endothelial morphology and function.  This together with other, biochemically-related factors, would determine the
focal nature of the disease.  It is thus geometry--and through geometry, hemodynamics--which we believe to be a factor in lesion localization.

*Acknowledgment*   The authors thank S.A. Altobelli, C.G. Caro and W.A.
Seed for their contributions to the work and ideas reflected in this
paper.  The authors also are appreciative of the support provided by
the National Science Foundation through Grant CME-80-01701.

## References

1. Mitchell JRA, Schwartz CJ (1965) Arterial Disease. Blackwell Scientific publishing Ltd, Oxford, England
2. Montenegro MR, Effen DA (1968) Topography of atherosclerosis in the
coronary arteries.  Lab Invest 18:126
3. Caro CG, Fitz-Gerald JM, Schroter RC (1971) Atheroma and arterial
wall shear:  observation, correlation and proposal of a shear dependent mass transfer mechanism for atherogenesis.  Proc R Soc Lond
(Biol) 177:109
4. Sinzinger H, Silberbauer K, Auerswald W (1980) Quantative investigation of sudanophilic lesions around the aortic ostia of human
fetuses, newborn, and children.  Blodd Vessels 17:44
5. Cornhill JF, Roach MR (1976)  A quantitative study of the localization of atherosclerotic lesions in the rabbit aorta.  Atherosclerosis 23:489
6. Kjaernes M, Svindland A, Walløe L, Wille SØ  Localization of early
atherosclerotic lesions in an arterial bifurcation in humans.  Acta
Path Microbiol Scand Sect A 89:35
7. Friedmann MH, Hutchins GM, Bargeron CB, Deters OJ, Mark FF (1981)
Correlation of human arterial morphology with hemodynamic measurements in arterial casts.  ASME J Biomech Engr 103:204
8. Cornhill JF, Levesque MJ, Nerem RM (1980) Quantitative study of the
localization of sudanophilic coeliac lesions in the White Carneau
pigeon.  Atherosclerosis 35: 103
9. Caro CG (1975) Mechanical factors in atherogenesis.  In: Hwang NCH,
Nørman NA (eds) Cardiovascular flow dynamics and measurements.  University Park Press, Baltimore, MD p 473
10. Nerem RM, (1981) Arterial fluid dynamics and interactions with
vessel walls.  In: Schwartz CJ (ed) Structure and function of the
circulation, Vol. 2 Plenum Press, NY p 719
11. Fry DL (1976) Hemodynamic forces in atherogenesis.  In: Scheinberg P
(ed) Cerebrovascular Diseases. Raven Press, NY p 77
12. Velican D, Velican C (1981) Accelerated atherosclerosis in subjects
with some minor deviations from the common type of distribution of
human coronary arteries.  Atherosclerosis 40:309

13. Somer JB., Evans G, Schwartz CJ (1972) Influence of experimental aortic coarctation on the pattern of aortic Evans blue uptake in vivo. Atherosclerosis 16:127
14. Schultz DL, Tunstall-Pedoe DS, Lee GJ, Gunning AJ, Bellhouse BJ (1969) Velocity distribution and transition in the arterial system. In: Wolstenholme GEW, Knight J (eds) Circulatory and Respiratory Mass Transport. J. and A. Churchill, London p 172
15. Seed WA, Wood NB (1971) Velocity patterns in the aorta. Cardiovascular Res. 5:319
16. Nerem RM, Seed WA, Wood NB (1972) An experimental study of the velocity distribution and transition to turbulence in the aorta. J. Fluid Mech. 52:137
17. Nerem RM, Rumberger JA, Jr, Gross DR, Muir WW, Geiger GL (1976) Hot-film coronary artery velocity measurements in horses. Cardiovascular Res. 10:301.
18. Wells MK, Winter DC, Nelson AW, McCarthy TC (1977) Blood velocity patterns in coronary arteries. ASME J Biomech Engr 99:26
19. Pedley TJ (1980) The fluid mechanics of large blood vessels. Cambridge Univ. Press, Cambridge, England
20. Walburn FJ, Stein PD (1982) Shear rate at the wall in a symmetrically branched tube simulating the aortic bifurcation. Biorheology 19:307
21. Fry DL (1969) Certain histological and chemical responses of the vascular interface to acutely induced mechanical stress in the aorta of the dog. Circ Res 24:93
22. Caro CG, Nerem RM (1973 Transport of $^{14}$C-4-cholesterol between serum and wall in perfused dog common carotid artery. Circ Res 32:187
23. Nerem RM, Mosberg AT, Shwerin WD (1975) Transendothelial transport of $^{131}$I-albumin. Biorheology 12:31
24. Chien S, Lee MML, Laufer LS, Handley DA, Weinbaum S, Caro CG, Usami S (1981) Effects of oscillatory mechanical disturbance on macromolecular uptake by arterial wall. Arteriosclerosis 1:326
25. Thibault LE, Fry DL (1980) Hydrodynamically induced wall shear stress effects on Evans blue dye uptake. In: Nerem RM, Guyton JR (eds) Hemodynamics and the Arterial Wall. University of Houston, Houston, TX p 34
26. Crawford DW, Back LH, Cole MA (1980) In vivo measurements of the boundary layer oxygen gradient in the normal dog femoral artery. In: Nerem RM, Guyton JR (eds) Hemodynamics and the arterial wall. University of Houston, Houston, TX p 67
27. Forstrom RJ, Voss GO, Blackshear PL Jr, (1974) Fluid dynamics of particle (platelet) deposition for filtering walls: relationship to atherosclerosis. ASME Fluids Eng 96:168
28. Nerem RM, Levesque MJ, Cornhill JF (1981) Vascular endothelial morphology as an indicator of blood Flow. ASME J Biomech Engr 103:172
29. Dewey CF, Bussolari SR, Gimbrone MA, Davies PF (1981) The dynamic response of vascular endothelial cells to fluid shear stress. ASME J Biomech Engr 103:177
30. Wright HP (1972) Mitosis patterns in aortic endothelium. Atherosclerosis 15:93

# Role of Connective Tissue in the Arterio-Atherosclerotic Process. Interest of a Cell-Matrix Directed Pharmacology

L. Robert, W. Hornebeck, and A. M. Robert

## Introduction

Vascular wall of all sizes from capillaries to the large arterial
trunks contain cells and intercellular matrix variable in quantity
(cell/matrix ratio), and also in quality (nature and relative amount
of matrix macromolecules). Capillaries contain basement membranes
elaborated by endothelial cells and perhaps pericytes. Basement membranes are known to be composed of several matrix macromolecules,
such as collagen type IV, laminin, fibronectin, heparan-sulphate
proteoglycans and some other less well characterised glycoproteins
(1, 2, 3). The large vessel walls such as the aorta contain several
differentiated cell types such as the endothelial cells, smooth
muscle cells, fibroblasts and probably also migrating cells such as
monocytes-macrophages. Such vessels contain also large amounts of
intercellular matrix macromolecules and the cell/matrix ratio is
often much in favor of the intercellular matrix. Several laboratories
invested a great effort in the isolation and characterisation of the
intercellular matrix components of vascular wall. It is beyond the
scope of this presentation to review this rapidly growing field.
Instead we shall describe shortly some of those experiments which
enlighten the intricate interrelationship between cells and the
intercellular matrix elements of the vascular wall.

Table 1. Distribution of intercellular matrix macromolecules in small
and large vascular walls

| Class of matrix macromolecules | Capillary wall (basal lamina) | Large arterial wall (aorta) |
|---|---|---|
| I. Collagens | Type IV (V) | Types I, III, IV, V, SC |
| II. Elastin | Absent | Present in media |
| III. Proteoglycans | PG-heparan sulphate | PG-heparan-sulphate -dermatan-sulphate -chondroitin-sulphates hyaluronate |
| IV. Structural glycoproteins | Laminin, fibro- nectin (entactin, protein P) | Microfibrils*, fibronec- tin, laminin. Four other glycopro- teins (3) with MW-s of $3.5 \ 10^4 KD$ ; $5 \ 10^4 KD$ ; $1.5 \ 10^5 KD$ ; $2.0 \ 10^5 KD$. |

* "Microfibrils" present in the intima and in the elastic fibers
of the media were shown to contain probably 2 to 3 different
glycoproteins.

Schematically, we can divided these matrix macromolecules into four
classes : (a) the collagen class and (b) the elastic fibers form
the fibrous proteins, (c) proteoglycans and (d) structural glycopro-

teins constitute the "amorphous" matrix elements. Proteoglycans are
mostly present in the interfibrillary space and structural glycoproteins assure the cohesion between the cell membranes and the intercellular matrix. They also appear to play a role in the vectorial
(oriented) biosynthesis of elastic and perhaps also collagen fibers.
Table 1 shows the distribution of these four classes of intercellular matrix macromolecules in capillaries and large arteries.

## Regulation of the Synthesis and Degradation of Matrix Macromolecules

The experiments performed in several laboratories, over the last
years, showed that these intercellular matrix macromolecules are
synthesised very early during the ontogenetic development of the
embryo in a well defined sequential fashion, starting appearantly
with the structural glycoproteins (laminin, fibronectin) and the
basement membrane collagens (4, 5). The morphogenesis of the vascular
wall is based on this sequential expression of the structural genes
coding for the matrix macromolecules, in variable quality and quantity according to the type of vessel wall. These matrix components
interact in the extracellular space and define by these interactions
the morphology and microarchitecture of the vessel wall. The differentiated cells will then "live" in their microenvironment composed
of the matrix elements they synthesise according to their genetic
"program" (Figure 1).

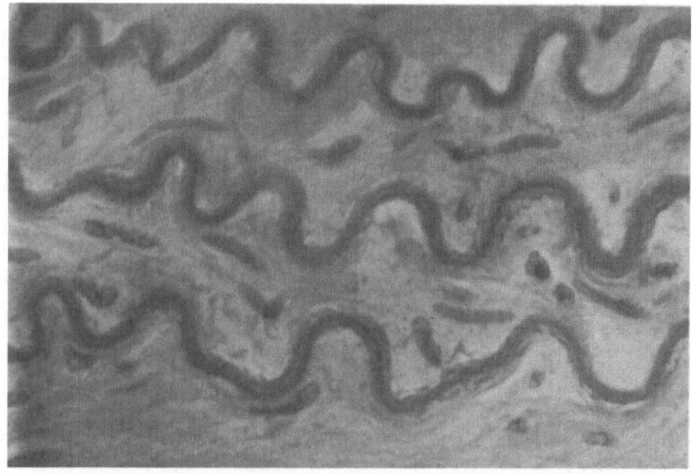

Fig. 1. Microphotography of a normal rabbit aorta-media. The smooth
muscle cells are relatively far apart, embedded in the intercellular
matrix they synthesise and secrete according to their normal "program" of differentiation. The integrity of the elastic fibers appears
to be an important factor in the maintenance of their normal environment

Although this "program" of biosynthesis appears to be genetically
determined, it is also under the influence of environmental factors
such as the nutritional factors, molecular and cellular elements of
the circulating blood and are also influenced by the action of
hormons, growth factors,and neuro-transmitters. All these influences
may produce deviations from the normal "program" of biosynthesis.

The formation of the atherosclerotic plaque is an example of a perturbation of the normal "program" of matrix biosynthesis. Arteriosclerosis, as observed during the aging of the arterial wall, may well be the result to a large extent of the genetic "program" itself (6).

We studied previously the action of lipoproteins on the biosynthetic activity of smooth muscle cells in aorta explants from normal rabbits (7). It appeared that collagen synthesis was selectively enhanced, all other incorporations were inhibited. When aorta explants of hyperlipidemic (cholesterol fed) rabbits were studied with a similar technique, they appeared to exhibit a higher biosynthetic activity for collagen and several other matrix macromolecules than control aortas (8). This oversynthesis of matrix macromolecules is appearant in the plaque formation where the migrating smooth muscle cells produce in a disordered fashion collagen, elastin and several other matrix macromolecules. We also studied another type of experimental arteriosclerotic model which is obtained by the immunisation of rabbits with $\kappa$-elastin in complete Freund's adjuvant (9). In this model strongly calcified arteriosclerotic plaques are produced with no or little lipid deposition. The arteries of these immunised rabbits exhibit a decreased incorporation rate when incubated with radioactive precursors (8). Table II shows this opposite effect of cholesterol feeding and elastin immunisation on the incorporation of $^{14}$C-lysine in fibrous elastin by rabbit aorta explants.

Table 2. Comparison of two different athero-arteriosclerotic models on the incorporation of $^{14}$C-lysine in fibrous elastin and on the elastase-type protease activity of rabbit aorta. I = high cholesterol diet. II = immunization with $\kappa$-elastin peptides. Average values for the number of animals indicated in parenthesis ± SEM (from JACOB et al.(8

| | Elastase-type activity (Suc-Ala)$_3$-pNa) ng panc. el. equivalents per mg DNA | Elastin biosynthesis cpm incorporated in the elastase extract of aorta per mg DNA x $10^{-3}$ |
|---|---|---|
| I - A. Control (7) | 60.4* ± 9.8 | 17.3 ± 4.6 |
| B. Cholesterol (6) | 130* ± 18.3 | 20.6 ± 2.6 |
| RATIO B/A | 2.2 (S) | 1.2 |
| | | |
| II - A. Control (7) | 130** ± 23.4 | 17.1 ± 0.70 |
| B. $\kappa$-elastin immunized rabbits (7) | 434** ± 111.2 | 6.0 ± 2.0 |
| RATIO B/A | 3.3 (S) | 0.35 (S) |

* determined on $MgCl_2$-extract
** determined on guanidinium-chloride extract.
The statistical variations between control and treated animals were evaluated by the Mann-Whitney distribution free test. S = significant difference ($\alpha < 0.01$).

In both models we could show however that the common feature is a strong increase of the elastase-type protease activity of the aorta extracts (8). This enzyme was recently isolated and characterised in our laboratory and shown to be a membrane-bound serine protease (10, 11, 12). Its biosynthesis in rat aorta smooth muscle cell cultures was recently studied with D. Bréchemier (13). The activity of the enzyme increased with passage number and with the *in vitro* age of the culture. The enzyme may well have an important biological role other than pathological elastolysis which appears to be triggered by the release of the enzyme, appearently (among other possible factors) by interaction with LDL (13, 14). This increase of elastase-type activity in smooth muscle cells may well explain the conspicuous decrease of elastic fibers in the elastin-immunized rabbit aorta (Fig. 2).

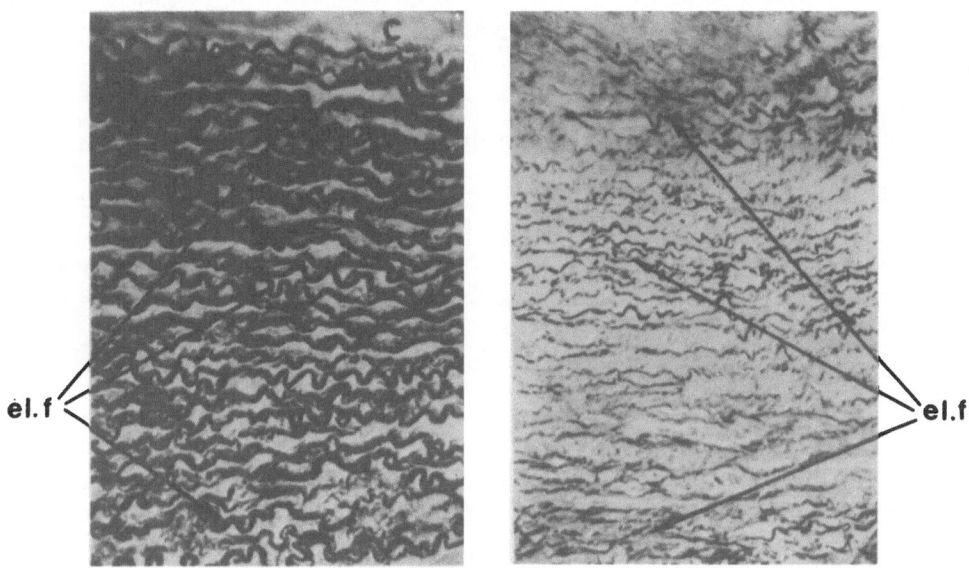

Fig. 2. Orcein-stained sections of the aorta of a normal rabbit (left) and of a rabbit immunised for 2 months with κ-elastin peptides in complete Freund's adjuvant. Notice the strong decrease of elastic fibers (from Godeau et al. (14))

Another elastase-type protease was recently isolated in our laboratory from human skin fibroblasts and shown to be a metallo-enzyme (12, 15). When injected into the skin of a rabbit or when applied to frozen skin sections, this enzyme hydrolyses elastic fibers as efficiently as leucocyte elastase (Fig. 3). These results lend support to the hypothesis of C. Frances et al. (15) attributing the disappearance of dermal elastic fibers and fibronectin in lychen *Sclerosus atrophicus* to the increase and liberation of this fibroblast-derived elastase-type protease. This enzyme may well be involved also in the progressive lysis of the elastic fibers of the superficial dermis in humans. This process shown in Fig. 4 was shown by Bouissou and collegues to proceed in a parallel fashion to elastolysis in the aorta and is strongly accelerated in diabetic and atherosclerotic patients (16). Skin biopsy is therefore a helpful tool in the evaluation of the progression of the arterial lesion. The above-mentioned cellular elastase-type enzymes act not only on the elastin component of elastic fibers but also on the "microfibrils". These modifications may be related to the increased deposition of cholesterol-esters in dermal matrix macromolecules, again in parallel with their deposition in cells and matrix of the arterial wall.

374

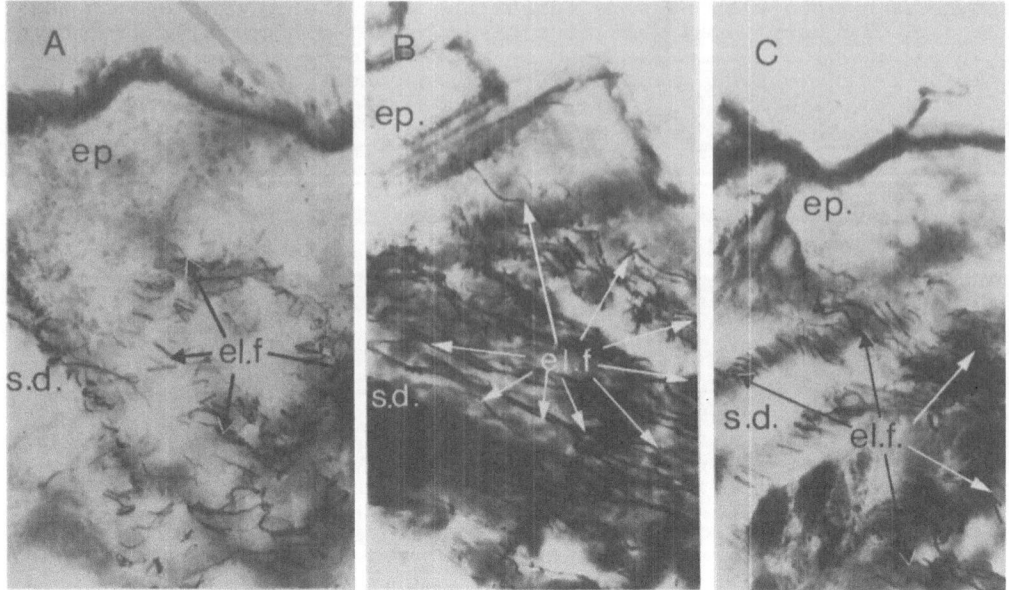

Fig. 3. Histological disappearance of elastic fibers components in the superficial dermis of rabbit six hours after elastase-type enzyme injections. (A) Intradermal injection of 30 μg of purified human leukocyte elastase. (B) Injection of sterile physiological saline. (C) Injection of 75 μg or partially purified human vulvar fibroblast elastase-type enzyme. Modified orcein staining technique. ep = epidermis ; sd = superficial dermis ; el.f = elastic fibers (arrows). Magnification 1,000 x. Elastic fibers : fibers with thickness comprised between 4-7 μm. (from Godeau et al. (15))

Another potential source of elastase-type proteases was identified recently in blood serum lipoproteins (17). All three fractions of serum lipoproteins isolated by ultracentrifugation (VLDL, LDL, HDL) contained elastase-type protease activity (Table 3). The protease present in HDL preparations was isolated and characterized and shown to be specifically associated with apo-$A_1$ (16). This enzyme was shown to cleave the apoproteins and may well play a role during the interaction between lipoproteins and arterial wall elements.

Another example of the deranged regulation of matrix macromolecule biosynthesis is the modification of the distribution of the different collagen types in atherosclerotic aortas. It was reported (18, 19) that collagen type I is increased in the plaque regions. Our own experiments performed on human post-mortem material with antibodies directed to collagens type I, III and to fibronectin as well as using the histochemical staining procedure of Junqueira (20) gave somewhat different results (21).

The early plaques as well as dissected areas of the media seem to be enriched in type III collagen and fibronectin which are codistributed and only the more evolved, aging plaques as well as the whole neo-intima of the arteriosclerotically modified human aorta appears to be enriched in type I collagen (Figure 4).

Table 3. Elastase-type activities determined on Suc(Ala)$_3$pNa of several lipoprotein fractions of human sera. Specific activity was determined in the following conditions : Buffer : 100 mM Tris-HCl, CaCl$_2$ 5 mM, Brij 35 0.1 %, NaN$_3$ 0.02 %, pH 8.0. Temperature : 37°C. Substrate concentration : 2.5 mM. Specific activity : nmole substrate hydrolysed per hour per mg of protein. % of total activity refers to the total elastase-type activity determined with the same substrate in the unfractionated sera. 1 μg of porcine pancreatic elastase (75 U/mg) hydrolyzed 245 nmoles of substrate in 1 hour under similar experimental conditions. The results represented the mean of 3 separate determinations. nd = not determined. (from JACOB et al.(8))

| Preparations | Serum number | | | |
|---|---|---|---|---|
|  | 1 | 2 | 3 | 4 |
| HDL 1.063<d<1.06 |  |  |  |  |
|   Spec. act. | 17.2 | 14.4 | 3.6 | 1.0 |
|   % of total | 5.9 | 23.0 | 4.0 | nd |
| LDL 1.006<d<1.063 |  |  |  |  |
|   Spec. act. | 9.42 | 11.8 | 2.1 | 0.56 |
|   % of total | 3.5 | 0.4 | 0.3 | nd |
| VLDL d<1.006 |  |  |  |  |
|   Spec. act. | 11.8 | 73.6 | 16.8 | 2.23 |
|   % of total | 3.3 | 7.6 | 3.6 | nd |
| Residual serum |  |  |  |  |
|   Spec. act. | 0.625 | 0.425 | 0.595 | nd |
|   % of total | 87.3 | 69.0 | 92.1 | nd |

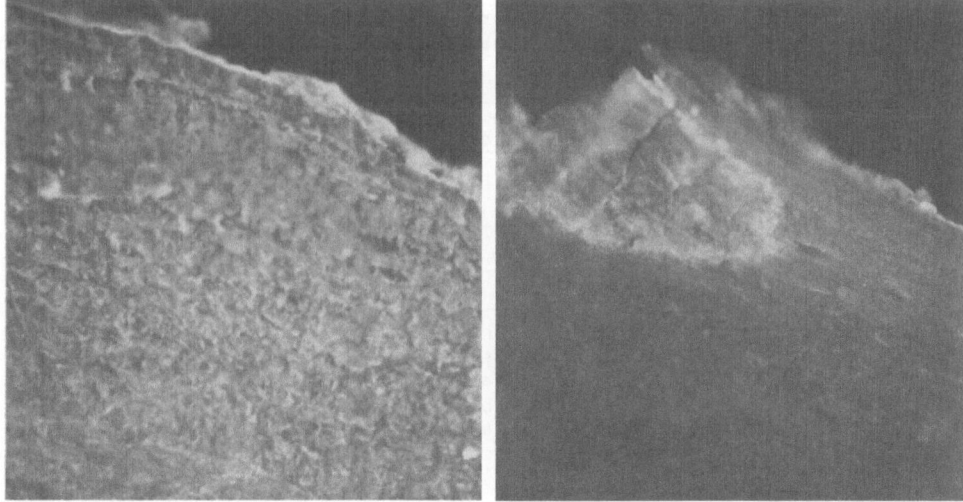

Fig. 4. Fibronectin in human atherosclerotic lesion, demonstrated by immunofluorescence techniques using rhodamin-stained anti-rabbit IgG antibodies. Left = relatively lesion free area of human aorta. Right = accumulation of fibronectin in the atherosclerotic lesion. Collagen type III shows the same localisation (from J. Labat-Robert et al. (21))

## Pharmacology of Matrix Biosynthesis and Cell-Matrix Interaction in the Vascular Wall

Pathological modification of matrix biosynthesis and/or degradation will result in a deranged cell-matrix interaction. Normal cell-matrix interaction, as determined by the "program" of biosynthesis of matrix macromolecules by differentiated vessel wall cells appears to be a prerequisit of the homeostasis of the vessel wall. Deranged cell-matrix interaction, as a result of the loss of membrane bound fibronectin, was shown to be a crucial factor in the anarchical behaviour of tumor cells (22, 23, 24). It appeared therefore interesting to investigate the possibility of pharmacologically modifying matrix biosynthesis and thereby cell-matrix interaction. The above summarized results rendered possible the study of pharmacologically active substances in model systems such as the cholesterol induced atheroma, and elastin-immun arteriosclerosis using quantitative morphometry and the *in vitro* explant (organ culture) or cell culture system by studying the modification of the biosynthetic pattern of matrix macromolecules produced by the smooth muscle cells.

We concentrated our attention on substances which cannot be considered primarily as hypolipidemic drugs. Table 4 summarizes the substances which were studied in our laboratory in this respect. Interesting results were obtained with several drugs. When calcitonin was administered during the immunization of rabbits with κ-elastin, it exerted a pronounced protective action against the development of immune arteriosclerosis (28).

Table 4. Drugs studied in our laboratory and shown to be able to modify the biosynthesis of matrix macromolecules by smooth muscle cells in rabbit aorta organ cultures or cell cultures using both *in vivo* or *in vitro* "treatment" of normal, cholesterol fed or κ-elastin immunised animals

| Drug | Matrix macromolecules most influenced | Observation and reference |
|---|---|---|
| Anthocyanosides and procyanidolic oligomers | Collagens, elastin | Increase cross-linking, resistance to collagenase and protect against its permeability increasing action (25, 26, 27). |
| Calcitonine | Decreased elastolysis (immun-atheroscler. model), decreased lipid matrix interaction (cholesterol ather. model, brain capillaries) | Mechanism of action yet unknown (28, 29) |
| α and β-blocking agents | Proteoglycans and collagen synthesis | Specific receptor mediated mechanism (?) (30, 31). |
| Colchicin | Proteoglycans ;inhibits increased collagen synthesis in cholesterol fed rabbit aorta. | Decreases also HDL/LDL+ VLDL ratio and lipid deposition in aorta,acts possibly through the modification of the "exportation" process (32) |

More recently, we investigated the action of calcitonin on the cholesterol induced atheroma in rabbits and found again a protective action at the level of the brain microvessels and also, to a lesser extent, at the level of the aorta (28, 29).

The demonstration of the increase of prostacyclin formation by Clopath and Sinzinger (33) as a result of calcitonin administration may be one of the factors explaining the above results.

Another group of substances studied include α and β-blocking drugs. We could show that α and β-blocking substances do modify the biosynthetic activity of smooth muscle cells in aorta explants. This was particularly pronounced at the level of proteoglycan and collagen biosynthesis.

Flavonoid-anthocyanoside type of substances such as the oligomers of procyanidol exert a different type of protective action on the vascular wall. This action was particularly clearcut at the level of the brain microvessels (25-27). Rabbits pretreated for 2 to 3 weeks with such drugs resisted intraventricular injection of collagenase which in untreated animals considerably increased the permeability of the blood brain barrier. It was previously demonstrated that this permeability increasing action of the collagenolytic enzymes is due to their attack of the basement membrane of brain microvessels accompanied by a strong increase of the pynocytotic activity of the endothelial cells (25-27).

It appears that the flavonoid-anthocyanoside type of substances act on the collagenous component of the vascular wall by increasing its resistance to collagenase.

Similar *in vivo-in vitro* experiments were also performed with colchicin (32). Rabbits treated with colchicin during cholesterol feeding had higher serum HDL/LDL+VLDL values and lower chylomicron content than cholesterol fed and untreated rabbits. But the most important modifications concerned the action of this drug on proteoglycan synthesis which may be related to the strongly decreased lipid deposition in the arterial wall of the treated rabbits (32). Details of these experiments are described elsewhere.

## Conclusions

Vessel wall cells during their differentiation follow a well defined "program" of biosynthesis of intercellular matrix macromolecules such as collagens, elastin, proteoglycans and structural glycoproteins. This "program" results in a specific matrix which represents the normal environment of vessel wall cells. A variety of factors can upset this specific cell-matrix interaction by modifying the normal "program" of matrix biosynthesis or by triggering degradative processes such as elastolysis. The athero-arteriosclerotic process is characterised by such an upset regulation of matrix biosynthesis and degradation. Drugs may be found which may specifically influence this process and thereby help to normalise matrix biosynthesis and cell-matrix interaction.

## Acknowledgements

The experiments described were supported by CNRS (GR N° 40), DGRST, INSERM, Fondation pour la Recherche Médicale Française and the Conseil Scientifique de l'Université Paris-Val de Marne. The efficient collaboration of the following collegues to these projects is thankfully acknowledged : Drs J. Labat-Robert, M. Moczar, G. Godeau, D. Bréchemier, M.P. Jacob, J.C. Derouette, C. Frances, M. Miskulin and G. Meimon.

## References

1.  Robert AM, Boniface R, Robert L (1979) Biochemistry and Pathology of Basement Membranes. Role in Diabetes. "Frontiers of Matrix Biology" S. Karger, Basel.
2.  Kefalides NA (1973) Structure and biosynthesis of basement membranes. In : Hall DA and Jackson DS (eds) Intern. Rev. Connective Tissue Res., Vol. 6, Academic Press, NY/London, p. 63-104
3.  Moczar M, Phan-Dinh-Tuy B, Robert L (1982) Structural glycoproteins from rabbit aortic media. Biochem J, submitted.
4.  Labat-Robert J (1981) Structural glycoproteins of connective tissue. In : Deyl, Adam (eds) Connective Tissue Research : Chemistry, Biology and Physiology, Alan R. Liss, Inc., NY, p. 233-246
5.  Garrone R (1981) The evolution of connective tissue. Phylogenetic distribution and moficiations during development. In : Connective Tissue Research : Chemistry, Biology and Physiology, Alan R. Liss, Inc., NY, p. 141-149.
6.  Robert B, Robert L (1973) Aging of connective tissues. General considerations. In : Robert L. (ed) Aging of Connective Tissues-Skin "Frontiers of Matrix Biology" Vol. 1, S. Karger, Basel, p. 1-45.
7.  Moczar M, Robert L (1976) Action of human hyperlipemic sera on the biosynthesis of intercellular matrix macromolecules in aorta organ cultures. Paroi Artérielle 3: 105-113.
8.  Jacob MP, Bréchemier D, Robert L, Hornebeck W (1982) Variation of elastase-type protease activity and elastin biosynthesis in rabbit aorta induced by cholesterol diet and immunization with elastin peptides. Artery, in print.
9.  Robert AM, Grosgogeat Y, Reverdy V, Robert B, Robert L (1971) Lésions artérielles produites chez le lapin par immunisation avec l'élastine et les glycoprotéines de structure de l'aorte. Etudes biochimiques et morphologiques. Atherosclerosis 13: 427-449.
10. Robert B, Derouette JC, Robert L (1974) Mise en évidence d'une protéase à activité élastolytique dans les extraits d'aortes humaines et animales. C.R. Acad. Sci. Paris 278: 3251-3254.
11. Hornebeck W, Derouette JC, Robert L (1975) Isolation, purification and properties of aortic elastase. FEBS Letters 58: 66-70.
12. Bréchemier D, Hornebeck W, Bourdillon MC, Blaes N, Crouzet B, Robert L (1980) Elastase-like proteases in rat aorta smooth muscle cells and fibroblasts. Artery 8: 342-347.
13. Bréchemier D, Robert L, Hornebeck W (1982) Isolation and characterisation of an elastase-type protease from rat aorta smooth muscle cells. Biochem J, submitted.
14. Godeau G, Lafuma Ch, Hornebeck W, Robert L (1982) Morphological and biochemical alterations of arterial and lung elastic tissue induced by immunisation with κ-elastin peptides, in preparation.

15. Godeau G, Frances C, Hornebeck W, Bréchemier D, Robert L (1982) Isolation and partial characterization of an elastase-type protease in human vulva fibroblasts : its possible involvment in vulvar elastic tissue destruction of patients with lichen *sclerosus et atrophicus*, J Invest. Dermatol. **78: 270-275**.
16. Jacob MP, Bellon G, Robert L, Hornebeck W, Ayrault-Jarrier M, Burdin J., Polonovski J (1981) Elastase-type activity associated with high density lipoproteins in human serum. Biochem Biophys Res Comm 103: 311-318.
17. McCullagh KG, Ehrhart LA (1974) Increased arterial collagen synthesis in experimental canine atherosclerosis, Atherosclerosis 19: 13-28.
18. Ehrhart LA, Holderbaum D (1977) Stimulation of aortic protein synthesis in experimental rabbit atherosclerosis. Atherosclerosis 27: 477-485.
19. McCullagh KG, Duance VC, Bishop KA (1980) The distribution of collagen types I, III and V (AB) in normal and atherosclerotic human aorta. J. Pathol 130: 45-55.
20. Junqueira LC, Bignolas G, Brentani R (1979) Picrosirius staining plus polarization microscopy, a specific method for collagen detection in tissue sections. Histochem J 11: 447-455.
21. Labat-Robert J, Szendroi M, Grimaud A, Godeau G, Robert L (1982) Codistribution of collagen type III and fibronectin in fresh human arterial lesion. in preparation.
22. Hynes RO, Destree AT, Perkins ME, Wagner DD (1979) Cell surface fibronectin and oncogenic transformation. J Supramol Structure 11: 95-104.
23. Vaheri A, Alitalo K, Hedman K, Kurkinen M, Saksela O, Vartio T (1980) Fibronectin and its loss in malignant transformation. In : Robert AM, Robert L (eds) Biochimie des Tissus Conjonctifs Normaux et Pathologiques, Vol. 2, Colloque CNRS, Paris N° 287 p. 249-254.
24. Labat-Robert J, Birembaut P, Robert L, Adnet JJ (1981) Modification of fibronectin distribution pattern in solid human tumors. Diagnostic Histopathology 4: 299-236.
25. Robert AM, Godeau G, Moati F, Miskulin M (1977) Action of anthocyanosides of *Vaccinium myrtillis* on the permeability of the blood brain barrier. J Med 8: 321-332
26. Kadar A, Robert L, Miskulin M, Tixier JM, Bréchemier D, Robert AM (1979) Influence of anthocyanoside treatment on the cholesterol induced atherosclerosis in the rabbit. Paroi Artérielle 5: 187-206.
27. Harsing J, Tixier JM, Kemeny A, Robert AM (1982) Effect of procyanidolic oligomers on the permeability of the blood-brain barrier. Arterial Wall, in print.
28. Robert L, Bréchemier D, Godeau G, Labat ML, Milhaud G (1977) Prevention of experimental immunarteriosclerosis by calcitonin. Biochem Pharmacol 26: 2129-2135.
29. Robert AM, Miskulin M, Godeau G, Tixier JM, Milhaud G (1982) Action of calcitonin on the atherosclerotic modifications of brain microvessels induced in rabbits by cholesterol feeding. Exper Mol Pathol 37: in print.
30. Moczar M, Migne J, Bruel J, Dimitrieff H, Wegrowski J, Robert L (1981) Effect of alpha-blocking agent, nicergoline and a beta blocking agent, acebutolol on the in vitro biosynthesis of the macromolecules of the intercellular matrix rabbit aortic media. Paroi Artérielle 7: 44
31. Berg RA, Moss J, Baum BJ, Crystal RG (1981) Regulation of collagen production by the β-adrenergic system. J Clin Invest 67: 1457-1462.

32. Wegrowski J, Harsing J, Godeau G, Robert AM, Moczar M (1982) Effect of colchicin on the cholesterol induced atherosclerosis of the rabbit. Arterial Wall, in print.
33. Clopath P, Sinzinger H (1980) Calcitonin increases porcine vascular prostacyclin formation. Prostaglandins 19: 1

# Arterial Wall Cells and Mitogens

R. Ross, E. Raines, and D. Bowen-Pope

In examining the pathogenesis of the lesions of atherosclerosis, we have been concerned principally about two cells derived from the artery: endothelium and smooth muscle, and their interactions with two cells from the blood: the platelet and the monocyte/macrophage (1,2). The platelet and the macrophage each can serve as important sources of mitogens, the platelet derived growth factor PDGF (3) and the macrophage derived growth factor MDGF (4), that are capable of stimulating arterial smooth muscle cells and fibroblasts to proliferate in cell culture.

Together with Dr. Thomas Wight, we have studied lesions of human atherosclerosis of the superficial femoral artery, fixed in the operating room at the time of removal during surgery, and have demonstrated that virtually all of the atherosclerotic lesions contain large numbers of smooth muscle cells and in most cases large numbers of lipid-laden macrophages. Together with Dr. A. Faggiotto we have observed a sequence of events in monkeys fed a high fat, high cholesterol diet in which macrophages appear under an intact endothelium in the form of a "fatty streak" within one month after placing the animals on the diet. These "foam cells" continue to increase in numbers until approximately four months, at which time breaks can be seen in the endothelium at junctional complexes. After five months on the diet, particularly in the abdominal aorta, iliac and femoral arteries, numerous areas were observed in which the endothelial cells had desquamated, leaving large elliptical-shaped patches devoid of endothelium in which platelet mural thrombi, together with adherent macrophages, were present overlying pre-existing lesions and adjacent to fatty streaks. Thus both platelets and macrophages are seen to interact relatively early in the development of the lesions of atherosclerosis, at least in the situation of chronic hypercholesterolemia.

## The Platelet Derived Growth Factor

The platelet derived growth factor has been purified essentially to homogeneity (5-7). It is a polypeptide of approximately 30,000 molecular weight consisting of two chains of 17,000 and 14,000 each, that are disulfide bonded. This peptide is cationic (pI 9.8) and binds to a specific high affinity cell surface receptor (Kd $10^{-11}$ M) (8,9). The numbers of receptors on arterial smooth muscle cells range from 80,000 to 40,000 per cell on monkey vs. human arterial smooth muscle cells (9). After PDGF binds to its specific cell surface receptor at 37 degrees C., the receptor-ligand complex is internalized by the cell and disappears from the surface. Within minutes after binding of PDGF to its receptor a tyrosine phosphokinase is activated that appears to be the receptor itself (L. Pike, et al., unpublished data). The PDGF receptor is a protein of approximately 164,000 molecular weight (10). Binding of PDGF to this receptor induces a host of intracellular events, some of which may be important to the genesis of the lesions of atherosclerosis. For example, after PDGF binds to its receptor there is a marked increase in phospholipid metabolism, in which the cellular content of phosphatidylinositol rapidly decreases. This is rapidly followed by an increase in the level of intracellular diglyceride which reaches a maximum within ten minutes and then begins to decrease. Following this increase and decrease in diglyceride, both monoglyceride and arachidonic acid increase in the culture medium (11). These changes suggest that binding of PDGF to its receptor rapidly activates a phospholipase type C activity that may have extensive ramifications in the metabolism of these cells.

Other phenomena that are activated by PDGF binding to the cell surface include increase in LDL binding (12), increase in pinocytosis (13), and increased protein and RNA synthesis. In addition to these responses, PDGF has been shown to be specifically chemotactic for cells such as smooth muscle (14), possibly explaining the intimal migration of medial smooth muscle cells at sites of endothelial injury, platelet adherence aggregation and release (15).

## Macrophage Derived Growth Factor

The macrophage derived growth factor has not yet been purified to homogeneity. A number of preliminary studies in our laboratory suggest that it is a different molecule from PDGF, in that antibodies directed against PDGF which completely inactivate PDGF have no effect on MDGF. MDGF appears to have different binding properties during chromatographic purification studies than those observed for PDGF. Future studies will determine the nature of this molecule, its binding properties to cells, and which cells are susceptible to this molecule in relation to those that respond to PDGF. Other studies remain to be performed to determine whether PDGF and MDGF are active in vivo. These studies will be critical if we are to further pursue the potential role of the two factors that may be released from platelets and macrophages in terms of the part they play in atherogenesis.

ACKNOWLEDGEMENT: This research was supported in part by grants from the U.S.P.H.S. nos. HL18645 and AM13970.

## References

1. Ross, R. and Glomset, J. New Engl. J. Med. 295:369-377, 420-425, 1976.
2. Ross, R. Arteriosclerosis: A Journal of Vascular Biology and Disease, Vol. 1, 293-311, 1981.
3. Ross, R. and Vogel, A. Cell 14:203-210, 1978.
4. Leibovich, S.J., and Ross, R. Am. J. Pathol. 84:501-513, 1976.
5. Heldin, C.H., Westermark, B., and Wasteson, A. Biochem. J. 193:907-918, 1981.
6. Deuel, T.F., Huang, J., Proffett, R.T., Chang, D., and Kennedy, B.B. J. Biol. Chem. 256:8896-8899, 1981.
7. Raines, E.W. and Ross, R. J. Biol. Chem., in press.
8. Bowen-Pope, D. and Ross, R. J. Biol. Chem., in press.
9. Heldin, C.H., Westermark, B., and Wasteson, A. Proc. Natl. Acad. Sci. U.S.A. 78:3664-3668, 1981.
10. Glenn, K., Bowen-Pope, D. and Ross, R. J. Biol. Chem., in press.
11. Habenicht, A.J.R., Glomset, J.A., King, W.C., Nist, C., Mitchell, C.D., and Ross, R. J. Biol. Chem., Vol. 256, No. 23, pp. 12329-12335, 1981.
12. Chait, A., Ross, R., Albers, J. and Bierman, E. PNAS 77, No. 7:4084-4088, 1980.
13. Davies, P.F. and Ross, R. J. Cell Biol. 79:663-671, 1978.
14. Grotendorst, G.R., Seppa, H.E.J., Kleinman, H.K., and Martin, G.R. Proc. Natl. Acad. Sci. U.S.A. 78:3669-3672, 1981.
15. Stemerman, M.B., and Ross. R. J. Exp. Med. 136:769-789, 1972.

# 2.1 Biology of Arterial Wall Cells

# The Microcarrier Co-Culture System:
# Interactions Between Endothelial and Smooth Muscle Cells In Vitro

P. F. Davies, C. Kerrn, and B. Eisenhaure

There is currently considerable interest in the interactions of vascular cells in relation to intimal smooth muscle cell (SMC) proliferation and lipoprotein metabolism. In vitro, medium conditioned by endothelial cells has been shown to contain factors which both stimulate (Gajdusek et al., 1980) and inhibit SMC proliferation (Castellot et al., 1981). Recently, Witte et al. (1982) have demonstrated modified LDL metabolism in fibroblasts exposed to endothelial cell conditioned medium and there have been reports of modification of low density lipoprotein (LDL) structural characteristics by endothelial cells (Henriksen et al., 1981), and by macrophages (Stein et al., 1981). Such modifications have resulted subsequently in altered patterns of interaction of the LDL with surface receptors of various cell types. Thus, by the use of conditioned media, some fascinating intercellular phenomena relating to cell growth and lipoprotein metabolsim are being uncovered.

In this laboratory, we are taking a slight different appraoch to studies of interactions between endothelium and SMC in culture. In addition to the use of conditioned medium, we are co-culturing vascular cells, that is, maintaining separate cell populations which are subsequently brought together to share the same culture medium. The rationale for this approach is as follows. It appears reasonable to postulate that local, potent interactions between endothelium and SMC may occur in situ. The simultaneous presence of both cell types offers the opportunity of metabolic cooperation between them. The close apposition of the two cell types and the small volume of interstitial fluid present in the intima and media of the artery may allow locally high concentrations of metabolites to exist under steady state conditions. In transposing this arrangement to an in vitro co-culture system it is diffcult to avoid considerable dilution of any putative factors because the ratios of cells to culture medium volume remains low, given the constraints imposed by conventional tissue culture. In order to improve the ratio of cells to medium volume, and hence minimise dilution effects, we have adapted and developed microcarrier culture of endothelium.

As shown in Figure 1, bovine aortic endothelial cells and human endothelial cells can be readily cultured to confluence on solid plastic microcarriers (Biosilon[R], NUNC, Denmark). The cells have been extensively characterised on this substratum and appear by criteria of cell growth, morphological appearance, ultrastructural characteristics, and certain physiological measurements to behave identically to their counterparts in conventional culture (Davies, 1981, 1982). At confluence, there are about 150 cells/microcarrier bead. The properties of microcarrier-borne endothelial cells which make them suitable for co-culture studies are: 1) they are an easily transferable substratum 2) they offer a high surface area to volume ratio for cell culture and 3) the solid plastic microcarriers are nonporous and therefore adsorption of metabolites within the microcarrier is avoided, as is a significant intra-bead aqueous volume. The co-culture system as shown in

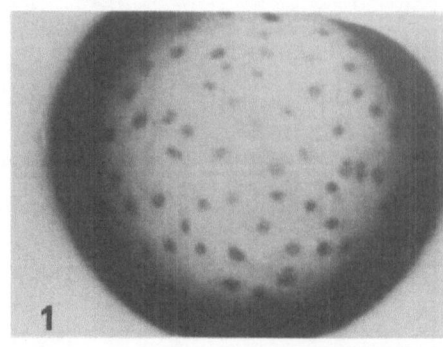

Fig. 1. Confluent bovine aortic endothelial cells cultured on solid plastic microcarriers (Biosilon[R]). Cell: bead ratio approx. 150:1. Hematoxylin stain, X 480

Figure 2 has recently been described (Davies and Kerr, 1982a). It consists of a target monolayer of SMC plated on to a petri dish surface above which is suspended a basket containing $2 \times 10^6$ endothelial cells cultured on microcarriers. Interchange of humoral factors between the two cell types can occur via a siliconised porous net (pore size 1 μm) which inhibits passage of cells. The juxtaposition of the two cell types is shown in Figure 3. In co-culture the appearance and viability of the endothelium on microcarriers is very good by both trypan blue exclusion (>90%) and lactate dihydrogenase release (<1% of LDH released by an equivalent lysed cell population). Over a four day period, some point-to-point bridging of cells occurred, but this represented a very small fraction of the total population.

## Stimulation of DNA Synthesis in Quiescent SMC by Co-culture with Endothelium

Bovine aortic SMC, subculture two, were maintained in plasma-derived serum (PDS; Vogel et al., 1980) in a quiescent stae of growth ($^3$H-thymidine index less than 6%) as shown in Figure 4a. After twenty-four hours in co-culture with endothelium on mocrocarriers, the labeling index rose to greater than 90% (Figure 4b). This high figure compares with maximum labeling indices using purified growth factors at high concentrations of 30-60% in these cells (Rutherford and Ross, 1976; Davies and Ross, 1980; Davies and Kerr, 1982b). In contrast, PDS conditioned by identical microcarrier cultures of endothelial cells resulted in variable labelling indices when added to smooth muscle cells. This variability ranged from toxicity at one extreme to as high as 42% labeled cells over a subsequent 24 hour incubation with $^3$H-thymidine. We conclude that with respect to SMC proliferation, there is a consistent and more potent stimulation when the cells are co-cultured with endothelium than when endothelial-conditioned medium is used. The mechanisms responsible for such an enhanced proliferative response in co-culture are discussed below.

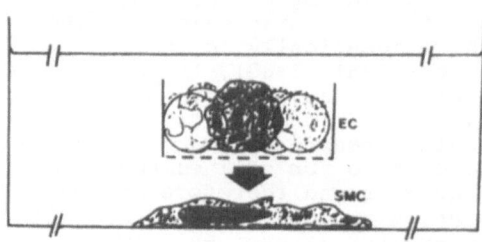

Fig. 2. Scheme for the co-culture of vascular endothelial cells with smooth muscle cell

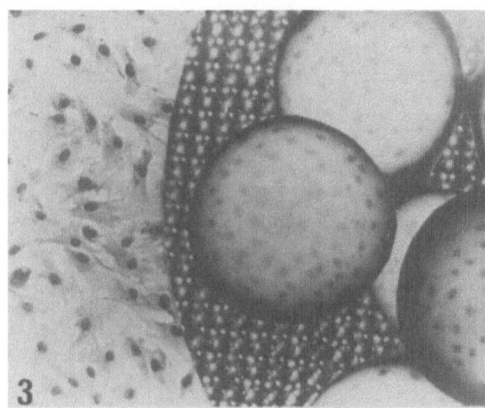

Fig. 3. Photomontage showing the spacial relationship between endothelial cells (microcarriers) and target smooth muscle cells in the co-culture system. Hematoxylin, X 250

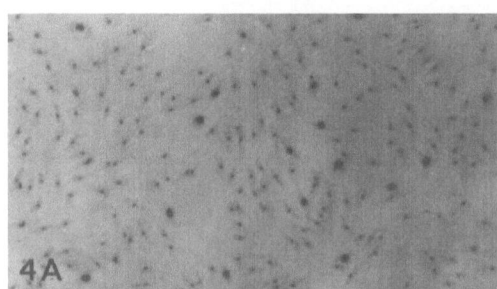 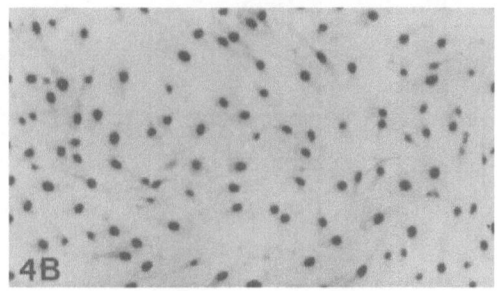

Fig. 4. Autoradiographic labelling of bovine aortic smooth muscle cell nuclei by $^3$H-thymidine. Cells were maintained quiescent in 5% plasma-derived serum. Fresh PDS (A) or PDS plus microcarrier cultures of bovine aortic endothelial cells (B) were then added. Labelling indices: A 5%; B 93%

## LDL Metabolism in Vascular SMC in Co-culture with Endothelium

The ease with which cell populations may be brought together for co-culture and then separated for individual analyses is illustrated in Figure 5. Using such an approach, endothelial and smooth muscle cells were separately pre-incubated with lipoprotein-deficient and growth factor-deficient medium prior to co-culture in the presence of iodinated LDL. Following incubation with $^{125}$I-LDL, the cell populations were separated for individual analyses of LDL binding, internalisation and degradation. Alterations in LDL metabolism in smooth muscle cells in co-culture with either microcarrier-bound endothelium or microcarrier-bound SMC (control), are summarised in Figure 6. Binding and degradation of LDL by the high affinity receptor system in vascular SMC was increased within 24 hours by co-culture with endothelium but not in co-culture with control SMC. After reaching a plateau by 30 hrs, it remained elevated throughout the duration of the experiment (to 50 hrs). The net internalisation of LDL and the rate of fluid endocytosis (measured independently) in the same cells revealed a progressive increase with time of co-culture with endothelium. LDL metabolism in the endothelial cells on the microcarriers remained unchanged by co-culture. We conclude that there was an endothelial specific stimulation of LDL metabolism in arterial SMC when the two populations were maintained in co-culture. It is quite conceivable that the effects of co-culture upon LDL metabolism occur secondary to the endothelial specific stimulation of cell cycle entry reported above; specific growth factors have been shown to stimulate LDL metabolism in their target cells (Chait et al., 1980; Witte and Cornicelli, 1980; Davies and Kerr, 1982b).

388

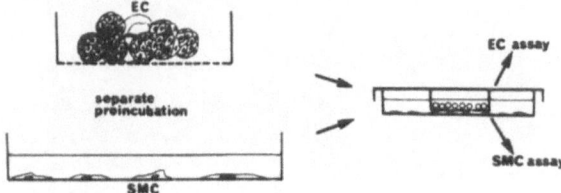

Fig. 5. Scheme for measurement of the effect of co-culture upon LDL metabolism in vascular cells. Following pre-incubation of separate cultures, $^{125}I$-LDL was added to the co-culture, after which the cell populations were separated for assay

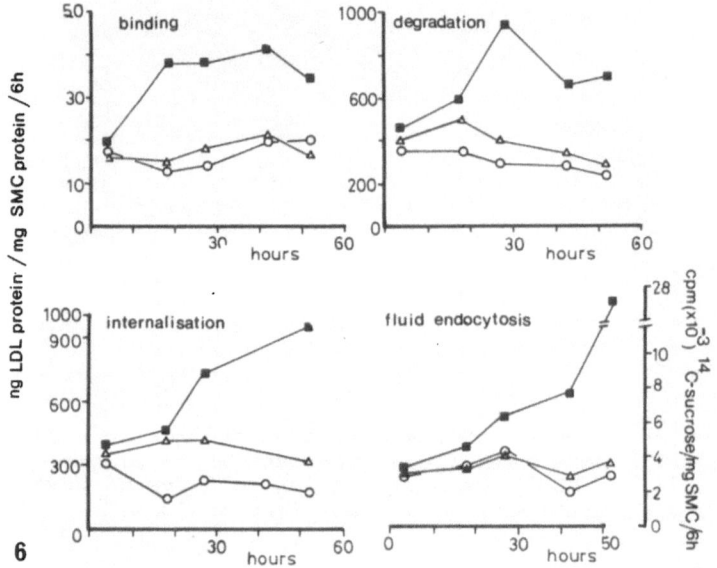

**6**

Fig. 6. Influence of microcarrier cultures of endothelial cells upon LDL metabolism in quiescent smooth muscle cells. Each point is the mean measurement over a 6 hour period. o SMC alone, △ SMC co-cultured with SMC (microcarriers), ■ SMC co-cultured with endothelial cells (microcarriers)

## Co-culture Allows the Potential for Multiple Interactions between Cell Populations

When medium conditioned by one cell population is collected then added to a second population, there is an inherent restriction of interpretation in terms of the interactions between the two cell populations. For example, first, there is no provision for signals or messages from the target cell to reach the cell which is conditioning the medium. Second, there is the possibility that short-lived potent factors produced by the conditioning cell may be inactive either because of short half life or by dilution when applied as conditioned medium to the target cell. Third, the separation of cell populations for the production of conditioned medium removes the normal checks and balances which presumably exist between two cell types such as endothelium and SMC residing so close together in vivo. By co-culturing the two cell populations, these restrictions are minimised.

In summary therefore, we would like to suggest that there exist important local interactions between endothelial cells and SMC which required the presence of both cell types, and which involve metabolic cooperation of a humoral nature between them. Such interactions may prove relevant both to the maintenance of vascular homeostasis and to the pathological changes associated with atherogenesis.

We are grateful to Drs. Ramzi Cotran and Michael Gimbrone and other members of the Department for helpful discussions. This work was supported by NIH grants HL24612 and HL22602.

## References

Castellot JJ, Addonizio ML, Rosenberg R, Karnovsky MJ (1981) Cultured endothelial cells produce a heparin-like inhibitor of smooth muscle cell growth. J Cell Biol 90: 372-379

Chait A, Ross R, Albers JJ, Bierman EL (1980) Platelet-derived growth factor stimulates activity of low density lipoprotein receptors. Proc Natl Acad Sci USA 77: 4084-4088

Davies PF, Ross R (1980) Growth-mediated, density-dependent inhibition of endocytosis in cultured arterial smooth muscle cells. Exptl Cell Res 129: 329-336

Davies PF (1981) Microcarrier culture of vascular endothelial cells on solid plastic beads. Exptl Cell Res 134: 367-376

Davies PF (1982) Microcarrier cultures in vascular endothelial research. Dev biol Stand 50: 125-137

Davies PF, Kerr C (1982a) Cocultivation of mammalian cells using microcarrier techniques: vascular endothelial and smooth muscle cells. Exptl Cell Res. in press

Davies PF, Kerr C (1982b) Modification of low density lipoprotein metabolism by growth factors in cultured vascular cells and human skin fibroblasts. Dependence upon duration of exposure. Biochim Biophys Acta. in press

Gajdusek C, DiCorelto P, Ross R, Schwartz SM (1980) An endothelial cell-derived growth factor. J Cell Biol 85: 467-472

Henriksen T, Mahoney EM, Steinberg D (1981) Enhanced macrophage degradation of low density lipoproteins previously incubated with cultured endothelial cells: recognition by receptors for acetylated low density lipoproteins. Proc Natl Acad Sci USA 78: 6499-6503

Rutherford RB, Ross R (1976) Platelet factors stimulate fibroblasts and smooth muscle cells quiescent in plasma to proliferate. J Cell Biol 69: 196-203

Stein O, Halperin G, Stein Y (1981) Interaction between macrophages and smooth muscle cells. Enhancement of cholesterol esterification in smooth muscle cells by media of macrophages incubated with acetylated LDL. Biochim Biophys Acta 665: 477-490

Vogel A, Ross R, Raines E (1980) Role of serum components in density-dependent inhibition of growth of cells in culture. J Cell Biol 85: 377-385

Witte LD, Cornicelli JA (1980) Platelet-derived growth factor stimulates low density lipoprotein receptor activity in cultured human fibroblasts. Proc Natl Acad Sci USA 77: 5962-5966

Witte LD, Cornicelli JA, Miller RW, Goodman DS (1982) Effects of platelet-derived and endothelial cell-derived growth factors on the low density lipoprotein receptor pathway in cultured human fibroblasts. J Biol Chem 257: 5392-5401

# Intermediate Filaments of the Vascular Wall

W. W. Franke and R. A. Quinlan

## Introduction

Intermediate-sized filaments (IF) are one major group of filaments
which constitute part of the cytoskeleton of vertebrate cells. Unlike
the situation for the other components of the cytoskeleton, the protein
composition of IFs of different cell types can vary considerably,
in different cell types and on the basis of the biochemical and
immunological characteristics of their constituent proteins, five
different cell specific IF subclasses have been identified (1-5).
Table 1 presents a summary.

Table 1. Different Types of Intermediate Filaments

| Protein Type | Subunit Poly-peptides (in one cell) | Molecular weight ($10^3$) | Isoelectric pH (denatured) | Occurrence |
|---|---|---|---|---|
| I. Cytokeratins | 2-8 | 40-68 | 5-8 | Epithelial cells |
| II. Vimentin | 1 | 57 | 5.3 | Non-epithelial cells, spec. mesenchymal cells, astrocytes, some myogenic cells, most cultured cell lines |
| III. Desmin | 1 | 53 | 5.4 | muscle cells, excl. one type of vascular smooth muscle cells |
| IV. Glia-Filament Protein | 1 | 51 | 5.6 | astrocytes |
| V. Neurofilament Protein | 3 | 210,160, 68 | 5.65,5.28 5.25 | neuronal cells |

For example, epithelial cells contain cytokeratin filaments, IF composed
of vimentin are primarily found in cells of mesenchymal origin, whereas
in muscle cells usually desmin filaments are found. The cell type specificity of IF has been of particular interest in diagnostic pathology for
the histogenesis of neoplasms (6).

There are situations where two IF classes can be co-expressed in the same cell. Cultured cells normally express, in addition to their cell-type IF class, vimentin filaments (7). Several examples of co-expression of two IF classes in situ have also been reported, this being for vimentin and desmin in the Z-line of skeletal muscle (8) and for vimentin and glial filament protein in astrocytes (9,10).
Visceral smooth muscle cells contain desmin as the predominant IF protein (11). By contrast many vascular smooth muscle cells of mammalian aortae have been reported to contain primarily vimentin (12,13). We have investigated further the IF composition of vascular smooth muscle cells.

## IF Composition of Vascular Smooth Muscle Tissue as Visualized by Immunofluorescence Microscopy

In addition to those cells which contain vimentin in the vascular wall of mammalian aorta, a type of smooth muscle cell is often found which contains both vimentin and desmin. Figure 1 shows the immuno-fluorescent staining of vimentin antibodies (left) and desmin anti-bodies (right) on frozen sections of bovine aorta.

There is clear preponderance of vimentin containing cells within the tunica intima and the inner regions of the tunica media, but in the central region of the tunica media, which is known to contain only smooth muscle cells (14,15), desmin positive cells arranged in the helical or circular tracts typical of smooth muscle cells are also seen. These cells appear to be also vimentin positive, and double immuno-

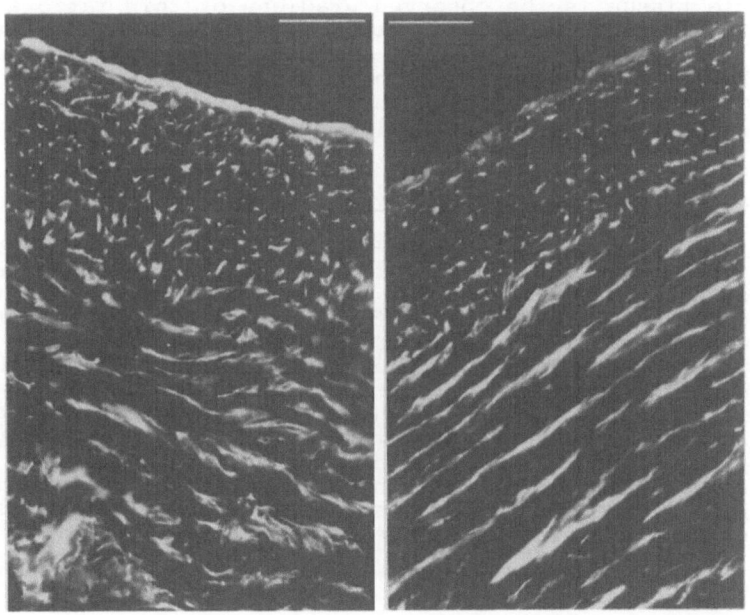

**Fig. 1.** Distribution of vimentin (left) and desmin (right) in bovine aorta shown by immunofluorescence microscopy (bars, 30 µm; L, lumen)

fluorescence studies have shown that the cells positive for desmin are
also positive for vimentin (16). Such cell types which express vimentin
and desmin are also found in the inner layers of the tunica media, but
here they are usually more sparsely distributed. The co-expression of
vimentin and desmin has also been claimed for the Z-line of avian and
mammalian skeletal muscle (for controversial views see 8,17) and in the
established cell line BHK-21, which is believed to be derived from
vascular smooth muscle tissue of the kidney (18). Some sublines of BHK-
21 cells express only vimentin (19). In the outer regions of the tunica
media of bovine aorta, where densely packed longitudinally orientated
smooth muscle cells are found, there is a third category of vascular
smooth muscle cells, those which are only desmin positive (16). In
other arteries of mammals, including human coronary arteries, variable
arrays of cells containing both vimentin and desmin are also observed
(16).

## Gel Electrophoretic Analyses

Different proportions of vimentin and desmin can be recovered from
vascular smooth muscle tissue, depending on the species and the
specific location in the vascular bed (13,18,20). In chick aorta, where
the arrangement of smooth muscle cells is different from that in
mammals (16), vimentin is usually predominant (Fig. 2a) but some desmin
is also found (16). In rat aorta, vimentin is again predominant (Fig.
2b, slot 1; slot 2c), but in bovine aorta both IF proteins appear in
almost equal amounts (Fig. 2b, slot 2d). In the tunica media of human
aorta desmin is hardly detectable (Fig. 2e), but here disproportionate
postmorten degradation by a $Ca^{2+}$ protease could not be excluded. A
further variability of the vimentin:desmin ratio in vascular smooth
muscle tissue is the observed gradient of this ratio along the length
of the aorta in mammals as studied in detail in the rat (20). Whether
the observed transition from a low to high desmin:vimentin ratio is
correlated with functional changes remains to be studied. Desmin is
also readily observed, together with vimentin, in certain smooth muscle
cells in smaller blood vessels.

## Chemical Cross-linking Studies

By the use of chemical cross-linking using cupric-o-phenanthroline-
mediated disulfide bridge formation of the single cysteine residue
present in both vimentin and desmin, heterodimers are found in vascular
smooth muscle tissue (Fig. 2f), indicative of the existence of
heteropolymer filaments (for details see 21). Vimentin and desmin have
a number of common sequence characteristics (22) and they appear to
have a similar steric arrangement in the IF. In myogenesis vimentin is
expressed before desmin in the presumptive myoblasts, and when desmin is
first seen to be expressed, the distributions of both proteins are
indistinguishable (17,23). This suggests that vimentin and desmin may
substitute for one another in certain situations. The functional
significance of the co-expression of vimentin and desmin in certain
smooth and skeletal muscle cells is unknown.

## Conclusions and Perspectives

The smooth muscle cell population in the vascular system can no longer
be considered homogeneous. Recent resultshave shown that three different smooth muscle cell types can be distinguished biochemically.

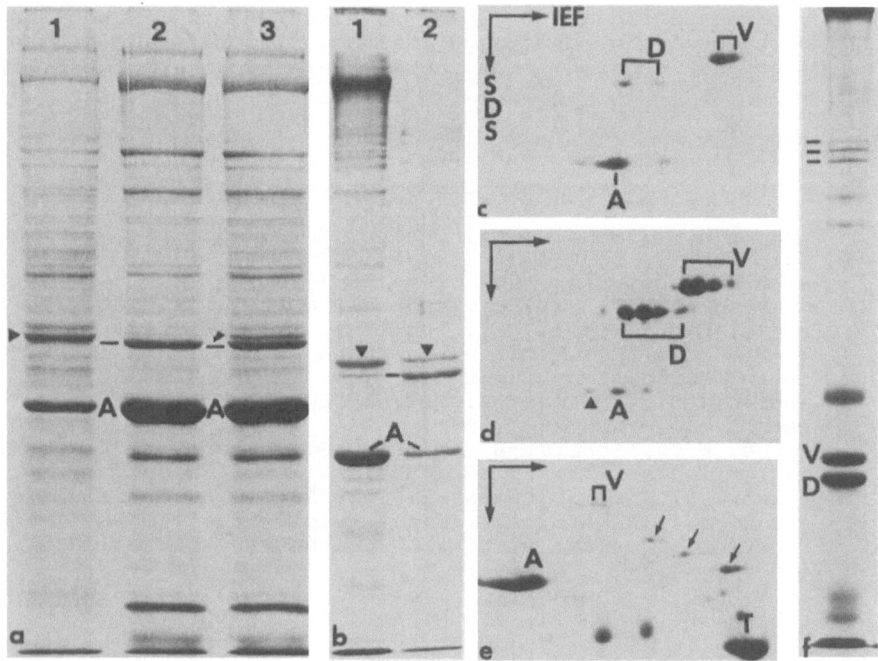

Fig. 2. Vimentin and desmin in aortic walls. (a) SDS-polyacrylamide
gel electrophoresis (PAGE) of cytoskeletal proteins from whole chicken
aorta (slot 1), gizzard (slot 2) and a mixture of the two preparations
(slot 3); arrowhead, vimentin; horizontal bar, desmin; A, actin. (b)
Vimentin (arrowhead) and desmin (bar) in cytoskeletal preparations from
aortic walls of rat (slot 1) and cow (slot 2). (c-e) Two-dimensional
gel electrophoresis (IEF, direction of isoelectric focusing; SDS,
second dimension electrophoresis in the presence of SDS) of cytoskeletal
material from aortic walls of rat (c) and cow (d) and total aortic
wall proteins of man (e); V, vimentin; D, desmin, A, $\alpha$-actin; T, tropo-
myosin; arrows in e, degradation products of vimentin. (f) SDS-PAGE of
cytoskeletal proteins from tunica media of bovine aorta after cross-
linking (for details see 21); V and D, monomeric vimentin and desmin;
horizontal triple bars, vimentin-vimentin dimer, vimentin-desmin hetero-
dimer, desmin-desmin dimer

These cell types are: 1. Those that express only vimentin IF; this
category includes cells of a cultured rat vascular smooth muscle
cell line, RVF-SM (24). 2. Those that express desmin as the only
major IF protein. 3. Those that express both vimentin and desmin.
The functions and implications of the existence of these different
smooth muscle cell types are as yet unclear. Recent work by Gabbiani
et al. (25) has suggested a biological difference in the response of
these different subclasses after endothelial injury in rat aortae;
here it appears that only the vimentin containing smooth muscle cell
subpopulation contributes to the resulting intimal thickening. Clearly
more experimental work on the characterization of these different
smooth muscle cell types in the vascular system is needed before one
can hope to understand the functional reason for the co-existence of
different smooth muscle cells in the same tissue.

394

Acknowledgments  We are indebted to Erika Schmid for her expert help and to the Deutsche Forschungsgemeinschaft for financial support. R.A.Q. is a stipendiate from the Alexander-von-Humboldt-Stiftung.

## References

1. Bennett, G.C., Fellini, S.A., Croop, J.M., Otto, J.J., Bryan, T. & Holtzer, H. Proc.Natl.Acad.Sci. USA 75, 4364-4368 (1978)
2. Franke, W.W., Schmid, E., Osborn, M. & Weber, K. Proc.Natl.Acad. Sci. USA 75, 5034-5038 (1978)
3. Lazarides, E. Nature 282, 249-256 (1980)
4. Anderton, B.H.T. Mus.Res. and Cell Mot. 2, 141-166 (1981)
5. Franke, W.W., Schmid, E., Schiller, D.L., Winter, S., Jarasch, E.-D., Moll, R., Denk, H., Jackson, B. & Illmensee, K. Cold Spring Harbor Symp.Quant.Biol. 46, in press (1982)
6. Gabbiani, G., Kapanci, Y., Barazzone, P. & Franke, W.W. Amer.J. Pathol. 104, 206-216 (1981)
7. Franke, W.W., Schmid, E., Winter, S., Osborn, M. & Weber, K. Exp.Cell Res. 123, 25-46 (1979)
8. Granger, B.L. & Lazarides, E. Cell 18, 1053-1063 (1979)
9. Yen, S.-H. & Fields, K.L. J.Cell Biol. 88, 115-126 (1981)
10. Schnitzer, J., Franke, W.W. & Schachner, M. J.Cell Biol. 90, 435-447 (1981)
11. Small, J.V. & Sobieszek, A. J.Cell Sci. 23, 243-268 (1977)
12. Gabbiani, G., Schmid, E., Winter, S., Chaponnier, C., De Chastonay, C., Vandekerckhove, J., Weber, K. & Franke, W.W. Proc.Natl.Acad.Sci. USA 78, 298-301 (1981)
13. Frank, E.D. & Warren, L. Proc.Natl.Acad.Sci. USA 78, 3020-3024 (1981)
14. Ross, R. & Klebanoff, S.J. J.Cell Biol. 50, 159-171 (1971)
15. Simionescu, N. & Simionescu, M. In: Histology (ed. L. Weis & R.O. Greep) p. 373. McGraw-Hill Book Company (1977)
16. Schmid, E., Osborn, M., Rungger-Brändle, E., Gabbiani, G., Weber, K. & Franke, W.W. Exp.Cell Res. 137, 329-340 (1982)
17. Bennett, G.S., Fellini, S.A., Toyama, Y. & Holtzer, H. J.Cell Biol. 82, 577 (1979)
18. Frank, E.D., Tuszynski, C.P. & Warren, L. Exp.Cell Res., in press (1982)
19. Tuszynski, C.P., Frank, E.D., Damsky, C.H., Buck, C.A. & Warren, L. J.Biol.Chem. 254, 6138-6143 (1979)
20. Osborn, M., Caselitz, J. & Weber, K. Differentiation 20, 196-202 (1981)
21. Quinlan R.A. & Franke, W.W. Proc.Natl.Acad.Sci. USA 79, in press (1982)
22. Geisler, N. & Weber, K. Proc.Natl.Acad.Sci. USA 78, 4120-4123 (1981)
23. Gard, D.L. & Lazarides, E. Cell 19, 263-275 (1980)
24. Franke, W.W., Schmid, E., Vandekerckhove, J. & Weber, K. J.Cell Biol. 87, 594-600 (1980)
25. Gabbiani, G., Rungger-Brändle, E., De Chastonay, C. & Franke, W.W., manuscript submitted

# A Putative Mechanism for the Conversion of Aortic Smooth Muscle Cells into Foam Cells that Bypasses the Autoregulatory LDL Receptor-Mediated Process

O. Stein and Y. Stein

The most prominent feature of atheromatosis is deposition of cholesteryl ester (CE) in the arterial wall. The origin of the arterial CE are plasma lipoproteins, yet the mechanisms involved in the intracellular accumulation of this CE have not been clarified completely. Smooth muscle cells, which constitute the main cellular population of normal aorta, become loaded with esterified cholesterol during development of atheroma and change into foam cells. Very often it is difficult to identify the foam cells as a SMC but careful morphological examination can still be quite helpful as demonstrated in Figs. 1 and 2 which are sections of rabbit aorta after 2 months of 1% cholesterol feeding. To reproduce such changes in culture, smooth muscle cells were exposed to LDL, the accepted donor of cellular CE. However, since LDL is taken up by SMC through a receptor-mediated process (1), accumulation of CE is prevented by autoregulation. The same is true also for β-VLDL (2) formed during feeding of high cholesterol diets. It is possible to induce CE accumulation in SMC by disruption of the autoregulation mechanism as was achieved by exposure of SMC to high concentrations of LDL in the presence of chloroquine, an inhibitor of lysosomal cholesteryl ester hydrolase (3). CE accumulation in SMC in culture will occur also when the donor LDL has been cationized and therefore taken up by a nonreceptor-mediated uptake (4). Since neither chloroquine nor cationized LDL are present in the atheromatous aorta *in situ*, the question still remains how does enrichment of smooth muscle cells with CE, and their conversion into foam cells occur during development of an atheroma.

The other cells which are present in an atheroma are macrophages. The macrophages in culture can be induced to accumulate cholesteryl ester by exposure to modified LDL or to β-VLDL because in these cells the receptor-mediated uptake is not auto-regulated (2). Recently we have developed a model system in which cultured peritoneal macrophages were loaded with cholesteryl ester by exposure to acetylated LDL and media conditioned with such macrophages were used to study their effect on cholesteryl ester deposition in SMC (5, 6). As shown in Fig. 3, the macrophage-conditioned medium was able to enhance cholesterol esterification and CE accumulation in SMC. This was not due to *de novo* synthesis of intracellular cholesterol, and the effect of enhanced CE accumulation in the SMC could be abolished by ether extraction of the medium (6). In further studies it became apparent that the induction of CE deposition in SMC was related to the enrichment of acetylated LDL with free cholesterol (FC), derived from cholesteryl ester hydrolysis in the macrophage and released back into the medium. Thus enriched acetylated LDL served as donor of FC to SMC, and the accumulation of esterified cholesterol was due to stimulation of intracellular ACAT activity.

To examine the capacity of nonmodified native lipoproteins to transport FC from cholesteryl ester enriched macrophages to cultured SMC or human skin fibroblasts (HSF), cholesteryl ester loaded cells were incubated with LDL and HDL. As seen in the table, cultured HSF responded to conditioned acetylated LDL as did the cultured SMC. Moreover, the other lipoproteins, i.e., LDL and to some extent also HDL, mimic the effect of acetylated LDL with respect to induction of cholesterol esterification in the HSF. Human HDL is not taken up avidly by a receptor-mediated process, but it could have become enriched in apolipoprotein E, secreted by the cultured macrophages (7). To determine whether apolipoprotein B-E receptors are responsible for the induction of cholesterol esterification by the macrophage-conditioned media studied, we have used also receptor-negative HSF from a donor homozygous for familial hypercholesterolemia (FHH-HSF). The macrophage-conditioned media containing the various lipoproteins induced cholesterol esterification in

TABLE 1.

Comparison of Media Supplemented with Human Plasma Lipoproteins, Added to Cholesteryl Ester (CE) Loaded Macrophages (MP), to Induce Cholesterol Esterification in Human Skin Fibroblasts (HSF) of Controls and of a Familial Homozygous Hypercholesterolemic (FHH) Patient

*Conditions:* Mouse peritoneal MP were cultured in Dulbecco-Vogt medium containing 10% calf serum for 24 h after plating; this medium was replaced by serum-free medium containing 1% bovine serum albumin and acetylated LDL, 50 µg protein/ml. After 72 h, this medium was collected and replaced by fresh medium containing 1% albumin and the indicated lipoproteins. 25 µg protein/ml of acetylated LDL had been used as 40-50% were taken up by the MP during subsequent 48 h; LDL and HDL concentration was 15 µg protein/ml. This medium was collected after 48 h and used for incubation with HSF. The HSF were placed at density $7 \times 10^4$ /30-mm petri dish in medium containing 10% fetal calf serum and [$^3$H]cholesterol and labeled for 72 h. The medium was removed, the cells washed thrice with PBS and postincubated in the indicated media. After 48 h the medium was collected, the cells washed and extracted. Following lipid extraction the amount of label recovered in CE was determined by TLC and total and esterified cholesterol by GLC. Zero time = petri dishes terminated prior to postincubation. Values are means ±S.E. of triplicate dishes of 4 experiments.

| HSF incubated with: | $^3$H label after 48 h postincubation (DPM) HSF | | Cellular cholesterol | |
| --- | --- | --- | --- | --- |
| | Total x $10^{-3}$ | CE x $10^{-2}$ | Total ($\mu g \cdot mg^{-1}$ protein) | Esterified |
| *Control HSF* | | | | |
| Medium added to MP, preloaded with CE, supplemented with: | | | | |
|     Acetylated LDL | 52 ± 4.7 | 129 ± 9 | 49.0 ± 1.6 | 14.4 ± 1.5 |
|     LDL | 50 ± 3.5 | 137 ± 10 | 53.3 ± 6.6 | 12.3 ± 0.9 |
|     HDL | 52 ± 3.6 | 72 ± 3 | 40.2 ± 3.4 | 7.8 ± 1.4 |
|   Albumin | 80 ± 10 | 10 ± 0.3 | 25.5 ± 2.1 | 1.3 ± 0.2 |
| Medium containing: | | | | |
|     Acetylated LDL | 41 ± 1.4 | 5 ± 0.6 | 36.2 ± 2.5 | 4.6 ± 0.2 |
|     LDL | 45 ± 1.8 | 16 ± 1.2 | 34.5 ± 0.9 | 4.4 ± 0.8 |
|     HDL | 30 ± 0.3 | 4 ± 0.4 | 22.6 ± 1.0 | 2.3 ± 0.4 |
| Zero time | 110 ± 10 | 17 ± 1.2 | 32.9 ± 1.6 | 4.3 ± 0.7 |
| *FHH-HSF* | | | | |
| Medium added to MP, preloaded with CE, supplemented with: | | | | |
|     Acetylated LDL | 33 ± 2.2 | 109 ± 18 | 67.3 ± 1.8 | 23.0 ± 1.3 |
|     LDL | 31 ± 1.2 | 70 ± 5.2 | 62.9 ± 2.5 | 19.4 ± 2.2 |
|     HDL | 32 ± 0.9 | 61 ± 6.8 | 48.6 ± 0.9 | 10.2 ± 0.8 |
|   Albumin | 48 | 5 | 39.7 | 5.1 |
| Medium containing: | | | | |
|     Acetylated LDL | 25 ± 1.2 | 6 ± 0.5 | 37.2 ± 1.3 | 5.7 ± 0.8 |
|     LDL | 28 ± 1.3 | 6 ± 0.5 | 40.7 ± 2.9 | 6.9 ± 1.2 |
|     HDL | 34 ± 1.4 | 4 ± 0.4 | 25.6 ± 0.5 | 3.6 ± 0.6 |
| Zero time | 87 ± 3.5 | 7 ± 0.7 | 30.5 ± 0.9 | 4.9 ± 0.8 |

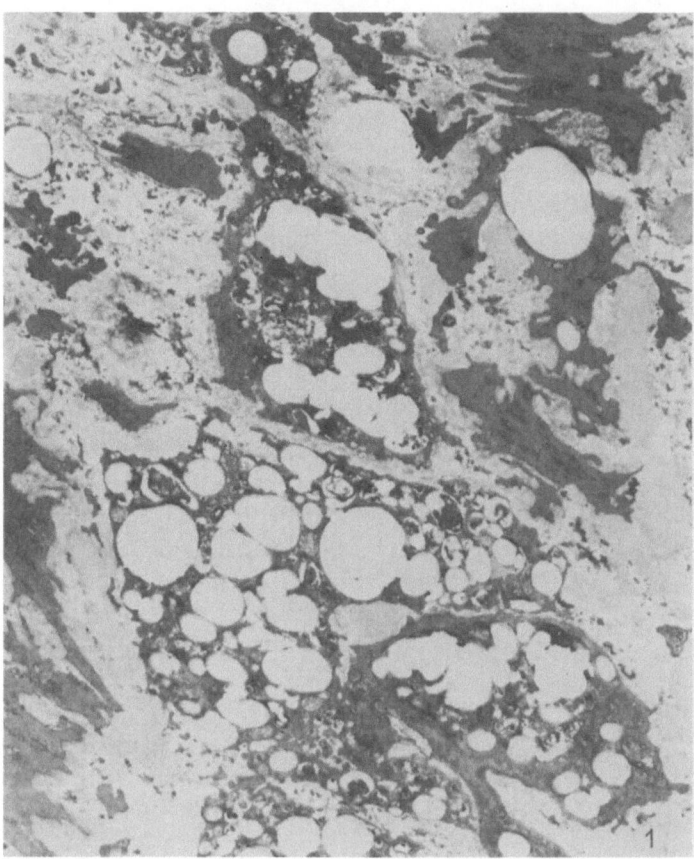

Fig. 1. Section of rabbit aorta after 2 months on 1% cholesterol diet. Numerous lipid-laden cells in the intima and outer media. Many of the lipid-laden cells retain the morphological appearance of smooth muscle cells

receptor-negative FHH-HSF to the same extent as in normal HSF (Table). Further studies have shown that HDL can perform a dual role: when added to CE-enriched MP it may serve as carrier and donor of FC to SMC; but when added to SMC during the induction of CE accumulation it can prevent the latter by competition with the cell for the surplus FC and thus fulfill its role as cholesterol acceptor, as was reported previously (8).

Conclusions

The present results describe a model system in which enrichment of SMC and HSF with CE can occur by bypassing receptor-mediated uptake of LDL or apoE rich lipo-proteins. Such a mechanism should not be susceptible to the autoregulation of an apo B-E receptor-mediated process and could explain how SMC can be changed into foam cells during induction of atheroma.

398

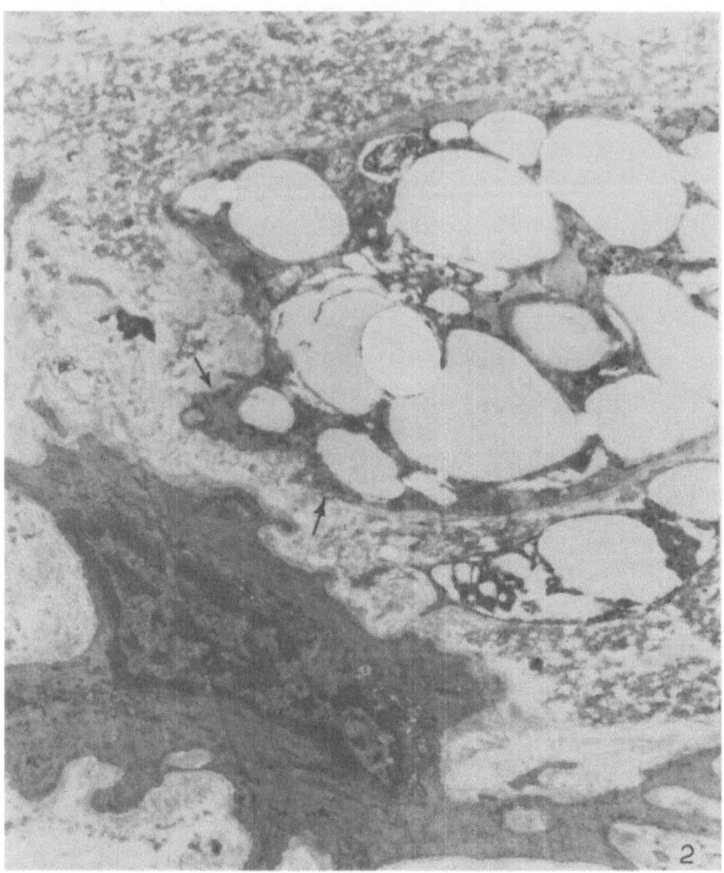

Fig. 2. Electron micrograph of atheromatous aorta showing one intact smooth muscle cell (SMC) and one foam cell which can still be identified as SMC by morphological criteria (arrows)

———————→

Fig. 3. MP were cultured in Dulbecco-Vogt medium containing 10% calf serum for 24–48 h. The medium was replaced by serum-free Dulbecco-Vogt medium, containing 1% bovine serum albumin. The concentration of acetylated LDL was 25 μg protein/ml and incubation was carried out for 72 h. The medium was collected, centrifuged for 10 min at 2000 rev/min and used for postincubation of SMC. Media derived from MP incubated without lipoproteins, as well as non-preincubated Dulbecco-Vogt medium, containing 1% bovine serum albumin, were supplemented with acetylated LDL, 25 μg protein/ml, and were used as controls. The SMC were plated at a density of $7 \cdot 10^4/30$ mm petri dish in medium containing 10% fetal calf serum and [$^3$H] cholesterol and labeled for 48–72 h. The medium was removed, the cell layer washed thrice with phosphate-buffered saline and postincubated in the presence of the indicated media. After 48 h the medium was collected, the cell layer washed and extracted. Following lipid extraction the amount of label recovered in cholesteryl ester was determined by TLC and the amount of total and esterified cholesterol by GLC. Zero time = petri dishes terminated prior to post incubation. Values are ± S.E. of triplicate dishes of six experiments. (Adapted from reference 6)

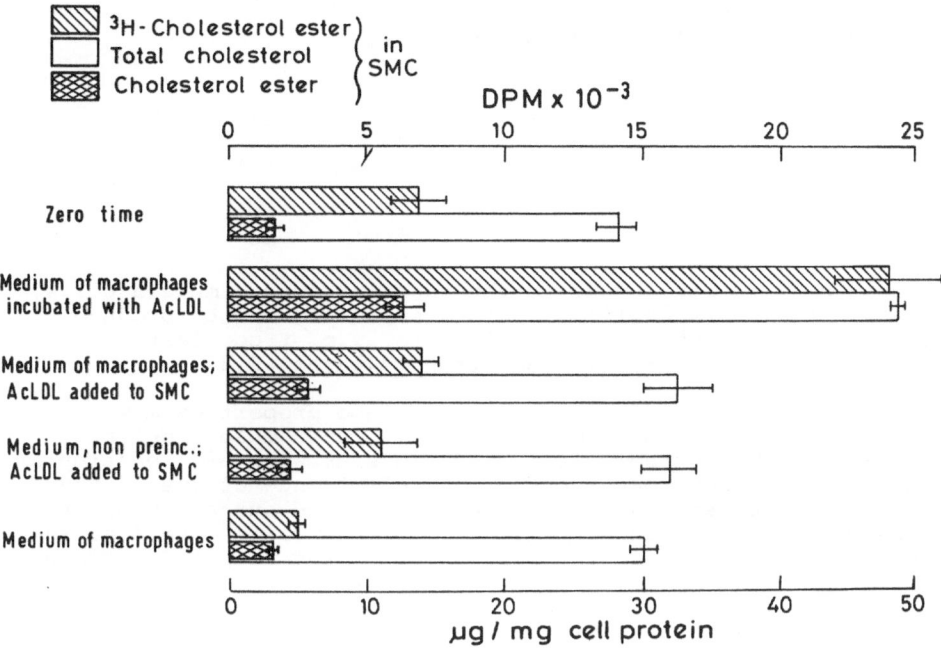

Fig. 3

References

1.  Brown MS, Kovanen PT, Goldstein JL (1981) Regulation of plasma cholesterol by lipoprotein receptors. Science 212: 628-635
2.  Goldstein JL, Ho, YK, Brown MS, Innerarity TL, Mahley RB (1980) Cholesteryl ester accumulation in macrophages resulting from receptor-mediated uptake and degradation of hypercholesterolemic canine β-very low density lipoproteins. J Biol Chem 255: 1839-1848
3.  Stein O, Vanderhoek J, Stein Y (1977) Cholesterol ester accumulation in cultured aortic smooth muscle cells. Atherosclerosis 26: 465-482
4.  Stein O, Halperin O, Stein Y (1979) Comparison of cholesterol egress from cultured cell enriched with cholesterol ester after exposure to cationized LDL or to LDL and chloroquine. Biochim Biophys Acta 573: 1-11
5.  Stein O, Halperin G, Stein Y (1981) Enhancement of cholesterol esterification in aortic smooth muscle cells by medium of macrophages conditioned with acetylated LDL. FEBS Letts 123: 303-307
6.  Stein O, Halperin G, Stein Y (1981) Interaction between macrophages and aortic smooth muscle cells: Enhancement of cholesterol esterification in smooth muscle cells by media of macrophages incubated with acetylated LDL. Biochim Biophys Acta 665: 477-490
7.  Basu SK, Brown MS, Ho YK, Havel RJ, Goldstein JL (1981) Mouse macrophages synthesize and secrete a protein resembling apolipoprotein E. Proc Natl Acad Sci USA 78: 7545-7549
8.  Stein Y, Glangeaud MC, Fainaru M, Stein O (1975) The removal of cholesterol from aortic smooth muscle cells in culture and Landschütz ascites cells by fractions of human high density apolipoprotein. Biochim Biophys Acta 380: 106-118

# Structure and Function of Arterial Smooth Muscle Cells

A. Kádár

Various functions are attributed to the vascular smooth muscle cells, as to maintain the contractility of the vessels (1) and to produce the precursors of connective tissue elements, i.e. tropoelastin, glycosaminoglycans, glycoproteins and tropocollagen (2,3).

Ultrastructural characteristics and cell surface properties may be indicative of the actual functional state of smooth muscle cells at a given time. Aging or pathological conditions as well as a particular physiological requirement may induce the predominance of one of these functions over the other. Changes of cell shape and surface properties alterations of the amount and localization of the various cell organelles are decisive factors in the assessment of the actual functional state of these cells.

It is supposed that primitive mesenchymal cells have a capacity to differentiate towards smooth muscle cells and have a proliferative tendency and a synthetic ability too (4). The above mentioned properties of arterial smooth muscle cells can be visualized in vivo as well as in vitro.

Two types of smooth muscle cells can be distinguished ultrastructurally representing the function of a smooth muscle cell. The "resting" of myofilaments whyle the smooth muscle cells actively engaged in extracellular matrix synthesis are the "modified" smooth muscle cells. The latter have an uneven surface, they are roundish, contain just a small amount of myofilaments and are characterized by an increased number of subcellular organelles (5,6) .

These phenotypic changes of smooth muscle cells i.e. the ability of synthetic type cells with a proliferating capacity to modify toward a contractile type was proven recently in cell cultures (7).

## References

1. Gabbiani G, Hirschel BJ, Ryan GB, Statkov PR, Majno G(1972) Granulation tissue as a contractile organ. A study of structure and function. J exp Med 135: 719-734
2. Ross R, Klebanoff SJ(1971) The smooth muscle cell. I. In vivo synthesis of connective tissue protein. J Cell Biol 50: 159-171
3. Kádár A(1979) The Elastic Fiber. VEB Gustav Fischer Verlag, Jena, Experimental Pathology, Suppl 5
4. Moss NS, Benditt EP(1970) Spontaneous and experimentally induced arterial lesion. I. An ultrastructural survey of the normal chicken aorta. Lab Invest 22: 166-182
5. Kádár A, Csonka É, Veress B, Chaldakov G, Bihari-Varga M(1977) Ultrastructural and functional aspects of vascular smooth muscle cells. In: Progress in Biochem Pharmacol, Karger, Basel p 84-87
6. Kádár A, Bihari-Varga M, Csonka É(1981) The synthesis, transport and excretion of connective tissue macromolecules by smooth muscle cells. Connective Tissue Res 8: 175-180
7. Chamley-Campbell JH, Campbell GR(1981) What controls smooth muscle phenotype? Atherosclerosis 40: 347-357

# Altered Growth Stimulation and LDL Degradation in Human Arterial Smooth Muscle Cells (ASMC) and Fibroblast (F) by Low Molecular Weight Serum Factors from Type II Diabetics

T. Koschinsky, C. Bünting and F. A. Gries

Effects of a prolonged exposure of arterial wall cells to an abnormal metabolic environment have been suspected as angiopathic factors in different metabolic diseases including diabetes. Altered growth and lipoprotein metabolism have been implicated but the nature of the pathogenic metabolic factors in non insulin dependent diabetics (NIDDM) is still unknown.

Serum factors from poorly controlled NIDDM stimulate growth in cultured human ASMC and F 20-50 % more than normal serum (p <0.001). The mitogenic potency of this diabetic serum type is related to low molecular weight compounds that can be completely recovered in the dialysate of Spectrapor 6 membrane (molecular weight cut off: 1000 daltons). The growth stimulation by dialyzed serum fraction is decreased to that of normal serum or dialyzed normal serum. Therefore, the relevance of serum factors as lipoproteins, growth hormone, platelet derived growth factor, insulin and insulin-like growth factor I and II for the increased growth stimulation of mesenchymal cells in type II diabetes is only of limited importance compared to these newly discovered diabetic serum growth factors of low molecular weight.

The low molecular weight compounds of diabetic serum are effective only in combination with serum factors of a molecular weight >12000 daltons that are essential for initiation and continuous stimulation of cellular growth. The growth effect of the original diabetic serum can be restored by recombining the low and higher molecular weight serum fractions (1, 2).

The diabetic serum fraction of low molecular weight is resistant to $95^\circ$C for 15 min., to $-20^\circ$C for at least 8 weeks, to pH 2-11 for 60 min. at $20^\circ$C, to treatment with pronase and trypsin and to extraction by chloroform/methanol. The growth stimulating activity of this serum fraction is reduced to 30-40 % by pretreatment with ß-glucosidase (2 mg/dialysate derived from 7 ml diabetic serum) for 200 min., $25^\circ$C, pH 6. There is a dose dependent linear growth stimulation of the low molecular weight fraction, when added in concentrations equivalent to 5-60 % serum.

2 fractions with growth stimulating activity can be separated after filtration of diabetic serum with Amicon PM 10 or YM 5 and subsequent chromatography on Biogel P6 (90 x 2.6 cm; flow rate 0.5 ml/min.; fraction: 5 ml/tube; eluent: .154 M NaCl). The first growth fraction eluted at tube 72-96 (tube 72 = vitamin $B_{12}$ (1350 D), tube 86 = glucose (180 D), tube 90 = NaCl (58 D) and the second growth fraction at tube 112-140, indicating hydrophobic or charged properties. These rather stable growth factors of nonpeptide nature with low molecular weight may easily penetrate into the arterial wall and thus contribute to the increased growth of ASMC in NIDDM.

The same type of diabetic serum decreased LDL-protein degradation (20-200 ug protein/test) by cathepsin D in human ASMC and F by 16-54 % compared to normal serum (p <0.01). This effect is also related to low molecular weight compounds (<12000 daltons) as the dialyzed diabetic serum fraction (>12000 daltons) did not differ anymore from normal serum in its effect on cathepsin D, and the recombination of both diabetic serum fractions restored the original serum effect. Optimal metabolic control of type II diabetes normalized the serum effects on growth (3) and LDL-protein degradation.

These low molecular weight compounds in serum from type II diabetics represent a new group of potentially angiopathic factors. They depend on the metabolic control of NIDDM and affect growth and lipoprotein catabolism by cathepsin D of cultured human ASMC and F in a way that might be relevant for the angiopathic development in NIDDM.


References

1) Koschinsky T, Bünting C, Schwippert B, Gries FA (1980) Increased growth stimulation of fibroblasts from diabetics by diabetic serum factors of low molecular weight. Atherosclerosis 37: 311-317
2) Koschinsky T, Bünting C, Schwippert B, Gries FA (1982) Studies on inherited and acquired metabolic disorders in cultured arterial smooth muscle cells and fibroblasts. Int. J. Obes. (in press)
3) Koschinsky T, Bünting C, Schwippert B, Gries FA (1981) Regulation of diabetic serum growth factors for human vascular cells by the metabolic control of diabetes mellitus. Atherosclerosis 39: 313-319

## 2.2  Growth Factors and the Arterial Wall

# Platelet-Derived Growth Factor: Properties and Biologic Activities

H. N. Antoniades and L. T. Williams

## Introduction

Normal cells in culture require the presence of clotted blood serum for growth
(1,2). In the absence of serum the cells become arrested in the $G_0/G_1$ phase of
the cell cycle. The readdition of serum stimulates DNA replication and cell proliferation (1,2). Attempts to identify the active component(s) in serum responsible for the growth of cells in culture led to the isolation and partial characterization of a new hormonal polypeptide growth factor from human serum which
appears to be indispensable for the growth of fibroblasts in culture (3). This
human serum-derived growth factor was shown to be a heat-stable(100°C), cationic
(pI 9.7) polypeptide unrelated to serum polypeptides with insulin-like activity
(3,4). It represented the major growth-promoting component in human serum since
its removal with cation-exchange resin rendered the serum incapable of supporting
the growth of fibroblasts (3).

## The Serum Growth Factor Derives from Platelets

Balk (5) initially reported that chicken embryo fibroblasts proliferated more
readily in culture medium supplemented with serum than with platelet-poor plasma.
These observations were confirmed and extended by other investigators who also
reported that extracts of platelets could restore the growth-promoting activity
of plasma (6-8). Subsequent studies have shown that the heat-stable, cationic
polypeptide growth factor which was initially isolated from human serum derived
from platelets (9). The serum growth factor was called platelet-derived growth
factor (PDGF). Subcellular fractionation of human platelets demonstrated that
PDGF is localized in the alpha granules (10). In vivo, PDGF is released selectively at the site of injury where at nanomolar concentrations it modulates the
growth, migration and metabolism of connective tissue cells.

## Structure of PDGF: Identification of Multiple Molecular Weight Forms

PDGF has been isolated from human serum (3), from human platelets (11-14) and
more recently from human platelet-rich plasma (15,16). It is a heat-stable, acid-
stable, cationic polypeptide. Unreduced PDGF consists of several active molecular
weight forms and the most prominent have been called PDGF-I and PDGF-II (12,15)
with molecular weights of about 32,000 and 35,000 respectively. PDGF-I was shown
to consist of two inactive reduced chains with molecular weights of about 15,000
and 18,000 (12). PDGF-II also consists of two inactive reduced chains with molecular weights of about 15,000 and 16,000 (12). It has been suggested that PDGF-
II derives from PDGF-I by proteolytic cleavage of the 18,000 molecular chain (12).
This suggestion may explain the reduction in the molecular weight of PDGF-II and
the reduction in the molecular weight of its 18,000 dalton subunit. Other possible explanations for the presence of multiple molecular weight forms of PDGF may
include a common precursor from which the various active PDGF molecules derive by
proteolysis. Such a possibility is supported by evidence for the presence of
several, distinct active PDGF molecules in the region of 30,000 to 35,000 daltons
(17). Demonstration of these multiple active forms of PDGF has been accomplished
in our laboratory by the development of a technique which allows the direct recovery and assay of active, unreduced PDGF from stained polyacrylamide gels
following preparative SDS-PAGE (12).

Biologic Functions of PDGF

Early studies emphasized primarily the growth promoting effects of PDGF in normal cells in culture. More recent studies have shown that PDGF exerts many other important functions such as stimulation of cell migration, cell metabolism and the modulation of cell membrane receptors. Target cells for these functions of PDGF include fibroblasts, smooth muscle cells, glial cells and neonatal mouse calvaria. Following is a brief account of these diverse functions of PDGF in cells in culture.

1. Effects on Cell Growth

PDGF appears to be indispensable for the growth of connective tissue cells in culture. As described above, platelet-poor plasma alone, or PDGF-depleted serum did not support the growth of these cells in culture. Addition of PDGF restored the ability of plasma and that of PDGF-depleted serum to stimulate DNA synthesis and cell division. In cultured fibroblasts, for optimal activity PDGF requires the synergistic action of other components present in plasma (18,19). Evidence has been presented which suggests that these plasma components belong to the family of polypeptides with insulin-like activity (20).

Unlike normal fibroblasts, viral transformed fibroblasts do not require PDGF for growth (21). These transformed cells can grow equally well in serum or in platelet-poor plasma (21).

2. Effects on Cell Migration

PDGF has been shown to stimulate the migration of cultured fibroblasts (22), smooth muscle cells (23,24) monocytes and neutrophils (25). There is no evidence linking the chemotactic effects of PDGF with those on DNA synthesis and cell proliferation. Other growth factors such as epidermal growth factor, fibroblast growth factor, nerve growth factor and insulin did not stimulate cell migration. Platelet factor 4, a polypeptide stored in the α-granules of platelets, has been shown to stimulate the migration of capillary pericytes and polymorphonuclear leukocytes (24,25).

3. Metabolic Effects

PDGF appears to regulate many diverse metabolic functions in cells in culture. For example, it stimulates amino acid transport, protein synthesis (26) and lipid synthesis (27-30) in cultured fibroblasts and in smooth muscle cells. It is a potent stimulant of prostacyclin production by vascular cells (31,32) and this effect is greatly potentiated by serotonin in cultured vascular smooth muscle cells (32). In neonatal mouse calvaria, PDGF stimulated bone resorption and this action appear to be mediated by the production of prostaglandin $E_2$ ($PGE_2$) (33). There is no evidence linking the metabolic activities of PDGF with its ability to stimulate DNA synthesis and cell division in cells in culture.

4. Modulation of Cell Membrane Receptors

Studies from several laboratories have shown that PDGF can modulate receptor binding of physiologically important components such as low density lipoprotein (LDL) (27-30) epidermal growth factor (34) somatomedin C (35), luteinizing hormone (36) and possibly serotonin (32). Modulation of LDL receptors appears to play an important role in the ability of PDGF to stimulate cholesterol ester synthesis in cultured fibroblasts and smooth muscle cells. Modulation of serotonin receptors by PDGF may account for the dramatic synergistic effects of these two platelet-released products in the production of prostacyclin by cultured vascular smooth muscle cells (32). Prostacyclin is a potent inhibitor of platelet aggregation. Its production by the PDGF-serotonin system may be part of the mechanism regulating platelet aggregation at the site of vascular injury.

## Recognition of PDGF Cell Membrane Receptors

Specific cell membrane receptors for PDGF have been demonstrated in cultures of mouse and human fibroblasts (37-39) and vascular smooth muscle cells (39,40). The reported number of PDGF receptors ranges from 50,000 to 350,000 sites per cell. Values for the apparent equilibrium dissociation constant for the binding of PDGF with its receptor were estimated at 1 nM (37), 0.1 nM (40) and 0.01 nM (39). Cell types unresponsive to PDGF were shown to be devoid of PDGF receptors (37-40).

## In Vivo Functions of PDGF

The ability of PDGF to stimulate the growth and migration of connective tissue cells and the migration of polymorphonuclear leukocytes indicates the important role of this hormonal growth factor in wound healing. Studies on the effect of PDGF on prostacyclin synthesis by cultured vascular cells, in the presence or absence of serotonin, provided new information on the possible role of PDGF in the regulation of platelet aggregation. The effects of PDGF on proliferation, migration and lipid metabolism of cultured aortic smooth muscle cells inspired a provocative new hypothesis for atherogenesis (41).

The work in the Authors' laboratories was supported by National Institutes of Health Grant CA 30101, The Council for Tobacco Research, USA, Inc., and the Milton Fund, Harvard Medical School. L.T. Williams is a recipient of an American Heart Association Clinician Scientist Award.

## References

1. Todaro G, Lazar G, Green H (1965) The initiation of cell division in a contact-inhibited mammalian cell line. J Cell Comp Physiol 66:325-334
2. Holley RW, Kiernan JA (1968) "Contact inhibition" of cell division in 3T3 cells. Proc Natl Acad Sci USA 60:300-304
3. Antoniades HN, Stathakos D, Scher CD (1975) Isolation of a cationic polypeptide from human serum that stimulates proliferation of 3T3 cells. Proc Natl Acad Sci USA 72:2635-2639
4. Scher CD, Stathakos D, Antoniades HN (1974) Dissociation of cell division stimulating capacity for Balb/c-3T3 from the insulin-like activity in human serum. Nature 247:271-281
5. Balk SD (1971) Calcium as a regulator of the proliferation of normal but not of transformed chicken fibroblasts in plasma containing medium. Proc Natl Acad Sci USA 68:271-275
6. Ross R, Glomset J, Kariya B, Harker L (1974) A platelet dependent serum factorthat stimulates the proliferation of arterial smooth muscle cells in vitro. Proc Natl Acad Sci USA 71:1207-1210
7. Kohler N, Lipton A (1974) Platelets as a source of fibroblast growth-promoting activity. Exp Cell Res 87:297-301
8. Westermark B, Wasteson AA (1976) A platelet factor stimulates human normal glial cells. Exp Cell Res 98:170-174
9. Antoniades HN, Scher CD (1977) Radioimmunoassay of a human serum growth factor for Balb/c-3T3 cells: Derivation from platelets. Proc Natl Acad Sci USA 74:1973-1977
10. Kaplan DR, Chao FC, Stiles CD, Antoniades HN, Scher CD (1979) Platelet α-granules contain a growth factor for fibroblasts. Blood 53:1043-1052
11. Antoniades HN, Scher CD, Stiles CD (1979) Purification of human platelet-derived growth factor. Proc Natl Acad Sci USA 76:1809-1813

408

12. Antoniades HN (1981) Human platelet-derived growth factor (PDGF): Purification of PDGF-I and PDGF-II and separation of their reduced subunits. Proc Natl Acad Sci USA 78:7314-7317
13. Heldin CH, Westermark B, Wasteson A (1979) Platelet-derived growth factor: Purification and partial characterization. Proc Natl Acad Sci USA 76:3722-3726
14. Heldin CH, Westermark B, Wasteson A (1981) Platelet-derived growth factor. Isolation by a large scale procedure and analysis of subunit composition. Biochem J 193:903-913
15. Deuel TF, Huang JS, Proffitt RT, Baenziger JU, Chang D, Kennedy BB (1981) Human platelet-derived growth factor. Purification and resolution into two active protein fractions. J Biol Chem 256:8896-8899
16. Raines EW, Ross R (1982) Platelet-derived growth factor I. High yield purification and evidence for multiple forms. J Biol Chem 257:5154-5160
17. Antoniades HN, Williams LT (1982) Human platelet-derived growth factor (PDGF): Structure and function. Fed Proc (in press)
18. Pledger WJ, Stiles CD, Antoniades HN, Scher CD (1977) Induction of DNA synthesis in Balb/c-3T3 cells by serum components: reevaluation of the commitment process. Proc Natl Acad Sci USA 74:4481-4485
19. Vogel A, Raines E, Kariya B, Rivest MJ, Ross R (1978) Coordinate control of 3T3 cell proliferation by platelet-derived growth factor and plasma components. Proc Natl Acad Sci USA 75:2810-2814
20. Stiles CD, Capone GT, Scher CD, Antoniades HN, Van Wyk JJ, Pledger WT (1979) Dual control of cell growth by somatomedins and platelet-derived growth factor. Natl. Acad Sci USA 76:1279-1283
21. Scher CD, Pledger WJ, Martin P, Antoniades HN, Stiles CE (1979) Tranforming viruses directly reduce the cellular growth requirement for a platelet-derived growth factor. J Cell Physiol 97:371-380
22. Seppa, H, Grotendorst G, Seppa S, Schiffmann E, Martin G (1982) Platelet-derived growth factor is chemotactic for fibroblasts. J Cell Biol 92:584-588
23. Grotendorst GR, Seppa HEJ, Kleinman HK, Martin GR (1981) Attachment of smooth muscle cells to collagen and their migration toward platelet-derived growth factor. Proc Natl Sci USA 78:3669-3672
24. Bernstein LR, Antoniades HN, Zetter BR (1982) Migration of cultured vascular cells in response to plasma and platelet-derived factors. J Cell Science (in press)
25. Deuel TF, Senior RM, Huang JS, Griffin GL (1982) Chemotaxis of monocytes and neutrophils to platelet-derived growth factor. J Clin Invest 69:1046-1049
26. Owen AJ, Geyer RP, Antoniades HN (1982) Human platelet-derived growth factor (PDGF) stimulated amino acid transport and protein synthesis by human diploid fibroblasts in plasma-free media. Proc Natl Acad Sci USA 79:3203-3207
27. Chait A, Ross R, Albers JJ, Bierman EL (1980) Platelet-derived growth factor stimulates activity of low density lipoprotein receptors. Proc Natl Acad Sci USA 77:4084-4088
28. Habenicht AJR, Glomset JA, Ross R (1980) Relation of cholesterol and mevalonic acid in the cell cycle in smooth muscle and Swiss 3T3 cells stimulated to divide by platelet-derived growth factor. J Biol Chem 255:5134-5140
29. Witte LD, Cornicelli JA (1980) Platelet-derived growth factor stimulates low density lipoprotein receptor activity in cultured human fibroblasts. Proc Natl Acad Sci USA 77:5962-5966
30. Leslie CC, Antoniades HN, Geyer RP (1982) Stimulation of phospholipid and cholesterol ester synthesis by platelet-derived growth factor in normal and homozygous familial hypercholesterolemia human skin fibroblasts. Biochim Biophys Acta 711:290-304

31. Coughlin SR, Moskowitz MA, Zetter BR, Antoniades HN, Levine L (1980) Platelet-dependent stimulation of prostacyclin synthesis by platelet-derived growth factor. Nature 288:600-602

32. Coughlin SR, Moskowitz MA, Antoniades HN, Levine L (1981) Serotonin receptor-mediated stimulation of bovine smooth muscle cell prostacyclin synthesis and its modulation by platelet-derived growth factor. Proc Natl Acad Sci USA 78:7134-7138

33. Tashjian A, Jr., Hohmann EL, Antoniades HN, Levine L (1982) Platelet-derived growth factor stimulates bone resorption vis a prostaglandin-mediated mechanism. Endocrinology (in press)

34. Wrann M, Fox CF, Ross R (1980) Modulation of epidermal growth factor receptors on 3T3 cells by platelet-derived growth factor. Science 210:1363-1364

35. Clemmons DR, Van Wyk JJ, Pledger WJ (1980) Sequential addition of platelet factor and plasma to Balb/c-3T3 fibroblast cultures stimulates somatomedin-C binding early in cell cycle. Proc Natl Acad Sci USA 77:6644-6648

36. Mondschein JS, Schomberg DW (1981) Growth factors moducate gonadotropin receptor action in granulosa cell cultures. Science 211:1179

37. Heldin CH, Westermark B, Wasteson A (1981) Specific receptors for platelet-derived growth factor on cells derived from connective tissue and glia. Proc Natl Acad Sci USA 78:3664-3668

38. Huang JS, Huang SS, Kennedy B, Deuel TF (1982) Platelet-derived growth factor I and II: Specific binding to responsive 3T3 cells. Fed Proc 41:899 (Abstract)

39. Bowen-Pope D, Ross R (1982) Platelet-derived growth factor II. Specific binding to cultured cells. J Biol Chem 257:5161-5171

40. Williams LT, Tremble P, Antoniades HN (1982) Vascular smooth muscle cell receptors for platelet-derived growth factor: Formation of a non-dissociable state of binding. Proc Natl Acad Sci USA (in press)

41. Ross R (1979) The pathogenesis in atherosclerosis. Mech Ageing Dev 9:435-440.

# Preparation and Characterisation of Platelet-Derived Growth Factor

C. N. Chesterman, T. Walker, K. Chamberlain and F. J. Morgan

## INTRODUCTION

Platelet-derived mitogenic activity, apparently specific for connective tissue cells, is the subject of interest for a number of reasons, not the least of which is possible involvement in the production of the initial lesions of atherosclerosis. It is not clear as to whether platelets release a number of mitogenically active proteins, but most investigation has centred on a cationic species which appears to represent the major activity and which is referred to as the platelet derived growth factor (PDGF).

It has been proposed that PDGF is a basic protein of MW about 30,000 composed of two polypeptide chains ($\sim$13 - 14,000 and $\sim$ 16,000 - 17,000) joined by disulphide bonds (1,2). Broad agreement with these proposals has been reached by others (3,4,5) but multiple forms have been isolated (MW 27,000 - 33,000) and their heterogeneity discussed (4,5,6). Possible explanations include differential glycosylation (4), proteolytic cleavage of the 33,000 species (4,5,6), proteolytic cleavage of a higher molecular weight precursor (5) or separate but similar gene products (4). As outdated platelet concentrates are commonly available, these have been the starting point for preparation studies of PDGF other than those reported by Heldin et al. (1,2,6). The leakage of platelet granule components into plasma during storage and the presence of plasma and platelet proteases are two factors which are likely to introduce artefacts when outdated platelets are used as a preparative source of PDGF.

In an effort to reduce artefacts to a minimum we have begun a programme to prepare PDGF from the release products of washed, freshly collected human platelets. We are simultaneously preparing PDGF from more readily available outdated platelet concentrates.

## MATERIALS And METHODS

### STARTING MATERIAL

#### A. Release products from fresh platelet concentrates

Platelet rich plasma (PRP) was prepared from acid/citrate/dextrose (ACD) anticoagulated whole blood and centrifuged at 250 g for 15 minutes at 4°C. Prostaglandin $E_1$ (PGE$_1$) at a concentration of 1 µg ml$^{-1}$ was added to the PRP and the platelets pelleted by centrifugation at 1200 g for 15 minutes at 4°C. The platelets were resuspended in Tyrode's buffer with PGE$_1$ 1 µg ml$^{-1}$ and washed three times at 4°C. The

washed platelets were resuspended in Tyrode's buffer containing thrombin (Parke Davis) 0.1 U ml$^{-1}$ and aprotinin 10 KIU ml$^{-1}$, warmed to 37°C
and mixed for 2 - 3 minutes until aggregation was apparent.  The supernatant release products (RP) were separated from the aggregated platelets by centrifugation at 4°C at 2200 g for 5 minutes.

## B.   Heparin-bound fraction from disrupted platelets

Outdated clinical platelet concentrates (more than 72 hours from collection) were freeze-thawed twice and centrifuged at 1200 g for 15
minutes.  The supernatant plasma was passed over heparin bound to 4%
agarose (heparin-sepharose, Pharmacia) at a ratio of approximately 4
litres plasma to 200 ml gel.  The gel was washed with 0.05 M phosphate
buffer pH 7.4 until the absorbance of the eluate was less than 0.5 at
230 nm, and mitogenic activity was eluted with 0.4 M NaCl in the same
buffer.

## PREPARATIVE PROCEDURE

Material from both RP of fresh platelets and the heparin-bound fraction
from outdated platelet concentrates were treated similarly in preparative steps essentially as described by HELDIN et al. (1).  After dialysis against 0.01 M NaCl buffer at pH 7.0 the active material was absorbed to CM-sephadex C-50 and eluted with either a gradient of increasing concentration of NaCl or by batchwise elution with 0.5 M NaCl.

Fractions with mitogenic activity were applied to a column of Cibacron
Blue-Sepharose in 1.0 M NaCl, 0.05 M phosphate, pH 7.4, which, after
thorough washing was eluted with 50% polyethylene glycol.  A final gel
chromatography step using Sephadex G 75 equilibrated in 1 M acetic acid
was employed.  Polypropylene containers and plastic columns were used
throughout.

Mitogenic activity was assayed by the stimulation of uptake of $^3$H-
thymidine into TCA-precipitable material in BALB/C 3T3 cells.  Human
plasma-derived serum (5% in DMEM) was used to maintain the cells prior
to and during the assay.  Radioimmunoassays (7) for platelet factor 4
and β-thromboglobulin was used to monitor preparative steps.

## ANALYTICAL TECHNIQUES

PDGF has been iodinated with $^{125}$I using a lactoperoxidase method (8).
Polyacrylamide gel electrophoresis in SDS has been performed using
15% gels (9).  Binding of $^{125}$I PDGF to 3T3 cells has been carried out
using a method similar to that described by HELDIN et al. (1).  The
incubations were carried out for 3 hrs at 4°C and inhibition of binding was tested by including RP from fresh platelets at a concentration
of 5 mg ml$^{-1}$.

High performance liquid chromatography (HPLC) has been carried out
using a Hewlitt Packard (model 1084B)  HPLC and employing conditions
essentially as described by JOHNSSON et al. (6).  Unpurified RP, partially purified PDGF and $^{125}$I-labelled, highly purified PDGF have been
subjected to HPLC.  Up to 400 μg protein in 1 M acetic acid was applied
to a Lichrosorb RP-8 column (10 μm particle size) equilibrated in 0.8 M
pyridine, 2 M formic acid, run with a flow rate of 0.5 ml min$^{-1}$, and
developed with a gradient of n-propanol.  The effluent was tested for
mitogenic activity or counted for radioactivity as appropriate.

## RESULTS And DISCUSSION

### Preparation from fresh platelet release products

The overall purification factor was $3 - 6 \times 10^3$ similar to that reported by HELDIN et al. (1) using similar techniques. The yield has varied but is of the order of 100 µg PDGF per 250 units of platelets. Despite the precautions taken to lessen the release of specific granules from the platelets during collection and centrifugation of the blood and in the subsequent platelet washing procedures there is up to 50% loss into the plasma and washing buffer as judged by RIA of β-thromboglobulin.

Electrophoresis in SDS polyacrylamide gels of $^{125}$I-PDGF resulted in two major components. A higher MW component (∿ 65,000) corresponds to bovine serum albumin (BSA) and is almost certainly an artefact of this labelling procedure, although aggregation of PDGF is a possibility.

The second component has consisted of either an apparent homogeneous peak of MW 30,000 or, in more recent preparations, a double peak representing MW 32,000 and 29,000 (Fig. 1, upper panel). In each case these peaks have been associated with mitogenic activity eluted from the gel when RP have been included with the electrophoresis. In addition, $^{125}$I-PDGF specifically bound (i.e. displaceable by RP) to BALB/C 3T3 cells and subsequently subjected to electrophoresis in the same conditions resulted in an identical pattern to the native material (Fig. 2, upper panel) with the loss of almost all the contaminating high MW protein.

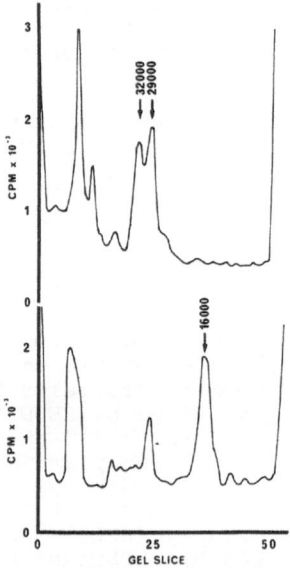

Fig. 1. The upper panel shows the profile of $^{125}$I radioactivity obtained from slices of 15% polyacrylamide gels after electrophoresis in SDS of $^{125}$I-PDGF purified from thrombin release products of washed platelets. In the lower panel the protein has been reduced in the presence of 1% β-mercaptoethanol

Only in the first preparation has there been two $^{125}$I-labelled bands
(∿ 15,000 and 12,000) when the $^{125}$I-PDGF was reduced with β-mercaptoethanol.  In other preparations a single band of $^{125}$I-labelled material
migrating in a position consistent with a MW 15,000 - 16,00 has been
recovered from the gels (Fig. 1, lower panel).  This was also seen
with the $^{125}$I-PDGF bound to the 3T3 cells (Fig. 2, lower panel).

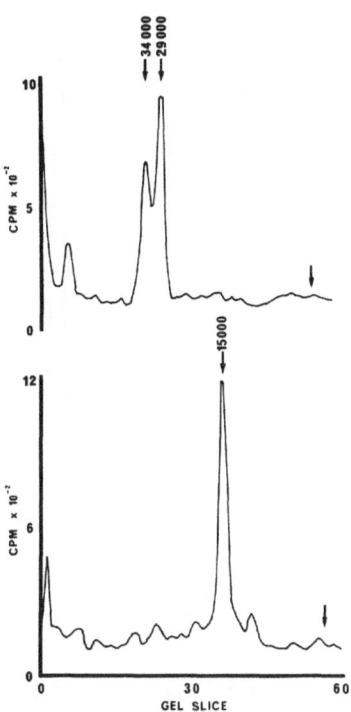

Fig. 2.  The upper panel shows the profile of $^{125}$I radioactivity after
electrophoresis as described in the legend to Fig. 1.  In this case the
$^{125}$I-PDGF has been layered over BALB/C 3T3 cells growing in multiwell
dishes, incubated at 4°C for 3 hrs before washing x 3 in cold PBS,
removal of the cells from the dish with a rubber policeman and finally
dissolution in 0.5 M NaOH + 2% SDS.  The lower panel shows the profile
of the protein reduced in 1% β-mercaptoethanol

The results of three separate HPLC analyses are shown together in
Fig. 3.  The profiles of mitogenic activity of 400 μg partially purified PDGF from outdated platelets (open columns) and of 400 μg fresh
platelet RP (hatched columns) are superimposed on the chromatographic
pattern of radioactivity obtained with an $^{125}$I-labelled preparation
of highly purified PDGF prepared from RP of fresh platelets.  The
iodinated PDGF had been rechromatographed on Sephadex G-100 in 1 M
acetic acid prior to HPLC in order to remove the high MW (∿ 65,000)
contaminant which appears to be a result of the labelling procedure
(see Fig. 1).  The major component from Sephadex G-100 chromatography
which eluted with an apparent MW ∿ 30,000 was applied to the HPLC
column with 233 μg RP as carrier.

The chromatographic patterns of mitogenic activity in the unlabelled
preparations and the $^{125}$I-labelled PDGF were similar.  The radioactive

414

peak coinciding with the biological activity contained 25% of the
total counts applied, the overall recovery being about 85%.

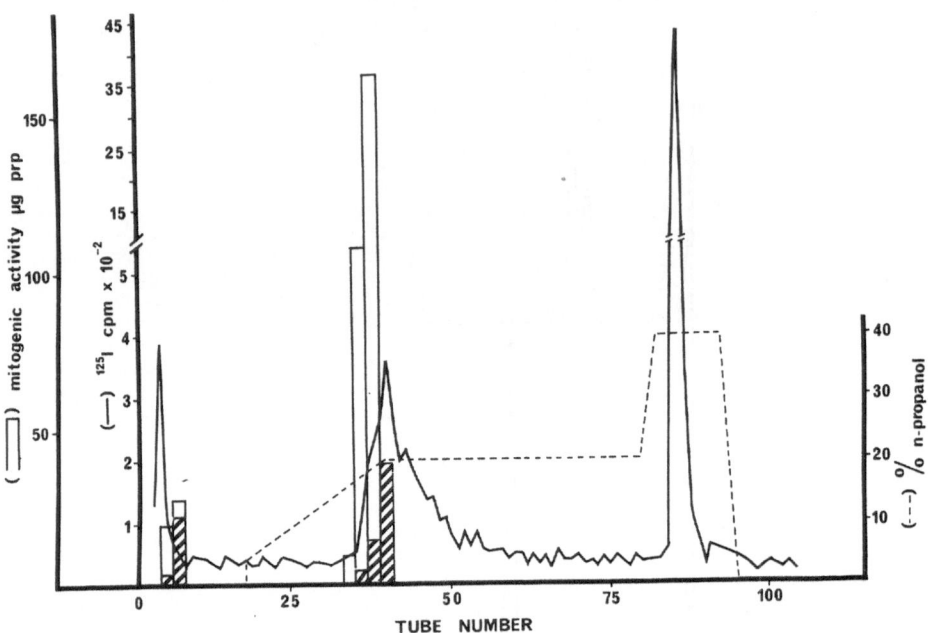

Fig. 3.  HPLC analysis of platelet-derived mitogenic activity from
fresh RP (▨), partially purified PDGF from outdated platelets (⊓) and
radioactive counts of [125]I-PDGF purified from fresh RP (—).  The profiles are from three separate experiments (see text).  The mitogenic
activity is expressed as equivalents of fresh platelet RP (prp)

Platelets release mitogenic activity when activated by a variety of
specific stimuli; the activity almost certainly residing in the α
granule.  We have used the platelet releasate resulting from the action of a "physiological" agonist in an attempt to define some of
the characteristics of this mitogen.  Our results therefore help to
verify a number of the findings reported with respect to PDGF.  While
proteolysis cannot be excluded (for example by thrombin itself) the
possibility was minimised by the use of fresh platelets, washed prior
to release, and by the inclusion of aprotinin in the medium.  The results support the broad findings of others using diverse starting
material ranging from disrupted fresh platelets (1,2) to outdated
concentrates (4,5).  Our preparation supports the contention of DUEUL
et al (4) that there are two authentic active protein fractions, perhaps only differing in carbohydrate content.  Our inability to define
two different subunit chains after reduction may reflect differential
labelling of two chains by [125]I-iodine or may suggest less size heterogeneity of the two chains than originally proposed (6).

## Preparation of PDGF from outdated platelet concentrates

The most pure preparation from this procedure has a specific activity of approximately 10% that of the PDGF derived from thrombin release products. The preparation has been subjected to analysis on HPLC as described above but no further studies performed until a more homogeneous preparation is obtained. During the preparative steps the mitogenic activity exhibits properties identical to that obtained from the fresh platelets.

## ACKNOWLEDGEMENTS

Natalie Fry and Nola Smedley provided expert technical assistance. This project is supported by a grant from the N.H. and M.R.C. of Australia.

## REFERENCES

1.   HELDIN C-H, WESTERMARK B, WASTESON A (1979)  Proc Natl Acad Sci USA 76: 3722-3726
2.   HELDIN C-H, WESTERMARK B, WASTESON A (1981)  Biochem J 193: 907-913
3.   ANTONIADES HN, SCHER CD, STILES CD (1979)  Proc Natl Acad Sci USA 76: 1809-1813
4.   DEUEL TF, HUANG JS, PROFFITT RT, BAENZIGER JU, CHANGE D, KENNEDY BB (1981)  J Biol Chem 256: 8896-8899
5.   RAINES EW, ROSS R (1982)  J Biol Chem 257: 5154-5160
6.   JOHNSSON A, HELDIN C-H, WESTERMARK B, WASTESON A (1981)  Biochem Biophys Res Comm 104: 66-74
7.   CHESTERMAN CN, McGREADY JR, DOYLE DJ, MORGAN FJ (1978)  Brit J Haemat 40: 489-500
8.   THORELL JI, JOHANSSON BC (1971)  Biochim Biophys Acta 251: 363-369
9.   LAEMMLI UK (1970)  Nature (Lond) 227: 680-685

# Effects of PDGF and Endothelial Cell Products on Cellular Lipid and Lipoprotein Metabolism in Human Fibroblasts

L. D. Witte, A. Cornicelli, K. P. Fairbanks, and DeWitt S. Goodman

## Introduction

Platelet-derived growth factor (PDGF) is a potent mitogen that has recently been purified and partly characterized (1-4). PDGF appears to be the principal growth factor in blood serum, may play an important role in the processes of wound healing and tissue repair, and may be involved in the pathogenesis of atherosclerosis (5). PDGF has been shown to have a number of effects on cells in culture, in addition to its effects on cell growth. These include a stimulation of prostaglandin synthesis (6), an apparent role in cellular chemotaxis (7), and an effect on the low density lipoprotein (LDL) receptor pathway and lipid metabolism of cells (8,9).

It is now well established that relationships exist between the processes of cell growth and of cholesterol synthesis and metabolism. Mammalian cells require cholesterol for new membrane synthesis. This cholesterol can be obtained by endogenous synthesis or from an exogenous source. Many cell types normally obtain cholesterol mainly from exogenous LDL via the LDL receptor pathway (10). Studies have indicated that LDL receptor activity is elevated in growing cells compared to quiescent cells (11). Furthermore, cell growth is blocked if cholesterol synthesis is inhibited and exogenous cholesterol is not available (12-14).

We now report the results of studies designed to explore in detail the effects of PDGF on both the LDL receptor pathway and on cholesterol biosynthesis in cultured human fibroblasts. Cholesterol synthesis rate was assessed by measuring the activitiy of 3-hydroxy-3-methylglutaryl coenzyme A (HMG-CoA) reductase, the rate limiting enzyme of cholesterol biosynthesis. In addition, studies with endothelial cell conditioned medium (ECCM), which contains both a potent mitogen (the EC-derived growth factor, or EDGF) (15,16), and an inhibitor of cellular LDL degradation (9), will be described.

## Methods

Extensive studies have been conducted to delineate the effects of PDGF on the various components of the LDL receptor pathway. The methods used have been described in detail (9). In brief, human fibroblasts were grown to near confluency, and then brought to quiescence and a state of LDL deprivation by 48 hours of culture in a medium that contained no lipoproteins and no PDGF. The cells were then exposed either to increasing concentrations of PDGF for 24 hours, or to a fairly high concentration of PDGF for increasing periods of time. At the end of the PDGF exposure period, assays were conducted for the metabolic parameters of interest. The parameters studied in various experiments included: specific LDL cell surface binding, LDL internalization, LDL degradation, HMG-CoA reductase, cholesterol esterification, DNA synthesis, and protein synthesis. $^{125}$I-LDL binding was assayed by measuring radioactivity released from intact cells by dextran sulfate at 4°C (or at 37°C). $^{125}$I-LDL binding, internalization, and degradation were measured conjointly after incubating cells with the $^{125}$I-LDL at 37°C. HMG-CoA reductase activity was assessed by determining the extent of conversion of substrate $^{14}$C-HMG-CoA into the product $^{14}$C-mevalonate. Cholesterol esterification was measured by incorporation of $^{14}$C-oleate substrate into cholesteryl oleate. DNA synthesis was assessed by measuring the incorporation of $^3$H-thymidine into DNA. Protein synthesis was measured by determining the incorporation of $^3$H-amino acids into cellular protein.

## PDGF and the LDL Receptor Pathway

Increasing concentrations of PDGF stimulated parallel increases in both DNA synthesis and $^{125}$I-LDL cell surface binding (9). The effect of PDGF was due entirely to an increase (up to 4.3-fold) in the number of receptor sites per cell, and not to a change in receptor affinity. Thus, the apparent $K_d$ remained at approximately 2.0 nM both in the absence and in the presence of PDGF.

We next sought to determine whether or not LDL bound by PDGF-stimulated cells was subsequently metabolized in the same manner as LDL bound by cells not treated with PDGF. This question was explored by measuring the effects of increasing levels of PDGF on cellular $^{125}$I-LDL binding, internalization, and degradation at 37°C. Approximately parallel, PDGF concentration-dependent increases in $^{125}$I-LDL binding, internalization, and degradation were observed throughout the PDGF concentration range studied. The ratios of internalized to bound $^{125}$I-LDL and of degraded to bound $^{125}$I-LDL were not changed in PDGF-stimulated compared to unstimulated cells. Thus, PDGF-stimulated cells appear to metabolize receptor-bound LDL in a manner that is both qualitatively and quantitatively identical with that seen with unstimulated cells.

It is well established that LDL internalization and degradation via the LDL receptor pathway is followed by a number of metabolic changes in the cell (10), including: (i) stimulation of cholesterol esterification (of acyl-CoA:cholesterol acyltransferase, or ACAT, activity); (ii) down-regulation (suppression) of LDL receptor activity; and (iii) suppression of HMG-CoA reductase activity. These effects are considered to be due to the free cholesterol made available to the cell after degradation of the LDL in the lysosome.

The effects of PDGF on these parameters were explored. ACAT activity was found to be stimulated to the same extent as was $^{125}$I-LDL binding when fibroblasts were treated with increasing concentrations of PDGF. Secondly, LDL receptor activity was markedly suppressed (down-regulated) by LDL both in PDGF-stimulated and in untreated cells. In the presence of PDGF, however, even at very high concentrations of LDL, the LDL receptor activity was not completely suppressed. The effects of PDGF on HMG-CoA reductase activity are discussed below. Taken together, these studies indicate that LDL cholesterol, taken in increased amounts into the PDGF-stimulated cell via the LDL receptor pathway, appears to become available normally and to have metabolic effects within the cell similar to those seen in quiescent cells.

## PDGF and HMG-CoA Reductase Activity

The effects of PDGF on HMG-CoA reductase activity were explored both in the absence and in the presence of LDL. In the absence of LDL, PDGF stimulated HMG-CoA reductase activity in a concentration-dependent manner, resulting in a 2-4-fold increase in reductase activity. Time course studies showed that this effect of PDGF on reductase activity was biphasic. Early after the addition of PDGF (4-8 hours) a large increase (3-4-fold) in reductase activity was observed. Reductase activity then declined, followed by a second, somewhat lesser increase at approximately 24 hours, concurrent with DNA synthesis.

It has been suggested (12-14) that mevalonate produced by HMG-CoA reductase may play two important roles in cell growth. First, conversion of the mevalonate to cholesterol can provide the sterol needed for new membrane synthesis during growth. Secondly, however, it has been suggested that there is also a non-sterol product of mevalonate which may be involved in trace quantities in the regulation of DNA synthesis and cell growth. In order to obtain information relevant to this concept, we conducted a detailed study of the effects of increasing concentrations of LDL on the time course of reductase stimulation by PDGF. We were particularly

interested to explore whether the two peaks of reductase stimulation (early, at
4-8 hours, and later, at about 24 hours) were differentially sensitive to inhibition by LDL. Five levels of LDL, from 2 to 200 μg/ml, were used. Increasing
concentrations of LDL throughout this concentration range produced progressive
decreases in reductase activity throughout the entire time period studied.
Roughly parallel inhibitions of reductase by LDL were seen in the early and later
peaks of enzyme stimulation. Even at 200 μg/ml, however, LDL was unable to completely suppress reductase activity at either time point (in the presence of PDGF).
This latter observation is consistent with the above suggestion that the mitogenically stimulated cell requires a mevalonate product in addition to cholesterol,
and that mevalonate itself would be required (12-14) to achieve complete reductase
suppression. The lack of a differential effect of LDL on the two peaks of reductase activity suggests that there is no evidence supporting a different mechanism
for regulation of the enzyme at the two time points.

Protein synthesis was also found to be increased by exposure to PDGF at the same
early and later time points. Time course studies of the effect of PDGF on the
LDL receptor had also previously shown an early (4-8 hours) increase in LDL binding,
with a further increase occurring at the time of DNA synthesis. These studies
suggest that stimulation of cells with PDGF results in both early (4-8 hours)
and later (at the time of DNA synthesis) effects on several possibly related
cellular metabolic parameters.


## Endothelial Cell Conditioned Medium and the LDL Receptor Pathway

Endothelial cells in culture release a potent mitogen, of potential significance
in atherogenesis. We used ECCM as a source of this mitogen. ECCM produced concentration-dependent and parallel increases in DNA synthesis and in $^{125}$I-LDL
binding that were both qualitatively similar to the increases produced by PDGF
(9). In contrast, a major difference between the effects of ECCM and PDGF was
seen when $^{125}$I-LDL internalization and degradation were examined. At higher
levels of ECCM, although LDL internalization was stimulated and appeared to take
place effectively, LDL degradation was inhibited. The inhibition of LDL degradation apparently led to a reduced liberation of LDL cholesterol, as evident from
studies carried out on the effects of ECCM on HMG-CoA reductase and on ACAT activities. Thus, ECCM-treated cells did not effectively increase cholesterol esterification or suppress reductase activity when LDL was present.

An assay was designed to measure the putative inhibitor of LDL degradation present
in ECCM, by determining the binding, internalization, and degradation of $^{125}$I-LDL
in human fibroblasts at 37°C. The amount of $^{125}$I-LDL degraded divided by the total
amount available for degradation in ECCM treated cells was compared to the similar
value obtained in non-treated cells. Using this value as an index of inhibition
(of LDL degradation), we conducted experiments to determine whether the mitogenic
effect of ECCM could be separated from the LDL degradation inhibitory effect.

On the basis of heat-stability the mitogenic effect of ECCM was found to be de-
stroyed at temperatures of 75°C and greater, while the inhibitory effect was
stable even at 100°C for 2 min. Utilizing specific molecular weight cut-off
membranes the size of the ECCM mitogen was found to be greater than 30,000
daltons, while the degradation-inhibitor appeared to be less than·2,000 daltons.
Finally, on Blue Sepharose affinity chromatography the mitogen in ECCM was found
to bind to the gel matrix, while the degradation-inhibitor did not bind. Therefore, on the basis of at least three criteria the mitogen and the LDL degradation-
inhibitor found in ECCM do not appear to be the same molecule and can, in fact,
be separated from each other.

## Concluding Remarks

The findings reported here may be of considerable potential significance with regard to the process of atherogenesis. In addition to PDGF's mitogenic effect, that can lead to arterial smooth muscle cell proliferation, PDGF has several effects on target cells that may promote lipid accumulation. Thus, as reported here, PDGF-stimulated cells did not show complete suppression of either HMG-CoA reductase or of LDL receptor number in the presence of large levels of LDL. These findings suggest that cells stimulated towards rapid growth by PDGF may also show enhanced LDL intake and enhanced cholesterol synthesis, even in the presence of excessive LDL.

The studies with ECCM suggest that endothelial cells may contribute in still another way to the processes of cell proliferation and lipid accumulation that occur in atherogenesis. Thus, endothelial cells can provide a mitogen, with metabolic effects similar to those seen with PDGF, but may also release an inhibitor of LDL degradation that may participate in the process of lipid accumulation. Whether these products of endothelial cells have in vivo physiological or pathophysiological significance can only await further investigation.

## Acknowledgements

This work was supported by NHLBI grant HL 21006 (SCOR in Arteriosclerosis)

## References

1.  Heldin, C-H., Westermark, B., and Wasteson, A. (1981) Platelet-derived growth factor. Isolation by large-scale procedure and analysis of subunit composition. Biochem. J. 193: 907-913
2.  Antoniades, H. N., Scher, C. D., and Stiles, C. D. (1979) Purification of human platelet-derived growth factor. Proc. Natl. Acad. Sci. U.S.A. 76: 1809-1813
3.  Deuel, T. F., Huang, J. S., Proffitt, R. T., Baenziger, J. U., Chang, D., and Kennedy, B.B. (1981) Human platelet-derived growth factor. Purification and resolution into two active protein fractions. J. Biol. Chem. 256: 8896-8899
4.  Raines, E. W., and Ross, R. (1982) Platelet-derived growth factor. I. High yield purification and evidence for multiple forms. J. Biol. Chem. 257: 5154-5160
5.  Ross, R. (1981) Atherosclerosis: A problem of the biology of arterial wall cells and their interactions with blood components. Arteriosclerosis 1: 293-311
6.  Coughlin, S. R., Moskowitz, M. A., Zetter, B. R., and Levine, L. (1980) Platelet-dependent stimulation of prostacyclin synthesis by platelet-derived growth factor. Nature 288: 600-602
7.  Grotendorst, G. R., Seppa, H. E., Kleinman, H. K., and Martin, G. R. (1981) Attachment of smooth muscle cells to collagen and their migration toward platelet-derived growth factor. Proc. Natl. Acad. Sci. U.S.A. 78: 3669-3672
8.  Chait, A., Ross, R., Albers, J. J., and Bierman, E. L. (1980) Platelet-derived growth factor stimulates activity of low density lipoprotein receptors. Proc. Natl. Acad. Sci. U.S.A. 77: 4084-4088.
9.  Witte, L. D., Cornicelli, J. A., Miller, R. W., and Goodman, DeW. S. (1982) Effects of platelet-derived and endothelial cell-derived growth factors on the low density lipoprotein receptor pathway in cultured human fibroblasts. J. Biol. Chem. 257: 5392-5401
10. Goldstein, J. L., and Brown, M. S. (1977) The low-density lipoprotein pathway and its relation to atherosclerosis. Ann. Rev. Biochem. 46: 897-930

11. Goldstein, J. L., and Brown, M. S. (1974) Binding and degradation of low density lipoproteins by cultured human fibroblasts. J. Biol. Chem. 249: 5153–5162.

12. Brown, M. S., and Goldstein, J. L. (1980) Multivalent feedback regulation of HMG CoA reductase, a control mechanism coordinating isoprenoid synthesis and cell growth. J. Lipid Res. 21: 505–517

13. Habenicht, A. J. R., Glomset, J. A., and Ross, R. (1980) Relation of cholesterol and mevalonic acid to the cell cycle in smooth muscle and Swiss 3T3 cells stimulated to divide by platelet-derived growth factor. J. Biol. Chem. 255: 5134–5140

14. Quesney-Huneeus, V., Wiley, M. H., and Siperstein, M. D. (1980) Isopentenyladenine as a mediator of mevalonate-regulated DNA replication. Proc. Natl. Acad. Sci. U.S.A. 77: 5842–5846

15. Gajdusek, C., DiCorleto, P., Ross, R., and Schwartz, S. M. (1980) An endothelial cell-derived growth factor. J. Cell Biol. 85: 467–472

16. Fass, D. N., Downing, M. R., Meyers, P., Bowie, E. J. W., and Witte, L. D. (1978) Cell growth stimulation by normal and von Willebrand porcine platelets and endothelial cells. Blood 52: Suppl. 1: 181 (abstr.)

## 2.3 HMG – CoA Reductase and Cell Metabolism

# Site of Action of LCAT in Plasma

P. J. Barter

When LCAT acts in human plasma the esterified cholesterol which is
formed is distributed throughout all lipoprotein fractions (1). In
mass terms, most is accommodated in the VLDL-LDL fraction (2). However, this does not necessarily indicate a direct incorporation of
LCAT-derived esterified cholesterol into all fractions, since human
plasma contains an esterified cholesterol transfer/exchange protein (3)
which promotes an equilibration of esterified cholesterol between all
lipoprotein fractions (4); esterified cholesterol incorporated into
any one lipoprotein fraction will become redistributed among all fractions. Thus, there are two potential pathways by which esterified
cholesterol of LCAT origin may be incorporated into a given lipoprotein
fraction: (i) as a direct incorporation from its site of synthesis and
(ii) as a transfer from another fraction as a consequence of the equilibration process.

According to a conventional view that LCAT acts only on HDL (5), an
incorporation of esterified cholesterol into VLDL and LDL may depend
totally on the process of equilibration and the transfer/exchange protein which promotes it. Recently, however, this view has been challenged. It has been proposed that, physiologically, LCAT exists as a
small molecular complex with apolipoproteins Al and D and that this
complex picks up free cholesterol from all lipoproteins; esterifies it
and incorporates a major proportion of the newly formed esterified
cholesterol directly into VLDL and LDL, bypassing the major HDL pool
(6). Such a view relegates the transfer/exchange protein to a minor
or non-existent role in terms of the incorporation of LCAT-derived
esterified cholesterol into VLDL and LDL.

## Which lipoprotein fractions are the immediate recipients of the esterified cholesterol formed in the LCAT reaction?

To address this issue, experiments have been designed to examine the
lipoprotein distribution of newly formed esterified cholesterol in a
system uncomplicated by concurrent equilibration of esterified cholesterol between the different lipoprotein fractions. This has been
achieved by taking advantage of the deficiency of esterified cholesterol transfer/exchange protein activity in pig plasma (7). Experiments have been performed with: (a) unseparated pig plasma and (b) a
reconstituted plasma containing human lipoproteins (separated from the
transfer/exchange protein by ultracentrifugation (4)) mixed with pig
lipoprotein-free plasma. To assess the potential of artefacts introduced by the ultracentrifugal separation of human lipoproteins, experiments have been performed also with: (c) unseparated human plasma
and (d) human lipoproteins reconstituted with human lipoprotein-free
plasma. Each preparation, plus a tracer amount of $^3$H-cholesterol, has
been incubated in vitro at 37°C, after which the various lipoproteins
have been isolated and assayed for esterified $^3$H-cholesterol. In the
absence of transfers between the different lipoprotein fractions in
mixtures (a) and (b), a recovery of esterified $^3$H-cholesterol is

indicative of an incorporation into that fraction directly from its
site of synthesis.

Table 1. Incubations of free [3]H-cholesterol with unseparated and with
reconstituted plasma

| Hours of Incubation | Percentage of total esterified [3]H-cholesterol recovered in VLDL + LDL | | | |
|---|---|---|---|---|
| | Human plasma | Pig plasma | Human lipoproteins + human lipoprotein-free plasma | Human lipoproteins + pig lipoprotein-free plasma |
| 1 | 14.4 | 13.6 | 12.8 | 10.6 |
| 3 | 21.8 | 13.0 | 25.3 | 9.9 |
| 6 | 34.7 | 13.1 | 31.1 | 11.9 |
| 24 | 59.4 | 14.2 | 57.7 | 9.3 |

Human plasma, pig plasma and a reconstituted "plasma" containing human
lipoproteins (density < 1.21 g/ml) mixed with either human or pig
lipoprotein-free plasma (density > 1.21 g/ml) were incubated at $37^{o}$C
with an ethanolic solution of free [3]H-cholesterol (4)). Each value
represents the mean of triplicate incubations in a single representative experiment. Comparable results have been obtained in two other
experiments.

In the case of unseparated human plasma and of human plasma reconstituted after ultracentrifugation, the lipoprotein distribution of esterified [3]H-cholesterol was virtually identical, indicating that the ultracentrifugation per se did not introduce a serious artefact. In each
case there was an initial recovery of esterified [3]H-cholesterol predominantly in HDL with subsequent redistribution to VLDL and LDL (Table
1); after 24 hours the specific activity of esterified cholesterol was
virtually identical in all fractions.

In the incubations which lacked transfer/exchange protein activity,
viz. pig plasma and human lipoproteins with pig lipoprotein-free plasma, the pattern of distribution was quite different from that when
the transfer/exchange protein was present. In each case, esterified
[3]H-cholesterol was recovered in both HDL and VLDL-LDL. However, the
relative proportions in each fraction did not vary with duration of
incubation. At physiological lipoprotein concentrations, whether
after one hour or 24 hours of incubation, 85-90% of the esterified [3]H-
cholesterol was recovered in HDL (Table 1). The proportion recovered
in VLDL-LDL, while constant in a given incubation mixture, was greater
in experiments in which the concentration of VLDL-LDL was increased
and less when the concentration of HDL was increased.

These results indicate that LCAT-derived esterified cholesterol is
incorporated into both VLDL-LDL and HDL directly from its site of
synthesis. But at physiological concentrations of lipoproteins the
major initial recipients are HDL.

Site of action of LCAT

Although the HDL fraction was the major initial recipient of the
esterified cholesterol formed in the LCAT reaction, finding that there

was a direct incorporation of some 10-15% into VLDL and LDL raises questions about the site of action of LCAT. Such a finding is compatible with either of two models (Fig. 1).

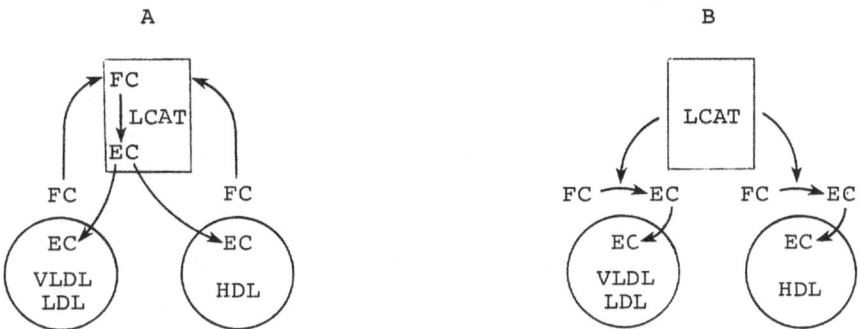

**Figure 1.** Alternate models for a direct incorporation of LCAT-derived esterified cholesterol into both HDL and VLDL-LDL

Model A proposes an action of LCAT within a small population of specific LCAT-substrate lipoproteins (possibly within the proposed LCAT-apo A1-apo D complex) from which esterified cholesterol is delivered directly to both HDL and VLDL-LDL by an unknown mechanism (possibly apo D acting as a transfer protein) which does not involve the esterified cholesterol transfer/exchange protein. Model B proposes that LCAT, either in isolation or as part of a complex with other proteins, acts directly on the free cholesterol in the surface monolayer of both HDL and VLDL-LDL, with the esterified cholesterol so formed being internalized into the lipoprotein core. It is possible to differentiate between these two models by performing in vitro incubations of plasma in which free $^{3}$H-cholesterol is introduced as a component of different lipoprotein fractions. Although the free $^{3}$H-cholesterol added as a component of one fraction redistributes rapidly between all fractions (8), complete equilibration is not instantaneous. During the first 30 minutes of incubation it is possible to examine the consequences of having marked differences in the specific activity of free cholesterol in one or other lipoprotein fraction. Model A, which proposes an action of LCAT which is remote from the major lipoprotein pools, predicts a relative incorporation of esterified $^{3}$H-cholesterol into VLDL-LDL and HDL which will be independent of differing free cholesterol specific activities in the two fractions. Model B predicts that the relative incorporation into VLDL-LDL and HDL will reflect their relative free cholesterol specific activities. For simplicity, the experiments described below were performed in a system containing only two lipoprotein fractions, LDL and HDL.

Preparations of isolated human and pig LDL and HDL were labelled with free $^{3}$H-cholesterol during two hour 37°C incubations. Other aliquots of the same lipoprotein preparations were subjected to identical incubation conditions without the addition of free $^{3}$H-cholesterol. Then in a typical experiment with pig plasma, small amounts of labelled pig LDL and unlabelled pig HDL were added to one aliquot of pig VLDL-deficient plasma, while a second aliquot received identical amounts of unlabelled LDL and labelled HDL. Comparable experiments were performed with mixtures of human LDL and HDL with pig lipoprotein-free plasma and with human VLDL-deficient plasma. These mixtures were then subjected to short periods of incubation at 37°C after which esterified $^3$H-cholesterol was measured in the total incubation mixture, in LDL and in HDL. LDL and HDL were separated both by ultracentrifugation and (more rapidly) by precipitation of LDL with heparin and manganese chloride (9). The method of separation did not influence the results; those shown in Table 2 represent LDL separated by ultracentrifugation.

Table 2. Incubations containing free $^3$H-cholesterol added as a component of LDL or HDL

| | | Increment in esterified $^3$H-cholesterol | | | |
|---|---|---|---|---|---|
| | | Total Incubation (% total $^3$H) | | Ratio $\frac{LDL}{Total\ Incubation}$ X 100 | |
| Incubation mixture | Time Interval (min) | Label added as LDL | Label added as HDL | Label added as LDL | Label added as HDL |
| Pig VLDL-deficient plasma | 0-10 | 0.5 | 3.3 | 21 | 4 |
| | 10-30 | 2.0 | 3.9 | 16 | 8 |
| | 30-180 | 12.9 | 14.4 | 13 | 13 |
| Human LDL, HDL plus pig lipoprotein-free plasma | 0-10 | 0.6 | 4.1 | 57 | 4 |
| | 10-20 | 0.9 | 2.0 | 40 | 16 |
| | 20-30 | 1.2 | 1.3 | 31 | 27 |
| | 30-120 | 6.7 | 7.3 | 28 | 29 |
| Human VLDL-deficient plasma | 0-10 | 0.5 | 2.1 | 29 | 2 |
| | 10-20 | 1.0 | 1.6 | 20 | 9 |
| | 20-30 | 1.2 | 1.2 | 13 | 17 |
| | 30-120 | 8.8 | 8.9 | 21 | 26 |

Pig or human VLDL-deficient plasma (d > 1.019 g/ml) or a mixture of human LDL (1.019-1.060 g/ml) and HDL (1.13-1.20 g/ml) with pig lipoprotein-free plasma (> 1.21 g/ml) were incubated with preparations of pig or human LDL or HDL prelabelled with free $^3$H-cholesterol. Each value represents the mean of triplicate incubations in a single representative experiment. Comparable results have been obtained in two other experiments.

In the case of both pig and human lipoproteins there were two consistent results during the first 10-20 minutes of incubation (Table 2). (a) The percentage of the added free $^3$H-cholesterol converted to esterified $^3$H-cholesterol in the total incubation mixture was much greater when it had been added as HDL than when added as LDL, clearly indicating a preferential esterification of HDL free cholesterol. (b) The percentage of the total esterified $^3$H-cholesterol which was recovered in LDL was much greater when the free $^3$H-cholesterol was added as LDL than when it was added as HDL. This result was apparent even in the incubations of human VLDL-deficient plasma in which, during the first 20 minutes, any equilibration of esterified cholesterol between HDL and LDL was insufficient to obscure an initial preferential incorporation of esterified $^3$H-cholesterol into one or other fraction. This finding essentially excludes Model A, but is consistent with Model B which proposes a direct action of LCAT on both LDL and HDL.

## Proposed scheme for the formation and distribution of esterified cholesterol in human plasma

Relating these present results to those in earlier studies of plasma esterified cholesterol transfers and exchanges (10-12), the following scheme is proposed. LCAT, perhaps as a component of the postulated LCAT-apo Al-apo D complex, interacts randomly with particles in all lipoprotein fractions. Because of the much greater number of HDL particles at physiological concentrations of lipoproteins, there is a predominance of such interactions within the HDL fraction. During an interaction free cholesterol on the lipoprotein surface is esterified and the esterified cholesterol so formed is internalized into the lipoprotein core. Since free cholesterol equilibrates between different lipoprotein fractions, a greater rate of esterification of HDL free cholesterol will create a concentration gradient down which free cholesterol will move from other lipoprotein fractions, so that, in net mass terms, the larger pool in the VLDL-LDL will contribute most of the free cholesterol for a reaction taking place predominantly in the HDL. In the absence of esterified cholesterol transfer/exchange protein activity, as in pig plasma, the process stops at this point with about 90% of the new esterified cholesterol in HDL and about 10% in VLDL-LDL (Table 1). However, in the presence of the transfer/exchange protein, as in human plasma, the much greater initial incorporation of esterified cholesterol into HDL creates a concentration gradient which drives a net mass transfer of esterified cholesterol from HDL to other fractions and, ultimately, to an even distribution between all fractions. In quantitative terms, a direct incorporation of 10% of LCAT-derived esterified cholesterol into human VLDL-LDL represents about 5-10 nmol/ml plasma/hour (5); by contrast, a molar transfer from human HDL to VLDL-LDL is of the order of 100-300 nmol/ml plasma/hour (10). Thus, although there may be a direct action of LCAT on VLDL-LDL, it may be concluded that transfers from HDL in the equilibration process mediated by the transfer/exchange protein represent the major pathway by which esterified cholesterol of LCAT origin is incorporated into human VLDL-LDL.

Acknowledgements  Miss A Stibbs and Miss J Berry are thanked for their technical assistance. This work was supported by grants from the National Health and Medical Research Council of Australia and from the National Heart Foundation of Australia.

## References

1. Akanuma T, Glomset J (1968) J Lipid Res 9: 620-626
2. Fielding CJ, Fielding PE (1981) J Biol Chem 256: 2102-2104
3. Pattnaik NM, Montes A, Hughes LB, Zilversmit DB (1978) Biochim Biophys Acta 530: 428-438
4. Barter PJ, Lally JI (1979) Metabolism 28: 230-236
5. Glomset JA (1968) J Lipid Res 9: 155-167
6. Fielding PE, Fielding CJ (1980) Proc Natl Acad Sci USA 77: 3327-3330
7. Barter PJ, Ha YC, Calvert GD (1981) Atherosclerosis 38: 165-175
8. Goodman D (1964) J Clin Invest 43: 2026-2036
9. Burstein M, Scholnick HR, Morfin R (1970) J Lipid Res 11: 583-595
10. Barter PJ, Jones ME (1980) Atherosclerosis 34: 67-74
11. Barter PJ, Jones ME (1981) J Lipid Res 21: 238-249
12. Hopkins GJ, Barter PJ (1980) Metabolism 29: 546-650

# The Isolation and Partial Characterisation of Two Lipid Transfer Proteins (LTP-I and LTP-II), Each of Which Facilitates the Transfer of Esterified Cholesterol, Triglyceride and Phospholipid Between Plasma Lipoproteins

G. D. Calvert and M. Abby

## A. Introduction

Although the overall composition of individual plasma lipoprotein
classes *in vivo* may be relatively constant, it can be shown (by
using radioactive tracer lipids) that the lipid components of lipoproteins are in a constant state of flux.  Cholesterol is esterified
predominantly in the high density lipoprotein (HDL) class by lecithin:
cholesterol acyltransferase (LCAT), and esterified cholesterol appears
to be transferred from HDL to very low density and low density lipoproteins (VLDL and LDL).  Phospholipid is also in flux; phosphatidylcholine forms a substrate for LCAT activity, with the resultant formation of lysophosphatidylcholine.  Throughout the day there are surges
in plasma triglyceride concentration, and the relative concentration
of triglyceride in lipoprotein particles varies.  Recent work has
shown that at least some of these lipid transfers are protein-mediated.

The bidirectional transfer of cholesteryl ester between human plasma
lipoproteins has been shown to be facilitated by a plasma protein
which has been called plasma cholesteryl ester transfer (or exchange)
protein (1-6).  This protein has been reported to have $M_r$ 80 000 and
pI 5.0 (2) or $M_r$ 130 000 and pI 5.2 (6).  The kinetics of cholesteryl
ester transfers have been extensively reported by Barter and
colleagues (7).

Transport between lipoproteins of the other major core lipid of plasma
lipoproteins, triglyceride, has also been shown to be facilitated by
a human plasma protein (8).  Whether or not triglyceride transfer
protein is the same as cholesteryl ester transfer protein has been a
moot question.  Because p-chloromercuriphenylsulphonate (PCMPS)
inhibits triglyceride transfer activity almost completely (at a concentration of 2 mM), whereas it has little effect on cholesteryl ester
transfer activity, it has been thought that the protein responsible
for the transfer of cholesteryl ester may differ from that responsible
for the transfer of triglyceride (9).

A human plasma phospholipid transfer protein has also been partially
purified and shown to have some of the characteristics of the cholesteryl ester transfer protein (6).  It has been suggested that apoli-
poprotein-D (apo-D) may also be required for cholesteryl ester transfer (10,11); however, apo-D has been shown to differ in several
respects from cholesteryl ester transfer protein (12).

We describe the isolation and some properties of two human plasma proteins (lipid transfer proteins, which we have designated LTP-I and
LTP-II) which facilitate cholesteryl ester, triglyceride and phospholipid transfer between plasma lipoproteins *in vitro*.

B.  Isolation of LTP-I and LTP-II

1.  Assay of lipid transfer activity

Lipid transfer activity was measured as the ability of protein fractions to accelerate the transfer of lipid tracer from LDL to HDL at
37°C.  The preparation of LDL labelled with [$^{14}$C]-triglyceride (12)
and with [$^3$H]-cholesteryl ester (4) has been previously described.
LDL labelled with unesterified cholesterol was prepared by incubating
cholesterol tracer in plasma in which LCAT was inhibited by 2 mM PCMPS,
then isolating LDL ultracentrifugally.  [$^{14}$C]-phosphatidylcholine-
labelled LDL was prepared by incubating phosphatidylcholine tracer in
ethanol with 100 volumes of human plasma at 37°C for 6 h, then purify-
ing the LDL fraction, labelled with [$^{14}$C]-phosphatidylcholine, by
ultracentrifugation.  The assay system for all measurements of lipid
transfer activity was similar, and adapted from reference (2).

2.  Isolation of LTP-I and LTP-II

One litre of human plasma, obtained from the blood transfusion service,
was made 25% saturated in ammonium sulphate.  Precipitated fibrinogen
was removed by centrifugation.  The supernatant was made 50% saturated
in ammonium sulphate, and the precipitated protein fraction containing
LTP was isolated by centrifugation.  The precipitate was solubilised in
water, dialysed to remove ammonium sulphate, and adjusted to salt
density 1.25 g/ml by the addition of NaBr.  After ultracentrifugation,
lipoproteins were removed by tube slicing.  The density > 1.25 g/ml
fraction, containing approximately 96% of plasma lipid transfer protein
activity, was subjected to hydrophobic interaction chromatography on
Phenyl-Sepharose.  Non-hydrophobic proteins were eluted with sodium
chloride, and hydrophobic proteins, including LTP, were eluted with
water.  The eluant was then adjusted to pH 4.5 with sodium acetate
buffer and subjected to CM-cellulose cation exchange chromatography in
4 M urea.  Lipid transfer activity was not retained by the column.  The
LTP-containing fractions were then applied to a DEAE-cellulose chromatography column at pH 6.2 in imidazole-HCl buffer with 4 M urea and
lipid transfer activity eluted with the same buffer containing a NaCl
gradient.  The active fractions were then chromatofocused in 4 M urea.

Those fractions eluting from the chromatofocusing column between pH
5.25 and 4.9 contained a protein which, on polyacrylamide gel in SDS,
had $M_r$ 67 000 - 70 000.  On isoelectric focusing, bands focused at pI
5.23, 5.13, 5.05 and 4.93.  This protein, which we have called lipid
transfer protein I (LTP-I), and which appeared as a single band on
alkaline polyacrylamide gel electrophoresis and polyacrylamide gel
electrophoresis in SDS, facilitated the transfer of cholesteryl ester,
triglyceride and phospholipid tracer from LDL to HDL.  The rate of
transfer was a function of the concentration of LTP-I in the assay
system.  The transfer of unesterified cholesterol was not measurably
affected by the presence of LTP-I (using incubation times as short as
5 minutes).

Those fractions eluting between pH 4.9 and 4.7 were concentrated and
fractions separated according to molecular weight by chromatography
on Sephacryl S-200, in 4 M urea.  Electrophoretically pure LTP-II was
obtained.  This had $M_r$ 55 000 and bands isofocused at pI 4.93, 4.88,
4.81, 4.73 and 4.68.  LTP-II facilitated the transfer of cholesteryl
ester, triglyceride and phospholipid to a degree dependent upon the
concentration of LTP-II in the assay incubation.  No concentration-
dependent effect on the transfer of non-esterified cholesterol tracer
was seen.

An antibody obtained to a mixture of LTP-I and LTP-II allowed us to demonstrate that LTP-I and LTP-II were immunochemically nonidentical.

LTP-I and LTP-II lipid transfer activities were modified by PCMPS (2 mM in incubation mixture) and 5,5' dithiobis-(2-nitrobenzoate) (DTNB, 1.4 mM). PCMPS reduced cholesteryl ester transfer by up to 36%, abolished triglyceride transfer activity, and increased phospholipid transfer activity by up to 15%. DTNB had no consistent effect on cholesteryl ester transfer, reduced triglyceride transfer activity by about 10% and increased phospholipid transfer activity by about 10%. The maximum effect of PCMPS and DTNB was on highly purified LTP. Assay conditions were not controlled sufficiently to allow us to distinguish quantitatively between the effect of inhibitors on LTP-I and LTP-II; nevertheless, the qualitative effect in all cases was similar. This would suggest that LTP-I and LTP-II have some structural features in common.

Purified LTP-I and LTP-II are stabilised in the presence of 4 M urea, retaining activity for at least 4 weeks at $4^{O}$C. In the absence of urea, highly purified LTP lost over 80% of its activity in 3 days at $4^{O}$C.

There was no evidence to suggest that LTP-I is a precursor of LTP-II, in that neither form of LTP changed into the other on storage in 4 M urea. The apparent $M_r$ of LTP-I and LTP-II was unchanged by reduction with β-mercaptoethanol in the presence of SDS.


C.  Conclusion


Clearly we are only beginning to understand the process of lipid trans- fer between plasma lipoproteins. We need to understand the biochem- istry of LTP-I and LTP-II, whether or not they act independently or in a complex *in vivo*, and the way in which they interact with plasma lipo- proteins. The identification of LTP-I and LTP-II gives us the poten- tial for novel investigations into the way in which lipids are trans- ported in the blood. The role of LTP in modifying the relationship between lipoproteins and cells is, as yet, unknown.

*Acknowledgments*  We thank Mr. Stan Bastiras, Mr. Andrew Fudge, Miss Helen Chalmers, Miss Jenny Fewster and Miss Helen Pederick for assistance at various stages of this investigation.

The work was supported by the National Heart Foundation of Australia.


References

1.  Zilversmit DP, Hughes LB, Balmer J (1975) Stimulation of choles- terol ester exchange by lipoprotein-free rabbit plasma. Biochim. Biophys. Acta 409: 393-398
2.  Pattnaik NM, Montes A, Hughes LB, Zilversmit DB (1978) Cholesteryl ester exchange protein in human plasma. Isolation and characteri- zation. Biochim. Biophys. Acta 530: 428-438

3. Barter PJ, Lally JI (1978) The activity of an esterified cholesterol transferring factor in human and rat serum. Biochim. Biophys.
   Acta 531: 233-236
4. Sniderman A, Teng B, Vezina C, Marcel YL (1978) Cholesterol ester
   exchange between human plasma high and low density lipoproteins
   mediated by a plasma protein factor. Atherosclerosis 31: 327-333
5. Marcel YL, Vezina C, Teng B, Sniderman A (1980) Transfer of
   cholesterol esters between human high density lipoproteins and
   triglyceride-rich lipoproteins controlled by a plasma protein
   factor. Atherosclerosis 35: 127-133
6. Ihm J, Harmony JAK, Ellsworth J, Jackson RL (1980) Simultaneous
   transfer of cholesteryl ester and phospholipid by protein(s)
   isolated from human lipoprotein-free plasma. Biochem. Biophys.
   Res. Comm. 93: 1114-1120
7. Barter PJ, Jones ME (1980) Kinetic studies of the transfer of
   esterified cholesterol between human plasma low and high density
   lipoproteins. J. Lipid Res. 21: 238-249
8. Barter PJ, Gooden JM, Rajaram OV (1979) Species differences in the
   activity of a serum triglyceride transferring factor. Atherosclerosis 33: 165-169
9. Hopkins GJ, Barter PJ (1980) Transfers of esterified cholesterol
   and triglyceride between high density and very low density lipoproteins: in vitro studies of rabbits and humans. Clin. Exp.
   Metab. 29: 546-550
10. Chajek T, Fielding CJ (1978) Isolation and characterization of a
    human serum cholesteryl ester transfer protein. Proc. Natl. Acad.
    Sci. USA 75: 3445-3449
11. Fielding PE, Fielding CJ (1980) A cholesteryl ester transfer com-
    plex in human plasma. Proc. Natl. Acad. Sci. USA 77: 3327-3330
12. Morton RE, Zilversmit DB (1981) The separation of apolipoprotein
    D from cholesteryl ester transfer protein. Biochim Biophys. Acta:
    350-355

# Besides Blockage of the Synthesis of HMG-CoA Reductase, Cycloheximide also Inhibits Its Degradation

W. Chen

## A. Introduction

A major rate-limiting step in the biosynthesis of cholesterol is the conversion of 3-hydroxy-3-methylglutaryl coenzyme A (HMG-CoA) to mevalonate (1, 2). The reaction is catalyzed by HMG-CoA reductase, an enzyme with a relatively short half-life. Incubation of mammalian cultured cells with several oxysterols, e.g., 25-hydroxycholesterol, inhibits the activity of HMG-CoA reductase, apparently by suppression of the synthesis of the enzyme (2, 3). In the presence of 25-hydroxycholesterol (2.5 uM) the reductase activity declines to less than a few percent of the controls within a few hours (4). Studies involving determination of HMG-CoA reductase activity after enucleation have suggested the existence of a rapidly turning-over system which are normally responsible for the inactivation and/or degradation of HMG-CoA reductase (5). In an attempt to further study this degradative system I have analyzed the effects of cycloheximide and 25-hydroxycholesterol, alone or in combination on the activity of the reductase.

## B. Materials and Methods

Chinese hamster ovary cells (CHO-K1) were grown in McCoy's 5a medium supplemented with 4 mg/ml of delipidated fetal bovine serum proteins (6). For experiments, actively proliferating cells were seeded at the density of $0.75 \times 10^6$ per 22 cm$^2$ culture dishes. They were grown for 1 or 2 days and treated with various reagents for different lengths of time as described. The activity of HMG-CoA reductase was determined in the sonicated lysates of cells by a previously published method (6, 7).

## C. Results and Discussion

### I. Effect of Cycloheximide on Protein Synthesis

Incubation of cells with cycloheximide (2 ug/ml) blocked the incorporation of [$^3$H]leucine into perchloric acid insoluble protein in CHO cells. After half an hour treatment the extent of inhibition reached 99% that of the control cells not treated with the drug. Therefore, the de novo synthesis of HMG-CoA reductase is presumably blocked rapidly and totally. Under the same condition 25-hydroxycholesterol (1 ug/ml) did not inhibit the incorporation of leucine into protein as previously reported (8).

## II.  Effect of Cycloheximide and 25-Hydroxycholesterol on HMG-CoA Reductase Activity

In the presence of cycloheximide or 25-hydroxycholesterol the decline in HMG-CoA reductase activity appears to conform to first order kinetics (for example, see Fig. 1).  The average half-life (± S.E.) of the enzyme activity in the presence of 25-hydroxycholesterol was 1.5 h ± 0.1 (8 experiments) and in the presence of cycloheximide, 5.1 h ± 0.6 (5 experiments).  Since it is usually assumed that cycloheximide suppresses HMG-CoA reductase by blocking the synthesis of protein, I investigated the effect of this reagent on the ability of 25-hydroxycholesterol to suppress the reductase activity.  When cells were treated simultaneously with cycloheximide and 25-hydroxycholesterol, the half-life of the enzyme activity was about 5 h, a value similar to that obtained with cycloheximide alone but significantly larger than that with 25-hydroxycholesterol alone.

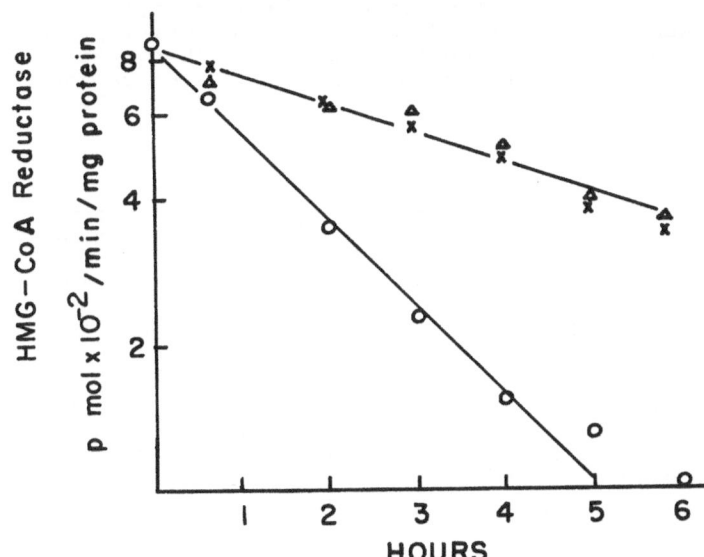

Fig. 1.  Effect of cycloheximide and 25-hydroxycholesterol treatment on HMG-CoA reductase activity.  CHO cells were incubated with 25-hydroxycholesterol (1 µg/ml) (0), cycloheximide (2 µg/ml) (Δ), or both together (X) for various lengths of time as indicated. Values represent means from triplicate cultures.  Standard errors are no more than 5% of the values shown

434

Abolishment of 25-hydroxycholesterol-mediated suppression of HMG-
CoA reductase activity by blockage of protein synthesis was also
observed in two other cell lines (mouse fibroblasts and Chinese
hamster lung cells) and with puromycin as inhibitor.  Preincubation of cells with cycloheximide or puromycin for 30 min or
longer totally eliminated the effect of 25-hydroxycholesterol on
the reductase activity (data not shown).  The ability of cycloheximide to block 25-hydroxycholesterol action on the reductase
appears to be at least partially reversible as demonstrated in an
experiment in which CHO cells were preincubated with cycloheximide for 2 h and then washed before incubation with 25-hydroxy-
cholesterol for 3 h.  As shown in Table 1, 25-hydroxycholesterol
has more suppressive effect on HMG-CoA reductase in those cultures
which were repeatedly washed to reduced cycloheximide concentration than in those not washed.  These washed cultures recovered
45% or 70% of protein synthesis 1/2 or 1 1/2 h respectively after
cycloheximide was washed off (data not shown).

Table 1. Reversible effect of cycloheximide on 25-hydroxycholes-
terol mediated suppression of HMG-CoA reductase activity.  Cycloheximide was removed from the cell culture by washing the monolayer
4 times with 4 ml volumes of warm phosphate buffered saline
(PBS).  Each value represents the mean ± S.E. from triplicate
cultures

| | HMGCoA reductase activity |
|---|---|
| | pmol/min/mg protein |
| Control | 648 ± 5 |
| Cycloheximide 2 h | 419 ± 12 |
| Cycloheximide 5 h | 373 ± 27 |
| 25Hydroxycholesterol 3 h | 100 ± 14 |
| Cycloheximide 2 h, then plus 25hydroxycholesterol 3 h | 462 ± 12 |
| Cycloheximide 2 h, then wash and incubate in fresh medium for 3 h | 522 ± 18 |
| Cycloheximide 2 h, then wash and incubate with 25-hydroxycholesterol, 3 h | 303 ± 16 |

D.   Concluding Remarks

The results reported herein are consistent with a hypothesis that
25-hydroxycholesterol inhibits the activity of HMG-CoA reductase
by repressing the synthesis of the enzyme, while cycloheximide
and puromycin suppress the enzyme synthesis and, in addition,
decrease the rate of enzyme degradation by inhibiting the synthesis of at least one of the components of the degradation system.
Thus the observed half-life of the enzyme activity in the presence
of 25-hydroxycholesterol is shorter than it is in the presence of

cycloheximide. Preincubation of the cells with cycloheximide before the addition of 25-hydroxycholesterol or simultaneous addition of cycloheximide with 25-hydroxycholesterol reduces the effect of the oxysterol on the level of HMG-CoA reductase because the rate of degradation of the enzyme has been diminished by the cycloheximide. Therefore, the apparent half-life of the enzyme activity under this condition was similar to that when cells were treated with cycloheximide alone. The results confirms our previous finding that the system which normally involves in the degradation of HMG-CoA reductase is short-lived (5), and they also indicate that at least one component of this degredative system is a protein with a half-life of not more than an hour. Evidence that cycloheximide inhibits the degradation of a specific protein (9) as well as of general intracellular proteolysis (10) have been recently demonstrated. However the datailed mechanism by which protein degradation was affected by inhibition of protein synthesis remains to be elucidated.

Acknowledgments   This research was supported by grant GM 22900 from the National Institutes of General Medical Sciences. Technical assistance was provided by Mr. Blaine A. Richards.

References

1.  Rodwell, VW, Nordstrom JL, Mitschelen JJ  (1976)  Regulation of HMG-CoA reductase.  Adv Lipid Res. 14: 1-7
2.  Kandutsch AA, Chen HW, Heiniger HJ  (1978)  Biological activity of some oxygenated sterols.  Science 201: 498-501
3.  Sinensky M, Torget R, Edwards PA  (1981)  Radioimmune precipitation of 3-hydroxy-3-methylglutaryl coenzyme A reductase from Chinese hamster fibroblasts, effect of 25-hydroxycholesterol. J Biol Chem 256: 11774-11779
4.  Kandutsch AA, Chen HW  (1974)  Inhibition of sterol synthesis in cultured mouse cells by cholesterol derivatives oxygenated in the side chain.  J Biol Chem 249: 6057-6061
5.  Cavenee WK, Chen HW, Kandutsch AA  (1981)  Regulation of cholesterol biosynthesis in enucleated cells.  J Biol Chem 256: 2675-2681
6.  Chen HW, Cavenee WK, Kandutsch AA  (1979)  Sterol synthesis in variant Chinese hamster lung cells selected for resistance to 25-hydroxycholesterol, cross resistance to 7-ketocholesterol, 20α-hydroxycholesterol, and serum. J Biol Chem 254: 715-720
7.  Chen HW  (1981)  The activity of 3-hydroxy-3-methylglutaryl coenzyme A reductase and the rate of sterol synthesis diminish in cultures with high cell density.  J Cell Physiol 108: 91-97
8.  Kandutsch AA, Chen HW  (1977)  Consequences of blocked sterol synthesis in cultured cells, DNA synthesis and membrane composition.  J Biol Chem 252: 409-415
9.  Reed BC, Ronnett GV, Lane MD  (1981)  Role of glycosylation and protein synthesis in insulin receptor metabolism by 3T3-L1 mouse adipocytes.  Proc Natl Acad Sci USA 78: 2908-2912
10. Amenta JS, Brocher SC  (1981)  Mechanisms of protein turnover in cultured cells.  Life Science 28: 1195-1208

# Intestinal HMG-CoA Reductase: Regulation and Function

E. F. Stange, A. Schneider, and H. Ditschuneit

## A. Introduction

As the putative key enzyme of cholesterol synthesis in the intestine as well as in other tissues, gut HMG-CoA reductase has been studied extensively in recent years. Despite these efforts, both the cellular localization and the regulation of the enzyme are still controversial.

Early work on cholesterol synthesis concluded that the majority of sterol was synthesized by the crypts rather than in the villi (1). Furthermore, the highest synthesis rates along the length of the gastrointestinal tract were found in the ileum. Similar studies on intestinal reductase confirmed this pattern of distribution, suggesting that the enzyme was indeed rate-limiting for sterol synthesis (2). Therefore, the concept arose that intestinal endogenous cholesterol served as a membrane component in actively proliferating crypt cells.

However, after proper precautions were taken to avoid inactivation of the villus cell reductase by the differential scraping procedure used hitherto, villus cells were found to be as active as crypt cells regarding both cholesterol synthesis from labelled precursors and reductase-specific activity (3,4). This view was obviously more consistent with the demonstration of a contribution of the intestinal wall to the serum cholesterol of several species.

Also, due to the increased synthesis of bile acids after cholesterol feeding in the rat, it was not clear whether dietary cholesterol or bile acids or both regulated intestinal sterol synthesis (1).

We therefore employed established techniques for isolating enriched epithelial cell fractions or organ culture whole pieces of gut mucosa to further investigate the role of the small intestine in cholesterol synthesis.

## B. Results and Discussion

### I. Cholesterol, Bile Acids and their Analogs

To reevaluate the effect of cholesterol feeding in a susceptible species which does not respond with an increased bile acid synthesis, we studied the effect of a 1% cholesterol diet fed for 2 days on intestinal HMG-CoA reductase in rabbits (4). Villus and crypt cell reductase in the jejunum were both suppressed to 26 and 28% of controls, respectively, whereas in the ileum the cholesterol suppression was less pronounced with 55 and 69% of controls. The effect was enhanced by longer feeding periods or by adding 5% coconut or corn oil to the cholesterol diet. Irrespective of the diet, specific reductase activity of villus cells was equal to or higher than in crypt cells.

Similarly, under the more controlled in vitro conditions of intestinal mucosal organ culture, cholesterol at concentrations exceeding 0.25 mM inhibited completely the induction of reductase observed in control cultures in cholesterol-free medium (5). On the other hand, oxygenated cholesterol derivatives such as 7-ketocholesterol and 25-hydroxycholesterol exerted a similar suppressive effect, although at 5 to 10-fold lower concentrations between 0.05 and 0.1 mM (6).

In sharp contrast, bile acids stimulated mucosal HMG-CoA reductase up to 3-fold when added to the medium in a concentration of 0.05 to 5.0 mM in the presence of 5% albumin to reduce their toxicity (5). This effect was seen with both predominant bile acids of the rabbit, glycocholic and glycodeoxycholic acid. Since the cholesterol content of the mucosa decreased after culture in medium containing bile acids, it is conceivable that their detergent effect led to a cholesterol depletion partly balanced by the increase in sterol synthesis. The suppression of canine mucosal reductase by bile acids reported previously (7) was short-lived and probably due to enhanced micellar absorption of residual cholesterol (8). Furthermore, the stimulatory action of bile acids was reproduced by the synthetic detergents Na- and glycofusidate (6), suggesting that the bile acid effect was indeed purely detergent and unphysiological.

Additional evidence for this hypothesis was obtained with mucosal cultures treated with cholesterol-bile acid micelles. In this instance, reductase was suppressed well below values at the start of the culture, similar to the effect of cycloheximide, a protein synthesis blocker (5). Therefore, cholesterol rather than bile acids appears to be the physiological luminal regulator of its mucosal synthesis.

## 2. Lipoproteins

Based on the work in various other cell cultures, such as fibroblasts or smooth muscle cells, we next defined the in vitro regulatory effects of homologous plasma lipoproteins on reductase in organ-cultured mucosa. Not unlike the effect in these other cell types, plasma LDL inhibited enterocyte reductase in a dose-dependent manner (9). However, the effective doses between 0.15 and 1.0 mM lipoprotein cholesterol were comparably high and full suppression of the enzyme could not be achieved. With both VLDL and HDL, the reductase response was biphasic, with 2 to 3-fold stimulation at 0.1-0.3 mM and a suppression at higher levels. Interestingly, this biphasic response to normal plasma HDL was converted to a dose-dependent reduction of the enzyme activity, when apoprotein E-rich HDL from cholesterol fed animals were used instead. Although a direct binding study is not possible in this biopsy tissue, the data are compatible with the presence of a B,E receptor in the basolateral membrane of the enterocyte. Since chylomicron remnants, which accumulate in the plasma of the cholesterol fed rabbit, were ineffective with respect to reductase regulation, probably both luminal cholesterol and plasma LDL and HDL represent the physiological regulator under this dietary condition.

## 3. Mevalonolactone and Compactin

Next it was of interest to look into the possibility that endogenously formed sterols feedback regulate their own synthesis. Employing two separate approaches, we enhanced endogenous sterol synthesis by adding mevalonolactone, a cholesterol precursor, to the medium, or, alternatively, blocked sterol formation by Compactin, a competitive HMG-CoA reductase inhibitor.

Unlike mevalonate, which was ineffective, mevalonolactone produced a dose-dependent suppression of the reductase at 0.1 - 10.0 mM by up to 62% of controls (10). On the other hand, Compactin induced the enzyme up to 240% at 0.5μg/ml, although the enzyme activity was latent in the presence of the inhibitor and demonstrable only after appropriate dilution of compactin during the reductase assay.

The effective suppression of the mucosal sterol synthesis was evident from a dose-dependent decrease in its cholesterol content. Moreover, the induction of latent enzyme activity was totally prevented by 10.0 mM mevalonolactone, but not by cholesterol. Under these conditions, therefore, cholesterol does not appear to be the only regulator, suggesting a multivalent regulation also in the intestine.

438

Finally, since the brush border enzyme alkaline phosphatase was significantly lower after culture in Compactin medium (but not in controls), it was of interest that HMG-CoA reductase was of importance for intestinal growth or differentiation. Later experiments demonstrated that this effect was prevented by adding cholesterol to the medium and was related to a growth inhibiting effect, since mucosal DNA also decreased when cholesterol synthesis was blocked.

## 4. Hormones

Since pancreatic, thyroid and adrenal hormones are known regulators of HMG-CoA reductase in the liver in vivo as well as in cultured hepatocytes (11), we studied their effect in the mucosal organ culture system (12). Surprisingly, both insulin and glucagon did not interfere with reductase activity in the rabbit mucosa. In contrast, triamcinolone significantly suppressed reductase in a dose-dependent fashion to 38% of controls after 24 h, but not after 2 h culture.

Alkaline phosphatase was induced after both periods, but the effect was more marked after 24 h. A parallel minor stimulation of both enzyme activities was noted in the presence of $10^{-9}$ M triiodothyronine, lower and very high concentrations were ineffective.

In view of the role of glucocorticoids as intestinal growth inhibitors and thyroid hormones as growth stimulators, we suggest that hormone induced changes in reductase reflect alterations of crypt membrane cholesterol synthesis, whereas the induction of alkaline phosphatase is mediated through an enhanced enterocyte regeneration and/or maturation. A similar pattern was also observed with gastrointestinal hormones, where secretin inhibited reductase in contrast to gastrin, cholecystokinin and somatostatin (unpublished data).

## 5. Interconversion through Phosphorylation/Dephosphorylation

Intestinal HMG-CoA reductase, much like the hepatic enzyme, has been shown to be interconvertible by phosphorylation/dephosphorylation both in the rat (13) and in the rabbit (8,9) under in vitro conditions. However, information on the importance of this mechanism in vivo as a short term regulatory control is not available. Although we observed an increase in the expressed activity of the reductase during the 24 h culture period, this activation state was not influenced by any of the hormones tested above. Interestingly, expressed and total reductase activity dissociated in the presence of bile acids (8); in all other instances mentioned above, only total enzyme activity was altered, even after shorter culture periods of 2 h.

Relation of HMG-CoA reductase to alkaline phosphatase in cultured intestine

| Treatment | Reductase | Alkaline phosphatase |
|---|---|---|
| Cholesterol | ↓ | 0 |
| 7-Ketocholesterol | ↓↓ | ↓ |
| 25-Hydroxycholesterol | ↓↓↓ | ↓ |
| Glycocholate | ↑↑ | ↓ |
| Glycodeoxycholate | ↑↑↑ | ↓ |
| Glycodeoxycholate + Cholesterol | ↓↓ | 0 |
| Mevalonolactone | ↓↓ | 0 |
| Compactin | ↑↑ | ↓↓ |
| Insulin | 0 | 0 |
| Glucagon | 0 | 0 |
| Triamcinolone | ↓ | ↑ |
| Triiodothyronine | ↑ | ↑ |
| Pentagastrin | 0 | 0-↓ |
| Secretin | ↓ | ↓ |

## C. Conclusion

I. HMG-CoA reductase is present in the intestine in an interconvertible active (de-phosphorylated) and inactive (phosphorylated) form. Both the expressed activity (de-termined in the presence of fluoride) and the total activity (determined in the pre-sence of endogenous or exogenous phosphatase) may dissociate during the isolation of enterocytes by EDTA chelation or during organ culture. However, the physiological importance of this potential regulatory process has not yet been established.

II. Supply of exogenous cholesterol by feeding experiments in vivo as well as in free, micellar or lipoprotein (LDL) form in cultured mucosa in vitro suppressed to-tal HMG-CoA reductase. Depletion of cellular cholesterol by bile acids and structur-ally similar detergents or specific inhibitors of sterol synthesis enhances reduct-ase activity. Therefore, the overall cholesterol balance appears to be a major de-terminant of mucosal reductase, suggesting a homeostatic control function.

III. Since specific inhibitors of HMG-CoA reductase decrease brush border alkaline phosphatase (see Table I) and mucosal DNA, the enzyme is vital for cellular differ-entiation and growth in culture. Furthermore, the divergent effects of glucocortic-oids and thyroid hormones on mucosal growth are reflected in the changes of reductase activity, suggesting that this enzyme is more important for growth than for differen-tiation.

## References

1. Dietschy JM, Siperstein MD (1965) Cholesterol synthesis by the gastrointestin-al tract: Localization and mechanisms of control. J. Clin. Invest. 44: 1311-1327
2. Shefer S, Hauser S, Lapar V, Mosbach EH (1972) HMG CoA reductase of intestinal mucosa and liver of the rat. J. Lipid Res. 13: 402-412
3. Merchant JL, Heller RA (1977) 3-Hydroxy-3-methylglutaryl coenzyme A reductase in isolated villous and crypt cells of the rat ileum. J. Lipid Res. 18: 722-733
4. Stange EF, Alavi M, Schneider A, Ditschuneit H, Poley JR (1981) Influence of dietary cholesterol, saturated and unsaturated lipid on 3-hydroxy-3-methyl-glutaryl CoA reductase activity in rabbit intestine and liver. J. Lipid Res. 22: 47-56
5. Stange EF, Schneider A, Alavi M, Ditschuneit H, Poley JR (1981) Effects of cholesterol and bile acids on HMG-CoA reductase and brush border enzymes in or-gan-cultured intestine. In: Paumgartner G, Stiehl A, Gerok W (eds) Bile Acids and Lipids, MTP Press, Lancaster, p 57-66
6. Stange EF, Schneider A, Preclik G, Alavi M, Ditschuneit H (1981) Regulation of 3-hydroxy-3-methylglutaryl CoA reductase by analogs of cholesterol and bile acids in cultured intestinal mucosa. Lipids 16: 397-400
7. Gebhard RL, Cooper AD (1978) Regulation of cholesterol synthesis in cultured canine intestinal mucosa. J. Biol. Chem. 253: 2790-2796
8. Stange EF, Schneider A, Preclik G, Ditschuneit H (1981) Bile acid induced inter-conversion of 3-hydroxy-3-methylglutaryl coenzyme A reductase in cultured intest-ine. Biochim. Biophys. Acta 666: 291-293
9. Stange EF, Alavi M, Schneider A, Preclik G, Ditschuneit H (1980) Lipoprotein regulation of 3-hydroxy-3-methylglutaryl coenzyme A reductase in cultured in-testinal mucosa. Biochim. Biophys. Acta 620: 520-527
10. Stange EF, Preclik G, Schneider A, Alavi M, Ditschuneit H (1981) Regulation of 3-hydroxy-3-methylglutaryl-CoA reductase by endogenous sterol synthesis in cul-tured intestinal mucosa. Biochim. Biophys. Acta 663: 613-620
11. Stange EF, Fleig WE, Schneider A, Nöther-Fleig G, Alavi M, Preclik G, Dit-schuneit H (1982) 3-Hydroxy-3-methylglutaryl CoA reductase in cultured hepa-tocytes. Atherosclerosis 41: 67-80

440

12. Stange EF, Preclik G, Schneider A, Seiffer E, Ditschuneit H (1981) Hormonal regulation of 3-hydroxy-3-methylglutaryl coenzyme A reductase and alkaline phosphatase in cultured intestinal mucosa. Biochim. Biophys. Acta 678: 202-206

13. Panini SR, Rudney H (1980) Short term reversible modulation of 3-hydroxy-3-
methylglutaryl coenzyme A reductase activity in isolated epithelial cells from
rat ileum. J. Biol. Chem. 255: 11633-11636

## 2.4 Phagocytosis in the Lesion

# Fluid-Phase Pinocytosis in Arterial Smooth Muscle Cells

D. E. Bowyer and E. M. Muir

Pinocytosis is the process by which cells take up materials from the extracellular environment. This can involve the specific recognition of a macromolecule by a receptor on the plasma membrane, followed by the interiorisation of the receptor-ligand complex (receptor-mediated pinocytosis, or the non-specific uptake of material present in the fluid entrapped within the forming pinosomes (non-specific fluid-phase pinocytosis). The functions of these processes include the uptake of nutrients and hormones, and possibly membrane surveillance. They may also be of significance in the pathological-overload of cells with extracellular substances. In atherosclerosis overload of arterial smooth muscle cells (SMC) with lipid, predominantly cholesterol and cholesteryl esters, is a characteristic feature of the foam cell (1). SMC take up low density lipoprotein (LDL) by both receptor-mediated and non-specific fluid-phase pinocytosis (2). Uptake by the receptor-mediated pathway, however, leads to the down regulation of receptors. It has been calculated that even under normal conditions, the concentrations of LDL to which SMC are exposed, would cause maximal suppression of the LDL receptor. Under such conditions the non-specific route may contribute significantly to the uptake of LDL (3). This route would become even more important under conditions in which the concentration of lipoproteins in the interstitial fluid is raised, for example hypercholesterolaemia or following loss of the endothelium. In view of the potential significance of the fluid-phase pathway in atherogenesis we have developed a method for its measurement in arterial SMC in culture, investigated the basic mechanisms involved, and begun to explore ways in which it may be modified.

## Methods

SMC were isolated from pig thoracic aortas and grown to confluence in Dulbecco's modified Eagles medium supplemented with antibiotics and 10% foetal calf serum, as described previously (4).

Pinocytosis was measured according to the method of Leake (5), samples containing radiolabelled sucrose, were assayed for radioactivity using $\beta$-scintillation counting and an internal standard was added to determine the efficiency of counting.

The mechanisms of pinocytosis were investigated by the use of metabolic inhibitors, antimicrotubular and antimicrofibrillar agents. Sodium fluoride, 2,4 dinitrophenol (DNP) 2-deoxyglucose, colchicine and vinblastine were dissolved in culture medium ; cytochalasin B was dissolved in dimethyl sulphoxide (final concentration 0.16% v/v) and oligomycin in ethanol (final concentration 1% v/v) and then diluted with culture medium to attain the final concentrations of anticytoskeletal agents shown. For measurements of pinocytosis confluent cultures were incubated at $37^{\circ}C$ in the presence of the inhibitors and $^{125}$I-labelled poly(vinylpyrrolidone) (PVP) for 4 h. Each experiment included a concurrent control incubation of SMC from the same sub-culture with $^{125}$I-labelled PVP but without modifier. Control cultures contained dimethyl sulphoxide in experiments with cytochalasin B, and ethanol in experiments with oligomycin. The ATP levels of SMC after incubation with metabolic inhibitors but without PVP was determined by the method of Pozzan (6).

The effect of cellular lipid composition was investigated by incubation of SMC with phospholipids of various composition or linoleic acid.
Liposomes of phospholipids were prepared by sonication in glass distilled water, under nitrogen and above their respective transition temperatures. The resulting preparations were sterilised by millepore filtration and the concentrations of phospholipid determined Linoleic acid was bound to defatted bovine serum albumin. Control cultures contained a similar concentration of albumin without bound fatty acid. In all experiments $^{125}$I-labelled PVP was added simultaneously with the lipid and incubated for 2 h.

444

The effects of lysosomal overload and anoxia were also investigated. Lysosomal overload was induced by incubating SMC in medium containing either chloroquine or sucrose for 72 h, [125]I-labelled PVP was present throughout the incubation. The accumulation of [125]I-labelled PVP was then measured. To measure release of PVP, SMC were incubated with PVP for 48 h, the medium removed, the cells extensively washed with Hank's balanced salt solution and reincubated with exactly 4 ml of medium containing either sucrose or chloroquine for 72 h. Under anoxic conditions, uptake and release of PVP were determined by a similar procedure, using a 2 h incubation.

## Results and Discussion

### Methods for Measurement of Fluid-phase Pinocytosis

The use of non-degradeable radiolabelled tracers has advantages over morphometric methods and the use of degradeable radiolabelled proteins, for the measurement of pinocytosis (4). In the present study we have compared the suitability of two commonly used non-degradeable tracers, namely radiolabelled sucrose and [125]I-labelled PVP. The latter has previously been shown to fulfil all the requirements of a tracer for pinocytosis in SMC ; its uptake is linear with time and proportional to the concentration in the incubation medium, showing that it neither stimulates nor inhibits pinocytosis, and it is retained within the cells for at least 48 h (5).
In contrast, the uptake of sucrose was non-linear with time (Figure 1a), accumulated sucrose was rapidly lost from the cells (Figure 1b) and a significant amount was able to enter cells at $4^{o}$C (22% of the amount accumulated at $37^{o}$C). Taken together, these results suggest that radiolabelled sucrose is able to enter cells by a non-pinocytic mechanism and is thus unsuitable as a tracer.

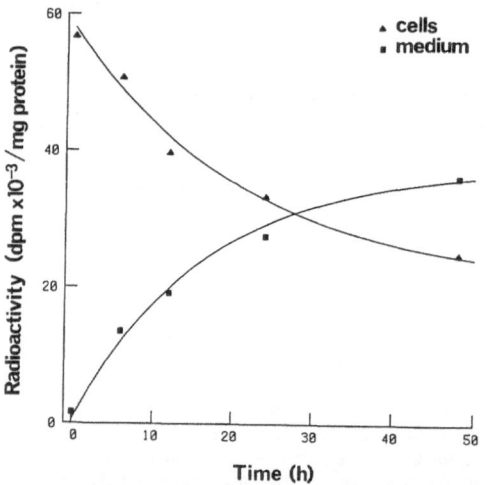

Release of previously accumulated sucrose from pig aortic SMC.
The values shown are the mean of 5 observations

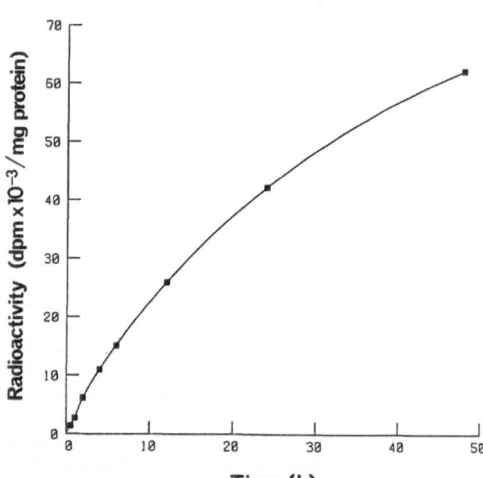

Accumulation of $^{3}$H-sucrose with time
Each point is the mean of 5 observations

### Mechanisms of Pinocytosis

Pinocytosis was found to be temperature dependent which probably reflects changes in membrane fluidity, as pinocytosis virtually ceased at a temperature close to the transition temperature of membrane lipids. Reduction of cellular ATP levels by treatment of the cells with metabolic inhibitors, caused a corresponding reduction in pinocytosis (Table 1), indicating that the process is energy-dependent. Incubation of the cells with the microtubular disruptive agents colchicine and vinblastine reduced pinocytosis to about half control values at all concentrations used. In contrast, the antimicrofibrillar agent cytochalasin B produced a concentration-dependent stimulation of pinocytosis (Table 2).

These results suggest a role of the microtubules in pinocytosis, possibly by their involvement in vesicle movement within the cell (7), which may be important in the membrane recycling necessary to maintain pinocytosis (8). Disruption of the micro-filaments may cause an increase in pinocytosis by relieving any constraint on invagination of the plasma membrane.

The data shown in the following tables represent the mean of 5 observations ± s.d.
*** denotes a significant difference compared to controls P <0.001 ; ** denotes P <0.01

Table 1. Effect of Metabolic Inhibitors on Cellular ATP levels and Pinocytosis

| Inhibitor | Concentration | ATP (% control) | Pinocytosis (% control) ± s.d.) |
|---|---|---|---|
| NaF | 5 µmol/l | 43 ± 5*** | 63 ± 5*** |
| 2 deoxglucose | 1 µmol/l | 70 ± 9*** | 87 ± 6** |
| Oligomycin | 29 µg/ml | 72 ± 8*** | 79 ± 5*** |
| 2,4 DNP | 5 µmol/l | 43 ± 5*** | 60 ± 4*** |

Table 2. Effect of Antimicrotubular and Antimicrofibrillar Agents on Pinocytosis

| Treatment | Concentration (µmol/l) | Pinocytosis (% control) |
|---|---|---|
| Colchicine | 1 | 54 ± 3*** |
| | 100 | 59 ± 4*** |
| Vinblastine | 1 | 57 ± 6*** |
| | 100 | 46 ± 7*** |
| Cytochalasin B | 5 | 104 ± 6 |
| | 20 | 186 ± 11*** |
| | 40 | 288 ± 7*** |

## Modifiers of Pinocytosis

A number of factors were found to modify pinocytosis including platelet factor rich serum (4), cellular lipid composition, lysosomal overload and anoxia.

### 1. Platelet-derived Growth Factor

An enhanced rate of PVP uptake was observed when SMC were incubated in medium supplemented with platelet factor rich serum as compared to platelet factor poor serum (4) This observation is an agreement with the enhanced uptake of radiolabelled sucrose by monkey SMC in the presence of purified platelet-derived growth factor (PDGF), and adds support to the suggestion that PDGF may have a dual role in atherogenesis, not only stimulating SMC proliferation but also enhancing lipid uptake by increasing the non-specific uptake of LDL (9).

### 2. Cellular Lipid Composition

The rate of pinocytosis may be dependent on the fluidity of the plasma membrane (10) thus the possibility of pharmacological modulation of the process by lipids which modify membrane fluidity, exists. The effects of a number of lipids were investigated, in particular polyunsaturated phosphatidylcholine (essential phospholipid) (EPL) which has been shown to exert a protective effect against atherosclerosis (11). Table 3 shows that of a range of lipids tested, only EPL was able to reduce pinocytosis. The effect was, however, dependent on the continued presence of EPL in the medium (12). Incubation of SMC with linoleic acid for a similar period did not effect pinocytosis although prolonged incubation resulted in a marked stimulation of pinocytosis (Table 3), probably produced by an increase in membrane fluidity as a result of incorporation of linoleic acid into membrane phospholipids. This suggests that the effect is not produced by incorporation of free linoleic acid into membrane phospholipids. Furthermore, the saturated derivative of EPL was less effective at reducing pinocytosis, which is consistent with EPL producing the effect by fusing with the plasma membrane as EPL, in contrast to its saturated derivative, is above its phase transition at $37^{\circ}C$ (13). Such fusion could have altered the physical properties of the plasma membrane and hence pinocytosis. These results raise the possibility that the protective effect that EPL exerts against atherosclerosis may be partly a result of its ability to reduce pinocytosis, and hence the uptake of LDL into SMC.

Table 3. Effect of Cellular Lipid Composition on Pinocytosis

| Treatment | Preincubation time with modifier | Concentration ($\mu g/ml$) | Pinocytosis (% control) |
|---|---|---|---|
| EPL | – | 100 | $72 \pm 4$ ** |
|  | – | 200 | $65 \pm 3$ *** |
| Saturated EPL | – | 100 | $107 \pm 4$ |
|  |  | 200 | $82 \ 1 \ 4$ *** |
| Linoleic Acid | – | 50 | $100 \pm 11$ |
|  | 4 days | 50 | $113 \pm 16$ |
|  | 7 days | 50 | $142 \pm 24$ *** |

## 3. Lysosomal Overload and Anoxia

SMC in the atherosclerotic lesion have been shown to be overloaded with lipid (1) and subjected to hypoxic conditions (14). We therefore measured PVP accumulation by SMC in which lysosomal overload had been induced by incubation with a high concentration of sucrose (15) or chloroquine (16), and by cells exposed to anoxic conditions. As there is some evidence that cells engorged with lipid may release their lysosomal contents (14), release of previously accumulated PVP under the above conditions, was also measured. It was found that SMC in which lysosomal overload had been induced, accumulated only approximately 40% of the $^{125}I$-labelled PVP accumulated by the controls, and that this was in part due to an increase in PVP release (Table 4). Anoxia produced a similar effect.

The reduction in pinocytosis could impair the functioning of the cells, for instance by reducing the uptake of nutrients or by affecting the normal turnover of plasma membrane components, which may determine their response to certain external stimuli such as mitogens(18). Furthermore, since intracellular PVP is known to be located within the lysosomes (D.S. Leake, personnal communication) the observed release of PVP raises the possibility that the conditions prevailing in atherosclerotic lesions may induce release of lysosomal enzymes, which would have important implications for the development of intimal injury and subsequent atherosclerosis.

Table 4. Effect of Anoxia and Lysosomal Overload on Accumulation and Release of PVP

| Treatment | Concentration ($\mu mol/l$) | Accumulation (% control) | Release (% control) |
|---|---|---|---|
| Anoxia (3,5h) |  | $50 \pm 4$ *** | $145 \pm 22$ *** |
| Chloroquine | 25 | $37 \pm 0.1$ *** | $142 \pm 9$ *** |
| Sucrose | $80 \times 10^3$ | $39 \pm 0.2$ *** | $142 \pm 2$ *** |

Acknowledgements

This work was supported by a grant from the British Heart Foundation

References

1. Coltoff-Schiller B, Goldfischer, S, Adamany AM, Wolinsky, H (1976) Endocytosis by vascular smooth muscle in vivo and in vitro  Am J Path 83: 45-60
2. Goldstein JL, Brown MS (1977) The low density lipoprotein pathway and its relation to atherosclerosis  Ann Rev Biochem 46: 897-930
3. Goldstein JL, Brown MD (1977) Atherosclerosis : the low density lipoprotein receptor hypothesis  Metabolism 26: 1257-1275
4. Muir EM (1981) Ph.D Thesis (Cambridge University)
5. Leake DS, Bowyer DE (1977) Quantitative studies of pinocytic uptake of $^{125}$I-labelled PVP by pig aortic smooth muscle cells in culture  Biochem Soc 5: 130-133
6. Pozzan T, Corps AN, Pontecurro CM, Hesketh TR, Metcalfe JC (1980) Cap formation by various ligands on lymphocytes shows the same dependence on high cellular ATP levels  Biochim Biophys Acta 602: 558-566
7. Allen RD (1975) Evidence for firm linkages between microtubules and membrane bounded vesicles  J Cell Biol 64: 497-503
8. Duncan R, Pratten MK (1971) Membrane economics in endocytic systems  J Theor Biol 66: 729-739
9. Davies PF, Ross R (1978) Mediation of pinocytosis in cultured arterial smooth muscle cells and endothelial cells by platelet derived growth factor  J Cell Biol 79: 663-671
10, Mahoney EM, Hamill AL, Scott WA, Cohn ZA (1977) Response of endocytosis to altered fatty acyl composition of macrophage phospholipid.  Proc Natl Acad Sci USA 74: 4895-4899
11. Samochowiec L, Kadibowska D, Rozewicka L, Kuza W, Szysska R (1976) Investigations in experimental atherosclerosis Part 2 : the effect of phosphatidyl-choline (EPL) in experimental changes in miniature pigs.  Atherosclerosis 23: 319-331
12. Bowyer DE, Fox JW, Muir EM (1979) Hemmung der endozytose in arteriellen glatten muskelzellen durch hochungesattigtes phosphatidylcholin Med Welt 30: 1447-1448
13. Pagano RE, Weinstein JN (1978) Interactions of liposomes with mammalian cells  A Rev Biophys Bioeng  7: 435-468
14. Niinikoski J, Heughan C, Hunt TK (1973) Oxygen tensions in the aortic wall of normal rabbits  Atherosclerosis 17: 353-359
15. Roberts AVS, Nicholls SDE, Williams KT, Lloyd JB (1976) Pinocytosis and intracellular proteolysis in experimentally induced lysosomal storage  Biochem Soc Trans 2: 1096-1098
16. Stein O, Halperin C, Stein Y (1979) Comparison of cholesterol egress from cultured cells enriched with cholesteryl ester after exposure to cationised LDL and chloroquine  Biochim Biophys Acta 573: 1-11
17. Stauber WT, Trout JJ, Schottelius BA (1981) Exocytosis of intact lysosomes from skeletal muscle after chloroquine treatment  Exp mol Path 34: 87-93
18. Maxfield FR, Davies PJA, Klempner L, Willingham ML, Pastan (1979) Epidermal growth factor stimulation of DNA synthesis is potentiated by compounds that inhibit its clustering in coated pits  Proc Natl Acad Sci USA  76: 5731-5735

# Interaction of Platelets, Macrophages and Lipoproteins in Relation to Atherogenes

A. J. Day, S. Preet Singh, K. Hudson, and S. Mojumder

Both macrophages and platelets have been considered as key cells in the cellular pathology of atherosclerosis for many years. Their suggested role however has been progressively modified as experimental data has emerged. Recent studies for example, have demonstrated the presence of receptors to modified LDL in macrophages (1,2) and have renewed early interest (3,4) in the reticulo-endothelial system in the formation of foam cells in early atherogenesis. Recent interest in platelets has centred on the involvement on prostacyclin and thromboxane on platelet aggregation and on the effect of platelet growth factors in the proliferation of arterial wall cells (5,6). There are a number of studies however which suggest that platelets might also promote cellular lipid accumulation and foam cell formation in the early lesion. Platelet thrombi injected *in vivo* stimulate the formation of macrophage foam cells (7,8). Where endothelial injury occurs (either by indwelling catheters or by repeated ballooning) platelet deposition is followed by the development of lipid containing cell lesions (9,10) with composition and metabolic characteristics of early atherogenesis (11). In the present study the interaction of platelets on various aspects of lipid uptake and metabolism in rabbit peritoneal macrophages is studied *in vitro* and some preliminary data on possible mechanisms for platelet involvement in foam cell formation suggested.

Three possible mechanisms can be postulated

1.  Platelets taken up by macrophages might stimulate cholesteryl ester accumulation in these cells by increasing their acyl cholesterol acyl transferase (ACAT) activity or decreasing their lysosomal cholesteryl ester hydrolase (LCEH) activity.

2.  Platelets, or factors released from platelets might influence receptor mechanisms for the uptake of low density lipoprotein in macrophages.

3.  Platelets might modify low density lipoprotein (for example by formation of malonyl dialdehyde LDL) so that its uptake by macrophages is facilitated (12).

These possible mechanisms for platelet-macrophage interaction are experimentally tested in the preliminary work described in the present paper.

In the first series of experiments the effect of platelets on the uptake of LDL and on the synthesis of cholesteryl ester by macrophages was studied. Human platelets were obtained from blood bank blood, and were suspended in calcium-magnesium free Hanks solution containing 1 $\mu$g/ml of $PGE_1$ and rabbit anti serum (prepared against human red cells 1:100 dilution) at a concentration of $2 \times 10^9$ platelets/ml. After the initial incubation, $5 \times 10^8$ platelets were added to petri plates containing rabbit peritoneal macrophages (13) incubated in Dulbecco's medium with 20% foetal calf serum together with $^{14}$C-labelled oleic acid and with or without 100 $\mu$g/ml of low density lipoprotein. After a further 10 to 12 hours incubation the macrophage/platelets were harvested, extracted and their chemical composition and the incorporation of $^{14}$C-labelled oleic acid into cholesteryl ester determined. Table 1 gives the data for one typical experiment.

Table 1.  Effect of Platelets on Cholesterol Ester Metabolism by Macrophages Stimulated with LDL[1]

|  | Platelets | *No LDL* Macrophages | Macrophages & Platelets | *Plus LDL* Macrophages | Macrophages & Platelets |
|---|---|---|---|---|---|
| Chemical Data |  |  |  |  |  |
| Protein (µg) | 1350 ± 50 | 890 ± 40 | 1960 ± 113 | 760 ± 30 | 1830 ± 50 |
| Cholesterol Ester % | - | 6.8 | 2.5 | 14.4 | 4.5 |
| $^{14}$C-Incorporation |  |  |  |  |  |
| Cholesterol Ester % | 0.5 ± 0.1 | 16.1 ± 0.6 | 10.3 ± 0.5[**] | 19.7 ± 0.7 | 12.3 ± 0.4[**] |

1.  Mean of 6 ± SEM
** p < 0.01

There is no evidence in either those cells which were incubated in the absence of LDL or in those incubated in the presence of LDL for any effect of platelets on either the accumulation of cholesteryl ester or of the incorporation of $^{14}$C-labelled oleic acid into cholesteryl ester in the macrophages.

Electron microscopy performed on the preparations of platelets, of macrophages alone and of macrophages and platelets indicated that platelets were taken up under these circumstances into lysosomes in the macrophages.

In view of these findings it was thought possible that platelets or their products might not reach the site of cholesterol esterifying and hydrolysing enzymes in the cells.  In further experiments therefore the effect of crude platelet homogenates on macrophage acyl cholesterol acyl transferase and lysosomal cholesteryl ester hydrolase activity was investigated.  ACAT activity was determined in microsomal preparations from rabbit macrophages (14) and LCEH activity in the 150000 g supernatant (15).  The data is given in Table 2.

Table 2.  Effect of Platelet Homogenate on Macrophage Cholesterol Esterifying and Hydrolysing Enzymes[1]

| Lysosomal Cholesterol Ester Hydrolase (pmol/min/mg protein) | | | | |
|---|---|---|---|---|
|  | *Control* | *+ Platelets* 20 | 100 | 200 |
| Experiment 1 | 247 ± 2 | 208 ± 15 | 261 ± 21 | 270 ± 13 |
| 2 | 266 ± 3 | - | 241 ± 9 | - |
| Acyl Cholesterol Acyl Transferase (pmol/min/mg protein) | | | | |
| Experiment 1 | 1.4 ± 1.4 | 0 | 0 | 0 |
| 2 | 12 ± 1 | - | 6 ± 3 | - |

1.  Mean of 3 ± SEM

An excess of platelet homogenate (equivalent of 20, 100, 200 platelets per macrophage in terms of cell numbers) was used in these studies.  There is no evidence even with a large excess of platelet homogenate for any reduction in macrophage LCEH activity or of any stimulation of macrophage ACAT activity by the platelet preparations.

The third mechanism for possible action of platelets (that is an effect on LDL in stimulating cholesteryl ester accumulation and foam cell formation) was investigated in a further series of experiments in which preliminary studies reported by Fogelman (12) were extended.  Low density lipoprotein (1.019 - 1.063) was prepared from normal pig serum and 5 mg of LDL protein in 0.5 ml saline plus 1 µg of arachidonic acid and 1.2 mg calcium chloride were incubated for 5 minutes in the dark at $37^o$.  A suspension containing $5 \times 10^{10}$ platelets in 2 ml Hanks solution was then added.  To this mixture was added 5 µg bradykinin and after a further 2 minutes 10 units of thrombin.  The mixture incubated in the dark for 1 hour.  At the end of this time the cells were

removed by centrifugation (2500 rpm for 30 minutes) and the supernatant containing
the LDL dialysed for at least 5 hours against 10 litres of 0.15 M sodium chloride
solution.  Controls were set up in which LDL was incubated but without addition of
the platelet suspension.  Macrophages plated out in petri plates at a concentration
of $5 \times 10^6$ cells per plate were then incubated with the LDL (either preincubated
with platelets or incubated alone) at a concentration of 100 µg/ml and in medium
consisting of Dulbecco's medium containing 10% foetal calf serum to which was added
$^{14}$C-labelled oleic acid.  After incubation for a further period of 16 hours the
macrophages were harvested and their chemical composition and the incorporation of
$^{14}$C-labelled oleic acid into cholesteryl ester determined.  Data is given in Table 3
for these experiments.

Table 3.  Modification of LDL by Platelets and its Subsequent Uptake and Metabolism
by Macrophages - 1 hr incubation[1]

|  | 1 hr Preincubation | |
|---|---|---|
|  | LDL Alone | LDL & Platelets |
| Chemical Data | | |
|   Protein (µg) | 278 ± 12 | 356 ± 12** |
|   Cholesterol Ester % | 24.0 ± 6.3 | 20.7 ± 5.0 |
| $^{14}$C-Incorporation | | |
|   Cholesterol Ester % | 5.9 ± 0.6 | 12.4 ± 0.6** |

1.  Mean of 6 ± SEM
** p < 0.01

In those cells where the LDL was preincubated with platelets for 1 hour the incorporation of fatty acid into cholesteryl ester was significantly increased.

It was thought that the effect of platelets in modifying LDL might be accentuated
by increasing the period of incubation so that in a subsequent experiment preincubation with platelets was extended to 16 hours and the LDL, either incubated alone or
incubated for 16 hours with or without platelets, then used for subsequent incubation
with macrophages.  The experiments were similar in all other respects to those
described above and the data is given in Table 4.

Table 4.  Modification of LDL by Platelets and its Subsequent Uptake and Metabolism
by Macrophages[1]

|  | 1 hr Preincubation | | 16 hr Preincubation | |
|---|---|---|---|---|
|  | LDL Alone | LDL & Platelets | LDL Alone | LDL & Platelets |
| Chemical Data | | | | |
|   Protein (µg) | 226 ± 11 | 200 ± 17 | 240 ± 8 | 144 ± 10 |
|   Cholesterol Ester % | 21.5 | 16.8 | - | - |
| $^{14}$C-Incorporation | | | | |
|   Cholesterol Ester % | 10.7 ± 0.3 | 13.9 ± 0.5** | 15.9 ± 0.5 | 9.1 ± 0.3** |

1.  Mean of 6 ± SEM
** p < 0.01

Results for the 1 hour incubation are essentially as described in Table 3 for the
previous experiment with an increase in the uptake and incorporation of fatty acid
into cholesteryl ester in those cells incubated with platelet LDL.  Where the LDL
was incubated without platelets for 16 hours its effect on the subsequent uptake
and incorporation of $^{14}$C-labelled oleic acid into cholesteryl ester in the macrophages was significantly greater than for the 1 hour preincubation.  On the other hand
where the LDL was incubated for 16 hours with platelets its effect on the subsequent
uptake and incorporation of $^{14}$C-labelled oleic acid into cholesteryl ester was
significantly less than was the case with the 16 hour LDL control.  Further experiments confirmed these findings.

It is apparent that changes occur to the LDL with 16 hours incubation compared to 1 hour incubation which increase its subsequent uptake by the macrophages and the resultant incorporation of $^{14}$C-labelled fatty acid into cholesteryl ester. On the other hand this effect is reduced by preincubation with platelets. The explanation for these preliminary findings can only be speculative at this stage. It is possible that the effect of platelets after 1 hour incubation is related to the formation of malonyl dialdehyde LDL and its subsequent uptake by macrophages as suggested originally by Fogelman et al (12). It appears possible however that there are other factors liberated from platelets which influence the spontaneous modification of LDL or which alter the uptake of the changed LDL by macrophages. It is clear that further work is necessary to pursue these possibilities.

*Acknowledgements*   We are grateful to Dr. Gordon Campbell, Department of Anatomy, University of Melbourne for carrying out the electron microscopy.

References

1. Goldstein J.L., Ho Y.K., Basu S.K. and Brown M.S. (1979) Binding site on macrophages that mediates uptake and degradation of acetylated low density lipoprotein, producing massive cholesterol deposition. Proc Natl Acad Sci USA  76:  333-337
2. Goldstein J.L., Ho Y.K., Brown M.S., Innerarity T.L. and Mahley R.W. (1980) Cholesteryl ester accumulation in macrophages resulting from receptor-mediated uptake and degradation of hypercholesterolemic canine - β-very low density lipoproteins.  J Biol Chem  255: 1839-1848
3. Day A.J. (1964) The macrophage system, lipid metabolism and atherosclerosis. J Atheroscler Res  4: 117-130
4. Day A.J. (1967) Lipid metabolism by macrophages and its relationship to atherosclerosis.  *In* "Advances in Lipid Research" (Ed. R. Paoletti and D. Kritchevsky) Academic Press  5: 185-207
5. Gryglewski R.J., Deminska-Kiec A., Zmuda A and Gryglewska T. (1978) Prostacyclin and thromboxane $A_2$ biosynthesis capacities of heart, arteries and platelets at various stages of experimental atherosclerosis in rabbits.  Atherosclerosis  31: 385-394
6. Ross R., Glomset J.A., Kariya B. and Harker L.A. (1974) A platelet-dependent serum factor that stimulates the proliferation of arterial smooth muscle cells *in vitro*. Proc Natl Acad Sci USA  71: 1207-1210
7. Chandler A.B. and Hand R.A. (1961) Phagocytized platelets; a source of lipids in human thrombi and atherosclerotic plaques.  Science  134: 946-947
8. Ardlie N.G. and Schwartz C.J. (1968) The organization and fate of autologous pulmonary emboli in hypercholesterolaemic rabbits.  J Path & Bact  95: 19-28
9. Moore S. (1979) Endothelial Injury and Atherosclerosis.  Exp Mol Pathol  31: 182-190
10. Minick C.R., Stemerman M.B. and Insull, W. (1977) Effect of regenerated endothelium on lipid accumulation in the arterial wall.  Proc Natl Acad Sci USA  74: 1724-1728
11. Day A.J., Bell F.P., Moore S. and Friedman R. (1974) Lipid composition and metabolism of thrombo-atherosclerotic lesions produced by continued endothelial damage in normal rabbits.  Circulation Res  34: 467-476
12. Fogelman A.M., Schechter I., Seager J., Hokom M., Child J.S. and Edwards P.A. (1980) Malondialdehyde alteration of low density lipoproteins leads to cholesteryl ester accumulation in human monocyte-macrophages.  Proc Natl Acad Sci USA  77: 2214-2218
13. Day A.J. and Fidge N.H. (1962) The uptake and metabolism of $C^{14}$-labelled fatty acids by macrophages *in vitro*. J Lipid Res  3: 333-338
14. Brecher P. and Chan C.T. (1980) Properties of acyl-CoA: cholesterol O-Acyl transferase in aortic microsomes from atherosclerotic rabbits.  Biochim Biophys Acta 617:  458-471
15. Brecher P., Pyun H.Y. and Chobanian A.V. (1977) Effect of atherosclerosis on lysosomal cholesterol esterase activity in rabbit aorta.  J Lipid Res  18: 154-163

# Role of Macrophage Foam Cells in Arterial Lesions

S.D.Fowler[1]

## Introduction

At some stage in their development, all atherosclerotic lesions contain foam cells.    These cells can be easily  identified by their
swollen cytoplasm filled with lipid inclusions.  Arterial foam cells
have been recognized since the early 1900's; their origin has been
variously attributed to endothelial cells, fibroblasts, smooth muscle cells, macrophages, or lymphocytes (Geer and Haust, 1972).  The
nature and origin  of arterial foam cells  has remained unresolved
even after the application  of electron microscopy to their study,
since the structural signs necessary for identification of cell type
are lost in the lipid overloaded cells.   A general consensus has
grown, however, that foam cells may be derived either from intimal
smooth muscle cells or from blood monocytes.

Recently, the question of the origin of foam cells has gained pro-
minance because the answer could determine whether foam cells are
considered as innocent bystanders in the disease process or as important contributors  to its genesis.   If foam cells are simply
transformed smooth muscle cells, their participation in lesion development may be a passive one.  Their lipid overloading could be
viewed as a sign  of cellular dysfunction  analogous to that of an
end-stage diseased organ.  If, however, foam cells are blood monocytes in disguise, their presence may signal that important biological events have taken place or are underway.

## Evidence for Foam Cells of Macrophage Origin

Direct evidence for foam cells with macrophage characteristics has
come from studies on cell populations isolated from atheromatous lesions (Fowler et al., 1979).  Two populations of lipid-containing
cells can be separated by Metrizamide density gradient centrifugation after digestion of atheromatous aortas with a mixture of collagenase and elastase enzymes  (Haley et al., 1977;  Fowler et al.,
1980).  One cell population equilibrates at high densities ($\rho$ = 1.10
- 1.14) and consists of recognizable smooth muscle cells with varying stages of lipid deposition.   A second  smaller population of
cells equilibrates at much lower densities ($\rho$ = 1.03 - 1.07).  These
cells appear as typical foam cells, and they possess great quantities of cholesterol and cholesteryl esters.   The low density foam
cells contain levels of catalase and lysosomal hydrolases comparable
to those measured in macrophages; the enzyme activities are substantially higher than those found in smooth muscle cells.  By rosetting
techniques, about 70% of the foam cells isolated from rabbit atheromatous aortas were found to possess Fc receptors (Fig. 1).   These
receptors have been found on all mononuclear phagocytes studied so

[1]Address:  Department of Pathology, School of Medicine, University
 of South Carolina, Columbia, South Carolina, 29208

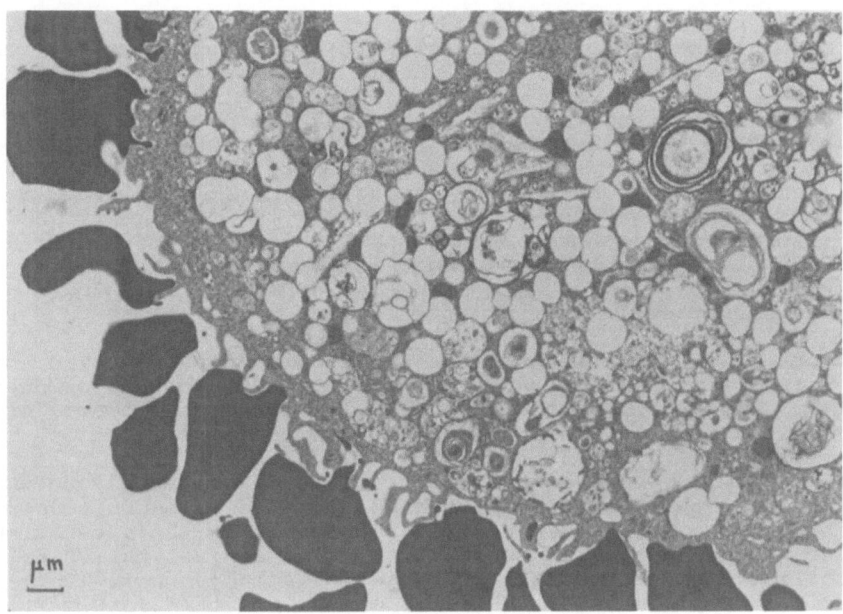

Fig. 1.    Demonstration of Fc receptors on foam cells.
Foam cells isolated from rabbit atheromatous aorta specifically bind IgG-coated erythrocytes.  Some bound erythrocytes can be subsequently interiorized and digested
by the foam cells.  For experimental details, see Fowler
et al., 1979.


far.  A smaller proportion of the foam cells exhibited C3 receptors
as well.  In addition, under appropriate conditions, the IgG-coated
erythrocytes could be interiorized and digested, providing evidence
that the foam cells act as phagocytes.

With similar techniques, Schaffner et al., (1980) observed both Fc
and C3 receptors on foam cells migrating out from cultured explants
of lesions taken from vessels of rabbits and monkeys.  These investigators also identified lysozyme, a well known macrophage enzyme,
in monkey foam cells.

Supporting these studies is a report by  Spraragan et al.,   (1969)
that {$^3$H}thymidine-labeled  blood monocytes  injected into rabbits
fed on cholesterol appeared in lesions as foam cells.  More recently, "foam cells" have been produced in culture by incubating macrophages with acetylated low density lipoproteins (Brown et al., 1979)
or β-very low density lipoprotein (Goldstein et al., 1980).

## Significance of the Macrophage Foam Cell

The above evidence strongly suggests that macrophages are present in
arterial lesions, and that they can be there in substantial numbers
under experimental conditions.   We know little about their activities in the lesions  but can speculate  about the  consequences of
their presence based on recent knowledge of the biology of mononuclear phagocytes (Van Furth, 1980).

454

Macrophages have long been recognized as scavenger cells.  This role
of macrophages is an integral part of the inflammatory response and
wound healing.  Membranous whorls and crystals of cholesterol are
commonly seen within lysosomes of arterial foam cells (Shio et al.,
1978, 1979), and they may be an indication that macrophages have migrated to the grumous core of lesions to scavenge decaying cells and
to remove oil-crystalline deposits of lipid.  This scavenger function could account for the generation of arterial foam cells from
mononuclear phagocytes.  Additionally, macrophages readily phagocytize denatured protein aggregates.  Complexes of plasma lipoproteins
with glycosaminoglycans or other matrix components of the artery
wall may be avidly taken up by macrophages.  This too could lead to
their intracellular lipid overloading.

More recently, numerous in vitro studies have revealed that macrophages secrete a wide variety of potent biological products (Table
1).  Many of these could potentially affect the course of developing
lesions and perhaps even function in lesion initiation.

For example, collagenase, elastase, and a proteoglycan-degrading enzyme are three neutral proteases secreted by macrophages that could
break down the key structural components of the arterial wall.  Macrophage elastase is especially active against native elastin fibrils.  Another neutral protease, plasminogen activator, forms plasmin from plasminogen.  Plasmin can affect the lysis of fibrin and
can activate components of complement.  Plasminogen activator may
also assist macrophages in their migration through tissues.  The secretion of these neutral proteases is induced by phagocytosis of
foreign particles or ingestion of immune complexes by macrophages;
prostaglandins act synergistically in stimulating macrophage secretion of collagenase.  The action of these proteases is modulated, in
a manner not yet clear, by $\alpha_2$-macroglobulin and other enzyme inhibitors. These inhibitors are also elaborated by macrophages.

Macrophages also release substantial quantities of lysosomal hydrolases into their surroundings.  If the pH falls in the microenvironment of the lesion,  these enzymes  could also effectively  degrade
collagen, elastin, and other matrix components and could even attack
arterial cells themselves.

TABLE 1.  MACROPHAGE SECRETION PRODUCTS POTENTIALLY AFFECTING ATHEROMATA

| NEUTRAL PROTEASES | COMPLEMENT COMPONENTS | BIOACTIVE LIPIDS |
|---|---|---|
| COLLAGENASE | C1 – C5 | PROSTAGLANDIN $E_2$ |
| ELASTASE | FACTOR B | PROSTAGLANDIN $I_2$ |
| PROTEOGLYCAN-DEGRADING ENZYME | FACTOR D | PROSTACYCLIN |
| PLASMINOGEN ACTIVATOR | ß1H | THROMBOXANE |
| | PROPERDIN | LEUKOTRIENE |
| ACID HYDROLASES | | HYDROXY-EICOSATETRAENEOIC ACIDS |
| | BINDING PROTEINS | PLATELET-ACTIVATING FACTOR |
| PROTEASES | | |
| LIPASES | FIBRONECTIN | |
| GLYCOSIDASES | TRANSFERRIN | REACTIVE METABOLITES OF OXYGEN |
| SULFATASES | APOLIPOPROTEIN E | SUPEROXIDE ANION |
| | | HYDROGEN PEROXIDE |
| OTHER ENZYMES | FACTORS REGULATING RESPONSES BY OTHER CELLS | HYDROXY RADICAL |
| | | SINGLET OXYGEN (?) |
| ARGINASE | MACROPHAGE GROWTH FACTOR | |
| LIPOPROTEIN LIPASE | ANGIOGENESIS FACTOR | |
| | MACROPHAGE INHIBITOR OF CELL PROLIFERATION | NUCLEOSIDES AND METABOLITES |
| | MACROPHAGE CHEMOTACTIC FACTOR | |
| ENZYME INHIBITORS | FACTOR STIMULATING COLLAGEN PRODUCTION | THYMIDINE |
| | FACTOR ENHANCING LDL RECEPTOR ACTIVITY | URACIL |
| $\alpha_2$-MACROGLOBULIN | | URIC ACID |
| PLASMIN INHIBITOR | | |

SOURCES:  DAVIES AND BONNEY, 1979; NATHAN ET AL., 1980

A cardinal feature of atherosclerosis is the migration of medial smooth muscle cells into the intima and the subsequent multiplication of these cells. It is now recognized that macrophages synthesize a potent growth promoting factor that acts on both fibroblasts and smooth muscle cells (Liebovich and Ross, 1976). Macrophages also produce chemotactic substances that attract other cells. Because of their position within the arterial wall, macrophages could thus possibly play an even more important role than platelets in the initiation of localized intimal proliferation of smooth muscle cells.

Macrophages release a variety of nonprotein substances of considerable potency. These could have important pathological consequences in arterial lesions.

One class of such substances is the arachidonic acid oxygen products. Prostaglandin $E_2$ and $I_2$ are synthesized in considerable quantities by macrophages, and in some circumstances prostacyclin or thromboxane may be produced as well. Leukotrienes and hydroxy-eicosatetraeneoic acids are also generated by macrophages. Production of all these compounds appears to be augmented when certain kinds of particles are phagocytized. The arachidonic acid derivatives could have multiple effects on arteries including modulation of smooth muscle contraction, histamine production, and arterial wall metabolism.

When triggered by a phagocytic stimulus, macrophages undergo a metabolic burst in which reactive metabolites of oxygen are generated. These are superoxide anion and hydrogen peroxide and possibly hydroxyl radicals and singlet oxygen as well. Such metabolites were recently shown to kill neoplastic cells (Nathan et al., 1979). Could they not kill proliferating smooth muscle cells as well? Alternatively, these reactive compounds could create oxidized derivatives of cholesterol and fatty acids that could have deleterious effects on cells that metabolize them.

Macrophages also generate large quantities of thymidine and other nucleoside metabolites, in part by degrading the DNA of dying cells. It is possible that proliferating smooth muscle cells could be sensitive to blockage of DNA synthesis by the macrophage nucleoside metabolites. In the microenvironment of the lesion, reduction in arginine concentrations by arginase, secreted by macrophages, could possibly also limit growth and function of arterial cells.

Whether significant immune reactions take place in arterial lesions is unknown. If they do occur, the presence of macrophages could markedly amplify their effects. Among the various immunoregulatory functions macrophages perform is the synthesis and secretion of all the major components of the complement system. Some of the degradation products of complement, such as C5a, are strongly chemotactic to macrophages. If they were generated in lesions, they could promote further accumulation of macrophages in vessels.

From the properties listed above, it is clear that macrophages could interact in arterial lesions in a variety of ways. However, not all mononuclear phagocytes exhibit these properties all the time. The state of activation of macrophges and the particular environmental setting in which they are found, appear to determine how many of their characteristics are expressed. Our challenge for the future will be to learn which of the manifold traits of macrophages are exhibited by these cells in the atheroma in vivo.

456

Acknowledgements

This work was supported in part by US Public Health Service Grants
HL-18157 and HL-24229 from the National Heart, Lung, and Blood In-
stitue and in part by a Grant-in-Aid from the New York Heart Association. Dr. Fowler is an Otto G. Storm Established Investigator of
the American Heart Association.

References

Brown, MS, Goldstein JL, Krieger M, Ho YK, Anderson RGW (1979) Re-
    versible accumulation of cholesteryl esters in macrophages in-
    cubated with acetylated lipoproteins. J. Cell Biol. 82: 597-613
Davis P, Bonney RJ (1979) Secretory products of mononuclear phago-
    cytes. A brief review. J. Reticuloendothel. Soc. 26: 37-47
Fowler S, Berberian PA, Shio H, Goldfischer S, Wolinsky H (1980)
    Characterization of cell populations from aortas of rhesus mon-
    keys with experimental atherosclerosis. Circ. Res. 46:520-530
Fowler S, Shio H, Haley NJ (1979) Characterization of lipid-laden
    aortic cells from cholesterol-fed rabbits. IV. Investigation
    of macrophage-like properties of arotic cell populations. Lab.
    Invest. 41: 372-378
Geer JC, Haust DA (1972) Smooth muscle cells in atherosclerosis.
    In: Pollack HS, Simms HS, Kirk DA (eds) Monographs on athero-
    sclerosis, Vol. 2 S. Karger, New York
Goldstein JL, Ho YK, Brown MS, Innerarity TL, Mahley RW (1980) Chol-
    esteryl ester accummulation in macrophages resulting from re-
    ceptor-mediated uptake and degradation of hypercholesterolemic
    canine β-very low density lipoproteins. J. Biol. Chem. 255:
    1839-1848
Haley NJ, Shio H, Fowler S (1977) Characterization of lipid-laden
    aortic cells from cholesterol-fed rabbits. I. Resolution of
    aortic cell populations by metrizamide density gradient centri-
    fugation. Lab. Invest. 37: 287-296
Liebovich SJ, Ross R (1976) A macrophage-dependent factor that sti-
    mulates the proliferation of fibroblasts in vitro. Am. J.
    Pathol. 84: 501-514
Nathan CF, Murray HW, Cohn ZA (1980) The macrophage as an effector
    cell. N. Eng. J. Med. 303: 622-626
Nathan CF, Silverstein SC, Brukner LH, Cohn ZA (1979) Extracellular
    cytolysis by activated macrophages and granulocytes. II. Hy-
    drogen peroxide as mediator of cytotoxicity. J. Exp. Med. 149:
    100-113
Schaffner T, Taylor K, Bartucci EJ, Fisher-Dzoga K, Beeson YH, Gla-
    gov S, Wissler RW (1980) Arterial foam cells with distinctive
    immunomorphologic and histochemical features of macrophages.
    Am. J. Pathol. 100: 57-74
Shio H, Haley NJ, Fowler S (1978) Characterization of lipid-laden
    aortic cells from cholesterol-fed rabbits II. Morphometric
    analyses of lipid-filled lysosomes and lipid droplets in aortic
    cell populations. Lab. Invest. 39: 390-397
Shio H, Haley, NJ, Fowler S (1979) Characterization of lipid-laden
    aortic cells from cholesterol-fed rabbits III. Intracellular
    localization of cholesterol and cholesteryl ester. Lab. In-
    vest. 41: 160-167
Spraragan SC, Giordano AR, Poon TP, Hamel H (1969) Participation of
    circulating mononuclear cells in the genesis of atheromata.
    Circulation 40 (Suppl. III): 24
Van Furth R, (ed) (1980) Mononuclear phagocytes: Functional aspects.
    Martinns Nijhoff BV, The Hague

# Chemotactic Responses of Monocyte-Macrophages.
# A Possible Mechanism for Their Migration into Atherosclerotic Lesions

R. G. Gerreti and J. A. Goss

## Role of the Monocyte in Early Atherogenesis

In previous studies (1,2) we have demonstrated that the earliest detectable lesions in swine fed a cholesterol/lard-enriched (C/L) diet develop in areas which take up intravenously-injected Evans blue dye (3). These lesions begin as microscopic foci of foam cells, and after some 15 wk on the C/L diet, cover much of these areas. Such lesions retain their fatty streak nature for up to 30-40 wk in swine with serum cholesterol levels of 400-600 mg/dl, although from about 15 wk onward, they extend topographically beyond areas of dye uptake (blue areas), into areas which are Evans blue negative (white areas), eventually encompassing much of the arch. Early lesions in blue areas are confined to the intima, exhibit little or no involvement of recognizable smooth muscle cells, and are characterized by large numbers of lipid-engorged foam cells (1). Moreover, these areas have been shown to be associated with the adherence of large numbers of blood monocytes to the endothelium, with subsequent penetration of the intima (2). This phenomenon is seen both prior to, and throughout the sequence of lesion development. The absence of morphologically-recognizable smooth muscle cells in these lesions, together with the presence of large numbers of lipid-filled cells which exhibit typical macrophage foam cell morphology at a time concomitant with adherence and intimal penetration by monocytes has led to the belief that the blood monocyte is the prime source of foam cells in these lesions. These fatty lesions are also characterized by the presence of large numbers of foam cells migrating through the endothelium. The direction of movement has been interpreted as being from the lesion into the lumen, based on the frequent presence of endothelial strands extending over the luminal aspect of migrating foam cells when viewed in the scanning electron microscope (4). Additionally, many migrating foam cells are ruptured on their luminal, aspect, leaving cytoplasmic veils empty of cytoplasm visible both in the scanning electron microscope and by transmission electron microscopy. It is unlikely that this appearance is artefactual, since the vessels are perfusion-fixed, and adjacent cells are intact. Rather, their appearance would suggest a possible rupturing of these turgid cells by shearing forces as they emerge from the vessel wall. The numbers of both adherent monocytes, and in particular, migrating foam cells increases with prolonged time on the atherogenic diet, and in later lesions, a 1:1 ratio of adherent monocytes:migrating foam cells exists (4). Despite the large numbers of migrating foam cells present on the surface of these lesions, there is a paucity of such cells in the circulating blood. As well, numerous degenerate foam cells can be found in the sinusoids of the liver and spleen. These findings again would suggest a migration of the cells from the lesion, with subsequent clearance from the circulation, as opposed to migration of blood lipophages into the arterial wall (4).

The results of these studies would indicate that the blood monocyte plays a role in lipid clearance in early atherogenesis, in that monocytes enter the arterial wall at pre-lesion and lesion stages, and are demonstrably phagocytic and accumulating lipid once they enter the vessel wall. At later stages, foam cells appear to migrate from these non-progressing fatty lesions. If one accepts this interpretation, it follows that in later fatty lesions, foam cell emigration is equal to monocyte immigration into the wall (assuming that all adherent monocytes enter the intima), since these cells on the lesion surface are in a 1:1 ratio. If this is the case, not only does the cellularity of the lesion remain constant, since efflux equals influx, but lipid is effectively cleared. The latter point may account for the non-progression of these lesions to fibrous plaques in arch regions, which have been shown to have little smooth muscle cell involvement (1,2). Thus it may be that the monocyte system represents an early line of resistance to atherogenesis rather than a pathologic response. This hypothesis is more tenable in view of the fact that macrophage foam cells appear to be enzymatically more capable of processing lesion lipid than medial smooth muscle cells, and secondly, it is the fibrous plaque which is resistant to regression. If one accepts this lipid clearance hypothesis, it follows that a mechanism may exist controlling the adherence and migration of monocytes into such areas known to be susceptible to early lesion formation. The present study was initiated to examine this possibility.

## Chemotactic Responses of Swine Monocytes

One potential mechanism controlling the influx of blood monocytes into arterial areas at sites prone to lesion formation is a chemotactic stimulus. In chemotaxis, cells directionally migrate along a gradient toward the source of a chemotactic factor, as opposed to the directionally-random migration of cells, or chemokinesis. We tested for chemotactic stimuli on swine monocytes in vitro using a 48-well modified Boyden blind well chamber. In such chambers, two wells are stacked one above the other, separated by a nucleopore filter with 5μm pore size (5). The lower wells are filled with buffer, or known or putative chemotactic factors to be tested, and the upper wells with a known number of monocytes in suspension. During an incubation period at $37^{O}$ C, monocytes attach to the upper side of the membrane and migrate through the pores in response to a gradient of the chemotactic factor (if present) set up across the nucleopore filter. At the end of incubation, the filters are fixed and stained, and the number of cells which have migrated to the bottom side of the filter are counted as a measure of the chemotactic response induced (5). Chemokinetic responses are differentiated from chemotactic responses by placing the factor to be tested in both wells at various concentrations, thus preventing formation of a gradient or producing negative or positive gradients, while still allowing for stimulation of random migration (chemokinesis) (6).

Using this system, we tested the response of monocytes from both normal (N) and hyperlipemic (H) swine against serum, plasma-derived serum, and extracts from homogenates of aortic blue, white, lesion and non-lesion areas. In all cases studied, regardless of the duration of C/L diet feeding from 6-30 wk, hyperlipemic serum elicited a greater migration of monocytes than did normolipemic serum, regardless of whether the monocytes were derived from N- or H-swine. The response was identical whether whole serum or plasma-derived serum was used.

The chemotactic response of monocytes to extracts from homogenates of the aortic arch of N-swine showed no difference between white and blue areas (Table I). However, blue area extracts from H-swine elicited a greater chemotactic response than white area extracts (Fig. 1) or thoracic aorta extracts from the same animal (Table I). This response was consistently two-to-four-fold greater toward blue area extracts, and was found to exist both at stages prior to the formation of grossly-visible lesions (6-9 wk C/L feeding) and after lesion formation (15-30 wk C/L feeding). The response to extracts of lesions was always greater than that to adjacent normal areas (Table I), regardless of the geographic location of the lesion in the aorta, and was generally greater than that to extracts of non-lesion blue areas from the same animal.

Table I. Chemotactic Responses of Swine Monocytes to Aortic Extracts

| Extract from | Monocytes/Field Migrated |
|---|---|
| Buffer | $7.22 \pm 1.3$ |
| 9 wk N-swine Blue area | $16.11 \pm 3.1$ |
| White area | $16.44 \pm 4.8$ |
| 9 wk H-Swine Blue area | $31.33 \pm 3.4$* |
| White area | $16.44 \pm 0.5$ |
| Thoracic White | $10.30 \pm 1.3$ |
| 15 wk Abdominal Lesion | $57.83 \pm 7.8$** |
| Non-lesion | $15.7 \pm 2.7$ |

\* Significantly different from adjacent white area extract ($p<.05$)
\*\* Significantly different from adjacent non-lesion area ($p<.05$)


Discussion

The results of these studies demonstrate the presence of a factor(s) chemotactic for monocytes in the aortic wall of swine at sites known to be predisposed to early lesion formation (1) compared to adjacent sites. Hyperlipemic serum is also chemotactic for monocytes from H-swine, and preliminary studies on the characterization of these factors suggest that this factor from serum and that from blue areas are the same. Moreover, only monocytes from H-swine respond chemotactically to this factor in blue area extracts. These findings would suggest that a chemotactic serum factor is present in hyperlipemia which may enter the vessel wall in blue areas, which are known to have characteristics of enhanced intimal accumulation of blood-borne macromolecules (7,8). The exact nature of the response mechanism is as yet unknown. However, based on our knowledge of other chemotaxis systems, intimal accumulation of such a factor may produce a gradient across the endothelium or activate receptor sites on the endothelium (9) to which the monocytes can respond chemotactically. The fact that only monocytes from H-swine are responsive suggests that the mechanism may be receptor-mediated, as has been shown to be the case for neutrophils (9) and other cell types (10). The high concentration of this factor in the serum would conceivably result in down-regulation or internalization of receptors on circulating monocytes which can be rapidly activated upon contact with the endothelium of blue areas (10). It has been demonstrated that such re-activation of chemotactic receptors from the down-regulated state can occur rapidly in response to gradients of less than 1%, although high concentrations of the same factor are inhibitory to chemotaxis (10). Monocytes from N-swine respond only chemokinetically, but not chemotactically, to blue area extracts, which would suggest that monocytes from N-swine either do not have this receptor, or that it is inactive or of very low affinity. Further studies are necessary to elucidate the nature of any chemotactic receptor in this system, and the means by which it is activated in the hyperlipemic state.

The existence of a chemotactic factor for monocytes in blue, but not white, areas at times prior to gross lesion formation is consistent with the focal and preferential penetration by monocytes of blue area intima at these stages of hyperlipemia (1,2) as well as with the accumulation of macrophage foam cells at slightly later times when lesions form (4). The fact that lesion extracts generally are more chemotactic than blue area extracts is also consistent with previous findings of greater numbers of monocytes adherent to the endothelium overlying lesions compared to blue areas (2). Similarly, the lower response to white area extracts correlates with the reduced incidence of monocyte penetration of white areas. These results thus support our contention that foam cells in early lesions in swine are primarily monocyte-derived, and indicate the existence of a mechanism whereby blood monocytes are attracted to sites predisposed to lesion formation. The initiating stimulus is unknown, but may relate to the enhanced accumulation of LDL in blue areas compared to white (11) at similar stages which could conceivably trigger a requirement for lipid clearance from these areas.

## References

1. Gerrity RG, Naito HK, Richardson M, Schwartz CJ (1979) Dietary-induced atherogenesis in swine. I. Morphology of the intima in pre-lesion stages. Am J Pathol 95: 775-793.
2. Gerrity EG (1981) Role of the monocyte in atherogenesis. 1. Transition of blood-borne monocytes into foam cells in fatty lesions. Am J Pathol 106: 19-28.
3. Gerrity RG, Richardson M, Somer JB, Bell FP, Schwartz CJ (1977) Endothelial cell morphology in areas of in vivo evans blue uptake in the young pig aorta. II. Ultrastructure of the intima in areas of differing permeability to proteins. Am J Pathol 89: 313-334.
4. Gerrity RG (1981) Role of the monocyte in atherogenesis. 2. Migration of foam cells from atherosclerotic lesions. Am J Pathol 106: 29-32.
5. Harvath L, Falk W, Leonard EJ (1980) Rapid quantitation of neutrophil chemotaxis: use of a polyvinylpyrrolidone-free polycarbonate membrane in a multiwell assembly. J Immunol Meth 37: 39-45.
6. Wilkinson PC, Allan RB (1978) Assay systems for measuring leukocyte locomotion: an overview. In: Gallin JI, Quie PG (eds) Leukocyte Chemotaxis. Raven Press, New York, p 1.
7. Bell FP, Adamson L, Schwartz CJ (1974) Aortic endothelial permeability to albumin: focal and regional patterns of uptake and transmural distribution of $^{131}$I-albumin in the young pig. Exp Mol Pathol 20: 57-68.
8. Bell FP, Gallus AS, Schwartz CJ (1974) Focal and regional patterns of uptake and the transmural distribution of $^{131}$I-fibrinogen in the pig aorta in vivo. Exp Mol Pathol 20: 281-292.
9. Hoover RL, Folger R, Haering WA, Ware BR, Karnovsky MJ (1980) Adhesion of leukocytes to endothelium: roles of divalent cations, surface charge, chemotactic agents and substrate. J Cell Sci 45: 73-86.

10. Snyderman R, Goetzl EJ (1981) Molecular and cellular mechanisms of leukocyte chemotaxis. Science 213: 830-837.
11. Feldman DL, Hoff HF, Gerrity RG (1982) Immuno-cytochemical localization of LDL in aortas of hyperlipemic swine. Fed Proc (in press).

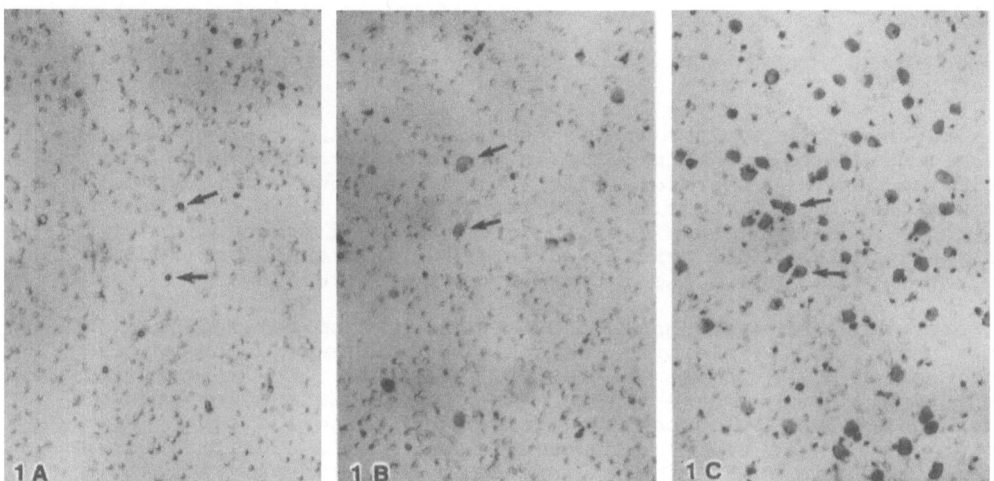

## Fig. 1.A,B

All figures are light photomicrographs (x625) of nuclepore filters from chemotaxis chambers stained with Haematoxylin and Wright's stains. Fig. 1a shows migration against buffer control. Most cells have not completely migrated through the filter, and can be seen only within pores (arrows). Fig. 1b demonstrates migration of monocytes (arrows) against Blue sepharose-bound extract of serum from a 9 wk N-swine. Fig. 1c illustrates migration of monocytes (arrows) against serum extract from a 9 wk H-swine, and shows many more monocytes migrated than in 1a or 1b. Compare figures with data in Table 1

# Macrophages in Coronary Artery and Aortic Intima and in Atherosclerotic Lesions of Children and Young Adults Up to Age 29[1]

H. C. Stary

## Introduction

This paper reports on the incidence, location, and fate of macrophages and macrophage foam cells in the coronary artery and aortic intima and in the atherosclerotic lesions of young human subjects. The work represents a preliminary report on one topic of a study now in progress and concerned with the evolution and progression of atherosclerosis in the coronary arteries and aortas of the population of New Orleans in the first 29 years of life.

The prevalence of macrophages and macrophage foam cells in the experimental atherosclerotic lesions of rabbits was demonstrated and reported by Anitschkow as early as 1913 (1). Their presence in the intimal fatty streaks of other species, including nonhuman primates and man, has also been recognized and acknowledged by many investigators. However, macrophage frequency and significance in human lesions is still widely disputed, and their part, if any, in the conversion of fatty streaks to fibrous plaques and in the continued growth of fibrous plaques is unknown.

## Methods

The data in this report are from a preliminary light and electron microscopic evaluation of the coronary arteries and aortas collected from human autopsy cases. Over the initial three years of the project we accumulated the coronary arteries and aortas of more than 400 subjects aged from fullterm birth to 29 years. In addition, we had available for study the coronary arteries of 50 young subjects from a feasibility study preceding the definitive study. The material is from males and females, blacks and whites, mainly the victims of accidents and homicides. The majority was autopsied at the corner's morgue of the City of New Orleans. Since these individuals were, in the main, healthy or at least unsymptomatic before they died, we have no information on their serum cholesterol levels during life. None had known lipoprotein abnormalities. From some we obtained postmortem blood for serum cholesterol determinations.

Only cases in which the interval between death and autopsy was relatively brief were used for 1-$\mu$m light microscopy and electron microscopy. Including the cases from the feasibility study, 276

---

[1]This work was supported by the National Institutes of Health, Grant HL-22739.

cases have been available so far for such studies. Various additional studies are being performed on tissues from the entire sample or on smaller subsamples, but the findings in this report are based only on the 1-μm and ultrathin section microscopy. We give the method we used to prepare the coronary arteries for study in another report on this project, elsewhere in this volume of the Symposium Proceedings (2). Preparation of the aorta differed. We removed, and immersion-fixed in osmium, multiple blocks of tissue from two standard locations in the descending thoracic and from one standard location in the abdominal aorta. Additional blocks were taken from lesions if counterparts did not occur in the standard aortic locations. All blocks were embedded in plastic. Quantitation of macrophages per unit area of nonatherosclerotic intima or lesion was by high-power light microscopy on 1-μm plastic-embedded sections. For confirmation of macrophage and macrophage foam cell identity vis-a-vis smooth muscle cells, and to confirm light microscopic quantiattions, we used electron microscopy. Quantitation of cell death was only by electron microscopy. Identification of cell types by electron microscopy was generally straightforward and reliable. Some intimal cells could not be classified by fine structural criteria. We feel confident, however, that we have correctly identified the majority.

## Definition of Macrophages and Macrophage Foam Cells

Macrophage. We apply the terms macrophage or intimal macrophage to monohistiocytic cells without lipid droplet inclusions (Fig. 1). The term intimal macrophage is used in preference to the term monocyte here since the cells in question occur in intimal tissue rather than in the blood and because there is experimental evidence that many are derived from local proliferation in the intima. The term macrophage is equivalent to the older term histiocyte which although possibly a better term is used less at the present. Macrophages have a range of fine structural appearances, all characteristic of this cell type, and determined by the functional state of the cell. Typically the cells are round, oval, or elongated, and not spindly like smooth muscle cells. The plasma membrane often has surface folds or ruffles which appear as numerous microvilli in cross-sections. The nucleus is kidney-shaped although this is not always apparent in ultrathin tissue sections. Lysosomes are not always present at every stage of activity but when present they are typically associated with a prominent Golgi apparatus and smooth ER. Bundles of thin filaments are most visible in the perinuclear region. Macrophages do not contain thick filaments and do not produce a basement membrane.

Macrophage Foam Cell. We apply the term macrophage foam cell or foam cell to cells with the fine structural characteristics of macrophages but containing lipid droplet inclusions (or the vacuoles left by them), independent of the number of the inclusions or vacuoles or the overall cell size (Figs. 2-4). Macrophages with inclusions generally encompassed the whole spectrum of transtional forms between macrophages and overloaded macrophage foam cells. Figs. 1-4 illustrate the spectrum of macrophage morphology within a single early lesion. Some of the features characteristic of macrophages are better developed in macrophage foam cells. The Golgi-smooth ER-lysosome

complex is generally very prominent and the plasma membrane has
microvilli more often. Cell size is variable. The frequent extremely
large size is associated with a large number of undigested droplet
inclusions. We have not used the term foam cell for smooth muscle
cells overloaded with lipid droplets. We use instead the term lipid-
laden smooth muscle cell. In our experience even extremely lipid-
laden smooth muscle cells retain some of their typical shape and
fine structural components that identify their cell type.


Results


Macrophages in Nonatherosclerotic Intima. Macrophages in the intima
of the coronary artery and aorta occurred in the first month of life
but they were infrequent up to about the middle of the second decade.
So far, we have not found intimal macrophages in every infant or
child. Earlier we had reported that intimal macrophages occurred
from the age of 5 years on. Having now data from a much larger sample of infants and children we find macrophages in the intima of
both the coronary artery and aorta of some of the youngest infants.
It is possible that more extensive sampling of the intima would
reveal intimal macrophages in all subjects. With infrequent exceptions, in the first 15 years of life, intimal macrophages occurred
in nonlesion intima as single and widely spaced cells, rather than
as groups of cells. Around and after the middle of the second decade of life, our sampling identified intimal macrophages in most
individuals, and their number per unit area of the intima increased.
The preferred location of intimal macrophages was the upper, glycosaminoglycan (GAG)-rich and smooth muscle cell-poor part of arterial
and aortic segments in which the intima was naturally thick.

Macrophages and Macrophage Foam Cells in Fatty Streaks. The term
fatty streak refers to the first gross visual appearance of early
atherosclerosis. Histologically in this type of lesion the fat was
stored either mainly in lipid-laden smooth muscle cells, or mainly
in macrophage foam cells, or more or less equally in both cell types.
There also was a quantitatively less important dusting of the extracellular matrix of the intima with lipid particles and organellar
debris from dead cells. Macrophages were always present in such
lesions. Their number varied greatly but there were always more
than in nonatherosclerotic intima. Neither the number of macrophages
nor the number of macrophage foam cells increased to correspond to
the thickness of the lesions as these generally progressed with
advancing age by accumulation of more smooth muscle cells, both
lipid-laden and without lipid, and more extracellular material. In
an earlier preliminary comment on this material we had reported
histologic evidence of coronary artery fatty streaks from about 15
years on. The more extensive data available now revealed small intimal macrophage foam cell accumulations in some of the youngest
children and infants, and as early as in the first month of life,
in both the coronary arteries and the aorta. The earliest accumulations consisted of small groups of macrophage foam cells floating in
the glycosaminoglycan-rich matrix of certain intimal segments. Un-
accompanied by lipid-laden smooth muscle cells or by extracellular
debris, the foam cell aggregates probably represent the first, grossly
invisible, chapter in the long story of human atherosclerosis development.

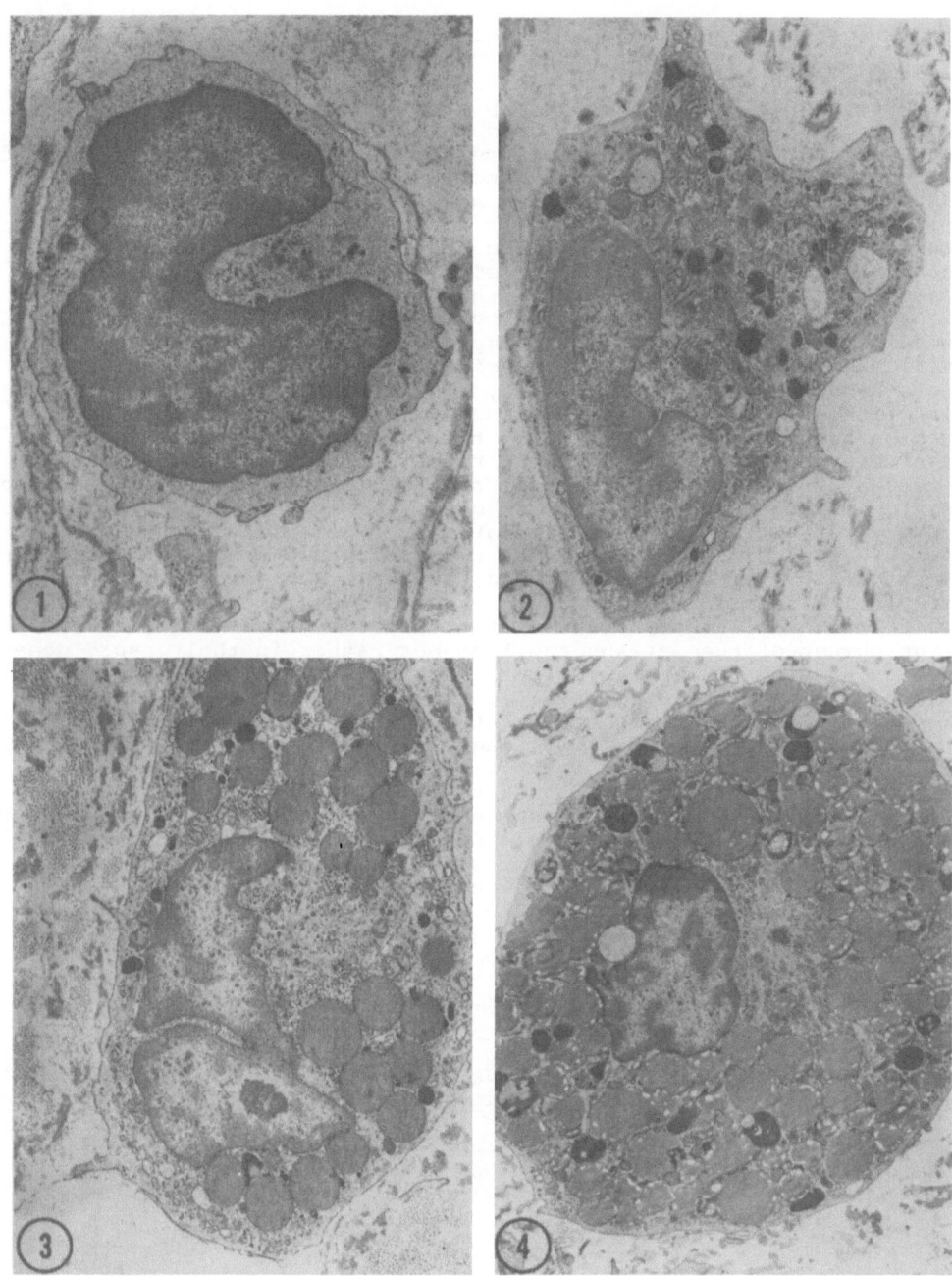

Figures 1-4. From a fatty streak type atherosclerotic lesion in the
proximal LAD of a 22-year-old man killed in an automobile (Case C-22).
Figure 1. Macrophage with few organelles (X 7000). Figure 2.
Macrophage with Golgi-SER-lysosomes and rare lipid droplet inclusions
(X 7000). Figure 3 (X 5000), and Figure 4 (X 3500). Macrophage foam
cells with Golgi-SER-lysosomes and many lipid droplet inclusions

Macrophages and Macrophage Foam Cells in Fibrous Plaques.  In 1-μm
and ultrathin sections, fibrous plaques consisted of all the components of fatty streaks plus enormous, at least microscopically,
accumulations of extracellular lipid particles, cholesterol crystals,
and the organelle remnants of dead cells.  (The accumulations are
known as necrotic cores in the literature.)  The hallmark of fibrous
plaques was, however, a greatly increased collagen component and a
massive increase in the number of RER-rich smooth muscle cells.  Ad-
joining the enormous extracellular accumulations were RER-rich smooth
muscle cells with or without lipid droplet inclusions rather than
macrophages and macrophage foam cells.  Macrophages and macrophage
foam cells were most numerous in the subendothelial space of the intima, and generally in regions above the extracellular accumulations.
Some foam cells were dead.  Our impression is that macrophages became
overloaded with cytoplasmic inclusions in the upper reaches of plaques,
where subsequently they also died.  Their remnants sagged in the
direction of the adventitia but instead of reaching it, and usually
even before finding an opening in the internal elastic lamina to
pass through, they accumulated near the base of plaques.  Since the
lifespan of overloaded macrophage foam cells is short, death of countless generations over a period of many years accounts for the eventual
enormity of extracellular accumulations.  The evidence then is that
necrosis in lesions occurs in the upper parts of plaques rather than
at the centers or bases of plaques, as the term necrotic core might
imply.  The significance of macrophages and macrophage foam cells
for the development of advanced atherosclerosis does not lie in a
large number of them at any one time but rather in their rapid generation and death.  Our material indicates that macrophages are the main
source of the necrotic material accumulated at the cores of plaques.
Smooth muscle cells, more resistant to death, provide the cellular
and connective tissue shell of plaques.

Smooth muscle cells and macrophages in their various modulations
were the only cell types we observed in the lesions of these children
and young adults.  Granulocytes did not play a part in human fatty
streaks or in early fibrous plaques.  In our experimental work with
primates we had not infrequently encountered some eosinophil and
neutrophil granulocytes in early lesions.

References

1.  Anitschkow N (1913) Über die Veränderungen der Kaninchenaorta bei
        experimenteller Cholesterinsteatose.  Beitr path Anat allgem
        Path 56: 379-404.
2.  Stary HC (1982) Structure and ultrastructure of the coronary
        artery intima in children and young adults up to age 29.
        Proc 6th Int Symp Atherosclerosis, Springer-Verlag, Berlin-
        Heidelberg-New York (this volume)

# 3 Lipoproteins – An Overview

# Structure-Function Relationships in the Plasma Lipoproteins

A. M. Gotto, Jr.

## A. Introduction

The plasma lipoproteins are macromolecular complexes consisting of apolipoproteins, phospholipids, cholesterol, cholesteryl esters and triglycerides.  A common model representing the structure of a plasma lipoprotein is illustrated in Figure 1.

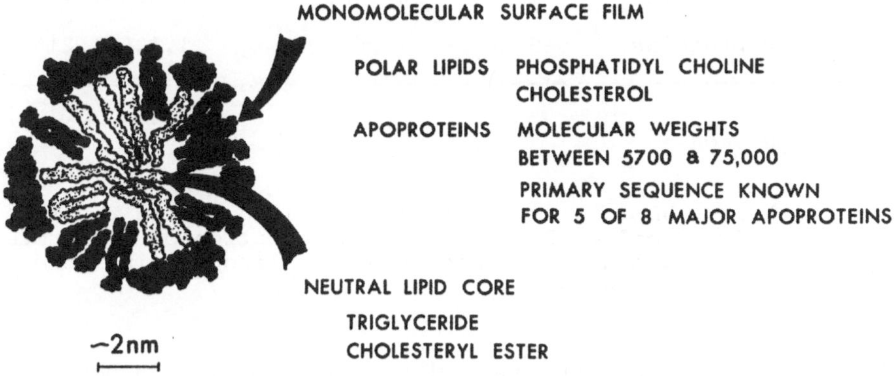

MONOMOLECULAR SURFACE FILM

POLAR LIPIDS  PHOSPHATIDYL CHOLINE
                CHOLESTEROL

APOPROTEINS  MOLECULAR WEIGHTS
                BETWEEN 5700 & 75,000

                PRIMARY SEQUENCE KNOWN
                FOR 5 OF 8 MAJOR APOPROTEINS

NEUTRAL LIPID CORE

TRIGLYCERIDE
CHOLESTERYL ESTER

~2nm

Fig. 1. The structure of $HDL_2$ obtained from space-filling models, adapted
from Verdery and Nichols (1).  The surface contains the polar components,
protein, phospholipid and cholesterol, whereas the core contains the
neutral lipids, mostly cholesteryl ester.  Copyright Baylor College of
Medicine, 1978

A lipoprotein will appear as a sphere when viewed as a negatively stained electron micrograph.  The surface of the particle consists of a monolayer of apolipoproteins and polar head groups of phospholipids (2).

The five classes of lipoproteins reflect the variation in size and
density from the chylomicrons, which contain a large lipid core rich
in triglyceride, to a subclass of the high density lipoproteins ($HDL_3$)
in which there is insufficient neutral lipid to form a central core.
Physical properties of the five classes are shown in Table 1.

Table 1. Physical properties of human plasma lipoprotein families

| | Electrophoretic Definition* | Particle Size | Daltons | Density |
|---|---|---|---|---|
| | | nm | | $g\ ml^{-1}$ |
| Chylo-microns | remain at origin | 75-1200 | >400,000,000 | <0.93 |
| VLDL | pre-β-lipo-proteins | 30-80 | 10-20,000,000 | 0.93-1.006 |
| IDL | slow pre-β-lipoproteins | 25-35 | 5-10,000,000 | 1.006-1.019 |
| LDL | β-lipoproteins | 18-25 | 2,300,000 | 1.019-1.063 |
| $HDL_2$ | α-lipoproteins | 9-12 | 360,000 | 1.063-1.125 |
| $HDL_3$ | α-lipoproteins | 5-9 | 175,000 | 1.125-1.210 |

*on paper
**on geon pevikon

On a molar basis, $HDL_3$ is the most abundant lipoprotein fraction and accounts for 70-80 mol % of the total concentration of lipoproteins in the plasma. Fasting concentrations of plasma lipoproteins in males vs. females are given in Table 2.

Table 2. Concentrations of major plasma lipoproteins in normal fasting humans

| | Males | | Females | |
|---|---|---|---|---|
| | μM | mol % | μM | mol % |
| VLDL | 0.1 | 0.7 | 0.04 | 0.2 |
| IDL | 0.04 | 0.3 | 0.03 | 0.1 |
| LDL | 1.6 | 10 | 1.3 | 6 |
| $HDL_2$ | 1.5 | 9 | 4.8 | 23 |
| $HDL_3$ | 12.7 | 80 | 15.1 | 71 |

The most remarkable difference between males and females is in $HDL_2$, in which the mol % in females is approximately three times as great as that in males. The $HDL_2$ subclass may represent the end product of the action of lipoprotein lipase on triglyceride-rich lipoproteins and it may be associated with increased protection against atherosclerosis (3). The proportion of protein in the lipoprotein classes is inversely related to particle size. On a molar basis, concentration of apoproteins is approximately the same in all classes except LDL. The molar concentration of apolipoproteins is 10-fold lower in LDL because the calculation is based on a high molecular weight of apoB (4).

## B. Structure-Function Relationships

I wish to refer to three aspects of structure-function relationships regarding the apolipoproteins. The first is lipid binding, the second is the role of apolipoproteins as ligands for binding to receptors on the surface of cells, and the third is the activation of enzymes involved in regulating lipoprotein metabolism.

We employ a nomenclature for apolipoproteins initially suggested by Alaupovic, which uses "A, B, C, D, E ..." to represent the subgroups. The apolipoprotein composition of the lipoproteins is shown in Table 3.

Table 3. Apoprotein composition of human plasma lipoproteins

|  | VLDL | IDL | LDL | HDL |
|---|---|---|---|---|
| | | mol % of total protein | | |
| apoA-I | | | | 45 |
| apoA-II | | | | 22 |
| apoB | 2 | 13 | 75 | |
| apoC-I | 8 | 26 | | 17 |
| apoC-II | 20 | 9 | | 2 |
| apoC-III | 60 | 41 | 22 | 7 |
| apoD | | | | 5 |
| apoE-II, III, IV | 9 | 13 | 3 | 1 |

The apoAs are found in chylomicrons and HDL. ApoB-100 is a major protein of LDL. ApoB-48 is a minor component of LDL and is made in the gut. The apoCs are made in the liver and are present in all of the lipoprotein families except LDL. ApoD is a minor constituent of HDL. ApoE is made in the liver and appears to be an important constituent of chylomicrons, VLDL, IDL and $HDL_2$ (5). The functions of a number of apolipoproteins are controversial (Table 4) or unknown (Table 5)(6-8).

Table 4. Plasma apolipoproteins whose function is controversial

|  | Function | Daltons | µM | Location |
|---|---|---|---|---|
| A-I | receptor-mediated uptake of HDL | 28,000 | 46 | HDL |
| A-II | activates hepatic lipase | 17,000 | 23 | HDL |
| C-III | inhibits uptake of apoE | 8,750 | 13 | HDL, LDL, IDL, VLDL |
| D | transfers cholesteryl ester | 20,000 | 5 | HDL |

Table 5. Plasma apolipoproteins with unknown function

|  | Source | Daltons | μM | Location |
|---|---|---|---|---|
| A-IV | intestine | 46,000 | 3 | chylomicrons |
| B-48 | intestine | 264,000 | ? | chylomicrons |
| C-III | liver | 8,750 | 13 | HDL, LDL, VLDL |
| $\alpha_2$-glyco-protein-I | ? | 54,000 | 0.3 | VLDL |
| Lp(a) | ? | ? | 1 | ? LDL |

## I. Lipid Binding

The central function of the apolipoproteins involves the binding of lipid. The analyses in model building studies of Segrest et al. in 1974 led to the proposal that the surface of an apolipoprotein contains specific lipid binding regions, called amphipathic helices, which have the ability to form alpha helices on binding lipid (9). As the apolipoproteins reside on the surface of the lipoprotein particle, the hydrophilic residues of the amphipathic helix would be oriented toward the hydrophilic exterior surface while the hydrophobic residues would be oriented toward the interior of the apolipoprotein. Thermodynamic studies of lipid binding by Pownall et al. have shown that the free energy of binding is related to the hydrophobicity of the apolipoprotein and probably derives from displacing hydrophobic regions from an aqueous to a more lipophilic environment in the interior of the lipoprotein particle (10). The energy change measured when binding occurs - that is, the magnitude of the free energy change - is always less than that predicted, even when corrections are made to account for the presence of hydrophilic residues on the exterior of the amphipathic helix. This finding has led to the concept that there is a gradation of polarity across the lipoprotein particle such that the outer part of the particle has a lesser degree of hydrophobicity than the inner part. These concepts are supported by studies of the energetics of apolipoprotein-phospholipid binding as performed by Pownall et al. (11). The determinants of lipid binding are summarized in Table 6.

We have identified the amphipathic helical lipid-binding regions in all of the apolipoproteins for which the secondary structure is known. Thus, available data collected to this point support the amphipathic helical structure. The exception would be apoB, for which the secondary structure or amino acid sequence is not yet known.

Table 6. Free energy of association, $\Delta G_a$, of lipid-associating peptides with DMPC

| Peptide | Measured | $\Delta G_a$ | |
|---|---|---|---|
| | | B & B calculated* | L calculated***** |
| | | kcal | |
| ApoC-III +0.3 M Gdm·Cl | -10 - 9.3 | -61 | +12.1 (-53) |
| RCM-A-II**** +0.3 M Gdm·Cl | - 8.0 - 7.2 - 6.2 | -66.6 | - 1.6 (-53.8) |
| LAP-16***** | - 6.5 | -16.7 | - 1.4 (-14.2) |
| LAP-20 | - 8.9 | -22.4 | - 4.4 (-17.8) |
| LAP-24 | - 9.5 | -28.1 | - 7.4 (-21.4) |

*Based upon Bull-Breese parameters (12) and $\Delta G_a = \Sigma \delta G$;
**Based upon Levitt parameters (13) and equation (4).
***Values in parentheses neglecting contribution of hydrophilic side chains.
****First value is for association with single bilayer vesicles and the second was obtained with multilayers.
*****Measured in 1.0 M NaCl.
******Values of $\delta G$; from (12) and (13).

## II. Cellular Uptake of Lipoproteins

A second function of the apolipoproteins is to modulate interaction of lipoproteins with receptors on the cell surface, thus regulating the cellular uptake of lipoproteins. This topic will be discussed in detail by other speakers at this symposium. Receptors for lipoproteins have been identified on many tissues, including endothelial cells, smooth muscle cells, fibroblasts and those of the liver and the adrenal cortex. Two apolipoproteins have been shown to serve as ligands for the recognition of lipoproteins by cellular receptors. One of these is apoB-100, the major protein of LDL (14). The second is apoE (15). Weisgraber and Mahley have characterized different amino acid substitutions in three isomorphic forms of apoE that may be separated by isoelectric focusing: apoE-2, E-3 and E-4 (16).

A pair of alleles specifies which isomorphs are present in a given individual. Thus, six different patterns are possible: E-2::E-2, E-3::E-3, E-4::E-4, E-2::E-3, E-2::E-4 and E-3::E-4. Approximately 1% of the population are homozygotes for the pattern E-2::E-2. This pattern has been found to be characteristic of dysbetalipoproteinemia, or type III hyperlipoproteinemia. Since type III is much less frequent that 1% of the population, other factors must influence the expression of the hyperlipidemia. Homozygotes for E-4::E-4 have been reported to have an increased frequency of type V hyperlipoproteinemia. (17) ApoE-2, apoE-3 and apO-4 reportedly differ in at least two amino acid residues involving cys/cys, cys/arg or arg/arg, respectively. The amino acid sequences of apoE-2 and apoE-3 are contrasted in Table 7.

474

Table 7. Amino acid sequences of the cysteine-containing CNBr peptides
of the E apoprotein*

---

Small peptide (17 residues)

E-3   Glu-Asp-Val-Cys-Gly-Arg-Leu-Val-Gln-Tyr-Arg-Gly-Glu-Val-Gln-Ala-Met
E-2                  Cys

Large peptide (89 residues)

E-3   Leu-Gly-Gln-Ser-Thr-Glu-Glu-Leu-Arg-Val-Arg-Leu-Ala-Ser-His-Leu-
E-2

E-3   Arg-Lys-Leu-Arg-Lys-Arg-Leu-Leu-Arg-Asp-Ala-Asp-Asp-Leu-Gln-Lys-
E-2

E-3   Arg-Leu-Ala-Val-Tyr-Gln-Ala-Gly-Ala-Arg-Glu-Gly-Ala-(Thr$_1$Ser$_2$Glx$_9$
E-2   Cys

E-3   Pro$_2$Gly$_6$Ala$_6$Val$_3$Ile$_1$Leu$_5$Trp$_1$Arg$_7$)-Met
E-2

---

* Adapted from (16)

According to this formulation, substitution of a single arginine, which
alters the charge on the protein, can profoundly alter the metabolism of
the apoE-containing lipoproteins.  Presumably, the arginine residue is
necessary for recognition of the apoprotein by lipoprotein receptors in
the liver (16).

III. Activation of Enzymes

A third structure-function relationship of the plasma apolipoproteins is
the activation of enzymes which regulate lipoprotein metabolism.  The
two enzymes to which I shall refer are lecithin:cholesterol acyltransferase (LCAT) and lipoprotein lipase.  LCAT requires either apoA-I or
apoC-I as an activator.  Based on our studies of amphipathic peptides,
we prepared a series of synthetic peptides to compare the relative
ability to bind lipid and to activate LCAT.  All of these peptides contain an amphipathic helix and are referred to as lipid-associating peptides.  The shortest contains 16 amino acid residues.  They do not contain the amino acid sequence of apoA-I or of the other naturally occurring
apolipoproteins.  The structure of LAP-20 is shown in Figure 2 (18).

SPACE FILLING MODEL & AMINO ACID
SEQUENCE OF MODEL PEPTIDE

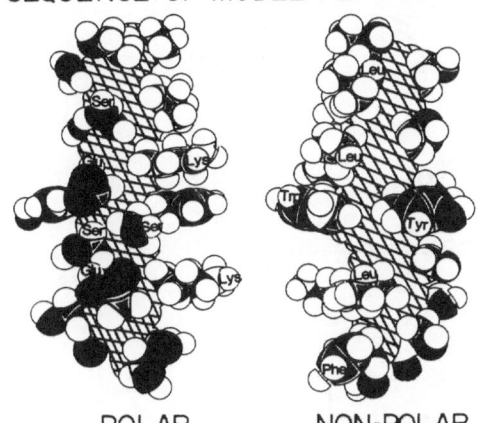

POLAR            NON-POLAR

Val-Ser-Ser-Leu-Leu-Ser-Ser-Leu-Lys-Glu-
Tyr-Trp-Ser-Ser-Leu-Lys-Glu-Ser-Phe-Ser

Figure 2. Synthetic peptide LAP-20, which has been shown to bind
phospholipid.  Copyright Baylor College of Medicine, 1978.

This peptide not only binds lipids; it also functions as an activator
of LCAT, although it does not serve as effectively as apoA-I.  The amino
acid sequences for the series of peptides known as LAP-16, -20 and -24
are shown below (19).

    val-ser-ser-leu-lys-glu-tyr-trp-ser-ser-leu-lys-glu-ser-phe-ser
                         LAP-16

    val-ser-ser-leu-leu-ser-ser-leu-lys-glu-tyr-trp-ser-ser-leu-lys-
                         glu-ser-phe-ser
                         LAP-20

    val-ser-ser-leu-leu-ser-ser-leu-leu-ser-ser-leu-lys-glu-tyr-trp-
                    ser-ser-leu-lys-glu-ser-phe-ser
                         LAP-24

These peptides differ in their content of leucine residues and in their
degree of lipid affinity.  The underlined residues indicate the substitutions between the peptides.  Pownall et al. have presented evidence
that the driving force for the binding of these peptides to lipid lies
in the transfer of hydrophobic amino acid chains from an aqueous to a
hydrophobic lipid environment (20).

Comparison of these peptides for their ability to bind lipid vs. activate LCAT has shown that the two phenomena are not directly correlated.
Although lipid binding is required for LCAT activation, not all of the
lipid binding peptides are able to activate LCAT (21).  It is apparent
that there is not a single specific amino acid sequence that determines
the ability to activate LCAT.  Figures 3a and 3b show comparisons
between lipid binding and LCAT activation.

476

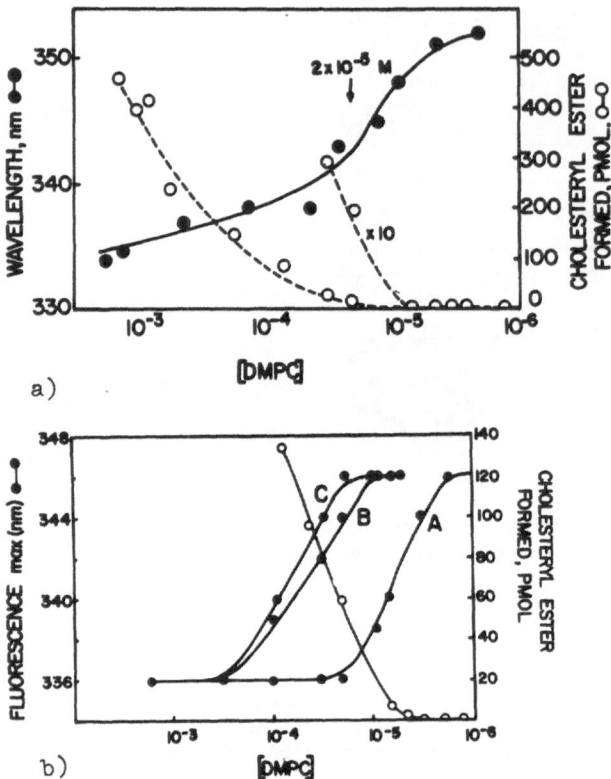

a)

b)

Figure 3. Effect of complex (peptide, dimyristoylphosphatidylcholine and $^3$H-cholesterol in a molar ratio of 1:20:0.4) concentration on LCAT activity and fluorescence. A complex of LAP-20 (3a) or LAP-24 (3b) was prepared. A stock solution of each was diluted to concentrations extending to $10^{-6}$M dimyristoylphosphatidylcholine and allowed to stand until no further change in fluorescence was observed < 2 hr. The fluorescence spectrum of each dilution was recorded and the fluorescence maximum plotted as a function of log concentration. For LCAT assays the same procedure was followed except that a 25 µl aliquot of the enzyme was added after 2 hr. The fluorescence shifts, from right to left, were in 0, 0.16 and 0.48 M Gdm Cl. LCAT activity was measured in the absence of Gdm Cl. Copyright Baylor College of Medicine, 1982.

Reversal of the sequence of lysine and glutamic acid in residues 16 and 17 in LAP-20 reduces the ability of the peptide to activate LCAT by 75% but does not substantially alter its ability to bind phospholipid (21). The precise structural determinants necessary for LCAT activation are currently under intensive study.

Previous studies involving solid phase peptide synthesis have helped to define the functional regions of apoC-II (22). In contrast to LCAT activation, the activator and lipid-binding regions occupy different sites of the protein (23). Region one, between residues 35 and 51, contains an amphipathic helix structure and is necessary for phospholipid binding (24). Residues 50-78 will activate lipoprotein lipase, even though they are unable to bind phospholipid (25). The two beta turns indicated in Figure 4 appear to be involved in increasing the rate of catalysis by lipoprotein lipase.

CALCULATED STRUCTURAL REGIONS OF APOC-II (35-78)

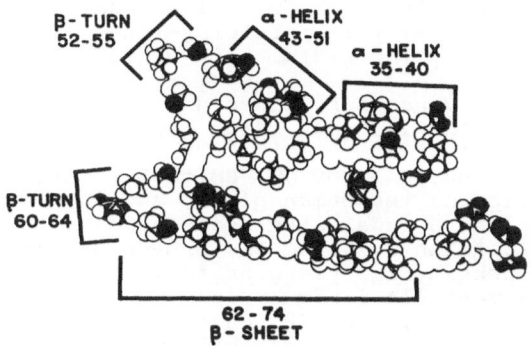

Figure 4. Proposed secondary structure of apoC-II (35-78). Copyright Baylor College of Medicine, 1981

Substitution of the tyrosine at residue 62 severely decreases the ability of apoC-II to activate lipoprotein lipase. We suggest that region 62-74 is involved in peptide-peptide interaction between apoC-II and lipoprotein lipase. Thus, unlike LCAT activation, activation of lipoprotein lipase does not appear to require high affinity hydrophobic binding of the apolipoprotein to either the surface of the lipoprotein or to an enzyme. A specific enzyme-activator association has been demonstrated by Smith et al. with the use of a synthetic fragment of apoC-II in which a dansyl residue is substituted on the amino terminal residue. They were able to demonstrate resonance energy transfer from tryptophan residues of lipoprotein lipase to the dansylated apoC-II peptide which does not contain tryptophan. The interaction could be demonstrated both in the absence of a substrate and in the presence of a nonhydrolyzable substrate (25).

C. Summary

In summary, there exist at least three important aspects of the structure-function relationship of apolipoproteins in the plasma lipoproteins. One involves lipid-binding, the second the uptake of lipoproteins by receptors on the surface of cells and the third the activation of the enzymes LCAT and lipoprotein lipase, which play crucial roles in the metabolism of the plasma lipoproteins. An understanding of the structure-function relationships of the plasma apolipoproteins may clarify their role in the regulation of lipoprotein metabolism. From this information, we may develop a better insight into the normal and aberrant mechanisms of lipid transport and into how this transport contributes to the pathophysiology of atherosclerosis.

References

1. Verdery RB, Nichols AV (1975) Arrangement of lipid and proteins in human serum high density lipoproteins: A proposed model. Chem Phys Lipids 14: 123-134

2.  Smith LC, Pownall HJ, Gotto AM Jr (1978) The plasma lipoproteins: Structure and metabolism.  Ann Rev Biochem 47: 751-777
3.  Patsch JR, Gotto AM Jr, Olivecrona T, Eisenberg S (1978) Formation of high-density lipoprotein$_2$-like particles during lipolysis of very low density lipoproteins in vitro.  Proc Natl Acad Sci USA 75: 4519-4523
4.  Smith R, Dawson JR, Tanford C (1972) The size and number of polypeptide chains in human serum low density lipoprotein.  J Biol Chem 247: 3376-3381
5.  Pownall HJ, Sparrow JT, Smith LC, Gotto AM Jr (1980) Structure and function of the human plasma apolipoproteins.  In: Gotto AM Jr, Smith LC, Allen B (eds) Atherosclerosis V, Springer-Verlag, New York, p 624
6.  Ose L, Roken I, Norum KA, Drevon CA, Berg T (1981) The binding of high density lipoproteins to isolated rat hepatocytes.  Scand J Clin Lab Invest 41: 63-73
7.  Sigurdsson G, Noel SP, Havel RJ (1979) Quantification of the hepatic contribution to the catabolism of high density lipoproteins in rats. J Lipid Res 20: 316-324
8.  Weisgraber KH, Bersot TP, Mahley RW (1978) Isolation and characterization of an apoprotein from the d<1.006 lipoproteins of human and canine lymph homologous with the rat A-IV apoprotein.  Biochem Biophys Res Commun 85: 287-292
9.  Segrest JP, Jackson RL, Morrisett JD, Gotto AM Jr (1974) A molecular theory of lipid-protein interactions in the plasma lipoproteins. FEBS Lett 38:247-253
10. Pownall HJ, Morrisett JD, Gotto AM Jr (1977) Composition-structure-function correlations in the binding of an apolipoprotein to phosphatidylcholine bilayer mixtures.  J Lipid Res 18: 14-23
11. Pownall HJ, Hickson D, Gotto AM Jr (1981) Thermodynamics of lipid-protein carboxymethlated apolipoprotein A-II from human plasma high density lipoprotein. J Biol Chem 256: 9849-9854
12. Bull HB, Breese K (1974) Surface tension of amino acid solutions: a hydrophobicity scale of the amino acid residues. Arch Biochem Biophys 161: 665-670
13. Levitt M (1976) A simplified representation of protein conformation for rapid simulation of protein folding.  J Mol Biol 104: 59-107
14. Brown MS, Kovanen PT, Goldstein JL (1981) Regulation of plasma cholesterol by lipoprotein receptors.  Science 212: 628-635
15. Sherrill BC, Innerarity TL, Mahley RW (1980) Rapid hepatic clearance of the canine lipoproteins containing the only E apoprotein by a high affinity receptor.  Identity with the chylomicron remnant transport process.  J Biol Chem 255:1804-1807
16. Weisgraber KH, Rall SC Jr, Mahley RW (1981) Human E apoprotein heterogeneity. Cysteine-arginine interchanges in the amino acid sequence of the apoE isoforms.  J Biol Chem 256:9077-9083
17. Ghiselli G, Schaefer EJ, Zeck LA, Gregg RE, Brewer HB Jr (1982) Increased prevalence of apolipoprotein E4 in type V hyperlipoproteinemia. (abstract) Clin Res 30: 291A
18. Pownall HJ, Hu A, Gotto AM Jr, Albers JJ, Sparrow JT (1980) Activation of lecithin:cholesterol acyltransferase by a synthetic model lipid-associating peptide.  Proc Natl Acad Sci USA 77: 3154-3158
19. Pownall HJ, Pao Q, Hickson D, Sparrow JT, Gotto AM Jr (1982) Thermodynamics of lipid-protein association in human plasma lipoproteins.  Biophys J 37: 175-177
20. Massey JB, Gotto AM Jr, Pownall HJ (1981) Thermodynamics of lipid-protein interactions: Interaction of apolipoprotein A-II from human plasma high density lipoproteins with dimyristoylphosphatidylcholine. Biochemistry 20: 1575-1584
21. Pownall HJ, Gotto AM Jr, Sparrow JT (1982) Correlation of the thermodynamics of lipid-protein interactions and the activation of LCAT by synthetic model apolipoproteins.  Submitted for publication.

22. Kinnunen PKJ, Jackson RL, Smith LC, Gotto AM Jr, Sparrow JT (1977) Activation of lipoprotein lipase by native and synthetic fragments. Proc Natl Acad Sci USA 74: 4848-4851
23. Smith LC, Kinnunen PKJ, Jackson RL, Gotto AM Jr, Sparrow JT (1978) Activation of lipoprotein lipase by native and synthetic peptide fragments of apolipoprotein C-II. In Carlson LA (ed) International Conference on Atherosclerosis, Raven Press, New York, p 269
24. Catapano AL, Kinnunen PKJ, Breckenridge WC, Gotto AM Jr, Jackson RL, Little JA, Smith LC, Sparrow JT (1979) Lipolysis of apoC-II deficient very low density lipoproteins: Enhancement of lipoprotein lipase action by synthetic fragments of apoC-II. Biochem Biophys Res Commun 89: 951-957
25. Smith LC, Voyta JC, Catapano AL, Kinnunen PKJ, Gotto AM Jr, Sparrow JT (1980) Activation of lipoprotein lipase by synthetic fragments of apolipoprotein C-II. Ann NY Acad Sci 348: 213-223

# Metabolism of Triglyceride-Rich Lipoproteins

R. J. Havel

Continuing advances in our understanding of the metabolism of chylomicrons and very low density lipoproteins (VLDL) in mammals have been
critically dependent upon new information about the structure and
function of apolipoproteins. This new information has come in substantial measure from the discovery of mutations affecting apolipoproteins or lipoprotein-receptors. Functions can now be ascribed to
each of the major groups of apolipoproteins (A, B, C and E) of nascent chylomicrons and VLDL. Here I will review chiefly recent research on the role of apolipoproteins B and E in the metabolism of
triglyceride-rich lipoproteins.

## Role of B Apolipoproteins

The discovery by Malloy and Kane of a young patient with some, but
not all of the clinical features of classical abetalipoproteinemia
(1, 2) led to the demonstration that the apolipoprotein B of chylomicrons differs structurally and antigenically from the apolipoprotein B of low density lipoproteins (LDL) (3). This demonstration
has become central to our new understanding of differences in the
metabolism of chylomicrons and VLDL. In all mammals evaluated to
date (humans, rats (4), rabbits (5), dogs (6), monkeys (7)), the major or sole apolipoprotein B secreted by the intestine has a lower
molecular weight than that of the predominant form of apolipoprotein
B in LDL. In the centile system proposed by Kane et al. (3), the
intestinal form of apo B is B-48 and that of LDL is B-100. These
forms of apo B differ in primary structure (3). They are antigenically related within species, but apo B-48 reacts variably to antisera raised to LDL (1, 4, 8). The patient with "normotriglyceridemic abetalipoproteinemia" discovered by Malloy and Kane, who has a
selective deletion of apo B-100, secretes apparently normal chylomicrons containing apo B-48 but is unable to secrete VLDL from the
liver, which (at least as found in blood plasma) contain only apo
B-100. Although the two proteins are obviously related structurally,
they evidently are under separate genetic control. One hypothesis
for the relationship between apo B-48 and apo B-100 is that they contain a common subunit necessary for assembly or secretion of nascent
triglyceride-rich particles. If so, the defect in the patient with
normotriglyceridemic abetalipoproteinemia that leads to deletion of
apo B-100 may lie in the synthesis of a second subunit or its linkage with the common subunit.

Although apo B-48 appears to be the distinctive form of apo B synthesized in the intestinal mucosa, it is not clear that the liver
synthesizes solely apo B-100. Indeed, in the rat, the liver synthesizes and secretes in VLDL substantial amounts of a protein with the
same apparent molecular weight as apo B-48, as well as apo B-100 (8 -
11). The rat may be unique in this respect, because apo B-100 is
clearly the major apo B secreted from perfused livers of guinea pigs

(12), rabbits (13) and monkeys (7), although small amounts of putative apo B-48 have been found in perfusates of rabbit livers (5). Apo B-48 is found in rat plasma LDL as well as VLDL (4, 8, 9, 11, 14), but the amount of apo B-48 relative to apo B-100 decreases with increasing density (8, 11). The turnover rate of apo B-48 in rat hepatic VLDL exceeds that of apo B-100 (9, 10), suggesting that at least some particles secreted from the liver contain only one form of apo B or the other.

Blood plasma of the patient with normotriglyceridemic abetalipoproteinemia contains virtually no LDL (2), suggesting that chylomicrons do not contribute normally to the formation of LDL. This concept receives support from studies in which the metabolism of radioiodinated B-48 of chylomicrons from intestinal lymph has been evaluated in intact rats (11). None of the apo B-48 appeared in a metabolically stable form in LDL, even though the ultracentrifugally separated LDL contained appreciable quantities of putative apo B-48. These results indicate that apo B-48 cannot be converted to apo B-100 and also suggest that the apo B-48 in rat plasma LDL arises from apo B-48 secreted by the liver.

In the rat, apo B-48 secreted in lymph chylomicrons is, like the component cholesteryl esters (15), rapidly removed from the blood by the liver as a component of chylomicron remnants (16). Most of the apo B of rat VLDL is also taken up by the liver, presumably as a component of VLDL remnants (17). On the basis of studies of the metabolism of apo B-48 and apo B-100 of plasma VLDL in the rat, Sparks and Marsh (14) have proposed that particles containing only apo B-48 are largely taken up by the liver as a component of VLDL remnants, whereas particles containing only apo B-100 are preferentially converted to LDL. However, in rabbits, hepatogenous VLDL contain very little if any apo B-48, yet only about 10% of VLDL particles are converted to LDL; the remainder appear to be taken up by the liver as VLDL remnants (18). Thus, in at least some mammals, the liver efficiently takes up VLDL remnants containing only apo B-100. In humans, most VLDL, which contain only apo B-100, are converted to LDL, but some remnant VLDL may be taken up by the liver and catabolized there, as in other mammals, particularly when VLDL concentrations are increased (19). The role of apo B components of chylomicrons and VLDL in the hepatic processing of remnants is discussed below.


Role of Apolipoprotein E


Important evidence for the function of apolipoprotein E in the metabolism of triglyceride-rich lipoproteins has also been derived from mutations of this protein. The human genetic polymorphism of apo E first described by Utermann and associates (20) is now recognized to reflect genetic polymorphism of the protein arising from a single locus (21) and to be caused by single amino acid substitutions (22). As deduced from isoelectric focussing electrophoresis in one or two dimensions, three common isoforms are recognized. Two of these, one (E-4) with arginine and the other (E-3) with cysteine at position 112 in the amino acid sequence of the protein, are associated with normal lipid and lipoprotein concentrations. The third, (E-2) with an additional cysteine-arginine substitution at various positions, or possibly with other point mutations, is associated with accumulation of chylomicron and VLDL remnants in blood plasma (22). As described below, amino acid substitutions in critical regions of the amino acid sequence lead to defective binding of apo E to lipoprotein receptors.

A crucial role for apo E in the metabolism of remnants of triglyc-eride-rich lipoproteins is supported by studies of remnant metabolism in rats. Apo E is secreted from the rat intestine at a negligible rate as compared with the secretion of apo B-48, apo A-I and apo A-IV, the principal apoproteins of nascent rat chylomicrons (23). Apo E, together with the several C apoproteins, is added to the surface of chylomicrons from high density lipoproteins (HDL) after secretion, mainly in exchange for phospholipids (24). This occurs to some ex-tent in the interstitial fluid of the intestinal villus, so that in-testinal lymph chylomicrons contain a substantial complement of apo E and apo C's. However, chylomicrons from intestinal lymph of rats treated for several days with large amounts of 17-α-ethinyl estradiol contain little E or C apoproteins, owing to the very low levels of these proteins in blood plasma (25). Addition of purified apo E to such chylomicrons in vitro renders the particles susceptible to rapid uptake of perfused rat livers, at a rate comparable to that of chy-lomicron remnants obtained from blood plasma of functionally evis-cerated rats injected with chylomicrons from intestinal lymph (25). Simultaneous addition of C and E apoproteins to chylomicrons from estradiol-treated rats yields particles that are poorly taken up by perfused livers. Since C and E apoproteins are present in plasma chylomicrons before their component triglycerides are largely hydrol-yzed by lipoprotein lipase, and the remnants produced thereby are de-pleted of C apoproteins as well as triglycerides and phospholipids, this result is consistent with other evidence (15, 26) that C apo-proteins prevent premature uptake of chylomicrons by the liver. Thus, it appears that apo E can contribute effectively to hepatic uptake of chylomicron remnants only when the concentration of C apoproteins on the particle surface has been sufficiently reduced. This effect appears to be common for the several C apoproteins (25). The spe-cial role of apo C-II in the action of lipoprotein lipase on chylo-micron triglycerides is clearly established by the exogenous hyper-lipemia that occurs when this protein is selectively lost as the re-sult of homozygosity for a single gene defect (27).

A role for apo E in the hepatic processing of chylomicron remnants is supported further by the observation that canine HDL that contain only apo E (apo E-HDL$_C$) compete for uptake of chylomicron remnants in perfused rat livers (28) and by the targeting to liver of artifi-cial triglyceride emulsions containing added apo E (26). Apparent opposing effects of apo E and C apoproteins are also observed with hepatogenous VLDL in the rat (15), consistent with the accumulation of both VLDL and chylomicron remnants in humans homozygous for the dysfunctional E-2 form of the protein.


Role of Hepatic Receptors in the Processing of Remnants


Several recent studies provide strong evidence that hepatic paren-chymal cells possess surface receptors whose properties closely re-semble the LDL receptors identified in a variety of cultured mamma-lian cells and that hepatic LDL receptors are important determinants of the efficiency with which LDL are removed from the blood (29). The discovery of an animal model of human familial hypercholesterole-mia, in which LDL receptors are deficient or functionally abnormal, has provided a unique opportunity to evaluate the role of hepatic LDL receptors in the metabolism of triglyceride-rich lipoproteins. In the homozygous WHHL rabbit discovered by Watanabe, hepatic as well as extrahepatic receptors are virtually undetectable (30 - 32). Plasma cholesterol and triglyceride levels are increased many-fold in these animals, and they have elevated levels of VLDL and IDL, as well as LDL (Table 1).

Table 1. Lipoprotein cholesterol, triglycerides and apo B levels in rabbits (mg/dl)

|  | Normal | | | WHHL | | |
|---|---|---|---|---|---|---|
|  | Cholesterol | Triglycerides | apo B | Cholesterol | Triglycerides | Apo B |
| VLDL | 17 | 129 | 10 | 110 | 154 | 25 |
| IDL | 8 | 14 | 7 | 116 | 78 | 64 |
| LDL | 12 | 16 | 16 | 218 | 146 | 168 |

As compared with normal rabbits, all of these lipoproteins are enriched in cholesteryl esters at the expense of triglycerides, and VLDL and IDL are enriched in apo B-100 and apo E at the expense of C apoproteins (Table 2).

Table 2. Properties of plasma lipoproteins in normal and WHHL rabbits

|  | VLDL | | IDL | | LDL | |
|---|---|---|---|---|---|---|
|  | Normal | WHHL | Normal | WHHL | Normal | WHHL |
| Cholesteryl esters/ triglycerides | 0.11 | 0.52 | 0.79 | 1.36 | 0.73 | 1.45 |
| Calculated diameter (Å) | 440 | 355 | 249 | 251 | 222 | 244 |
| Apoprotein B (% of total protein) | 41 | 55 | 72 | 82 | 91 | 91 |
| Electrophoretic mobility | Pre-β | Slow Pre-β | β | β | β | β |

Thus, lipoproteins with properties resembling VLDL remnants as well as LDL accumulate in WHHL rabbits (13). However, chylomicron remnants, which would be identified by the presence of apo B-48, do not. Hepatic uptake of cholesteryl esters and protein of chylomicron remnants occurs at a normal rate in WHHL rabbits and to the same extent as in unaffected rabbits (33). This observation provides strong evidence that the hepatic LDL receptor is not required for normal processing of chylomicron remnants. As with LDL, this uptake appears to occur via endocytosis into hepatic parenchymal cells. Thus, in rats, autoradiographic studies show that chylomicrons are taken up into endocytic vesicles of parenchymal cells which rapidly fuse to form multivescular body-like structures (16). After a few minutes, these organelles acquire lysosomal enzymes, leading to degradation of chylomicron lipids and protein. Although it seems likely that chylomicrons and LDL are processed via common endosomes, the normal processing of chylomicron remnants in WHHL rabbits strongly suggests that a distinct receptor is responsible for the process of adsorptive endocytosis of chylomicron remnants. Binding sites that recognize apo E but not apo B-100 have been found in crude liver membrane preparations from dog, swine and humans (34); these sites could represent the chylomicron remnant receptor. Binding of apo E to these sites requires calcium ion. No appreciable binding to such sites has been observed in liver membrane preparations from normal or WHHL rabbits, but EDTA-insensitive binding of chylomicron remnants can be observed (33). This binding is not specific for particles that contain apo E or apo B-48 and its role in hepatic uptake of chylomicron remnants is uncertain.

Apo B-48 could contribute to hepatic uptake of chylomicron remnants (14, 25). In vitro binding experiments with lymph chylomicrons from estradiol-treated rats have provided no evidence that apo B-48 can bind to the LDL receptor or to other receptors present in rat liver membrane preparations (35). Borensztajan and associates have provided evidence that apo B-48 is not required for normal hepatic uptake of cholesterol in chylomicron remnants (36). They digested all of the proteins of rat lymph chylomicrons with pronase and then incubated the treated chylomicrons with chylomicron-depleted rat plasma to transfer proteins other than apo B-48 to the particles. When injected into intact rats, labeled cholesteryl esters in the treated chylomicrons were rapidly taken up by the liver at a rate indistinguishable from that of untreated chylomicrons.

As described above, lipoproteins whose properties resemble those of VLDL remnants do accumulate in blood plasma of WHHL rabbits. Kita and associates have shown that apo B-100 is cleared slowly from VLDL in WHHL rabbits. The labeled protein is taken up much more slowly into the liver than in normal rabbits and a larger fraction eventually appears in LDL (37). Similar studies have been performed by Stoudemire and associates in fasted rabbits. In rabbits fasted for several days LDL and IDL levels increase several-fold, but unlike the situation in WHHL rabbits, VLDL levels change little. Receptor-dependent catabolism of LDL, assessed in vivo by injection of radio-iodinated LDL and methyl-LDL, is greatly reduced in fasted rabbits (18). As in WHHL rabbits, clearance of apo B-100 from VLDL is reduced in fasted rabbit and more accumulates in IDL than in fed animals. These results are consistent with the hypothesis that, unlike chylomicron remnants, VLDL remnants are normally processed in the liver predominantly by the LDL receptors. Since the salient difference between rabbit chylomicron and VLDL remnants resides in their unique B apoproteins, it is possible that apo B-100 interferes with recognition of apo E by the chylomicron remnant receptor. As with LDL, hepatic uptake of VLDL remnants in rats occurs via endocytosis into hepatocytes (16). This observation is consistent with, but clearly does not establish, a common receptor-dependent process.

Observations of the binding of apo E from patients with familial dysbetalipoproteinemia to LDL receptors in liver membrane preparations or on extrahepatic cell surfaces provide further insights into the role of this protein in the processing of remnant particles. Discoidal phospholipid complexes of rat and human apo E normally bind with high affinity to these receptors (38, 39) and are taken up rapidly by perfused livers of estradiol-treated rats (38). By contrast, such complexes of apo E from many patients with familial dysbetalipoproteinemia (phenotype E-2/2) bind poorly to LDL receptors (40) and are taken up slowly into the perfused livers (38). Since remnants of both chylomicrons and VLDL accumulate in plasma in familial dysbetalipoproteinemia, it seems likely that binding of apo E to both the chylomicron remnant receptor and the LDL receptor is impaired. However, the finding of grossly impaired binding of apo E to LDL receptors is not universal in patients with familial dysbetalipoproteinemia and the E-2/2 phenotype (40). In one patient whose apo E binds almost normally to LDL receptors, the second cysteine-arginine substitution occurs at a different site in apo E (residue 145) than in a

patient with apo E than binds poorly (residue 158) (22), yet both
patients have typical dysbetalipoproteinemia with comparable hyperlipoproteinemia and typical xanthomata.  A patient has also been discovered with typical dysbetalipoproteinemia whose plasma contains no
detectable apo E (41).  These observations strongly support the concept that apo E has a critical, rate-determining role in the uptake
of remnant particles by hepatic receptors.  Evidently, binding of
phospholipid complexes of apo E to LDL receptors in vitro does not
invariably reflect the dysfunctional property of the protein as it
exists in remnant particles.  Other evidence indicates that the disposition of apo E on lipoprotein particles critically influences the
uptake of these particles by the liver in vivo.  As described above,
addition of C apoproteins to triglyceride-rich lipoproteins can inhibit hepatic uptake.  In addition, it has been found that the hepatic uptake of rat HDL containing apo E is greatly influenced by the
manner of isolation of the particles.  Apo E in HDL obtained by ultracentrifugation (a procedure accompanied by loss of some apo E from
the particles) is rapidly taken up by the liver, whereas apo E in
HDL separated by gel chromatography is not (42).  Finally, uptake of
remnant particles by perfused rat livers occurs with considerably
higher efficiency than uptake of apo E in discoidal complexes (15,
38).  The determinants of these differences in the behavior of particles containing apo E are unknown, but could permit "fine tuning"
of the adsorptive endocytosis of apo E-containing particles by the
liver.

In humans with familial dysbetalipoproteinemia, the abnormal processing of VLDL remnants is associated with reduced levels of LDL and a
reduced rate of conversion of VLDL and intermediate density lipoproteins (IDL) to LDL (43).  This observation suggests that the process
of formation of LDL from VLDL may also involve binding of VLDL remnants to the hepatic LDL receptor.  Deckelbaum and associates have
proposed that exchanges of cholesteryl esters and triglycerides between VLDL and LDL could progressively reduce the amount of cholesteryl esters in LDL, that would otherwise contain excessive amounts
of this core lipid.  The surface of the LDL is concomitantly modified so that the acquired triglycerides can be removed by lipolysis
(44).  Ginsberg and associates have obtained evidence that the efficient conversion of VLDL remnants to LDL may involve the hepatic hep-
arin-releaseable lipase in monkeys (45).

Further research is required to delineate the steps normally involved
in the formation of LDL.  The cholesteryl esters of LDL in humans
(19) and rabbits (13) are derived from the action of lecithin-cholesterol acyltransferase.  The same is the case for much of the cholesteryl esters of VLDL in these species.  Therefore, the factors
that determine the efficiency with which VLDL-remnants and LDL are
taken up into the liver by adsorptive endocytosis are likely to be
important determinants of the extent to which these esters circulate
for sustained periods in the blood in association with atherogenic
lipoprotein particles.


Concluding Remarks


Apolipoprotein-mediated binding of lipoproteins to cell surface receptors is now recognized to have a key role in the terminal catabolism of chylomicrons and VLDL and may also be involved in the conversion of VLDL to LDL.  This brief review of recent advances in this

486

field highlights the importance of discoveries of inborn errors of metabolism affecting humans and experimental animals. Increasingly sophisticated methods of molecular and cell biology have made rapid exploitation of these discoveries possible, but the need to continue detailed evaluations of humans and animals with disorders of plasma lipoproteins is evident.

*Acknowledgments*  It is a pleasure to acknowledge the contributions of several past and present associates from San Francisco to the recent results reported (Y-s. Chao, L.S.S. Guo, R.L. Hamilton, D.A. Hardman, C.A. Hornick, A.L. Jones, J.P. Kane, L. Kotite, G. Renaud, J.P. Stoudemire, F.T. van't Hooft, and E.E.T. Windler; and of collaborators at the University of Texas in Dallas (D.W. Bilheimer, M.S. Brown, J.L. Goldstein, T. Kita and P.T. Kovanen). The personal research described was supported by a grant from the U.S. Public Health Service (HL-14237).

## References

1.  Malloy MJ, Kane JP (1979) Normotriglyceridemic abetalipoproteinemia: clinical and biochemical features of a new syndrome. Pediatr Res 11: 519
2.  Malloy MJ, Kane JP, Hardman DA, Hamilton RL, Dalal KB (1981) Normotriglyceridemic abetalipoproteinemia. Absence of the B-100 apolipoprotein. J Clin Invest 67: 1441-1450
3.  Kane JP, Hardman DA, Paulus HE (1980) Heterogeneity of apolipoprotein B: Isolation of a new species from human chylomicrons. Proc Natl Acad Sci USA 77: 2465-2469
4.  Krishnaiah KV, Walker LF, Borensztajn J, Schonfeld G, Getz GS (1980) Apolipoprotein B variant derived from rat intestine. Proc Natl Acad Sci USA 77: 3806-3810
5.  Hornick CA, Havel RJ, Kane JP  Unpublished observations.
6.  Frost PH, Havel RJ, Kane JP  Unpublished observations.
7.  Rudel LL  Personal communication.
8.  Elovson J, Huang YO, Baker N, Kannan R (1981) Apolipoprotein B is structurally and metabolically heterogeneous in the rat. Proc Natl Acad Sci USA 78: 157-161
9.  Wu A-L, Windmueller HG (1981) Variant forms of plasma apolipoprotein B. Hepatic and intestinal biosynthesis and heterogeneous metabolism in the rat. J Biol Chem 256: 3615-3618
10. Sparks CE, Marsh JP (1981) Catabolism of the B apolipoproteins of hepatic VLDL in the rat. Circulation 64: IV-102
11. van't Hooft FM, Hardman DA, Kane JP, Havel RJ (1982) Apolipoprotein B (B-48) of rat chylomicrons is not a precursor of the apolipoprotein of low density lipoproteins. Proc Natl Acad Sci USA 79: 179-182
12. Guo LSS, Hamilton RL, Ostwald R, Havel RJ (1982) Secretion of nascent lipoproteins and apolipoproteins by perfused livers of normal and cholesterol-fed guinea pigs. J Lipid Res 23: 543-555
13. Havel RJ, Kita T, Kotite L, Kane JP, Hamilton RL, Goldstein JL, Brown MS  Unpublished data.
14. Sparks CE, Marsh JB (1981) Metabolic heterogeneity of apolipoprotein B in the rat. J Lipid Res 22: 519-527
15. Windler E, Chao Y-s, Havel RJ (1980) Determinants of hepatic uptake of triglyceride-rich lipoproteins and their remnants in the rat. J Biol Chem 255: 5475-5480

16. Jones AL, Hornick CA, Renaud G, van't Hooft FM, Havel RJ
    Unpublished observations.
17. Faergeman O, Sata T, Kane JP, Havel RJ (1975) Metabolism of apo-
    protein B of plasma very low density lipoproteins in the rat.
    J Clin Invest 56: 1396-1403
18. Stoudemire JB, Renaud G, Havel RJ (1982) Hypercholesterolemia
    in fasting rabbits: reduction of receptor-dependent low density
    lipoprotein catabolism. Circulation  In press.
19. Havel RJ, Goldstein JL, Brown MS (1980) Lipoproteins and lipid
    transport. In: Bondy PK, Rosenberg LE (eds) Metabolic Control
    and Disease 8th ed, WB Saunders, Philadelphia, pp. 393-494
20. Utermann G, Jaeschke M, Menzel J (1975) Familial hyperlipopro-
    teinemia Type III: deficiency of a specific apolipoprotein (apo
    E-III) in the very low density lipoproteins. FEBS Lett 56: 352-
    355
21. Havel RJ (1982) Familial dysbetalipoproteinemia: new aspects of
    pathogenesis and diagnosis. In: Havel RJ (ed) Medical Clinics
    of North America on Lipid Disorders, WB Saunders, Philadelphia,
    66: 441-454
22. Mahley RW, Rall SC, Jr, Innerarity TL, Weisgraber KH  This volume.
23. Imaizumi K, Fainaru M, Havel RJ, Vigne J-L (1978) Origin and
    transport of the A-I and arginine-rich apolipoproteins in mesen-
    teric lymph of rats. J Lipid Res 19: 1038-1046
24. Imaizumi K, Fainaru M, Havel RJ (1978) Composition of proteins
    of mesenteric lymph chylomicrons in the rat and alterations pro-
    duced upon exposure of chylomicrons to blood serum and serum
    proteins. J Lipid Res 19: 712-722
25. Windler E, Chao Y-s, Havel RJ (1980) Regulation of the hepatic
    uptake of triglyceride-rich lipoproteins in the rat. J Biol Chem
    255: 8303-8307
26. Shelburne F, Hanks J, Meyers W, Quarfordt S (1980) Effect of
    apoproteins on hepatic uptake of triglyceride emulsions in the
    rat. J Clin Invest 65: 652-658
27. Breckenridge WC, Little JA, Steiner G, Chow A, Poapst M (1978)
    Hypertriglyceridemia associated with deficiency of apolipopro-
    tein C-II. N Engl J Med 298: 1265-1273
28. Sherrill BC, Innerarity TL, Mahley RW (1980) Rapid hepatic clear-
    ance of the canine lipoproteins containing only the E apoprotein
    by a high affinity receptor. Identity with the chylomicron rem-
    nant transport process. J Biol Chem 255: 1804-1807
29. Brown MS, Kovanen PT, Goldstein JL (1981) Regulation of plasma
    cholesterol by lipoprotein receptors. Science 212: 628-635
30. Tanzawa K, Shimada Y, Kuroda M, Tsujita Y, Arai M, Watanabe H
    (1980) WHHL-rabbit: a low density lipoprotein receptor-deficient
    animal model for familial hypercholesterolemia. FEBS Lett 118:
    81-84
31. Kita T, Brown MS, Watanabe Y, Goldstein JL (1981) Deficiency
    of low density lipoprotein receptors in liver and adrenal gland
    of the WHHL rabbit, an animal model of familial hypercholesterol-
    emia. Proc Natl Acad Sci USA 78:2268-2272
32. Attie AD, Pittman RC, Watanabe Y, Steinberg D (1981) Low densi-
    ty lipoprotein receptor deficiency in cultured hepatocytes of
    the WHHL rabbit. J Biol Chem 256: 9789-9792
33. Kita T, Goldstein JL, Brown MC, Watanabe Y, Hornick CA, Havel
    RJ (1982) Hepatic uptake of chylomicron remnants in WHHL rabbits:
    a mechanism genetically distinct from the low density lipopro-
    tein receptor. Proc Natl Acad Sci USA 79: 3623-3627
34. Mahley RW, Hui DY, Innerarity T, Weisgraber KH (1981) Two inde-
    pendent lipoprotein receptors on hepatic membranes of dog, swine,
    and man. Apo-B, E and apo E-Receptors. J Clin Invest 68: 1197-
    1206

488

35. Havel RJ, Kovanen PT, van't Hooft FM, Goldstein JL, Brown MS Unpublished data.
36. Borensztajn J, Getz GS, Padley RJ, Kotlar TJ (1982) The apoprotein B-independent hepatic uptake of chylomicron remnants. Biochem J 204: 609-612
37. Kita T, Brown MS, Bilheimer DW, Goldstein JL (1982) Delayed clearance of very low density and intermediate density lipoproteins with enhanced conversion to low density lipoprotein in WHHL rabbits. Proc Natl Acad Sci USA  In press.
38. Havel RJ, Chao Y-s, Windler EE, Kotite L, Guo LSS (1980) Isoprotein specificity in the hepatic uptake of apolipoprotein E and the pathogenesis of familial dysbetalipoproteinemia. Proc Natl Acad Sci USA 77: 4349-4353
39. Windler EET, Kovanen PT, Chao Y-s, Brown MS, Havel RJ, Goldstein JL (1980) The estradiol-stimulated lipoprotein receptor of rat liver: a binding site that mediates the uptake of rat lipoproteins containing apoproteins B and E. J Biol Chem 255: 10464-10471
40. Schneider WJ, Kovanen PT, Brown MS, Goldstein J, Utermann G, Weber W, Havel RJ, Kotite L, Kane JP, Innerarity TL, Mahley RW (1981) Familial dysbetalipoproteinemia. Abnormal binding of mutant apoprotein E to low density lipoprotein receptors of human fibroblasts and membranes from liver and adrenal of rats, rabbits, and cows. J Clin Invest 68: 1075-1085
41. Ghiselli G, Schaefer EJ, Gascon P, Brewer HB (1981) Type III hyperlipoproteinemia associated with apolipoprotein E deficiency. Science 214: 1239-1241
42. van't Hooft F, Havel RJ (1982) Metabolism of apolipoprotein E in plasma high density lipoproteins from normal and cholesterol-fed rats. J Biol Chem  In press.
43. Chait A, Albers JJ, Brunzell JD, et al. (1977) Type-III hyperlipoproteinemia ("Remnant removal disease"). Insight into the pathogenic mechanism. Lancet 1: 1176-1178
44. Deckelbaum RJ, Eisenberg S, Oschry Y, Butbul E, Sharon I, Olivecrona T (1982) Reversible modification of human plasma low density lipoproteins toward triglyceride-rich precursors. A mechanism for losing excess cholesterol esters. J Biol Chem 257: 6509-6517
45. Goldberg JJ, Le N-A, Paterniti JR, Jr, Ginsberg HM, Brown WV (1981) Effect of inhibition of hepatic triglyceride lipase on very low density lipoprotein apoprotein B catabolism in Macaca fasicularis.  Clin Res 29: 539A

# Apolipoprotein E and Cholesterol Metabolsim

R. W. Mahley, S. C. Rall, Jr., T. L. Innerarity, and K. H. Weisgraber

Our knowledge and understanding of the structure and function of apolipoprotein E (apoprotein E or apo-E) have progressed rapidly in the 9 years since it was first identified by the Shores (1). The role of apo-E in mediating the interaction between certain lipoproteins and the lipoprotein receptors on various cells has been well established. In this capacity, apo-E plays a part in mediating the cellular uptake of lipoproteins, the redistribution or degradation of the lipid and protein moieties, and the regulation of the plasma concentrations of specific lipoproteins. This may be particularly crucial in overall cholesterol homeostasis as it relates to the uptake of cholesterol-rich lipoproteins (e.g., chylomicron remnants, β-VLDL, and HDL-with apo-E) by the liver (for review see 2). This discussion will review some of the findings relating to apo-E metabolism, as well as the latest data concerning the structure and function of apo-E.

Apoprotein E is a constituent of several different lipoproteins. It is found in VLDL, chylomicrons, and chylomicron remnants. In addition, it occurs in a subclass of HDL referred to as HDL-with apo-E. (The major subclass of HDL lacks the E apoprotein and is referred to as typical HDL or HDL-without apo-E (2).) When isolated and purified from the lipoproteins of man and various animals, apo-E displays striking homology (Fig. 1). It is a 34,000 to 37,000 molecular weight glycoprotein characteristically containing from 10 to 12 mol% of the amino acid arginine — hence, the original designation of this protein as the arginine-rich apoprotein.

The different roles of apo-E in lipoprotein metabolism should be discussed in light of the following points: 1) that apo-E-enriched lipoproteins are induced by cholesterol feeding in a variety of animals, including man; 2) that apo-E mediates hepatic clearance of certain lipoproteins; and 3) that apo-E mediates the interaction of certain lipoproteins by the LDL (apo-B,E) receptor, a function it has in common with apo-B (for review see 2-4).

Let's consider the first point — that apo-E-enriched lipoproteins are induced by cholesterol feeding in a variety of animals. In studies of rabbits, dogs,

490

swine, rats, monkeys, and man, apo-E has been shown to become a major protein constituent of two different lipoproteins after cholesterol feeding. The two lipoproteins are β-VLDL and HDL$_c$. The β-VLDL are cholesteryl ester-rich lipoproteins that appear in the d < 1.006 ultracentrifugal fraction. They have β-electrophoretic mobility, unlike the pre-β–migrating VLDL that normally are present in this fraction (2-4). The HDL$_c$ are also cholesteryl ester-rich lipoproteins. They are formed in the plasma or extracellular space from typical HDL that have acquired apo-E and become enriched in cholesterol (Fig. 2). The typical HDL can accept cholesterol from peripheral cells (e.g., fibroblasts, smooth muscle cells, and macrophages), as described in various studies (5-7). It appears that the cholesterol is esterified by LCAT, resulting in the production of the cholesteryl ester-rich HDL$_c$.

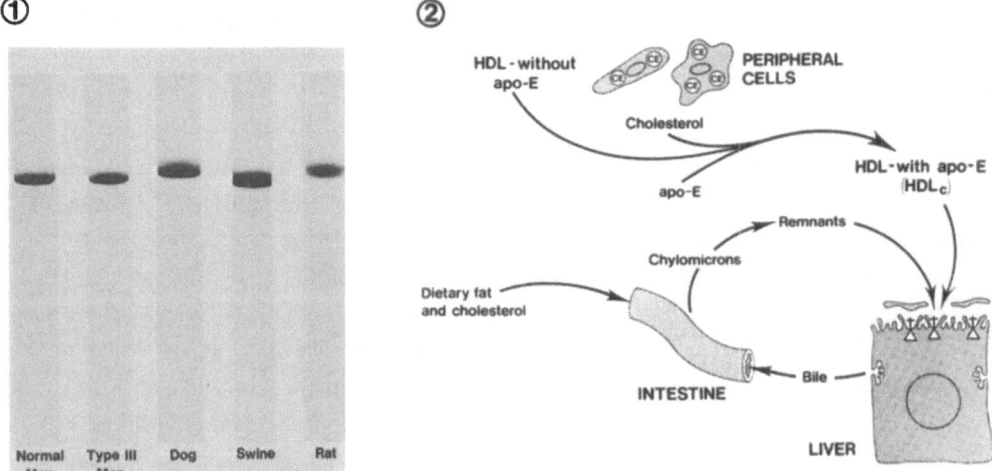

Fig. 1. Comparison of the electrophoretic mobility (11% SDS gels) of apoprotein E isolated from the various species

Fig. 2. Diagram illustrating the conversion of HDL-without apo-E (typical HDL) to HDL-with apo-E (HDL$_c$) as they acquire cholesterol from peripheral cells. The HDL-with apo-E are recognized by hepatic lipoprotein receptors. Chylomicron remnants are cleared from the plasma by the liver via the same receptor-mediated process responsible for HDL$_c$ uptake. (Reproduced with permission from Ref. 2.)

One of the functions of HDL$_c$ may be to transport cholesterol from peripheral tissues to the liver for excretion. The hepatic recognition of the HDL$_c$ would be mediated by apo-E (for review see 2-4). The feasibility of this scheme is supported by the recent findings of Basu et al. (8), who demonstrated that cholesterol-loaded macrophages can release large quantities of cholesterol, and that they can also synthesize and secrete large quantities of apo-E.

The use of HDL$_c$ in both <u>in vivo</u> turnover studies and <u>in vitro</u> liver perfusion studies has helped to establish the importance of apo-E in mediating hepatic clearance of plasma lipoproteins (2). In these studies, HDL$_c$ were rapidly and efficiently cleared from the plasma by the liver via a receptor-mediated uptake process (9,10). Furthermore, the hepatic uptake process described for HDL$_c$ appears to be identical to the high affinity process responsible for chylomicron remnant clearance by the liver (11). Consequently, it is now generally agreed that apo-E is one of the prime determinants in mediating chylomicron remnant uptake by the liver (for review see 2,9,12-14).

Like apoprotein B, apo-E mediates the interaction between certain lipoproteins and the apo-B,E receptors of various cells. The apo-B,E receptor interacts not only with LDL containing apo-B, but also with HDL containing apo-E (2,3,15,16). It has been shown that LDL and HDL-with apo-E interact with the same receptor sites, and that both these apo-B- and apo-E-containing lipoproteins have similar roles in regulating intracellular cholesterol metabolism.

The importance of, and similarity between, apo-B and apo-E were established by studies in which specific amino acid residues of these apoproteins were chemically modified; such alterations resulted in the loss of receptor binding activity (9,17,18). A limited number of arginine and lysine residues of lipoproteins containing apo-B and apo-E were subjected to selective chemical modification (Fig. 3). When arginine residues were modified by cyclohexanedione, receptor binding activity was blocked (17). Likewise, when lysine residues were altered by reductive methylation or other modification procedures, the lipoproteins were incapable of binding (18). The importance of these residues in mediating apoprotein-receptor interaction will be discussed later.

Recently, our attention has focused on the detailed structure of the apo-E in order to define more precisely the nature of its interaction with receptors. Before discussing its structure, however, we need to consider certain general characteristics of apo-E. Human apoprotein E occurs as three major forms, which can be separated and visualized by isoelectric focusing on acrylamide gels (Fig. 4) (19,20). These include the E2, E3, and E4 isoforms. An important genetic disease, Type III hyperlipoproteinemia, has helped to unravel the story concerning these isoforms (21). Utermann et al. (22,23) were the first to recognize that the Type III disorder is associated with an abnormality of the E isoforms.

Subjects with this disease possess only the E2 isoform. Recently, Zannis and Breslow analyzed the distribution of the various E isoforms in family studies and proposed a genetic model (24,25). Their model suggests that the synthesis of apo-E is under the control of three independent alleles located at a single gene locus, and that each allele codes for a major isoform (the E2, E3, or E4). Consequently, the model predicts the existence of three homozygous and three heterozygous phenotypes. The minor isoforms arise as a result of post-translational glycosylation of the major isoforms. The E2, E3, and E4 isoforms differ from each other by a single charge (Fig. 4).

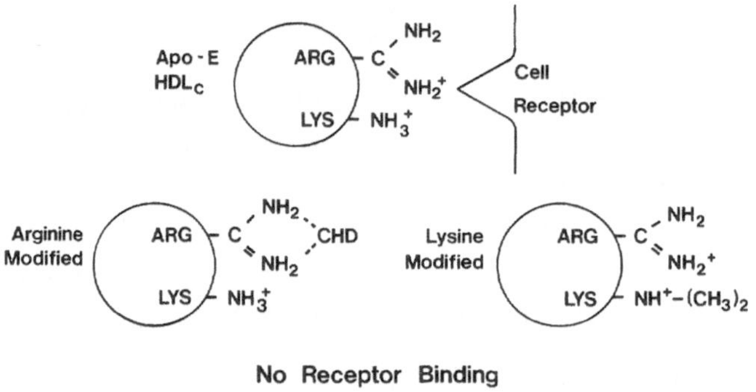

No Receptor Binding

Fig. 3. Schematic diagram illustrating the role of lysine and arginine residues in mediating the interaction of apo-E $HDL_c$ with lipoprotein receptors. Their role may be either direct or indirect. Selective chemical modification of either the lysine or arginine residues abolishes the binding activity of lipoproteins containing apo-E or apo-B

Since the genetic model predicts that structural differences would exist among the major isoforms, we undertook a sequence analysis of apo-E from subjects homozygous for the E2, E3, and E4 isoforms. As shown in Fig. 5, apo-E2 is a single polypeptide chain of 299 amino acids with a molecular weight of 34,200 (26). Two residues of cysteine were found in E2, at positions 112 (site A) and 158 (site B). The sequence of apo-E3 was identical in every respect to E2, except that at position 158 (site B) there was a residue of arginine instead of cysteine. Apoprotein E4 contained no cysteine and had arginine at both residues 112 and 158. The sites at which the cysteine/arginine interchanges occurred are listed in Fig. 4. The relative charge differences among the three major isoforms were explained by single amino acid substitutions involving the cysteine/arginine interchanges.

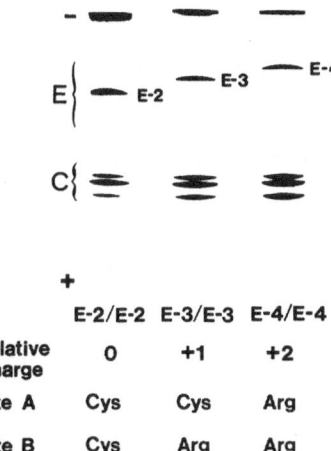

|  | E-2/E-2 | E-3/E-3 | E-4/E-4 |
|---|---|---|---|
| Relative Charge | 0 | +1 | +2 |
| Site A | Cys | Cys | Arg |
| Site B | Cys | Arg | Arg |

Fig. 4. Isoelectric focusing gels of VLDL from subjects homozygous for E2, E3, and E4. The differences in the sequence among these proteins at site A (residue 112) and site B (residue 158) are summarized. The cysteine/arginine interchanges explain the known charge differences

It was of interest to investigate the effect of these amino acid substitutions on the known function of apo-E — its ability to interact with lipoprotein receptors. To compare the receptor activity, the E2, E3, and E4 isoforms were separately recombined with phospholipid and tested for their ability to compete with LDL for binding to the apo-B,E receptors on fibroblasts. As shown in Fig. 6, apo-E3 and apo-E4 competed strongly — and in a similar manner — with iodinated LDL for the fibroblast receptor (20). The equal binding activity of E3 and E4 indicated that the arginine/cysteine interchange at site A was not important in modulating the binding activity of these isoforms; recall that E3 possessed a cysteine residue at site A (residue 112), whereas E4 had an arginine at this site. However, apo-E2 from a Type III hyperlipoproteinemic subject (D.R.) competed poorly with LDL for the receptor binding, suggesting that the amino acid substitution of cysteine for arginine at site B was of critical importance; recall that E3 and E4 both had arginine at site B (residue 158). We postulated that a positive charge at site B (residue 158) may be necessary for the binding of apo-E to the apo-B,E receptor. Therefore, we undertook studies to convert the cysteine residue at site B in E2 to a positively charged amino acid, using the reagent cysteamine. Cysteamine reacts with cysteine, converting the cysteine to a lysine analogue having a positive charge.

```
                           1
           H₂N-Lys-Val-Glu-Gln-Ala-Val-Glu-Thr-Glu-Pro-Glu-Pro-Glu
                                                               |
                                                              Leu
                                            20
           Ala-Leu-Glu-Trp-Arg-Gln-Gly-Ser-Gln-Trp-Glu-Thr-Gln-Gln-Arg
           |
           Leu                                 40
           Gly-Arg-Phe-Trp-Asp-Tyr-Leu-Arg-Trp-Val-Gln-Thr-Leu-Ser-Glu
                                                                     |
                       60                                           Gln
           Arg-Leu-Glu-Gln-Thr-Val-Gln-Ser-Ser-Leu-Leu-Glu-Glu-Gln-Val
           |
           Ala
           Leu-Met-Asp-Glu-Thr-Met-Lys-Glu-Leu-Lys-Ala-Tyr-Lys-Ser-Glu
                                                           80        |
                                                                    Leu
           Leu-Arg-Ala-Arg-Thr-Glu-Glu-Ala-Val-Pro-Thr-Leu-Gln-Glu-Glu
           |
           Ser                  100
           Lys-Glu-Leu-Gln-Ala-Ala-Gln-Ala-Arg-Leu-Gly-Ala-Asp-Met-Glu
                         120                                        |
                                                                   Asp
           Met-Ala-Gln-Val-Glu-Gly-Arg-Tyr-Gln-Val-Leu-Arg-Gly-Cys-Val
           |
           Leu                                                    140
           Gly-Gln-Ser-Thr-Glu-Glu-Leu-Arg-Val-Arg-Leu-Ala-Ser-His-Leu
                                                                     |
                                                                    Arg
           Lys-Gln-Leu-Asp-Asp-Ala-Asp-Arg-Leu-Leu-Arg-Lys-Arg-Leu-Lys
           |
           Cys 160
           Leu-Ala-Val-Tyr-Gln-Ala-Gly-Ala-Arg-Glu-Gly-Ala-Glu-Arg-Gly
                             180                                    |
                                                                   Leu
           Arg-Gly-Gln-Glu-Val-Leu-Pro-Gly-Leu-Arg-Glu-Arg-Ile-Ala-Ser
           |
           Val                        200
           Arg-Ala-Ala-Thr-Val-Gly-Ser-Leu-Ala-Gly-Gln-Pro-Leu-Gln-Glu
                   220                                              |
                                                                   Arg
           Met-Glu-Glu-Met-Arg-Ala-Arg-Leu-Arg-Glu-Gly-Trp-Ala-Gln-Ala
           |
           Gly
           Ser-Arg-Thr-Arg-Asp-Arg-Leu-Asp-Glu-Val-Lys-Glu-Gln-Val-Ala
                                                               240  |
                                                                   Glu
           Gln-Leu-Arg-Ile-Gln-Gln-Ala-Gln-Glu-Glu-Leu-Lys-Ala-Arg-Val
           |
           Ala              260
           Glu-Ala-Phe-Gln-Ala-Arg-Leu-Lys-Ser-Trp-Phe-Glu-Pro-Leu-Val
                         280                                        |
                                                                   Glu
           Ala-Gln-Val-Lys-Glu-Val-Leu-Gly-Ala-Trp-Gln-Arg-Gln-Met-Asp
           |
           Ala                                               299
           Val-Gly-Thr-Ser-Ala-Ala-Pro-Val-Pro-Ser-Asp-Asn-His-COOH
```

Fig. 5.  Amino acid sequence of apo-E2 from subject D.R.  See Ref. 26 for details of the structure

Cysteamine treatment of apo-E3 had no effect on its binding activity (Fig. 7) (20).  However, cysteamine treatment of apo-E2 resulted in a considerable increase in binding activity.  Although full activity was not established in the apo-E2 by cysteamine treatment, the experiment nonetheless demonstrated the importance of having a positive charge at site B.

Up to this point in our studies, we had demonstrated that E2, E3, and E4 differed at two sites — site A (residue 112) and site B (residue 158).  The calculated gene frequency from the population studies indicated that E3 homozygosity was the most common phenotype, and that apo-E3 was most likely the parent form of apoprotein E.  Therefore, apo-E2 differed from apo-E3 by a single amino acid substitution at site B, with apo-E2 having a cysteine residue substituted for an arginine. On the other hand, apo-E4 differed from apo-E3 at site A. Apoprotein E4 contained arginine at this site, whereas apo-E3 had a cysteine residue. Thus, the E2 and E4 isoforms could have arisen as a result of a point mutation involving a single nucleotide change in the gene for E3.

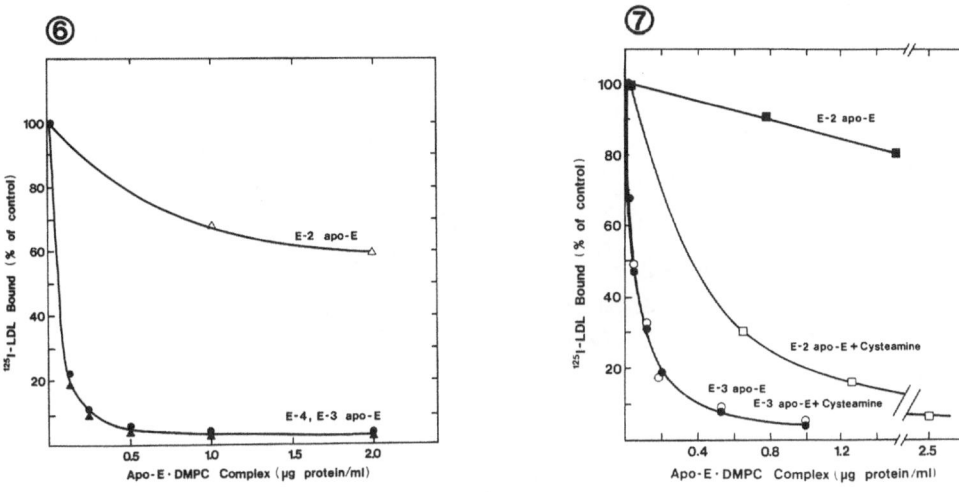

Fig. 6. Ability of apo-E·DMPC complexes from subjects homozygous for E2 (Δ; subject D.R.), E3 (▲), and E4 (●) to compete with human [125]I-LDL for binding at 4°C to normal human fibroblasts. (Reproduced with permission from Ref. 20.)

Fig. 7. Comparison of the ability of control (untreated) and cysteamine-modi-fied apo-E·DMPC complexes to compete with [125]I-LDL for binding to normal human fibroblasts. Untreated E2 apo-E·DMPC (■); cysteamine-treated E2 apo-E·DMPC (□); untreated E3 apo-E·DMPC (●); cysteamine-treated E3 apo-E·DMPC (○). (Reproduced with permission from Ref. 20.)

The substitution at site B in E2 has been shown to be critical for binding. The results suggested that a crucial region of the apo-E molecule responsible for receptor binding should be in the region of residue 158. To pursue this possi-bility, the apo-E from an E3 homozygote was subjected to cyanogen bromide cleavage, and each fragment was tested for binding activity. We found that the active fragment, composed of 93 amino acid residues, was located near the middle of the sequence (27). This fragment included residue 158. Of special interest, as shown in Fig. 8, was a portion of the active fragment of apo-E consisting of approximately 20 amino acids that would be predicted to form an α-helix. This region was enriched in lysine and arginine residues. When the lysine or arginine residues were chemically modified, in the same manner we had previously modified the whole apo-E, the binding activity was abolished. (Note that site B may be very close structurally to this cluster of arginine and lysine residues.) This region of the apo-E molecule has been extensively studied and its role in receptor binding elucidated (27).

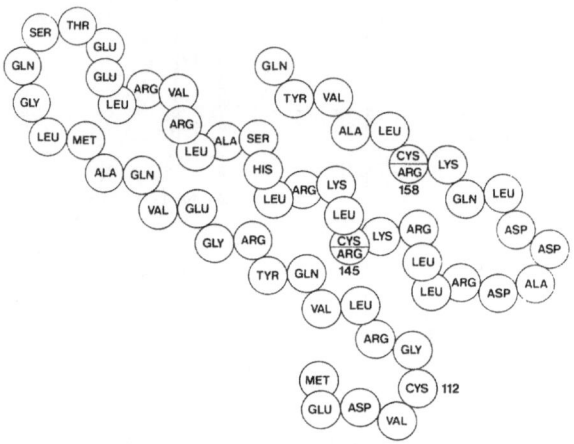

**Fig. 8.** A portion of the apo-E sequence from the region of the molecule determined to be involved in receptor binding. Two sites of substitution known to effect binding are at residues 145 (W.M. apo-E2) and 158 (D.R. apo-E2)

To gain additional insight into the structure-function relationships of apo-E, we recently extended our analysis to other individuals with Type III hyperlipoproteinemia. Results from a collaborative study showed a marked difference in the binding activities of apo-E2 from various Type III subjects (28). In a further study, the apo-E of three of these subjects (D.R., J.T., and W.M.) was analyzed in detail — both with respect to binding activity and amino acid sequence (29). All three subjects were classic Type III hypercholesterolemic patients; all were homozygous for E2; and all had two cysteine residues per mole of E2. The apo-E from D.R., who served as the source of apo-E for the sequence and binding studies cited above, was markedly defective, whereas W.M. apo-E demonstrated considerable binding activity (but did not reach a normal level in our studies) (29).

We asked ourselves if these differences in binding activity could be explained by an analysis of the structure of the protein. To determine this, a partial sequence analysis of the apo-E from subjects J.T. and W.M was performed (29). We found that the apo-E from W.M. had two cysteine residues; however, one of the cysteines appeared at a new site (site C, residue 145). Residue 145 in both normal apo-E3 and D.R. apo-E was arginine. Therefore, a new allele ($\epsilon$2*) for apo-E, also involving a cysteine/arginine interchange, had been observed. Furthermore, at site B there was a residue of arginine, as observed for this site in apo-E3. We concluded that the apo-E2 of W.M. and D.R. differed from one another at two sites — B and C. The substitution of cysteine for arginine in the apo-E2 of W.M. occurred in the same region of the molecule we identified as significant for the purpose of binding to the apo-B,E receptor.

The apo-E of J.T. was also revealing. This subject was found to be genotypically heterozygous, and had one allele that was identical to that of D.R. ($\epsilon$2) and one that was identical to that of W.M ($\epsilon$2*) (29). It is significant that the binding activity of J.T. apo-E was intermediate between that of D.R. and W.M. A summary of the structural relationships among these forms of apo-E is depicted in Fig. 9.

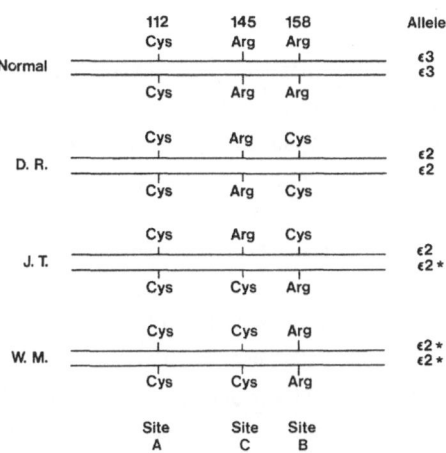

<u>Fig. 9.</u> Schematic summary of the apo-E2 sequence and allelic (genotypic) relationships among subjects D.R., J.T., and W.M. The normal apo-E3 is given for comparison. The numbers 112, 145, and 158, corresponding to sites A, C, and B, respectively, are residue numbers in the apo-E polypeptide chain. (Reproduced with permission from Ref. 29.)

Our studies indicate that we must update our information on apo-E alleles. There are three sites of substitution that must be considered (residues 112,

145, and 158), and four alleles ($\epsilon$4, $\epsilon$3, $\epsilon$2, and $\epsilon$2$^*$) rather than three. (It is predictable that others will be found.) Apoprotein E4 is characterized by an absence of cysteine, whereas E3 contains one residue of cysteine. Both E2 and E2$^*$ possess two residues of cysteine per mole; however, they occur at different sites. Despite the fact that subjects D.R. and W.M. were homozygous for E2, as determined by isoelectric focusing, the nature of their defects was different. Furthermore, the severity of the abnormality in receptor binding activity was different, with E2 being more defective than E2$^*$ (29).

However, Type III hyperlipoproteinemia has an added degree of complexity. Many subjects homozygous for E2 are hypolipidemic or normolipidemic, although their plasma usually contains $\beta$-VLDL. The questions are: What form of apo-E2 do these individuals have? Where are the cysteine residues? Is the receptor binding activity normal or abnormal? The apo-E from a 40-year-old male, who had the E2 phenotype but was normolipidemic (plasma cholesterol, 180 mg/dl), was extensively studied (30). Partial sequence analysis revealed that his E2 was identical to that of D.R. — the cysteine residues were at site A (residue 112) and B (residue 158). Furthermore, the receptor binding activity of his apo-E was markedly defective and was identical to that of D.R.'s apo-E.

These results indicate that the nature of a defect or abnormality in protein structure can predict in vitro receptor binding activity, shedding light on the region of the apo-E molecule responsible for binding activity. However, in considering the clinical expression of the disease, other factors that play upon or modulate the effects of the E2 protein defect on lipoprotein metabolism are involved. The nature of these other factors, however, is open to speculation.

The role of apo-E in mediating lipoprotein interaction with specific receptors has been established. Through the use of selective chemical modification of specific amino acid residues of lipoproteins, we have gained insight into the importance of the lysine and arginine residues in this process. This insight has been expanded by structure-function studies of mutant forms of apo-E. These studies have revealed important information concerning the genetic heterogeneity of the apo-E isoforms, focusing attention on the importance of a specific region of apo-E in the binding process.

## References

1. Shore VG, Shore B (1973) Heterogeneity of human plasma very low density lipoproteins. Separation of species differing in protein components. Biochemistry 12: 502-507

2. Mahley RW (1982) Atherogenic hyperlipoproteinemia: The cellular and molecular biology of plasma lipoproteins altered by dietary fat and cholesterol. In: Havel RJ (ed) Medical Clinics of North America: Lipid Disorders. WB Saunders, Philadelphia, PA, pp 375-402

3. Mahley RW (1978) Alterations in plasma lipoproteins induced by cholesterol feeding in animals including man. In: Dietschy JM, Gotto AM Jr, Ontko JA (eds) Disturbances in Lipid and Lipoprotein Metabolism. American Physiological Society, Bethesda, MD, pp 181-197

4. Mahley RW (1981) Cellular and molecular biology of lipoprotein metabolism in atherosclerosis. Diabetes 30 (Suppl 2): 60-65

5. Ho YK, Brown MS, Goldstein JL (1980) Hydrolysis and excretion of cytoplasmic cholesteryl esters by macrophages: Stimulation by high density lipoprotein and other agents. J Lipid Res 21: 391-398

6. Stein Y, Glangeaud MC, Fainaru M, Stein O (1975) The removal of cholesterol from aortic smooth muscle cells in culture and Landschutz ascites cells by fractions of human high-density apolipoproteins. Biochim Biophys Acta 380: 106-118

7. Bates SR, Rothblat GH (1974) Regulation of cellular sterol flux and synthesis by human serum lipoproteins. Biochim Biophys Acta 360: 38-55

8. Basu KS, Brown MS, Ho YK, Havel RJ, Goldstein JL (1981) Mouse macrophages synthesize and secrete apoprotein resembling apolipoprotein E. Proc Natl Acad Sci USA 78: 7545-7549

9. Mahley RW, Innerarity TL, Weisgraber KH (1980) Alterations in metabolic activity of plasma lipoproteins following selective chemical modifications of the apoproteins. Ann NY Acad Sci 348: 265-277

10. Mahley RW, Innerarity TL, Weisgraber KH, Oh SY (1979) Altered metabolism (in vivo and in vitro) of plasma lipoproteins after selective chemical modification of lysine residues of the apoproteins. J Clin Invest 64: 743-750

11. Sherrill BC, Innerarity TL, Mahley RW (1980) Rapid hepatic clearance of the canine lipoproteins containing only the E apoprotein by a high affinity receptor. Identity with the chylomicron remnant transport process. J Biol Chem 255: 1804-1807

12. Havel RJ (1980) Lipoprotein bioysnthesis and metabolism. Ann NY Acad Sci 348: 16-29

13. Brown MS, Kovanen PT, Goldstein JL (1981) Regulation of plasma by lipoprotein receptors. Science 212: 628-635

14. Attie AD, Pittman RC, Steinberg D (1982) Hepatic catabolism of low density lipoprotein mechanisms and metabolic consequences. Hepatology 2: 269-281

15. Innerarity TL, Mahley RW (1978) Enhanced binding by cultured human fibroblasts of apo-E-containing lipoproteins as compared with low density lipoproteins. Biochemistry 17: 1440-1447

16. Pitas RE, Innerarity TL, Arnold KS, Mahley RW (1979) Rate and equilibrium constants for binding of apo-E HDL$_c$ (a cholesterol-induced lipoprotein) and low density lipoproteins to human fibroblasts: Evidence for multiple receptor binding of apo-E HDL$_c$. Proc Natl Acad Sci USA 76: 2311-2315

17. Mahley RW, Innerarity TL, Pitas RE, Weisgraber KH, Brown JH, Gross E (1977) Inhibition of lipoprotein binding to cell surface receptors of fibroblasts following selective modification of arginyl residues in arginine-rich and B apoproteins. J Biol Chem 252: 7279-7287

18. Weisgraber KH, Innerarity TL, Mahley RW (1978) Role of the lysine residues of plasma lipoproteins in high affinity binding to cell surface receptors on human fibroblasts. J Biol Chem 253: 9053-9062

19. Weisgraber KH, Rall SC Jr, Mahley RW (1981) Human E apoprotein heterogeneity: Cysteine-arginine interchanges in the amino acid sequence of the apo-E isoforms. J Biol Chem 256: 9077-9083

20. Weisgraber KH, Innerarity TL, Mahley RW (1982) Abnormal lipoprotein receptor-binding activity of the human E apoprotein due to cysteine-arginine interchange at a single site. J Biol Chem 257: 2518-2521

21. Fredrickson DS, Goldstein JL, Brown MS (1978) The familial hyperlipoproteinemias. In: Stanbury JB, Wyngaarden JB, Fredrickson DS (eds) The Metabolic Basis of Inherited Disease, 4th edition. McGraw-Hill, New York, NY, pp 604-655

22. Utermann G, Jaeschke M, Menzel J (1975) Familial hyperlipoproteinemia Type III: Deficiency of a specific apolipoprotein (apo E-III) in the very-low-density lipoproteins. FEBS Lett 56: 352-355

23. Utermann G, Langenbeck U, Beisiegel U, Weber W (1980) Genetics of the apolipoprotein E system in man. Am J Hum Genet 32: 339-347

24. Zannis VI, Breslow JL (1980) Characterization of a unique human apolipoprotein E variant associated with Type III hyperlipoproteinemia. J Biol Chem 255: 1759-1762

25. Zannis VI, Breslow JL (1981) Human very low density lipoprotein apolipoprotein E isoprotein polymorphism is explained by genetic variation and post-translational modification. Biochemistry 20: 1033-1041

26. Rall SC Jr, Weisgraber KH, Mahley RW (1982) Human apolipoprotein E: The complete amino acid sequence. J Biol Chem 257: 4171-4178

27. Innerarity TL, Friedlander EJ, Rall SC Jr, Weisgraber KH, Mahley RW (1982) Identification of the region of apolipoprotein E responsible for lipoprotein receptor binding. Circulation: In press

28. Schneider WJ, Kovanen PT, Brown MS, Goldstein JL, Utermann G, Weber W, Havel RJ, Kotite L, Kane JP, Innerarity TL, Mahley RW (1981) Familial dysbeta-lipoproteinemia: Abnormal binding of mutant apoprotein E to low density lipoprotein receptors of human fibroblasts and membranes from liver and adrenal of rats, rabbits, and cows. J Clin Invest 68: 1075-1085

29. Rall SC Jr, Weisgraber KH, Innerarity TL, Mahley RW (1982) Structural basis for receptor-binding heterogeneity of apolipoprotein E from Type III hyperlipoproteinemic subjects. Proc Natl Acad Sci USA: In press

30. Rall SC Jr, Weisgraber KH, Innerarity TL, Mahley RW, Assmann G (1982) Identical structural and receptor binding defects in apolipoprotein E2 from hypo-, normo-, and hypercholesterolemic subjects. Circulation: In press

# Selective Removal of Plasma Low-Density Lipoproteins by Combined Extracorporeal Plasma Separation-Immunoadsorption

W. Stoffel, C. Bode, H. Borberg, M. Tauchert, K. Oette, and M. Fuchs**

Familial hypercholesterolemia (Type IIa - hyperlipoproteinemia) is being observed in its hetero- and less frequent in its homozygous form. The disease is characterized by high serum cholesterol concentrations in the range between 400 and up to 1000 mg/dl serum.

The genetic defect has been established: a defect LDL-receptor prohibits the receptor mediated uptake of LDL and thereby the regulation of cholesterol synthesis at the HMG-CoA-reductase level[1]. This abnormal cholesterol metabolism leads to the deposition of cholesterol and its esters, leads in the skin to the formation of xanthelasm, around tendon, and joints as xanthomata and in the arterial wall to atherosclerotic plaques, which in many cases reduces the individual's life span considerable; in homozygous patients below 20 years[2]. Sniderman reported in 1980 that apo B concentrations correlate much better with coronary infarction than total cholesterol[3].

It is not surprising that surgical techniques such as the portocaval shunt and conservative treatments aim at lowering the deleterious influence of persisting high LDL-serum concentrations. Among the presently used treatments plasmapheresis since 1975 is the most common technique[4]. Although plasmapheresis and also Heparin-Sepharose affinity absorption as intermittent method do lower serum cholesterol levels and do lead to the deprivation of cholesterol pools as reported by Thompson[4], both methods, but particularly plasmapheresis remove all plasma components, good or bad, the immunoglobulin and HDL in addition to LDL. Albumin restores the colloidosmotic pressure but cannot substitute for the other plasma components removed. Hypochromic anemia after prolonged plasmapheresis has been reported[5]. Synthetic plasma substitution induces a secondary hypercholesterolemia. Plasma exchange on the other hand carries the enigma of hepatitis infection. But beyond these arguments the costs of plasmapheresis exchange are a serious drawback in the lifetime treatment of the type IIa patients.

The Heparin-Sepharose affinity adsorption reported by Lupien et al.[6] lowers LDL levels by no more than 30 % but this adsorbens also eliminates components of the complement and the clotting system.

We have elaborated recently a very specific, rapid and efficient method for the removal of apo B-containing serum lipoproteins, LDL and VLDL, first in experiments in vitro and then in animal experi-

ments[7]. After careful studies and the approval by the ethic commis-
sion of our University this new approach was adapted to the treatment
of homo- and heterozygous patients with heriditary (familial)hyper-
cholesterolemia[8].

The principle of the method is the following: Monospecific human LDL-
antiserum was raised for mass-production in sheep, immunized with
human serum LDL, homogenous by the common biochemical (density, pro-
tein- and lipid composition, electron microscopy) and immunological
criteria (single precipitation line in double immunodiffusion and
immunoelectrophoresis). Monospecific LDL-antibodies were isolated by
a single chromatographic step: antiserum was poured over a LDL-Sepha-
rose CL-4B column to which LDL was covalently linked via cyanogen
bromide activated Sepharose. The monospecific antibodies were likewise coupled in a multiattachment to cyanogen bromide activated Sepharose CL-4B or CL-6B. Two columns with a volume of 400 ml each were
prepared and dedicated to each of the six patients presently being
treated.

Whereas the pig-experiment required a shunt-operation between the ca-
rotis artery and the jugular vein to obtain an effective blood flow,
the blood flow in the extracorporeal circulation of the patient was
between the cubital veins of both arms. The patient's blood, with
heparin and citrate as anticoagulants, enters at a rate of 60 to 80
ml/min the blood cell separator. The plasma, free of any corpuscular
elements, passes over the anti-LDL-Sepharose bed and recombines, now
free from LDL and VLDL, with the blood concentrate to enter the cubital vein of the opposite arm. Plasma flow-rate is around 30-40 ml.
The capacity of the anti-LDL-column of 400 ml with a void volume of
250-300 ml is  around 4-6 g LDL-cholesterol. The saturation of the
immunoadsorbent can be monitored by carotenes (carrot juice), fed to
the patient the evening before the treatment. The two affinity columns
are successively used. While one column serves as immunoadsorbent,
the LDL-loaded column is being desorbed with 0.2M glycine pH 2.8 and
neutralized again for subsequent use. With this arrangement every
LDL-cholesterol level can be adjusted in the patient's blood.

In the meantime the complete procedure of immunoadsorption and
column restauration has been automatized.

In the following figures the results of our observations and experiences are summarized:

Figure 1 a,b demonstrate the kinetics of the LDL-removal during the
immunoadsorption from the blood of a heterozygous child, 14 years of
age. Within  2-3 hours the total cholesterol concentration is lowered
to about 100 mg/dl by the extensive removal of LDL. On the average
the patient's total plasma passes twice to three times over the im-
munoadsorbens-bed during the time-course of the treatment. About 10-
15 g LDL are bound to the immunoadsorbent.

Provided a proper treatment of the anti-LDL-Sepharose ·columns (steri-
lity, acid medium only for the short LDL-desorption interval), we
have used our columns for more than 18 months without any loss of
the capacity.

The immediate and long term effects of the immunoadsorption are demonstrated in fig. 2 and table 1 summarizes the clinical data.

504

Figure 1a.

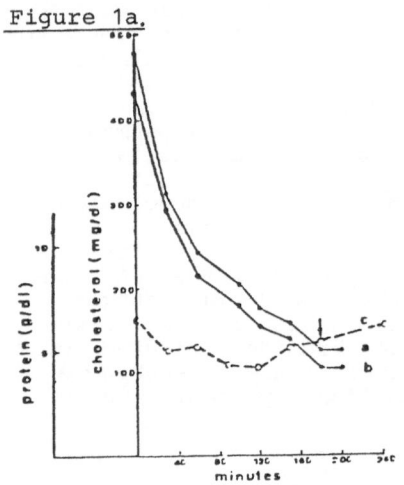

Time-course of changes of
a = total cholesterol,
b = LDL + VLDL and
c = plasma protein in plasma line before entering
immunoadsorption column

Figure 1b.

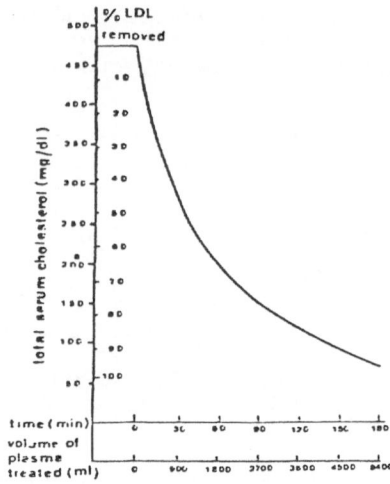

Absolute concentration change
and percentage removal of LDL-
cholesterol by immunoadsorbent
column.
Plasma flow-rate: 30 ml/min

Table 1.

CLINICAL DATA AND RESULTS

| | | Total plasma cholesterol levels | | | | | Removed‡ | | |
|---|---|---|---|---|---|---|---|---|---|
| Patient | Steady state* (mg/dl) | Before treat-ment† (mg/dl) | After treat-ment (mg/dl) | Mean between treat-ments (mg/dl) | Interval between treat-ments (weeks) | LDL (g) | Choles-terol (g) | Re-moved choles-terol (%)¶ |
| 1 | 260± 30 | 260 | 115 | 203 | 3 | 9 | 4·4 | 56 |
| | | 290 | 130 | 176 | 2 | 9·5 | 4·8 | 55 |
| | | 221 | 99 | 169 | 3 | 7·5 | 3·6 | 55 |
| | | 236 | 108 | | | 7·5 | 3·6 | 55 |
| 2 | 470± 15 | 472 | 112 | 223 | 2 | 14 | 7·0 | 76 |
| | | 334 | 153 | 283 | 4 | 11 | 5·3 | 54 |
| | | 412 | 180 | 285 | 3 | 15 | 7·3 | 56 |
| | | 390 | 138 | 247 | 1 | 11 | 5·3 | 65 |
| | | 355 | 113 | 241 | 2 | 11·5 | 5·7 | 68 |
| | | 368 | 146 | 251 | 2 | 10 | 5·0 | 60 |
| | | 356 | 133 | 251 | 2 | 12 | 6·3 | 63 |
| | | 369 | 158 | 241 | 2 | 10 | 4·7 | 57 |
| | | 324 | 119 | 207 | 1 | 11 | 5·4 | 63 |
| | | 294 | 95 | 197 | 1 | 9 | 4·3 | 68 |
| | | 296 | 112 | 278 | 5 | 7·5 | 3·7 | 62 |
| | | 443 | 164 | | | 13 | 6·4 | 63 |
| 3 | 500± 20 | 448 | 171 | 228 | 0·5 | 11 | 5·3 | 62 |
| | | 285 | 88 | 183 | ? | 8 | 3·9 | 69 |
| | | 276 | 103 | 150 | 0·5 | 10 | 4·9 | 63 |
| | | 196 | 53 | | | 6 | 3·0 | 74 |

Figure 2.

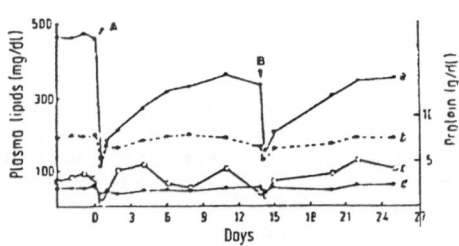

Immediate and longer term effects
of extracorporeal removal of LDL.
A and B = consecutive treatments.
a = total cholesterol, b = total
protein, c = triglycerides,
d = HDL-cholesterol

*Lowest level under medical ma-
nagement. †Immediately before
extracorporeal removal of LDL.
‡LDL and cholesterol concentrations recovered from the columns
upon regeneration of the immunoadsorbent. ¶Removed cholesterol as a percentage of total
cholesterol before treatment.

The most unexpected observations of extensive and careful studies,
first in pig and then in man, were

1) that we did not observe any "bleeding" of the immunoadsorbent
   column, which would lead to an immune answer by the patient; no
   patient ever showed anti-sheep anti-LDL antibodies[9].

2) the complement system is not activated by the immunoadsorbens
   which we prepared (C3 and C5).

3) The patients tolerated the procedure over a period of less than
   three hours very well with no adverse subjective disturbances.

What is the influence on the patient's cholesterol metabolism and
how does the bile secretion of neutral and acidic sterols respond
during the time-course of a four week experiment under the conditions of a closed metabolic ward?

The daily dietary intake and the daily total acidic and neutral fecal sterol excretion were determined and from their difference the
de novo synthesis of cholesterol estimated (mg x day$^{-1}$) while the
two siblings were in a metabolic steady state for a period of two
weeks. The same parameters were determined during a period of three
weeks with immunoadsorption-treatments at day 7, 14 and 21.

The in-patients' caloric intake consisted of liquid formula meals
adjusted to maintain a constant body weight within 1 kg.

Isolation of fecal neutral- and acidic sterols were performed as
described previously and gas-liquid chromatographic separations[10],
identifications and quantitations were performed after derivati-
zations as trifluoroacetyl derivatives which proved to be much superior to trimethylsilyl derivatives so far used.

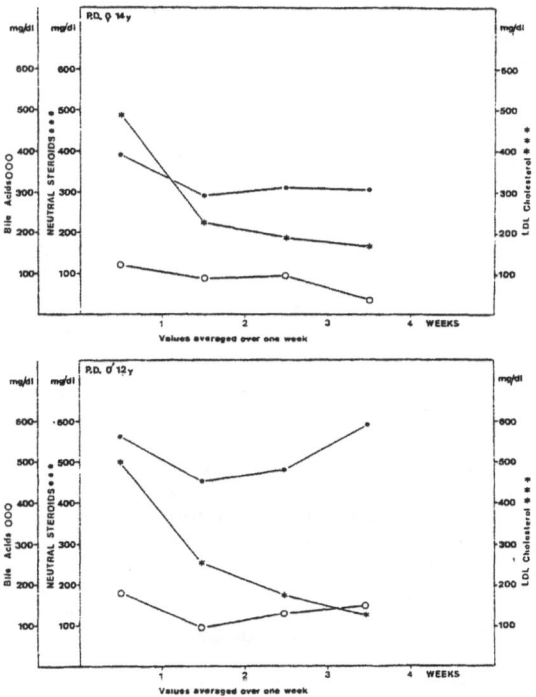

Figure 3 demonstrates the correlation of neutral and acidic
sterol concentrations and serum
LDL-cholesterol concentrations
under constant dietary cholesterol uptake.

Fig. 3. Serum LDL-concentrations
versus fecal neutral steroid and
bile acid concentrations during
a 4 weeks cholesterol balance
study of two heterozygous sibb-
lings. Daily concentrations were
averaged over one week.
Upper diagram: 14 year old girl,
lower diagram: 12 year old boy

The weekly LDL-apheresis reduced the LDL-cholesterol concentration from 500 mg/dl to an average concentration of about 250 mg/dl for the first week, 170 mg/dl after the second and 130 mg/dl after the third week. Fecal neutral steroid concentrations ranged between 570 mg/day in the first and 460 mg/day and 490 mg/day in the second and third, and 600 mg/day in the fourth week; acidic sterols were between 180 mg and 100 mg/day, Table 2.

Table 2.

| week | P.D. ♂ 12 y | | | P.D. ♀ 14 y | | |
|------|-------------------|---------------|-----|-------------------|---------------|-----|
|      | neutral steroids | bile acids | LDL | neutral steroids | bile acids | LDL |
| 1.   | 570 | 175 | 501 | 390 | 123 | 488 |
| 2.   | 455 | 95  | 251 | 292 | 86  | 227 |
| 3.   | 487 | 129 | 171 | 308 | 90  | 197 |
| 4.   | 600 | 151 | 133 | 304 | 33  | 171 |

Neutral and acidic fecal steroids (mg/d) and serum LDL-concentrations (mg/dl) averaged over the period of one week.

Therefore our conclusion, irrespective of the lacking knowledge of the de novo synthesis rate of cholesterol during this period, is that the constant fecal efflux of neutral and acidic sterols and the hormons removal of LDL-cholesterol by immuno-adsorption can only be explained by the depletion of cholesterol pools. Indeed this can be followed visually by the considerable reduction of the palpable tuberous and tendon xanthomas over the olecranon and achilles tendon and in the interdigital skin.

The patients' coronary atherosclerosis has been verified by coronary angiography and controls will be carried out in due time.

In summary: A new continuous extracorporeal method, which bases on the selective elimination of apo B-containing serum lipoproteins, VLDL and LDL, has been elaborated and is currently successfully applied in the treatment of homo- and heterozygous heriditary (familial) hypercholesterolemia. Future coronary angiographic controls will prove whether a depletion of cholesterol deposits in the artery wall gradually occurs as observed for skin and tendon xanthomata and xanthelasm and as the morphological basis of the subjective improvement of angina pectoris.

Needless to stress that our approach will be the basis for the selective removal of any pathological or pathogenic serum or plasma component.

References

1. Brown M S & Goldstein J L (1976) N Engl J Med 294: 1386-1390
2. Fredrickson D S & Lees R S (1966) Chapter 22 in the Metabolic Basis of Inherited disease, ed. Stanbury J B, Wyngaarden J B & Fredrickson D S. McGraw-Hill Book Company 2nd Edition: 429
3. Sniderman A D, Carew T E & Steinberg D (1975) J Lipid Res 16: 293-299
4. Thompson G R, Lowenthal R & Myant N B (1975) Lancet i: 1208-1211
5. Berger G M B, Miller J L, Bounici F, Jaffa H S & Dubovsky D V (1976) Am J Med 65: 243-251
6. Lupien P J, Moorjani S & Awad J (1976) Lancet: 1261-1265

7. Stoffel W & Demant Th (1981) Proc Nat Acad Sci 78: 611-615
8. Stoffel W, Greve V & Borberg H (1981) Lancet: 1005-1007
9. Ovary Z (1964) Passive cutaneous anaphylaxis in applied immuno-logical methods. Blockwall, Oxford: 294
10. Miettinen T A, Ahrens E H jr & Grundy S M (1965) J Lipid Res 6: 411-424

# 3.1 Structural and Metabolic Aspects of Lipoproteins

# Apolipoprotein Mutants and Apolipoprotein Disorders

## G. Assmann

A high degree of increased differentiation has come to the field of
genetic dyslipoproteinemia. Most of the classical lipoprotein phenotypes have been shown to be genotypically heterogenous or subject to
allelism. Characterization of the various apolipoproteins, of cellular lipoprotein receptors and of enzymes catalyzing intravascular
changes in lipoproteins has permitted the identification of the underlying molecular defect in a number of inborn errors of lipoprotein
metabolism. This short summary describes abnormalities in lipoprotein
metabolism where the molecular defect can be directly traced to mutations of apolipoproteins. They are called apolipoprotein disorders
here and are defined as diseases in which the etiology and pathophysiology are directly related to a structural defect or a defect in
biosynthesis or secretion of an apolipoprotein (Table 1). With the
recent availability of screening techniques there is an explosive
growth in the detection of apolipoprotein mutants. In certain cases
apolipoprotein variants have been described without pathological
complications. However, there is little doubt  that subtle changes in
metabolism may exist even in these, as it is very possible that more
sophisticated methods may be required to precisely determine the
effects involved here.

Table 1. Apolipoprotein disorders

| Apolipoprotein | Defect |
| --- | --- |
| A-I | Tangier disease |
| | Apo A-I Milano variant |
| | Apo A-I Marburg, Giessen variants |
| | Apo A-I Münster 1-3 variants |
| A-IV | Apo A-IV Giessen variant |
| | Apo A-IV Münster variants |
| B | recessive abetalipoproteinemia |
| | homozygous hypobetalipoproteinemia |
| | normotriglyceridemic abetalipoproteinemia |
| C | apolipoprotein C-II deficiency |
| E | apolipoprotein E-2 homozygosity |
| | a. dysbetalipoproteinemia |
| | b. familial type III hyperlipoproteinemia |

## 1. Tangier disease

Tangier disease was first described by FREDRICKSON in 1961 and is
named for Tangier Island, Virginia, where the patients first known
to have the disease lived. The most striking clinical symptom in
Tangier disease is substantial enlargement and yellow-orange discolo-
ration of the tonsils. In addition, splenomegaly is seen in most
patients, as is peripheral neuropathy. The disease is characterized
by the following laboratory findings: 1. low plasma cholesterol concentrations ( < 100 mg/dl) and normal or elevated plasma triglycerides;
2. nearly total absence of high density lipoproteins (HDL) in plasma
in conjunction with altered chemical composition of other plasma
lipoproteins; 3. concentration of cholesteryl esters in numerous
organs, primarily in the macrophages of tonsils, lymph nodes, thymus,
bone marrow, liver, spleen and rectal mucosa. In addition to the storage of cholesteryl esters there is an accumulation of lipids in
Schwann cells and intestinal smooth muscle cells. Arterial smooth

512

muscle cells or other cells of the arterial wall are not affected.
Arteriosclerosis is not a clinical symptom of this disease. The combination of low plasma cholesterol and enlarged, yellow-orange tonsils is characteristically indicative of Tangier disease.

The biochemical cause of analphalipoproteinemia is probably a structural defect in apolipoprotein A-I. This apolipoprotein is present
in the serum of Tangier patients at a concentration of 1 % of the
normal concentration. In contrast to normal apolipoprotein A-I, which
is detected as a component of HDL falling almost exclusively in the
density range of 1.063-1.21 g/ml KBr, Tangier apolipoprotein A-I is
found in the fraction >1.21 g/ml. Isolated Tangier Apo A-I shows loss
of the ability to reassociate with normal HDL. Storage of cholesteryl
esters in the macrophages must be considered a direct consequence of
the analphalipoproteinemia. As yet no definitive statement can be
made regarding why, in spite of the complete absence of normal HDL,
arteriosclerosis is not seen as a complication in Tangier disease.

## 2. Structural variants of apolipoprotein A-I

Structural variants of Apo A-I can be identified in native serum by
isoelectric focusing (fig. 1). In our own studies of 1000 patients
subjected to coronary angiography, three different familial apolipoprotein A-I structural variants were discovered (Apo A-I Münster 1-3)
Normal Apo A-I in the probands in these families was reduced to
approximately 50 % of the normal serum concentration, though there
was no indication of hypoalphalipoproteinemia. Apparently, despite
the defective structure of the apolipoprotein A-I Münster 1-3, the
physicochemical properties (protein-protein interaction, protein-
lipid interaction) are intact, such that functional deficiencies
in terms of altered HDL concentration are absent. This is in contrast
to findings in patients with the apo A-I Milano variant where hypoalphalipoproteinemia is a feature of the apolipoprotein defect.

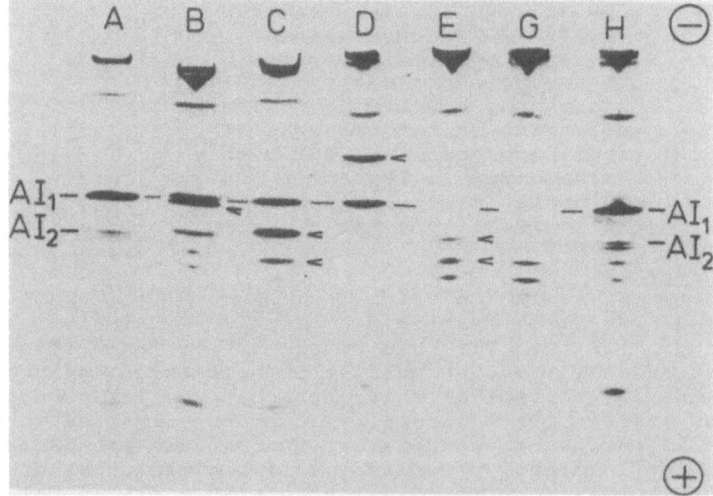

Fig. 1. Illustration of apolipoprotein A-I structural variants
(using isoelectric focusing of native serum). Gels A and H.: normal
serum; gel B: apolipoprotein A-I Münster-1 variant; gel C: apolipoprotein A-I Münster-2 variant; gel D: apolipoprotein A-I Münster-3
variant; gel E: apolipoprotein A-I Milano variant; Gel G: Tangier
disease

## 3. Structural variants of apolipoprotein A-IV

Such variants have been identified in a limited number of cases. The clinical significance is as yet unknown.

## 4. Abetalipoproteinemia

The disease described in a Jewish girl by BASSEN and KORNZWEIG in 1950 is, analogous to FRIEDRICH'S ataxia and fat malabsorption syndrome, characterized by retinitis pigmentosa, acanthocytosis and neurological symptoms. The diagnosis is confirmed by exremely low levels of cholesterol ($<$ 100 mg/dl) and triglycerides ($<$ 30 mg/dl) and the total absence of apolipoprotein B-containing lipoproteins (chylomicrons, VLDL, LDL, Lp(a)). On the basis of family studies, two forms of abetalipoproteinemia can be distinguished, on the one hand, recessive abetalipoproteinemia (autosomal recessive inheritance) and, on the other hand, the homozygous form of hypobetalipoproteinemia. In the case of recessive abetalipoproteinemia the parents of the probands exhibit normal concentrations of apolipoprotein B and LDL, while in the other case both parents have extremely low apolipoprotein B levels. The precise biochemical defect responsible for the apolipoprotein B deficiency is not yet known. Apolipoprotein B cannot be detected immunologically either in plasma or the intestinal mucosa (site of synthesis of chylomicrons).

## 5. Normotriglyceridemic abetalipoproteinemia

In this variant, in contrast to the classical form of abetalipoproteinemia, triglycerides are resolved in the intestine and chylomicrons formed and secreted. The intestinal synthesis of apolipoprotein B-48 is evidently not affected. However, as a consequence of selective inhibition of hepatic synthesis of apolipoprotein B-100, neither VLDL, nor LDL are present in plasma. Normotriglyceridemic abetalipoproteinemia is associated with only very modest neurological changes. This metabolic defect, although reported only once to date is, in the case of further confirmation, an indication of the fact that apolipoprotein B-100 and apolipoprotein B-48 are under separate genetic control. Furthermore, it may be assumed that chylomicron apolipoprotein B (B-48) is not a precursor of LDL apolipoprotein B (B-100).

## 6. Apolipoprotein C-II deficiency

In the case of hyperchylomicronemia it is imperative that a check be made to see whether the serum apolipoprotein C-II concentration is normal. Clear semiquantitative results are generally available by urea-polyacrylamide gel electrophoresis or isoelectric focusing of lipoproteins $<$ 1.006 g/ml in density; immunochemical tests (radioimmunoassay, immunoelectrophoresis) with monospecific antibodies confirm the diagnosis. To date, an apolipoprotein C-II deficiency as the cause of reduced lipoprotein lipase activity with consecutive hyperchylomicronemia has been described in only a very few cases. Just as in familial lipoprotein lipase deficiency, hyperchylomicronemia is seen as early as childhood and leads to similar clinical complications, particularly acute pancreatitis. In contrastto familial lipoprotein lipase deficiency, neither xanthomatosis nor heptomegaly have been observed to date in patients with apolipoprotein C-II deficiency. The few cases described up to now do not permit generalizations with reference to clinical complications of this disease.

## 7. Apolipoprotein E-2 homozygosity

In the case of apolipoprotein E-2 homozygosity (approximately 1 % of the population) there is resultant dysbetalipoproteinemia as a consequence of disturbed catabolism of chylomicron remnants and IDL. In the lipoprotein electrophoresis, ß-VLDL are found in the d < 1.006 g/ml supernatant (i.e. dysbetalipoproteinemia), VLDL cholesterol is elevated, LDL cholesterol and total cholesterol are reduced. The abnormal ß-VLDL have the following properties: a. spherical particles 250 A in diameter on average (normal VLDL: approximately 400 A); b. float in $S_F$-range 20-60 (normal VLDL: $S_F$ 20-400); c. rich in cholesterol (normal VLDL: triglyceride-rich); d. high apolipoprotein E concentration; e. no normal apolipoprotein E (i.e. Apo E-3 or Apo E-4), only defective apolipoprotein E (Apo E-2) present. It is assumed that the ß-VLDL are metabolic products of the chylomicrons (i.e. chylomicron remnants) or VLDL (i.e. VLDL remnants). Evidently, as a result of a structural mutation of apolipoprotein E-3 yielding apolipoprotein E-2 the remnants of the triglyceride-rich molecules are not properly recognized by the hepatic apoprotein E receptor and thus accumulate in the plasma. Apparently, more than one mutation exists causing the apolipoprotein E-2 phenotype. Arginine-cysteine interchanges may occur at different sites in the molecule not affecting the charge and the isoelectric focusing behavior, but possibly affecting the function of this apolipoprotein.

It has not been possible to date to determine whether apo E-2 homozygosity causing dysbetalipoproteinemia per se is associated with an increased coronary risk. In our own studies of a group of patients who underwent coronary angiography, apolipoprotein E-2 homozygosity occurred with similar frequency among those with coronary heart disease than among unaffected patients or within the general population (tab. 2). The low number of cases does not permit any conclusion as to whether apolipoprotein E-2 may be considered a biochemical indicator of increased coronary risk. One to two percent of the patients with apolipoprotein E-2 homozygosity progress to a condition characterized by severe early coronary arteriosclerosis, peripheral arteriosclerosis and xanthomatosis: type III hyperlipoproteinemia.

Table 2. Apolipoprotein E polymorphism and coronary heart disease

| | frequency of apolipoprotein E phenotypes | | | | | |
| --- | --- | --- | --- | --- | --- | --- |
| | E-3 | E-2 | E-4 | E-2/E-4 | E-2/E-3 | E-3/E-4 |
| coronary sclerosis present (coronary angiography on 385 patients) | 61.3 | 1.6 | 2.1 | 2.3 | 11.2 | 21.6 |
| coronary sclerosis absent (coronary angiography on 365 patients) | 57.3 | 1.4 | 1.4 | 2.5 | 16.4 | 21.1 |
| company employees (n=1000) (from periodic check-ups) | 62.7 | 0.8 | 2.3 | 3.0 | 11.0 | 20.2 |

## 8. Familial type III hyperlipoproteinemia

Familial type III hyperlipoproteinemia was described initially in 1967 by FREDRICKSON et al. Employing a combination of ultracentrifugation and lipoprotein electrophoresis, these authors discovered abnormal VLDL in the plasma of this type, which did not exhibit the usual pre-ß mobility, but rather ß mobility. These abnormal lipoproteins were designated "ß-VLDL" or "floating ß-lipoproteins", which yield a broad ß-band in the electrophoresis of native serum ("broad ß disease"). Later studies by HAVEL and KANE showed a high concentration of apolipoprotein E in the ß-VLDL. In 1975, UTERMANN et al. described the genetic defect of type III hyperlipoproteinemia as an increase in Apo E-2 with simultaneous absence of Apo E-3 and Apo E-4. ZANNIS and

BRESLOW in 1979 introduced a triallelic model for Apo E (E-N, E-D and E-4), corresponding to six different genotypes and phenotypes in the population. Consequently, apolipoprotein E-2 homozygosity corresponds to the genotype E-D/E-D. In 1981, WEISGRABER et al. identified a structural mutation of apolipoprotein E-3 as a biochemical defect of type III hyperlipoproteinemia.

Only 2 % of all patients with the apolipoprotein genotype E-D/E-D (homozygous for Apo E-2) develop clinical signs of type III hyperlipoproteinemia. Type III hyperlipoproteinemia becomes manifest when, in addition to Apo E-2 homozygosity, there is either a further inborn error of lipid metabolism present (e.g. familial hypercholesterolemia, familial hypertriglyceridemia, familial combined hyperlipidemia, polygenic hypercholesterolemia) or there is a secondary hyperlipoproteinemia (e.g. in hypothyroidism) present. Obviously, under these circumstances, that is apolipoprotein E-2 homozygosity combined with increased biosynthesis of VLDL or reduced catabolism of LDL, the condition in question is extreme dysbetalipoproteinemia causally related to atherosclerosis and xanthomatosis.

The diagnosis of familial type III hyperlipoproteinemia (frequency approximately 1:5000) can be confirmed on the basis of the clinical findings (xanthomata of the hand lines, tuberous xanthomata, intermittent claudicatio, coronary heart disease) and the biochemical findings (Apo E-2 homozygosity, ß-VLDL, hyperlipidemia with elevated cholesterol and triglycerides). The early occurrence of coronary heart disease and/or peripheral vascular occlusion (often before age 40) are frequent complications of this disorder of lipid metabolism.

The differentiation of apolipoprotein E-2 homozygosity from type III hyperlipoproteinemia is at present possible only on the basis of clinical observations. Of particular clinical interest is the question of which patients, if any, with apolipoprotein E-2 homozygosity have an increased coronary risk. In any case, apolipoprotein E-2 homozygosity occurs in the population with a frequency of 1 % and is characterized by dysbetalipoproteinemia which, at least in a number of patients, is accompanied by the early onset of coronary sclerosis. Between type III hyperlipoproteinemia with extreme elevation of ß-VLDL and apolipoprotein E-2 homozygosity with low serum cholesterol levels and slight elevation of ß-VLDL there is an entire spectrum of metabolic anomalies whose relationship to coronary sclerosis is in need of explanation.

References
1. Menzel, H.J., Kladetzky, R.G., Assmann, G.
   One-step screening method for the polymorphism of apolipoproteins A-I, A-II and A-IV.
   J. Lipid. Res., in press (1982)
2. Menzel, H.J., Kövary, P.M., Assmann, G.
   Apolipoprotein A-IV polymorphism in man.
   Clin. Gen., in press (1982)
3. Assmann, G., Menzel, H.J.
   Apolipoprotein disorders.
   La Ricerca Clin. Lab. 12, 63, 1982
4. Assmann, G.
   Lipoproteine und Atherosklerose.
   Schattauer Verlag, Stuttgart, New York, 1982
5. Herbert, P.N., Assmann, G., Gotto, A.M.,Jr.,Fredrickson,D.S.
   Familial Lipoprotein Deficiency:Abetalipoproteinemia,Hypobetalipoproteinemia,and Tangier Disease.In:The Metabolic Basis of Inherited Disease,Stanburg et al.,eds.,Mc Graw-Hill,New York 5th ed.,chapter 29, p. 589, 1982

# Determination of Plasma Apolipoprotein Profiles

P. Alaupovic

## Introduction

Rapid advances in the chemistry and metabolism of plasma apolipoproteins have already
produced a considerable impact on the existing conceptual views about the plasma lipoprotein system.  They have shifted the attention from lipid to protein constituents and emphasized the significance of apolipoproteins as the most probable determinants of the structural stability and functional specificity of lipoprotein particles (1, 2).  While the discovery of new apolipoproteins and their wide distribution
throughout the density spectrum have revealed a new dimension in the complexity of
plasma lipoproteins, the recognition of apolipoproteins as unique constituents and
specific markers of a great variety of lipoprotein particles has provided a convenient and simple means for their identification and classification (1-3).  According
to this view, plasma lipoprotein system consists of a mixture of lipoprotein families
which are differentiated and characterized on the basis of their constituent apolipoproteins.  Lipoprotein families which contain a single apolipoprotein are referred to
as <u>simple</u> or <u>primary lipoprotein families</u>; these lipoprotein families represent the
simplest lipoprotein forms of the system.  Lipoprotein families which contain two or
more apolipoproteins are called <u>complex</u> or <u>secondary lipoprotein families</u> (2, 3).  It
has now become possible by use of specific  immunological procedures to identify individual lipoprotein families and to monitor their formation, interactions and degradation irrespective of their size, hydrated density or lipid composition.

If one assumes that the optimal functioning of lipid transport processes depends on
and is expressed by certain characteristic concentrations of simple and complex lipoproteins (primary and secondary lipoprotein families), any perturbations of this
macromolecular system will result in changed concentrations of simple and complex
lipoprotein particles commensurate with the type and extent of underlying metabolic
defect or environmental influence.  Therefore, various deranged states of lipid
transport may be identified and characterized by distinct profiles of simple and
complex lipoproteins or their corresponding apolipoprotein concentrations.  The determination of apolipoprotein concentrations or <u>apolipoprotein profiling</u> can be defined as "an attempt to express in quantitative apolipoprotein terms the simple and
complex lipoproteins which are characteristic of normal or deranged states of lipid
transport".  Since a simple methodology for isolating and separating simple and complex lipoproteins is still not available, the present aim of apolipoprotein profiling
is to determine the apolipoprotein concentrations in whole plasma and to evaluate
their biochemical and clinical significance.

## Assays for Quantification of Apolipoproteins

It has become obvious from the outset, that, due to the complexity of lipoproteins,
the development of reliable assays for quantitative determination of apolipoproteins
had to be based on highly specific and sensitive immunological procedures (4).  During the last ten years, such procedures developed for most, if not all, well characterized apolipoproteins include radioimmunoassay (5-12), radial immunodiffusion (13-
15) and electroimmunoassay (16-19).  More recently, enzyme immunoassays (20, 21) and
immunonephelometric measurements (22-24) of apolipoproteins have also been developed.
Each of these immunoassays has some inherent advantages and drawbacks.  Some of the
problems encountered in immunoassays of apolipoproteins are due to physical-chemical
properties peculiar to lipoproteins, while others can be traced down to limitations
of individual assays.  A partial list of such difficulties includes differences in
the physical state of apolipoproteins in standards and samples, differences in the
immunoreactivity of apolipoproteins present in both simple and complex lipoproteins,

masking of antigenic sites, polymorphism of apolipoproteins, lack of adequate standards, variations in the affinity of antisera, differences in assay conditions, quality control and technical skill. However, despite these problems and difficulties, the similarity and agreements between reported data are more prevalent than discrepancy and disagreements.

Apolipoprotein Profiles of Whole Plasma

Preliminary results on apolipoprotein profiling of normolipidemic children and adults have already revealed some significant differences in the apolipoprotein levels related to ontogeny, age, sex and environmental influences. The apolipoprotein profile of cord plasma is characterized by low levels of apolipoproteins (Apo) A-I, A-II, B and D and normal levels of apolipoproteins C-I, C-II, C-II and E when compared to adult levels (25). However, soon after the birth, the levels of apolipoproteins A-I, A-II, B and D increase markedly reaching almost the adult levels. A very interesting and characteristic effect of age is that related to concentrations of ApoB (Table 1; data only presented for males). After 5 years of age, the levels of ApoB slowly decrease to reach the lowest concentrations during the puberty. After puberty, the

Table 1. Apolipoprotein profiles of normolipidemic children and adults

| Subjects | Age | Apolipoproteins | | | | |
|---|---|---|---|---|---|---|
| | | A-I | B | C-II | C-III | E |
| | Years | | | mg/dl | | |
| Cord plasma (n = 30) | – | 67 (13) | 27 (9) | 3.3 (1) | 5.2 (1.9) | 8.5 (3.6) |
| Children (n = 13) | 0.5- 4 | 115 (24) | 92 (33) | 1.9 (0.3) | 5.6 (1.7) | 10.3 (2.7) |
| Children (n = 10) | 5- 9 | 130 (17) | 72 (12) | 2.1 (0.2) | 5.7 (1.1) | 8.8 (1.5) |
| Children (n = 7) | 10-14 | 134 (16) | 58 (14) | 2.5 (0.9) | 7.0 (2.5) | 8.0 (2.6) |
| Children (n = 5) | 15-19 | 109 ( 8) | 78 (11) | 2.6 (0.8) | 5.3 (1.1) | 7.2 (1.7) |
| Adults (n = 55) | 20-39 | 123 (17) | 96 (27) | 2.7 (0.6) | 7.3 (2.3) | 10.2 (2.6) |
| Adults (n = 40) | 40-59 | 133 (16) | 110 (23) | 3.1 (1.0) | 8.4 (2) | 10.1 (3.0) |
| Adults (n = 5) | ≥ 60 | 141 (29) | 121 (28) | – | 7.8 (0.4) | 11.3 (1.6) |

Means (S.D.)

ApoB concentrations show a gradual increase which then continues into adulthood. The levels of ApoA-peptides, ApoC-peptides and ApoE seem to stabilize during or immediately after puberty. After puberty, female children have higher levels of ApoA-I and ApoA-II than male children. Female children also seem to have higher levels of apolipoproteins B, C-III and E than male children at any age interval from 5-19. The apolipoprotein profiles of normolipidemic, asymptomatic men and women, 20-76 years of age, were determined in three population groups including Oklahoma City, Oklahoma; London, England; and Göteborg, Sweden. In all three populations, the levels of apolipoproteins A-I, B, C-II and C-III were higher than in cord plasma or plasma samples from children (Table 1; data only presented for males from Oklahoma City). There was practically no difference between adults and children in the levels of apolipoproteins A-II, D, E and F. Although there were no statistically significant differences between three populations in the levels of plasma cholesterol and triglyceride, women from the London group had significantly higher levels of ApoE and lower levels of ApoA-I than women from Oklahoma City. Similarly, men from London had significantly higher levels of ApoC-III and ApoE than men from Oklahoma City. In each population sample, women had higher levels of ApoA-I and lower levels of ApoC-III than men. In samples from Oklahoma City and Göteborg, women also tend to have lower levels of ApoB, but higher levels of ApoE than men. A study on the effect of age on apolipoprotein concentrations in men and women from the Oklahoma City area indicated slight increases in the levels of apolipoproteins A-I, B, C-III and E up to the middle of the fifth decade with a subsequent plateau or even slight decline.

Studies from this and other laboratories have indicated that apolipoprotein profiles of dyslipoproteinemic states can be grouped into three main categories:

      1. Profiles characterized by the absence of an apolipoprotein(s)
      2. Profiles characterized by the deficiency of an apolipoprotein
      3. Profiles characterized by hyperapolipoproteinemia

There are now four recognized dyslipoproteinemias characterized by the absence of an immunologically-detectable apolipoprotein. ApoB is the missing apolipoprotein in abetalipoproteinemia (26), ApoC-II in the ApoC-II deficiency (27), ApoE in the ApoE-deficiency disease (28) and ApoA-I and ApoC-III in a newly reported metabolic disorder of lipid transport (29, 30). In this category, the determination of apolipoprotein profile represents an absolute diagnostic criterion for identifying and differentiating lipid transport disorders.

The second category encompasses apolipoprotein profiles of Tangier disease, hypobetalipoproteinemia and lecithin:cholesterol acyltransferase (LCAT) deficiency. These apolipoprotein profiles have already been described (31). Briefly, Tangier disease is characterized by very low levels of ApoA-I and ApoA-II, hypobetalipoproteinemia by low levels of ApoB and the LCAT deficiency by low levels of apolipoproteins A-I, A-II and B. Although apolipoprotein profiles in this category do not represent an absolute diagnostic criterion, they are still characteristic enough to be used as a means for identifying and differentiating lipid transport disorders.

The third category of apolipoprotein profiles is characterized by significantly increased levels of one or several apolipoproteins. This category is the largest group of dyslipoproteinemias and includes all of the primary and secondary hyperlipoproteinemias. Although it is not possible to present and discuss in detail the results of apolipoprotein profiling in this large group of dyslipoproteinemias, it suffices to report that preliminary data indicate the occurrence of certain characteristic patterns in apolipoprotein profiles of primary hyperlipoproteinemias (18, 31). The first of these patterns is characterized by low levels of apolipoproteins A-I, A-II and B and increased levels of ApoC and ApoE (phenotype I). The hallmark of the second pattern is a proportional increase in the levels of all three ApoC-peptides and ApoE (phenotypes III and IV). The third pattern is characterized by a significant increase of ApoB (phenotypes IIa and IIb), and the fourth by a specific increase in the levels of ApoC-III (phenotype IV and IIb). Although the determination of apolipoprotein concentrations in this category of lipid transport disorders does not provide an absolute diagnostic criterion, it offers very useful clues about the chemical nature of accumulating lipoprotein particles, and, indirectly, about the underlying biochemical derangements. Apolipoproteins A-I and A-II occur mainly as simple lipoprotein particles characterized either by the sole presence of A-I (LP-A-I) or by the presence of both A-I and A-II (LP-A). Changes in the concentrations of apolipoproteins A-I and A-II affect mainly these two types of lipoprotein particles. A significant increase in the levels of ApoB without concomitant increases in the levels of ApoC and/or ApoE indicates an increased concentration of lipoprotein B (LP-B) particles, a simple lipoprotein family characteristic of low-density lipoproteins. An elevation of ApoC-III levels without commensurate increases in the concentrations of ApoC-I and ApoC-II reflects the presence of lipoprotein C-III (LP-C-III), a triglyceride- and cholesterol ester-rich lipoprotein particle which contains ApoC-III as the sole protein; these particles first isolated from patients with chronic renal failure (32) occur in the very low- and low-density regions.  On the other hand, a simultaneous elevation of all ApoC-peptides, ApoB and ApoE is sugges-tive of the accumulation of various triglyceride-rich particles (LP-B:C:E) which contain these apolipoproteins as integral constituents of their protein moieties; these complex lipoprotein families occur mainly at densities less than 1.006 g/ml. Complete lipolysis of these particles yields triglyceride-poor simple lipoproteins LP-B, LP-C and LP-E.  A partial lipolysis of triglyceride-rich LP-B:C:E particles may generate a variety of lipoprotein species such as LP-B:E, LP-C:E, LP-B:E, etc. These products of partial hydrolysis occur mainly within a density range of 0.96-1.019 g/ml.  We suggest that accumulation of some of these simple and complex lipo-proteins, as expressed by the apolipoprotein profiles, reflects the most common met-abolic defects of lipid transport.  The elevated levels of LP-B particles may result either from their overproduction or impaired removal (defective receptor pathway). The disproportionate increase of ApoC-III may result from the overproduction of tri-glyceride-rich LP-C-III particles, although a simultaneous underutilization of these particles cannot be ruled out.  The increased levels of ApoC and ApoE and the re-duced levels of ApoA and ApoB seem to indicate impaired catabolic processes of tri-glyceride-rich lipoproteins such as delayed removal or decreased lipolysis.

Most of the secondary hyperlipoproteinemias, with the possible exception of liver diseases (31), are also characterized by one of the four patterns identified in pa-tients with primary hyperlipoproteinemias (33).  For example, patients with insulin-independent diabetes and patients with chronic renal failure have increased levels of ApoC-III as the most characteristic feature of their apolipoprotein profiles.  On the other hand, patients with poorly controlled insulin-dependent diabetes have slightly lower levels of ApoA-I, but significantly higher levels of ApoB, ApoC-I, ApoC-III and ApoE than the normal subjects (31, 33).  Thus, in both types of dia-betes, there is an accumulation of triglyceride-rich lipoproteins.  However, they differ qualitatively and quantitatively from one another.  Patients with nephrotic syndrome have highly elevated levels of ApoB and moderate elevations of ApoC and ApoE.  Like in familial hypercholesterolemia, the high B/C-III and B/E ratios in-dicate an elevated concentration of LP-B particles.  In addition, there is also an increased accumulation of some triglyceride-rich particles with ApoC and ApoE as the constituents of their protein moieties.  The presence of these lipoprotein spe-cies may be due to both increased hepatic synthesis and defective catabolism.

The usefulness of apolipoprotein profiling has been further enhanced by a number of recent studies which have shown that apolipoprotein levels may be better predictors of coronary artery disease than lipid levels (34-37).  A more detailed account of these studies is presented elsewhere in this volume.

Since most dyslipoproteinemic states are characterized by changed concentrations of simple and complex lipoprotein families, development of simple procedures for their separation seems to be one of the most important goals for further refinement of apolipoprotein profiling.  Apolipoprotein profiles of simple and complex lipoproteins may, indeed, be of considerable clinical importance as a new means for classifying disorders of lipid transport and as an efficient device for monitoring the progress of therapeutic interventions.

## References

1. Osborne JC, Jr, Brewer HB, Jr (1977) The plasma lipoproteins. Adv. Protein Chem 31:253-337
2. Alaupovic P (1982) The role of apolipoproteins in lipid transport processes. Ric Clin Lab 12:3-21
3. Alaupovic P (1972) Conceptual development of the classification systems of plasma lipoproteins. Protides Biol Fluids Proc Colloq 19:9-19
4. Herbert PN, Bausserman LL, Henderson LO, Heimen RJ, LaPiana MJ. Church EC, Shulman RS (1978) Apolipoprotein quantitation. In: Peters H (ed) The Lipoprotein Molecule. Plenum Press, New York, p 35-56

5.  Schonfeld G, Leès RS, George PK, Pfleger B (1974) Assay of total plasma apolipoprotein B concentration in human subjects. J Clin Invest 53:1458-1467
6.  Fainaru M, Glangeau MC, Eisenberg S (1975) Radioimmunoassay of human high density lipoprotein apoprotein A-I. Biochim Biophys Acta 386:432-443
7.  Karlin JB, Juhn DJ, Starr JI, Scanu AM, Rubenstein AH (1976) Measurement of human high density lipoprotein apolipoprotein A-I in serum by radioimmunoassay. J Lipid Res 17:30-37
8.  Schonfeld G, Chen J-S, McDonnell WF, Jeng I (1977) Apolipoprotein A-II content of human plasma high density lipoproteins measured by radioimmunoassay. J Lipid Res 18:645-655
9.  Kashyap ML, Srivastava LS, Chen C-Y, Perisuth G, Campbell M, Lutmer RF, Glueck CJ (1977) Radioimmunoassay of human apolipoprotein C-II. A study in normal and hypertriglyceridemic subjects. J Clin Invest 60:171-180
10. Blum CB, Aron L, Sciacca R (1980) Radioimmunoassay studies of human apolipoprotein E. J Clin Invest 66:1240-1250
11. Mackie A, Caslake, ML, Packard CJ. Shepherd J (1981) Concentration and distribution of human plasma apolipoprotein E. Clin Chim Acta 116:35-45
12. Suarez BK, Schonfeld G (1981) Characterization of apolipoprotein E (ApoE): Apoprotein levels in the various ApoE phenotypes. J Clin Endocrinol Metab 53:435-438
13. Cheung MC, Albers JJ (1977) The measurement of apolipoprotein A-I and A-II levels in men and women by immunoassay. J Clin Invest 60:43-50
14. Sistonen P, Enholm C (1980) On the heritability of serum high density lipoprotein in twins. Am J Hum Genet 32:1-7
15. Polz E, Kotite L, Havel RJ, Kane JP, Sata T (1980) Human apolipoprotein C-I: Concentration in blood serum and lipoproteins. Biochem Med 24:229-237
16. Kahan J, Sundblad L (1969) Immunochemical determination of β-lipoproteins. Scand J Clin Lab Invest 24:61-68
17. Fager G, Wiklund O, Olofsson S-O, Norfeldt P-I, Vedin A, Bondjers G. (1980) Quantitation of human serum apolipoprotein A-I by electroimmunoassay. Studies on some techniques for standardization of the assay and determination of serum apolipoprotein A-I levels in a random population sample of middle-aged men. Scand J Clin Lab Invest 40:451-460
18. Alaupovic P, Curry MD, McConathy WJ (1978) Quantitative determination of human plasma apolipoproteins by electroimmunoassays. In: Carlson LA, Paoletti R, Sirtori CR, Weber G (eds.). International Conference on Atherosclerosis, Raven Press, New York, p 109-115
19. Calvert GD, Yates RA, Roeger DC (1979) Electroimmunoassay of a subunit protein in a macromolecular complex (apolipoprotein B in human plasma very low density lipoprotein); implications for other electroimmunoassays. Clin Chim Acta 97:135-142
20. Fruchart JC, Desreumaux C, Dewailly P, Sezille G, Jaillard J, Carlier Y, Bout D, Capron A (1978) Enzyme immunoassay for human apolipoprotein B, the major protein moiety in low-density- and very-low-density lipoproteins. Clin Chem 24:455-459
21. Holmquist L (1980) Quantifation of human serum very low density apolipoproteins C-I, C-II, C-III and E by enzyme immunoassay. J Immunol Meth 34:243-251
22. Ballatyne FC, Williamson J, Shapiro D, Caslake MJ, Perry B (1978) Estimation of apolipoprotein B in man by immunonephelometry. Clin Chem 24:788-792
23. Heuck CC, Schlierf G (1979) Simplified immunonephelometric quantitation of apolipoprotein B in hyperlipoproteinemic serum. Clin Chem 25:782-785
24. Weinstock N, Bartholome M, Seidel D (1981) Determination of apolipoprotein A-I by kinetic nephelometry. Biochim Biophys Acta 663:279-288
25. McConathy WJ, Lane DM (1980) Studies on the apolipoproteins and lipoproteins of cord serum. Pediatr Res 14:757-761
26. Salt HB, Wolff OH, Lloyd JK, Fosbrooke AS, Cameron AH, Hubble DV (1970) On having no beta lipoprotein. A syndrome comprising a beta-lipoproteinemia, acanthocyatosis and steatorrhea. Lancet 2:325-329
27. Breckenridge WC, Little JA, Steiner G, Chow A, Poapst M (1978) Hypertriglyceridemia associated with deficiency of apolipoprotein C-II. N Engl J Med. 298:1265-1273

28. Ghiselli G, Schafer EJ, Gascon P, Brewer HB, Jr (1981) Type III hyperlipoproteinemia associated with apolipoprotein E deficiency. Science 214:1239-1241
29. Schaefer EJ, Heaton WH, Wetzel MG, Brewer HB, Jr (1982) Plasma apolipoprotein A-I absence associated with a marked reduction of high density lipoproteins and premature coronary artery disease. Arteriosclerosis 2:16-26
30. Norum RA, Lakier JB, Goldstein S, Angel A, Goldberg RB, Block WD, Noffze DK, Dolphin PJ, Edelglass J, Bogorad DD, Alaupovic P (1982) Familial A-I and C-III deficiency and precocious coronary disease. N Engl J Med 306: in press
31. Alaupovic P (1980) Structure and function of plasma lipoproteins with particular regard to hyperlipoproteinemias and atherosclerosis. Ann Biol Clin 38:83-93
32. Attman P-O, Gustafson A, Alaupovic P, Knight C, Wang C-S, Bass H (1980) Abnormalities of plasma lipoprotein system in patients with chronic renal failure (CRF). Circulation 62 Part II:180
33. Alaupovic P, McConathy WJ, Curry MD, Fesmire JD (1982) Characterization of dyslipoproteinemias by apolipoprotein profiles. In: Noseda G, Fragiacomo C, Fumagalli R, Paoletti R (eds). Lipoproteins and Coronary Atherosclerosis, Elsevier Biomedical Press, Amsterdam, p 135-144
34. Avogaro P, Bittolo Bon G, Cazzolato G, Quinci GB (1979) Are apolipoproteins better discriminators than lipids for atherosclerosis. Lancet 1:901-903
35. Vergani C, Trovato G, Dioguardi N (1978) Serum total lipids, lipoproteins cholesterol, apoproteins A and B in cardiovascular disease. Clin Chim Acta 87:127-133
36. Kladetzky RG, Assman G, Walgenbach S, Tauchert P, Helb HD (1980) Lipoprotein and apoprotein values in coronary angiography patients. Artery 7:191-205
37. Sniderman A, Shapiro S, Marpole D, Skinner B, Teng B, Kwiterovich PO, Jr (1980) Association of coronary atherosclerosis with hyperapobetalipoproteinemia [increased protein but normal cholesterol levels in human plasma low density (β) lipoproteins]. Proc Natl Acad Sci USA 77:604-608

# The Plasma Cholesterol: Cholesterol-Ester Cycle

S. Eisenberg and B. Perret

Three years ago, at the V International Symposium on Atherosclerosis (1), we have presented evidence that both LDL and HDL are metabolic products of the core and surface domains of triglyceride-rich lipoproteins. The data can be summarized as follows: Triglyceride-rich lipoproteins (chylomicrons and VLDL) are primary secretory products of intestinal and hepatic cells. In the plasma, the two lipoproteins interact with lipoprotein lipases at luminal surfaces of endothelial cells and deliver triglyceride-fatty acids to tissues. The reaction leaves behind a triglyceride-depleted lipoprotein that contains non-hydrolyzable core lipids (cholesterol esters) and residual triglycerides. As well, the post-lipolysis particles remain with excess of surface constituents, phospholipids, free cholesterol and apoproteins. Our experiments indicated that the metabolism of non-triglyceride molecules in chylomicrons and VLDL is best described along two pathways: a core pathway, and a surface pathway (2, 3). Along the core pathway, the lipoprotein cholesterol ester and residual triglyceride molecules together with apo B and sufficient quantities of phospholipids and free cholesterol form remnant particles or LDL (4). Along the surface pathway, HDL precursors are formed (4, 5). These precursors are converted to spherical HDL by the activity of the LCAT system and accumulation of cholesterol ester molecules.

The lipoprotein system is also modified by movement of single lipid and protein molecules. Such movements — exchange or transfer — involve phospholipids, apo A's, apo C's, apo E's, free cholesterol, cholesterol esters and triglycerides. In the present communication we describe new experiments on the movement of free and esterified cholesterol between lipoproteins. These experiments led us to suggest the presence in plasma of a cholesterol - cholesterol ester cycle which is responsible for major remodelling of all plasma lipoproteins.

Most plasma cholesterol enters the circulation in unesterified form and is associated with newly synthesized lipoproteins, mainly chylomicrons and VLDL. More free cholesterol is acquired from cell membranes. During the course of lipolysis, free cholesterol is displaced from the triglyceride-rich lipoproteins, and is distributed among "cholesterol acceptors" present near the sites of lipolysis. Three such potential acceptors should be considered: circulating blood cells (red and white cells and platelets), endothelial and tissue cells and plasma lipoproteins. In a recent study we investigated the possible role of these three systems as potential acceptors for lipolysis-generated cholesterol (6). The study included determinations of rates of cholesterol exchange and rates of in vitro (or in situ) lipolysis-induced cholesterol transfer from biosynthetically labeled rat plasma VLDL to freshly prepared human blood cells, to the isolated perfused rat hearts or to HDL. The exchange of [3H]cholesterol between VLDL and HDL was much faster than between VLDL and cells, probably reflecting the different organization of lipids in lipoproteins as compared to cell membranes. With lipolysis, we found avid and rapid transfer of cholesterol from VLDL to HDL but none to circulating blood cells, and only minimal to tissues. We have therefore concluded that nearly all of the lipolysis-generated cholesterol remains in the lipoprotein system. According to Glomset and Norum (7), this amounts to 2.6-4-2 g cholesterol per day, far in excess of total body cholesterol synthesis ($\sim 1$ g/day) and of dietary cholesterol (0.3-0.5 g/day). The lipoprotein system then must deal with very large amounts of cholesterol each day.

The molecular mechanism(s) responsible for transfer of cholesterol from lipolyzed VLDL to HDL (and by implication, lack of transfer to cells), are currently under investigation. As for the exchange process, we suspect that they reflect basic differences in lipid organization between lipoproteins and cells. Alternatively, they may reflect the mode of cholesterol transfer. For example, it is possible that the cholesterol moves together with phospholipids and apoproteins as a structured "surface remnant", that fuses with other lipoproteins but not with cells. Of interest, more recently we have found that LDL may also serve as acceptor for cholesterol, and that on a free cholesterol basis is a better acceptor than HDL (B. Perret and S. Eisenberg, unpublished). Yet, as free cholesterol is further metabolized in HDL, LDL apparently serves in this cycle a role of an intermediary acceptor for the cholesterol generated by lipolysis.

Regardless of mechanism of cholesterol transport, it is commonly believed that the further metabolism of cholesterol occurs in HDL via the LCAT reaction. In many animal species, however, HDL-cholesterol esters are transferred to lower density lipoproteins. This reaction is catalyzed by a specific transfer protein present in plasma of some species including humans (8) but absent from the plasma of other species, for instance the rat (9). The reaction was originally demonstrated in human plasma by Nichols and Smith (10), who observed in incubated human plasma transfer of cholesterol esters from HDL to VLDL and of triglycerides from VLDL to HDL. In humans, as much as 80% of the LCAT-derived cholesterol esters may be transferred from HDL to lower density lipoproteins (11) and constitute their major source of cholesterol esters. This reaction (or series of reactions) is therefore responsible for major re-modelling of core-composition of all plasma lipoproteins.

An experimental system for the study of core-lipid transfer among lipoproteins was recently constructed and evaluated by us (12). The system was based on rat plasma devoid of cholesterol ester and triglyceride transfer activities supplemented with either rat plasma HDL labeled biosynthetically with [$^3$H]cholesterol esters and [$^{14}$C]unesterified cholesterol or with rat plasma VLDL labeled with [$^{14}$C]-palmitate triglycerides. The rat plasma system retained its LCAT activity. Cholesterol ester and triglyceride transfer were initiated by the addition of human plasma protein fraction of d > 1.21 g/ml. The system thus allowed a study of the LCAT and the core-lipid transfer reactions separately or in combination. It also allowed a study of transfer of existing cholesterol esters (in the HDL) and of cholesterol esters formed during the incubation period. The absence of core-lipid transfer in rat plasma was confirmed. In this system (devoid of transfer activity) about 90% of the cholesterol esters formed during the time of incubation remained in HDL. In the presence of transfer activity, about 50% of the HDL cholesterol esters (existing and the newly formed ones) moved to lower density lipoproteins, predominantly VLDL, and some of the VLDL-triglycerides moved to HDL. Transfer of cholesterol esters from HDL caused an increase in LCAT activity of the system, although transfer was independent of LCAT activity. Comparison of transfer of existing (pre-formed) cholesterol esters and of newly formed LCAT derived cholesterol esters indicated that they were almost identical.

524

In this system therefore, LCAT-derived cholesterol esters first accumulated in HDL and only afterwards were transferred to VLDL. By calculation, it was possible to show that more than one half of the cholesterol esters that were transferred from HDL were replaced by triglycerides. The reaction therefore resulted in considerable change of the core-lipid composition of the lipoprotein. VLDL became poor in triglycerides and rich in cholesterol esters, whereas HDL lost cholesterol esters but accumulated triglycerides.

Core lipid transfer occurs also between VLDL and LDL, and LDL becomes cholesterol ester poor, and triglyceride rich following incubation with VLDL and core-lipid transfer protein(s) (13). Addition of lipoprotein lipase to the incubation system — or incubation of the triglyceride-enriched LDL with the lipase — resulted in triglyceride hydrolysis and net loss of core lipids (cholesterol esters and triglycerides) from the lipoprotein. The combined activity of core-lipid transfer and lipase therefore results in major remodelling of the cholesterol ester rich lipoproteins (LDL and HDL).

Can similar reactions affect HDL? The answer to this question is in the affirmative. We have recorded almost identical phenomena with HDL from patients with abetalipoproteinemia (14), and more recently with $HDL_2$ isolated from normolipidemic humans (unpublished). In both instances we have observed the two stages described above: exchange of HDL cholesterol esters for VLDL-triglycerides followed by hydrolysis of the exchanged triglycerides with lipoprotein lipase.

## PLASMA CHOLESTEROL – CHOLESTEROL ESTER CYCLE

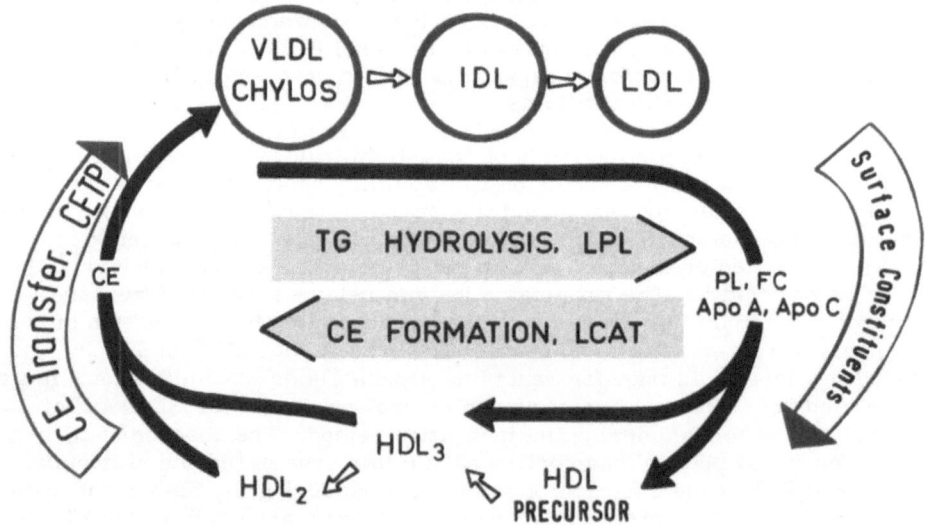

Fig. 1

The experiments discussed here established the presence of a cholesterol-cholesterol ester cycle in human plasma (Figure 1). The cycle starts with generation of unesterified cholesterol (together with other surface constituents) from lipolyzed triglyceride-rich lipoproteins and transfer of this cholesterol to LDL and HDL. This cholesterol becomes esterified in HDL by the LCAT reaction and thereby $HDL_3$ is formed. With generation of more cholesterol, $HDL_3$ may become transformed to $HDL_2$. Concomitantly, in humans, cholesterol ester molecules are transferred to chylomicrons and VLDL allowing continued activity of the LCAT. At the same time, however, triglycerides are transferred to HDL (and LDL). These triglycerides can be hydrolized and are irreversibly lost from the lipoprotein. The activity of the cholesterol ester transfer and the cholesterol ester for triglyceride exchange reactions followed by triglyceride hydrolysis thus results in limitation and reduction of size of the cholesterol ester-rich lipoproteins (LDL and HDL) and accumulation of cholesterol esters in triglyceride-rich lipoproteins. The profile of a lipoprotein system in an individual is therefore determined by the sum of several metabolic processes, including flux of triglycerides through the plasma, rates of triglyceride hydrolysis and of cholesterol esterification, distribution of core-lipids among lipoproteins and irreversible catabolism of lipoprotein particles. It is only when all the above-mentioned interactions are considered, that the variation of the plasma lipoprotein system among individuals can be explained.

The concepts described here are strongly supported by many clinical and laboratory observations. Three examples of lipoprotein systems that can be fully explained by these concepts deserve special attention. The first is the HDL system in patients with severe hypertriglyceridemia. In these patients, the HDL cholesterol levels are low, and the HDL is enriched with triglycerides. In some instances we and others have observed a triglyceride : cholesterol ratio in HDL above 1.0 (normal, less than 0.2)! In some patients, most HDL is present in a subpopulation which is smaller and denser than $HDL_3$. These findings together are consistent with increased activity of the cholesterol ester transport, and the cholesterol ester-triglyceride exchange systems with slow but progressive hydrolysis of the exchanged triglycerides. The second is abetalipoproteinemia, a disease where acceptors for cholesterol esters are absent from the plasma, although LCAT sctivity and the cholesterol ester transfer protein(s) are present. In this disease we have found that about two thirds of the plasma (and therefore HDL) cholesterol are present in an abnormally light and large-sized HDL subpopulation which we designate $ABL-HDL_2$. The source of cholesterol in this disease is apparently cell membranes. With the accumulation of LCAT derived cholesterol esters and in the absence of acceptors for these molecules, the size of HDL increases above the limits imposed in normals, and the abnormally big $ABL-HDL_2$ is formed. The third example is the lipoprotein system in the rat, an animal species devoid of cholesterol ester transfer and cholesterol ester-triglyceride exchange activities. In this species we have observed that the only HDL population present in plasma is $HDL_2$, and there is total absence of $HDL_3$ (15). These two last examples are compatible with interruption of the cholesterol cholesterol ester cycle at the cholesterol ester transfer site of the cycle.

References

1. Eisenberg S (1980) The origin in plasma of low density and high density lipoproteins. Atherosclerosis V: 146-151
2. Eisenberg S (1980) Plasma lipoproteins interconversion. Ann NY Acad Sci 348: 30-47

3. Eisenberg S, Chajek T, Deckelbaum RJ (1981) The plasma origin of low density and high density lipoproteins. In: Parnow B, Carlson L (eds) Metabolic Risk Factors in Ischemic CV Disease, Raven Press, NY, pp 56-67

4. Deckelbaum RJ, Eisenberg S, Fainaru M, Barenholz Y, Olivecrona T (1979) In vitro production of human plasma very low density lipoprotein-like particles. A model for very low density lipoprotein catabolism. J Biol Chem 254: 6079-6087

5. Chajek T, Eisenberg S (1978) Very low density lipoprotein. Metabolism of phospholipids, cholesterol, and apolipoprotein C in the isolated perfused rat heart. J Clin Invest 61: 1654-1665

6. Perret BP, Eisenberg S, Chajek-Shaul T, Deckelbaum RJ, Olivecrona T (1982) Free cholesterol distribution during in vitro lipolysis of rat plasma very low density lipoprotein. Lack of a role for blood and heart cells. Submitted for publication

7. Glomset JA, Norum KR (1973) The metabolic role of lecithin:cholesterol acyltransferase: Perspective from pathology. Adv Lipid Res 11: 1-65

8. Pattnaik NM, Montes A, Hughes LB, Zilversmit DB (1978) Cholesterol ester exchange protein in human plasma. Isolation and characterization. Biochim Biophys Acta 530: 428-438

9. Barter PJ, Lally JI (1978) The activity of an esterified cholesterol transferring factor in human and rat serum. Biochim Biophys Acta 531: 233-236

10. Nichols AV, Smith L (1965) Effect of very low density lipoprotein on lipid transfer in incubated plasma. J Lipid Res 6: 206-210

11. Nestel PK, Reardon M, Billington T (1979) In vivo transfer of cholesterol esters from high density lipoproteins to very low density lipoproteins in man. Biochim Biophys Acta 573: 403-407

12. Eisenberg S (1982) The plasma cholesterol ester transfer reaction. Evaluation of an experimental system and mechanism of transfer between high density (HDL) and very low density (VLDL) lipoproteins. Submitted for publication

13. Deckelbaum R, Eisenberg S, Oschry Y, Olivecrona T (1982) Reverse modification of human plasma low density lipoprotein toward triglyceride rich precursors: A mechanism for losing excess cholesterol ester. J Biol Chem. In press

14. Deckelbaum RJ, Eisenberg S, Oschry Y, Blum C (1981) Abnormal high density lipoproteins in abetalipoproteinemia. Relevance to normal HDL formation (Abstract) Arteriosclerosis 1: 392

15. Oschry Y, Eisenberg S. Rat plasma lipoproteins. Re-evaluation of a lipoprotein system in an animal devoid of cholesterol ester transfer activity. J Lipid Res. In press

# Pathogenesis of Secondary Hyperlipoproteinemia

G. Middelhoff, W. Därr, and G. Schettler

## 1. Introduction

Secondary hyperlipoproteinemias are those disorders of lipid metabolism, generally characterized by hyerlipoproteinemia (HLP) phenotypes II or IV, which occur in the course of various parenchymal, endocrinological or infectious diseases or during certain nutritional, toxicological or pharmacological manipulations. They are--by definition--reversible with successful treatment of the underlying defect (1). They are equally attractive for clinicians and biochemists for several reasons: 1) they are very common; 2) they provide valuable diagnostic and therapeutical information for the physician; 3) they are potentially atherogenic, at least with chronic diseases such as diabetes mellitus or kidney ailments; 4) secondary HLP represent, because of their inducibility, "natural models" for studies of pathogenesis of lipid and lipoprotein disorders.

Secondary hyperlipoproteinemias are characterized by either quantitative alterations of plasma lipoproteins leading to uncomplicated hyperlipoproteinemias, or by qualitative alterations leading to dyslipoproteinemias with the detection of abnormal lipoproteins in the plasma compartment. Taking these phenomena and the basic physiological aspects of lipid and lipoprotein metabolism into account three basic principles for the pathogenesis of these disorders can be postulated: 1) increased synthesis and/or secretion of normal or abnormal lipoproteins; 2) disturbed catabolism of these lipoproteins; 3) physicochemical mechanisms. A combination of these pathomechanisms is possible.

This paper presents results from our recently performed studies with patients who suffer from different, clinically relevant secondary hyperlipoproteinemias and puts these data into perspective with the relevant literature.

## 2. Methods

Lipoproteins were prepared from EDTA-plasma after an overnight fast by conventional sequential ultracentrifugation (2) or by zonal ultracentrifugation (3). Lipid analyses, were performed with enzymatic test kits or modified micromethods; bile acids (BA) were analyzed either enzymatically or by GLC (4). Apo A-AI and apo-AII were measured by RIA (solid phase method (5)) or by radial immunodiffusion with commercially available plates. Apo-B was determined by RID with commercial plates or by nephelometry (6). The apolipoprotein patterns in the individual lipoprotein fractions were analyzed by densitometry after PAGE or IEF procedures.

Bile acids were incubated with plasma or native lipoproteins using standard procedures (buffer of physiological ionic strength and neutral pH; 37 $^\circ$C; incubation for 60 min.), the resulting complexes were isolated and separated from unbound material by means of ultracentrifugation, dialysis or gel chromatography techniques. Subsequent stoichiometrical analyses were performed as outlined above. The urinary lipids were extracted with the Folch procedure, the urinary lipoproteins were isolated by ultracentrifugation after concentration of the dialyzed material by lyophilization. The recoveries of protein and cholesterol ranged from 85 - 95 %. Electron microscopy was performed with the negative staining technique and 2 % phosphotungstate solutions.

### 3.1. Cholestatic Liver Disease and Hyperlipoproteinemia

In previous studies (7) we had described an abnormal HDL in patients with acute viral hepatitis which was characterized by substantial cholestasis. This HDL showed an abnormal mobility and lipid stainability in lipoprotein electrophoresis due to an altered lipid and apolipoprotein composition: it was triglyceride- and cholesterol-depleted, phospholipid- and bile acid-rich and apo-AI-poor. The normal AI/AII-ratio of total HDL had dropped from around 3.2 to below 2.0. The AI- and AII-values in plasma as measured by RIA were slightly depressed. We also found, after separation of lipoprotein X from the LDL density range, a TG- and BA-rich LDL. These alterations were fully reversible with complete clinical recovery. Subsequent studies showed that similar changes occurred in the acute phase of biliary obstruction. The absolute levels of BA in in plasma in intra- and extrahepatic cholestasis are comparable with similar ratios of di-/trihydroxycholanic acids and allow no differential diagnosis of these two conditions.

In order to define the mechanism of the observed AI-dissociation from native HDL in cholestasis, we performed a systematic in vitro-study by incubating the major physio-logically occuring bile acids (BA) and normal, native HDL. The result of a typical experiment with glycochenodeoxycholate as the ligand is shown in Fig. 1.

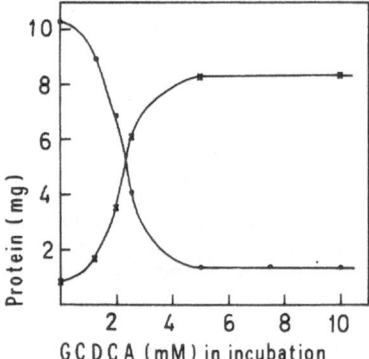

Fig. 1. Incubation of native HDL with glycochenodeoxycholic acid and subsequent isolation of lipoprotein-free material (d 1.21 g/ml - infranate; crosses) from lipoprotein-containing material (d 1.21 g/ml - supernate; circles)

An increase of the BA concentration in the medium leads to a splitting-off of protein from the lipoprotein-containing material (d1.21-supernate). The two curves intersect at that BA concentration (2.3 mM) which corresponds to the critical micellar concentration (CMC) of this BA described by other investigators (8). We analyzed the split off proteins and found that below the CMC of any BA only AI and the C-peptides, together with any contamination of albumin, were lost from HDL. The reduced AI/AII-ratios are summarized for glycocholate in Table 1. The ratios obtained in vitro compare well with those from typical patients. AI can be recovered in the d1.21-infranate in almost lipid-free, BA-rich form. Under these conditions also Lp-X-positive material could be seen. Above the CMC HDL is disrupted as documented by electron microscopy and similar AI/AII-ratios in both compartments.

Preliminary data suggest that AI has a substantially higher affinity towards bile acids than its counterpart AII. A comparison of the different BA established the following order of efficiency as detergents towards HDL: Chenodeoxycholete = deoxycholate ⟩ cholate ⟩ ursodeoxycholate. The taurine conjugates are more effective than the corresponding glycine compounds. We established that all lipoprotein fractions bind BA,

Table 1. AI/AII-ratios in BA-rich HDL

|  | Condition |  | AI/AII |
|---|---|---|---|
| in vitro | Control |  | 3.4 |
|  | GCA | 2.5 mM | 3.12 |
|  | GCA | 4.0 mM | 1.97 |
|  | GCA | 8.0 mM | 1.96 |
| in vivo | Patient I |  | 1.59 |
|  | Patient II |  | 1.97 |
|  | (GCA = glycocholic acid) |  |  |

but with different affinities and that HDL is quantitatively highly important as BA carrier. The binding of BA involves obviously two distinct mechanisms, for both during in vitro-binding and after in vivo-isolation it is possible to remove up to 50 % of the isolated BA by simple dialysis techniques.

In summary, the data clearly stress the importance of physicochemical mechanisms in the genesis of abnormal lipoproteins during cholestasis due to the detergent-like actions of BA in vivo. Similar observations for Lp-X, the abnormal lipoprotein in the LDL-density range in cholestatic liver disease (9), could thus be extended and confirmed. Furthermore, the decline of the CE fraction both in plasma and isolated lipoproteins (data not shown) point to an impairment of the LCAT-reaction as reported (10). The presence of TG-rich LDL indicate a catabolic defect as measured in various parenchymal liver diseases with markedly depressed HTGL-activities (11). Thus, in cholestatic liver disease, various pathophysiological mechanisms are operative simultaneously, leading to profound alterations of the plasma lipoproteins.

## 3.2. Nephrotic Syndrome and Hyperlipoproteinemia

In the animal model of the nephrotic syndrome (NS) substantial losses of lipoproteins via the kidney paired with plasma lipoprotein changes have been described (12). Similar data concerning the human, adult NS are scanty and partly contradictory (13, 14). Pertinent information is desirable if we consider that HDL might possess an anti-atherogenic potential and many authors claim an increased prevalence of premature atherosclerosis in patients suffering from NS. Our study was thus designed to answer these questions.

We measured the type and amount of lipiduria and lipoproteinuria and correlated these data with the plasma lipoproteins. 23 adult patients with stable NS were studied. The leading, bioptically ensured diagnoses of the underlying kidney disease were perimembranous glomerulonephritis (n = 7) and mesangial proliferative glomerulonephritis (n = 6). Due to the daily proteinuria (borderline value 3 g/dl) and the plasma albumin levels (borderline value 4 g/dl) two groups of patients were formed. Their biochemical plasma parameters are summarized in Table 2. Of the patients with the less serious form of the disease 4 suffered from secondary hyperlipoproteinemia phenotype IV. Among the severely ill patients only 1 showed normal plasma lipid levels. Plasma triglycerides are elevated to a comparable amount in both groups. LDL-cholesterol and apo-B show a gradual increase with the severity of disease; thus it was possible to calculate strong negative correlation coefficients between these parameters and plasma albumin (r = -0.82 for LDL-C and r = -0.80 for apo-B). HDL-cholesterol is markedly depressed in both groups, apo-A (and also apo-AI) is almost identical in controls and patients. These values indicate an altered HDL-composition, as shown in Fig. 2: HDL of nephrotic patients is relatively protein-rich and cholesterol- and phospholipid-depleted.

Table 2. Biochemical parameters of patients with nephrotic syndrome

|  |  | Controls (n = 10) | mild NS (n = 10) (M ± SD) | serious NS (n = 13) |
|---|---|---|---|---|
| Triglycerides | mg% | 62 ± 25 | 168 ± 99 | 217 ± 101 |
| Phospholipids | mg% | 246 ± 55 | 270 ± 64 | 374 ± 72 |
| Cholesterol | mg% | 151 ± 20 | 211 ± 35 | 318 ± 69 |
| LDL-cholesterol | mg% | 78 ± 20 | 130 ± 28 | 228 ± 70 |
| Apolipoprotein B | mg% | 55 ± 11 | 110 ± 33 | 167 ± 59 |
| HDL-cholesterol | mg% | 60 ± 6 | 47 ± 11 | 45 ± 15 |
| Apolipoprotein A | mg% | 248 ± 14 | 257 ± 37 | 261 ± 56 |
| Albumin | g% | 5.4 ± 0.5 | 4.4 ± 0.2 | 2.6 ± 0.9 |
| Proteinuria | g/24 h | 0.056 ± 0.043 | 1.87 ± 1.09 | 5.86 ± 2.88 |

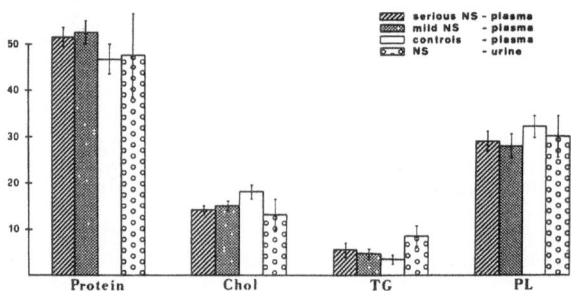

Fig. 2. Compositional analysis (in % of total lipoprotein mass) of HDL from nephrotic patients (plasma and urine) and controls (plasma)

Concerning the urinary excretion of lipids and lipoproteins, the cholesteroluria and phospholipiduria correlate strongly with the proteinuria (r = 0.84 for Chol, r = 0.83 for PL). No apo-B could be detected with immunological procedures in the urine. After conventional ultracentrifugation of the concentrated urine only HDL-like material was detected as validated by compositional analyses (Fig. 2), immunological techniques yielding AI/AII-ratios of 5.1 + 1.7 and electron microscopy of the HDL-subfractions isolated by zonal ultracentrifugation. Free, e.g. not lipoprotein-bound apo-AI was not found in the urine. The absolute amount of apo-HDL in the urine lies between 3 and 72 mg/d with a curvi-linear relationship between proteinuria and lipoproteinuria (r = 0.74).

In summary, taking the plasma pool of apo-HDL of 10 g into account, the renal HDL-loss in human NS seems to be without major pathophysiological significance. This is in contrast to the animal model, the aminoglycoside nephrosis of the rat (12). HDL is not substantially altered in its composition and physicochemical properties in the kidney and during urinary passage. An increased synthesis of lipoproteins and disturbances of the catabolism of the TG-rich lipoproteins in nephrotic patients have been described (15, 16). Our finding of increased VLDL and HDL particle numbers and an abnormal, TG-rich LDL (data not shown) confirm these reports. Thus, as in the case of cholestatic liver disease, a combination of several factors seems to be involved in the pathogenesis of secondary hyperlipoproteinemia in nephrosis.

### 3.3. Obesity and Hyperlipoproteinemia

Obesity is associated with various metabolic disturbances including a high prevalence of hyperlipoproteinemia, in general phenotype IV. Many authors define this disorder of lipid metabolism as secondary in nature. The underlying molecular defects, however, are not known. In an ongoing clinical study we investigate the effect of weight reduction by total fasting under metabolic ward conditions. We are specifically interested how plasma lipoproteins in grossly obese patients with combined hyperlipoproteinemia (phenotype IV) are affected. So far 3 patients have completed the trial. Concomitant with a mean weight loss of 10 % within 4 weeks plasma lipid levels normalized (mean values: TG from 439 to 145, Chol from 290 to 220 mg/dl), mean LDL-Chol from 174 to 148 mg/dl, and HDL-Chol from 30 to 24 mg/dl. The LDL-/HDL-ratio deteriorated from 5.8 to 6.1 (normal value 1.55) reflecting the abnormal and non-correctable cholesterol distribution over the various lipoprotein fractions in these patients. In tandem with the drop of HDL-chol, the apo-AI- and apo AII-levels in plasma decreased. A stoichiometrical analysis of HDL before and after weight reduction confirmed that its composition did not change. This was validated by zonal centrifugation analysis. At the beginning of the study, when phenotype IV is still present, basically no $HDL_2$ can be detected in the plasma. With successful weight reduction and complete normalization of plasma lipid levels HDL drops, but a normal $HDL_2$-$HDL_3$-pattern does not reappear. Data about a longer follow-up of these patients is still lacking. The activity of the lipolytic enzymes was neither measured in the plasma compartment nor in the adipose tissue. The fact that the abnormal cholesterol distribution cannot be normalized in obese hyperlipoproteinemic patients during "successful" weight reduction points to some underlying metabolic or structural defect independent of the energy balance of these subjects and could be of possible primary importance. This conclusion is supported by recent data from Söbris et al. (17) who detected no decrease of the highly elevated adipose tissue lipase activity after successful treatment of overweight, hyperlipoproteinemic patients.

In summary, hyperlipoproteinemia in at least some obese patients is characterized by a disturbed cholesterol distribution with high LDL and low HDL and mainly $HDL_2$ levels. An increased synthesis of VLDL in the liver and an impaired catabolism of TG-rich lipoproteins has been found by other investigators. Thus, as for the two other forms of secondary hyperlipoproteinemia described above, a multifactorial defect is operative in the pathogenesis of overt hyperlipidemia in obesity. A reassessment of this disturbance as a secondary form of hyperlipoproteinemia has to be considered on the basis of the presented data.

### 4. Conclusions

A detailed study of patients with various forms of secondary hyperlipoproteinemia reveals that alterations of plasma lipoproteins reflect multiple defects in the regulation of lipid metabolism as well as a multifactorial pathogenesis of these disturbances. An increased synthesis of normal and/or abnormal lipoproteins may coincide with disturbances of the catabolism of these particles due to alterations of the enzyme systems. This again, might be aggravated by certain physicochemical mechanisms not operative under normal conditions. The importance of the lipoproteins as carriers of certain substrates or substances is stressed by the data presented. Finally, a detailed analysis of the mechanisms involved might lead to a complete reassessment of the disease under study. The clinical implications of these findings stem from the obvious need to treat those groups of patients who have secondary hyperlipoproteinemias characterized by a high prevalence of premature atherosclerosis.

### References

1. Klose G, Windler E, Greten H (1982) Befunde zur Pathogenese sekundärer Hyperlipoproteinämien. In: Fortschritte in der Inneren Medizin, Kommerell B, Hahn P, Kübler W, Mörl H, Weber E (ed) Springer-Verlag Berlin Heidelberg New York,

p. 170-177

2. Havel RJ, Eder HA, Bragdon JH (1955) Distribution and chemical composition of ultracentrifugally separated lipoproteins in human serum. J Clin Invest 34: 1345-1354

3. Patsch JR, Gotto AM (1979) Separation and analysis of HDL subclasses by zonal ultracentrifugation. In: Report of the High Density Lipoprotein Methodology Workshop. Lippel K (ed) NIH Publ. 79-1661: 310-324

4. Fröhling W, Stiehl A (1976) Bile salt glucuronides: Identification and quantitative analysis in the urine of patients with cholestasis. Europ J Clin Invest 6: 67-74

5. Riesen W, Mordasini R, Middelhoff G (1978) Quantitation of the two major apoproteins of human high density lipoproteins by solid phase radioimmunoassay. FEBS Letters 91: 35

6. Heuck CC, Middelhoff G (1978) Vergleichende Untersuchung der Bestimmung von Apolipoprotein B. Fresenius Z Anal Chem 290: 127-128

7. Middelhoff G, Mordasini R, Stiehl A, Greten H (1979) A bile-acid-rich high density lipoprotein (HDL) in acute hepatitis. Scand J Gastroent 14: 267-272

8. Igimi H, Carey MC (1980) pH-solubility relations of chenodeoxycholic and ursodeoxycholic acids: physical-chemical basis for dissimilar solution and membrane phenomena. J Lipid Res 21: 72-90

9. Manzato E, Fellin R, Baggio G, Walch S, Neubeck W, Seidel D (1976) Formation of lipoprotein-X. Its relationship to bile compounds. J Clin Invest 57: 1248-1260

10. Sabesin SM, Hawkins HL, Kuiken L, Ragland JB (1977) Abnormal plasma lipoproteins and lecithin-cholesterol acyltransferase deficiency in alcoholic liver disease. Gastroenterology 72: 510-518

11. Klose G, Windelband J, Weizel A, Greten H (1977) Secondary hypertriglyceridemia in patients with parenchymal liver disease. Europ J Clin Invest 7: 557-562

12. Gherardi E, Vecchia L, Calandra S (1980) Experimental nephrotic syndrome in the rat induced by puromycin aminonucleoside, plasma and urinary lipoprotein. Exp Mol Pathol 32: 128

13. DeMendoza SG, Kashyap ML, Chen CJ, Lutmo RF (1976) High density lipoproteins in nephrotic syndrome. Metabolism 25: 1143

14. Felts JM, Mayerle JA (1975) Urinary loss of plasma high density lipoprotein - a possible cause of hyperlipidemia of the nephrotic syndrome. Circulation 50: III

15. Oetliker O, Mordasini R, Lütschg J, Riesen W (1980) Lipoprotein metabolism in nephrotic syndrome in childhood. Pediat Res 14: 64

16. Kekki M, Nikkilä E (1971) Plasma triglyceride metabolism in adult nephrotic syndrome Europ J Clin Invest 1: 345

17. Söbris R, Petersson BG, Nilsson-Ehle P (1981) Effects of weight reduction on plasma lipoproteins and adipose tissue metabolism in obese subjects. Europ J Clin Invest 11: 491-498

# Surface Organization of the Apolipoproteins of Plasma High Density Lipoproteins and Relevance to Functions

A. M. Scanu and C. Edelstein

Little is known on the organization of the apolipoproteins on the plasma high density lipoproteins (HDL) surface and on the factors controlling the mass distribution of these apolipoproteins and their role in HDL structure and function. In a previous study using as a model system canine HDL, we showed that apo A-II

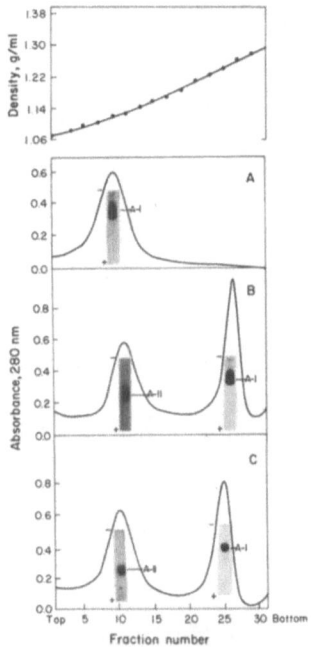

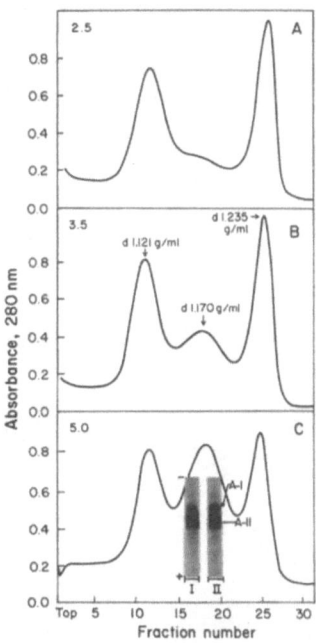

Fig. 1. Density gradient ultracentrifugal profiles of canine HDL (A) and of products obtained upon incubation of this lipoprotein with double-(B) and single-chain (C) apo A-II at the initial apo A-II apo A-I weight ratio of 1.3. The incubations were carried out at room temperature for 30 minutes in 0.15 M NaBr, 0.05% EDTA, pH 8.0 and the products separated by density gradient centrifugation in NaBr solutions (d 1.078-1.298 g/ml) for 66 hours at 14°C. The insets show SDS gel patterns of the peaks which were recorded at 280 nm. The top profile is a plot of the fraction number vs density (g/ml) of the gradient formed during centrifugation

Fig. 2. Density gradient profiles of the products obtained upon incubation of canine HDL with excess amounts of double-chain apo A-II. (A) Apo A-II:HDL apo A-I weight ratio, 2.5; (B) ratio, 3.5; (C) ratio, 5. The inset shows SDS gel patterns of the combined fractions identified by bars. Incubations and centrifugal procedures were as in Fig. 1

534

because of its greater affinity for the hydrophilic-hydrophobic interface, can
displace apo A-I from the HDL surface in a process which is not attended by a
loss of lipids (1). We have now experimental evidence that the monomeric form
of apo A-II, either reduced and carboxymethylated (RCM) human apo A-II or rhesus
apo A-II, exhibit the same action. Fig. 1 shows the density gradient ultracentrifugation profile of an incubated mixture of canine HDL and human lipid-free apo
A-II (B) or its monomeric counterpart (RCM apo A-II) (C). In this example the
experimental conditions were chosen so that the amount of human apo A-II in the
system was just enough to occupy the surface of canine HDL according to previous
theoretical considerations (2,3). It is evident that in both cases at the end
of the centrifugal run all of the apo A-II banded in the HDL region whereas the
displaced apo A-I was near the bottom of the gradient.

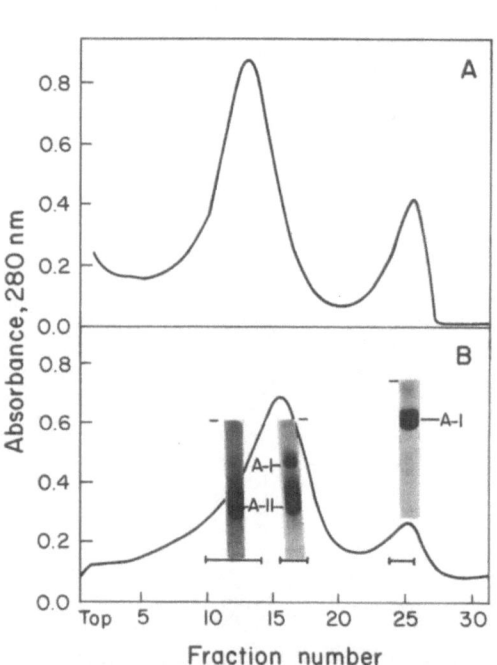

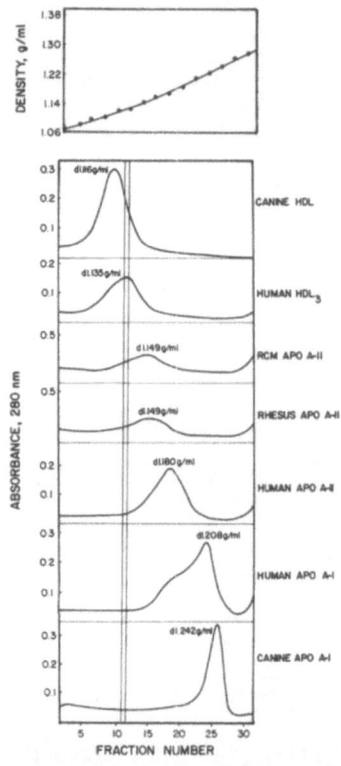

Fig. 3. Density gradient profiles of the
products obtained after incubation of
canine HDL with excess amounts of single-
chain (RCM) apo A-II. (A) apo A-II:HDL
apo A-I weight ratio, 2.5; (B) ratio, 5.0.
The inset shows SDS gel patterns of the
pooled fractions within bars. Identical
results were obtained when rhesus single-
chain apo A-II was used. Experimental
conditions were the same as in Fig. 1

Fig. 4. Density gradient ultracentrifugation profile of human HDL$_3$
and various forms of apo A-I and
apo A-II. The gradient conditions
were the same as described in legend
to Fig. 1. The top profile shows a
plot of the fraction number vs density (g/ml) of the NaBr density
gradient formed during centrifugation

In later studies, we have examined the effect of adding various amounts of apo
A-II in excess of the estimated maximal occupancy of this apoprotein for the HDL
surface (4). In such instances, three peaks were resolved, one corresponding to
HDL, one representing lipid free apo A-I and an intermediate one containing a
lipid free apo A-I-apo A-II complex as determined by chemical, immunochemical
and electrophoretic analysis. The intermediate peak increased as the apo A-II:
HDL ratio increased. Rather surprising was the light density of this intermed-

iate peak (d 1.170 g/ml) in view of the fact that it did not contain lipids. When RCM apo A-II (a single chain polypeptide) replaced double chain human apo A-II in the system, the intermediate peak appeared as a shoulder of the main HDL peak and contained both apo A-I and apo A-II in a complex separable by column chromatography. The density of this complex was lighter than that involving the double-chain apo A-II. We suspected that in the high salt gradient used, apo A-II (double-chain), apo A-II (single-chain) and apo A-I sedimented at a different rate. To corroborate these assumptions, lipid-free human and canine apo A-I, human and rhesus apo A-II as well as RCM human apo A-II, were spun in the same gradient used for the separation of the lipoprotein-apoprotein mixture. After 66 hours, the apoproteins occupied a position in the gradient which was proportional to their molecular weight. The one having the smaller mass sedimented at a slower rate (Fig. 4). To assess whether equilibrium conditions were reached, we placed a mixture of human HDL$_3$ and human apo A-II at different positions in the gradient (see arrows in Fig. 5). After 66 hours, the banding of

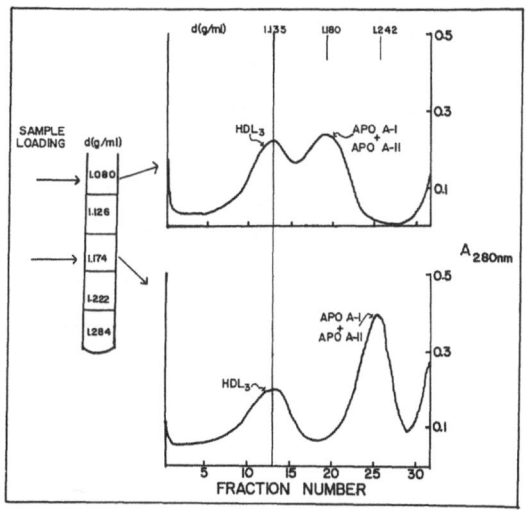

Fig. 5. Density gradient ultracentrifugation profile of a mixture of human HDL$_3$ and human apo A-II. Effect of position of sample loading. Human HDL$_3$ (0.5 mg) was incubated for 30 minutes at room temperature with human apo A-II (1 mg) and the products resolved by density gradient centrifugation as in Figure 1. After 66 hours of centrifugation, the gradient position of the HDL band is identical in both panels, but not that of the apo A-I:apo A-II complex

HDL$_3$ was uneffected by the initial positioning of sample loading on the gradient, whereas the band corresponding to the apo A-I:apo A-II complex was markedly affected indicating that equilibrium conditions for these apoproteins had not been reached. We attribute this phenomenon to a preferential hydration of the apoproteins in the salt medium used and in particular apo A-II or any complex involving this apoprotein. Of significance is the observation that under the ultracentrifugal conditions used in our studies, the banding of the apo A-II monomer coincided with that of HDL.

The above studies invite several comments. In the first place, apo A-II effectively competes with apo A-I for the HDL surface to the point that it becomes the sole component of it. After surface saturation is reached, HDL no longer takes up apo A-II; its excess remains in solution and forms a mixed complex with the displaced apo A-I in stoichiometries which appear to be controlled by the differences in affinity between apo A-II and apo A-I for the HDL surface and by their intrinsic capacity to self associate in solution. When studied in high salts, these apoproteins undergo preferential hydration, a process which impairs their sedimentation behavior in a gravitational field to the extent that in a salt gradient such as that used in our studies, the position of the apo A-II monomer approximates that of the HDL particles. From the above, it is apparent that the occupancy and mass ratios of the two major apoproteins of HDL are influenced by the properties of these apoproteins in solutions and by their affinity for the hydrophilic-hydrophobic surface. An extrapolation of these findings to physiological conditions can only be entertained on a speculative basis. The competition of apo A-II vs apo A-I at the HDL surface has been shown to be a factor in the regulation of the in vitro activity of the enzyme lecithin-cholesterol acyltransferase owing to the fact that apo A-II removes from the lipoprotein surface apo A-I (5,6) which specifically activates this enzyme. The occurence of a complex between apo A-I and apo A-II when both of these apoproteins are free in solution may be attributed to a role played by apo A-I in facilitating the solubility of apo A-II in plasma and its metabolism. The mass ratio between apo A-I and apo A-II in HDL may also have relevance to cell function. Studies from this laboratory have shown that when HDL is incubated in vitro with leukocytes, apo A-II but not apo A-I undergoes extensive hydrolysis, resulting in an HDL particle with different structural properties and likely function (7,8).

To sum up, we have obtained experimental evidence that apo A-I and apo A-II compete against each other at the hydrophilic-hydrophobic interface but associate with each other when in solution. It is our belief that these physico-chemical events may have relevance to biological processes involving the movement of apoproteins from the HDL surface to other amphiphilic surfaces or to an aqueous environment. Our studies have also unraveled a previously unrecognized hydrodynamic behavior of these apoproteins in high salt solutions probably related to their high degree of hydration. It follows that isopycnic banding conditions must be carefully checked in studies involving density gradient ultracentrifugation of lipoproteins and apolipoproteins. This also points at the need for utilizing complementary techniques in these systems.

The work in the Authors' laboratory was supported by USPHS Grant HL 18577.

## References

1. Lagocki PA, Scanu AM (1980) In vitro modulation of the apolipoprotein composition of high density lipoproteins: displacement of apolipoprotein A-I from HDL by apolipoprotein A-II. J Biol Chem 255: 3701-3706
2. Shen BW, Scanu AM, Kezdy FJ (1977) The structure of human serum lipoproteins inferred from compositional analyses. Proc Natl Acad Sci 74: 837-841
3. Edelstein C, Kezdy FJ, Scanu AM, Shen BW (1979) Apolipoproteins and the structural organizationof plasma lipoproteins: human plasma high density lipoprotein-3. J Lip Res 20: 143-153
4. Edelstein C, Halari M, Scanu AM (1982) On the mechanism of the displacement of apo A-I and apo A-II from the high density lipoprotein surface: effect of concentration and molecular forms of apo A-II. J Biol Chem (in press)
5. Chung J, Abano D, Fless G, Scanu AM (1979) Isolation, properties and mechanism of in vitro action of lecithin cholesterol acyltransferase. J Biol Chem 254: 7456-7464
6. Scanu AM, Lagocki P, Chung J (1980) Effect of apolipoprotein A-II on the structural of high density lipoproteins: relationship to the activity of lecithin cholesterol acyltransferase in vitro. Proc N Y Acad Sci 348: 160-173
7. Ritter MC, Scanu AM (1980) Structural changes in human serum high density lipoprotein-3 attending incubation with blood leukocytes. J Biol Chem 255: 3763-3769
8. Polacek D, Scanu AM (1982) Polymorphonuclear cells from human peripheral blood but not lymphocytes, monocytes nor monocyte-derived macrophages cause the in vitro hydrolysis of apolipoprotein A-II of serum high density lipoproteins. Trans Assoc Amer Physicians (in press)

# Receptor Interactions of Human Apolipoprotein E

K. H. Weisgraber, S. C. Rall, Jr., T. L. Innerarity, and R. W. Mahley

## Introduction

Apolipoprotein E (apo-E) is a 34,000 to 37,000 molecular weight protein that occurs in several classes of plasma lipoproteins in humans and in a variety of animals. This apoprotein plays a central role in plasma cholesterol transport and metabolism (1). It is one of the apoproteins responsible for determining lipoprotein interaction with the apo-B,E (LDL) receptor on fibroblasts and other peripheral cells (2,3). In addition, apo-E appears to be one of the key proteins mediating lipoprotein recognition and uptake by hepatic receptors (4,5).

Apoprotein E is a heterogeneous protein displaying several immunochemically related isoforms on isoelectric focusing gels. These isoforms are commonly designated as E1, E2, E3, and E4, and they differ progressively from E1 to E4 by a single positive charge. According to the currently accepted genetic model, the apo-E heterogeneity results from a combination of two independent factors: 1) heritable alterations in the protein, resulting from three independent alleles acting at a single gene locus, and 2) post-translational glycosylation of the major isoforms with the addition of one or more negatively charged sialic acid residues (6). Each allele codes for a major isoform — i.e., E2, E3, or E4. Thus, the model predicts three homozygous (E2/E2, E3/E3, E4/E4) and three heterozygous (E2/E3, E2/E4, E3/E4) phenotypes. In a given individual, the minor isoforms, including E1, arise from post-translational glycosylation of one of the major isoforms.

The pathological lipid disorder, Type III hyperlipoproteinemia (primary dysbetalipoproteinemia), has been associated with subjects phenotypically homozygous for apo-E2 (6,7,8). A characteristic feature of this disorder is impaired remnant clearance, which may result from the defective binding ability of apo-E2 (9,10). To determine if structural differences in the apo-E molecule are related to impaired function, we initiated studies of the structure-function relationships of apo-E with regard to receptor interaction.

## Structure-Function Relationships

By carrying out an amino acid sequence analysis, we have determined that the three major isoforms of apo-E differ only in their cysteine and arginine contents, with E2, E3, and E4 containing 2, 1, and 0 residues of cysteine per mole, respectively. The cysteine/arginine interchanges occur at two sites in the E molecule, site A (residue 112) and site B (residue 158), and are responsible for the charge differences between the major isoforms (Fig. 1). Other than at these sites, the proteins are identical. These results establish that the genetic influence on apo-E is at the level of the structural gene (11,12).

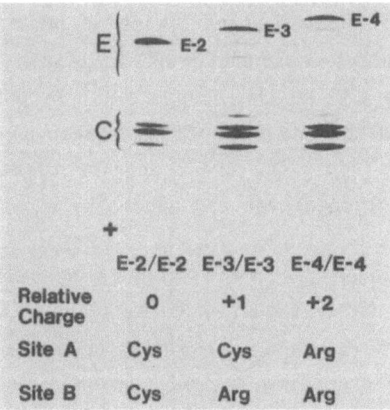

Fig. 1. Isoelectric focusing on polyacrylamide gels of the VLDL from subjects homozygous for apo-E2, E3, and E4. A summary of the amino acid substitutions that occur in three forms at site A (residue 112) and site B (residue 158) and the effect of these substitutions on the relative charge differences among the three forms of apo-E is shown in the table below the gels

In order to determine the effect of these amino acid interchanges on apo-E receptor interactions, we examined the ability of various apo-E·phospholipid complexes to compete with $^{125}$I-labeled LDL ($^{125}$I-LDL) for receptor sites on cultured fibroblasts. These studies demonstrated that both apo-E4 and apo-E3 competed effectively and equally in displacing LDL from receptors, indicating that the cysteine/arginine interchange at residue 112 (site A, Fig. 1) had no effect on receptor interaction. In marked contrast, the apo-E2 from the Type III hyperlipoproteinemic subject D.R., which was used for the sequence analysis, was markedly defective in its ability to displace LDL (∿1% of the ability of E3 or E4).  This demonstrated that the cysteine/arginine interchange at residue 158 (site B, Fig. 1) had a profound effect on receptor binding (10).  The importance of the positive charge at residue 158 was established using β-mercaptoethylamine (cysteamine).  This reagent converts neutral cysteine residues to positively charged lysine analogues via disulfide bond formation.  Cysteamine treatment of apo-E2 resulted in a 10- to 20-fold increase in binding activity.  However, cysteamine treatment of E3 and E4 had no effect on receptor binding.

The situation with Type III apo-E2 is more complicated.  Although several E3 preparations from different subjects showed essentially identical binding activity, the apo-E2 from Type III subjects was not equally defective (13). Examination of apo-E2 preparations from a number of Type III subjects disclosed a heterogeneity in binding activity ranging from 1 to 50% of the E3 activity. Results of the analysis of three subjects (D.R., J.T., and W.M.) are illustrated in Fig. 2.  D.R. served as the source of apo-E2 on which the total sequence was determined.  It is important to note that although J.T. and W.M. apo-E2 showed considerable binding activity, it was still deficient relative to E3.  In addition, cysteamine treatment resulted in increased receptor binding.  Partial sequence analysis of W.M. apo-E revealed a structural heterogeneity within the E2/2 phenotype, resulting from a new, fourth form of apo-E and a new apo-E allele ( ε 2*) (14).  W.M. apo-E2 differed from D.R. apo-E2 in that one of the cysteine/arginine substitutions was at a new site, residue 145 (Table I).  At residue 112, the apo-E from both subjects had cysteine.

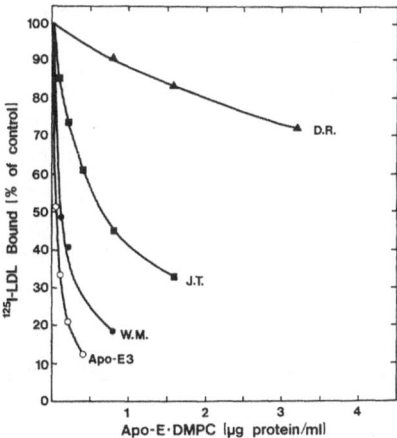

<u>Fig. 2.</u>  Ability of apo-E·DMPC complexes to compete with human [125]I-LDL for binding to normal human fibroblasts.  Complexes were prepared from the apo-E of subjects D.R. (▲), J.T. (■), W.M. (●), and from the apo-E of a subject homozygous for apo-E3 (○).  (Reproduced with permission from Ref. 14.)

Table I. Structural relationship of the four forms of apo-E

| Subject | Allele | Residue 112 | Residue 145 | Residue 158 |
|---------|--------|-------------|-------------|-------------|
| D.R.(E2/2) | $\epsilon 2$ | cysteine | arginine | cysteine |
| W.M.(E2/2) | $\epsilon 2\ast$ | cysteine | cysteine | arginine |
| E3/3 | $\epsilon 3$ | cysteine | arginine | arginine |
| E4/4 | $\epsilon 4$ | arginine | arginine | arginine |

Analysis of the apo-E2 from subject J.T. revealed that although he was phenotypically an E2 homozygote, his apo-E was approximately an equal mixture of both the D.R. and W.M. apo-E2 forms. Thus, J.T. was genotypically a heterogyzote.

The sequence data from the apo-E2 of the three Type III subjects then correlates with the binding activity heterogeneity (Fig. 2). Subject D.R., who was genotypically homozygous for the $\epsilon 2$ allele, had the most defective apo-E2 with respect to binding activity ($\sim$1% of the activity of E3). Subject W.M., who was genotypically homozygous for the $\epsilon 2\ast$ allele, had less defective apo-E2 ($\sim$50% of the activity of E3). The apo-E2 of J.T., who was genotypically heterozygous with one $\epsilon 2$ (D.R.) and one $\epsilon 2\ast$ (W.M.) allele, demonstrated binding activity intermediate between that of D.R. and W.M. apo-E2 ($\sim$10% of E3). Thus, it appears that the cysteine for arginine substitution at residue 158 was more deleterious than the substitution at residue 145. These results require modification of the genetic model for apo-E to include a fourth apo-E allele ( $\epsilon 2\ast$), which specifies for apo-E2$^{\ast}$ (14).

Previously, we established that a limited number of arginine and lysine residues are involved in the interaction between the B and E apoproteins and the apo-B,E receptor (15,16). Visual inspection of the amino acid sequence of apo-E reveals that there is a relatively high concentration of basic residues located near the center of the molecule: 35% of the lysine and arginine residues occur between residues 134 and 191, a region that represents only 19% of the total sequence (Table II).

Table II. Basic region of apo-E3

$^{134}$Arg-Val-Arg-Leu-Ala-Ser-His-Leu-Arg-Lys-Leu-Arg-Lys-Arg-Leu-Leu-Arg-Asp$^{151}$

$^{152}$Ala-Asp-Asp-Leu-Gln-Lys-Arg-Leu-Ala-Val-Tyr-Gln-Ala-Gly-Ala-Arg-Glu-Gly$^{169}$

$^{170}$Ala-Glu-Arg-Gly-Leu-Ser-Ala-Leu-Arg-Glu-Arg-Leu-Gly-Pro-Leu-Val-Glu-Gln$^{187}$

$^{188}$Gly-Arg-Val-Arg$^{191}$

It is noteworthy that the two cysteine for arginine substitutions that had a deleterious effect on receptor binding activity also occur in this area of the molecule — at residue 145 (E2*) and residue 158 (E2). The cysteine/arginine interchange that occurs at residue 112 lies outside this region and does not affect binding activity.

In summary, several lines of evidence strongly suggest that there is a specific region of apo-E involved in the interaction between apo-E and the apo-B,E (LDL) receptor. This region of the molecule is enriched in lysine and arginine residues and contains the cysteine for arginine substitution sites that have a deleterious effect on receptor activity.

Acknowledgements   The authors wish to thank Dr. Thomas P. Bersot for obtaining plasma from patients and volunteers. We wish to acknowledge the excellent technical assistance of Ms. Kay Arnold, Mr. Reed Harris, Ms. Jana Seymour, and Mr. David Begert. In addition, we wish to thank Mr. Russell Levine for editorial assistance, Mr. Richard Wolfe for manuscript preparation, and Ms. Gwen Watson for illustrations.

## References

1.   Mahley RW (1978) Alterations in plasma lipoproteins induced by cholesterol feeding in animals including man. In: Dietschy JM, Gotto AM Jr, Ontko JA (eds) Disturbances in Lipid and Lipoprotein Metabolism. American Physiological Society, Bethesda, MD, pp 181-197
2.   Innerarity TL, Mahley RW (1978) Enhanced binding by cultured human fibroblasts of apo-E-containing lipoproteins as compared with low density lipoproteins. Biochemistry 17: 1440-1447
3.   Mahley RW, Innerarity TL (1978) Properties of lipoproteins responsible for high affinity binding to cell surface receptors of fibroblasts and smooth muscle cells. In: Kritchevsky D, Paoletti R, Holmes WL (eds) Drugs, Lipid Metabolism, and Atherosclerosis. Plenum Press, New York, NY, pp 99-127
4.   Sherrill BC, Innerarity TL, Mahley RW (1980) Rapid hepatic clearance of the canine lipoproteins containing only the E apoprotein by a high affinity receptor. Identity with the chylomicron remnant transport process. J Biol Chem 255: 1804-1807
5.   Hui DY, Innerarity TL, Mahley RW (1981) Lipoprotein binding to canine hepatic membranes: Metabolically distinct apo-E and apo-B,E receptors. J Biol Chem 256: 5646-5655

6.   Zannis VI, Breslow JL (1981) Human very low density lipoprotein apolipopro-
     tein E isoprotein polymorphism is explained by genetic variation and post-
     translational modification. Biochemistry 20: 1033-1041

7.   Utermann G, Jaeschke M, Menzel J (1975) Familial hyperlipoproteinemia Type
     III: Deficiency of a specific apolipoprotein (apoE-III) in the very-low-
     density lipoproteins. FEBS Lett 56: 353-355

8.   Pagnan A, Havel RJ, Kane JP, Kotite L (1977) Characterization of human very
     low density lipoproteins containing two electrophoretic populations: Dou-
     ble pre-beta lipoproteinemia and primary dysbetalipoproteinemia. J Lipid
     Res 18: 613-622

9.   Havel RJ, Chao Y-S, Windler EE, Kotite L, Guo LSS (1980) Isoprotein speci-
     ficity in the hepatic uptake of apolipoprotein E and the pathogenesis of
     familial dysbetalipoproteinemia. Proc Natl Acad Sci USA 77: 4349-4353

10.  Weisgraber KH, Innerarity TL, Mahley RW (1982) Abnormal lipoprotein recep-
     tor-binding activity of the human E apoprotein due to cysteine-arginine
     interchange at a single site. J Biol Chem 25: 2518-2521

11.  Weisgraber KH, Rall SC Jr, Mahley RW (1981) Human E apoprotein heterogen-
     eity: Cysteine-arginine interchanges in the amino acid sequence of the
     apo-E isoforms. J Biol Chem 256: 9077-9083

12.  Rall SC Jr, Weisgraber KH, Mahley RW (1982) Human apolipoprotein E: The
     complete amino acid sequence. J Biol Chem 257: 4171-4178

13.  Schneider WJ, Kovanen PT, Brown MS, Goldstein JL, Utermann G, Weber W,
     Havel RJ, Kotite L, Kane JP, Innerarity TL, Mahley RW (1981) Familial dys-
     betalipoproteinemia: Abnormal binding of mutant apoprotein E to low dens-
     ity lipoprotein receptors of human fibroblasts and membranes from liver and
     adrenal of rats, rabbits, and cows. J Clin Invest 68: 1075-1085

14.  Rall SC Jr, Weisgraber KH, Innerarity TL, Mahley RW (1982) Structural basis
     for receptor-binding heterogeneity of apolipoprotein E from Type III hyper-
     lipoproteinemic subjects. Proc Natl Acad Sci USA: In press

15.  Mahley RW, Innerarity TL, Pitas RE, Weisgraber KH, Brown JH, Gross E (1977)
     Inhibition of lipoprotein binding to cell surface receptors of fibroblasts
     following selective modification of arginyl residues in arginine-rich and B
     apoproteins. J Biol Chem 252: 7279-7287

16.  Weisgraber KH, Innerarity TL, Mahley RW (1978) Role of the lysine residues
     of plasma lipoproteins in high affinity binding to cell surface receptors
     on human fibroblasts. J Biol Chem 253: 9053-9062

# Effects of Hormones on Plasma Lipoprotein Concentrations

B. M. Wolfe

Hormonal regulation of lipoprotein transport in the blood continues to intrigue scientific investigators. I shall briefly review some aspects of current knowledge of the subject. An influence of sex hormones on lipoproteins was noted by Russ, Eder and Barr. They reported that plasma from young women contains more alpha-lipoprotein, but less beta-lipoprotein than men of comparable age (1). Subsequent studies have shown that a variety of both natural and synthetic estrogens in therapeutic doses influence lipoprotein concentrations.

Table 1. Effects of Estrogens on Serum Lipoprotein Levels

| Hormone | Experimental Group | Lipoprotein Class | Effect | Reference |
|---|---|---|---|---|
| Estradiol (2 mg/day) | Postmenopausal women | HDL-cholesterol | Increase 10-15% | Wallentin *et al* (2) |
| Estradiol (2 mg/day) | Postmenopausal hypercholester-olemic women | LDL-cholesterol | Decrease 22% | Tikkanen *et al* (3) |
| Conjugated equine estrogens (1.25 mg/day) | Postmenopausal women | VLDL-triglycerides | Increase 59% with doubling production | Glueck *et al* (4) |
| Ethinyl-estradiol (20 µg/day) | Oöphorectomized women | VLDL-triglycerides | Increase | Gustafson *et al* (5) |

Administration of the major human natural estrogen 17 β-estradiol increases serum high density lipoproteins (HDL), but lowers low density lipoproteins (LDL) in postmenopausal women. Glueck *et al* have shown that the elevation of total triglycerides and very low density (VLDL)-triglycerides induced in postmenopausal women by conjugated equine estrogens can be explained by the doubling of VLDL production (4). Very small amounts of ethinyl-estradiol (20 µg/day) have been reported to elevate triglycerides in oöphorectomized women; however, the progestin norethindrone quickly abolishes the increment in triglycerides (5).

Bradley *et al* have drawn attention to the reduction of HDL-cholesterol induced by norethindrone acetate (6). Cheng, in our laboratory, has examined the effects of low dose norethindrone acetate (2.5 mg/daily for 3 weeks) in two normolipidemic postmenopausal women (7). Compared to control values obtained from the same subject either before or 5 weeks after the period of norethindrone acetate treatment, fasting concentrations of HDL-cholesterol fell 19-43%, LDL-cholesterol fell 7-22%, total cholesterol fell 12-16%, and total triglycerides fell 16-40%. Turnover of [$^3$H]-VLDL-triglycerides was estimated at the end of each treatment and control period after pulse-injection of [2-$^3$H]glycerol. These studies were done under steady state conditions during

544

the last 12 hours of a 16-hour isocaloric intravenous infusion of glucose (1100 kcalories/m$^2$ body surface/day).  In this glucose-fed state
the concentration of plasma VLDL-triglycerides was 42-83% lower during norethindrone acetate treatment versus control values in the same
subject.  The fall in plasma VLDL-triglycerides was attributable to a
26-79% decrease in VLDL-triglyceride production.  In similar studies
in the glucose-fed state in miniature swine, we found that comparable
doses of norethindrone acetate decreased the mean VLDL-triglyceride
concentration by 42%.  The hypolipemic effect of norethindrone acetate
was attributable to a 60% decrease in hepatic triglyceride secretion
(8).

Table 2. Effects of Various Progestins on Serum Lipoprotein Levels

| Hormone | Experimental Group | Lipoprotein or lipid class | Effect | Reference |
|---|---|---|---|---|
| Norethindrone acetate (5 mg/day) | Women | HDL-cholesterol | Decrease 19-43% | Bradley et al (6) |
| Norethindrone acetate (100 µg/kg body wt$^{0.75}$/day) | Miniature swine | VLDL-triglycerides | Decrease 42% with 60% fall in production | Wolfe & Grace (8) |
| Norgestrel (75 µg/day) | Premenopausal women | Total triglycerides | Decrease 22% | Spellacy et al (9) |
| Norgestrel (75 µg/day) | Premenopausal women | Total cholesterol | Decrease 10% | Eckstein et al (10) |
| D-norgestrel (4 µg/kg body wt$^{0.75}$/day) | Female rats | VLDL-triglycerides | Decrease 20% with decrease in hepatic micro-somal GPAT | Khokha & Wolfe (11) |

Norgestrel is another widely used progestin.  It is more potent on a
weight basis than norethindrone acetate.  In conventional doses employed for contraceptive purposes, norgestrel has been reported to
lower both serum triglycerides (9) and cholesterol (10).  Khokha and
Wolfe (11) have examined the action of the active isomer D-norgestrel
in female rats receiving this steroid for 14 days and have observed
that VLDL-triglycerides were 20% lower in D-norgestrel-treated rats
than in matched controls.  The fall in serum VLDL-triglycerides corr-
esponded to a significant (27%) decrease in hepatic microsomal glycerol phosphate acyltransferase (GPAT) in the livers of rats receiving
D-norgestrel.  Thus the triglyceride- and HDL-lowering effects of progestins contrast markedly with those of estrogens.

Although the relationship of hypothyroidism to the genesis of clinical
coronary artery disease remains controversial, the effects of thyroid
hormones on lipoprotein levels are becoming increasingly well-defined.
Walton et al demonstrated that hyperthyroidism lowered LDL protein-
levels by increasing catabolism (12).  Abrams and Grundy found that
both LDL- and HDL-cholesterol were lower in thyrotoxic versus euthyroid
patients, despite increased cholesterol synthesis in the latter (13).
Likewise, triglyceride levels in thyrotoxic patients are decreased as
compared to values in the same subject when euthyroid (14).  Lack of
thyroid hormone leads to elevation of LDL-cholesterol in association
with decreased fecal neutral steroid excretion (13).  LDL protein

catabolism is reduced in both hypothyroid human subjects (12) and
rats (15). The elevated VLDL levels in hypothyroidism are attributable to impaired removal, because VLDL transport decreases (16).
Hypothyroidism appears to diminish catabolism of both VLDL and LDL.

Table 3. Effects of Thyroid Hormones on Lipoprotein Levels

| Experimental Group | Lipoprotein or lipid class | Effect | Reference |
|---|---|---|---|
| Thyrotoxic patients | LDL | Decreased compared to euthyroid value, with increased catabolism | Walton *et al* (12) |
| Thyrotoxic patients | LDL-cholesterol | Decreased 34%, despite increased cholesterol synthesis | Abrams *et al* (13) |
| Thyrotoxic patients | HDL-cholesterol | Decreased 20% | Abrams *et al* (13) |
| Thyrotoxic patients | Total triglycerides | Compared to euthyroid value, mean level and production decreased | Nikkilä *et al* (14) |
| Hypothyroid patients (obese) | LDL-cholesterol | Increased 25%, decreased fecal neutral steroids | Abrams *et al* (13) |
| Hypothyroid rats | LDL-cholesterol | Increased 86%, decreased LDL removal | Sykes *et al* (15) |
| Hypothyroid patients (non-obese) | VLDL-triglycerides | Increased 36%, lower VLDL triglyceride transport compared to euthyroid value | Abrams *et al* (16) |

Massive hyperlipemia in acute insulin deficiency is well-known, but
rare. Some more common effects are listed in Table 4. Acute insulin
deficiency (17) and ketoacidosis (18) lead to increased triglyceride
levels through increased production; however, noninsulin-dependent
diabetes may also be associated with increased production (18).
Chronic deficiency elevates VLDL, while decreasing LDL and HDL (19).

Table 4. Effects of Insulin Deficiency on Lipoprotein Levels

| Experimental Group | Lipoprotein or lipid class | Effect | Reference |
|---|---|---|---|
| Dogs given anti-insulin serum | VLDL-triglycerides | Increase 2-fold, with 5-fold increase in secretion | Balasse *et al* (17) |
| Ketoacidotic patients | Total triglycerides | Increase 6-fold, with trebling of production | Nikkilä *et al* (18) |
| Chronic diabetic rats | VLDL-triglycerides | Increase 3-fold, due to impaired removal | Van Tol (19) |
| Chronic diabetic rats | $LDL_2$-cholesterol | Decrease 23% | Van Tol (19) |
| Chronic diabetic rats | HDL-cholesterol | Decrease 20% | Van Tol (19) |

546

Improved diabetic.control through insulin therapy has been reported
to decrease VLDL-triglyceride by 70% and LDL-cholesterol by 20%, while
increasing HDL-cholesterol by as much as 60% (20) or as little as 15%.
(21). However, studies by Chait *et al* in a hyperinsulinemic, hyperlipemic woman with partial lipodystrophy before and during diazoxide
administration indicate that diazoxide-induced lowering of insulin
concentration may be accompanied by reduction of both VLDL production
and concentration (22). This is compatible with indirect evidence
correlating VLDL production with insulin concentration (23).

Evidence is also accumulating that lipoprotein concentration and/or
transport may also be influenced by gastric inhibitory polypeptide
(24), norepinephrine (25), parathormone (26), glucagon (27), and
corticosteroids (27).

REFERENCES

1.  Russ EM, Eder HA, Barr DP (1951) Protein-lipid relationships in
    human plasma. Am J Med 11:468-479
2.  Wallentin L, Larsson-Cohn U (1977) Metabolic and hormonal effects
    of post-menopausal oestrogen replacement treatment. Acta Endocr
    86:597-607
3.  Tikkanen JM, Kuusi T, Vartiainen E, Nikkilä EA (1979) Treatment
    of post-menopausal hypercholesterolaemia with estradiol. Acta
    Obstet Gynaecol Scand Suppl 88:83-88
4.  Glueck CJ, Fallat RW, Scheel D (1975) Effects of estrogenic com-
    pounds on triglyceride kinetics. Metabolism 24:537-545
5.  Gustafson A, Svanborg A (1972) Gonadal steroid effects on plasma
    lipoproteins and individual phospholipids. J Clin Endocr Metab
    35:203-207
6.  Bradley DD, Wingerd J, Petitti DB, Krauss RM, Ramcharon S (1979)
    Serum high-density-lipoprotein cholesterol in women using oral
    contraceptives, estrogens and progestins. N Engl J Med 299:17-20
7.  Cheng DCH (1979) Hypolipidemic effects of norethindrone acetate
    and of soy protein. M.Sc Thesis. The University of Western Ont-
    ario, London, Canada
8.  Wolfe BM, Grace DM (1979) Norethindrone acetate inhibition of
    splanchnic triglyceride secretion in conscious glucose-fed swine.
    J Lipid Res 20:175-182
9.  Spellacy WN, Buhi WC, Birk SA (1974) Norgestrel and carbohydrate-
    lipid metabolism: glucose, insulin and triglyceride changes dur-
    ing six months time of use. Contraception 9:615-625
10. Eckstein P, Whitby M, Fotherby K, Butler C, Mukherjee TK, Burnett
    JBC, Richards DK, Whitehead TP (1972) Clinical and laboratory
    findings in a trial of norgestrel, a low-dose progestogen-only
    contraceptive. Br Med J 3:195-200
11. Khokha R, Wolfe BM (1982) Hypotriglyceridemic action of d-norges-
    trel in rats. Proceedings 6th International Symposium on Athero-
    sclerosis, Berlin
12. Walton KW, Scott PH, Dykes PW, Davies JWL (1965) The significance
    of alterations in serum lipids in thyroid dysfunction. II Alter-
    ations of the metabolism and turnover of $^{131}$I-low density lipo-
    proteins in hypothyroidism and thyrotoxicosis. Clin Sci 29:217-
    238
13. Abrams JJ, Grundy SM (1981) Cholesterol metabolism in hypothy-
    roidism and hyperthyroidism in man. J Lipid Res 22:323-338
14. Nikkilä EA, Kekki M (1972) Plasma triglyceride metabolism in
    thyroid disease. J Clin Invest 51:2103-2114
15. Sykes M, Cnoop-Koopmans WM, Julien P, Angel A (1981) The effects
    of hypothyroidism, age, and nutrition on LDL catabolism in the
    rat. Metabolism 30:733-738

16. Abrams JJ, Grundy SM, Ginsberg H (1981) Metabolism of plasma triglycerides in hypothyroidism and hyperthyroidism in man. J Lipid Res 22:307-322
17. Balasse EO, Bier DM, Havel RJ (1972) Early effects of anti-insulin serum on hepatic metabolism of plasma free fatty acids in dogs. Diabetes 21:280-288
18. Nikkilä EA, Kekki M (1973) Plasma triglyceride transport kinetics in diabetes mellitus. Metabolism 22:1-22
19. Van Tol A (1977) Hypertriglyceridemia in the diabetic rat. Defective removal of serum very low density lipoproteins. Atherosclerosis 26:117-128
20. Paisey R, Elkeles RS, Hambley J, Magill P (1978) The effects of chlorpropamide and insulin on serum lipids, lipoproteins and fractional triglyceride removal. Diabetologia 15:81-85
21. Calvert GD, Graham JJ, Mannik T, Wise PH, Yeates RA (1978) Effects of therapy on plasma-high-density-lipoprotein-cholesterol concentration in diabetes mellitus. Lancet ii:66-68
22. Chait A, Janus E, Mason AS, Lewis B (1979) Lipodystrophy with hyperlipidaemia: The role of insulin in very low density lipoprotein over-synthesis. Clin Endocr 10:173-178
23. Olefsky JM, Farquhar JW, Reaven GM (1974) Reappraisal of the role of insulin in hypertriglyceridemia. Am J Med 57:551-560
24. Wasada T, McCorkle K, Harris V, Kawai K, Howard B, Unger RH (1981) Effect of gastric inhibitory polypeptide on plasma levels of chylomicron triglycerides in dogs. J Clin Invest 68:1106-1107
25. Basso LV, Havel RJ (1970) Hepatic metabolism of free fatty acids in normal and diabetic dogs. J Clin Invest 49:537-547
26. Ljunghall S, Lithell H, Vessby B, Wide L (1978) Glucose and lipoprotein metabolism in primary hyperparathyroidism. Effects of parathyroidectomy. Acta Endocr 89:580-589
27. Lewis B (1976) In The Hyperlipidemias, Blackwell Scientific Publications, Oxford, p.160

# 3.2 Lipoprotein Receptors

# Monoclonal Antibody as a Probe for Structural and Functional Studies of the LDL Receptor

U. Beisiegel, M. S. Brown, W. J. Schneider, R. G. W. Anderson, and J. L. Goldstein

Familial hypercholesterolemia (FH) is a naturally-occurring human model for the study of atherosclerosis. Subjects who are heterozygous for this autosomal dominant trait have 2-fold elevations in the plasma level of LDL-cholesterol from birth and develop atherosclerosis in the fourth and fifth decades. Subjects who are homozygous for the genetic defect have 6 to 10-fold elevations of LDL-cholesterol from the time of intrauterine life and develop fulminant atheriosclerosis with myocardial infarctions usually occurring before age 20.

The primary defect in familial hypercholesterolemia involves the gene encording the LDL receptor. This receptor is produced by body cells when they require cholesterol for synthesis of membranes, steroid hormones, or bile acids. Circulating plasma LDL binds to the receptor and is taken into the cell and digested, liberating its cholesterol for metabolic use. The LDL receptor serves two functions in the body: 1) it provides a major route for the degradation of plasma LDL, and 2) it supplies cholesterol to sterol-requiring cells.

FH heterozygotes produce half the normal number of active LDL receptor molecules. Homozygotes produce 0-20 percent of the normal number of active LDL receptors. As a result of this receptor deficiency, plasma LDL cannot be degraded efficiently, the lipoprotein accumulates to high levels in plasma, and atherosclerosis occurs.

## Preparation of Monoclonal Antibody

To gain further insights into the structure and function of the LDL receptor and to learn more about how mutations affect its function, we have prepared monoclonal antibodies directed against the receptor. We used techniques that were pioneered by Kohler and Milstein. To prepare the monoclonal antibody, we injected mice with a partially purified preparation of LDL receptors obtained from the adrenal cortex of the cow, a rich source of receptors. Splenic lymphocytes from the immunized mice were fused with the SP2/0 line of mouse myeloma cells. Hybrid cells producing antibodies to the LDL receptor were selected on the basis of the ability of the antibodies to bind to the partially purified LDL receptor. Several clones of antibody-producing cells were obtained.

One of the clones of antibody-producing cells was studied in detail. The monoclonal antibody produced by this clone is designated IgG-C7. It is of the IgG 2b subclass. The antibody reacts with human and bovine LDL receptors, but not with rabbit, dog, hamster, rat, or mouse receptors.

552

## Structural and Functional Studies

In normal human fibroblasts 125-I-labeled IgG-C7 binds in molar a-
mounts that are equivalent to the molar amounts of 125-I-LDL bound.
A similar molar equivalency is observed for the binding of IgG-C7
and LDL to the purified bovine adrenal receptor. This suggests that
the LDL receptor has one IgG-C7 binding site for each LDL binding
site.

In six of eight patients with homozygous FH, whose cells failed to
bind 125-I-LDL, there was no binding of 125-I-IgG-C7. However, in
the other two receptor-negative patients, there were appreciable
amounts of binding of 125-I-IgG-C7.

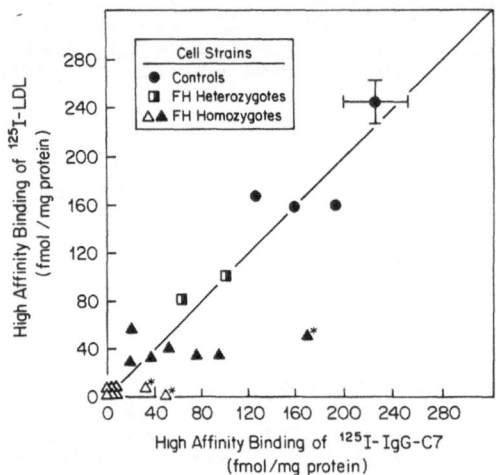

Fig. 1.

High affinity binding of
125-I-LDL and 125-I-la-
beled monoclonal antibo-
dy against LDL receptor
IgG-C7 at 4°C to monolay-
ers of normal and mutant
fibroblasts expressing
different amounts of LDL
receptor activity.
The diagonal line repre-
sents the theoretical va-
lues expected for 1 to 1
stoichiometric binding of
125-I-LDL and 125-I-IgG

We believe that these latter two patients have inherited at least
one mutant allele that produces an altered receptor that cannot
bind LDL, but retains the ability to bind the monoclonal antibody.
Studies are now in progress to determine the structural basis for
the alteration in the properties of the LDL receptor in these
cross-reacting mutants.

## References

Beisiegel,U., Schneider,W.J., Goldstein,J.L., Anderson,R.G.W., and
Brown,M.S. (1981) Monoclonal antibodies to the LDL receptor as probes for study of receptor-mediated endocytosis and the genetics of
familial hypercholesterolemia. J.Biol.Chem. 256: 11923-11931.

Goldstein,J.L., and Brown,M.S. (1981) The LDL receptor defect in
familial hypercholesterolemia: Implications for pathogenesis and
therapy. Med.Clin.N.Amer. 66: 335-362

Schneider,W.J., Beisiegel,U., Goldstein,J.L., and Brown,M.S. (1982)
Purification of the low density lipoprotein receptor, an acidic
glycoprotein of 164,000 molecular weight. J.Biol.Chem. 257: 2664-
2673.

# The Role of Receptors in Apolipoprotein B Metabolism

C. J. Packard, J. Shepherd, and H. R. Slater

## Introduction

A new perspective on lipoprotein metabolism has been gained from the
identification and characterisation of specific high affinity lipoprotein receptors. These are located on cell membranes and serve to
facilitate and control the ingress of lipoprotein cholesterol into
the cell. They exhibit two important properties. First, they are
subject to autoregulation so that when cellular cholesterol requirements rise, the receptors are stimulated to promote lipoprotein assimilation. Conversely, when the cell is replete with the sterol, receptor activity is suppressed. Second, they demonstrate a high degree
of ligand specificity which derives from selective interaction between
the receptor and apoproteins on the surface of lipoproteins. Two
polypeptides, apolipoproteins B and E, have been implicated in this
recognition process and two distinct membrane receptor activities
have also been identified (1,2,3,4). One seems to be confined to
hepatocytes and apparently operates as an efficient mechanism for the
cellular assimilation of chylomicron remnants. The other which appears to be identical to the fibroblast receptor of Goldstein and
Brown (1) is widely distributed throughout the tissues of the body
and plays an important role in the metabolism of low density lipoproteins (LDL).

In this discussion we confine our attention to the activity of the
latter. Our experimental approach is based on the observation that
receptor-lipoprotein interaction can be abolished by chemical modification of the arginyl residues on the lipoprotein with 1,2 cyclohexanedione (6). This treatment produces modified particles whose
catabolism is restricted to pathways which do not involve the agency
of the receptor. By comparing plasma clearances and tissue uptakes
of the native and chemically treated lipoproteins it is therefore
possible to obtain an estimate of the activity of the receptor pathway
*in vivo* (7,8,9).

## Animal Studies

A rabbit model has been used to show that the receptor pathway does
operate *in vivo* and is subject to the same autoregulatory phenomena
observed in fibroblasts grown in culture. Native LDL is cleared from
the plasma of control rabbits consistently faster than simultaneously
injected CHD/LDL; and kinetic analysis of their clearance rates indicates that under normal conditions, 44% of total LDL catabolism occurs
by the receptor route. (Figure 1)

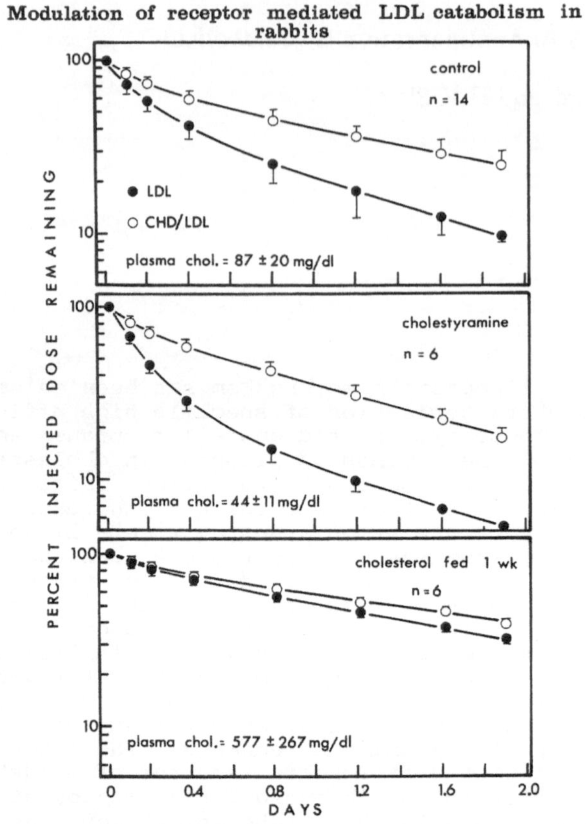

## Modulation of receptor mediated LDL catabolism in rabbits

Figure 1. The metabolism of $^{125}I$-LDL and $^{131}I$-CHD/LDL was examined in three groups of rabbits. Following injection of the tracers in rapid sequence, plasma samples were obtained at intervals over the next two days. Clearance curves (mean ± 1SD) were constructed for each tracer and were analysed by curve peeling. In the control animals maintained on a standard rabbit chow diet, receptor mediated catabolism accounted for 44% of total LDL clearance. Following cholestyramine administration (2 g/d for 14 d) to a second animal group, this value rose to 62% while cholesterol feeding (1% cholesterol added to the diet) reduced it to 20%

Measurement of the relative uptakes of these tracers by rabbit tissues shows that the pathway is widespread (8) and that the liver has a singularly important role in its operation (Figure 2). Similar conclusions were reached by Kovanen et al. (5) using a radioassay to determine tissue receptor activity.

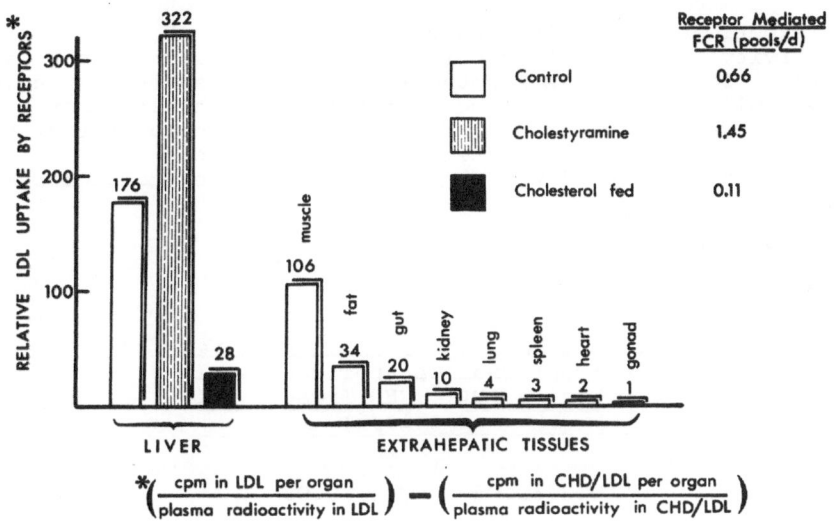

Figure 2.   At the end of the turnover studies described in Figure 1 the radioactivity present in a range of the animals' tissues was measured and expressed
relative to the plasma radioactivity as outlined above.   In the liver, more than
95% of the radioactivity was TCA precipitable while in other tissues this value
ranged from 80-95%.   The uptake values shown above represent whole organ uptake of
LDL.   Although the adrenal gland was most active per gram tissue, in whole organ
terms the liver was quantitatively more important

Autoregulation is central to the function of the receptor pathway *in
vitro* and is also in evidence *in vivo* when cholesterol metabolism is
perturbed.   This was achieved in our experimental model either by
depleting the animal (and particularly its liver) of the sterol by
administration of the bile acid sequestrant cholestyramine or by feeding cholesterol to expand tissue sterol pools.   Treatment with the
drug increased receptor mediated LDL catabolism from the plasma
(Figure 1) and promoted uptake of the lipoprotein into the liver
(Figure 2).   No other tissue showed this kind of response.   Cholesterol
feeding suppressed the activity of the receptor pathway.   The difference in the plasma clearance rates of native and cyclohexanedione
treated LDL was virtually eliminated as was receptor mediated tissue
uptake of the lipoprotein.   We concluded from the above observations
that LDL catabolism was linked to cholesterol homeostasis through
the agency of the high affinity LDL receptor both in the cell and in
the whole animal.

## Human Studies

The animal experiments described above indicate that modulation of LDL
receptor activity may be an appropriate means of regulating plasma
LDL cholesterol levels. This hypothesis was validated for man using
an approach similar to that pursued in rabbits. In healthy normal
subjects the fractional clearance of native LDL exceeded that of the
cyclohexanedione-modified lipoprotein (7) so that approximately one
third of the plasma LDL pool was removed daily by the receptor route
(Table 1).

Table 1.

| Subjects/treatment | Fractional Catabolic Rate of | |
|---|---|---|
| | Native LDL | CHD Treated LDL |
| | (pools/d) | |
| Normal (n=10) | 0.34±0.05 | 0.20±0.03 |
| Normal, cholesterol fed (n=6) | 0.29±0.06 | 0.18±0.03 |
| Type II, control (n=7) | 0.26±0.04 | 0.19±0.03 |
| Type II, bezafibrate treated (n=7) | 0.30±0.04 | 0.19±0.02 |
| FH hetero, control (n=5) | 0.19±0.05 | 0.15±0.03 |
| FH hetero, cholestyramine (n=5) | 0.24±0.04 | 0.17±0.04 |

Expansion of the circulating cholesterol pool by feeding cholesterol
supplemented diets (6 eggs/day, ie about 1500 mg cholesterol/day)
lowered significantly the fractional clearance of native LDL without
affecting that of the cyclohexanedione treated lipoprotein. Thus
the observed rise in plasma LDL was accompanied by a fall in its
receptor mediated catabolism. Similarly, subjects suffering from
primary Type II hyperlipoproteinaemia or from its more specific form,
familial hypercholesterolaemia (FH), also presented with defective
LDL receptor activity which in this instance probably caused their
disease. Receptor mediated catabolism of the lipoprotein was reduced
in these subjects to 30-50% of normal (7,10,11). An attempt was therefore made to promote their receptor activity using two drugs. The
effect of the first, cholestyramine, has already been described in
rabbits. When prescribed to a group of five FH heterozygotes it effectively lowered circulating LDL by promoting its plasma clearance
via the receptor pathway, and consideration of the animal studies
suggests that this increased activity is primarily located in the
liver, consonant with the known effects of cholestyramine on hepatic

cholesterol metabolism. Similarly, partial ileal bypass surgery also increases the drain on the hepatic cholesterol pool and other workers have shown that this procedure increases receptor mediated LDL catabolism (12).

Bezafibrate lowered circulating LDL cholesterol by stimulating the activity of the LDL receptor pathway. This raised the fractional clearance of LDL by this route towards normal in seven Type II hypercholesterolaemic subjects. Although the mechanism of this effect is not completely clear, experiments in rats indicate that the drug inhibits hepatic cholesterologenesis and thereby may produce a fall in hepatocyte cholesterol levels. If this action also occurs in man it may trigger a rise in membrane receptor activity in order to satisfy cellular cholesterol requirements and cause the increase in receptor mediated LDL catabolism which we observed.

Finally, it is now clear that the high circulating LDL concentrations characteristic of hypothyroidism derive primarily from defective expression of receptor activity (13). Thyroxine replacement therapy alleviates this defect, producing an increase in LDL receptor activity and lowering the plasma concentration of the lipoprotein to normal.

## Conclusions

The data presented above, we believe, demonstrates that the high affinity LDL receptor pathway originally described in fibroblasts plays an important role in LDL metabolism in both animals and man. Its activity *in vivo* is affected by genetic, environmental and hormonal factors, and it is possible by pharmacologic intervention to restore receptor function towards normal in subjects in whom it is impaired.

*Acknowledgements*   This work was supported by grants from the Scottish Home and Health Department (K/MRS/50/C429) and from the British Heart Foundation (81/6).

## References

1.  Goldstein J L, Brown M S (1977) The low density lipoprotein pathway and its relation to atherosclerosis. Ann Rev Biochem 46: 897-930
2.  Brown M S, Goldstein J L (1978) General scheme for regulation of cholesterol metabolism in mammalian cells. In: Distrubances in Lipid and Lipoprotein Metabolism; editors Dietschy J M, Gotto A M and Ontko J A. American Physiological Society, Bethesda, Md, pp 173-180
3.  Mahley R W and Innerarity T L (1978) Properties of lipoproteins responsible for high affinity bind to cell surface receptors of fibroblasts and smooth muscle cells. Adv Exp Med Biol 109: 99-127
4.  Mahley R W, Hui D Y, Innerarity T L, Weisgraber K H (1981) Two independent lipoprotein receptors on hepatic membranes of dog, swine and man. J Clin Invest 68: 1197-1206

5.  Kovanen P T, Basu S K, Goldstein J L and Brown M S (1979) Low
    density lipoprotein receptors in bovine adrenal cortex II. Low
    density lipoprotein binding to membranes prepared from fresh tis-
    sue.  Endocrinology 104: 610-616
6.  Mahley R W, Innerarity T L, Pitas R E, Weisgraber K H, Brown J H,
    Gross E (1977) Inhibition of lipoprotein binding to cell surface
    receptors of fibroblasts following selective modification of arg-
    inyl residues in arginine rich and B apoproteins.  J Biol Chem
    252: 7279-7287
7.  Shepherd J, Bicker S, Lorimer A R, Packard C J (1979) Receptor
    mediated low density lipoprotein catabolism in man.  J Lipid Res
    20: 999-1006
8.  Slater H R, Packard C J, Bicker S, Shepherd J (1980) Effects of
    cholestyramine on receptor mediated plasma clearance and tissue
    uptake of human low density lipoprotein in the rabbit.  J Biol
    Chem 255: 10210-10213
9.  Slater H R, Packard C J, Shepherd J (1982) Measurement of receptor
    independent lipoprotein catabolism using 1,2 cyclohexanedione-
    modified low density lipoprotein.  J Lipid Res 23: 92-96
10. Shepherd J, Packard C J, Bicker S, Lawrie T D V, Morgan H G (1980)
    Cholestyramine promotes receptor mediated low density lipoproteins
    catabolism.  N Engl J Med 302: 1219-1222
11. Stewart J M, Packard C J, Lorimer A R, Boag D E, Shepherd J (1982)
    Effects of bezafibrate on receptor mediated and receptor independ-
    ent low density lipoprotein catabolism in type II hyperlipoprotein-
    emic subjects.  Atherosclerosis (in press).
12. Spengel F A, Jadhav A, Duffield R G M, Wood C B, Thompson G R
    (1981) Superiority of partial ileal bypass over cholestyramine in
    reducing cholesterol in familial hypercholesterolemia.  Lancet
    768-770
13. Thompson G R, Soutar A K, Spengel F A, Jadhav A, Gavigan S P,
    Myant N B (1981) Defects of receptor mediated low density lipo-
    protein catabolism in homozygous familial hypercholesterolemia
    and hypothyroidism in vivo.  Proc Natl Acad Sci, USA 78: 2591-2595

# Factors Influencing Receptor-Mediated Low Density Lipoprotein Catabolism

G. R. Thompson

In 1974 Brown and Goldstein showed that cultured skin fibroblasts from patients with homozygous familial hypercholesterolaemia (FH) lacked the low density lipoprotein (LDL) receptors which were present in normal fibroblasts. Since then a vast literature has accumulated on the topic of the LDL receptor, which has now been identified in a variety of other cells and tissues *in vitro* including arterial smooth muscle cells, endothelial cells, lymphocytes, monocytes, adrenal cortex, ovary and liver. The relevance of the LDL receptor to atherosclerosis and its importance in regulating the plasma cholesterol level (2) have been reviewed in detail by the Dallas group. The characteristic features of this saturable, high affinity mechanism for LDL uptake into cells are that it has a greater affinity for apoE than for apoB, and that binding is abolished if these apoproteins have their lysine or arginine residues modified or by addition of EDTA to the incubation medium or pretreatment of cell membranes with pronase (2). Recently Schneider *et al* (3) reported the partial purification of the LDL receptor from bovine adrenal cortex, which appears to be an acidic protein with a molecular weight in the region of 163,000. Thus an impressive body of evidence exists concerning the cell biology and biochemistry of the LDL receptor *in vitro*. The chief purpose of this communication is to review briefly *in vivo* evidence for the functional existence of LDL receptors in man and experimental animals and to examine the manner in which their expression is influenced by genetic, hormonal and environmental factors.

## Quantitating Receptor-Mediated LDL Catabolism *in vivo*

Mahley *et al* (4) showed that coupling the arginine groups of apoB with cyclohexanedione prevented receptor-mediated binding of LDL *in vitro*. Subsequently they (5) and Shepherd *et al* (6) exploited this observation to develop a means of quantitating receptor-mediated LDL catabolism *in vivo*. By simultaneously injecting both native and blocked LDL, the one labelled with $^{125}I$, the other with $^{131}I$, it was possible to quantitate both total (native) and receptor-independent (blocked) LDL catabolism by analysing the plasma decay curves of the two tracers. The results of this type of approach suggest that up to 50% of LDL is catabolized via the LDL receptor in rats and monkeys (5) and roughly one-third in humans (6). Neither Shepherd and colleagues nor we ourselves have encountered any adverse reactions during administration of cyclohexanedione-blocked LDL to man. Also, despite the fact that the chemical reaction is reversible *in vitro* (5) there is no evidence that uncoupling of cyclohexanedione from LDL occurs *in vivo* (6, 7).

## Factors Influencing Receptor-Mediated LDL Catabolism

### Genetic

It had long been known that LDL catabolism was decreased in FH but
Shepherd *et al* (6) were the first to provide *in vivo* evidence that
this defect specifically affected the receptor-mediated pathway. Their
findings of a partial defect in heterozygotes were substantiated by our
subsequent demonstration (7) that receptor-mediated LDL catabolism in
homozygotes was virtually nil, both before and after plasma exchange
(Fig. 1).   This confirms that the defect is primary and not secondary
to saturation of a normal receptor-mediated clearance mechanism by an
expanded LDL pool resulting from increased synthesis.   Recent unpublished data (Harders-Spengel *et al*) show that receptor-mediated binding
of LDL by liver membranes is reduced by approximately 50% in FH heterozygotes compared with control subjects.   This finding, if confirmed
in homozygotes, together with evidence from other sources that the
liver is the major site of LDL catabolism (8) suggests that accessory
liver transplantation merits serious consideration as a possible,
definitive treatment for homozygous FH.   The development of the
WHHL-rabbit by Watanabe and colleagues which lacks hepatic receptors
for LDL (9) should enable this approach to be tested experimentally.

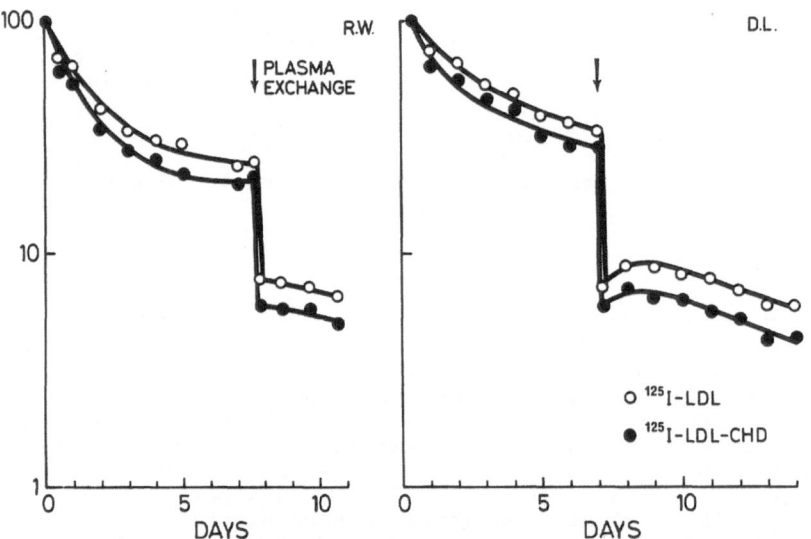

Fig. 1. Plasma radioactivity curves of $^{125}I$-LDL and $^{131}I$-LDL-cyclohex-
anedione (CHD) in two FH homozygotes.  Note the parallelism of the two
curves and the fact that $^{131}I$-LDL-cyclohexanedione is, if anything,
cleared more rapidly than $^{125}I$-LDL which is the reverse of the normal
situation.  Calculation of the respective fractional catabolic rates
of native and blocked LDL showed that receptor-mediated catabolism was
virtually nil and uninfluenced by plasma exchange

## Hormonal

It is known that administration of ACTH increases the number of LDL
receptors expressed in adrenal cortical cells of rodents (10) and that
LDL cholesterol is used for steroid synthesis by such cells.
Whether FH homozygotes respond normally to an ACTH stimulus remains
to be determined.

Chait and colleagues have shown that both insulin (11) and tri-iodo-
thyronine (12) increase the number of LDL receptors expressed by cultured skin fibroblasts when each is added to the incubation medium.
It has long been recognized that hypercholesterolaemia is a feature of
hypothyroidism and that both this manifestation and the underlying
defect of LDL catabolism improve on treatment with thyroid hormone.
Recently we took the opportunity to determine receptor-mediated and
-independent LDL catabolism in one such patient and found a defect of
both pathways, especially the former, which improved markedly after
the patient had been rendered euthyroid (7).

Pharmacological doses of oestrogens have been shown to have a striking
effect in stimulating the uptake and degradation of LDL by rat liver
(13).        This process appears to be receptor-mediated (14) and involves hepatocytes rather than Kupffer cells (15).  Whether an analogous
effect is exerted by physiological amounts of oestrogen in humans remains uncertain, although there is some evidence that pre-menopausal
females catabolize LDL more efficiently than post-menopausal females
and males (16).

## Nutritional and Age-Related Factors

Mahley and colleagues have recently published data obtained in pigs and
dogs which demonstrate the existence of two distinct types of lipoprotein receptor in the liver (17), which they term apoE and apoB,E
receptors.  The latter is synonomous with the LDL receptor whereas apoE
receptors do not bind LDL but have a high affinity for apoE-containing
lipoproteins, including the remnant particles which result from the
hydrolysis of triglyceride-rich lipoproteins.  According to these
authors apoB,E receptors are expressed in the livers of growing animals
but not in those of adults unless these had been previously fasted.
Conversely, hepatic apoB,E receptors were suppressed in growing animals
by cholesterol feeding and in this respect resemble the LDL receptor of
fibroblasts.  However, the apparent absence of expression of these
receptors in adult human liver (17) is difficult to reconcile with evidence that a significant proportion of LDL is catabolized via the receptor pathway in man and that, in animals at least, the liver is the major
site in the body where this process occurs.  Further data are needed
before this important question can be resolved.

## Therapeutic Influences

Shepherd *et al* (18) were the first to show that administration of the
anion-exchange resin cholestyramine to patients with heterozygous FH
promoted receptor-mediated LDL catabolism.  A similar response was observed in dogs given the resin colestipol, and this was shown to be
accompanied by an increase in receptor-mediated binding of LDL by liver
membranes (19).  This effect of colestipol was magnified if the dogs
were concomitantly given the HMG-CoA reductase inhibitor mevinolin.
The most likely explanation for these findings is that stimulation of
bile acid synthesis by anion-exchange resins results in an increased

562

demand for cholesterol within the hepatocyte, which is normally met from both exogenous and endogenous sources. Inhibition of cholesterol synthesis by mevinolin diminishes the contribution from endogenous cholesterol and thus promotes further the uptake of exogenous (LDL) cholesterol, presumably via hepatic apoB,E receptors. Similarly, the increased excretion and synthesis of bile acids which accompanies partial ileal bypass is even more marked than that induced by cholestyramine and has been shown to result in a correspondingly greater increase in receptor-mediated LDL catabolism in FH heterozygotes who have undergone this procedure (20). An analogous response has been observed in Rhesus monkeys following partial ileal bypass (21), as illustrated in Fig. 2.

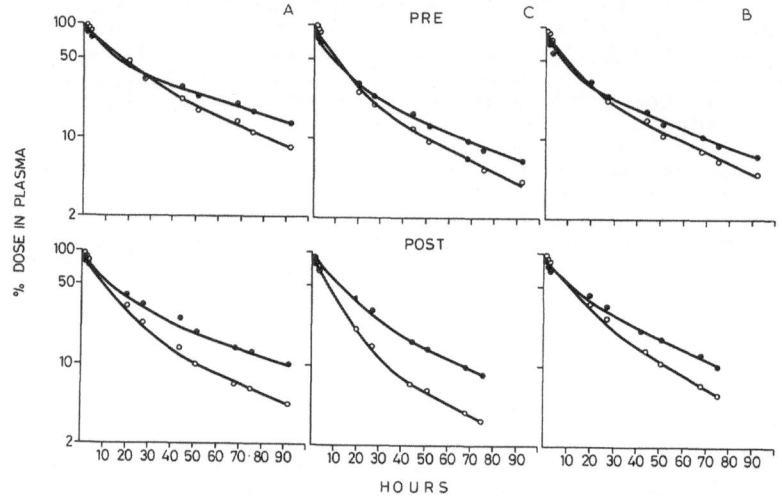

Fig. 2. Plasma radioactivity curves after injection of simian [125]I-LDL (○) and [131]I-LDL-cyclohexanedione (●) into three Rhesus monkeys before and six weeks after partial ileal bypass. Note the widening of the gap between the two tracers, indicating an increase in receptor-mediated LDL catabolism (from Spengel et al, reference 21)

Post-mortem studies in one of the animals killed during a third turnover study six months after partial ileal bypass showed that most of the extravascular radioactivity present at the time of death was in the liver, of which more than 80% appeared to have been taken up by the receptor-mediated pathway. In both man and monkey, partial ileal bypass was accompanied by appreciable decreases in serum cholesterol, of the order of 30%, which supports the concept that receptor-mediated catabolism plays an important role in regulating LDL levels in the body.

References

1. Brown MS, Goldstein JL (1974) Familial hypercholesterolemia: Defective binding of lipoproteins to cultured fibroblasts associated with impaired regulation of 3-hydroxy-3-methylglutaryl coenzyme A reductase activity. Proc Natl Acad Sci 71: 788-792
2. Brown MS, Kovanen PT, Goldstein JL (1981) Regulation of plasma cholesterol by lipoprotein receptors. Science 212: 628-635
3. Schneider WJ, Goldstein JL, Brown MS (1981) Partial purification and characterization of the low density lipoprotein receptor from bovine adrenal cortex. J Biol Chem 255: 11442-11447

4. Mahley RW, Innerarity TL, Pitas RE, Weisgraber KH, Brown JH, Gross E (1977) Inhibition of lipoprotein binding to cell surface receptors of fibroblasts following selective modification of arginyl residues in arginine-rich and B apoproteins. J Biol Chem 252: 7279-7287

5. Mahley RW, Weisgraber KH, Melchior GW, Innerarity TL, Holcombe KS (1980) Inhibition of receptor-mediated clearance of lysine and arginine-modified lipoproteins from the plasma of rats and monkeys. Proc Natl Acad Sci USA 77: 225-229

6. Shepherd J, Bicker S, Lorimer AR, Packard CJ (1979) Receptor-mediated low density lipoprotein catabolism in man. J Lipid Res 20: 999-1006

7. Thompson GR, Soutar AK, Spengel FA, Jadhav A, Gavigan SJP, Myant NB (1981) Defects of receptor-mediated low density lipoprotein catabolism in homozygous familial hypercholesterolemia and hypothyroidism *in vivo*. Proc Natl Acad Sci USA 78: 2591-2595

8. Pittman RC, Attie AD, Carew TE, Steinberg D (1982) Tissue sites of catabolism of rat and human low density lipoproteins in rats. Biochim Biophys Acta 710: 7-14

9. Kita T, Brown MS, Watanabe Y, Goldstein JL (1981) Deficiency of low density lipoprotein receptors in liver and adrenal gland of the WHHL rabbit, an animal model of familial hypercholesterolaemia. Proc Natl Acad Sci USA 78: 2268-2272

10. Kovanen PT, Goldstein JL, Chappell DA, Brown MS (1980) Regulation of low density lipoprotein receptors by adrenocorticotropin in the adrenal gland of mice and rats *in vivo*. J Biol Chem 255: 5591-5598

11. Chait A, Bierman EL, Albers JJ (1979) Low density lipoprotein receptor activity in cultured human skin fibroblasts. J Clin Invest 64: 1309-1319

12. Chait A, Bierman EL, Albers JJ (1979) Regulatory role of triiodothyronine in the degradation of low density lipoprotein by cultured human skin fibroblasts. J Clin Endocr Metab 48: 887-889

13. Chao Y, Windler EE, Chen GC, Havel RJ (1979) Hepatic catabolism of rat and human lipoproteins in rats treated with 17α-ethinyl estradiol. J Biol Chem 254: 11360-11366

14. Windler EET, Kovanen PT, Chao Y-S, Brown MS, Havel RJ, Goldstein JL (1980) The estradiol-stimulated lipoprotein receptor of rat liver. A binding site that mediates the uptake of rat lipoproteins containing apoproteins B and E. J Biol Chem 255: 10464-10471

15. Chao Y-S, Jones AL, Hradek GT, Windler EET, Havel RJ (1981) Autoradiographic localisation of the sites of uptake, cellular transport and catabolism of low density lipoproteins in the liver of normal and estrogen-treated rats. Proc Natl Acad Sci USA 78: 597-601

16. Hurley PJ, Scott PJ (1970) Plasma turnover of $S_f$ 0-9 low-density lipoprotein in normal men and women. Atherosclerosis 11: 51-76

17. Mahley RW, Hui DY, Innerarity TL, Weisgraber KH (1981) Two independent lipoprotein receptors on hepatic membranes of dog, swine and man. J Clin Invest 65: 1197-1206

18. Shepherd J, Packard CJ, Bicker S, Lawrie TDV, Morgan HG (1980) Cholestyramine promotes receptor-mediated low-density-lipoprotein catabolism. N Engl J Med 302: 1219-1222

19 Kovanen PT, Bilheimer DW, Goldstein JL, Jaramillo JL, Brown MS (1981) Regulatory role for hepatic low density lipoprotein receptors *in vivo* in the dog. Proc Natl Acad Sci USA 78: 1194-1198

20. Spengel FA, Jadhav A, Duffield RGM, Wood CB, Thompson GR (1981) Superiority of partial ileal bypass over cholestyramine in reducing cholesterol in familial hypercholesterolaemia. Lancet 2: 768-770

21. Spengel FA, Harders-Spengel K, Duffield R, Wood C, Myant NB, Thompson GR (1982) The effect of partial ileal bypass on receptor-mediated uptake and catabolism of low density lipoprotein in the Rhesus monkey. Res Exp Med (Berl) in press

# Rat and Human Lipoprotein Utilization by Cultured Rat Ovary Granulosa Cells

D. B. Weinstein, K. Nakamura, and J. R. Schreiber

In the rat, the four-day estrous cycle requires a continuous program of cellular proliferation and differentiation. In each cycle, follicles initiate growth with the oocyte increasing in size and the initiation of mitotic division of the granulosa cell layer. Follicular development is controlled by the presence and number of receptors for gonadotropin and steroid hormones (FSH, LH, estrogen and testosterone). FSH induces the appearance of more FSH receptors and LH/hCG and prolactin receptors on the granulosa cells (1). FSH also induces the appearance of aromatose enzymes which are required for aromatization of androgens to estrogens by granulosa cells. As the follicle matures FSH stimulates the synthesis and secretion of progestins (progesterone and 20-α-dihydroprogesterone). The granulosa cells maintain progestin synthesis during the ovulating and luteal phases of the cycle. Cholesterol is the precursor of progestin production via an FSH-induced mitochondrial side chain cleavage pathway which forms pregnenolone, which is then converted to progesterone and 20-α-dihydroprogestin.

Plasma lipoproteins provide a source of exogenous cholesterol for extrahepatic tissues (2) and under physiological conditions the major cholesterol carrying lipoprotein in the rat is high density lipoprotein (HDL). ANDERSEN and DIETSCHY (3) have demonstrated that the continuous availability of plasma lipoprotein cholesterol, rather than de novo synthesis, is the requirement for maintenance of steroid hormone production by rat adrenal and gonadal cells in vivo. Their study indicated a preferential utilization of HDL in steroidogenic tissues of the rat. Specific binding sites for rat HDL have been dmonstrated in interstitial tissue isolated from rat testis (4). It has been demonstrated both in rat ovary and testis dispersions and rat gonadal cell culture systems that plasma lipoproteins increase gonadotropin-stimulated steroid hormone production (5-8).

Our studies on lipoprotein-stimulated steroidogenesis in rat granulosa cell cultures (9, 10) incorporates three major advantages compared to previous in vitro models. First, the granulosa cells are isolated from immature, hypophysectomized female rats so that the ovaries have not been recently exposed to pituitary gonadotropins (FSH, LH, prolactin). The animals are implanted with capsules containing diethylstilbestrol (DES) which triggers granulosa cell proliferation in synchronous fashion in every follicle of the ovaries. After 5-7 days the ovaries are removed and the enlarged preantral follicles are punctured to release approximately $1 \times 10^6$ viable granulosa cells per ovary without the use of degradative enzymes. Second, the granulosa cells from these follicles can be cultured in serum-free medium and differentiation with the same time course as they do in vivo, i.e., they contain a full complement of functional FSH receptors and the administration of FSH in vitro stimulates aromatase activity as well as the formation of functional LH/hCG and prolactin receptors (11). Androgen, in combination with FSH, stimulates progesterone and 20-α-dihydroprogesterone production (12). Third, these studies were carried out in serum-free (lipoprotein-free) medium, thus providing an opportunity to examine the effects of lipoproteins on granulosa cell function and differentiation.

## METHODS

Granulosa cells were cultured as previously described (9, 10) in serum-free McCoy's 5a medium supplemented with penicillin, streptomycin, and 2 mM L-glutamine in a humidified 95% air - 5% $CO_2$ incubator at 37°C. Human lipoprotein in the density range 1.019-1.063 g/ml (LDL) and rat and human lipoprotein in the density range 1.090-1.21 (HDL) were isolated by preparative ultracentrifugation. Radioiodinated lipoproteins were prepared using the iodine monochloride method of MACFARLANE (13) and $^{125}I$-lipoprotein degradation products in the medium were measured as previously described (9). Unmetabolized $^{125}I$-lipoprotein and free $^{125}I$-iodide were removed from 1 ml medium by the addition of 50 µl of 5 mg/ml albumin, 250 µl of 50% TCA and 400 µl of 5% AgNO$_3$ followed by centrifugation and filtration. The supernatant radioactivity is a measure of lipoprotein degradation. The physiologic end point of these studies of the interaction of granulosa cells and lipoproteins is progestin hormone synthesis. Progesterone and 20-α-dihydroprogesterone (the major progestin products) secreted into the medium were measured, after ether extraction by specific radioimmunoassay (9, 10).

RESULTS

We first examined the effect of added human and rat lipoproteins on progestin production by the rat granulosa cells. Granulosa cells were cultured for two days in the presence or absence of stimulating hormones (50 ng/ml oFSH + $10^{-7}$M androstenedione). The medium was removed and the cells were recultured for 2 days in the presence or absence of added lipoproteins. In the absence of stimulatory hormones, the granulosa cells produced no progestin product either in the presence or absence of added lipoprotein. The addition of FSH plus androstenedione stimulated the production of approximately 220 ng/ml 20-α-dihydroprogesterone and 16 ng/ml progesterone in the absence of lipoproteins. The addition of increasing log concentrations of human HDL, human LDL, and rat HDL to cells previously stimulated by FSH and androstenedione resulted in a linear increase in the production of both 20-α-dihydroprogesterone and progesterone to a maximum 3-5 fold increase. On the basis of lipoprotein protein concentration, human HDL and human LDL are equally effective cholesterol donors. At low concentrations (10 and 30 µg/ml), human HDL and rat HDL were similarly effective but at the higher concentration, rat HDL was less effective than human HDL in stimulating progestin production. These results demonstrate a direct action of lipoproteins on progestin production by FSH + androgen-primed granulosa cells cultured in serum-free medium. On the basis of these results, it seems likely that all the lipoproteins tested can provide cholesterol substrate to cultured granulosa cells in which the progestin biosynthetic pathway has been induced by hormone pretreatment.

In the analysis of human LDL utilization by these cultured granulosa cells, the possible influence of DES must be considered. Before culture, granulosa cell proliferation was stimulated by placing DES capsule in the immature rat. KOVANEN et. al. (14) have reported that pharmacologic doses of 17α-ethinyl estradiol cause a marked lowering of plasma lipoprotein levels in the rat due to enhanced liver uptake secondary to increased LDL binding sites. To test whether the utilization of human LDL by the cultured granulosa cells was due to DES pretreatment, we tested the effect of lipoproteins on progestin production by cultured granulosa cells from intact 26 day old female rats not given exogenous estrogen. Again, human LDL and human HDL were equally effective in stimulating progestin production, indicating that pharmacologic estrogen treatment is not necessary for LDL utilization by these granulosa cells.

We next investigated the degradation of $^{125}I$-labeled rat and human lipoproteins by rat ovary granulosa cells. The cells were obtained from DES-stimulated hypophysectomized immature female rats and were cultured in serum-free medium for 2 days. $^{125}I$-labeled lipoproteins were then added. The granulosa cells degraded the $^{125}I$-labeled lipoproteins to acid-soluble products, mainly monoiodotyrosine. The degradation of $^{125}I$-labeled rat HDL was a saturable, high affinity process (Km = 21 µg protein/ml). Degradation of rat HDL is a specific process since degradation was not inhibited by the presence of unlabeled human LDL. In studies measuring both rat $^{125}I$-HDL degradation and progestin (progesterone plus 20-α-dihydroprogesterone) production by the same granulosa cell cultures, the cholesterol potentially made available to the cells by rat HDL degradation could account for almost 90% of the cholesterol substrate necessary for the measured increment in progestin production(Table 1). The degradation of human $^{125}I$-HDL is also a specific, saturable and high affinity process (Km = 20 µg protein/ml). However, in contrast to human $^{125}I$-LDL, the degradation of human $^{125}I$-HDL can provide only 20% of the cholesterol substrate necessary for the measured increment in progestin production (Table 1). Granulosa cells can also degrade human $^{125}$I-LDL by a saturable, high affinity process (Km = 8 µg protein/ml), but LDL degradation can be inhibited significantly by a 10-fold excess of unlabeled human HDL. The degradation of human $^{125}$I-LDL can potentially provide twice the cholesterol necessary for increased progestin production (Table 1).

Table 1. Summary of lipoprotein degradation and progestin production by cultured rat granulosa cells

| Lipoprotein | | Degradation | | Progestin Production | |
|---|---|---|---|---|---|
| | Km[a] | Vmax[b] (lipoprotein protein) | Vmax[b] (lipoprotein cholesterol) | Km[a] | Vmax[b] |
| Rat $^{125}$I-HDL | 21±8 | 435±98 | 174±40 | 19±4 | 195±56 |
| Human $^{125}$I-HDL | 20±2 | 91±29 | 34±11 | 32±11 | 235±15 |
| Human $^{125}$I-LDL | 8±3 | 256±15 | 435±25 | --- | 222±48 |

a.  µg lipoprotein protein/ml, causing 1/2 maximal stimulation
b.  ng/2 X $10^5$ cells/24 hrs maximal degradation or production

Treatment of the granulosa cells with pronase (1-20 µg/ml) for 30 minutes at 37°C inhibited human $^{125}$I-LDL degradation by more than 80%, but actually enhanced rat $^{125}$I-HDL, indicating that the pathways which account for the degradation of LDL and HDL by the cells are separate.


We have also used radiolabeled human and rat lipoproteins to study the mechanisms by which hormones stimulate granulosa cell steroid production. It has been shown previously that androgens synergistically augment FSH-stimulated progestin production by cultured rat ovary granulosa cells (15). While it has been demonstrated that this androgen effect is androgen receptor-mediated (16), the mechanism by which androgen stimulates progestin production remains unknown. This interaction is interesting since FSH binds to cellular membrane receptor while androgen binds cytoplasmic receptors. In the absence of FSH and androgen, 2 X $10^5$ granulosa cells degraded basal levels (50-100 ng lipoprotein protein/24 hours) of added $^{125}$I-lipoproteins. These unstimulated cells produced no measurable 20-α-dihydroprogesterone. The addition of $10^{-7}$M androstenedione, testosterone, or 5α-dihydrotestosterone in the absence of FSH had no effect on lipoprotein degradation or 20-α-dihydroprogesterone production. FSH addition alone stimulated lipoprotein degradation by 50 to 300%, while the addition of androgen synergistically augmented the FSH-stimulated degradation of rat and human lipoproteins. The increase in lipoprotein degradation due to FSH alone or FSH plus androgen was associated with increased 20-α-dihydroprogesterone production. FSH was relatively more effective in stimulating lipoprotein degradation while androgen synergized with FSH to be a relatively better stimulator of progestin production. The addition of 10-fold excess cyproterone acetate (an antiandrogen) inhibited the testosterone effect, suggesting that the testosterone effect on lipoprotein degradation and progestin production is mediated via the granulosa cell androgen receptor. We have thus demonstrated that androgen, in combination with FSH, augments the steroidogenic pathway of the granulosa cell from the utilization of lipoproteins to the production of progestin end-products. The data suggest that FSH stimulated the degradation of lipoproteins and the uptake of lipoprotein cholesterol while androgen plus FSH stimulates the conversion of cellular cholesterol to progestin hormone products.

## DISCUSSION

The model system described in this report of cultured rat ovary granulosa cells which differentiate in serum-free medium, offers a unique opportunity to study the interactions of a steroidogenic cell with both HDL and LDL. These cells can be prepared for culture without the use of enzymes so that observed effects on lipoprotein uptake and/or degradation are due to the cells themselves and not to contamination of cell surfaces with residual enzymes such as collagenase or proteases. These cells are able to utilize both LDL and HDL by separate mechanisms which likely involve separate receptor-mediated processes.

The utilization of lipoprotein cholesterol by granulosa cells can be easily monitored by measuring progestin products which accumulate in the medium. Such comparisons of HDL degradation leading to cholesterol substrate provision and steroid hormone production have provided insight about the mechanism which regulates high-affinity uptake of HDL in steroidogenic tissues. First, rat granulosa cells degrade rat HDL via a specific, saturable process whose $K_m$ is identical within experimental limits to the $K_m$ of progestin production suggested that these 2 processes are directly linked. Second, the specificity and affinity of HDL degradation in granulosa cells from the ovary are similar to those observed for the rat testis cell membrane receptor for rat HDL. Third, granulosa cells differentially recognize rat and human HDL as indicated by a four-fold higher degradation rate of rat HDL. It is not known whether the difference is solely due to apoprotein differences in the two species of HDL, although CHEN and REAVEN (personal communication) have recently shown that apoprotein A-I is the mediator of high-affinity binding to the testis HDL receptor. Fourth, the cells make 5 times more progestin than can be accounted for by the cholesterol made available to the cell by degradation of human HDL. GWYNNE and HESS (17) have reported a similar discrepancy (4-fold) between degradation of human HDL apoprotein and cholesterol uptake in cultured rat adrenal cells. This suggests that human HDL binds to a high-affinity receptor on rat steroidogenic cells but may not be internalized as a whole particle or that the particles may be taken into the cells with cholesterol utilization following a path distinct from that of apoprotein degradation and/or removal from the cells. It should be noted that the extent of degradation of the $^{125}$-I HDL particles may be an underestimate of the true rate of uptake and processing of HDL particles since CHEN and REAVEN (personal communication) have recently described that chemical derivatization of tyrosine residues in HDL proteins inhibits HDL binding to testis membranes. Similarly, we have observed on our studies that unlabeled HDL and HDL labeled with $^{125}$I by the ICl method do not provide identical amounts of cholesterol precursor for steroidogenesis when presented to cells at identical lipoprotein particle concentrations. Thus, tyrosine residues may play a major role in the uptake pathway mediated by HDL receptors.

Granulosa cells are able to differentiate normally under the culture conditions we have described, thus allowing an examination of the effect of the various lipoprotein classes on this differentiation process. Finally, the interaction of quite different trophic agents on these granulosa cells, such as FSH and androgen, can be examined using radiolabeled lipoproteins so that individual mechanisms of action can be examined in detail. The physiological significance of lipoprotein interaction with ovarian follicle granulosa cells is unknown, since blood vessels do not penetrate the follicle basement membrane until vascularization occurs at the corpus luteum state. Studies with luteal cells indicate that interactions similar to those described for granulosa cells and plasma lipoproteins are important for regulation of progestin production. The definitive studies to demonstrate lipoprotein-stimulated steroidogenesis and gonadal control mechanisms will await the use of in vivo data.

## ACKNOWLEDGMENTS

We wish to thank Drs. Aaron Hsueh and Gregory Erickson for help in completion of these studies. This work was supported by the NIH Research Project Grant HD-12303 and the Atherosclerosis SCOR program HL 14197-10.

## References

1. Savard K (1973) The biochemistry of the corpus lutem. Biol. Reprod. 8: 183-202
2. Brown MS, Goldstein JL (1976) Receptor-mediated control of cholesterol metabolism. Science 191: 150-154
3. Andersen JM, Dietschy JM (1978) Relative importance of lipoproteins in the regulation of cholesterol synthesis in the adrenal gland, ovary and testis of the rat. J. Biol. Chem. 253: 9024-9032
4. Chen Y-DI, Kramer FB, Reaven GM (1980) Identification of specific high density lipoprotein binding sites in rat testis and regulation of binding by human chronic gonadotropin. J. Biol. Chem. 255: 9162-9167
5. Quinn PG, Dombrausky LJ, Chen Y-DI, Payne AH (1981) Serum lipoproteins increase testosterone production in hCG-desentized leydig cells. Endocrinology 109: 1790-1792
6. Rosenblum MF, Huttler CR, Strauss JF (1981) Control of sterol metabolism in cultured rat granulosa cells. Endocrinology 109: 1518-1527
7. Nimrod A (1981) On the synergistic action of adrogen and FSH on progestin secretion of cultured rat granulosa cells. Mol. Cell. Endrocrinol. 21: 51-62
8. Schreiber JR, Weinstein DB, Hsueh AJW (1982) Lipoproteins stimulate androgen production by cultured rat testis cells. J. Steroid Biochem. 16: 39-43
9. Schreiber JR, Hseuh AJW, Weinstein DB, Erickson GF (1980) Plasma lipoproteins stimulate progestin production by rat ovarian granulosa cells cultured in serum-free medium. J. Steroid Biochem. 13:1009-1014
10. Scheiber, JR, Nakamura K, Weinstein DB (1982) Degradation of rat and human lipoproteins by cultured rat ovary granulosa cells. Endocrinology 110: 55-63
11. Erickson GF, Wang C, Hseuh AJW (1979) FSH-induction of function LH receptors in granulosa cells cultured in a chemically-defined medium. Nature 279: 336-338
12. Nimrod A, Lindner HA (1976) A synergistic effect of androgen on the stimulation of progesterone secretion by FSH in cultured rat granulosa cells. Molec. Cell Endocrinol. 5: 315-320
13. MacFarlane AS (1958) Efficient trace-labeling of proteins with iodine. Nature 182: 53
14. Kovanen P, Brown MS, Goldstein JL (1979) Increased binding of low density lipoprotein to liver membranes from rats treated with 17$\alpha$ ethinyl estradiol

15. Leung PCK, Armstrong DT (1979) Estrogen treatment of immature rats inhibits ovarian androgen production in vitro. Endocrinology 104: 1411-1417
16. Schreiber JR, Reid R, Ross GT (1976) A receptor-like testosterone-binding protein in ovaries from estrogen-stimulated hypohysectomized immature female rats. Endocrinology 98: 1206-1213
17. Gwynne JT, Hess B (1980) The role of high density lipoprotein in rat adrenal cholesterol metabolism and steroidogenesis. J. Biol. Chem. 254: 11367-11371

# 3.3 Regulation of Lipoprotein Synthesis and Secretion

# Contribution of Apoprotein B Production Rate in the Regulation of Lipoprotein Levels in Man

Y. A. Kesaniemi and S. M. Grundy

## Introduction

There is a wide range in plasma total and low density lipoprotein (LDL) cholesterol in the general population, but factors determining this variability are poorly understood. The work of GOLDSTEIN and BROWN (1) has demonstrated that clearance of LDL is mediated in part by specific receptors for LDL on the surface of cells. The importance of LDL receptors in regulating LDL concentrations is illustrated by the genetic disorder, familial hypercholesterolemia (FH), which is characterized by a deficiency of receptors and marked elevations in LDL levels. Beyond this disorder, however, little is known about control of LDL concentration in patients with various cholesterol levels. One possibility is that LDL levels over the wide "normal" range may be controlled primarily through the metabolism of apolipoprotein B, the almost exclusive apoprotein of LDL (apoLDL). For this reason, we have examined synthetic and clearance rates of apoLDL and their role in regulating LDL concentrations in a group of subjects showing a broad range in levels from low-normal to mildly-elevated. The purpose of the study was to determine whether production or clearance of LDL is the major factor controlling LDL concentrations.

## Methods

Sixteen patients with plasma cholesterol from low normal to mildly elevated were studied in the metabolic unit on a standardized diet of mixed solid food and liquid formula containing 40% of calories as fat. Total cholesterol ranged from 162 to 322 mg/dl. Four patients had plasma cholesterol levels above the 95th percentile for the corresponding age and sex group according to the Lipid Research Clinics Program Prevalence Study (2). The plasma triglyceride values ranged from 78 to 244 mg/dl and all the values fell below the 95th percentile (2). LDL-cholesterol varied from 104 to 231 mg/dl, and in two patients values exceeded the 95th percentile for the general population. None of the patients appeared to have FH because of lack of marked hypercholesterolemia, tendon xanthomas, or history of unusually premature coronary heart disease; also family histories of these abnormalities were absent. After the patients had been on the diet for 10 days to 2 weeks, LDL (D= 1.025-1.060 g/ml) was isolated and iodinated with $^{125}I$. $^{125}I$-LDL was injected intravenously and blood samples and urine specimens collected for 14-21 days. The kinetic parameters for LDL turnover were calculated according to MATTHEWS model (3). The fractional catabolic rate (FCR) was measured independently by relating the daily urinary excretion rate of $^{125}I$ radioactivity to the $^{125}I$ radioactivity in plasma (U/P ratio). The rate of apoLDL synthesis was calculated by multiplying the apoLDL pool size with FCR. The apoLDL pool size was calculated from the measured plasma volume and from the measured concentration of plasma apoLDL.

## Results

The apoLDL concentrations among the 16 patients ranged from 74 to 167 mg/dl. The FCR for apoLDL as calculated from the plasma radioactivity die-away curve ranged from 0.236 to 0.441 day$^{-1}$. Similar results were obtained when FCR was calculated from U/P ratios. No significant correlation could be found between plasma apoLDL concentrations and FCR (r=0.10). In contrast, synthetic rates varied from 9.5 to 29.2 mg/day/kg ideal weight (IW) and were correlated positively with plasma apoLDL concentrations (r=0.74;p<0.001). A high correlation between plasma apoLDL levels and synthetic rates also was found among the 12 subjects whose total cholesterol concentrations fell below the 95th percentile for age and sex (r=0.74; p<0.01). In addition, significant correlations were observed between synthetic rate of apoLDL and a) LDL-cholesterol (r=0.50; p<0.05, b) LDL protein/cholesterol ratio (r=0.55; p<0.05), and c) plasma total triglycerides (r=0.52; p<0.05). Almost significant were the relations between apoLDL synthesis and d) plasma total cholesterol (r=0.45; p<0.08), e) VLDL-triglycerides (r=0.47; p<0.06) and f) total body weight (r=0.43; p<0.10). None of these 6 parameters were correlated significantly with FCR of apoLDL (r=-0.25, -0.28, 0.28, -0.20, 0.19 and 0.01, respectively). The relations between concentrations and synthesis of apoLDL were examined in another way in Table 1. The patients were divided into 3 groups according to their apoLDL concentrations: Group I (apoLDL < 100 mg/dl), Group II (apoLDL = 100-130 mg/dl), and Group III (apoLDL > 130 mg/dl). In these groups, mean levels of apoLDL increased significantly from 83 to 122 to 149 mg/dl; LDL-cholesterol rose significantly from 131 to 169 to 201 mg/dl; and synthetic rates for apoLDL increased significantly from 11.6 to 17.0 to 23.8 mg/day/kg IW. In contrast, the FCR of apoLDL remained unchanged (0.319, 0.288, and 0.334, respectively).

**Table 1.** Plasma lipids and kinetic parameters for $^{125}$I-ApoLDL turnover studies as subgrouped according to the plasma ApoLDL concentration (mean±SEM)

| Group (No) | Total Chol | Total TG | LDL Chol | Plasma ApoLDL | ApoLDL FCR | ApoLDL synthesis | |
|---|---|---|---|---|---|---|---|
| | | mg/dl | | | day$^{-1}$ | mg/day/kgIW | mg/day/kg |
| I (4) | 209+19 | 145+36 | 131+12 | 83+5[a] | 0.319+0.031 | 11.6+1.2[a] | 11.5+1.2 |
| II (6) | 250+9 | 168+14 | 169+4[a] | 122+2[a] | 0.288+0.021 | 17.0+0.9[a] | 14.6+1.0[a] |
| III (6) | 285+10[a,b] | 205+10 | 201+8[a,b] | 149+5[a,b] | 0.334+0.027 | 23.8+1.8[a,b] | 20.5+2.3[a,b] |

[a]Significantly higher than I (p<0.02 or less)
[b]Significantly higher than II (p<0.05 or less).

## Concluding Remarks

In this study subjects with plasma cholesterol levels from low-normal to mildly-elevated were examined to evaluate the role of apoLDL synthesis and catabolism in regulation of plasma apoLDL and LDL-cholesterol concentrations. The major finding was that concentrations of apoLDL and LDL-cholesterol over a broad range of LDL levels were regulated mainly by synthetic rates of apoLDL (4). Our findings in subjects whose LDL-cholesterol varied over the normal range differ from those in patients with FH in that their FCR did not decrease with increasing LDL levels. The most notable feature of the patients of this study was a broad range of synthetic rates of apoLDL that correlated closely with apoLDL concentrations. These rates varied from 9.5 to 29.5 mg/day/kgIW (8.6 to 26.9 mg/day/kg) in patients whose LDL-cholesterol levels ranged from 104 to 231 mg/dl. It is interesting to compare these production rates to those reported previously for normocholesterolemic subjects by other workers. Table 2 shows kinetic parameters of LDL-turnover in normal subjects for previous studies. Although types of subjects, diets and other conditions varied to some extent among the different reports, the comparisons are of interest nevertheless.

Table 2. Kinetics of LDL-B (apoLDL) turnover in normal subjects - review of previous studies

| Reference | No | LDL-apoB (apoLDL) mg/dl | LDL-FCR day$^{-1}$ | LDL-apoB(apoLDL) synthesis mg/day/kg |
|---|---|---|---|---|
| Bilheimer et al (5) | 6 | 48±6 | 0.450±0.072 | 8.0±0.7 |
| Garnick et al (6) American Indians | 10 | 52±3 | 0.432±0.01 | 7.3[a] |
| Janus et al (7) | 7 | 55[a] | 0.310±0.04 | 7.7±1.7 |
| Nestel et al (8) Vegetarians | 7 | 57±14 | 0.648 | 9.1±2.3 |
| Sigurdsson et al (9) | 6 | 67±12[a] | 0.397±0.097[a] | 11.7±2.0[a] |
| Reardon et al (10) | 3 | 70±20[a] | 0.287±0.045[a] | 8.3±2.5[a] |
| Calvert et al (11) | 5 | 74±14[a] | 0.308±0.078[a] | 10.2[a] |
| Nestel et al (12) | 5 | 76±35[a] | 0.400±0.17[a] | 12.1±1.6[a] |
| Garnick et al (6) White Americans | 5 | 77±4 | 0.411±0.01 | 13.7[a] |
| Shephard et al (13) | 8 | 80±13 | 0.322±0.035 | 11.5±1.9 |
| Packard et al (14) | 4 | 81±4 | 0.287±0.057 | 8.7±1.7 |
| Nestel et al (8) Non-Vegetarians | 6 | 84±20 | 0.552[a] | 11.8±0.6 |
| Packard et al (15) | 5 | 98±16 | 0.312±0.029 | 11.6±1.6 |
| Walton et al (16) | 8 | 108±20[a] | 0.302±0.095[a] | 14.3±6.0[a] |

[a] Calculated or estimated from the published data.

The results of the present study for low apoLDL levels (Table 1) fit well with previous findings(Table 2). Most previous studies have been done in subjects in the "low-normal" range of apoLDL and LDL cholesterol. Even in this range, however, there appears to be a fairly good correlation between apoLDL(LDL-B) levels and production rates (r=0.77;n=14; p<0.001) (Table 2) whereas apoLDL(LDL-B) concentrations are not correlated with FCR(-0.39;n=14). Unfortunately, few studies have been done in subjects in the "high-normal" range for comparison, but as shown by the present work (Table 1) correlations noted at lower concentrations appear to extend to higher ones as well.

An important question concerning the source of LDL in subjects of the present study can be raised. First, LDL might be derived from the catabolism of VLDL; and second, it could be the product of direct synthesis. PHILLIPS et al (17) have reported a positive correlation between VLDL-triglycerides and LDL-cholesterol in subjects with total triglycerides over the normal range. In our study, apoLDL synthesis was significantly related to plasma total triglycerides and almost significantly to VLDL-triglycerides; this observation also suggests that VLDL concentrations (and perhaps VLDL synthesis rates) partially regulate LDL concentrations. In patients with FH, however, a significant portion of LDL appears to arise by direct secretion

(VLDL-independent synthesis of LDL) (18,19). Our recent studies (20) suggest that subjects with LDL levels in the high normal range also have a considerable portion of their LDL-B secreted directly, independently of VLDL-B secretion. In addition, we found a negative correlation between direct LDL-B secretion and VLDL -B production rate whereas total apoprotein B synthesis (VLDL-B plus direct LDL-B) was correlated positively with direct LDL-B secretion. These findings together with previous reports (18,19) suggest that when apoprotein B production rate remains low-normal apoB is secreted with triglyceride-rich core, but when apoB synthesis is increased part of apoprotein B will be secreted as cholesterol-ester containing particles. Whether cholesterol and/or triglyceride synthesis regulates how apoB is secreted is not known.

Although the synthesis of LDL-B generally seems to regulate the plasma LDL-B (apoLDL) and LDL-cholesterol concentrations in subjects with serum cholesterol from low normal to mildly elevated there may be populations with disproportionally high LDL-B synthesis rates as compared to plasma LDL levels. We have studied $^{125}$I-apoLDL turnover in normolipidemic men with a well-documented coronary heart disease (status post coronary artery by-pass grafting) and in age, sex and plasma lipid matched controls (21). The patients with coronary heart disease had considerably higher apoLDL synthesis rates than control subjects, even though LDL cholesterol concentrations were on the same level. However, the FCRs for apoLDL were also higher in coronary heart disease patients than in controls. These findings show that some individuals with high apoLDL production rate can still maintain normal LDL concentrations by increasing LDL clearance. The results of this study also suggest that the rate of flux of apoprotein B through LDL may affect atherogenesis independent of LDL concentrations.

## References

1. Goldstein JL, Brown MS (1977) The low density lipoprotein pathway and its relation to atherosclerosis. Ann Rev Biochem 46:897-930.
2. The Lipid Research Clinics Program Epidemiology Committee. (1979) Plasma lipid distributions in selected North American populations: The Lipid Research Clinics Program Prevalence Study. Circulation 60: 427-439.
3. Matthews CME (1957) The theory of tracer experiments with $^{131}$I-labelled plasma proteins. Phys Med Biol 2:36-53.
4. Kesaniemi YA, Grundy SM (1982) The significance of low density lipoprotein production in the regulation of plasma cholesterol level in man. J Clin Invest (In press).
5. Bilheimer DW, Goldstein JL, Grundy SM, Brown MS (1975) Reduction in cholesterol and low density lipoprotein synthesis after portacaval shunt surgery in a patient with homozygous familial hypercholesterolemia. J Clin Invest 56:1420-1430.
6. Garnick MB, Bennett PH, Langer T (1979) Low density lipoprotein metabolism and lipoprotein cholesterol content in southwestern American Indians. J Lipid Res 20:31-39.
7. Janus ED, Nicoll AM, Turner PR, Magill P, Lewis B (1980) Kinetic bases of the primary hyperlipidaemias: studies of apolipoprotein B turnover in genetically defined subjects. Europ J Clin Invest 10:161-172.
8. Nestel PJ, Billington T, Smith B (1981) Low density and high density lipoprotein kinetics and sterol balance in vegetarians. Metabolism 30:941-945.
9. Sigurdsson G, Nicholl A, Lewis B (1975) Conversion of very low density lipoprotein to low density lipoprotein. A metabolic study of apolipoprotein B kinetics in human subjects. J Clin Invest 56:1481-1490.
10. Reardon MF, Fidge NH, Nestel PJ (1978) Catabolism of very low density lipoprotein B apoprotein in man. J Clin Invest 61:850-860.
11. Calvert GD, James HM (1979) Low-density lipoprotein turnover studies in man. Evaluation of the integrated rate equations method, use of a whole-body radioactivity counter, and the problem of partial denaturation. Clin Sci 56:71-76.

12. Nestel PJ, Reardon M, Fidge NH (1979) Sucrose-induced changes in VLDL-and LDL-B apoprotein removal rates. Metabolism 28:531-535.
13. Shephard J, Packard CJ, Grundy SM, Yeshurun D, Gotto AM Jr, Taunton OD (1980) Effects of saturated and polyunsaturated fat diets on the chemical composition and metabolism of low density lipoproteins in man. J Lipid Res 21:91-99.
14. Packard CJ, Shephard J, Joerns S, Gotto AM, Taunton OD (1980) Apolipoprotein B metabolism in normal, type IV and type V hyperlipoproteinemic subjects. Metabolism 29:213-221.
15. Packard CJ, Third JLHC, Shephard J, Lorimer AR, Morgan HG, Lawrie TDW (1976) low density lipoprotein metabolism in a family of familial hypercholesterolemic patients. Metabolism 25:995-1006.
16. Walton KW, Scott PJ, Dykes PN, Davies JWL (1965) The significance of alterations in serum lipids in thyroid dysfunction. II. Alterations of the metabolism and turnover of 131-I-low-density lipoproteins in hypothyroidism and thyrotoxicosis. Clin Sci 29:217-238.
17. Phillips NR, Havel RJ, Kane JP (1981) Levels and interrelationships of serum and lipoprotein cholesterol and triglyceridies. Association with adiposity and the consumption of ethanol, tobacco, and beverages containing caffeine. Arteriosclerosis I:13-24.
18. Soutar AK, Myant NB, Thompson GR (1977) Simultaneous measurement of apolipoprotein B turnover in very low-and low-density lipoproteins in familial hypercholesterolemia. Atherosclerosis 28:247-256.
19. Janus ED, Nicoll A, Wootton R, Turner PR, Magill PHJ, Lewis B (1980) Quantitative studies of very low density lipoprotein: conversion to low density lipoprotein in normal controls and primary hyperlipidaemic states and the role of direct secretion of low density lipoprotein in heterozygous familial hypercholesterolaemia. Europ J Clin Invest 10:149-159.
20. Kesaniemi YA, Beltz WF, Grundy SM (1981) Role of direct secretion of low density lipoprotein in causation of primary hypercholesterolemia. Arteriosclerosis 1:366a.
21. Kesaniemi YA, Grundy SM (1982) Overproduction of low density lipoprotein (LDL) in normolipidemic coronary heart disease (CHD) patients. Clin Res 30:526a.

# Measurements of C Apoprotein Kinetics in Man

P. J. Nestel, N. H. Fidge and M. W. Huff

There have been few in vivo studies of C apoprotein metabolism in
man. Berman et al. (1) have carried out analyses of total C apoprotein kinetics following reinjection of radiolabelled VLDL. The
simulated model resembled that for VLDL B apoprotein metabolism,
comprising a series of 4 delipidation steps of the triglyceride-
rich particles during which C peptides become transferred to HDL,
producing a final IDL particle which retains a small fraction of
the original VLDL C apoprotein. The model did not identify the
lipoprotein with which the C peptides entered the circulation,
both VLDL and HDL fitting the data, but removal of C protein
appeared to occur with HDL. The major aspects of this in vivo
model coincided with findings observed consistently during the
in vitro lipolysis of VLDL, and with studies of isolated cells
and organs.

A later report from this group (2) discussed the faster removal
rate of the C than of the A peptides, from plasma HDL in 2 normal
subjects. If C apoprotein was removed predominantly within HDL,
then the above discrepancy suggested either that C peptides were not
cleared as part of intact HDL particles, but removed independently
from the lipoprotein, or that the C and A proteins were not distributed uniformly among the HDL subclasses.

Our laboratory has developed techniques that have allowed more
precise descriptions of the kinetics of individual C peptides in
normal and in hyperlipidemic subjects (3). The methodology is
based on the determination of the specific radioactivity-time
curves of the three major C peptides following their reinjection
within triglyceride-rich particles.

Following reinjection of VLDL radiolabelled C apoproteins redistribute
rapidly between VLDL and HDL so that isotopic equilibrium, demonstrated by the similar specific radioactivities of the corresponding
peptides in VLDL and HDL, is reached within a few hours in a normal
subject. The initial exchange of C apoproteins within the plasma
and possibly also with a smaller extravascular pool such as lymph,
gives rise to a two-pool system. In other subjects, especially
in those with hypertriglyceridemia who have greatly expanded
intravascular pools of C apoproteins, largely within VLDL, the
removal of radioactivity is more commonly monoexponential. The C
apoproteins are therefore metabolized mainly within a single homogeneous pool (for each C peptide) and appear to reside mainly within
the plasma. It is also clear that the three major C apoproteins
have similar fractional removal rates (half-time of removal
averaging just under 30 hours in normal subjects not eating fat).
This implies similar sites and modes of catabolism and closely
related functions. As suggested by other work the CII and CIII
peptides might act in unison, the former initiating the dismantling
of triglyceride-rich particles while the latter ensures that the
particle is not prematurely removed from the circulation.

TABLE 1. Kinetic parameters of C apoprotein metabolism in normolipidaemic and hypertriglyceridaemic subjects and in 6 normal men before and 10 days after a carbohydrate-rich diet

| Subjects | Apoprotein CII | | | Apoprotein CIII1 | | | Apoprotein CIII2 | | |
|---|---|---|---|---|---|---|---|---|---|
| | Mass mg/kg | FCR[†] hr$^{-1}$ | Flux[†] mg/kg/d | Mass mg/kg | FCR hr$^{-1}$ | Flux mg/kg/d | Mass mg/kg | FCR hr$^{-1}$ | Flux mg/kg/d |
| Normal (n=8) | 1.8 | 0.029 | 1.2 | 4.5 | 0.027 | 2.6 | 3.7 | 0.026 | 2.4 |
| Hypertri- glyceridaemic (n=7) | 4.8 | 0.013 | 1.5 | 12.7 | 0.013 | 3.7 | 8.2 | 0.014 | 2.5 |
| Normal (n=6) | .86 | 0.029 | 0.60 | 1.93 | 0.025 | 1.15 | 1.78 | 0.026 | 1.13 |
| Normal (n=6) (high carbo- hydrate) | 1.39 | 0.027 | 0.89 | 3.21 | 0.026 | 1.99 | 2.59 | 0.031 | 1.92 |

†FCR - irreversible fractional removal rate; Flux = production rate

The table shows 1) that all C peptides are higher in hypertriglyceridaemia due to diminished FCR; 2) that after a high carbohydrate diet, the rise in C peptides in normal subjects is due to increased flux.

We have shown kinetically that C apoprotein mass increases with rising plasma triglyceride levels (Table 1). In subjects with established hypertriglyceridemia this appears to be due entirely to reduced removal. In a large group of subjects with various forms of hypertriglyceridemia, the synthetic rates for all C peptides were not greater than in normal subjects (3). Over-production of C apoprotein does not therefore accompany hyper-triglyceridemia, in contrast to the increased formation of VLDL B protein, indicative of increased secretion of particles. This might conceivably contribute to the persistence of hypertrigly-ceridemia though in our subjects there was no reduction in the apo-CII:apo-CIII ratio as reported by some workers.

We have however observed an increase in C apoprotein production when hypertriglyceridemia was induced with carbohydrate-rich diets (Table 1; 4). When normal individuals eat such a diet there is an increase in triglyceride production resulting in moderate hypertriglyceridemia which does not usually persist beyond a few weeks. As in our previous studies (5) the expansion in VLDL B apoprotein pool size was due to increased formation of VLDL B (or number of VLDL particles) and also to reduced fractional removal. By contrast the mass and pool size of each C apo-protein rose significantly in response to increased production rather than to diminished removal.

The question arises whether a rise in C apoprotein production is required to handle the increased formation of triglyceride since hypertriglyceridemia does not occur in the heterozygous

578

form of apo-CII deficiency, despite half-normal CII levels. On the other hand with overproduction of VLDL triglyceride much more C apoprotein may be required to limit the degree of hypertriglyceridemia. Whereas the increased pool size of C apoproteins of hypertriglyceridemic subjects was due entirely to decreased removal, with carbohydrate loading expansion in C peptide pool size was related to increased production. Hypertriglyceridemia may therefore reflect failure to increase C apoprotein production and carbohydrate-induced hypertriglyceridemia may persist only if C apoprotein formation fails to match triglyceride overproduction.

A second set of studies was designed to perturb the metabolism of the C apoproteins by inducing maximal lipolysis with infusions of heparin. However, even when triglyceride-rich particles were catabolized rapidly the rates of loss of the individual C apoproteins were proportional to their initial concentrations in the particles. The findings in one subject are shown in Figure 1: the rates of transfer of radiolabelled C apoproteins from the triglyceride-rich lipoproteins to HDL were identical for the three C peptides. The consistency of this finding, firstly in the metabolic steady state, then during overproduction due to dietary carbohydrate and finally during rapid catabolism, demonstrates the functional unity of these proteins.

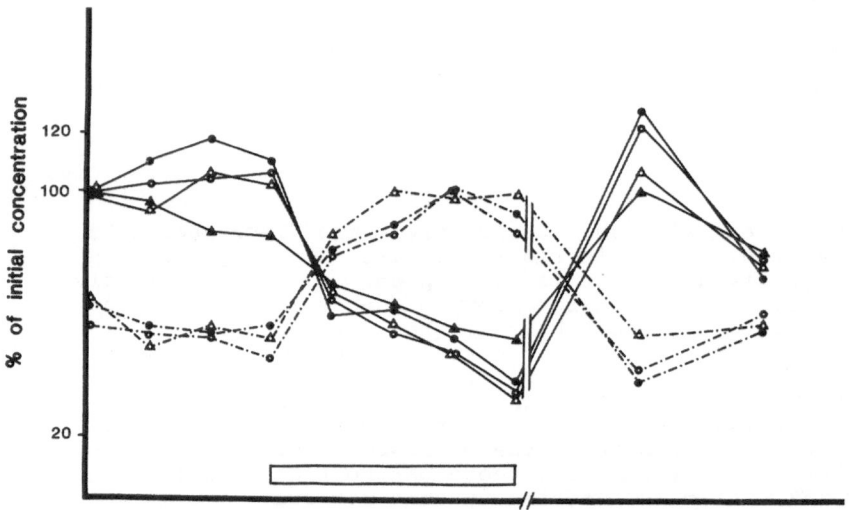

Fig.1. Percentage redistribution of triglyceride (TG) and C apoproteins (CII, CIII$_1$ and CIII$_2$) between triglyceride-rich lipoprotein (TGRL) and high density lipoprotein (HDL) during and after heparin infusion (shown by rectangular block). ▲ = plasma triglyceride; ● = apo CII; ○ = apo CIII$_1$; △ = apo CIII$_2$; TGRL = ——— ; HDL = —·—· .

A most interesting finding to arise from the heparin studies was that of an alternative catabolic pathway for the C apoproteins. When heparin was infused into four severely hypertriglyceridemic subjects, the loss of C apoproteins from triglyceride-rich particles was far greater than could be recovered within HDL, the discrepancy being as great as 90-95%. Substantial

catabolism of C apoprotein can therefore be analogous to the
"shunt" pathway we had described for VLDL B apoprotein, where
up to 75% of remnants can be removed without conversion to LDL (6).
These findings may apply only in cases of severe hypertriglyceridemia but raise the important question whether this lack of conservation of C apoproteins might exacerbate the severity of the hyperlipoproteinemia.

References

1.  Berman M, Hall M, Levy RI, Eisenberg S, Bilheimer DW, Phair RD
    and Goebel RH (1978)  Metabolism of apo B and apo C lipoproteins
    in man: Kinetic studies in normal and hyperlipoproteinemic
    subjects  J Lipid Res 19: 38-56
2.  Schaefer EJ, Foster DM, Jenkins LL, Lindgren FT, Berman M,
    Levy RI and Brewer HB Jr (1979)  The composition and metabolism
    of high density apoprotein subfractions  Lipids 14: 511-520
3.  Huff MW, Fidge NH, Nestel PJ, Billington T and Watson B (1981)
    Metabolism of C-apolipoproteins: kinetics of CII, CIII$_1$ and
    C-III$_2$, and VLDL-apolipoprotein B in normal and hyperlipo-
    proteinemic subjects  J Lipid Res 22: 1235-1246
4.  Huff MW and Nestel PJ (1982)  Metabolism of apolipoproteins CII,
    CIII$_1$, CIII$_2$ and VLDL-B in human subjects consuming high carbo-
    hydrate diets  Metabolism (in press)
5.  Nestel PJ, Reardon MF and Fidge NH (1979)  Very low density
    lipoprotein-B apoprotein kinetics in human subjects  Cir Res
    45: 35-41
6.  Reardon MF, Fidge NH and Nestel PJ (1978)  The catabolism of
    very low density lipoprotein B apoprotein in man  J Clin Invest
    61: 850-860

# Regulation of Rat Liver Apolipoprotein E mRNA and Cloning of Its cDNA

J. M. Taylor, C. Fukazawa, S. C. Rall, Jr., K. H. Weisgraber, R. W. Mahley, and J. W. McLean

Apolipoprotein E (apo-E) is an arginine-rich glycoprotein of approximately 35,000 molecular weight that is an abundant component in several classes of mammalian plasma lipoprotein particles (for review see 1). It is a major secretory product of the liver, but may also be produced by other tissues in significant quantities. Metabolic studies indicate that apo-E plays a central role in plasma cholesterol transport and uptake by various tissues (for review see 2). Apolipoprotein E interacts with specific cell surface receptors, which then mediate cellular uptake of associated lipoprotein particles. Several genetic variants of human apo-E have been described, some of which show a great deal less receptor binding than normal apo-E (2,3,4). The complete amino acid sequence of human apo-E has recently been reported by Rall, Weisgraber, and Mahley (5). They have also found that the three major isoforms of apo-E differ in their amino acid sequences, a result of arginine/cysteine interchanges at two sites in their peptide chains. These differences correlate with altered receptor binding activity shown by some variants (5,6).

The recent advances made in determining apo-E structure, function, and metabolism emphasize the importance of understanding the detailed molecular mechanisms involved in the regulation of apo-E production and the control of the expression of its gene. A central component in the expression of a mammalian structural gene is the messenger RNA (mRNA), which codes for the protein and determines its production. An understanding of apo-E biosynthesis would be considerably enhanced by the availability of a specific complementary DNA (cDNA) hybridization probe for mRNA quantitation and sequence determination. This communication reports the preparation and partial characterization of rat apo-E cDNA, as well as a preliminary study of the expression of its corresponding mRNA. The following procedures have been widely described by investigators, and we have previously reported the details of the experimental protocols as employed in our laboratory (7).

The first step in this analysis involved the partial purification of apo-E mRNA. Total poly(A)-containing RNA was isolated from normal rat liver and translated in a mRNA-dependent cell-free protein-synthesizing system derived from rabbit reticulocyte lysate, with [³H]leucine included to radioactively label the translation products of exogenous mRNA (7). Following translation, newly synthesized proteins corresponding to the precursors of total plasma proteins produced by liver mRNA, as well as apo-E, were immunoprecipitated with specific antibodies and examined by gel electrophoresis and fluorography (Fig. 1A). The apo-E precursor protein could be identified as a major peptide product of the liver, with a molecular weight of about 34,000.

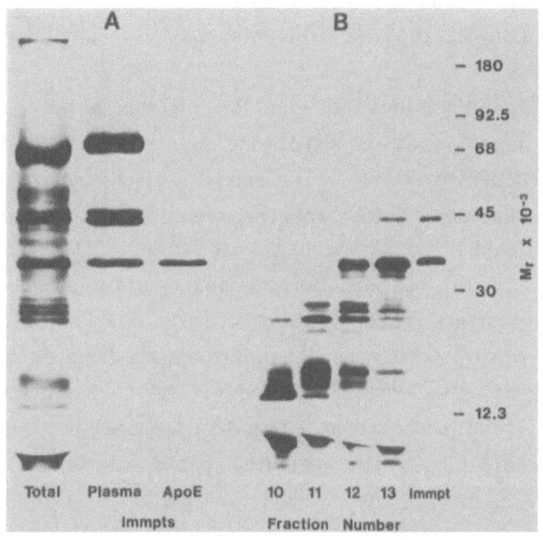

Fig. 1. Translation products of rat liver mRNA. Panel A shows the translation products of total poly(A)-containing RNA, immunoprecipitated with antibodies to total plasma proteins, and immunoprecipitated with antibodies to apo-E. Panel B shows the translation products of RNA of fractions from the upper portion of a sucrose gradient, and an immunoprecipitate of fraction 13 translation products with antibody to total plasma proteins

To enrich for apo-E mRNA, the liver poly(A)-containing RNA was sedimented through an isokinetic sucrose gradient and collected in fractions. The fractions were analyzed by cell-free translation, followed by gel electrophoresis; two RNA fractions were found to be especially enriched for apo-E mRNA (Fig. 1B). A mRNA fraction was then employed as a template for double-stranded cDNA (ds-cDNA) synthesis by reverse transcriptase. The 3'-ends of the ds-cDNA were tailed with oligo(dC), and the tailed ds-cDNA was inserted into the PstI restriction endonuclease site in the ampicillin resistance gene of the plasmid pBR322 that had previously been tailed with oligo(dG). The bacterial host E.

582

<u>coli</u> RRI was then transformed with this hybrid DNA, and about 1000 ampicil-
lin-sensitive, tetracycline-resistant transformants were selected. Transformants were screened by colony filter hybridization with [32]P-labeled cDNA to mRNA
fractions enriched and deficient in apo-E mRNA. A recombinant DNA plasmid
(pALE124), containing a ds-cDNA of about 900 base pairs in length, was identified as a possible candidate for containing the apo-E sequence. In order to
facilitate the subsequent examination and use of this cDNA sequence, it was
subcloned into the bacteriophage M13mp7. Recombinant bacteriophages containing
the coding strand (M13ALE124m) and the complementary noncoding strand
(M13ALE124c) were identified.

To determine the identity of the apo-E candidate plasmid, M13ALE124c DNA was
immobilized on a nitrocellulose filter and hybridized to total liver poly(A)-
containing RNA. The specifically bound RNA was eluted and then translated in
the cell-free protein-synthesizing system, and the translation product was
identified as apo-E by immunoprecipitation and gel electrophoresis. The identity of the apo-E recombinant plasmid was reconfirmed by a partial nucleotide
sequence determination of the ds-cDNA insert. This nucleotide sequence was
employed to predict the corresponding amino acid sequence of a portion of the
rat apo-E protein. The rat amino acid sequence was then compared to the previously determined protein sequences of human apo-E (5) and dog apo-E (S.C.
Rall, Jr., K.H. Weisgraber, and R.W. Mahley, unpublished results).

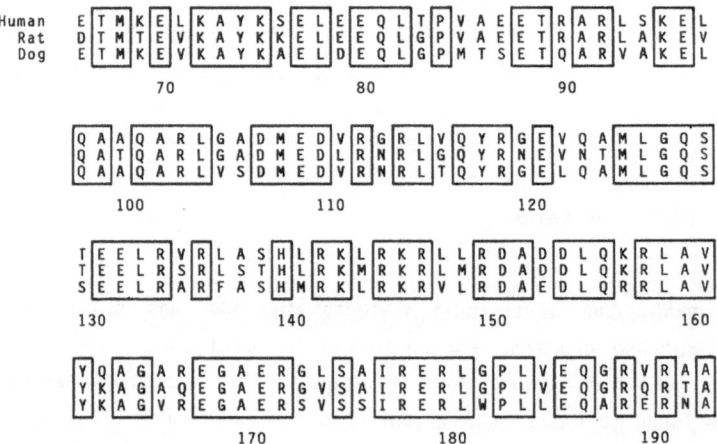

Fig. 2. Partial amino acid sequence of human, rat (predicted), and dog apo-E.
The boxes enclose residues that are identical among the three species. The
numbers correspond to the human sequence

583

Figure 2 shows that there is a relatively high homology among the three amino acid sequences, confirming the identity of the rat apo-E plasmid. In the region illustrated, 65% of the amino acid residues are identical in all three proteins. The relatively high conservation of sequence suggests that this region of the apo-E is important in the function of the protein. In this regard, it has been shown that the arginine residues at positions 145 and 158 (Fig. 2) are interchanged with cysteine residues in certain isoforms of human apo-E (5). Furthermore, these residues are important in the interaction between apo-E and its specific cell surface receptor (6).

The size of rat apo-E mRNA, as well as the relative level of this mRNA, were investigated by cDNA hybridization to RNA blots. Total poly(A)-containing RNA from normal liver was denatured with glyoxal, resolved by electrophoresis through agarose gels, and transferred by blotting to a nitrocellulose filter. The RNA was then hybridized to a $^{32}$P-labeled cDNA (prepared from M13ALE124m) and examined by autoradiography. The apo-E mRNA was found to be about 1300 nucleotides in length (Fig. 3A, lane 1). When an examination was made of liver RNA, prepared from diabetic rats 72 h after alloxan treatment, apo-E mRNA levels were found to be increased about 1.6-fold above normal levels (Fig. 3A, lane 2).

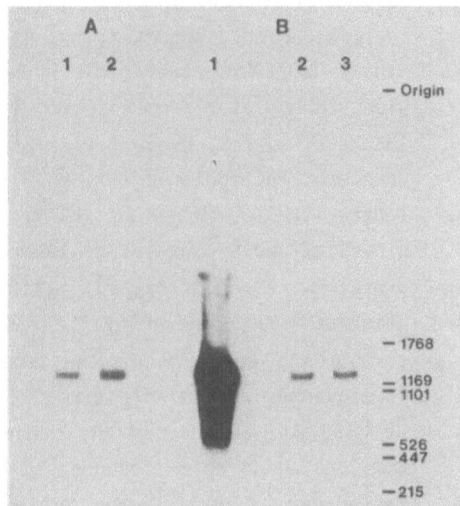

Fig. 3. Apo-E mRNA length and quantitation. The autoradiogram shows the results of hybridization of $^{32}$P-labeled cDNA to equal amounts of poly(A)-containing RNA from normal liver (A,1), 72 h alloxan-diabetic liver (A,2), normal liver (B,1), normal intestine (B,2), and 72 h alloxan-diabetic intestine (B,3). Different exposure times were used to develop the autoradiograms in panels A and B. They were quantitated by densitometry scanning. Nucleotide lengths of molecular weight markers are indicated

Apolipoprotein E mRNA was detected in the small intestine, but at a level about 100-fold less than that found in the liver (Fig. 3B). These results confirm the report (8) that apo-E may be produced by the intestine — though in very low amounts. The availability of a specific cloned hybridization probe for apo-E should now permit an investigation into the mechanisms involved in apo-E production.

Acknowledgements    We are grateful to Drs. Leonard S. Jefferson and Daniel E. Peavy for thoughtful discussions. A portion of this research was supported in part by Grant AM31615 from the National Institutes of Health to JMT, Public Health Service International Research Fellowship TW02849 to JWM, and a fellowship from the Juvenile Diabetes Foundation to JWM.

## References

1.  Mahley RW (1978) Alterations in plasma lipoproteins induced by cholesterol feeding in animals including man. In: Dietschy JM, Gotto AM Jr, Ontko JA (eds) Disturbances in Lipid and Lipoprotein Metabolism. American Physiological Society, Bethesda, MD, pp 181-197
2.  Mahley RW (1982) Atherogenic hyperlipoproteinemia: The cellular and molecular biology of plasma lipoproteins altered by dietary fat and cholesterol. In: Havel RJ (ed) Medical Clinics of North America: Lipid Disorders. WB Saunders, Philadelphia, PA, pp 375-402
3.  Innerarity TL, Mahley RW (1978) Enhanced binding by cultured human fibroblasts of apo-E-containing lipoproteins as compared with low density lipoproteins. Biochemistry 17: 1440-1447
4.  Weisgraber KH, Innerarity TL, Mahley RW (1982) Abnormal lipoprotein receptor-binding activity of the human E apoprotein due to cysteine-arginine interchanges at a single site. J Biol Chem 257: 2518-2521
5.  Rall SC Jr, Weisgraber KH, Mahley RW (1982) Human apolipoprotein E: The complete amino acid sequence. J Biol Chem 257: 4171-4178
6.  Weisgraber KH, Rall SC Jr, Mahley RW (1981) Human E apoprotein heterogeneity: Cysteine-arginine interchanges in the amino acid sequence of the apo-E isoforms. J Biol Chem 256: 9077-9083
7.  Ricca GA, Hamilton RW, McLean JW, Conn A, Kalinyak JE, Taylor JM (1981) Rat $\alpha_1$-acid glycoprotein mRNA. J Biol Chem 256: 10362-10368
8.  Windmueller HG, Wu A-L (1981) Biosynthesis of plasma apolipoproteins by rat small intestine without dietary or biliary fat. J Biol Chem 256: 3012-3016

# Effect on LP-X on Hepatic Cholesterol Synthesis

A. K. Walli and D. Seidel

Cholestasis causes changes in the pattern of plasma lipoproteins which reflect abnormal liver function. Cholestatic hypercholesterolemia is one of the oldest known forms of hypercholesterolemia in humans. The associated increase in the content of unesterified cholesterol is found in lipoprotein-X, a unique lipoprotein characteristic of obstructive jaundice. It floats at a density of 1.063 g/ml during ultracentrifugation and is characterized by its high content of phospholipid and unesterified cholesterol and the absence of apo-B, the major apoprotein of LDL. It exists in the form of a vesicle with an albumin core, its precursors are synthesized in liver and normally excreted in bile. During biliary obstruction this lipid material refluxes into plasma to form LP-X. (1) Even though LP-X is rich in cholesterol, it is surprising that cholesterol circulating in the form of LP-X does not exert feedback control through HMG-CoA reductase on hepatic cholesterol synthesis during cholestasis. (2)

Liver plays an important role in the regulation of cholesterol metabolism and some of the factors controlling hepatic cholesterol biosynthesis can be summarized as follows: (I) Composition and size of the bile pool (II) Hormonal regulation via cyclic AMP (III) Fluidity of the microsomal membrane and its influence on synthesis or activation of microsomal enzymes (IV) Circadian rhythm (V) Dietary status (VI) Biological age (VII) Enterohepatic circulation of bile salts and cholesterol (VIII) Intracellular enzymes and metabolic status (IX) Exchange of membrane cholesterol of the tissue with plasma lipoproteins (X) Negative feed-back due to dietary cholesterol regulated by the receptors for apo-B or apo-E or both.

During cholestasis factors I, VII and X are disturbed. Various conflicting explanations have been offered to explain the increased hepatic cholesterogenesis in cholestasis. Kattermann and Creutzfeldt (3) suggested that cholestasis alters hepatic metabolism in such a way that cholesterol feed-back is impaired at the cellular level. Weis and Dietschy (4) showed that diminished supply of lymph lipoprotein due to interruption of the enterolymphatic circulation during cholestasis causes increased hepatic cholesterol synthesis. They were able to correct this defect by infusion of lymph lipoproteins. However Cooper and Ockner (5) did not observe the complete suppression of enhanced hepatic cholesterol synthesis in biliary obstruction by infusion of lymph lipoproteins. The possibility that other factors such as LP-X may exert an influence on hepatic cholesterol metabolism remains open. Since the appearance of LP-X is a consistent feature of cholestasis, studies on its site of uptake, its effect on the activity of HMG-CoA reductase and on the uptake of chylomicron remnants in the liver were undertaken, in order to clarify the hypercholesterolemia of cholestasis.

## Methods

### Isolation and Labelling of LP-X

In order to establish the site of LP-X uptake, LP-X was isolated from human bile by a combination of ultracentrifugation and Cohn fractionation (6). After checking its purity by chemical, electrophoretic and immunochemical analysis, it was iodinated in the albumin moiety with $^{125}$I-Iodine by the standard iodination technique. It was then dialyzed and recentrifugated for 20 hours at d 1.065 g/ml to remove any traces of free iodine and albumin. Before use the preparation was again dialyzed and checked for purity.

### Liver Perfusion Technique

Livers were perfused after isolation with Krebs-Ringer-bicarbonate buffer containing 2.5% albumin and 10% hemoglobin in the form of human erythrocytes in a recirculating system.

### Isolated Hepatocytes

Hepatocytes were prepared by the technique of collagenase perfusion. They were incubated in Krebs-Ringer-bicarbonate buffer containing 4% albumin at 37°C.

### Isolated Lymphocytes

Lymphocytes were isolated from heparinized blood over lymphoprep gradient. They were then incubated in RPMI medium containing 10% foetal calf serum. After 2 hours of incubation unattached cells were incubated in the fresh medium.

### Fibroblasts

Fibroblasts derived from normal subjects were maintained in Dulbecco's minimal essential medium with 25 mM $NaHCO_3$, 20 mM Hepes buffer, pH 7.4 and 10% foetal calf serum. Cultures between 5 to 10 passages were used for experiments.

## Results and Discussion

### Clearance of LP-X from Plasma

For in vivo experiments rats were anaesthatized with Evipan natrium and 1 ml $^{125}$I LP-X (about 2-3 mg free cholesterol) was injected into the saphenous vein. As seen in Fig. 1 LP-X disappears very rapidly from the circulation. The disappearance of $^{125}$I LP-X is similar to the long term decay curve obtained in rats which have been injected with un-labelled LP-X. (1)

### Uptake of LP-X in vivo, in Isolated Perfused Livers, Isolated Hepato-cytes, Lymphocytes and Monolayer Cultures of Fibroblasts

Measurement of $^{125}$I-activity in various organs after the administration of $^{125}$I LP-X shows that most of the radioactivity is found in the spleen. When rats were injected with $^{125}$I LP-X, the amount of radioactivity found in the spleen was 7-fold greater on a g wet weight basis than that found in liver at 60 min.after injection (Fig. 2). Measurement of the radioactivity at various time intervals shows that this high activity in spleen was maintained even 24 h after injection of $^{125}$I LP-X. A small amount of radioactivity was found in other organs, such as pan-

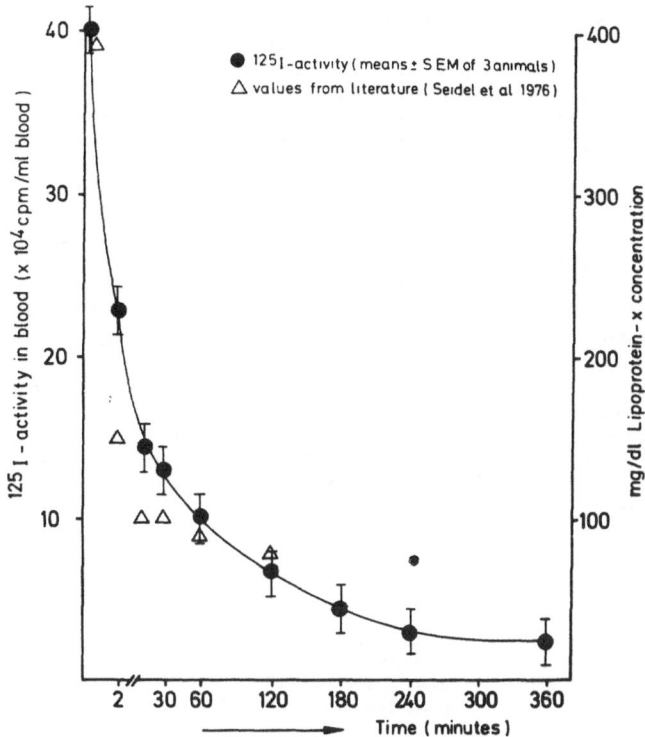

<u>Fig. 1.</u>
Kinetics of removal of $^{125}$I LP-X from blood.
Rats were injected with 1 ml of $^{125}$I LP-X (2-3 mg cholesterol) in saphenous vein and blood was removed at various time intervals to measure $^{125}$I-radioactivity

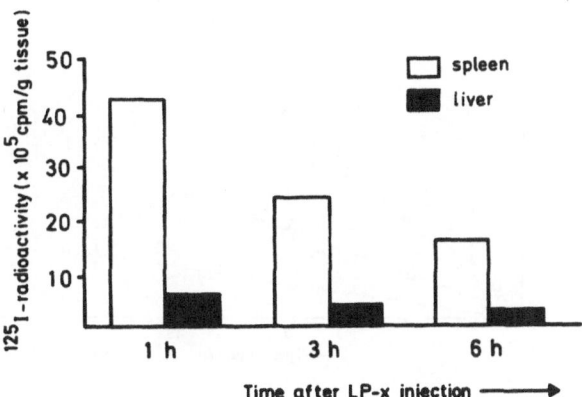

<u>Fig. 2.</u>
Distribution of $^{125}$I-radioactivity in liver and spleen after administration of $^{125}$I LP-X (2-3 mg cholesterol)

588

creas, kidney, lung, heart and muscles. In contrast, after injection
of 125 I-albumin a small but equal amount of radioactivity was found
in the liver and spleen. These results clearly show that in rats LP-X
is mainly taken up the spleen and that the amount of LP-X removed from
the circulation by the liver is only a small fraction of that removed by
the spleen. Experiments with isolated perfused livers showed that when
125 I LP-X is added to the perfusion medium, it is removed by the liver
to only a small extent, but within minutes. However when hepatocytes
were isolated from these perfused livers, it was observed that only
a small percentage of the 125I activity found in the liver was present
in parenchymal cells. Instead it was mainly present in the non-parenchymal cells. These in vitro experiments substantiate the results of
the in vivo experiments, showing that the spleen and non-parenchymal
liver cells remove LP-X from the circulation.

The binding and uptake of $^{125}$ I LP-X by lymphocytes, fibroblasts and
hepatocytes was concentration dependent but did not reach saturation
kinetics (Fig. 3). Hepatocytes and fibroblasts bound only a small
fraction of the amount bound by lymphocytes. This again stresses the
importance of non-hepatic cells such as lymphocytes in the removal of
LP-X.

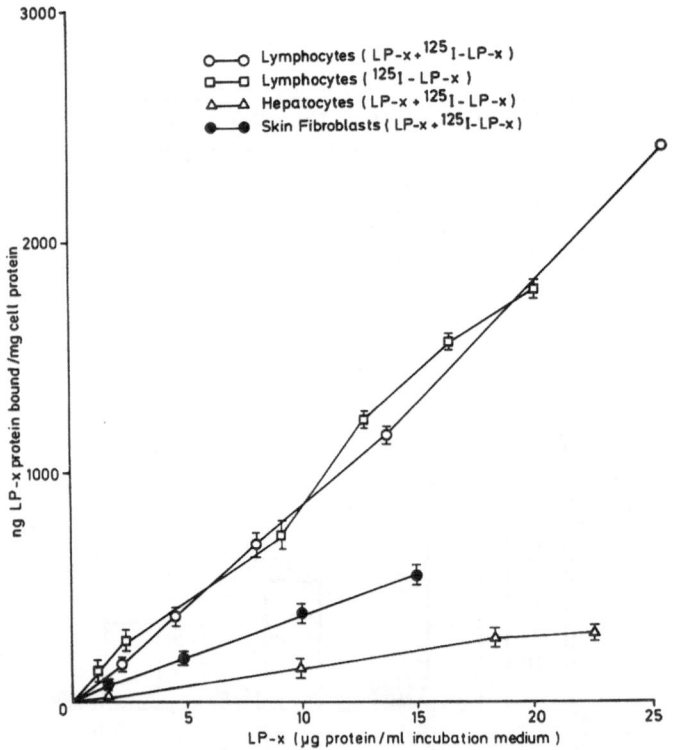

Fig. 3.
Binding and uptake of LP-X by isolated hepacytes, lymphocytes and
monolayer cultures of fibroblasts. Cells were incubated with 125I LP-X
( 1.48x10$^4$ cpm/μg LP-X protein) and unlabelled LP-X. Incubations were
carried out at 37°C for 120 min

## LP-X and HMG-CoA reductase activity

Parallel to the binding or uptake of LP-X by lymphocytes, suppression of the activity of HMG-CoA reductase similar to that with LDL was noted in these cells. Lymphocytes isolated from the blood of cholestatic patients also contained very low activity of HMG-CoA reductase as compared to controls (0-11.5 pmol as compared to 55 pmol/mg protein/h). However addition of LP-X to the perfusion medium caused a 5-fold increase in the activity of HMG-CoA reductase in microsomes of these livers (Fig. 4). An increase in the activity of the enzyme was also noted in microsomes of hepatocytes incubated with LP-X. In vitro incubation of isolated hepatic microsomes with LP-X resulted in the suppression of the enzyme activity in a concentration dependent manner. This increase in the activity of HMG-CoA reductase by LP-X is not specific for hepatic tissue. Inclusion of LP-X in media of monolayer cultures of fibroblasts, either in the presence of foetal calf serum or lipoprotein deficient serum, increases the activity of the reductase. These data suggest that in those cells which poorly bind or take up LP-X, a leaching of cellular cholesterol might occur.

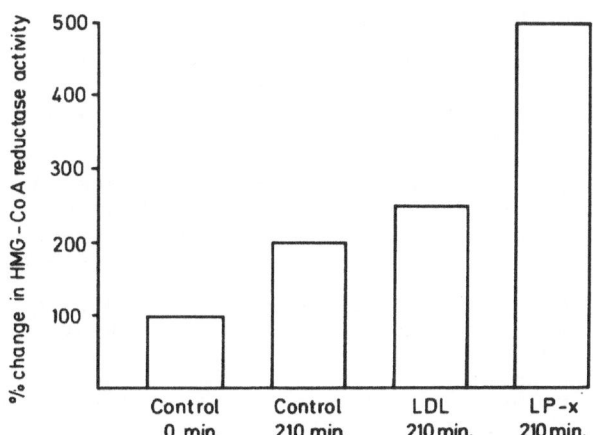

Fig. 4.
Effects of LP-X or LDL on the activity of HMG-CoA reductase in isolated perfused rat livers. LDL or LP-X was added to the medium after 30 min equilibration period (37 mg cholesterol/dl medium)

## LP-X and Uptake of Chylomicron Remnants by Liver

It is well established that hepatic tissue almost completely removes chylomicron remnants from the circulation. In the presence of LP-X in the perfusion medium the removal of [14]C cholesteryl oleate labelled remnants was significantly reduced (about 50% of control). The liver tissue also had about 50% of the [14]C-activity as compared to controls. Similarly isolated hepatocytes bound about 50% of the [14]C-labelled remnants, as compared to those without LP-X. Thus both the reduced uptake of remnants and probably leaching of cellular cholesterol due to the high phospholipid content of LP-X may play a major role in enhanced cholesterol synthesis in cholestatic liver and result in hypercholesterolemia.

The pathobiochemical features of cholestatic hypercholesterolemia may be summarized as follows:
1. Physicochemical conversion of biliary lipid micelles into the LP-X vesicle after reflux of bile into the plasma.
2. Disturbed triglyceride hydrolysis of plasma lipoproteins through unphysiological apoprotein binding on the LP-X vesicle.
3. Disturbed enterohepatic circulation of bile acids and cholesterol.
4. Lack of inhibition of hepatic cholesterol biosynthesis by chylomicron remnants in the presence of LP-X.
5. Inability of liver to take up cholesterol in the form of LP-X.
6. Leaching of hepatic cellular cholesterol by LP-X, possibly because of its high ratio of phospholipid to cholesterol.

## Acknowledgements

This study was supported by the Deutsche Forschungsgemeinschaft ( S FB 89, Cardiology - D 3400 Göttingen FRG).

We are thankful to Miss Christina Wiese and Miss Sylvia Kumm for excellent technical assistance.

## References

1. Seidel D, Buff HU, Fauser U, Bleyl U (1976) On the metabolism of lipoprotein-X. Clin.Chim.Acta 66:195-207
2. Liersch M, Baggio G, Heuck CC, Seidel D (1977) Effect of lipoprotein-X on hepatic cholesterol synthesis. Atherosclerosis 26: 505-514
3. Kattermann R, Creutzfeldt W (1970) The effect of experimental cholestasis on the negative feed-back regulation of cholesterol synthesis in rat liver. Scand J Gastroenterol 5: 337-342
4. Weis JH, Dietschy JM (1971) Presence of an intact cholesterol feed back mechanism in the liver in biliary stasis. Gastroenterology 61: 77-84
5. Cooper AD, Ockner RK (1974) Studies of hepatic cholesterol synthesis in experimental acute biliary obstruction. Gastroenterology 66: 586-595
6. Manzato E, Fellin R, Baggio G, Walch S, Neubeck W, Seidel D (1976) Formation of lipoprotein-X, its relation to bile compounds. J. clin. Invest. 57: 1248-1260

# 3.4 Apolipoproteins

# Apolipoprotein Research: A Multidisciplinary Task

G. M. Kostner

The situation in apolipoprotein research has escaped from an easy to survey field. Not only that the quantity of individual apolipoproteins (apo-Lp) recognised today has passed the number of 20, there is a great variety of specialists of different disciplines involved in this task. Chemists and biochemists have separated and purified nonidentical peptides and subunits. To give a brief overview of the state of the art, I have listed the best known apo-Lp of human serum in Table 1.

Table 1. Apolipoproteins of human serum

| Apolipoprotein | Mol. weight x $10^{-3}$ | Major density class |
|---|---|---|
| AI:$AI_1$-$AI_5$ | 28.5 | HDL |
| AII | 17.5 | ($HDL_2$), $HDL_3$ |
| AIII | ApoD | |
| A-IV | 46.0 | d.1.21 bottom |
| A-V | 50 | d.1.21 bottom |
| B-100 | 550 | LDL |
| B-48 | 275 | chylomicrons |
| CI: $CI_{1,2}$ | 7.0 | chylom. VLDL, (HDL) |
| CII: $CII_{0,1}$ | 8.5 | " |
| CIII:$CIII_{0-4}$ | 8.5 | " |
| D | 22 | $HDL_3$, VHDL |
| E:$E^{2-4}$, s2, s3, (s4) | 36.0 | VLDL, IDL, $HDL_C$ |
| F | 30 | HDL |
| G | 72 | VHDL, d.1.21 bottom |
| H ($\beta_2$-G-I) | 54 | chylom., d.1.21 bottom |
| PRP (Pro-rich) | 74 | d.1.21 bottom |
| SAA (Thr-poor) | 10; 20; ... | HDL |
| "$D_2$" | 7.0 | HDL |
| E-AII complex | 46.0 | $HDL_C$ |
| (a) | >500 | $HDL_1$, SPB |

Even for insiders of the field it is hard sometimes to keep up with nomenclature and newly detected subspecies. Certainly something needs to be done with that respect. To clarify matters I have chosen the ABC nomenclature of Alaupovic (1) wherever possible without committing myself to pretend that all these apo-Lp necessarily form their own Lp-families in the classical sense.

Some of these apo-Lp served as model substances for physico-chemists to study lipid:protein interactions as well as three dimensional structures of lipid-protein associates. We have profited a great deal from these investigations not only in pure theoretical terms but certainly also the implication of the results for enzyme-substrate interactions as well as activations of lipases and transferases. These achievements also helped another group of investigators to reveal metabolic para-

594

meters as well as pool sizes and distributions of individual apo-Lp.
With that respect we must admit that we are still at the beginning
of understanding the significance of all different subspecies for the
lipid metabolism in man. There are still major apo-Lp, e.g. AII or
Lp(a) among others whose function remained obscure until todate.

Just recently we have learned that apo-Lp are formed and partially also
secreted in the form of precursors (2) giving rise to distinct isoforms.
Posttranslational processing without doubt plays a fundamental role in
the final manufacture of apo-Lp as we find them in the blood stream.
Genetic defects such as $E^3$-deficiency, Tangier disease and others attracted specialists in this field to get involved with molecular-bio-
logical problems which certainly bear implications for atherogenesis.
In close connection with this field, studies are undertaken to elucidate the receptor mediated lipoprotein metabolism. Today we know
3 different kinds of lipoproteins which are bound, internalized and
degraded via the Brown Goldstein mechanism: ApoB (3), ApoE (4) and
Lp(a) (5). The number of publications in this field has grown exponen-
tionally over the past few years and there is little doubt that receptors not only govern the cholesterol metabolism to a decisive extent,
but also are of major importance for the biosynthesis of steroids in
hormonal glands. At the moment we are only at the beginning to understand all mechanisms involved in controlling these systems.

Receptor studies without doubt have fertilized epidemiologists by providing a working point to survey risk and anti-risk factors for atherosclerosis. Today it is not sufficient anymore to type any dyslipoproteinemia according to Fredrickson, one of our fathers in this field; now
we want to know whether or not someone is receptor negative, deficient,
homozygous or heterozygous $E^3$, CII or B-100 deficient and many things
more. To obtain such answers, clinical chemists have provided tools to
study apo-Lp patterns and concentrations and to trace defects on a
cellular level.

It cannot be expected that in a workshop like this with restrictions
in time and space, to focus on all of these problems. Nevertheless I
have tried to compile a number of specialists of different disciplines,
not necessarily to solve all open questions but rather to give a basis
for discussion as well as stimulations for future research.

Acknowledgments   Some of the studies mentioned in this article have been
supported by the Fonds zur Förderung der wissenschaftlichen Forschung.

References

1. Alaupovic P (1971) Apolipoproteins and Lipoproteins. Atherosclerosis
   13.: 141-146
2. Zannis VI, Kurnit DM, Brewlow JL (1982) Hepatic apoA-I and apo-E and
   intestinal apoA-I are synthesized in precursor isoprotein forms by
   organ cultures of human fetal tissues. J biol Chem 257: 536-544
3. Goldstein JL, Brown MS (1976) The LDL pathway in human fibroblasts:
   A receptor mediated mechanism for the regulation of cholesterol
   metabolism. Curr Topics in Cell Regulation II, 147 pp Acad press
4. Mahley RW, Hui DY, Innerarity TL (1981) Two independent lipoprotein
   receptors on hepatic membranes of dog, swine and man. J clin Invest
   68: 1197-1206
5. Krempler F, Kostner GM, Roscher A, Sandhofer F (1982) Binding of
   Lp(a) to surface receptors of cultured human fibroblasts. J clin
   Invest in the press

# Significance of Apolipoproteins for the Biochemical Profile of Atherosclerosis

P. Avogaro, G. Bittolo Bon, F. Belussi, G. Cazzolato, and E. Pontoglio

The experimental induction in animals of a pattern similar to human
atherosclerosis through a cholesterol-enriched diet and the finding
of high plasma cholesterol levels in population groups at high risk
for coronary disease suggested a close link between human atherosclerosis and hyperlipidemia. This underlies the "lipid hypothesis"
of atherogenesis. A contributory factor in this were the epidemiological surveys that have flourished in recent years, all of which
have pointed to a lipid parameter or to a ratio between lipid parameters as the best biochemical marker of coronary risk. From time
to time total cholesterol (1), LDL-C (2), HDL-C (3) and the LDL-C/
HDL-C ratio (4) have taken turns as the best discriminator of coronary risk. If we look however to studies performed in large series
of atherosclerotic patients we can observe that a hyperlipidaemic
state is not frequently recorded. Gotto et al. (5) have recorded
a significant plasma cholesterol gradient with advancing coronary
occlusion, but the values were always within normal confidence
limits. Goldstein et al (6) had observed a hyperlipidemia in only
31 % of their series of 500 survivors. It appears therefore that
only a small number of patients show an hyperlipemic pattern when
the analysis is limited to the plasma lipid levels. Some interestig
data have been obtained by a study we conducted (7-9) on a large
series of myocardial infarct survivors taken as a paradigm of human
atherosclerosis. The upshot of that study was: 1) that on the evidence of the plasma lipid parameters (C, TG, LDL-C, HDL-C) only
a relatively small proportion of patients were beyond the 95th
percentile of a normal population; 2) if the plasma levels of apolipoproteins B, A-I and A-II were considered as well as the plasma
lipid parameters, only 2 patients out of the 344 studied were completely normal; 3) the apoB levels and the apoB/apoA-I and apoB/
total cholesterol ratios seemed to be the best discriminators between patients and controls. Our study had limitations having been
conducted on patients who had already had an infarct. Following
studies, however, performed on a large series of coronary disease
patients investigated with angiography (10,11) yielded perfectly
equivalent values, thereby confirming the importance of apolipoprotein B and/or apoA-I. Hence the challenge to ask a new classification of hyperlipidemias connected with human atherosclerosis (12)
that would assess jointly some plasma lipid and some apolipoprotein levels. In a provisional scheme we have suggested some possibilities were purely speculative, such as the possibility of an
isolated increase of apoB and of an isolated deficiency of apoA-I.
Recently Sniderman et al. (13) and Kwiterovich et al. (14) provided
evidence of a human atherosclerosis. Franceschini et al. (15) singled
out the apoB-VLDL levels as the best discriminator. Vergani et al.
(16), Laskier et al. (17) and Schaefer et al. (18) have found
severe coronary atherosclerosis, associated with an isolated apoA-
I deficiency. The mosaic thus outlined suffers a relevant limitation
as the value of apolipoproteins as prognostic risk factors is

presently unknown. To date there is the isolate contribution of Ishikawa et al. (19), who in 12 cases of death from coronary disease
had previously identified a significant reduction of apoA-I. In
their case of an isolated hyper-apoB condition Kwiterovich et al.
(14)' could demonstrate a normal receptorial control of HMG-CoA
reductase. The inclusion of determinations of the main apolipoproteins, especially apoB and apoA-I, in a modern classification
of human atherosclerosis-related hyperlipidemia thus seems appropriate. A modern classification, to be of help in clinical practice, must include the determination of total cholesterol, triglycerides, LDL-C, HDL-C, apoB, apoA-I and apo-E. It is also to be
hoped that epidemiological surveys of atherosclerosis related conditions will comply with the above indications.

## References

1. KANNEL W.B., DAWBER T.R., KAGAN A., REVOTSKIE N., STOKES J.
   Factors or risk in the development  of coronary heart disease.
   Six years follow-up experience. Ann. Int. Med. 1961; 55; 33-50

2. KANNEL W.B., CASTELLI W.P., GORDON T., MAC NAMARA P.M. Serum
   cholesterol, lipoproteins and the risk of coronary heart disease:
   The Framingham Study. Ann. Int. Med. 1971; 74: 1-12

3. CASTELLI W.P., DOYLE J.Y., GORDON T.G., HAMES C.G., HJORTLAND M.C.
   HULLEY S.B., KAGAN A., ZUKEL W.J. HDL-Cholesterol and other
   lipids in coronary heart disease. The Cooperative Lipoprotein
   Phenotyping Study. Circulation 1977; 55: 767-772

4. KANNEL W.B, CASTELLI W.P. Is the serum total cholesterol an
   anachronism? Lancet 1979; ii: 950-951

5. GOTTO A.M., GORRY G.A., THOMPSON J.R., COLE J.S., TROST R.,
   YESHURUN D., DE BAKEY M.E. Relationship between plasma lipid
   concentrations and coronary artery disease in 496 patients.
   Circulation 1977; 56: 875-883

6. GOLDSTEIN J.L., HAZZARD W.R., SCHROTT H.G., BIERMAN E.L., MOTULSKY
   G., LEVINSKI M.J., CAMPBELL E.D. Hyperlipidemia in Coronary Heart
   Disease. I. Lipid Levels in 500 survivors of myocardial infarction.
   J. Clin. Invest. 1973; 52: 1533-1543

7. AVOGARO P., CAZZOLATO G., BITTOLO BON G:, BELUSSI F. Levels and
   chemical composition of $HDL_2$ $HDL_3$ and other major lipoprotein
   classes in survivors of myocardial infarction. Artery 1979; 5:
   495-508

8. AVOGARO P., BITTOLO BON G., CAZZOLATO G., QUINCI G.B. Are apolipo
   proteins better discriminators than lipid for atherosclerosis?
   Lancet 1979; i: 901-903

9. AVOGARO P., CAZZOLATO G., TARONI G., BELUSSI F. Chemical
   composition of ultracentrifugal fractions in different patterns
   of human atherosclerosis. Atherosclerosis 1977; 26: 163-172

10. KLADETZKY R.G., ASSMANN G., WALGENBACH S., TAUCHERT P., HELB H.D.
    Lipoprotein and apoprotein values in coronary angiography patients.
    Artery 1980; 7: 191-205

11. RIESEN W., MORDASINI R., SALZMANN C. a. GURTNER H.P. Apoproteins in angiographically documented coronary heart disease In Lipoproteins and Coronary Atherosclerosi (Noseda C., Fragiacomo C., Fumagalli R. and Paoletti R. Eds). Elsevier Biomedical Amsterdam 1982, 129

12. AVOGARO P., BITTOLO BON G., CAZZOLATO G. Need for new classification of lipoprotein derangements in human atherosclerosis. Lancet 1981; $i$: 1257

13. SNIDERMAN A., SHAPIRO GL, MARPOLE D., SKINNER B., TENG B., KWITEROVICH P.O. Jr. Association of coronary atherosclerosis with hyperapobetalipoproteinemia (increased protein but normal cholesterol levels in human plasma low density (B) lipoproteins). Proc. Natl. Acad. Sci. USA 1980; 77: 604-608

14. KWITEROVICH P., SNIDERMAN A,. FORTE T., BACHORIK P., CHATTERJEE S. Familial hyperapobetalipoproteinemia in a Amish Kindred. Arteriosclerosis (abs) 1981; 1: 87

15. FRANCESCHINI G., BONDOLIA., MANTERO M., SIRTORI M., TATTONI G., BIASI G., SIRTORI C.R. Increased apoprotein B in very low density lipoproteins of patients with peripheral vascular disease Arteriosclerosis 1982; 2: 74-80

16. VERGANI C., BETTALE G. Familial hypo-alpha-lipoproteinaemia. Clin. Chim. Acta 1981; 114: 45-52

17. LAKIER J., GOLDSTEIN S., NORUM R., BLOCK W., GOLDBERG R. Premature atherosclerosis associated with apolipoprotein A-I deficiency, Detroit type. Atherosclerosis (abs) 1981: i: 367a

18. SCHAEFER E.J., HEATON W.H., WETZEL M.G., BREWER H.B. Jr. Plasma apolipoprotein A-I absence associated with a marked reduction of high density lipoproteins and premature coronary artery disease. Arteriosclerosis 1982; 2: 16-26

19. ISHIKAWA T., FIDGE N., THELLE D.S., FORDE O.H., MILLER N.E. The Trømso Heart Study: Serum apolipoprotein A-I concentration in relation to future coronary heart disease. Europ. J. Clin. Invest. 1978; 8: 179-182

# Regulation of Lipoprotein Gene Expression

L. Chan, T. Antalis, M. H. Lin-Su, P. Cheung, and Y. C. Lin-Lee

## Introduction

The application of molecular biology in the study of apolipoprotein biosynthesis
has been a relatively recent event. About six years ago, our laboratory initiated
a series of studies on the biosynthesis of an apolipoprotein, apoVLDL-II, in a
model system (1-5). This apoprotein was synthesized in the cockerel liver at a
very low basal level. It was induced to become a major protein secreted by the
liver when estrogen was administered to this animal. While the observations in this
system were interesting and might help elucidate the mechanism of action of estrogen
in the liver, there was no known mammalian counterpart to apoVLDL-II. We have
thus extended our studies and have performed experiments on the biosynthesis of two
well-characterized mammalian apolipoproteins, apoE and apoA-I.

## Translation of Rat apoE in vitro

Total RNA was isolated from rat liver by a modification of the guanidine-HCl method
of Cox (6). Polyadenylated RNA was purified from the preparation by oligo(dT)
cellulose chromatography (7). It was translated in vitro in an mRNA-dependent
wheat germ system (8) and the nuclease-treated reticulocyte lysate system (9) by
using [$^{35}$S]methionine as an amino acid precursor. A product, designated preapoE,
was specifically precipitated by a rabbit anti-rat apoE serum and accounted for
1.0 - 1.5% of the total radiolabeled peptides. It migrated as a single band of
radioactivity on SDS gels with an apparent molecular weight similar to that of
mature plasma apoE.

Our results confirmed and extended the previous report by Hay and Getz (10) that an
apoE-like product was produced when rat liver mRNA was translated in vitro. Both
our study (11) and those of Getz and co-workers (10,12) strongly suggested that
preapoE contained an NH$_2$-terminal signal peptide. However, the apparent similarity
in size between preapoE and plasma apoE was puzzling and initially unexplained.

We next added signal peptidase (in the form of dog pancreatic microsomal membranes)
in the translation reaction and analyzed the translation product under these conditions. We found that a slightly smaller (by about 500 daltons) immunoprecipitated
apoE was produced. Since plasma apoE is a glycoprotein (13), we studied the effect
of the microsomal membranes on the sensitivity of the product to endoglycosidase H,
an enzyme which cleaves between the two N-acetylglucosamine units of a mannose-rich
core region in serum-type glycoproteins (14). We found that the microsomal membranes
converted the preapoE from an endoglycosidase H-resistant to an enzyme-sensitive
species. Our experiments suggest that processing of preapoE at the endoplasmic
reticulum takes place by the cotranslational removal of a signal peptide and core
glycosylation of the cleaved protein. It is likely that the apoprotein subsequently
undergoes further modification in the form of peripheral glycosylation and trimming,
possibly in the Golgi apparatus, before being secreted as the mature plasma apolipoprotein. The latter fortuitously assumes an apparent molecular weight similar to
that of the initial translation product (11).

## Translation of Rat apoA-I in vitro

We have performed similar translation studies on rat apoA-I mRNA in vitro (15). We found that the initial translation product, designated preapoA-I, was cotranslationally cleaved in vitro by dog pancreatic microsomal membranes. Independent studies by Stoffel et al. (16) indicated that an 18 amino acid signal peptide was cleaved cotranslationally. Subsequently, Gordon et al. (17) showed that in the case of rat intestinal apoA-I, a pro-segment of 6 amino acids might be subseqeuntly cleaved before the "mature" plasma protein was produced.

Signal peptides in presecretory apolipoproteins were first found in avian apoVLDL-II (3,5) and have subseqeuntly been described in avian (2) and mammalian apoA-I (15-17) and mammalian apoE (10-12). It is not clear how the nascent apoprotein, with its phospholipid binding amplipathic helix (18), avoids being "stuck" to the outer layer of the endoplasmic reticulum, thus impeding translocation of the nascent peptide into the cisternae (5).

## Translation of Baboon and Human apoA-I and apoE

Since we are ultimately interested in the biochemistry of apolipoprotein biosynthesis in the higher primate and in man, we have extended our studies in the rat to similar studies in the baboon and man. Baboon and human liver polyadenylated RNAs were translated in the nuclease-treated reticulocyte lysate in vitro, by using [$^{35}$S]methionine as an amino acid precursor. ApoA-I and apoE immunoreactive products were precipitated by antisera to the human apoproteins. As shown in Figure 1, both the baboon and the human translation products were recognized by the anti-

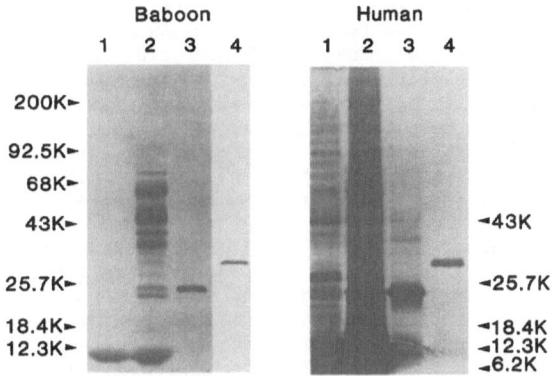

Fig. 1. Translation in vitro of baboon (left) and human (right) apoA-I and apoE mRNA. Total hepatic polyadenylated RNA was translated in a rabbit reticulocyte lysate system in vitro by using ($^{35}$S)-methionine as a labeled amino acid precursor. Immunoprecipitation was carried out with monospecific antisera against human apoE and apoA-I. Products were analyzed by 5-15% acrylamide slab gel in sodium dodecyl sulfate, and visualized by fluorography. Lane 1: blank translation (no mRNA added), lane 2: total translation product; lane 3: immunoprecipitated ($^{35}$S)apoA-I; lane 4: immunoprecipitated ($^{35}$S)apoE

sera. ApoA-I mRNA appeared to represent approximately 1%, whereas apoE mRNA approximately 0.3-0.5%, of the total translational activity from both species. Interestingly, the initial translation products, preapoA-I and preapoE, both behaved very much like the corresponding rat preproteins. Namely, on SDS gels, baboon and human preapoA-I had apparent molecular weights slightly larger (by about 2,000 daltons) than the corresponding plasma protein whereas the preapoEs appeared to migrate with an identical $R_f$ as plasma apoE. It is likely that glycosylation and modification of the processed apoE might similarly account for this interesting coincidence.

## Regulation of Rat Apolipoprotein mRNA in Liver and Intestine

Studies in our laboratory on feeding rats with a high cholesterol diet coupled with the antithyroid drug, propylthiouracil, produced a two- to three-fold increase in the plasma cholesterol and apoE in this animal. Quantitation of hepatic apoE concentration indicated that apoE mRNA activity also increased three-fold, concomitant with a similar increase in apoE synthesis in liver slices studied in vitro. These observations suggest that dietary cholesterol regulates apoE synthesis at a pretranslational level (19).

Similar studies performed in the intestine showed that a high cholesterol diet (without propylthiouracil) stimulated apoA-I and apoE mRNA activities (20). We also demonstrated for the first time that apoE is definitely synthesized in the rat intestine, albeit at a very low rate.

## Molecular Cloning of Mammalian Apolipoprotein cDNAs

The translation studies were interesting and indicated that apoE and apoA-I synthesis were regulated by dietary cholesterol. However, while most of the changes were pretranslational, the experiments did not differentiate between transcriptional from posttranscriptional effects of the diets. To more precisely localize the level of regulation of apolipoprotein synthesis, we needed a specific DNA hybridization probe. We therefore proceeded to clone the double-stranded cDNA for the apoproteins. Double-stranded cDNA was synthesized to total rat liver mRNA by the enzyme reverse transcriptase. After $S_1$ nuclease treatment, the dscDNA was tailed with approximately 15 deoxycytidine residues. It was annealed to the plasmid pBR322 which had been opened by the enzyme Pst I and tailed with approximately 15 deoxyguanosine residues. The hybrid plasmid was use to transform E. coli strain RR1. The recombinant plasmids were subsequently amplified and grown up by standard techniques. Screening for specific DNA clones was performred by the technique of hybrid-translation (21). Thus far, four clones for apoE have been identified by this method. Simultaneous nucleotide sequence analysis of the clones and amino acid sequence analysis of rat apoE are in progress to definitely confirm the identity of the clones.

Acknowledgments  We thank Dr. W.A. Bradley, J.P. Moore, J. Wasetis, M. Holtgrefe for helpful discussion and technical assistance. This work was supported by grants HL-23470 and SCOR grant HL-27341 from the U.S. National Institutes of Health.

## References

1. Chan L, Jackson RL, O'Malley BW, Means AR (1976) Synthesis of very low density lipoproteins in the cockerel: effects of estrogen. J Clin Invest 58:368-379
2. Chan L, Bradley WA, Jackson RL, Means AR (1980) Lipoprotein synthesis in the cockerel liver: effects of estrogen on hepatic polysomal messenger RNA activities for the major apoproteins in very low and high density lipoproteins and albumin, and evidence for precursors to these secretory proteins. Endocrinology 106:275-283

3. Chan L, Bradley WA, Means AR (1980) Amino acid sequence of the signal peptide of apoVLDL-II, a major apoprotein in very low density lipoproteins. J Biol Chem 255:10060-10063

4. Chan L, Dugaiczyk A, Means AR (1980) Molecular cloning of the gene sequences of a major apoprotein in avian very low density lipoproteins. Biochemistry 19:5631-5637

5. Dugaiczyk A, Inglis AS, Strike PM, Burley RW, Beattie WG, Chan L (1981) Comparison of the nucleotide sequence of cloned DNA coding for an apoprotein (apoVLDL-II) from avian blood and the amino acid sequence of an egg yolk protein (apovitellenin I): Equivalence of the two sequences. Gene 14:175-182

6. Cox RA (1968) The use of guanidium chloride in the isolation of nucleic acids. Methods Enzymol 12:120-129

7. Aviv H, Leder P (1972) Purification of biologically active globin messenger RNA by chromatography on oligothymidylic acid-cellulose. Proc Natl Acad Sci USA 69:1408-1412

8. Davis JW, Aalbers AMJ, Stuiks EJ, Van Kammen A (1977) Translation of cowpea mosaic virus RNA in a cell-free extract from wheat germ. FEBS Lett 77:265-269

9. Pelham HRB, Jackson RJ (1976) An efficient mRNA-dependent translation system from reticulocyte lysates. Eur J Biochem 67:247-256

10. Hay R, Getz GS (1979) Translation in vivo and in vitro of proteins resembling apoproteins of rat plasma very low density lipoprotein. J Lipid Res 20:334-348

11. Lin-Lee YC, Bradley WA, Chan L (1981) mRNA-dependent synthesis of rat apolipoprotein E in vitro: cotranslational processing and identification of an endoglycosidase H-sensitive glycopeptide intermediate. Biochem Biophys Res Commun 99:654-661

12. Getz GS, Hay R, Reardon C (1980) Biosynthesis of rat apolipoprotein E. In: Gotto AM, Smith LC, Allen B (eds) Atherosclerosis V: 156-159. Springer-Verlag New York Inc

13. Weisgraber KH, Mahley RW, Assmann G (1977) The rat arginine-rich apoprotein and its redistribution following injection of iodinated lipoproteins into normal and hypercholesterolemic rats. Atherosclerosis 28:121-140

14. Tarentino AL, Maley F (1974) Purification and properties of an endo-$\beta$-N-acetylglucosaminidase from Streptomyces griseus. J Biol Chem 249:811-817

15. Lin-Su MH, Lin-Lee YC, Bradley WA, Chan L (1981) Characterization, cell-free synthesis and processing of apolipoprotein A-I from rat high density lipoproteins. Biochemistry 20:2470-2475

16. Stoffel W, Blobel G, Walter P (1981) Synthesis in vitro and translocation of apolipoprotein A-I across microsomal vesicles. Eur J Biochem 120:519-522

17. Gordon JI, Smith DP, Andy R, Alpers DH, Schonfeld G, Strauss AW (1982) The primary translation product of rat intestinal apolipoprotein A-I mRNA is an unusual preproprotein. J Biol Chem 257:971-978

18. Segrest JP, Jackson RL, Morrisett JD, Gotto AM (1974) A molecular theory to lipid-protein interactions in the plasma lipoproteins. FEBS Lett 38:247-253

19. Lin-Lee YC, Tanaka Y, Lin CT, Chan L (1981) Effects of an atherogenic diet on apolipoprotein E biosynthesis in the rat. Biochemistry 20:6474-6480

20. Tanaka Y, Lin-Lee YC, Lin-Su MH, Chan L (1982) Intestinal biosynthesis of apolipoproteins in the rat: apoE and apoA-I mRNA translation and regulation. Metabolism (in press)

21. Ricciardi RP, Miller JS, Roberts BE (1979) Purification and mapping of specific mRNAs by hybridization-selection and cell-free translation. Proc Natl Acad Sci USA 76:4927-4931

# Apolipoprotein AIV Metabolism in Man

H. Noel, F. and P. J. Nestel

Apoprotein AIV is characterised by an unusual distribution amongst
lipoproteins.  A major component of lymph chylomicrons and very low
density lipoprotein, it resides almost entirely unassociated with
lipoproteins in the vascular compartment.  A major source of AIV
peptide appears to be the intestine, although recent studies have
suggested that at least some AIV is produced by rat liver and in
this respect it may be significant that rat HDL contains AIV.
Whether AIV peptide is made by human liver is not yet known,
although if present it represents only a small proportion of the
total mass of human HDL.

A role for apo-AIV in triglyceride transport is suggested by its
association with chylomicrons which transport a huge load of
ingested fat each day.  In abetalipoproteinemia, the plasma levels
of AIV are approximately half those of normal subjects [1] and Green
et al [2] showed that the elevation of urinary triglyceride following ingestion of fat in subjects with chyluria was accompanied by a
significant increase in triglyceride AIV apoprotein.  Windmueller
and Wu [3] however found that, in the rat, ingestion of dietary fat
altered only the secretory route, and not the production rate of
AIV apoprotein.  In glucose fed animals, more AIV was shunted by
the portal system but after fat feeding more appeared in the lymph
associated with triglyceride rich lipoprotein (TGRL).  Thus the
fact that lymphatic transport of AIV is greatly increased by fat
feeding in rats [4] may not imply increased production of the apoprotein, but mere redirection into either transport system as
required.

A putative physiological role for AIV apoprotein should therefore
take into account its coexistence with lymph chylomicrons of gut
origin and in their absence, the lipoprotein free fraction of
plasma or lymph, and in addition a possible involvement (from rat
studies [5] ) of HDL in the scheme.

To investigate this proposal, we have studied the kinetics and fate
of AIV apoprotein in man, by administering radioiodinated AIV peptide as a component of chylomicrons, plasma lipoprotein free fraction (LFF) or HDL, to suitable subjects.  AIV apoprotein was purified
from human chylomicrons (obtained from lymph of chylothorax patients),
by preparative SDS-gel electrophoresis;  AIV peptide was then
labeled with $^{125}$I and incorporated by in vitro exchange into the
appropriate fractions which were separated from unbound $^{125}$I-AIV
by ultracentrifugation at their respective densities.  Aliquots
were incubated with buffered saline to determine their stability,
or with plasma to measure the extent of in vitro exchange.  The
labeled AIV present in all fractions, comigrated with unlabeled AIV,
as shown in Fig.1.

When lymph chylomicrons containing $^{125}$I-labeled AIV apoprotein was
administered to normolipemic subjects, 95% of the label was removed
from TGRL within 5 min and transferred to both HDL and LFF fractions.
However, 90% of the radioactivity remained with chylomicrons after
incubation with saline, and 60% remained following in vitro

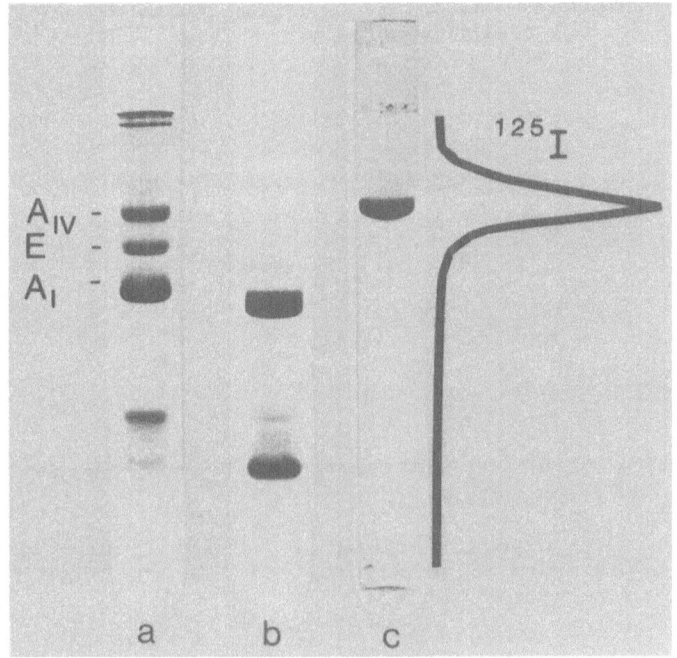

<u>Fig.1.</u> SDS-polyacrylamide gel (15%) separation of (a) lymph chylo-
micron (b) HDL and (c) purified AIV apoprotein. After iodination
and incorporation of $^{125}$I-AIV peptide into any fraction, most of the
label was found in gel slices associated only with AIV, as shown in
tracing of $^{125}$I counts on right

incubation with plasma for 1 hr. In hypertriglyceridemic subjects
however, 31% of $^{125}$I remained with chylomicrons after reinjection
and transfer from this fraction was significantly retarded compared
to normolipemic subjects. The plasma T½ of AIV in both groups was
similar however, (25-28 hr). Redistribution of labeled AIV apoprotein between lipoproteins is shown for both groups in Fig. 2.

Specific radioactivity (SA) of AIV peptide was determined using
measurements of total radioactivity and electroimmunoassay to
quantitate AIV mass in each fraction. The SA of HDL-AIV was
approximately 10 fold that of LFF-AIV, and although AIV mass of TGRL
was too low to allow accurate immunoassay, estimates indicate that
TGRL-AIV SA were at least equal to and probably higher than HDL-AIV
SA. This suggests that AIV has a high affinity for both lipoproteins
and is transferred from chylomicrons to a limited pool of HDL which
becomes rapidly labeled and saturated and the remainder transfers to
the larger mass of LFF-AIV apoprotein. There was no indication of
equilibration in SA between HDL and LFF.

The relationship between HDL- and LFF-AIV was investigated further
by separately injecting both fractions, intercalated with $^{125}$I-AIV
apoprotein, into volunteers. Most label remained with HDL, but a
time dependent transfer of AIV into TGRL and LFF occurred, reaching
a peak at approximately 10 hr following HDL/$^{125}$I-AIV administration.

604

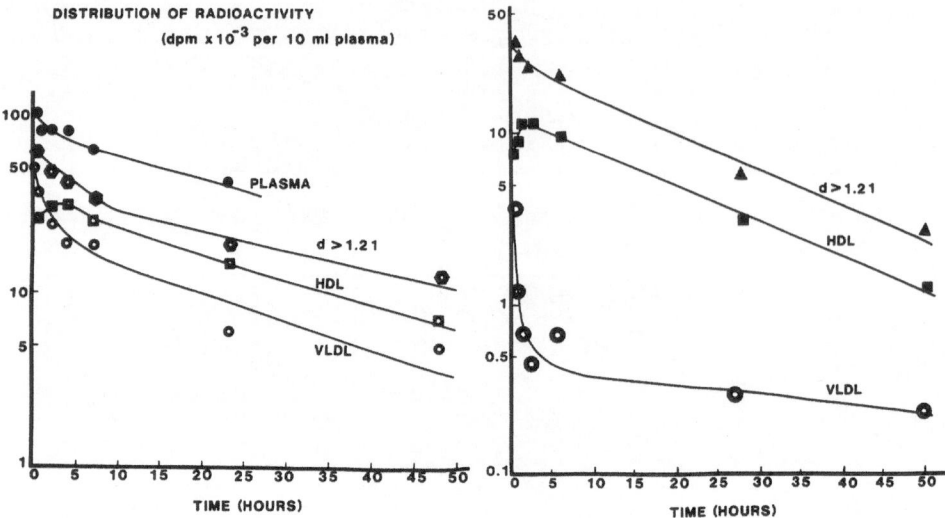

DISTRIBUTION OF RADIOACTIVITY
(dpm x10$^{-3}$ per 10 ml plasma)

Fig. 2.   Redistribution of label following administration of
chylomicron/$^{125}$I-AIV into (left) a hypertriglyceridemic and (right)
a normolipemic subject


The SA of AIV in HDL and in TGRL also remained at least 10 x higher
than in LFF, supporting the hypothesis of a greater affinity of AIV
for the former fractions.   When LFF/$^{125}$I-AIV was given, the SA of
HDL-AIV was 20 x and TGRL-AIV 10 x higher than LFF within 30 min
after injection (Fig. 3) further supporting the hypothesis.   The
flux of AIV, measured in one hyperlipemic subject, was approximately
20 mg/kg/day, suggesting that the peptide is produced in moderately
large quantities compared to other apoproteins.

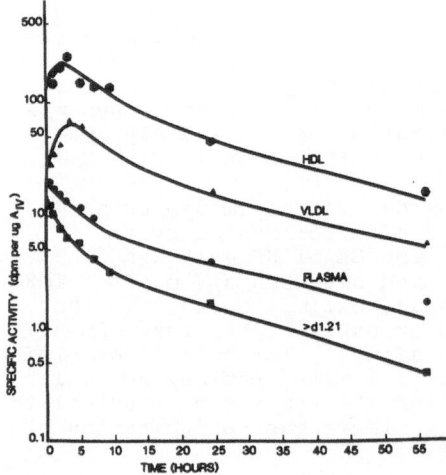

Fig. 3.   Specific activity of AIV apoprotein in HDL, VLDL and
LFF following injection of LFF/$^{125}$I-AIV

These studies suggest that HDL or a complex in this density range, plays a prominent role in human AIV metabolism. The physiological significance of this role is not clear, particularly since human HDL is notoriously low in AIV, compared to rat, in which we have previously shown that HDL probably plays an important function. In this animal there appeared to be a precursor product relationship between LFF and HDL-AIV pools (5). Since nascent HDL in perfusates from rat liver contain AIV apoprotein, it is possible that newly secreted human HDL contains AIV, but this may rapidly transfer to other fractions, possibly in exchange for other apoproteins, (e.g. C or E apoproteins) or lipid during triglyceride transport and exchange. HDL is quantitatively most important and turned over much more rapidly in the rat than in man, and increased AIV levels may be associated with greater fat transport tasks required of this lipoprotein in this species.

Nevertheless, immunoassay measurements in this laboratory showed that approximately 5% of human plasma AIV is present in HDL and subfractionation may reveal a higher proportion in one fraction, specifically involved in certain lipid transport tasks, than in others. Further studies are continuing to explore the function of this unique amphipathic apoprotein.

## References

1.    Green PHR, Glickman RM, Riley JW and Quinet E (1980) Human apolipoprotein AIV. Intestinal origin and distribution in plasma. J Clin Invest 65: 911-919
2.    Green PHR, Glickman RM, Saudek CD, Blum CD and Tall AR (1979) Human intestinal lipoproteins. Studies in chyluric subjects. J Clin Invest 64: 233-242
3.    Windmueller HG and Wu A (1981) Biosynthesis of plasma apolipoproteins by rat small intestine without dietary or biliary fat. J Biol Chem 256: 3012-3016

4.    Krause BR, Sloop CH, Castle CK and Roheim PS (1981) Mesenteric lymph apolipoproteins in control and ethinylestrodiol-treated rats: a model for studying apolipoproteins of intestinal origin. J Lipid Res 22: 610-619

5.    Fidge NH (1980) The redistribution and metabolism of iodinated apolipoprotein AIV in rats. Biochem Biophys Acta 619: 129-141

# Mechanism of Action of Lipoprotein Lipase: Role of Apolipoprotein C-II[1]

R. L. Jackson, K. Shirai, J. A. K. Harmony, and D. Quinn

## Introduction

Lipoprotein lipase (LpL) is a key enzyme in the catabolism of triglyceride-rich lipoproteins, chylomicrons and very low density lipoproteins (VLDL) (Nilsson-Ehle et al., 1980; Quinn et al., 1982). The characteristic features of LpL are inhibition by molar sodium chloride, activation by apolipoprotein C-II (apoC-II), a constituent of VLDL and high density lipoproteins (HDL), and an alkaline pH-optimum (pH 8.0–8.5). The importance of LpL and apoC-II in lipoprotein metabolism is best described by the fact that a deficiency of these proteins results in hypertriglyceridemia.

The physiological site of action of LpL is the luminal surface of the capillary endothelium where the enzyme is bound to the endothelial cell surface through ionic interaction with cell-associated glycosaminoglycans. Based on LpL binding studies with cultured bovine endothelial cells, Cheng et al. (1981) and Shimada et al. (1981) have suggested that the LpL receptor is heparan sulfate.

The LpL substrate is a high aggregate weight triglyceride-rich lipoprotein. Chylomicrons and VLDL contain a core of the neutral lipids (triglycerides and cholesteryl esters) surrounded by a monolayer surface of proteins and polar lipids (mostly phosphatidylcholine, sphingomyelin and unesterified cholesterol). LpL catalyzes the hydrolysis of the sn-1 and sn-3 ester bonds of triacylglycerols and the sn-1 ester bond of phosphatidylcholine and phosphatidylethanolamine. Limited information is available concerning the chemical steps of LpL catalysis. For simplicity, we suggest that LpL action consists of the following steps: (1) binding of LpL to the lipoprotein interface; (2) formation of an interfacial Michaelis complex between the substrate and the active site of the enzyme; (3) chemical catalysis of the hydrolysis of the ester bond; and (4) release of products from the active site. The purpose of this report is to review the possible mechanism by which apoC-II enhances LpL catalysis with particular emphasis given to each of the proposed chemical steps. We present a model for apoC-II stimulation of LpL catalysis consistent with the formation of an apoC-II-induced Michaelis complex between substrate and enzyme.

## Interaction of LpL and Lipid Interface

Since apoC-II is a lipid-binding protein and associates with lipid at the lipoprotein interface, one possible mechanism by which apoC-II enhances LpL catalysis is by specific interaction with LpL at the lipid interface such that the concentration of the enzyme is increased. However, based on several lines of evidence, this explanation seems unlikely. The most convincing evidence against this mechanism is that synthetic fragments of apoC-II corresponding to residues 50–78 do not associate with lipid and yet they are activators of LpL with triglyceride emulsions (Kinnunen et al., 1977), apoC-II-deficient VLDL (Catapano et al., 1979) and monomolecular films of trioctanoylglycerol (Smith et al., 1980).

[1] This work was supported by U.S. Public Health Service grants HL 22619 and HL 23019. D.M.Q. is supported by the Lipid, Atherosclerosis and Nutrition Training Grant HL 07460. J.A.K.H. is an Established Investigator of the American Heart Association.

Shirai et al. (1981) showed that LpL binds to sonicated vesicles of dipalmitoyl phosphatidylcholine even in the absence of apoC-II; the addition of apoC-II does not increase the amount bound. Bengtsson and Olivecrona (1980) reported similar results with triglyceride emulsions. Jackson et al. (1980) also studied the interaction of LpL with monomolecular films of 1,2-didecanoylglycerol in the presence and absence of apoC-II. ApoC-II is not required for the accumulation of LpL at the lipid interface. In the presence of apoC-II, there is an increase in the LpL-catalyzed hydrolysis of diglycerides. However, the amount of enzyme at the monolayer is less than when apoC-II was absent. Taken together, these findings suggest that apoC-II does not facilitate the interaction of LpL with the lipid interface.

## Interfacial Activation of LpL

Quinn et al. (1982) and Shirai et al. (1982a, b, c) have suggested that the binding of LpL to a lipid interface changes the catalytic properties of the enzyme, possibly through a conformational change. When LpL catalyzes the hydrolysis of water-soluble substrates, i.e., p-nitrophenylbutyrate (PNPB), apoC-II acts as a partial noncompetitive inhibitor of the LpL-catalyzed hydrolysis of PNPB. Inhibition occurs by the formation of a 1:1 complex of LpL and apoC-II with a dissociation constant of $0.6 \pm 0.2$ μM; this value compares to 0.5 μM for the interaction of a dansyl fragment of apoC-II (residues 43-78) and LpL (Smith et al., 1982). In the absence of apoC-II, addition of sonicated vesicles of dipalmitoylphosphatidylcholine (DPPC) enhances the LpL-catalyzed hydrolysis of PNPB 8-fold (Shirai and Jackson, 1982); the enhancing effect is specific for the gel state of the lipid. ApoC-II acts as a competitive inhibitor of the LpL-catalyzed hydrolysis of PNPB when the enzyme is associated with the lipid vesicle. Quinn et al. (1982) have analyzed the kinetics of inhibition and have suggested that apoC-II and LpL form a 1:1 complex with a dissociation constant of 0.13 μM. This value for the interaction of apoC-II and LpL at the lipid interface is 50-fold smaller than the dissociation constant (6.5 μM) for the interaction of apoC-II and DPPC (Cardin et al., 1982). Shirai et al. (1982b) also incorporated 0.5 mol % trioleoylglycerol into sonicated vesicles of DPPC and reported that the addition of apoC-II inhibited the LpL-catalyzed hydrolysis of PNPB; there was a corresponding reciprocal increase in the hydrolysis of trioleoylglycerol. These results suggest that apoC-II not only increases the catalytic rate for triglycerides but also determines the substrate specificity of LpL. This alteration in specificity is probably associated with a conformational change in the enzyme. Evidence for a conformational change has also been provided by using specific antiserum (Shirai et al., 1982). Fab fragments prepared from rabbit anti-bovine milk LpL inhibit the LpL-catalyzed hydrolysis of substrate. Preincubation of the enzyme with apoC-II or substrate (trioleoylglycerol emulsion, VLDL or phosphatidylcholine vesicles) prior to adding the Fab fragments does not prevent inhibition by the Fab fragments. However, addition of both apoC-II and substrate prevents inhibition, suggesting a cooperative protective effect.

## Kinetic Model for the Activator Role of ApoC-II in LpL Catalysis

Based on these data, we conclude that LpL first binds to a lipid interface and that the lipid associated enzyme then interacts with apoC-II forming a 1:1 complex. The formation of the complex is associated with binding of substrate to the active site. Scheme I presents a model for apoC-II stimulation of LpL.

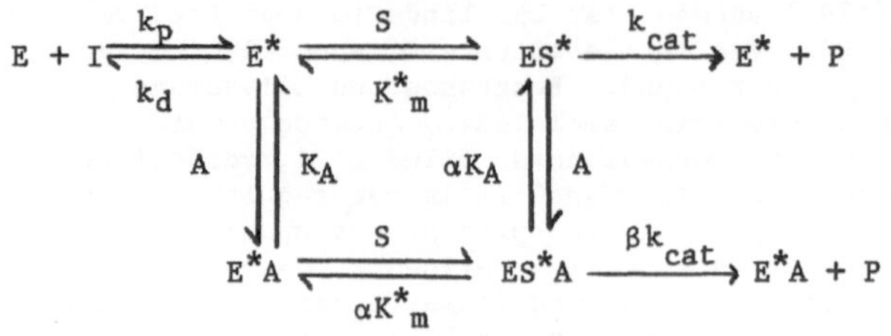

$$E + I \underset{k_d}{\overset{k_p}{\rightleftharpoons}} E^* \underset{K^*_m}{\overset{S}{\rightleftharpoons}} ES^* \xrightarrow{k_{cat}} E^* + P$$

$$A \downarrow\uparrow K_A \qquad \alpha K_A \downarrow\uparrow A$$

$$E^*A \underset{\alpha K^*_m}{\overset{S}{\rightleftharpoons}} ES^*A \xrightarrow{\beta k_{cat}} E^*A + P$$

<u>Scheme I</u>

In this scheme, E = LpL; I = lipoprotein interface; E* = LpL bound to the substrate-containing particle interface, but with unoccupied active site; S = triglyceride or phospholipid substrate; ES* = Michaelis complex of LpL and S; P = products; $K_A$ = dissociation constant of LpL-apoC-II complex, with units molecules area$^{-1}$; $\alpha$ = factor by which $K^*_m$ and $K_A$ are changed when LpL and apoC-II interact, $0 < \alpha \leqslant 1$; $\beta$ = factor by which $k_{cat}$ is changed when LpL and apoC-II interact, $\beta > 1$.

The mechanism given in Scheme I suggests that there are two possible routes to product formation, one involving apoC-II (ES*A) and the other occurring in the absence of apoC-II (ES*). In this scheme, apoC-II, is considered a nonessential activator of the LpL-catalyzed hydrolysis of lipid substrates. This view is, consistent with the fact that substrate turnover can occur, albeit at a lower rate, in the absence of apoC-II. Furthermore, apoC-II is not required for catalysis of hydrolysis of short-chained, water-soluble lipids.

The effect of apoC-II on the kinetic parameters $K_m$ and $V_{max}$ has been determined for the LpL-catalyzed hydrolysis of apoC-II deficient triglyceride-rich lipoproteins. Matsuoka et al. (1981) determined the kinetic parameters with human apoC-II deficient VLDL and purified bovine milk LpL. Maximal hydrolysis of VLDL-triglycerides occurs with 2.5 µg apoC-II per mg triglyceride. Over the triglyceride range of 0.5 to 3.0 mM, apoC-II has little effect on the apparent $V_{max}$. However, the apparent $K_m$ of the enzyme for VLDL-triglycerides decreases from 7.8 mM to 1.0 mM. Similar results were obtained by Fitzharris et al. (1981) using guinea pig VLDL; the major effect of apoC-II is to decrease the apparent $K_m$ by 4-fold. Quinn et al. (1982) have proposed a steady-state kinetic derivation based on the mechanism of Scheme I.

If $\alpha \ll 1$, and therefore interaction between LpL and apoC-II induces a large reduction in $K^*_m$ then $(1 + A/\alpha K_A) \gg 1$ when $(1 + A/K_A) \simeq 1$ and Equations 1 and 2 simplify to describe the dependence of $V_{max}$ and $K_m$ on apoC-II:

$$V^{app}_{max} = \frac{k_{cat}\, E_T\, S(1 + \frac{\beta A}{\alpha K_A})}{K^*_m + S(1 + \frac{A}{\alpha K_A})} \qquad (1)$$

and

$$K^{app}_m = \frac{k_d}{k_p} \frac{K^*_m\, S}{K^*_m + S(1 + \frac{A}{\alpha K_A})} = \frac{k_d}{k_p} \frac{[K^*_m/(1 + \frac{A}{\alpha K_A})]S}{K^*_m/(1 + \frac{A}{\alpha K_A}) + S} \qquad (2)$$

Equation 2 casts the dependence of $K_m^{app}$ in two ways. The rightmost way of expressing the dependence of $K_m^{app}$ on apoC-II emphasizes that addition of apoC-II causes $K_m^*$ to decrease. Thus, the higher the apoC-II concentration, the more the distribution of LpL at the particle surface is shifted toward the interfacial Michaelis complex $ES^*A$. Hence, one of the effects of apoC-II on LpL-catalyzed hydrolysis of lipid substrates is to increase the active site occupation factor $S/(K_m^* + S)$. Since $V_{max}$ also contains the occupation factor, $V_{max}$ may be increased because apoC-II increases the occupation factor, in addition to the potential effect of apoC-II on $k_{cat}$ expressed by $\beta$.

If $K_m^* \ll S(1 + A/\alpha K_A)$ and $\beta = 1$, then equations 1 and 2 reduce to:

$$V_{max} = k_{cat} E_T \quad \text{and} \quad K_m^{app} = \frac{k_d}{k_p} \frac{K_m^*}{1 + \dfrac{A}{\alpha K_A}} \quad (3)$$

Equation 3 predicts no effect on $V_{max}$ but a reduction in $K_m$ on addition of apoC-II, which agrees with the effect discussed above of apoC-II on the bovine milk LpL-catalyzed hydrolysis of VLDL-triglycerides.


## Acknowledgment

We gratefully acknowledge the assistance of Ms. Janet Simons in preparing the manuscript for publication.


## References

Bengtsson G, Olivecrona T (1980) Lipoprotein lipase: Some effects of activator proteins. Eur J Biochem 106: 549-555

Cardin AD, Jackson RL, Johnson JD (1982) 5-Dimethylaminonaphthalene-1-sulfonyl 3-aminotyrosyl apolipoprotein C-III: Preparation, characterization and interaction with phospholipid vesicles. J Biol Chem 257: 4987-4992

Catapano AL, Kinnunen PKJ, Breckenridge WC, Gotto AM, Jackson RL, Little JA, Smith LC, Sparrow JT (1979) Lipolysis of apoC-II deficient very low density lipoproteins: Enhancement of lipoprotein lipase action by synthetic fragments of apoC-II. Biochem Biophys Res Commun 89: 951-957

Cheng C-F, Oosta GM, Bensadoun A, Rosenberg RD (1981) Binding of lipoprotein lipase to endothelial cells in culture. J Biol Chem 256: 12893-12898

Fitzharris TJ, Quinn DM, Goh EH, Johnson JD, Kashyap ML, Srivastava LS, Jackson RL, Harmony JAK (1981) Hydrolysis of guinea pig nascent very low density lipoproteins catalyzed by lipoprotein lipase: Activation by human apoli poprotein C-II. J Lipid Res 22: 921-933

Jackson RL, Pattus F, de Haas G (1980) Mechanism of action of milk lipoprotein lipase at substrate interfaces: Effects of apolipoproteins. Biochemistry 19: 373-378

Kinnunen PKJ, Jackson RL, Smith LC, Gotto AM, Sparrow JT (1977) Activation of lipoprotein lipase by native and synthetic fragments of human plasma apoli poprotein C-II. Proc Natl Acad Sci USA 74: 4848-4851

Matsuoka N, Shirai K, Johnson JD, Kashyap ML, Srivastava LS, Yamamura T, Yamamoto A, Saito Y, Kumagai A, Jackson RL (1981) Effects of apolipoprotein C-II on the lipolysis of very low density lipoproteins from apoC-II deficient patients. Metabolism 30: 818-824

Nilsson-Ehle P, Garfinkle AS, Schotz MC (1980) Lipolytic enzymes and plasma lipoprotein metabolism. Ann Rev Biochem 49: 667-693

Quinn D, Shirai K, Jackson RL (1982) Lipoprotein lipase: Mechanism of action and role in lipoprotein metabolism. In: Holman R (ed) Progress in Lipid Research. Pergamon Press, Oxford (In press)

Quinn DM, Shirai K, Jackson RL, Harmony JAK. Lipoprotein lipase-catalyzed hydro
    lysis of water-soluble p-nitrophenyl esters. Inhibition by apolipoprotein C-II.
    (Submitted)
Shimada K, Gill P-J, Silbert JE, Douglas WHJ, Fanburg BL (1981) Involvement of
    cell surface heparin sulfate in the binding of lipoprotein lipase to
    cultured endothelial cells. J Clin Invest 68: 995-1002
Shirai K, Matsuoka N, Jackson RL (1981) Interaction of lipoprotein lipase with
    phospholipid vesicles: Role of apolipoprotein C-II and heparin. Biochim
    Biophys Acta 665: 504-510
Shirai K, Jackson RL (1982a) Lipoprotein lipase-catalyzed hydrolysis of
    p-nitrophenyl butyrate: Interfacial activation by phospholipid vesicles.
    J Biol Chem 257: 1253-1258
Shirai K, Wisner DA, Johnson JD, Srivastava LS, Jackson RL (1982b) Immunological
    studies on bovine milk lipoprotein lipase: Effects of Fab fragments on
    enzyme activity. Biochim Biophys Acta (In press)
Shirai K, Jackson RL, Quinn DM. Reciprocal effect of apolipoprotein C-II on the
    lipoprotein lipase-catalyzed hydrolysis of p-nitrophenyl butyrate and
    trioleoylglycerol. (Submitted)
Smith LC, Voyta JC, Catapano JC, Kinnunen PKJ, Gotto AM, Sparrow JT (1980)
    Activation of lipoprotein lipase by synthetic fragments of apolipoprotein
    C-II. Ann NY Acad Sci 348: 213-223
Smith LC, Voyta JC, Kinnunen PKJ, Gotto AM, Sparrow (1982) Lipoprotein lipase
    interaction with synthetic N-dansyl fragments of apolipoprotein C-II.
    Biophys J 37:174-175

# Human Apolipoprotein Mutants

G. Utermann

The protein moiety of plasma lipoproteins consists of several distinct polypeptides called apolipoproteins. These proteins serve different specific functions in lipid transport including enzymatic cofactor activity, recognition of cell surface receptors and exchange of cholesterylesters between lipoproteins. Mutants of apolipoproteins will be excellent probes to study structure-function relationships of these proteins. Mutations affecting the function of apolipo-proteins may perturb lipoprotein metabolism and result in certain forms of genetic dys- or hyperlipoproteinemia that might be termed apolipoproteinopathies (1).

The recent development of screening procedure for apolipoprotein mutants has resulted in the detection of (a) genetic polymorphism of apolipoprotein E (b) genetic polymorphism of apolipoprotein A IV and (c) rare mutants of apolipoprotein A I.

Polymorphism of Apolipoprotein E

The human E apoprotein exhibits genetic polymorphism that may be demonstrated by 1D- or 2D-techniques of isoprotein analysis (2,3,4, Fig.1). Six common apo E phenotypes designated apo E-2/2, E-3/3, E-4/4, E-4/3, E-4/2 and E-3/2 exist in the population (3,4 for nomenclature see ref.5). Extended family studies have established that these phenotypes are controlled by three autosomal codominant alleles Є2, Є3 and Є4 at the apo E structural gene locus (3,4). The differences between apo E isoforms E2, E3 and E4 reside in the primary structure of the protein and are the result of arginine - cysteine interchange at two different sites (6).

The alleles at the apo E gene locus contribute to the normal variance of plasma cholesterol, triglyceride, apo B and apo E concentrations in the population (7, G.Utermann unpublished results) and have frequencies in hyperlipidemics and patients with myocardial infarc-tion that are significantly different from those in unrelated healthy blood donors or patients with other disorders (Table 1). This suggests that apo E genes are among the genetic risk factors for atherosclerosis.

Homozygotes for the Є2 allele (phenotype E-2/2) invariably present with a lipoprotein phenotype that is characterized by 1. presence of cholesterol-rich VLDL, 2. presence of beta-VLDL and 3. subnormal concentrations of LDL (= primary dysbetalipoproteinemia). There is however considerable variability in the phenotypic expression of the dyslipoproteinemia that relates to (a) the particle distribution along the VLDL/chylomicron → IDL/remnant → LDL cascades and (b) the wide distribution of lipid levels that range from subnormal cholesterol to excessive hyperlipidemia (hyperlipoproteinemia type III; 2,7,8,9).

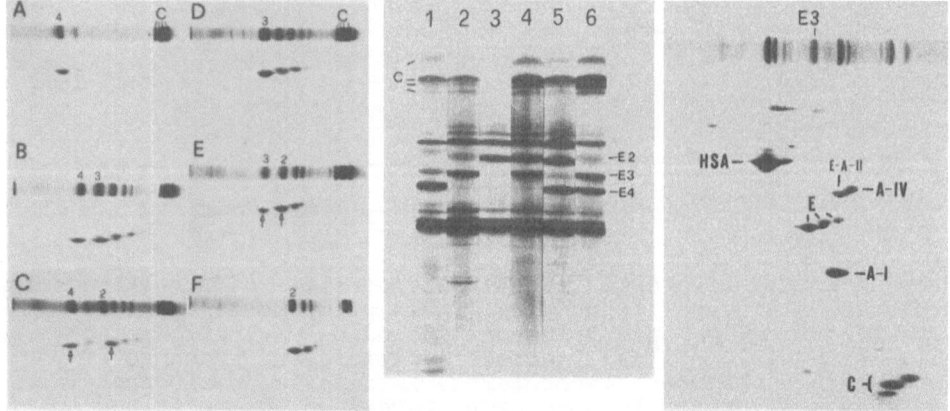

Fig.1 Left: 2D-electrophoresis of apo VLDL from the six apo E phenotypes -4/4 (A), -4/3 (B), -4/2 (C), -3/3 (D), -3/2 (E) and -2/2 (F). Focusing gels showing the separation in the first dimension are inserted at the top of each panel. Middle: Electro-focusing of apoproteins from heparin/Mg$^{++}$ precipitated lipoproteins showing the six common apo E phenotypes. Positions of the major apo E isoforms are labeled. Right: 2D-electrophoresis of apolipo-proteins from heparin/Mg$^{++}$ precipitated lipoproteins (phenotype E-3/3). The separation in the first dimension is shown at the top. Note that there is no overlap of coprecipitated proteins with the major apo E isoform

The present concept to explain the phenotypic differences among E-2/2 homozygotes assumes that the expression at the lipoprotein level of the $\mathcal{E}$2 genes is modulated by other independent factors e.g. genes and/or environment (9). However biochemical heterogeneity that is not recognized by electrofocusing may also contribute to the observed phenotypic differences between E-2/2 subjects.

The apo E protein from some patients with hyperlipoproteinemia type III and phenotype E-2/2 is a non-functional mutant that does not bind to LDL-receptors, thus explaining the accumulation of remnant lipoproteins in the patients plasma and the tendency for dyslipoproteinemia in heterozygotes for the $\mathcal{E}$2 allel (10).

Table 1.  Association between Apo E Genes, Hyperlipidemia, and Myocardial Infarction

|  | $\mathcal{E}$2 present (%) | | $\mathcal{E}$2 absent (%) | | Significance[1] |
|---|---|---|---|---|---|
| Controls | 149 | (14,5) | 882 | (85.5) | $x^2_{df}1 = 9,72$ |
| Hyperlipid-emics | 54 | (22,6) | 182 | (77.4) | $0.005 > p > 0.001$ |
|  | $\mathcal{E}$4 present (%) | | $\mathcal{E}$4 absent (%) | | |
| Controls | 280 | (27,2) | 751 | (72.8) | $x^2_{df}1 = 4,806$ |
| M.J. | 115 | (22,0) | 408 | (78.0) | $0.05 > p > 0.025$ |

[1]Woolf procedure

## Polymorphism of Apolipoprotein A IV

Apo A IV mutants may be demonstrated by a simple two-step procedure that combines agarose gel electrophoresis in detergent with electro-focusing of the prepurified apoproteins (1). However one mutant previously designated A IV-Marburg (1) may be missed by this technique due to the similar isoelectric point of the variant with a minor apo A I isoform (A $I_2$). Depending on the conditions of focusing, the A IV-Marburg variant may be masked by A $I_2$.

To overcome this problem we have used immunofixation with anti apo A IV to demonstrate A IV isoforms. With this technique most individuals (~88%) in the german population present with one major apo A IV isoform with an apparent pI in 6M urea of 5.50 (A IV-1; Fig. 2). About 10% of individuals exhibit an additional more alkaline isoform of apparent pI 5.53 (A IV-2) that is identical with the variant previously designated A-IV-Marburg. Rarely this alkaline isoform is the only one present in an individual. In less than 1% of the population still other rare A IV isoforms were detected that have apparent pI's of 5.55 (A IV-3) and 5.47 (A IV-4).

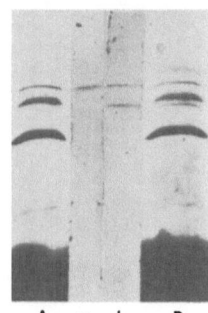

A   a   b   B

**Fig. 2.** Electrofocusing of apolipoproteins from an apo A IV 1-1 homozygous (A, a) and from an apo A IV 3-1 heterozygous individual (B, b). A, B: coomassie blue staining; a, b: immunofixation with anti apo A IV. Only part of the gel in the vicinity of apo A I and A IV isoforms is shown

No individual had more than 2 of these isoforms. In combination with the segregation data from family studies this suggests that a genetic polymorphism of apo A IV exists in man, that is controlled by at least 4 different autosomal codominant alleles, probably at the apo A IV structural gene locus. Two of these alleles (A $IV^1$, A $IV^2$) are common in the population whereas others are rare (A $IV^3$, A $IV^4$). Some of the apo A IV variants described probably are identical with those recently observed by Menzel et al. (10).

No association of any of the A IV genes with dyslipoproteinemia has yet been detected. However more extended studies especially on homozygotes for the rare alleles are needed. Possibly such mutants could provide the key for understanding the function of apo A IV that at present is not known.

## Mutants of Apolipoprotein A I

Four probands heterozygous for a mutant of apolipoprotein A I were detected by screening of 2282 unrelated individuals (frequency ~1/600). Three individuals had a phenotypically identical variant designated A I-Marburg (1). All three probands with apo A I-Marburg had hypertriglyceridemia (TG > 250 mg/dl) and subnormal HDL-cholesterol

( <30 mg/dl) but no other lipoprotein abnormalities. The kindreds
of two probands with A I-Marburg were studied (Fig. 3). The family
data are consistent with an autosomal codominant inheritance of
the trait (11). Analysis of the plasma lipid- and lipoprotein-
levels in relation to the A I phenotype were complicated by the high
prevalence of diabetes mellitus and hypothyroidism in the M-kindred
and of hyperlipidemia in both kindreds. No consistent relationship
between plasma lipoprotein patterns and the mutant A I could be
demonstrated. Rather the mutant A I and the dyslipoproteinemia
seem to co-exist independently in these kindreds. The apo A I
mutant and genetic apo E phenotypes segregate independently,
indicating, that the structural gene loci for apo A I and apo E
are not closely linked (11).

One proband with an alkaline mutant of apo A I (A I-Giessen; Ref.1)
had no dyslipoproteinemia, nor had any of his blood relatives with
the mutant isoform hyper- or dyslipoproteinemia. However the isolated
mutant A I isoform of the heterozygous proband had lost the ability
to activate lecithin-cholesterol acyltransferase and hence is a
non-functional mutant (P.Soltys, J.Haas, G.Utermann, unpublished).

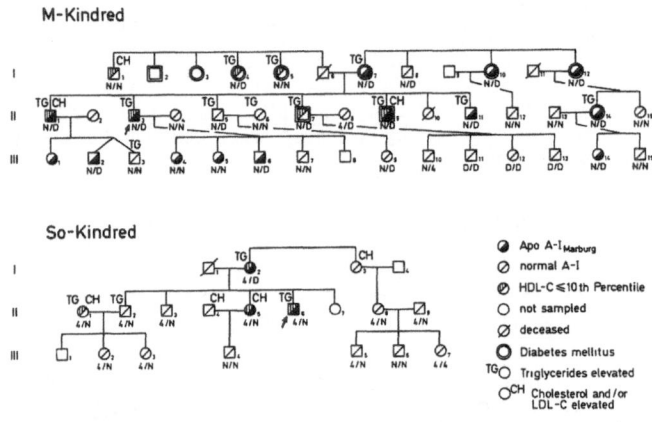

Fig. 3. Pedigrees of kindreds with apo A I-Marburg. Apo E phenotypes are indicated under the symbols (apo E nomenclature according to ref. 4, N = E3, D = E2)

References

1. Utermann G, Feussner G, Franceschini G, Haas J, Steinmetz A
   (1982) Genetic variants of group A apolipoproteins. Rapid
   methods for screening and characterization without ultracentrifugation. J.Biol.Chem. 257: 501-507
2. Utermann G, Hees M, Steinmetz A (1977) Polymorphism of apolipoprotein E and occurance of dysbetalipoproteinemia in man.
   Nature 269: 604-607
3. Zannis VI, Just PW, Breslow JL (1981) Human apolipoprotein E
   isoprotein subclasses are genetically determined. Am. J. Hum.
   Genet. 33: 11-24

4. Utermann G, Steinmetz A, Weber W (1982) Genetic control of human apolipoprotein E polymorphism: comparison of one- and two-dimensional techniques of isoprotein analysis. Hum. Genet. in press
5. Zannis VI, Breslow JL, Utermann G, Mahley RW, Weisgraber KH, Havel RJ, Goldstein JL, Brown MS, Schönfeld G, Hazzard WR, Blum C (1982) Proposed nomenclature of apo E isoproteins, apo E genotypes and phenotypes. J.Lipid Res. in press
6. Weisgraber KH, Rall SC jr, Mahley RW (1981) Human E apoprotein heterogeneity: Cysteine-arginine interchanges in the amino acid sequence of the apo E isoforms. J.Biol.Chem. 256: 9077-9081
7. Utermann G, Pruin N, Steinmetz A (1979) Polymorphism of apolipoprotein E. III. Effect of a single polymorphic gene locus on plasma lipid levels in man. Clin.Genet. 15: 63-72
8. Utermann G, Canzler H, Hees M, Jaeschke M, Mühlfellner G, Schoenborn W, Vogelberg KH (1977) Studies on the metabolic defect in Broad-ß disease (hyperlipoproteinemia type III). Clin.Genet. 12: 139-154
9. Utermann G, Vogelberg KH, Steinmetz A, Schoenborn W, Pruin N, Jaeschke M, Hees M, Canzler H (1979) Polymorphism of apolipoprotein E. II. Genetics of hyperlipoproteinemia type III. Clin. Genet. 15: 37-62
10. Schneider WJ, Kovanen PT, Brown MS, Goldstein JL, Utermann G, Weber W, Havel RJ, Kotite L, Kane JP, Innerarity TL, Mahley RW (1981) Familial dysbetalipoproteinemia: Abnormal binding of mutant apoprotein E to LDL receptors of human fibroblasts and membranes from liver and adrenal of rats, rabbits, and cows. J.Clin.Invest. 68: 1075-1085
11. Menzel HJ, Kladetzky RG, Assmann G (1982) One-step screening method for the polymorphism of apolipoproteins A-I, A-II and A-IV. J.Lipid Res. in press
12. Utermann G, Steinmetz A, Paetzold R, Wilk J, Feussner G, Kaffarnik H, Mueller-Eckhardt Ch, Seidel D, Vogelberg KH, Zimmer F (1982) Apolipoprotein A I-Marburg: Studies on two kindreds with a mutant of human apolipoprotein A I. Hum. Genet. submitted

# 3.5 Lipolytic Enzymes

# Use of Specific Antibodies in the Study of the Function of Lipoprotein Lipase

A. Bensadoun and S. R. Behr

## A. Introduction

There is, at present, extensive evidence (1) that lipoprotein lipase (LPL, glycerol ester hydrolase, EC 3.113) is the enzyme responsible for the hydrolysis of triglycerides in chylomicrons and very low density lipoproteins (VLDL). The functional LPL is an exoenzyme associated with the surface matrix of vascular endothelial cells (1, 2). Recent equilibrium-binding data of highly purified avian LPL to culture bovine endothelial cells, demonstrate the presence of a class of high affinity sites (11). The action of LPL on VLDL leads to the removal of triglyceride from the particle core and to the loss of some surface constituents, mainly phospholipid, cholesterol and apolipoprotein C. It has been shown, in vitro, that "LDL-like particles" are formed from VLDL in the presence of milk LPL (3). The site of transformation of these particles to LDL lipoproteins comparable to circulating LDL is still unknown. The surface constituents leaving the VLDL particle during lipolysis have been shown to become associated with subclasses of HDL classes (4). Therefore, the process of lipolysis leads to the generation of new lipoproteins and to changes in the chemical composition and physical properties of pre-existing circulating lipoproteins. Recently, the use of highly specific inhibitors of LPL namely, antibodies against avian adipose tissue LPL, has provided direct experimental evidence, in vivo, that LPL is indispensible for the hydrolysis of VLDL triglyceride. Anti-LPL serum injected into roosters quantitatively blocks the catabolism of VLDL triglyceride, plasma LDL levels decrease exponentially and the chemical composition of LDL is altered. Simultaneously, the HDL particles become smaller and more dense (5). The immunological inhibition of LPL has provided a means of isolating large quantities of newly secreted VLDL which accumulate in the plasma compartment. In addition, the inhibition of LPL in vivo provides a method determining the rate constants of LDL removal under non-steady state conditions. In this report these methods have been exploited to explain the increased plasma VLDL and LDL cholesterol which result from cholesterol feeding in roosters and to explain the existence of a VLDL-independent pathway of LDL synthesis.

## B. Preparation of Anti-Lipoprotein Lipase Serum

To obtain valid results it is essential to ensure that the polyclonal antiserum employed is monospecific. This was accomplished by immunizing goats with highly purified adipose tissue LPL (7). Purity of the antigen was established by slab gel electrophoresis in the presence of SDS and urea, and by isoelectric focusing. Immunoglobulin fractions prepared from these antisera quantitatively inhibit partially purified LPL from adipose, heart and liver tissues, but do not inhibit the NaCl-resistant liver lipase (7). Immunodiffusion experiments with purified anti-LPL immunoglobulins showed a single precipitation line against crude extract of chicken adipose tissue concentrated by ammonium sulfate precipitation. A line of identity was seen between this crude preparation and highly purified LPL (8).

## C. VLDL Secretion Rate in Normal and Cholesterol-Fed Animals

The mean concentration of plasma cholesterol in roosters on a cholesterol-free diet is 64 ± 10 mg/100 ml plasma. After at least three weeks on a diet containing 1% cholesterol and 5% corn oil in grow mash, the mean plasma cholesterol was 193.5 ±

114 mg/100 ml. Animals with plasma cholesterol higher than 130 mg/100 ml were selected for experiments discussed below. These animals had VLDL and LDL cholesterol
concentrations of respectively 164 ± 120 mg and 89 ± 27 mg/100 ml plasma. These
values are 540 and 6-fold higher than those measured in control animals in VLDL and
LDL respectively. VLDL secretion rates were measured by quantitative inhibition of
LPL (Fig. 1). The hourly rate of secretion of VLDL triglyceride in cholesterol-fed
roosters was 96.6 ± 25.5 mg/100 ml plasma/hr. This is more than twice the mean rate
of VLDL triglyceride production in control roosters fed a diet of 5% corn oil in
grow mash (42.8 ± 9.2 mg/100 ml/hr). The chemical composition of the newly secreted
VLDL differed significantly from VLDL produced in a normal fed rooster. The proportion of unesterified cholesterol increased from 4.9 to 9.2%, cholesterol esters from
2.0 to 9.8% and phospholipids from 5.2 to 13%, while the percentage of triglyceride
dropped from 79.6 to 60%. Since the newly secreted VLDL particle is enriched in
cholesterol, VLDL cholesterol secretion rates are 3.8-fold higher in cholesterol-fed
animals (Fig. 1).

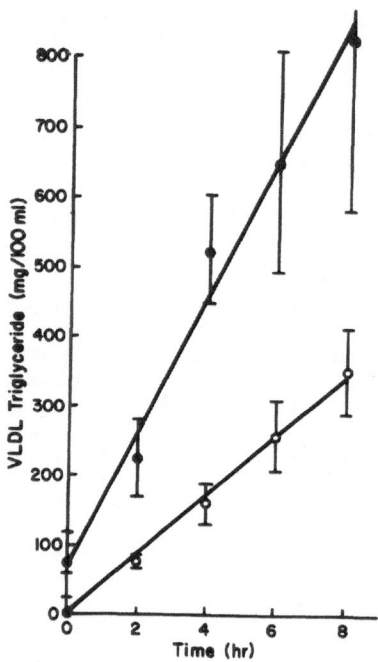

FIGURE 1. VLDL triglyceride production. VLDL triglyceride concentration was determined in plasma from
fasted roosters injected with anti-
LPL serum and fed a 1% cholesterol,
5% corn oil diet (n = 4), or a control diet containing 5% corn oil
(n = 5). LPL activity was inhibited
for the entire duration of the experiment by hourly injections of
anti-LPL. 1% cholesterol, 5% corn
oil diet, ●—●; control diet o—o

## D. VLDL Secretion by Extra-Hepatic Tissues

VLDL secretion rates by the small intestine in roosters fed low cholesterol diet
were estimated by inhibiting LPL in functionally hepatectomized roosters. The
rate of VLDL cholesterol production was 2.2 ± 0.2 mg/100 ml plasma/hr. This represents 28% of VLDL cholesterol secretion of sham-hepatectomized rooster. In cholesterol-fed roosters, the small intestine accounted for approximately the same proportion of the total VLDL influx.

## E. LDL-Catabolism

In roosters fed a cholesterol-free diet, inhibition of LPL leads to a decrease in LDL concentration (5) by a first-order process ($K = 0.29$ hr$^{-1}$). In the cholesterol-fed animals, it was of interest to ask whether a VLDL-independent pathway of LDL synthesis exist. Direct synthesis of LDL by the liver has been demonstrated in hypercholesterolemic rats (9) and in the isolated perfused pig liver (10). If indeed direct secretion of LDL occurs, one would expect that as the VLDL dependent pathway of LDL synthesis is inhibited by anti-LPL serum, a new steady state of LDL concentration would be established. Figure 2 illustrate the catabolism of LDL in a cholesterol-fed rooster. It is of interest that the first-order rate constant which accounts for removal of over 80% of LDL cholesterol is very similar to that determined in animals fed a cholesterol-free diet. The VLDL-independent pathway of LDL synthesis ($a = 1.4$ mg cholesterol/100 ml plasma/hr) accounts for less than 10% of the total LDL flux (23 mg cholesterol/100 ml plasma/hr).

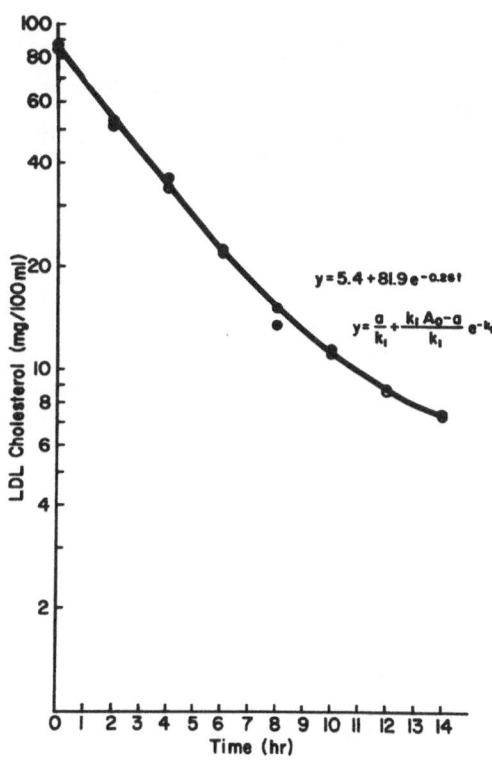

FIGURE 2. Effect of anti-LPL serum on LDL concentration in a rooster fed a 1% cholesterol, 5% corn oil diet. The experimental points were fitted by repeated iterations to a model which assumes first-order removal of plasma LDL and a constant secretion of LDL by a VLDL-independent pathway of synthesis. Model, $dy = -K_1 y dt + a dt$, where $y$ is LDL concentration; $K_1$, first-order rate constant; $a$, secretion rate of LDL by VLDL-independent pathway of LDL synthesis. Integration of this equation gives =

$$y = \frac{a}{K_1} + \frac{K_1 A_0 - a}{K_1} e^{-K_1 t}$$

Where $A_0$ is the LDL concentration at $t = 0$. Calculated values o—o; experimental points ●—●

The present findings indicate that the enlarged LDL pool size in the cholesterol-fed animal is not due to a defective catabolic rate, but rather to an increased LDL flux which results from a greatly enhanced VLDL-cholesterol secretion rate. The 3.8-fold increase in VLDL-cholesterol secretion in response to cholesterol feeding suggest that some of the cholesterol-enriched particles which accumulate in plasma might be derived from hepatic and intestinal VLDL. The previous experiments illustrate that the inhibition of LPL in vivo is a convenient means of determining VLDL secretion rates by the liver and the intestine, and of analyzing parameters of LDL catabolism.

622

F.  References

1.  Robinson DS  (1970)  Comprehensive Biochemistry.  Florkin M, Stortz EH (eds)
    Elsevier, Amsterdam, pp 51-116
2.  Borensztajn J, Robinson DS  (1970)  The effect of fasting on the utilization
    of chylomicron triglyceride fatty acids in relation to clearing factor lipase
    (lipoprotein lipase) releasable by heparin in the perfuse rat heart.  J Lipid
    Res  11:  111-117
3.  Deckelbaum RJ, Eisenberg S, Fainaru M, Borenholz Y, Olivecrona T  (1979)   In
    vitro production of human plasma low density lipoprotein-like particles.  J
    Biol Chem  254:  6079-6097
4.  Patsch JR, Gotto AM, Olivecrona T, Eisenberg S  (1978)  Formation of high den-
    sity lipoprotein$_2$-like particles during lipolysis of very low density lipopro-
    teins in vitro.  Proc Natl Acad  75:  4519-4523
5.  Behr SR, Patsch JR, Forte T, Bensadoun A  (1981)  Plasma lipoprotein changes
    resulting from immunologically blocked lipolysis.  J Lipid Res  22:  443-451
6.  Kompiang IP, Bensadoun A, Yang MWW  (1976)  Effect of an anti-lipoprotein li-
    pase serum on plasma triglyceride removal.  J Lipid Res  17:  498-505
7.  Bensadoun A, Kompiang IP  (1979)  Role of lipoprotein lipase in plasma trigly-
    ceride removal.  Fed Proc 38:  2622-2626
8.  Cheung AH, Bensadoun A, Cheng CF  (1978)  Direct solid phase radioimmunoassay
    for chicken lipoprotein lipase.  Anal Biochem  94:  346-357
9.  Noel SP, Nong L, Dolphin PJ, Dory L, Rubinstein D  (1979)  Secretion of choles-
    terol-rich lipoproteins by perfused livers of hypercholesterolemic rats.  J
    Clin Invest  64:  674-683
10. Nakaya N, Chung BH, Patsch JR, Taunton OD  (1977)  Synthesis and release of low
    density lipoproteins by the isolated perfused pig liver.  J Biol Chem  252:
    7530-7533
11. Cheng CF, Oosta GM, Bensadoun A, Rosenberg RD  (1981)  Binding of lipoprotein
    lipase to endothelial cells in culture.  J Biol Chem  256:  12893-12898

# The Role of Hepatic Triglyceride Lipase in Primates

I. J. Goldberg, N.-A. Le, J. R. Paterniti, Jr., H. N. Ginsberg, F. T. Lindgren, and W. V. Brown

## INTRODUCTION

The catabolism of very low density lipoproteins (VLDL) and production of low density lipoproteins (LDL) has been postulated to proceed via the actions of the enzyme lipoprotein lipase (LPL) bound to the luminal surface of capillary endothelial cells. A genetic deficiency of this enzyme exists in humans with Type I Hyperlipoproteinemia. These subjects have been shown to catabolize VLDL (Quarfordt et al. 1970) and convert VLDL to LDL (Nicoll et al. 1980). Thus, it is unlikely that LPL in humans is the sole enzyme capable of converting VLDL to LDL. In addition, an intermediate step in this pathway, the conversion of IDL and small VLDL ($S_f$ 12-60) to LDL ($S_f$ 0-12) primarily occurs across the splanchnic bed in man (Turner et al. 1981). It has therefore been postulated that hepatic triglyceride lipase (HTGL), a liver enzyme with both triglyceride hydrolase (LaRosa et al. 1972) and phospholipase activities (Ehnholm et al. 1975) is involved in the production of LDL in primates.

While HTGL can hydrolyze VLDL triglyceride in vitro, in vivo studies of this enzyme have been limited to the rat, an animal in which most VLDL is removed from the circulation without conversion to LDL (Faegerman et al. 1975). In studies performed in rats with antibody inhibition of HTGL, VLDL triglycerides and phospholipids showed marked increases (Jansen et al. 1979, Grosser et al. 1981). In addition, HDL phospholipid increased. Although in one study (Grosser et al. 1981), the changes in VLDL clearly preceded those in HDL, in the other study (Jansen et al 1979) an increase in $HDL_2$ phospholipids was the initial change noted. In the latter study, no change was noted in the metabolism of injected radiolabelled HDL suggesting that HTGL altered the lipid but not the apoprotein components of HDL. In a third study, an increase in HDL phospholipids was also noted (Kuusi et al. 1979), but the injection of whole antiserum in that study may have accounted for the differences in the results.

## VLDL METABOLISM DURING ACUTE INHIBITION OF HEPATIC TRIGLYCERIDE LIPASE

The physiologic role of HTGL has been investigated in a primate model, the cynomolgus monkey. Our objectives were to produce an HTGL deficient animal and to document alterations that occur in the composition and mass of the major lipoprotein classes. In addition, since an increase in the mass of VLDL, as noted in the rat, may be due to either an increase in the production or a decrease in the catabolism of that lipoprotein, the removal and conversion of intravenously injected radiolabeled homologous VLDL apolipoprotein-B to IDL and LDL was assessed during saline and immunologic blockade of HTGL.

An antiserum to purified human HTGL was prepared in a goat. IgG preparations of goat anti-human HTGL serum and nonimmune goat serum were immunoabsorbed against preheparin plasma. In vitro, the anti-HTGL IgG inhibited cynomolgus monkey HTGL activity, but not LPL activity. In vivo inhibition of HTGL activity after intravenous infusion of this IgG was confirmed by assay of lipase activity in liver tissue obtained by percutaneous biopsies.

We have reported changes in the kinetics of VLDL apolipoprotein-B after acute inhibition of HTGL in the cynomolgus monkey, suggesting a decrease in the catabolism of VLDL and a decrease in its conversion to LDL (Fig. 1) (Goldberg et al. 1981). Similar alterations were not produced during control studies using nonimmune goat IgG preparations.

This research was supported by grants HL28765, HL23077, HL 22967, HL 18574, HL 06157 and HL 07343 from the National Institutes of Health.
IJG is the recipient of a Clinician-Scientist Award from the American Heart Association and its local affiliate, the New York Heart Association.

624

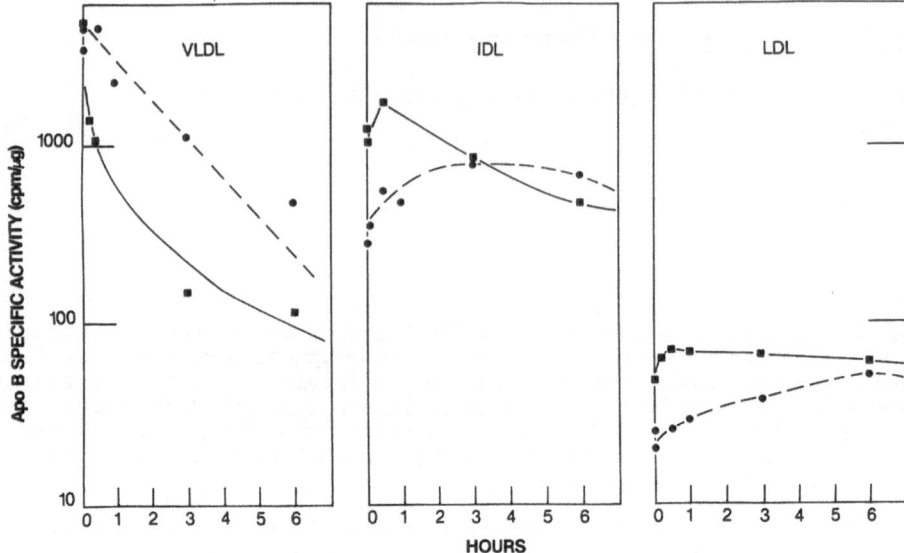

Figure 1. Comparison of VLDL apolipoprotein-B metabolism before and during infusion of anti-HTGL IgG in the cynomolgus monkey. The identical homolgous VLDL preparation labeled with either $^{125}$Iodine or $^{131}$Iodine was intravenously injected in a single animal on two consecutive days, the first during infusion of saline (●—●) and the second after a bolus of anti-HTGL IgG (20mg/kg) followed by a three hour infusion of an equal quantity of anti-HTGL IgG (●----●). Specific activities of apolipoprotein-B in VLDL, IDL and LDL were performed as previously reported (Le et al., 1978)

Changes in lipoprotein mass obtained using isopycnic ultracentrifugation demonstrated a 60-300% increase in VLDL triglyceride (d<1.006) after a three hour intravenous infusion of anti-HTGL IgG in three monkeys . VLDL phospholipids also increased 50-380%. Dramatic changes in the total mass of VLDL ($S_f$ 20-400) was also demonstrated by analytic ultracentrifugation (Table 1). Animals receiving nonimmune goat IgG showed no increase in VLDL mass.

Table 1. VLDL mass before and after a 3 hour infusion of anti-HTGL or nonimmune goat IgG in the cynomulgus monkey determined by analytic ultracentrifugation

| Time (Hours) | 0 | 3 |
|---|---|---|
| Animals Receiving Anti HTGL IgG | | |
| A | 3 | 9 |
| B | 4 | 66 |
| C | 8 | 43 |
| D | 2 | 66 |
| | | |
| Animals Receiving Nonimmune IgG | | |
| A | 1 | 1 |
| B | 0 | 0 |
| C | 32 | 0 |

## HDL MASS AFTER INHIBITION OF HEPATIC TRIGLYCERIDE LIPASE

In three animals, a modest increase in HDL$_2$ phospholipids was noted three hours after infusion of anti-HTGL IgG. Control animals infused with nonimmune IgG showed similar changes. These results obtained by isopycnic ultracentrifugation were confirmed by analytic ultracentrifugation (Figures 2 and 3).

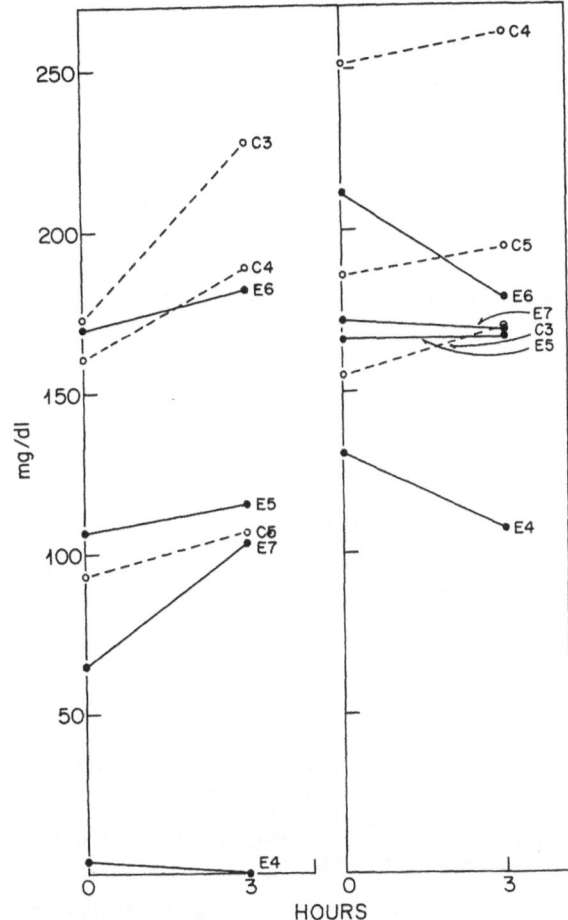

Figure 2. HDL mass determined by analytic ultracentrifugation in cynomolgus monkeys before and after receiving anti-HTGL IgG (●—●) or nonimmune IgG (o---o). HDL$_2$ mass is shown in the left panel and HDL$_3$ mass in the right panel

626

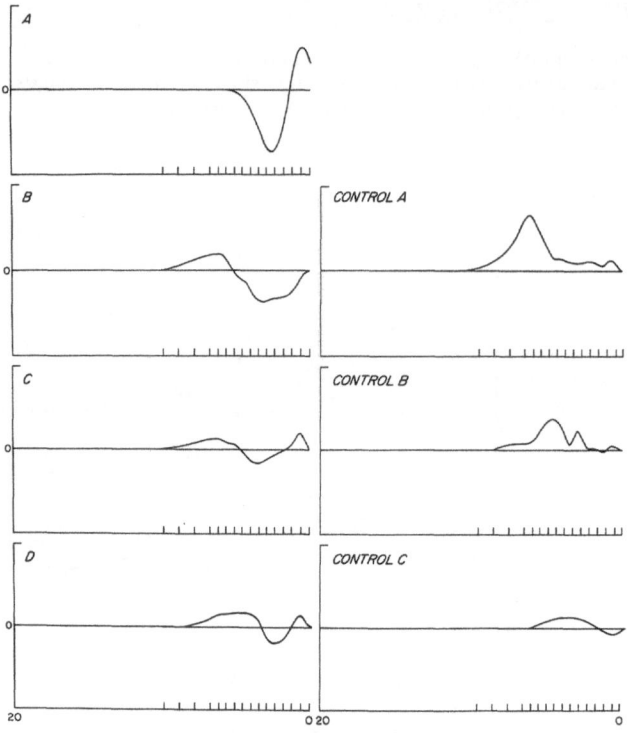

Figure 3. Difference plots of HDL masses obtained by subtracting initial mass from that obtained after a 3 hour infusion of anti-HTGL (A,B,C,D) or nonimmune (control A,B,C,) IgG into different cynomolgus monkeys. Deflections above the zero line indicate an increase in mass, while those below the line indicate a decrease

DISCUSSION

The increase in VLDL mass and the decrease in VLDL apolipoprotein-B catabolism during inhibition of HTGL in the cynomolgus monkey demonstrate that HTGL is involved in VLDL catabolism in this primate. Since lipoprotein lipase was not inhibited in these studies, VLDL catabolism continued during HTGL inhibition. Chylomicrons are a poor substrate for HTGL, but individual VLDL particles may be degraded by either of these two enzymes. Alternatively, a subclass of VLDL, perhaps those deficient in apo-CII, may be the preferred substrate for hepatic triglyceride lipase. These may be either nascent particles or those that have undergone a partial digestion by LPL.

In previous studies performed in the rat, changes in HDL were emphasized, and, as a result, the major role of the enzyme was postulated to be in conversion of $HDL_2$ to $HDL_3$. With HTGL inhibition in the cynomolgus monkey, we observed a small but consistent increase in $HDL_2$ mass and decrease in $HDL_3$ mass. However, control animals similarly showed an increase in $HDL_2$. The changes in HDL were much less striking than those observed in VLDL. These alterations in HDL mass may have been secondary to the decrease in the metabolism of the lower density lipoproteins. Catabolism of VLDL via LPL has been shown to result in the transfer of lipids to HDL (Eisenberg and Olivecrona 1979). We hypothesize that excess surface coat removed from VLDL by HTGL action may not be handled in a similar manner. The generation of these surface coat components within the liver could result in direct uptake of those lipids by the hepatocytes. This may occur via the receptor for apolipoprotein E. Thus, the hydrolysis of VLDL by HTGL would not increase HDL lipids. Inhibition of HTGL would necessitate VLDL hydrolysis proceeding via LPL, thus producing a secondary increase in the transfer of surface components to HDL.

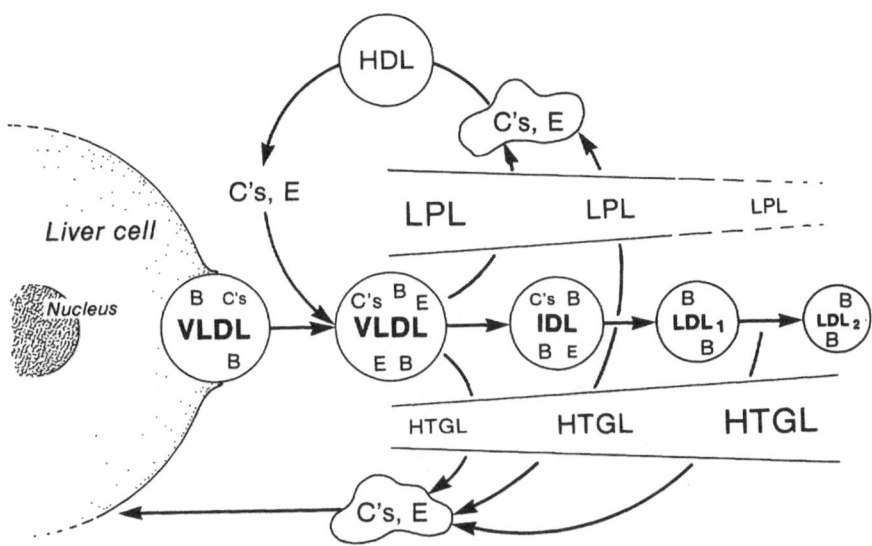

Figure 4. Postulated roles of hepatic triglyceride lipase and lipoprotein lipase in catabolism of VLDL and generation of HDL. Both enzymes may have a parallel function in catabolism of VLDL but the preferred substrate for lipoprotein lipase may be the larger lipoproteins with sufficient apolipoprotein $C_{II}$ to fully activate that enzyme. HTGL may become the more predominant hydrolytic enzyme of lipoproteins of decreasing size. Surface components generated in peripheral tissues during this process are then transferred to HDL. Hydrolysis of VLDL, IDL, and larger LDL by hepatic triglyceride lipase may also produce excess surface coat which is removed by the liver without its being transferred to HDL. Thus lipoprotein lipase but not hepatic triglyceride lipase action would lead to an increase in HDL levels

REFERENCES

1.  Ehnholm C, Shaw W, Greten H, Brown WV (1975) Purification from human plasma of a heparin released lipase with activity against triglyceride and phospholipids. J Biol Chem 250:6750-6761

2.  Eisenberg S, Olivecrona T (1979) Very low density lipoprotein. Fate of phospholipids, cholesterol and apolipoprotein C during lipolysis in vitro. J Lipid Res 20:614-623

3.  Faegerman O, Sata T, Kane JP, Havel RJ (1975) Metabolism of apoprotein B of plasma very low density lipoproteins in the rat. J Clin Invest 56:1396-1403

4.  Goldberg IJ, Le NA, Paterniti JR, Ginsberg HN, Brown WV (1981) Effect of inhibition of hepatic triglyceride lipase on very low density apoprotein-B catabolism in Macaca fasicularis. Clin Res 29:539A, (Abstract)

5.  Grosser J, Schrecker O, Greten H (1981) Function of hepatic triglyceride lipase in lipoprotein metabolism. J Lipid Res 22:437-442

6.  Jansen H, vanTol A, Hulsmann WC (1980) On the metabolic function of heparin releasable liver lipase. Biochem Biophys Res Commun 92:53-59

7.  Kuusi T, Kinnunen PKJ, Nikkila EA. (1979) Hepatic endothelial lipase antiserum influences rat plasma low and high density lipoproteins in vivo. FEBS Lett 104:384-388

8.  LaRosa JE, Levy RI, Windmueller HG, Fredrickson DS (1972) Comparison of the triglyceride lipase of liver, adipose tissue and postheparin plasma. J Lipid Res 13:356-363

9.  Le NA, Melish JS, Roach BC, Ginsberg HN, Brown WV (1978) Direct measurement of apoprotein B specific activity in [125]I labeled lipoproteins. J Lipid Res 19:578-584

10. Nicoll AB, Lewis B (1980) Evaluation of the roles of lipoprotein lipase and hepatic lipase in lipoprotein metabolism in vivo and in vitro studies. Eur J Clin Invest 10:489-495

11. Quarfordt SM, Frank A, Shames DM, Berman M, Steinberg D (1970) Very low density lipoprotein triglyceride transport in Type IV Hyperlipoproteinemia and the effects of carbohydrate rich diets. J Clin Invest 49:2281-2297

12. Turner PR, Miller, NE, Cortese L, Hazzard W, Coltart J, Lewis B (1981) Splanchnic metabolism of plasma apolipoprotein B. Studies of artery-hepatic vein differences of mass and radiolabel in fasted human subjects. J Clin Invest 67:1678-1686

# Function of Hepatic Endothelial Lipase in Lipoprotein Metabolism

T. Kuusi, E. A. Nikkilä, M. J. Tikkanen, M.-R. Taskinen, and C. Ehnholm

## Introduction

Two lipolytic enzymes are released into the circulation by intravenous administration of heparin, lipoprotein lipase (LPL) from adipose and muscle tissue, and hepatic endothelial lipase (HEL) from vascular endothelium of the liver (1). The function of LPL in the degradation of triglyceride-rich lipoproteins is well documented whereas the role of HEL in the lipoprotein metabolism is less certain. The present paper summarizes the data which indicate that HEL is the main phospholipase in postheparin plasma having a physiological function in the degradation of HDL2 phospholipids and probably in the conversion of HDL2 to HDL3-like particles.

## Lipolytic activities of hepatic endothelial lipase

Initially purified as triglyceride lipase, hepatic lipase was shown to be also a phospholipase (2) and monoacylglycerol hydrolase (3). The co-purification of these lipolytic activities suggested that they could be due to a single enzyme. This possibility was further supported by our finding (4) that the three lipolytic activities are closely correlated in postheparin plasma after inactivation of the LPL activity by specific antiserum. Therefore, identical results are obtained using any of these lipids as a substrate for HEL. About 70 to 80% of all phospholipase activity which is released into human circulation by heparin is inhibited by anti-HEL serum showing that most phospholipase activity comes from the vascular bed of the liver (4,1). This addresses an important role for HEL in the hydrolysis of circulating lipoprotein phospholipids.

## Consequences of selective inactivation of hepatic endothelial lipase in rat

A large body of evidence on the role of HEL in plasma lipoprotein metabolism has been obtained from studies in rats where the HEL activity has been specifically blocked by antibodies, and the subsequent changes in lipoproteins have been recorded. A few years ago we showed that inhibition of HEL by antiserum in vivo in rats led to an increase in the level of HDL phospholipids and cholesterol (5). Thereafter, similar approach has been used by others and the rise of HDL and particularly HDL2 phospholipids by antiserum treatment has been confirmed (6,7,8). Accumulation of also VLDL (6,7) and IDL (8) has been described, but these observations have not been made in all studies. On the other hand, the in vivo uptake of either CM, VLDL or their remnants by perfused rat livers is unaffected by removal of HEL by a heparin-preperfusion (9,10) Thus it is possible that the modified catabolism of VLDL may be secondary to impairment of HDL degradation in HEL-inactivated rats. We have tested the possible function of HEL in the removal of chylomicrons from the circulation in rat. One group of animals was given anti-HEL rabbit γ-globulins while the other received normal rabbit γ-globulins. Thereafter rat lymph chylomicrons were infused intravenously for 30 min to both groups and the lipoproteins were isolated thereafter. The average removal of chylomicron triglyceride was similar in anti-HEL

This work was supported by grants from Nordisk Insulinfond and Sigrid Juselius Foundation. The skilfull technical assistance of Mrs Sirkka Mannelin and Ms Paula Teräväinen is gratefully acknowledged.

and control animals. HDL2 phospholipids were increased significantly more in anti-HEL treated rats, which was the only significant difference found between the two groups (Kuusi T et al., to be published). This result is consistent with the view that phospholipids of the infused chylomicrons had been transferred to HDL2 but their removal had been blocked by inactivation of HEL in vivo.

## Function of hepatic endothelial lipase in lipoprotein metabolism of man

Direct proof on the role of HEL in the plasma lipoprotein metabolism of man is difficult to obtain. There is, however, much circumstantial clinical evidence to indicate that HEL is involved in the catabolism and regulation of plasma HDL2. First, if plasma HDL2 were degraded by HEL there should be an inverse relationship between HDL2 and HEL under condition where LPL, also regulating HDL2 shows minor variation. We have studied this kind of situation in a group of military academy cadets (11) who were all physically fit, of similar age and ate same diet. Their postheparin plasma LPL activity showed less variation than LPL in a free-living unselected population. In this cohort a negative correlation was found between HDL2 and postheparin plasma HEL activity. This finding supports the hypothesis obtained from rat studies that HEL is important in the regulation of plasma HDL2 also in man, and that it is responsible for the removal of HDL2 lipids.

A situation analogous to the inactivation of HEL by antibodies is a HEL deficient man. We have analyzed the HDL profile of a 32 year old man with the postheparin plasma HEL activity of only about 10% of the normal average. He is of normal weight and has a normal plasma lipoprotein pattern apart from elevated HDL cholesterol (59 mg/dl). The LPL and LCAT activities are normal. The rate zonal separation of his HDL2 and HDL3 is shown in Fig. 1 (subject 1). Compared with a 26 year old female who has normal HEL activity in her postheparin plasma (subject 3) the HDL2 concentration is much elevated in the man with HEL deficiency. For comparison, we have analyzed the HDL zonal profile of a female who has HEL activity between those of the two others. Thus, these three normolipidemic subjects who have similar LPL and LCAT but widely different HEL activities show completely different HDL subfraction distribution as judged from the rate zonal profiles. The high HDL2/HDL3 ratio of subject 1 suggests that depression of HEL activity in man results in a similar change of HDL subfractions as that found in rats after blocking of HEL with a specific antibody.

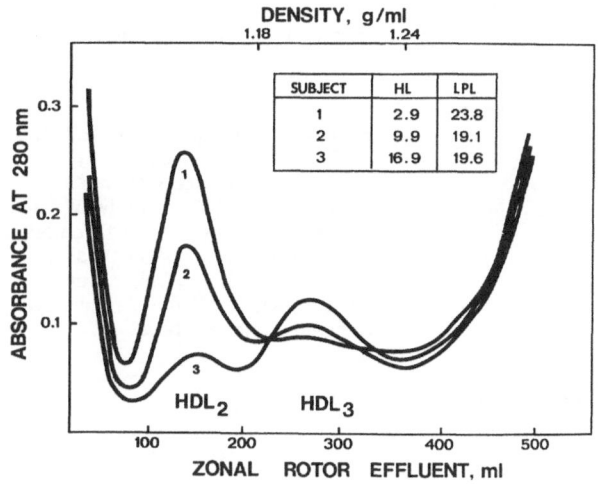

Figure 1. Zonal ultracentrifugation of HDL from subjects with similar LPL and LCAT but different HEL activities

630

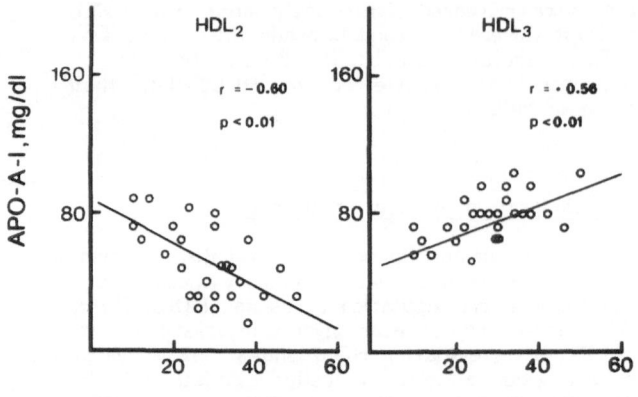

Figure 2. Relationship between the apolipoprotein A-I of HDL subfractions and postheparin plasma hepatic endothelial lipase activity

HEPATIC LIPASE ACTIVITY
$\mu mol \cdot h^{-1} \cdot ml^{-1}$

We have previously suggested that HEL could convert HDL2 to HDL3 by removing phospholipids and cholesterol from the former particle. (12). This would allow the HEL to act in concert with LPL to form an HDL shuttle (or cycle) serving in the transport of cholesterol. The finding that the subject with deficient HEL activity not only had unusually high HDL2 but also a very low level of HDL3 supports the above concept. However, we were not able to demonstrate a significant positive correlation between any of HDL3 lipids and the postheparin plasma HEL activity in the military students mentioned above (11). Since the HDL cycle hypothesis actually implies that HDL2 lipids are partially removed by HEL but the apoproteins are left in the particle a correlation should in fact be sought between the apoprotein A-I in the HDL subfractions of the military student material. The results are shown in Fig. 2. Apart from the inverse relationship between the HDL2 apo A-I concentration and HEL activity the study revealed also a significant positive correlation between HDL3 apo A-I content and the postheparin plasma HEL activity. The absence of correlation between HDL3 lipid levels and HEL activity can be explained by a selective delipidation of HDL2 by HEL converting the HDL2 to a particle with less lipid but with intact apo A-I content and floating in the HDL3 density range. Thus one could not anticipate to find major changes in HDL3 lipid levels along with increasing or decreasing HEL activity.

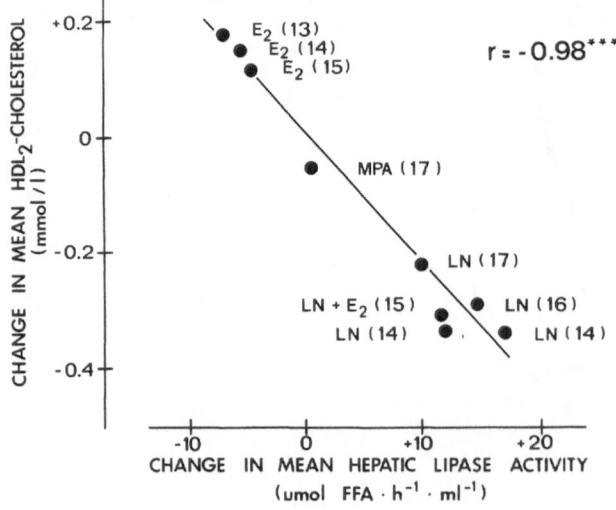

Figure 3. Changes in HDL2 and HEL activity induced by sex steroids. The mean changes in HDL2 and HEL activity are taken from references indicated in parentheses. E2, Estradiol; LN, levo-norgestrel; MPA, medroxy-progesterone acetate

Changes in hepatic endothelial lipase and HDL2 induced by sex steroids

Additional evidence for the function of HEL in HDL metabolism has been obtained from studies where HEL activity is changed without influencing other lipolytic enzymes. Such a situation, widely studied in our laboratory, is the treatment with different steroid hormones (13-17). Estradiol (E2) decreases the postheparin plasma HEL activity and causes an increase in HDL (13) and HDL2 (14,15) cholesterol whereas levonorgestrel (LN), a progestin with androgenic activity, increases postheparin plasma HEL activity and causes an opposite change in HDL2 cholesterol (14-17). On the other hand, medroxyprogesterone acetate (MPA), a progestin with less androgenic activity, does not cause significant changes in either HEL activity or in HDL2 cholesterol (17). None of these hormones influences the LPL or LCAT activities. Fig. 3 summarizes the results of our studies with sex steroids showing the mean changes in HEL activity and HDL2 cholesterol (13-17). It is remarkable that a strikingly linear relationship exists between the changes induced in these two variables by steroid hormones under conditions where no changes occurred in other lipoproteins or lipolytic enzymes. We have therefore suggested that the major effects of steroid hormones on plasma HDL2 cholesterol are mediated by induction or suppression of HEL activity (15).

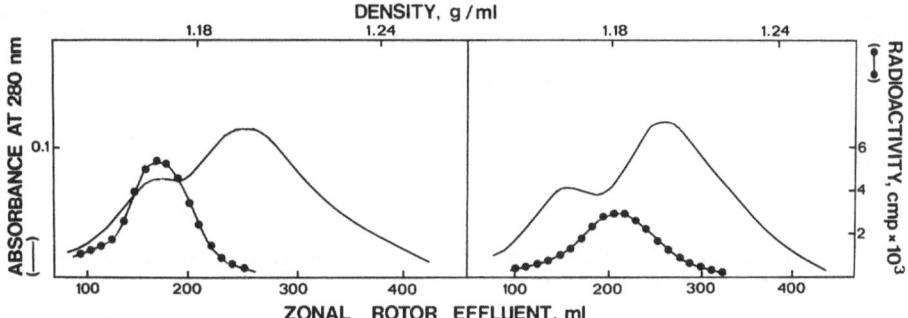

Figure 4. Zonal ultracentrifugation of HDL2 before and after hydrolysis by hepatic lipase. HDL2 (0.25 mg phospholipid) labelled with 1-($^3$H)oleyl-2-palmitoyllecithin was incubated with heat-inactivated (left) or intact (right) HEL in 1% albumin for six hours at +37°C, followed by the addition of total HDL (d 1.063-1.21 g/ml) and zonal ultracentrifugation. Only the HDL profile is shown (albumin was present at d>1.25)

Hydrolysis of HDL2 by hepatic endothelial lipase

The selective hydrolysis of HDL2 phospholipids by HEL has been demonstrated recently (18,19). Thus, HDL2 is the preferred substrate lipoprotein of HEL also in vitro (18). We have also studied the hydrolysis of HDL2 phospholipids by HEL in vitro with particular emphasis on the zonal behaviour of HDL2 after incubation with either heat-inactivated or intact HEL purified from postheparin plasma. Although there were only minor changes in the zonal flotation pattern of normal HDL2 after incubation with HEL (18) the HDL2 taken from subject 2 (in Fig. 1) with 50% decreased HEL activity, had increased density as a consequence of a 20% hydrolysis of phospholipids by HEL (Fig. 4). Thus, HDL2 of a low-HEL person lost enough lipids to change its ultracentrifugal properties upon incubation with purified HEL without any hepatic cholesterol uptake. This indicates that HEL partly regulates the subfraction distribution of HDL

Conclusions: Hepatic endothelial lipase accounts for most phospholipase activity in postheparin plasma, which suggests an important function for the enzyme in lipoprotein phospholipid metabolism. Inactivation of HEL in rats by antiserum increases the phospholipid content of HDL (HDL2) suggesting a role for HEL particularly in the catabolism of HDL2 phospholipids. Human plasma HDL2 is inversely

632

related to postheparin plasma HEL activity. On the other hand, HDL3 apolipoprotein A-I is positively related to HEL activity. These correlations support the idea that HEL degrades HDL2 converting it to HDL3. Alterations induced in postheparin plasma HEL activity by different sex steroid treatments cause reciprocal changes in HDL2. Finally, incubation of HDL2 with purified HEL leads to formation of particles with higher density in zonal ultracentrifugation analysis. These results strongly support the concept that HEL has an important function in the regulation of plasma HDL subfraction distribution and of the plasma levels of HDL2.

REFERENCES
1. Kuusi T, Nikkilä EA, Virtanen I, Kinnunen PKJ (1979) Localization of the heparin releasable lipase in situ in the rat liver. Biochem J 181:245-246
2. Ehnholm C, Shaw W, Greten H, Brown WV (1975) Purification from human plasma a heparin-releasable lipase with activity against triglyceride and phospholipids. J Biol Chem 250:6756-6761
3. Kuusi T, Kinnunen PKJ, Ehnholm C, Nikkilä EA (1979) A simple purification procedure for rat hepatic lipase. FEBS Lett 98:314-318
4. Kuusi T, Nikkilä EA, Taskinen M-R, Somerharju P, Ehnholm C (1981) Hydrolysis of phospholipids, monoglycerides and triglycerides by human postheparin plasma hepatic lipase. Clin Chim Acta in press
5. Kuusi T, Kinnunen PKJ, Nikkilä EA (1979) Hepatic endothelial lipase antiserum influences rat plasma low and high density lipoproteins in vivo. FEBS Lett 104:384-388
6. Jansen H, van Tol A, Hülsmann WC (1980) On the metabolic function of heparin-releasable liver lipase. Biochem Biophys Res Comm 92:53-59
7. Grosser J, Schrecker O, Greten H (1981) Function of hepatic triglyceride lipase in lipoprotein metabolism. J Lipid Res 22:437-442
8. Murase T, Itakura H (1981) Accumulation of intermediate density lipoprotein in plasma after intravenous administration of hepatic triglyceride lipase antibody in rats. Atherosclerosis 39:293-300
9. Kuusi T (1979) Heparin-releasable lipase of rat liver. Purification of the enzyme and studies on its function in lipoprotein metabolism. Thesis, University of Helsinki 1979
10. Suri BS, Targ ME, Robinson DS (1981) The removal of partially metabolized very-low-density lipoproteins by perfused rat liver. Biochem J 196:787-794
11. Kuusi T, Saarinen P, Nikkilä EA (1980) Evidence for the role of hepatic endothelial lipase in the metabolism of plasma high density lipoprotein2 in man. Atherosclerosis 36:589-593
12. Nikkilä EA, Kuusi T, Taskinen M-R (1980) Role of lipoprotein lipase and hepatic endothelial lipase in the metabolism of high density lipoproteins: A novel concept on cholesterol transport in HDL cycle. In: Metabolic risk factors in ischemic CV disease. B. Pernow and L.A. Carlson, eds. Raven Press, New York, pp 205-215
13. Tikkanen MJ, Kuusi T, Vartiainen E, Nikkilä EA (1979) Treatment of postmenopausal hypercholesterolemia with estradiol. Acta Obstet Gynecol Scand Suppl 88: 83-88
14. Tikkanen MJ, Nikkilä EA, Kuusi T, Sipinen S (1982) Effect of female sex hormones on lipoprotein lipids and postheparin plasma lipase activities. Acta Endocrinol 99:630-635
15. Tikkanen MJ, Nikkilä EA, Kuusi T, Sipinen S (1981) Changes in serum high density lipoprotein (HDL2 and HDL3) lipids and lipolytic enzyme activities during estrogen and progestin treatment. J Clin Endocrinol Metab in press
16. Tikkanen MJ, Kuusi T, Nikkilä EA, Sipinen S (1981) Reduction of plasma high-density lipoprotein2 cholesterol and increase of postheparin plasma hepatic lipase activity during progestin treatment. Clin Chim Acta 115:63-71
17. Tikkanen MJ, Nikkilä EA, Kuusi T, Sipinen S (1982) Differential effects of two progestins on plasma high density lipoprotein (HDL2) and postheparin plasma hepatic lipase activity. Atherosclerosis 40:365-369
18. Shirai K, Barnhart RL, Jackson RL (1981) Hydrolysis of human plasma high density lipoprotein2 phospholipids and triglycerides by hepatic lipase. Biochem Biophys Res Comm 100:591-597
19. Groot PHE, Jansen H, van Tol A (1981) Selective degradation of the high density lipoprotein-2 by heparin-releasable liver lipase. FEBS Lett 129:269-273

# Genetic Regulation of Lipoprotein Lipase

M. C. Schotz, O. Ben-Zeev, R. C. LeBoeuf, and A. J. Lusis

We are currently using a biochemical-genetic approach to examine aspects of the nature and regulation of lipoprotein lipase (LPL). This enzyme which hydrolyzes the triglyceride core of chylomicrons and VLDL plays a key role in the formation of circulating low density and high density lipoproteins (1). However, factors controlling its metabolic regulation and its differential expression in various tissues are not well understood. We have chosen the mouse as a model organism, since the utility of the mouse in genetic analysis is well established and hundreds of inbred strains are available. We describe here genetic variations affecting LPL expression in heart and adipose tissues. The results suggest that the enzyme in the two tissues is under independent genetic control.

## Genetic variation

A survey of inbred strains of mice for variations in LPL expression in heart and adipose tissues revealed differences in strains C57BL/6 and BALB/c. The specific activity of LPL in the heart of C57BL/6 was twice that found in BALB/c. On the other hand, the specific activity of LPL in the inguinal adipose of C57BL/6 was about half that noted in BALB/c (Table 1).

## Enzyme structure versus enzyme activity

These genetic variations in LPL specific activities could result from differences in enzyme structure, which could alter the activity per molecule of LPL, or from differences in the number of LPL molecules. We have searched for possible structural variations of the enzyme by comparing the thermal stability and substrate affinity of the enzyme in the two strains.

Thermal stability is probably the most sensitive measure of variations in enzyme structure. It has been estimated that 50-70% of all single amino acid substitutions in an enzyme result in a detectable change in enzyme thermal stability (2). However, detailed comparisons of the kinetics of heat inactivation of LPL revealed no differences in the thermal stability of LPL between the two strains.

The apparent $K_m$ values of heart LPL in C57BL/6 and BALB/c did not differ significantly (2.8 and 2.5 mM triglyceride, respectively). However, a significant difference was observed in the case of adipose LPL, with C57BL/6 exhibiting an apparent $K_m$ of 3.8 mM triglyceride compared with 1.1 mM for BALB/c. This difference in $K_m$ could account for the difference in adipose LPL specific activity observed between the strains. The altered $K_m$ of LPL between the strains presumably reflects a structural variation in either the LPL molecule or in a molecule affecting its catalytic activity. Titration studies using specific antibody would provide more conclusive evidence concerning the nature of these variations.

## Inheritance patterns

$F_1$ progeny derived from crosses between C57BL/6 and BALB/c exhibited specific activities of LPL in heart which were intermediate between the parental values,

634

indicating codominant inheritance. In adipose tissue, on the other hand, the LPL
specific activities and apparent $K_m$ values of $F_1$ progeny resembled more closely
one parent, C57BL/6 (Table 1). This suggests the possibility of dominant/recessive
inheritance.

The segregation patterns of LPL were examined using recombinant inbred (RI) lines
rather than conventional backcross analysis. A recombinant inbred line is constructed by starting with the $F_2$ generation of 2 inbred lines such as C57BL/6
and BALB/c. The animals in each subsequent generation are inbred by brother/sister
mating for at least 20 generations to obtain a set of RI lines. During this process the parental genes become scrambled and new combinations of the parental
genes are fixed in the RI strains. In other words, genes which are initially
homozygous are recombined and finally made homozygous again in the RI lines as a
result of inbreeding. RI lines provide several advantages over conventional backcross analysis for determination of genetic linkage and analysis of complex traits
(3).

Table 1. LPL Specific Activity in Heart and Inguinal Adipose Tissue in Parental
and Recombinant Inbred Strains

| PARENTAL STRAIN | LPL SPECIFIC ACTIVITY (mU/mg PROTEIN) | |
| --- | --- | --- |
| | HEART | ADIPOSE |
| C57BL/6 = B | $13.4 \pm 0.9$ | $5.9 \pm 1.2$ |
| BALB/c = C | $5.7 \pm 1.4$ | $10.6 \pm 2.1$ |
| $F_1$ | $10.2 \pm 1.0$ | $7.2 \pm 1.5$ |
| RI STRAINS | | |
| D | 13.2(B) | 5.6(B) |
| E | 10.4(B) | 6.4(B) |
| G | 7.1(C) | 5.9(B) |
| H | 13.8(B) | 9.8(C) |
| I | 11.6(B) | 4.4(B) |
| J | 7.5(C) | 12.6(C) |
| K | 7.2(C) | 9.4(C) |

Values given are the mean obtained from 5-8 female mice of each strain, C57BL/6By
and BALB/cBy, which were fasted overnight. Standard deviations are given only
for the parental strains. LPL activity was determined (4); one milliunit represents release of one nanomole of free fatty acid per minute. The symbols "B" and
"C" denote values similar to the parental strains, C57BL/6 or BALB/c, respectively.

Table 1 shows the distribution of heart and adipose LPL specific activities among
7 RI strains derived from C57BL/6 (B) and BALB/c (C). Heart and adipose LPL specific activity for each RI strain resembled that of one parent or the other. This
suggests that the LPL specific activities in each tissue are determined by single

major genes. If multiple genes were involved in either variation, new combinations of these genes present in the RI strains would produce nonparental LPL values.

## Independent genetic control of heart and adipose LPL

If the variations in heart and adipose LPL were determined by the same genetic locus, then the RI strains would retain the parental combinations of LPL specific activities (that is, high heart and low adipose activities or low heart and high adipose activities). Although the parental combinations of LPL were observed in 5/7 RI strains, two of the strains (G and H) exhibited recombinant phenotypes. This indicates that the LPL expressed in the two tissues is under the control of separate unlinked genes.

## Prospects

In contrast to the extreme clinical disorders seen in human subjects with genetic deficiencies of LPL or its cofactor apo-C-II, enzyme mutants in the mouse involving relatively small changes in activity could be detected. The characterization of such mutants should yield important information about the genes that are involved in the final expression of LPL, including genes that determine the enzyme's structure, production, localization and degradation. Ultimately, it may be possible to analyze the possible involvement of genetic variation among these genes in diseases such as atherosclerosis.

## Acknowledgements

This study was supported in part by grants from the Veterans Administration Wadsworth Medical Center and NIH HL16577, HL07386, and AM27008.

## References

1. Nilsson-Ehle P, Garfinkel AS, Schotz MC (1980) Lipolytic Enzymes and Plasma Lipoprotein Metabolism. Ann. Rev Biochem 49: 667-693
2. Paigen K (1971) The Genetics of Enzyme Realization. In: Rechcigl M Jr (ed), Enzyme Synthesis and Degradation in Mammalian Systems, University Park Press, Karger, Basel, pp 1-44
3. Taylor BA (1978) Recombinant Inbred Strains:Use in Gene Mapping. In: Morse HC (ed), Origins of Inbred Mice, Academic Press, New York, pp 423-438
4. Nilsson-Ehle P, Schotz MC (1976) A Stable Radioactive Substrate Emulsion for Assay of Lipoprotein Lipase. J. Lipid Res. 17: 536-541

# Lipoprotein Lipase: Apolipoprotein C-II Interactions Studied by Fluorescence and Monoclonal Antibodies

L. C. Smith, J. C. Voyta, M. F. Rohde, P. K. J. Kinnunen, A. M. Gotto, Jr., and J. T. Sparrow

## A. Introduction

Lipoprotein lipase is a triglyceride hydrolase present on the capillary endothelium. This enzymatic hydrolytic process is the key event for removal of triglyceride in chylomicrons and very low density lipoproteins (VLDL). The chylomicrons and VLDL are too large to penetrate the openings of the vascular and endothelium for direct access to the cells, except for arterial macrophages (1), which synthesize and secrete lipoprotein lipase. Apolipoprotein C-II (apoC-II), a 78 amino acid protein found in chylomicrons, VLDL and high density lipoproteins (HDL) is metabolically important as the activator for lipoprotein lipase. The precise molecular mechanism by which apoC-II enhances triglyceride hydrolysis by the enzyme is not yet known. Previous work from this laboratory (2, 3) with synthetic fragments of apoC-II has shown that only the carboxyl third of the activator is required for enhancement of triglyceride by lipoprotein lipase.

ApoC-II, like other apolipoproteins, undergoes changes in secondary protein structure when combined with phosphatidylcholine (4). The circular dichroic spectrum and the blue-shifted tryptophan fluorescence spectrum are consistent with extensive $\alpha$-helix content as an amphipathic structure, oriented at the lipid-water interface (5). In this putative structure, the bipolar regions of apoC-II have the nonpolar amino acid side chains which interdigitate with the lipid molecules of the surface film and the neutral core of the lipoprotein. The charged, polar amino acid side chains contribute to the structured aqueous interface through hydrogen bonding with water molecules. Since lipoprotein lipase also can undergo hydrophobic association with phospholipids (6), as indicated by blue-shifted tryptophan fluorescence and flotation of the enzyme with VLDL (7), it seems probable that the interaction of the enzyme with the apoprotein activator involves extensive lateral protein:protein interactions.

Initial support for the importance of apoprotein:enzyme association has been obtained with monomolecular surface films of apoC-II (8). In the absence of lipid, apoC-II forms a stable surface film with a conformation that is biologically active, as shown by the ability of the isolated apoprotein surface film to activate lipoprotein lipase. When apoC-II and lipoprotein lipase are allowed to interact in the absence of lipid, a stable apoprotein:enzyme forms at the interface. This surface film complex can be isolated by physical transfer from one subphase to another. To study this interaction in the presence of a substrate structure which is more closely related to the physiological substrates and to eliminate the possibility that apoC-II acts only by restructuring the substrate interface to enhance lipoprotein lipase binding without a direct apoprotein:enzyme interaction, we have prepared apoC-II fragments which contain the fluorescent dimethylaminonaphthylsulfonyl (DNS) group only on the amino terminal residue. Since these synthetic peptides have no tryptophan residues, it is possible to monitor interaction between the activator and the enzyme by resonance energy transfer (9) from the tryptophan groups of the enzyme to the dansyl peptide if the interaction distance is less than 5 nm. The affinity of the activator and the enzyme can be readily determined both in the presence and absence of a lipid-water interface. The ability of monoclonal antibodies against lipoprotein lipase to disrupt with the interaction of the fluorescent peptide with the enzyme was also studied as an independent index of the nature of the role of apoC-II.

637

## B. Materials and Methods

Bovine milk lipoprotein lipase was purified by the method of Kinnunen (10). Synthetic apoC-II peptides were made was described previously (2, 11) except that the DNS group was incorporated on the amino terminal by acylation of the amino terminal group before peptide cleavage from the solid phase support. Homogenous peptides were obtained by reversed phase chromatography (12). The phospholipid vesicles, which contained the nonhydrolyzable lipid ethers, β-0-hexydecyl-γ-0-octadec-9-enyl-DL-lecithin,trioctadec-9-enylglyceryl ether and cholesterol in molar ratios of 1:0.02:0.05, were prepared by the method of Batzri and Korn (13). The solvent was removed by centrifugation through buffer-depleted Sephadex G-50 columns (14). The relative increase in fluorescence of 490 nm upon excitation at 280 nm, with or without vesicles, was measured on a SLM Model 400 proton counting spectrofluorimeter. Equations for the calculation of $K_a$ value are given elsewhere (15). Data was examined by analysis of the following equation:

$$F = \frac{K_a\ ([P_t] - F[E_t])}{1 + K_a([P_t] - F[E_t])}$$

where F is the ratio of the enzyme:peptide complex divided by the total enzyme concentration and is equivalent to the value of the relative fluorescence of 490 nm at each experimental peptide concentration constant, $P_t$ is the total peptide concentration, $E_t$ is the total enzyme concentration. Values for $K_a$ were obtained by a nonlinear squares fit of equation 1.

Monoclonal antibodies (16) against bovine milk lipoprotein lipase were generated by fusing spleen cells from immunized BALB/c mice with two myeloma cell lines, P3X63AG8.653 and S194/5.XX0.BU.1. Ten cell lines producing antibodies were established, five from each myeloma. The hybridoma lines were used to prepare murine ascites fluid. The monoclonal antibodies were fractionated by ammonium sulfate precipitation. A cyanogen bromide digest of lipoprotein lipase was subjected to analytical SDS gel electrophoresis for an electrophoretic blot onto nitrocellulose, on which fragments were visualized by monoclonal antibodies (17).

## C. Results

The presence of the dansyl group on the amino terminal fragment had little effect on the ability of synthetic peptide to activate lipoprotein lipase. The magnitude of the activation of modified peptides was essentially the same as that produced by the respective unmodified apoC-II fragments (18). To avoid changes in surface composition and properties produced by enzymatic hydrolysis of lipids during binding experiments, vesicles containing non-hydrolyzable lipids were used. It was established in separate experiments that substitution of ether-containing phosphatidylcholine had no effect on trioleylglycerol hydrolysis (19). Both DNS-apoC-II peptides and lipoprotein lipase bound to the vesicles independently . There was an incremental increase in the $K_a$ values for enzyme:activator association with increasing peptide chain length (Table 1).

| Peptide | Association Constant No Lipid | With Vesicles | Relative Activation of Lipoprotein Lipase |
|---|---|---|---|
| ApoC-II-DNS(64-78) | $0.04 \times 10^6\ M^{-1}$ | $0.4 \times 10^6\ M^{-1}$ | 0 |
| ApoC-II-DNS(60-78) | $0.3 \times 10^6\ M^{-1}$ | $0.8 \times 10^6\ M^{-1}$ | 60% |
| ApoC-II-DNS(55-78) | $0.3 \times 10^6\ M^{-1}$ | $1.2 \times 10^6\ M^{-1}$ | 80% |
| ApoC-II-DNS(50-78) | $0.3 \times 10^6\ M^{-1}$ | n.d. | n.d. |
| ApoC-II-DNS(43-78) | $0.5 \times 10^6\ M^{-1}$ | $22.0 \times 10^6\ M^{-1}$ | 100% |

638

The values for the association constant increased about an order of magnitude between apoC-II-DNS(55-78) and apoC-II-DNS(43-78). By contrast, in the absence of lipid, the interaction of the apoC-II-DNS peptides with lipoprotein lipase had no chain length dependence after a 10-fold increase in $K_a$ when apoC-II-DNS(64-78) was extended by 4 amino acids. Competitive displacement of apoC-II-DNS(55-78) by apoC-II(55-78) and the lack of energy transfer from DNS peptides to unrelated proteins such as albumin demonstrated the specificity for the interaction.

Three of the four monoclonal antibodies tested disrupted the interaction between apoC-II-DNS(60-78) and lipoprotein lipase, as judged by the decrease in DNS fluorescence polarization. Monoclonal antibodies which disrupted the interaction also recognized 17,000 molecular weight CNBr fragment of lipoprotein lipase as determined by electrophoretic transfer analysis, suggesting the apoC-II recognition site occurs on this part of lipoprotein lipase.

D. Discussion

The demonstration of the interaction of apoC-II-DNS peptides in a 1:1 stoichiometry with lipoprotein lipase and the results with monoclonal antibodies to lipoprotein lipase reinforce our previous suggestions that the activation of lipoprotein lipase involves specific protein:protein interaction involving the carboxyl terminal third of apoC-II. This same chain length dependence of both energy transfer between the enzyme and the DNS peptide at the lipid-water interface and of the peptide activation of the lipoprotein lipase catalysis strongly supports this view. The 10-fold increase, in the absence of lipid, of the affinity of the activator peptide with the enzyme when residues 60-64 are included emphasizes the importance of this sequence region of apoC-II. The loss in the ability to activate when other amino acids were substituted for Tyr$_{62}$ in apoC-II(55-78) had clearly identified the role of this putative β-turn in the mechanism of activation (3). It does not seem possible to reconcile these results with a mechanism of activation whereby the activator peptide only produces an alteration of the substrate interface without a direct interaction with the enzyme.

The hypertriglyceridemia produced by the familial absence of apoC-II (20) clearly demonstrates the physiological importance of the activator. The spectroscopic demonstration of protein:protein association indicates that an understanding of the control of lipoprotein lipase by apoC-II most likely require physiochemical studies of the activator:enzyme complex. Whether or not apoC-II facilitates the kinetics of phospholipid binding by lipoprotein lipase remains for future study.

The present results were obtained by spectroscopic methods in a well-defined system. It is a direct measure of the strength of interaction of lipoprotein lipase and apoC-II. The values calculated for the association constant for the apoC-II-(DNS) peptide: lipoprotein lipase complex in the presence of phospholipid vesicles are about the same as those obtained by analysis of kinetic data (21) but are lower by orders or magnitudes than other reported values (22, 23). The $K_a$ for the activator:enzyme interaction deduced from kinetic measurements involves additional assumptions about the rates of catalysis and of product release, which may account for the different reported values.

E. Summary

The molecular mechanism by which apoC-II enhances lipoprotein lipase catalysis of triglycerides is unknown but involves direct protein:protein interactions.

F. Acknowledgements

Support for this work was provided by Welch Q-343, HHD grants HL-15648, HL-27341, HL-17269, EPA R80-8773, and the Paulo Foundation, Helsinki, Finland.

## G.  References

1.  Taylor K, Elner V, Kluskens L, Zarins CK, Glasgov S (1981)  Mononuclear phago-cytes in foam cell lesions and in the artery wall of normal animals.  Arterio-sclerosis 1:  357a
2.  Kinnunen PKJ, Jackson RL, Smith LC, Gotto AM, Sparrow JT (1977)  Activation of lipoprotein lipase by native and synthetic fragments of human plasma.  Proc Natl Acad Sci USA  74:  4848-4851
3.  Smith LC, Voyta JC, Catapano AL, Kinnunen PKJ, Gotto AM, Sparrow JT (1980)  Activation of lipoprotein lipase by synthetic fragments of apolipoprotein C-II.  Ann NY Acad Sci  348:  213-221
4.  Morrisett JD, Jackson RL, Gotto AM (1977)  Lipid-protein interactions in the plasma lipoproteins.  Biochim Biophys Acta  472:  93-133
5.  Segrest JP, Morrisett JD, Jackson RL, Gotto AM (1974)  A molecular theory of lipid-protein interactions in the plasma lipoproteins.  FEBS Lett 38:  247-253
6.  Voyta JC, Kinnunen PKJ, Smith LC - unpublished experiments
7.  Fielding CJ, Fielding PE (1976)  Mechanism of salt-mediated inhibition of lipo-protein lipase.  J Lipid Res  17:  248-256
8.  Miller AL, Smith LC (1973)  Activation of lipoprotein lipase by apolipoprotein glutamic acid.  J Biol Chem  248:  3359-3362
9.  Stryer L (1978)  Fluorescence energy transfer as a spectroscopic ruler.  Ann Rev Biochem  47:  819-846
10.  Kinnunen PKJ (1977)  Purification off bovine lipoprotein lipase with the aid of detergent.  Med Biol  55:  187-191
11.  Edelstein MS, McNair DS, Sparrow JT (1981)  The conversion of solid phase pep-tide synthesizers to computer control.  In:  Rich DH, Gross E (eds) Peptides: Synthesis - Structure - Function, Proceedings of the Seventh American Peptide Symposium, Rockford, IL, pp 217-220
12.  Hancock WS, Capra JD, Bradley WA, Sparrow JT (1981)  The use of reversed-phase high-performance liquid chromatography with radial compression for the analysis of peptide and protein mixtures.  J Chrom  206:  59-70
13.  Batzri S, Korn ED (1973)  Single bilayer liposomes prepared without sonication.  Biochem Biophys Acta  298:  1015-1019
14.  Fry DW, White JC, Goldman ID (1978)  Rapid separation of low molecular weight solutes without dilution.  Anal Biochem  90:  809-815
15.  Voyta JC, Wainio P, Kinnunen PKJ, Gotto AM, Sparrow JT, Smith LC (1982)  Lipo-protein lipase interaction with synthetic N-dansyl-apolipoprotein C-II peptides.  Submitted for publication
16.  Kohler G, Milstein C (1975)  Continuous cultures of fused cells secreting anti-body of predefined specificity.  Nature  256:  495-497
17.  Towbin H, Stachelin T, Gordon J (1979)  Electrophoretic transfer of proteins from polyacrylamide gels to nitrocellulose sheets:  Procedure and some applica-tions.  Proc Natl Acad Sci USA  76:  4350-4354
18.  Catapano AL, Kinnunen PKJ, Breckenridge WC, Gotto AM, Jackson RL, Little JA, Smith LC, Sparrow JT (1979)  Lipolysis of apoC-II deficient very low density lipoproteins:  Enhancement of lipoprotein lipase action by synthetic fragments of apoC-II.  Biochem Biophys Res Commun  89:  951-957
19.  Jacobs GW, Charlton SC, Catapano AL, Hoff HF, Smith LC (1982)  Model plasma lipoproteins:  A stable reproducible triglyceride-rich microemulsion, a protein-free model of very low density lipoproteins.  Submitted for publication
20.  Breckenridge WC, Little A, Steiner G, Chow A, Poapst M (1978)  Hypertriglyceri-demia association with deficiency of apolipoprotein C-II.  New Engl J Med  298: 1265-1273
21.  Bengston G, Olivecrona T (1979)  Apolipoprotein C-II enhances hydrolysis of monoglycerides by lipoprotein lipase, but the effects is abolished by fatty acids.  FEBS Lett  106:  345-348
22.  Chung J, Scanu AM (1973)  Isolation, molecular properties, and kinetic charac-terization of lipoprotein lipase from rat heart.  J Biol Chem  252:  4202-4209
23.  Fielding CJ, Fielding PE (1977)  The activation of lipoprotein lipase by lipase co-protein (apoC-2).  In:  Polonovski J (ed) Cholesterol and Lipolytic Enzymes, Masson Publishing Co, NY, NY, pp 165-172

# 4 Thrombosis

# Arachidonic Acid Metabolism in Human Platelets

A. J. Marcus

## Introduction

Arachidonic acid (20:4) is classified as "essential" for human nutrition since long-term ingestion of a diet deficient in this compound
results in a disease entity (1).  In mammals, arachidonate is either
obtained from the diet or  synthesized from another essential fatty
acid, linoleic (18:2) by the process of chain elongation and desatura-
tion.  We first described the presence of 20:4 in human platelets in
1962 (2).

Arachidonic acid is the most important precursor of stable prostaglandins ($PGE_2$, $PGF_{2\alpha}$), thromboxane $A_2$ ($TXA_2$), prostacyclin ($PGI_2$)
and hydroxy acids-which include new compounds in leukocytes of great
interest--the leukotrienes.  In general, the metabolites formed from
arachidonic acid can be classified as lipid autacoids because they act
locally in tissues and in proximate surrounding structures.  In addition,
the effects of prostanoids are usually transient and they are synthesized mainly in response to cell perturbation.  This is in contrast
to the actions of hormones which are usually synthesized in different
locations than the target tissues which they set into motion.  An arachidonic  acid metabolite may exert a stimulatory effect on one tissue
and inhibit another.  This effect may be a reflection of the interaction
of the metabolite with cellular adenylate cyclase or the presence of a
specific receptor for a given eicosanoid on the cell.

The pharmacologic approach to inhibition or stimulation of arachidonic
acid transformation is currently an important facet of basic and applied
research.  It involves such medical specialties as reproductive physiology, gastro-intestinal mobility and secretion, cardiovascular and renal
function, rheumatology, modulation of the inflammatory response and inhibition of platelet adhesion, aggregation and release.

Research in arachidonic acid metabolism has passed through three phases:
a)  a clinical observation made 50 years ago by a gynecologist, b) several decades of basic biochemical research involving chemical characterization and synthesis of arachidonic acid metabolites and c) attempts
to correlate biological effects of eicosanoids with the pathogenesis of
several unexplained disease states.  Inhibition or stimulation of the
formation of arachidonic acid derivatives may eventually be important
in the prevention and treatment of disabling diseases such as peptic
ulcer, hypertension, renal failure, asthma, psoriasis, congenital heart
disease and thrombosis (3,4).

## Mobilization of Arachidonic Acid in Platelets

In 1969 we reported that there was very little free arachidonic acid in platelets (5). It thus follows that synthesis of eicosanoids requires release of esterified 20:4 which is present mainly in the platelet phospholipid fraction. Release of 20:4 from platelet phospholipids is a calcium-dependent step and occurs via mechanical or appropriate biochemical perturbation of the platelet surface. Availability of free 20:4 results in activation of platelet cyclooxygenase and lipoxygenase. This can be demonstrated in vitro by adding arachidonate exogenously to a platelet suspension. Such addition will be followed by synthesis of thromboxane A$_2$ and hydroxy acids within seconds, and the platelets will aggregate.

Platelet phosphatidyl inositol (PI) contains an abundance of 20:4 (5) and is probably a major source of this fatty acid for thromboxane and hydroxy acid synthesis. Thus, stimulation of platelets with thrombin results in transient accumulation of diglyceride catalyzed by the action of a phospholipase C which is specific for phosphatidyl inositol (6,7). Cleavage of the arachidonate from diglyceride by a diacylglycerol lipase has been demonstrated in platelets (6). Studies by Broekman et al in our laboratory (8,9) have demonstrated an increase in platelet lysophosphatidylethanolamine upon stimulation. Broekman and colleagues have also shown that most of the free fatty acids such as arachidonate liberated several seconds following platelet stimulation are probably derived from phospholipids other than PI (9). Billah and Lapetina (10) have recently provided additional information concerning release of arachidonate upon platelet stimulation. They demonstrated, with the use of a modified, acidic extraction procedure, the presence of lyso PI, the formation of which is catalyzed by a phospholipase A$_2$. They maintain that platelet PI is also degraded by a phospholipase C. This phospholipase C degrades PI to a 1,2-diacylglycerol which then becomes phosphorylated to phosphatidic acid.

Research on the phospholipase step in liberation of free 20:4 is important since inhibition of this enzyme may result in pharmacologic control of the arachidonic acid pathway in the modulation of thrombosis and possibly atherosclerosis. Figure 1. depicts the derivatization of arachidonic acid in platelets and endothelial cells as currently understood.

## The Cyclooxygenase Reaction

As already mentioned platelet cyclooxygenase is a substrate-activated enzyme. Cyclization and oxygenation of 20:4 requires 1 heme molecule for 2 subunits of enzyme, molecular oxygen, a hydroperoxide activator and free arachidonate. The first product formed from 20:4 and oxygen is PGG$_2$ which is a 15-hydroperoxy endoperoxide. However, the cyclooxygenase enzyme also possesses peroxidase activity and therefore the 15-hydroxy derivative, PGH$_2$ rapidly forms. Our knowledge of this series of reactions is based mainly on the pioneering studies of Samuelsson (11).

The requirement for molecular oxygen by cyclooxygenase is a step which can be measured in the laboratory. Stimulation of platelets by thrombin, collagen or arachidonic acid is followed by an abrupt, transient

increase in oxygen consumption which can be correlated at the onset
of the platelet aggregation response (12). This "burst" of oxygen
consumption does not occur if the platelet donor has recently ingested
acetyl salycylic acid (ASA). Platelet cyclooxygenase is irreversibly
inactivated by ASA and no recovery from this step is possible since
platelets cannot synthesize protein. Inhibition of cyclooxygenase
activity by non-steroidal anti-inflammatory agents--especially ASA is
a very important aspect of arachidonic acid research.

Platelet Lipoxygenase

In addition to cyclooxygenase,which is particulate, platelets contain a
soluble cytoplasmic enzyme which catalyzes conversion of arachidonate
to 12-hydroperoxy-eicosatetraenoic acid (12-HPETE) and this is followed
by formation of 12-hydroxy-eicosatetraenoic acid (12-HETE). 12-HPETE is
unstable and therefore has been difficult to evaluate in vitro as an
agonist or chemotactic agent. 12-HETE is stable and may have less biological activity than 12-HPETE. The precise function of these platelet
lipoxygenase products is unknown although they are chemotactic for polymorphonuclear leukocytes.

It is rather unfortunate that functional pa rameters of platelet lipoxygenase products have not as yet been clarified. This is because following aspirin ingestion platelet 12-HETE production increases. In fact,
so long as free 20:4 is available, platelet lipoxygenase will continue to
catalyze formation of 12-HETE. It is of interest that in leukocytes,
the lipoxygenase catalyzes formation of 5-hydroperoxy-eicosatetraenoic
acid. 5-HPETE is the precursor of leukotrienes.

Role of the 20:4 Pathway in Platelet Aggregation and Secretion

Addition of a stimulus such as thrombin to platelets results in an immediate shape change and aggregation response. The initial wave of
aggregation is followed by a second phase which is irreversible and
induced mainly by secretion of adenosine diphosphate (ADP) from intracellular platelet granules. The latter reactions are termed "platelet
release".

Thromboxane $A_2$ synthesis is involved in the reactions described above.
Addition of thrombin results in activation of phospholipases C and $A_2$
which renders free 20:4 available for cyclooxygenation and lipoxygena-
tion. Endoperoxides and thromboxane form as do hydroxy acids but the
latter probably do not play a direct role in the aggregation response.
Thromboxane $A_2$ causes calcium mobilization which in turn induces ADP
release from the platelet. $TXA_2$ also inhibits adenylate cyclase which
results in a fall in cyclic AMP levels. Released ADP then induces aggregation of other platelets arriving at the site (platelet recruitment). Thromboxane $A_2$ itself is also released from the platelet and
this also serves to "recruit" additional platelets into the aggregate
(4,13).

646

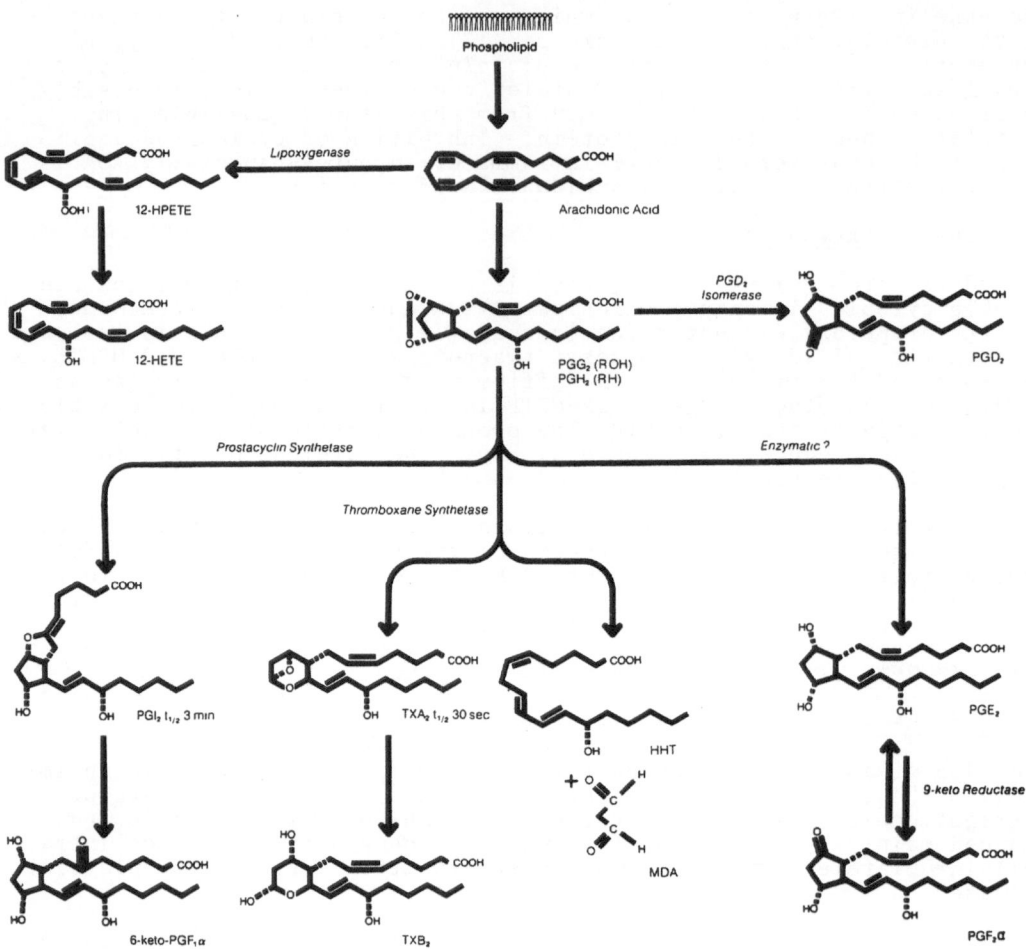

Figure 1. Composite diagram of arachidonic acid metabolism in platelets and endothelial cells. The essential fatty acid, arachidonate, is important in the regulation of platelet,endothelial cell and leukocyte function. The enzymic transformation of arachidonic acid in platelets, endothelial cells and leukocytes is a response to cell stimulation or perturbation. Arachidonic acid is released from cell phospholipid by the action of phospholipases which are currently under study in various laboratories. The precise subcellular localization of the phospholipid

donor for arachidonate is not known. Aspirin or indomethacin will inhibit cyclization of arachidonate. All products of the cyclooxygenase pathway must pass through the endoperoxide stage. The endproducts are qualitatively and quantitatively different in each tissue in which they are formed, depending upon which enzymes are present for further processing the endoperoxides. The endothelial cell transforms endoperoxides to $PGI_2$ whereas the platelets process endoperoxides to $TXA_2$. Endothelial cells can also utilize platelet endoperoxides for the formation of $PGI_2$. Recently products of the lipoxygenase pathway have assumed new importance--mainly because of the elucidation of the structure and function of leukotrienes (not shown). The lipoxygenase pathway in platelets continues to function in the setting of aspirin or indomethacin inhibition of the cyclooxygenase. This may have important but as yet unknown implications.

## Classification of Platelet Stimuli

We find it useful to think of platelet stimuli in terms of their capacity to induce an "oxygen burst", aggregation response, serotonin (5-HT) release and $TXA_2$ synthesis. These responses probably all reflect the ability of the stimulus to mobilize intracellular platelet calcium. This classification approach can be amplified to a broad spectrum of platelet agonists and has been conceptualized as the "basic platelet reaction" by Holmsen (14).

ADP elicits a strong biphasic aggregation response in platelet-rich plasma (PRP) but 5-HT release averages 30% and a burst of oxygen consumption as we measure it is not detectable (12). AGEPC (also known as PAF--Platelet-Activating-Factor) in our experience is similar to ADP in its effects on human PRP (15); thus, AGEPC induces 5-HT release in the vicinity of 30% although a strong biphasic aggregation response occurs. AGEPC does not produce a burst of oxygen consumption in human PRP. Addition of collagen to PRP results in a strong aggregation response which is accompanied by 60% 5-HT release. Furthermore, collagen promotes a burst of oxygen consumption and thromboxane production in human PRP.

The work in the Author's laboratory was supported by grants from the Veterans Administration, the National Institutes of Health (HL 18828-07 SCOR, RR 05396), the New York Heart Association, and the A.R. Krakower Foundation.

## References

1. Burr GO, Burr MM(1929) A new deficiency disease produced by the rigid exclusion of fat from the diet. J. Biol. Chem. 82:345-367
2. Marcus AJ, Ullman HL, Safier LB, Ballard HS (1962) Platelet phosphatides: their fatty acid and aldehyde composition and activity in different clotting systems. J. Clin Invest. 41: 2198-2212
3. Marcus AJ (1979) The role of prostaglandins in platelet function. In: Brown EB (ed) Progress in Hematology, vol 11,Grune and Stratton, New York, pp.147-171
4. Gorman RR, Marcus AJ (1981) Prostaglandins and cardiovascular disease. Current Concepts--A Scope Publication, Upjohn Company, Kalamazoo, Michigan
5. Marcus AJ, Ullman HL, Safier LB (1969) Lipid Composition of subcellular particles of human blood platelets. J. Lipid Res. 10:108-114
6. Bell RL, Kennerly DA, Stanford N, Majerus PW (1979) Diglyceride lipase: a pathway for arachidonate release from human platelets.

Proc. Natl. Acad. Sci. U.S.A.  76:3238-3241

7. Rittenhouse-Simmons S  (1979) Production of diglyceride from phosphatidylinositol in activated human platelets. J. Clin. Invest. 63: 580-587

8. Broekman MJ, Ward JW, Marcus AJ (1980) Phospholipid metabolism in stimulated human platelets.  Changes in phosphatidylinositol, phosphatidic acid, and lysophospholipids. J. Clin. Invest. 66: 275-283

9. Broekman MJ, Ward JW, Marcus AJ (1981) Fatty acid composition of phosphatidylinositol and phosphatidic acid in stimulated platelets: persistence of arachidonyl-stearyl structure. J. Biol. Chem. 256: 8271-8274

10. Billah MM, Lapetina EG (1982) Formation of lysophosphatidylinositol in platelets stimulated with thrombin or ionophore A23187. J. Biol. Chem. 257:5196-5200

11. Samuelsson B (1965) On the incorporation of oxygen in the conversion of 8,11,14-eicosatrienoic acid to prostaglandin $E_1$. J. Amer. Chemical Soc. 87: 3011-3013

12. Bressler NM, Broekman MJ, Marcus AJ (1979) Concurrent studies of oxygen consumption and aggregation in stimulated human platelets. Blood 53: 167-178

13. Marcus AJ (1982) Platelet aggregation. In: Colman RW, Hirsh J, Marder VJ, Salzman EW (eds) Hemostasis and Thrombosis: Basic Principles and Clinical Practice, J.B. Lippincott, Philadelphia,PA, pp. 380-389

14. Holmsen H (1982) Biochemistry of the platelet:  energy metabolism. In:  Colman RW, Hirsh J, Marder VJ, Salzman EW (eds) Hemostasis and Thrombosis:  Basic Principles and Clinical Practice, J.B. Lippincott, Philadelphia, PA, pp. 431-443

15. Marcus AJ, Safier LB, Ullman HL, Wong KTH, Broekman MJ, Weksler BB, Kaplan KL (1981)  Effects of acetyl glyceryl ether phosphorylcholine on human platelet function in vitro. Blood 58:1027-1031

# Factors Influencing the Growth, Stability and Fate of Arterial Thrombi

H. R. Baumgartner, H. Kuhn, and T. B. Tschopp

Arterial thrombi grow in the presence of flowing blood. As they grow, the shear forces which tend to remove them also increase, at least as long as the circulating blood volume and vessel diameter remain unchanged. Thus whether an artery eventually occludes or how large a thrombus grows before it breaks off and embolizes into the microvasculature, depends on thrombus stability. The growth of thrombi and the rate of their embolisation has been studied by several investigators in the microvasculature in vivo (Begent and Born, 1970; Arfors et al 1976). Thrombogenesis in larger arteries is difficult to study in vivo under controlled conditions, since the artery wall is not translucent and optical observation not possible. We therefore developed in vitro and ex vivo perfusion systems (Baumgartner 1973, Baumgartner et al 1980c) which mimic the sequence of events observed in vivo and allow to study thrombogenesis under well controlled flow conditions. In this assay our results obtained in collaboration with other laboratories are summarized with regard to thrombus growth and thrombus stability under conditions of arterial blood flow.

## METHODS

Perfusion of citrated blood in vitro. Blood anticoagulated with 15-20 mM sodium citrate is recirculated at 37°C by a pump from a reservoir through an annular chamber on whose core the subendothelial surface of rabbit aorta is exposed to the flowing blood back into the reservoir (Baumgartner and Muggli 1976).

Perfusion of native blood ex vivo. In human volunteers and patients (Baumgartner 1976, Weiss et al 1978) blood is directly sampled from an antecubital vein through the annular chamber at a preselected flow rate by a pump. In rabbits (Baumgartner 1979) blood is recirculated from a carotid artery through the annular chamber into a jugular vein. Blood flow is kept constant at a preselected flow rate by a peristaltic pump between chamber and jugular vein.

Estimation of thrombus growth. Two different approaches are used:

1. Morphometry of thrombi in 0.8 μm thick cross sections of the exposed rabbit aorta after standardized fixation. The two most important parameters are the cross sectional thrombus area per surface length and the maximum thrombus height (average of the three tallest thrombi in a cross section). The former corresponds to the total thrombus mass (volume) per surface area (Baumgartner et al 1980c) and correlates excellently with the number of $^{51}$Cr labelled platelets deposited per

surface area (Tschopp 1977).

2. The <u>pressure difference</u> which develops between the entrance and the exit of the chamber was more recently established for monitoring the obstruction of the chamber by growing thrombi. Our results show that this pressure difference is a more sensitive parameter than the reduction of blood flow in our ex vivo perfusion set up in rabbits (Baumgartner and Kuhn in preparation).

## RESULTS AND DISCUSSION

### Thrombus growth
The most important factors influencing thrombus growth include blood flow and wall shear rate; the functional state of platelets, the clotting system and possibly leucocytes, vessel wall thrombogenicity and vessel wall thromboresistance. Results obtained by modifying platelets and plasma coagulation shall not be discussed here.

### 1. Blood flow (wall shear rate)
Two independent mechanisms control the <u>adhesion of platelets</u> to the vessel wall and also affect subsequent thrombus formation. Firstly, platelets must get from the blood to the vicinity of the vessel wall (platelet transport). Secondly, platelets which arrive at the vessel wall must react and bind to the vessel wall (platelet reaction). Rheological considerations and experimental evidence indicate that the rate of platelet adhesion is dependent on blood flow, more precisely on the wall shear rate (Baumgartner 1973, Turitto et al 1979b). The wall shear rate is proportional to the ratio of blood flow velocity to vessel diameter. It is thus highest in arterioles or stenosed arteries and lowest in large veins (Turitto and Baumgartner 1982). Perfusion experi-

Table 1.

Shear rate dependence of thrombus growth

| Blood flow rate ml/min | Shear rate $s^{-1}$ | n | Citrated blood Thrombus area $\mu m^2/\mu m$ | Max.thrombus height $\mu m$ | n | Native blood Thrombus area $\mu m^2/\mu m$ | Max.thrombus height $\mu m$ |
|---|---|---|---|---|---|---|---|
| 5 | 325 | | n.d. | n.d. | 7 | 1.3±0.6 | 42±14 |
| 10 | 650 | 13 | 0.6±0.1 | 12± 1 | 12 | 2.1±0.5 | 53± 7 |
| 20 | 1300 | 5 | 1.5±0.6 | 29± 8 | 14 | 11 ±2 | 90±14 |
| 40 | 2600 | 5 | 3.4±0.7 | 46± 7 | 13 | 17 ±3 | 137±18 |
| 160 | 10000 | 6 | 9.6±3.7 | 70±12 | | n.d. | n.d. |

Values are means ± SE

Thrombus area per subendothelial surface length and maximal thrombus heights were determined morphometrically after 3 min exposure time of subendothelium to flowing rabbit blood in vitro and ex vivo.

Table 2.

Shear rate dependence of chamber obstruction

| Blood flow rate ml/min | Shear rate $s^{-1}$ | n | 15 min perfusion time | |
|---|---|---|---|---|
| | | | pressure difference between chamber entrance and exit mm Hg | decrease in flow rate % |
| 5 | 325 | 6 | 44± 9* | 0 |
| 10 | 650 | 6 | 60± 9 | 3 |
| 20 | 1300 | 6 | 187±21 | 10 |
| 40 | 2600 | 11 | 273±22 | 18 |

* mean ± SE

Native rabbit blood was perfused through an annular chamber at the flow rates indicated. The blood was recirculated from a carotid artery through the chamber and a roller pump back into a jugular vein. Subendothelium of a 2 cm long segment of rabbit aorta was exposed on the rod of the chamber to the flowing blood. Blood pressure was monitored at the entrance and the exit of the chamber, flow at the exit.

ments using rabbit and human blood established that the rate of platelet adhesion to subendothelium is proportional to the wall shear rate, up to about 1000 $s^{-1}$. At higher shear rates no further increase in adhesion was observed (Turitto and Baumgartner 1979, Turitto et al 1980). These experimental observations are in agreement with rheological considerations indicating that platelet adhesion is predominantly transport controlled at low shear and reaction controlled at higher shear rates (Turitto et al 1979b). This is consistent with the fact that platelet adhesion defects are more readily apparent at high than at low shear rates (Weiss et al 1978, Baumgartner et al 1980b).

For thrombus growth the situation is far more complex from a theoretical point of view since thrombi themselves change the flow pattern and may create turbulent flow in their vicinity. However, experimental evidence clearly demonstrates that the thrombus growth rate also increases with the shear rate (Table 1). Unlike the rate of platelet adhesion which levels off at a shear rate of about 1000 $s^{-1}$ in citrated blood, the thrombus growth rate continues to increase up to unphysiological high shear rates of 10000 $sec^{-1}$ even with citrated blood (Table 1). At present we have no explanation for this phenomenon and postulate that thrombi which grow rapidly must be more stable than those growing slowly (see below).

The results presented in table 1 are based on morphometric measurements. Recent experiments demonstrated that the development of thrombi on subendothelium in our annular chamber can also be monitored by measuring blood pressure at the entrance and the exit of the chamber (Baumgartner and Kuhn in preparation). The pressure at the entrance of the chamber corresponds to the arterial blood pressure of the rabbit and usually remains constant throughout an ex vivo perfusion experiment.

The pressure at the exit of the chamber decreases to negative values with perfusion time. The pressure difference between entrance and exit correlates with the morphometrically measured thrombus volume attached to the subendothelial surface. Table 2 shows that the pressure difference which developed within 15 min perfusion of native blood is much greater at high than at low flow rate indicating that the chamber occludes more rapidly at high than at low shear rate. Results obtained by measuring a pressure difference after 15 min perfusion (Table 2) thus correspond to those obtained by measuring thrombus volumes and thrombus heights after 3 min (Table 1): thrombi grow more rapidly with increasing shear rate. This implies that at constant blood flow rates thrombi will grow more rapidly in stenosed than in healthy arteries.

Red blood cells markedly enhance platelet adhesion to subendothelium (Baumgartner et al 1971). At a shear rate of 800 $sec^{-1}$ the rate of platelet adhesion from whole blood was approximately 50 times that from platelet rich plasma. Theoretical consideration indicate that this difference can be fully explained by the physical role of the red cells which enhance platelet transport towards the vessel wall by their oscillation in flowing blood (Turitto and Baumgartner 1975). At much higher shear rates humoral factors, such as ADP possibly released by the red cells (Hellem 1960), may also become important (Turitto and Weiss 1980).

2. Vessel wall thrombogenicity

Vessel wall thrombogenicity has been little investigated. It is established that the vessel wall can generate and release substances which inhibit platelet adhesion to subendothelium (see vessel wall thromboresistance). Vessel wall thrombogenicity depends on physical and chemical properties of the surface exposed to the blood and may also depend on thrombogenic substances, such as tissue factor or factor VIII/von Willebrand factor generated by the vessel wall. The comparatively smooth subendothelial surface of rabbit aorta can be modified to a brush-like surface by digestion with α chymotrypsin. Thereby the amorphous basement membrane like material and microfibrils are removed and what remains is an internal elastic lamina with numerous collagen fibrils protruding into the lumen (Baumgartner 1977). Perfusion experiments demonstrated that this surface is more thrombogenic than intact subendothelium. On the latter surface thrombus formation peaks at about 5-10 min and then the thrombi disappear again. On α chymotrypsin-digested subendothelium the thrombi continue to grow and do not break off since they are anchored to the vessel surface by the collagen fibrils which are observed within the platelet masses (Baumgartner 1977). Thus a rough surface with free collagen fibrils appears to be more thrombogenic than a smooth one. On the other hand, the chemical composition of the exposed surface also plays an important role: intact endothelium, artificial surfaces (Turitto et al 1979a) and even basement membrane collagens are less thrombogenic than type I and type III collagen fibrils (Santoro and Cunningham 1981).

3. Vessel wall thromboresistance

The lining of intact vascular endothelial cells constitutes a perfect thromboresistant surface. Some of the factors which contribute to this important property have been identified. They include the negative cell charge, a special proteoglycan coat and the ability of endothelial cells to generate prostacyclin, the most potent platelet inhibitor, and plasminogen activator (Gimbrone 1976). However, thromboresistance

is far from beiing fully understood. For example, inhibition of prostacyclin generation by high doses of aspirin does not cause increased
adherence of platelets to endothelium (Tschopp and Baumgartner 1981).
Recent observations in our laboratory indicate, on the other hand, that
the level of prostacyclin production by smooth muscle cells of the
media may be an important regulator of thrombosis on damaged vessels
which have lost their endothelial lining. Thus a correlation was found
between the ability of aortas from different species to generate
prostacyclin and the thrombogenicity of their aorta after endothelial
denudation in vivo. On subendothelium of guinea pig aorta which produces
only small amounts of prostacyclin significantly more thrombi developed
than on rat aorta which is known to generate large amounts of prostacyclin. The rabbit was intermediate. In addition, rat aorta subendothelium was rendered much more thrombogenic by inhibition of prostacyclin generation with aspirin (Tschopp and Baumgartner 1981). Similar
results were obtained in perfusion chamber experiments: Significantly
more platelets adhered to and significantly more thrombi formed on
subendothelium from rabbits treated with aspirin than on subendothelium
from untreated rabbits (Baumgartner and Tschopp 1979; Baumgartner et
al 1980a; Baumgartner et al 1982). Prostacyclin is probably not the
only substance produced by the vessel wall which may regulate the
complex interactions between platelets, the coagulation system and the
vessel wall.

Thrombus stability
It has been known for a long time that arterial thrombi may break off
when they have grown to a certain size and reattach further downstream
or embolize into the microvasculature (Baumgartner et al 1976). Thrombus
stability is a very relevant factor in thrombogenesis since it determines - among other factors - to which size a thrombus grows before it
breaks off or whether it will eventually develop an occluding thrombus.
Despite the obvious importance and probably due to the methodological
difficulties to investigate thrombus stability, very little is known
at present about the factors which control and regulate thrombus stability. It is only recently that we are beginning to gain some insight
by analysing the time course of thrombogenesis under strictly controlled

Table 3.

Thrombus growth rate and thrombus stability

| Blood flow rate ml/min | Shear rate $s^{-1}$ | Perfusion time (min) | | | | |
|---|---|---|---|---|---|---|
| | | 1 | 3 | 5 | 10 | 20 |
| | | Maximal thrombus height (µm) | | | | |
| 10 ml/min | 50* | O | O | O | O | O |
| 10 ml/min | 650 | 1.8±0.6 | 12± 1.1 | 12± 3.1 | 12± 3 | O |
| 40 ml/min | 2600 | 15 ±3.3 | 46± 7.2 | 41±11 | 22± 2.8 | 13± 5.5 |
| 160 ml/min | 10000 | 25 ±6.6 | 70±12 | 58±10 | 35±11 | 30±10 |

* annular chamber with a wider annular gap space
Values are means ± SE. Four to thirteen experiments were performed per
point.

Citrated rabbit blood was perfused through annular chambers at the
flow rates and for the time periods indicated. The maximal thrombus
height is the average of the three tallest thrombi in a specimen.

blood flow conditions. So far, the thrombus growth rate and a number
of clotting factors appear to influence the stability of thrombi.

1. Thrombus growth rate
As indicated above,the thrombus growth rate increased with the shear
rate. In other words thrombi grow more rapidly at high flow rates.
This is again evident from table 3 at 1 and 2 min perfusion time. The
results presented in table 3 also demonstrate that - independent of
flow rate - thrombus heights peak at 3min. Then thrombi start to break
down and what remains after prolonged perfusion is a monolayer of
platelets covering the subendothelial surface (Baumgartner 1973,
Turitto and Baumgartner 1979, Turitto et al 1980). The fact that thrombi,
independent of height, begin to desaggregate at the same time indicates that an intrinsic mechanism exists which relaxes the platelet
thrombi after 3 min. Surprisingly, the thrombi which grow at low shear
reverse more rapidly than those which grow at high shear (Table 3),
despite the fact that the shear forces which tend to remove thrombi
are much greater at high shear rate. We therefore postulate that thrombi
which grow more rapidly are more stable than those which grow slowly
in flowing citrated blood. The mechanism for this increased stability
is unknown at present.

2. Clotting factors
The perfusion of native blood avoiding any anticoagulation enables us
to investigate the interaction between platelets and the coagulation
system in thrombogenesis on subendothelium and to assess the relative
importance of the various clotting factor  for thrombus stability by
investigating patients with defined clotting factors deficiencies
(Weiss et al 1981). In collaboration with Weiss and Turitto we are
currently investigating patients with severe deficiency of fibrinogen,
factor XII, factor XI, factor X, factor IX, factor VIII/AHF, factor VII
and factor V. It appears that plasma fibrinogen, factor XII and factor
XI are less important for thrombus stability than factors VIII/AHF and
IX (Weiss, Turitto, Vicic and Baumgartner in preparation). Thus thrombin
generation in the microenvironement of the growing thrombus appears to
be more important for thrombus stability than the actual formation of
fibrin from plasma fibrinogen.

Fate of thrombi
There are two basically different fates of arterial thrombi, Firstly,
a thrombus remains where he originated and is organized by adjacent
smooth muscle cells. Secondly, a thrombus breaks off, dissolves, re-
attaches further down-stream or embolizes into the microvasculature.
There is ample evidence for both mechanisms.

1. Organisation of thrombi
It has always been accepted that occlusive thrombi are organized and
possibly recanalised. However there is also unequivocal evidence that
mural arterial thrombi in experimental animals (Moore 1973, Jorgensen
et al 1967, Pearson et al 1979a) as well as man (Friedman 1971, Pearson
et al 1979b) may be organized by smooth muscle cells of the vessel wall.
Thereby the thrombotic masses are incorporated into the vessel wall
and thus contribute to the progression of arteriosclerosis. Interestingly, the smooth muscle cells of organized human arterial thrombi
have monoclonal characteristics (Pearson et al 1979b) whereas those
experimentally induced in the hybrid hare are polyclonal (Pearson et
al 1979a).

## 2. Embolisation and/or dissolution
Small platelet thrombi which break off may desaggregate in the flowing
blood and pass through the microvasculature without causing any damage.
Larger and stabler emboli, depending on their size, may obstruct
smaller or larger vessels of the microvasculature and cause circumscribed ischemia.

There is some evidence that detached platelet aggregates may adhere
again to the vessel wall further down-stream and even cause endothelial
injury (Mustard et al 1970). Perfusion experiments demonstrated that
platelets or platelet aggregates derived from up stream thrombi may
adhere to surfaces which by themselves develop few adherent platelets
(Baumgartner et al 1976). Activated platelets may thus adhere to surfaces which are not attractive for normally circulating platelets.

### Conclusion
By using new approaches for the investigation of thrombogenesis we are
gaining new insights into the complex interplay between the vessel wall,
blood flow, platelets and coagulation. The exposure of vascular surfaces to blood flowing under well controlled conditions and the careful subsequent analysis of cellular and plasmatic depositions on the
exposed surface may help us to bridge the gap between sophisticated
test tube experiments and the much more complex situation in vivo. It
enables us for the first time to compare anticoagulants and platelet
inhibitors in the same system and may also help us to identify novel
compounds for the prevention of thrombosis and eventually arteriosclo-
rosis.

### References

Arfors, K.E., Cockburn, J.S. and Gross, J.F. (1976): Measurement of
growth rate of laser-induced intravascular platelet aggregation and the
influence of blood flow velocity. Microvasc. Res. 11, 79-88

Baumgartner, H.R. (1973): The role of blood flow in platelet adhesion,
fibrin deposition and formation of mural thrombi. Microvasc. Res. 5,
167-179

Baumgartner, H.R. (1976): Effects of anticoagulation on the interaction of human platelets with subendothelium in flowing blood. Schweiz.
Med. Wochenschr. 106, 1367-1368

Baumgartner, H.R. (1977): Platelet interaction with collagen fibrils
in flowing blood. I. Reaction of human platelets with α chymotrypsin
digested subendothelium. Thrombos. Haemostas. 37, 1-16

Baumgartner, H.R. (1979): Effects of acetylsalicylic acid, sulfinpyrazone and dipyridamole on platelet adhesion and aggregation in flowing
native and anticoagulated blood. Haemostasis 8, 340-352

Baumgartner, H.R. and Muggli, R. (1976): Adhesion and aggregation:
morphological demonstration and quantitation in vivo and in vitro. In:
"Platelets in Biology and Pathology", J.L. Gordon (ed.), Elsevier/North
Holland Biomedical Press, New York, pp. 23-60

Baumgartner, H.R., Muggli, R. and Tschopp, T.B. (1980a): Interaction of platelets with subendothelium in flowing blood. In: "Platelets - Cellular Response Mechanism and their Biological Significance", A. Rotman, F.A. Meyer, C. Gitler and A. Silberberg (eds.), John Wiley & Sons Ltd., New York, pp. 17-28

Baumgartner, H.R., Muggli, R. and Tschopp, T.B. (1982): Antiplatelet drugs and the interactions between platelets, fibrin and components of the vessel wall. In: "Advances in Pharmacology and Therapeutics II", H. Yoshida, Y. Hagihara and S. Ebashi (eds.), Pergamon Press, Oxford, pp. 21-29

Baumgartner, H.R., Muggli, R., Tschopp, T.B. and Turitto, V.T. (1976): Platelet adhesion, release and aggregation in flowing blood: effects of surface properties and platelet function. Thrombos. Haemostas. 35, 124-138

Baumgartner, H.R., Stemerman, M.B. and Spaet, T.H. (1971): Adhesion of blood platelets to subendothelial surface: distinct from adhesion to collagen. Experientia 27, 283-285

Baumgartner, H.R. and Tschopp, T.B. (1979): Platelet interaction with aortic subendothelium (SE) in vitro: locally produced PGI$_2$ inhibits adhesion and formation of mural thrombi in flowing blood. Thrombos. Haemostas. 42, 6

Baumgartner, H.R., Tschopp, T.B. and Meyer, D. (1980b): Shear rate dependent inhibition of platelet adhesion and aggregation on collagenous surface by antibodies to human factor VIII/von Willebrand factor. Brit. J. Haematol. 44, 127-139

Baumgartner, H.R., Turitto, V.T. and Weiss, H.J. (1980c): Effect of shear rate on platelet interaction with subendothelium in citrated and native blood. II. Relationship among platelet adhesion, thrombus dimensions, and fibrin formation. J. Lab. Clin. Med. 95, 208-211

Begent, N. and Born, G.V.R. (1970): Growth rate in vivo of platelet thrombi, produced by iontophoresis of ADP, as a function of mean blood flow velocity. Nature 227, 926-930

Friedman, M. (1971): The coronary thrombus: its origin and fate. Hum. Pathol. 2, 81-128

Gimbrone, M.A. (1976): Culture of vascular endothelium. In: "Progress in Hemostasis and Thrombosis 3", T.H. Spaet (ed.), Grune & Stratton, New York, pp. 1-28

Hellem, A.J. (1960): The adhesiveness of human blood platelets in vitro, Scand. J. Clin. Lab. Invest. 12, Suppl. 51

Jørgensen, L., Rowsell, H.C., Hovig, T. and Mustard, J.F. (1967): Resolution and organization of platelet-rich mural thrombi in carotid arteries of swine. Amer. J. Path. 51, 681-719

Moore, S. (1973): Thromboatherosclerosis in normolipemic rabbits. A result of continued endothelial damage. Lab. Invest. 29, 478-487

Mustard, J.F., Jørgensen, L. and Packham, M.A. (1970): Formed elements as a source of vascular injury. Thrombos. Diathes. Haemorrh. 40, Suppl. 137-144

Pearson, Th.A., Dillman, J., Solez, K. and Heptinstall, R.H. (1979): Monoclonal characteristics of organising arterial thrombi: significance in the origin and growth of human atherosclerotic plaques. Lancet 8106, 7-11

Pearson, Th.A., Dillman, J., Williams, K.J., Wolff, J.A., Adams, R., Solez, K. and Heptinstall, R.H. (1979a): Clonal characteristics of experimentally induced atherosclerotic lesions in the hybrid hare. Science 206, 1423-1425

Santoro, S.A. and Cunningham, L.W. (1981): The interaction of platelets with collagen. In: "Platelets in Biology and Pathology - 2". J.L. Gordon (ed.), Elsevier/North Holland Biomedical Press, New York, pp. 249-264

Tschopp, Th.B. (1977): Aspirin inhibits platelet aggregation on, but not adhesion to, collagen fibrils: an assessment of platelet adhesion and deposited platelet mass by morphometry and $^{51}$Cr-labeling. Thrombos. Res. 11, 619-632

Tschopp, T.B. and Baumgartner, H.R. (1981): Platelet adhesion and mural platelet thrombus formation on aortic subendothelium of rats, rabbits, and guinea pigs correlate negatively with the vascular $PGI_2$ production. J. Lab. Clin. Med. 98, 402-411

Turitto, V.T. and Baumgartner, H.R. (1975): Platelet interaction with subendothelium in a perfusion system: physical role of red blood cells. Microvasc. Res. 9, 335-344

Turitto, V.T. and Baumgartner, H.R. (1979): Platelet interaction with subendothelium in flowing rabbit blood: effect of blood shear rate. Microvasc. Res. 17, 38-54

Turitto, V.T. and Baumgartner, H.R. (1982): Platelet-surface interactions. In: "Hemostasis and Thrombosis, basic principles and clinical practice", R.W. Colman, J. Hirsh, V.J. Marder and E.W. Salzman (eds.), J.B. Lippincott Company, Philadelphia, pp. 364-379

Turitto, V.T., Muggli, R. and Baumgartner, H.R. (1979a): Platelet adhesion and thrombus formation on subendothelium, epon, gelatine and collagen under arterial flow conditions. ASAIO J. 2, 28-34

Turitto, V.T. and Weiss, H.J. (1980): Red blood cells: their dual role in thrombus formation. Science 207, 541-543

Turitto, V.T., Weiss, H.J. and Baumgartner, H.R. (1979b): Rheological factors influencing platelet interaction with vessel surfaces. J. Rheol. 23, 735-750

Turitto, V.T., Weiss, H.J. and Baumgartner, H.R. (1980): The effect of shear rate on platelet interaction with subendothelium exposed to citrated human blood. Microvasc. Res. 19, 352-365

658

Weiss, H.J., Turitto, V.T. and Baumgartner, H.R. (1978): Effect of
shear rate on platelet interaction with subendothelium in citrated and
native blood. I. Shear dependent decrease of adhesion in von Willebrand's disease and the Bernard-Soulier syndrome. J. Lab. Clin. Med.
92, 750-764

Weiss, H.J., Turitto, V.T. and Baumgartner, H.R. (1981): Platelet-
fibrin deposition on subendothelium in congenital bleeding disorders.
Thrombos. Haemostas. 46, 249

# Biosynthesis and Some Biological Properties of Prostaglandins and Leukotrienes

S. Hammarström

## Introduction

Prostaglandins and leukotrienes are oxygenated derivatives of arachidonic acid and certain other polyunsaturated fatty acids. They cause a number of biological effects including alterations of blood pressure, changes in blood platelet aggregation, stimulation of macromolecular permeability in the microcirculation and induction of leukocyte locomotion. In this chapter, some characteristics of the enzymes and reactions leading to prostaglandin and leukotriene biosynthesis and some biological properties of the leukotrienes will be briefly reviewed.

## Biosynthesis of Prostaglandin Endoperoxides

Prostaglandin endoperoxides (1,2) are labile intermediates in the biosynthesis of prostaglandins (3) and thromboxanes (4). The structures and proposed mechanism of formation of prostaglandins $G_2$ and $H_2$ from arachidonic acid are shown in Fig. 1. The reactions in this figure

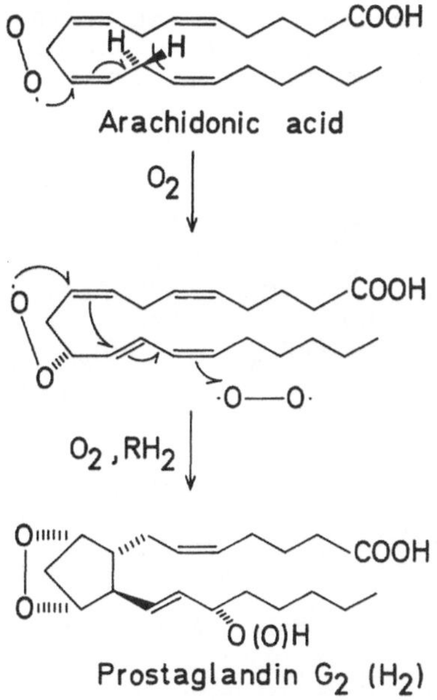

Arachidonic acid

$O_2$

$O_2$, $RH_2$

Prostaglandin $G_2$ ($H_2$)

Fig. 1. Proposed mechanism for the conversion of arachidonic acid to prostaglandin endoperoxides (prostaglandins $G_2$ and $H_2$)

are catalyzed by a single membrane bound glycoprotein called prostaglandin endoperoxide synthase (EC 1.14.99.1) (5-8). It consists of
two identical subunits of molecular weight ca. 70,000 which together
bind two molecules of heme. Heme is required for enzymatic activity
both in the cyclooxygenase reaction leading to formation of prostaglandin $G_2$ and in the peroxidase reaction in which prostaglandin $G_2$
is converted to prostaglandin $H_2$. The subcellular localization of
the enzyme has been determined using immunohistochemical techniques
(9,10). The results showed a dense localization on endoplasmatic reticulum and nuclear membranes in 3T3 fibroblasts and more precisely on
the cytoplasmic side of the endoplasmatic reticulum of sheep vesicular
glands. Mechanistic studies on prostaglandin biosynthesis have been
performed using $^{18}O$ labeled oxygen gas and precursor acids labeled at
specific positions with tritium or carbon 14 ((1,11). The data indicated that the initial step in the transformation is stereospecific
removal of a hydrogen from carbon atom 13. Subsequently, one molecule
of oxygen attaches to the acid, first at C-11 and then at C-9 to form
an endoperoxide group (see Fig. 1). This leads to the formation of a
bond between C-8 and C-12 to give a cyclopentane group and finally
introduction of a second molecule of oxygen as a hydroperoxy group
at C-15 in prostaglandin $G_2$. Next, the hydroperoxy group is reduced
to give prostaglandin $H_2$.

## Transformations of Prostaglandin Endoperoxides

The reactive endoperoxide prostaglandin $H_2$ is a common precursor of
all prostaglandins and thromboxanes of the two-series and of 12-hydroxy-
5,8,10-heptadecatrienoic acid (HHT, Fig. 3). Separate enzymes catalyze
the conversions of prostaglandin $H_2$ into the five primary products
shown in Fig. 2.

Prostaglandin D synthase converts prostaglandin $H_2$ to prostaglandin $D_2$.
It has been purified to homogeniety from rat brain cytosol and consists
of a single polypeptide with a molecular weight of ca. 80,000. The enzyme is stabilized by thiols but does not require glutathione for activity (12).

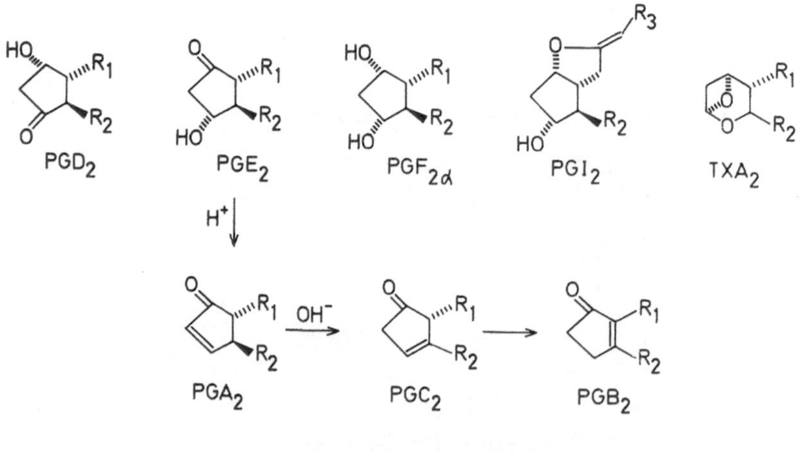

Fig. 2. Prostaglandins Formed from the Endoperoxide Prostaglandin $H_2$

Prostaglandin E synthase (EC 5.3.99.3) converts prostaglandin $H_2$ to prostaglandin $E_2$. The partially purified enzyme from bovine vesicular gland microsomes (13) is labile (half-life at $25^{\circ}C$: 30 min). Various thiols including glutathione protected the enzyme from inactivation. Glutathione was also required as a cofactor for the reaction.

Enzymes catalyzing the formation of prostaglandins $A_2$, $B_2$ and $C_2$ from prostaglandins $E_2$, $C_2$ and $A_2$, respectively (Fig. 2) have been partially purified from rabbit blood serum (14,15).

Prostaglandin $F_\alpha$ synthase activity was present in microsomes from guinea pig uteri. The enzyme was remarkably heat stable (80% of the activity remained after 10 min at $100^{\circ}C$). Neither glutathione nor NADPH stimulated the conversion of prostaglandin $H_2$ to prostaglandin $F_{2\alpha}$ by the uterine microsomes (16).

Prostaglandin I (or prostacyclin) synthase has been partially purified from aortic microsomes (17). Recently, spectral evidence has been presented suggesting that this enzyme contains thiolate bound heme and resembles cytochrome P-450 in this way (18).

Thromboxane synthase from human (19) and bovine platelets (20) has been partially purified from microsomes. After solubilization with Triton X-100 the enzyme was separated from prostaglandin endoperoxide synthase by chromatography on DEAE cellulose. An interesting property of the enzyme is that it converts prostaglandin $H_2$ to a mixture of thromboxane $A_2$ and 12-hydroxy-5,8,10-heptadecatrienoic acid (HHT, Fig. 3, (21)). The formation of HHT involves cleavage of the cyclopentane group in prostaglandin $H_2$ between C-8 and C-9 and between C-11 and C-12. Carbon atoms 9, 10 and 11 are eliminated as malondialdehyde and a double bond is formed between C-8 and C-9 (originally C-12) in the $C_{17}$ acid. Endoperoxides lacking a $\Delta^5$ double bond are transformed predominantly according to the latter reaction to $C_{17}$ hydroxy acids. This is true e.g. for prostaglandins $H_1$ and $\Delta^4$-$H_1$ (see Fig. 3). This demonstrates a strikingly specific requirement for a cis double bond at precisely the $\Delta^5$ position to permit the thromboxane forming reaction

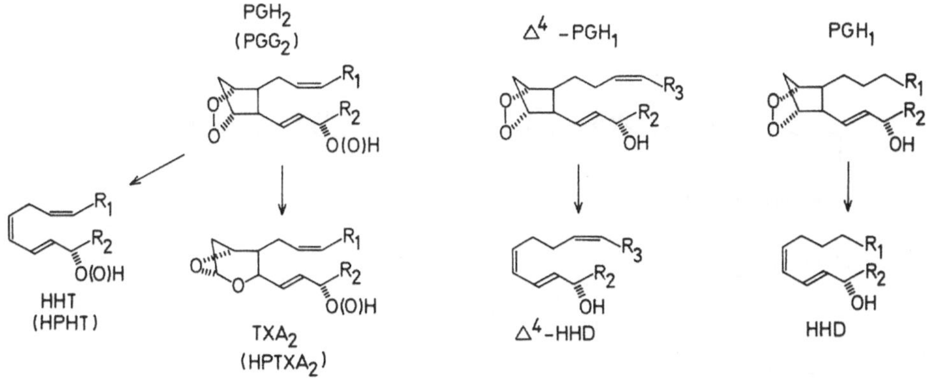

Fig. 3. Conversion of Prostaglandin Endoperoxides to Thromboxanes and $C_{17}$ Hydroxy Acids by Thromboxane Synthase (From Ref. 22)

to occur (22). Prostaglandin $G_2$, which like prostaglandin $H_2$ has a double bond at this position was transformed into a mixture[2] of 15-hydroperoxythromboxane $A_2$ and 12-hydroperoxy-5,8,10-heptadecatrienoic acid (Fig. 3, (23)).

## Leukotrienes: Discovery, Structure Elucidation and Biosynthesis

Leukotrienes were first described in 1938 as a component of lung per-fusates causing characteristic contractions of guinea pig intestine (24). This factor was referred to as "slow reacting substance" (SRS) or "SRS of anaphylaxis" (SRS-A) until 1979 when its chemical structure was reported (25,26). At that time the term leukotriene was introduced as a trivial name indicating a structural feature (conjugated triene) and cellular sources of SRS (basophilic leukemia cells, neutrophilic leukocytes and cells related to leukocytes, e.g. mast cells and masto-cytoma cells).

The originally characterized SRS, leukotriene $C_4$, is a glutathione containing derivative of arachidonic acid. The tripeptide is linked as a thioether to the fatty acid and is adjacent to a hydroxyl group and the conjugated triene (Fig. 4). These structural features sugges-ted that leukotriene $C_4$ was formed by addition of glutathione to an epoxide. An appropriate epoxide had been described (27) shortly before

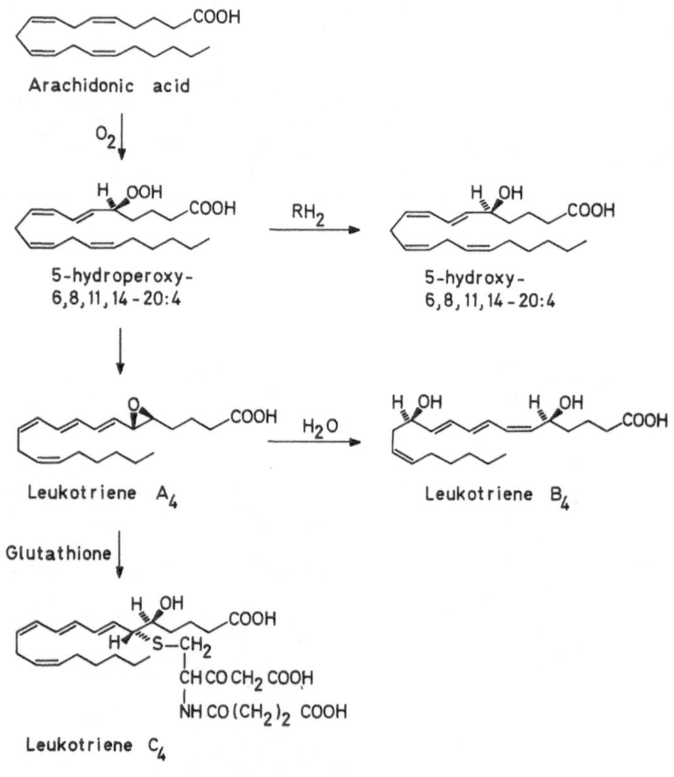

Fig. 4. Structures and Biosynthesis of Leukotrienes

the structure of leukotriene $C_4$ was reported (25,26). The biosynthetic pathway shown in Fig. 4 was originally postulated in the papers on the structure of leukotriene $C_4$ (25,26) and has subsequently been verified experimentally (28,29). The epoxide in Fig. 4 (leuktriene $A_4$) seems to be formed from arachidonic acid by two enzymatic reactions: The first one is catalyzed by a calcium dependent lipoxygenase (30,31) which converts arachidonic acid to a hydroperoxy acid by introducing a mole- cule of $O_2$ at C-5. A conjugated diene is formed during this reaction. The product is either reduced to a hydroxy acid which cannot be further transformed to leukotrienes or it is converted to the epoxide. The latter reaction involves elimination of hydrogen from C-10 and of OH from the hydroperoxy group. This leads to the formation of a conjugated triene (at $\Delta^{7,9,11}$) with an allylic epoxide group (at C-5, C-6). Enzy- matic conversion of leukotriene $A_4$ to leukotriene $C_4$ (Fig. 4) has been demonstrated using suspensions of murine mastocytoma cells (28,29), rat basophilic leukemia cells (28) and human peripheral leukocytes (29). In this reaction the sulfhydryl group of glutathione opens the epoxide group at C-6 in an $S_N 2$ type of reaction.

An alternative conversion of leukotriene $A_4$ to a 5,12-diol (leukotriene $B_4$, Fig. 4) occurs in polymorphonuclear leukocytes (27,32). This reac- tion involves addition of OH (from water) to C-12, isomerization of the triene (to $\Delta^{6,8,10}$) and opening of the epoxide at C-6. The enzymes of leukotriene biosynthesis have not yet been resolved or purified and con- sequently little information is available on their properties.


## Metabolism of Leukotrienes


Leukotriene C is metabolized rapidly *in vitro* and *in vivo* by sequential degradation of the peptide part (33,34). Elimination of the amino ter- minal glutamic acid yields leukotriene D (Fig. 5). This reaction is

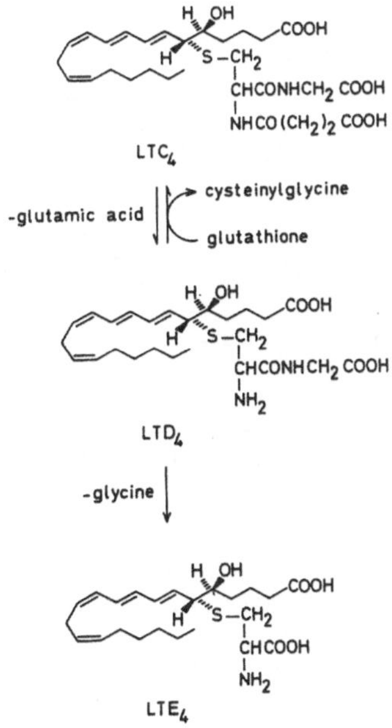

Fig. 5. Metabolism of Leukotriene $C_4$

catalyzed by the membrane bound enzyme γ-glutamyl transpeptidase. The reaction is reversible and the $K_m$ for leukotriene $C_4$ (5.6 µM) is similar to the $K_m$ for glutathione, another substrate for this enzyme (35). Leukotriene $D_4$ is further transformed to leukotriene $E_4$ (Fig. 5) by elimination of the carboxyl temrinal glycine residue. A particulate dipeptidase from kidney and other tissues catalyzes this reaction (36). Leukotriene $B_4$ is converted by polymorphonuclear leukocytes to 20-hydroxy and 20-carboxyleukotriene $B_4$ (37).


## Cardiovascular and Respiratory Effects of Leukotrienes


Leukotrienes $C_4$, $D_4$, and $E_4$ stimulate the smooth muscles of lung parenchymal strips and trachea from several species including man (e.g. 38,39). When administered intravenously or as aerosols, leukotriene $C_4$ increased the insufflation pressure in guinea pigs (38) and the transpulmonary pressure in anesthetized monkeys (40). The latter effect was due to reduced pulmonary compliance rather than increased resistance, indicating that the effect was primarily due to contractions of the peripheral parts of the lungs. Following administration into the right atrium of monkeys, leukotriene $C_4$ also had pronounced cardiovascular effects (40). Initially (30-60 sec after injection) the

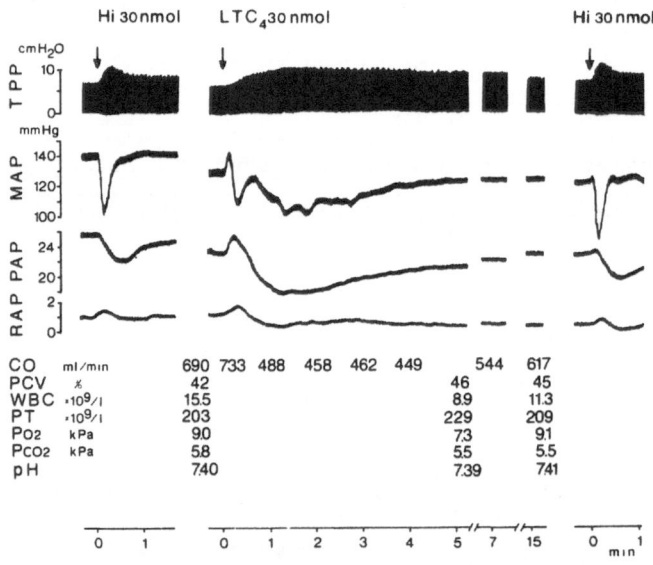

Fig. 6. Effects of leukotriene $C_4$ and histamine, injected into the right atrium of an artificially ventilated monkey. (From Ref. 40)

mean systemic pressure (MAP, Fig. 6), the pulmonary arterial pressure (PAP) and the right atrial pressure (RAP) were transiently elevated. These effects were followed by a more prolonged hypotension (5-15 min). In addition, the cardiac output (CO) was reduced, the hematocrit (PCV) and platelet count (PT) somewhat increased and the white blood cell count (WBC) considerably reduced.

## Microvascular Effects of Leukotrienes

Leukotrienes $C_4$ and $D_4$ have pronounced microvascular effects as judged by experiments using the hamster cheek pouch model (41). After a transient vasoconstriction (maximum after 90 sec) especially of terminal arterioles, leakage of FITC labeled dextran occurs at the postcapillary venules (Fig. 7). The vasoconstrictor effect of leukotriene $C_4$ might

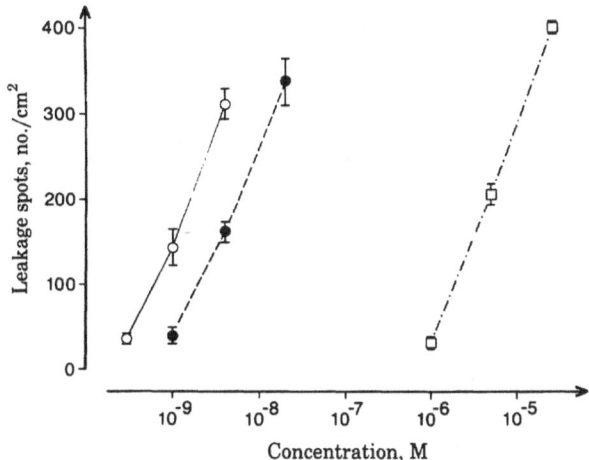

**Fig. 7.** Effects of leukotriene $C_4$ (o——o) and leukotriene $D_4$ (●---●) and histamine (□---□) on vascular permeability of the hamster cheek pouch. (from Ref. 41)

contribute to the hypertension and the effect on vascular permeability to the hypotension (by reduced venous return) shown in Fig. 5. In addition to these effects, leukotrienes $C_4$ and $D_4$ decrease coronary blood flow and left ventricular contractile force in isolated guinea pig hearts (42).


## Effects on Leukocytes

The biological effects of amino acid containing leukotrienes (e.g. leukotrienes $C_4$, $D_4$, and $E_4$) differ from those of diol leukotrienes (e.g. leukotriene $B_4$). The latter does not have direct effects on airway smooth muscles or vascular permeability. On the other hand, leukotriene $B_4$ has effects on leukocyte behaviour which are not shared by amino acid containing leukotrienes. These effects include stimulation of directional and random motion of leukocytes (43), stimulation of leukocyte adhesion to endothelial cells of postcapillary venules ((41), Fig. 8) and induction of lysosomal enzyme release from leukocytes (44).

666

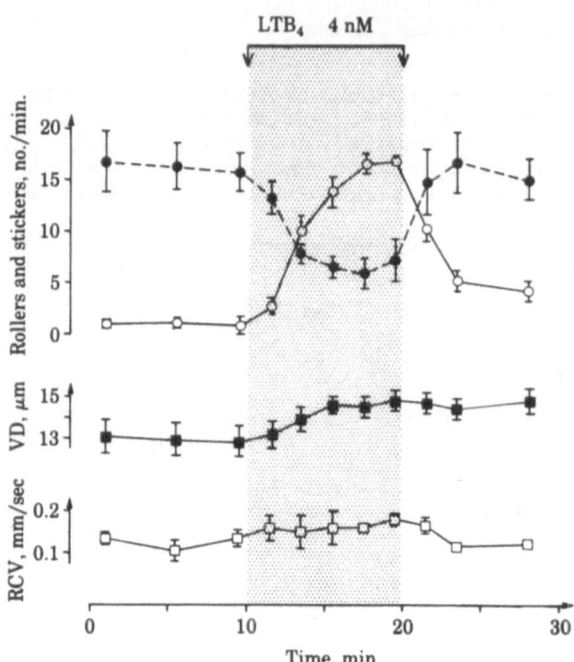

**Fig. 8.** Effect of leukotriene $B_4$ on the numbers of leukocytes rolling (●---●) and sticking to the vessel wall (o——o) in a postcapillary venule of the hamster cheek pouch. (From Ref. 41)

**Acknowledgments**  The work in the author´s laboratories was supported by grants from the Swedish Medical Research Council (project 03X-5914).

## References

1. Samuelsson, B (1965) On the incorporation of oxygen in the conversion of 8,11,14-eicosatrienoic acid to prostaglandin $E_1$. J Am Chem Soc 87:3011-3013
2. Hamberg M, Svensson J, Wakabayashi T, Samuelsson B (1974) Isolation and structure of two prostaglandin endoperoxides that cause platelet aggregation. Proc Natl Acad Sci USA 71:345-349
3. Bergström S, Ryhage R, Samuelsson B, Sjövall J (1963) The structures of prostaglandin $E_1$, $F_{1\alpha}$ and $F_{1\beta}$. J Biol Chem 238:3555-3564
4. Hamberg M, Svensson J, Samuelsson B (1975) Thromboxanes: a new group of biologically active compuonds derived from prostaglandin endoperoxides. Proc Natl Acad USA 72:2994-2998
5. Miyamoto T, Ogino N, Yamamoto S, Hayaishi O (1976) Purification of prostaglandin endoperoxide synthetase from bovine vesicular gland microsomes. J Biol Chem 251:2629-2636
6. Hemler M, Lands WEM, Smith WL (1976) Purification of the cyclooxygenase that forms prostaglandins. J Biol Chem 251:5575-5579
7. van der Ouderaa FJ, Buytenek M, Nugteren DH, van Dorp DA (1977) Purification and characterization of prostaglandin endoperoxide

synthetase from sheep vesicular glands. Biochim Biophys Acta 487: 315-331

8. Ohki S, Ogino N, Yamamoto S, Hayaishi O (1979) Prostaglandin hydroperoxidase as an integral part of prostaglandin endoperoxide synthetase from bovine vesicular gland microsomes. J Biol Chem 254:829-836

9. Rollins TE, Smith WL (1980) Subcellular localization of prostaglandin forming cyclooxygenase in Swiss mouse 3T3 fibroblasts by electron microscopic immunocytochemistry. J Biol Chem 255:4872-4875

10. Smith WL, Wilkin GP (1977) Immunochemistry of prostaglandin endoperoxide forming cyclooxygenases: the detection of cyclooxygenases in rat, rabbit, and guinea pig kidneys by immunofluorescence. Prostaglandins 13:873-892

11. Hamberg M, Samuelsson B (1967) On the mechanism of the biosynthesis of prostaglandins $E_1$ and $F_{1\alpha}$. J Biol Chem 242:5336-5343

12. Shimizu T, Yamamoto S, Hayaishi O (1979) Purification and properties of prostaglandin D synthetase from rat brain. J Biol Chem 254:5222-5228

13. Ogino N, Miyamoto T, Yamamoto S, Hayaishi O (1977) Prostaglandin endoperoxide E isomerase from bovine vesicular gland microsomes, a glutathione requiring enzyme (1977) J Biol Chem 252 890-895

14. Polet H, Levine L (1975) Partial purification and characterization of prostaglandin A isomerase from rabbit serum. Arch Biochem Biophys 168:96-103

15. Polet H, Levine L (1975) Metabolism of prostaglandins E, A, and C in serum. J Biol Chem 250:351-357

16. Wlodawer P, Kindahl H, Hamberg M (1976) Biosynthesis of prostaglandin $F_{2\alpha}$ from arachidonic acid and prostaglandin endoperoxides in the uterus. Biochim Biophys Acta 431:603-614

17. Wlodawer P, Hammarström S (1980) Conversion of prostaglandin endoperoxides by prostacyclin synthase from pig aorta. Prostaglandins 19:969-976

18. Ullrich V, Castle L, Weber P (1981) Spectral evidence for the cytochrome P 450 nature of prostacyclin synthetase. Biochem Pharmacol 30:2033-2036

19. Hammarström S, Falardeau P (1977) Resolution of prostaglandin endoperoxide synthase and thromboxane synthase of human platelets. Proc Natl Acad Sci USA 74:3691-3695

20. Yoshimoto T, Yamamoto S, Okuma M, Hayaishi O (1977) Solubilization and resolution of thromboxane synthesizing system from microsomes of bovine blood platelets. J Biol Chem 252:5871-5874

21. Diczfalusy U, Falardeau P, Hammarström S (1977) Conversion of prostaglandin endoperoxides to $C_{17}$-hydroxy acids catalyzed by human platelet thromboxane synthase. FEBS Lett 84:271-274

22. Diczfalusy U, Hammarström S (1979) A structural requirement for the conversion of prostaglandin endoperoxides to thromboxanes. FEBS Lett 105:291-295

23. Hammarström S (1980) Enzymatic synthesis of 15-hydroperoxythromboxane $A_2$ and 12-hydroperoxy-5,8,10-heptadecatrienoic acid. J Biol Chem 255:518-521

24. Feldberg W, Kellaway CH (1938) Liberation of histamine and formation of lysolecithin-like substances by cobra venom. J Physiol (London) 94:187-226

25. Murphy RC, Hammarström S, Samuelsson B (1979) Leukotriene C: a slow reacting substance from murine mastocytoma cells. Proc Natl Acad Sci USA 76:4275-4279

26. Hammarström S, Murphy RC, Samuelsson B, Clark DA, Mioskowski C, Corey EJ (1979) Structure of leukotriene C: identification of the amino acid part. Biochem Biophys Res Commun 91:1266-1272

27. Borgeat P, Samuelsson B (1979) Arachidonic acid metabolism in polymorphonuclear leukocytes: unstable intermediate in the formation of dihydroxy acids. Proc Natl Acad Sci USA 76:3213-3217

28. Hammarström S, Samuelsson B (1980) Detection of leukotriene $A_4$ as

an intermediate in the biosynthesis of leukotrienes $C_4$ and $D_4$.
FEBS Lett 122:83-86

29. Rådmark O, Malmsten C, Samuelsson B (1980) Leukotriene $A_4$: enzymatic conversion to leukotriene $C_4$. Biochem Biophys Res Commun 96:1679-1687

30. Jakschik BA, Sun FF, Lee LH, Steinhoff M (1980) Calcium stimulation of a novel lipoxygenase. Biochem Biophys Res Commun 95:103-110

31. Borgeat P, Samuelsson B (1979) Arachidonic acid metabolism in polymorphonuclear leukocytes: effects of ionophore A23187. Proc Natl Acad Sci USA 76:2148-2152

32. Rådmark O, Malmsten C, Samuelsson B, Clark DA, Goto G, Marfat A, Corey EJ (1980) Leukotriene A: stereochemistry and enzymatic conversion to leukotriene B. Biochem Biophys Res Commun 92:954-961

33. Hammarström S (1981) Metabolism of leukotriene $C_3$ in the guinea pig. Identification of metabolites formed by lung, liver and kidney. J Biol Chem 256:9573-9578

34. Hammarström S, Bernström K, Örning L, Dahlén SE, Hedqvist P (1981) Rapid in vivo metabolism of leukotriene $C_3$ in the monkey Macaca irus. Biochem Biophys Res Commun 101:1109-1115

35. Örning L, Hammarström S (1982) Kinetics of the conversion of leukotriene C by γ-glutamyl transpeptidase. Biochem Biophys Res Commun 106:1304-1309

36. Bernström K, Hammarström S (1981) Metabolism of leukotriene D by porcine kidney. J Biol Chem 256:9579-9582

37. Hansson G, Lindgren JÅ, Dahlén SE, Hedqvist P, Samuelsson B (1981) Identification and biological activity of novel ω-oxidized metabolites of leukotriene $B_4$ from human leukocytes. FEBS Lett 130:107-112

38. Hedqvist P, Dahlén SE, Gustafsson L, Hammarström S, Samuelsson B (1980) Biological profile of leukotrienes $C_4$ and $D_4$. Acta Physiol Scand 110:331-333

39. Dahlén SE, Hedqvist P, Hammarström S, Samuelsson B (1980) Leukotrienes are potent constrictors of human bronchi. Nature 288:484-486

40. Smedegård G, Hedqvist P, Dahlén SE, Revenäs B, Hammarström S, Samuelsson B (1982) Leukotriene $C_4$ affects pulmonary and cardiovascular dynamics in monkey. Nature 295:327-329

41. Dahlén SE, Björk J, Hedqvist P, Arfors KE, Hammarström S, Lindgren JÅ, Samuelsson B (1981) Leukotrienes promote plasma leakage and leukocyte adhesion in postcapillary venules: In vivo effects with relevance to the acute inflammatory response. Proc Natl Acad Sci USA 78:3887-3891

42. Levi R, Burke JA, Corey EJ (1982) SRS-A, leukotrienes and immediate hypersensitivity reactions of the heart. Adv. Prostaglandin, thromboxane and leukotriene Res 9:215-222

43. Palmblad J, Malmsten C, Udén AM, Rådmark O, Engstedt L, Samuelsson B (1981) Leukotriene $B_4$ is a potent and stereospecific stimulator of neutrophil chemotaxis and adherence. Blood 58:658-661

44. Feinmark SJ, Lindgren JÅ, Claesson HE, Malmsten C, Samuelsson B (1981) Stimulation of human leukocyte degranulation by leukotriene $B_4$ and its ω-oxidized metabolites. FEBS Lett 136:141-144

# Interactions Between Lipoproteins and PGI$_2$ Under Physiologic and Pathophysiologic Conditions

W. Förster

## A. Introduction

Nordøy et al. (1) have proved that LDL inhibit generation of an
antiplatelet principle by cultured arterial endothelial cells and
suggested it to be a PGI$_2$-like substance. Starting out from these
results we have been carring out systematic studies (2-8) to
assess our working hypothesis that interactions between lipoproteins (LP) and prostacyclin (PGI$_2$) could be relevant to the pathogenesis of atherosclerosis.

## B. Methods

LP were isolated from serum of healthy men and women and from
insulin dependent diabetics of type 1 mean age 21.6 $\pm$ 1.8 years,
duration of diabetes 7.8 $\pm$ 2.0 years and more than 40 years,
respectively. The patients suffering 7.8 years from diabetes received 30 ml/day linseed oil for 4 weeks in addition to their normal diet. LP were isolated from serum by ultracentrifugation and
ultrafiltration according to earlier described methods (2,3) and
quantified by estimation of the cholesterol part of LP. The LP
were incubated with the microsomal fraction of pig aorta and the
reaction was started by addition of PGH$_2$. The isolation and determination of 6-keto-PGF$_{1\alpha}$ by GLC using PGF$_{1\alpha}$ as internal standard was carried out according the method described earlier (3).
Data were statistically analyzed, a P value of $< 0.05$ was considered as significant. The in vitro effects of LDL and HDL on the
transformation of PGH$_2$ to PGI$_2$ were investigated in physiological
concentrations of 0.1-2.0 mg LP-cholesterol/ml.

## C. Results and Discussion

First we investigated the influence of LDL and HDL taken from men and women (4) and from premenopausal and postmenopausal women. If there are relevant correlations between LP and PG, such mutual relations should also exist to the known epidemiological datas concerning the incidence of heart infarction. LDL derived from the blood of male persons inhibited the $PGI_2$ synthesis concentration-dependent (Fig.1).

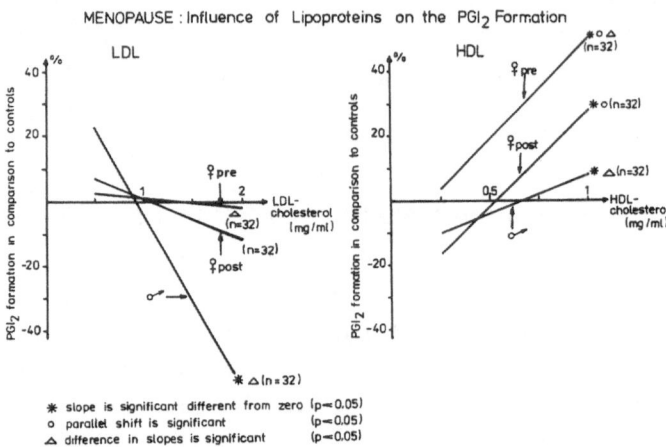

**Fig. 1.** Interactions between lipoproteins and $PGI_2$ under physiologic and pathophysiologic conditions

There was, however, no inhibition of the $PGI_2$ synthesis by LDL derived from the blood of premenopausal women, not even in the highest concentration used. But LDL taken from the blood of post-menopausal women had in higher concentrations a tendency to inhibit the $PGI_2$ synthesis, though less than LDL of men. HDL behaves contrary: HDL taken from the blood of male persons had only in the highest concentration used a tendency to $PGI_2$ stimulation, whereas HDL from premenopausal women increasingly enhanced the $PGI_2$ synthesis, in the highest concentration used by about 50 %. HDL taken from the blood of postmenopausal women stimulated the $PGI_2$ synthesis by not more than maximal 20 %. As it was seen with the LDL, the effect of the postmenopausal HDL approximates to that of the HDL from male persons. These results correlate with those by Gordon et al. in the Framingham Study (9).

Investigations of the last years (1o,11) revealed a disturbed
ratio $PGI_2/TXA_2$ in patients with diabetes mellitus. On the other
hand, it is wellknown that diabetics tend to develop atherosclerotic and thrombotic disorders. Therefore we wanted to know if
there are correlations between LP and the $PGI_2$ synthesis also under
these pathophysiological conditions. The determination by GLC of
the fatty acid patterns of the plasma phospholipids from diabetic
patients with 7.8 years disease duration resulted in an increased
proportion of $C_{18:0}$ and a slightly increased proportion of $C_{20}:5$
(EPA). The shares of oleic and linoleic acids were slightly diminished. The inhibitory action of LDL obtained from diabetic males
with a disease period more than 4o years on the $PGI_2$ biosynthesis
was markedly enhanced in comparison with results with LDL from
diabetics suffering 7.8 years or healthy persons. Similar tendencies were seen with HDL from female diabetics. Both groups  showed
a parallel shift of the dose-response curves into the inhibitory
range. HDL from female diabetics suffering more than 4o years did
not stimulate the $PGI_2$ synthesis even in the highest concentration
investigated (Fig.2). All patients suffering more than 4o years
from diabetes mellitus showed distinct signs of macroangiopathic
diseases.

DIABETES DURATION: Influence of Lipoproteins on the $PGI_2$ Synthesis

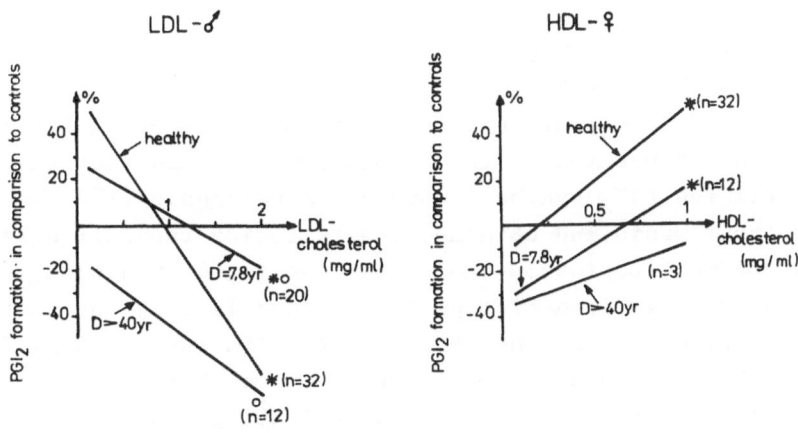

* slope is significant different from zero (p< 0,01)

o parallel shift is significant (p<0,01)

Fig. 2. Interactions between lipoproteins and $PGI_2$ under physiologic
and pathophysiologic conditions

To reveal the influence of polyunsaturated fatty acids, the group
of diabetics with a disease period of 7.8 years was given 30 ml/day
linseed oil additionally to their normal diet during four weeks.
In the control group of healthy persons kept on the same diet not
only the proportion of $\alpha$-linolenic acid in the phospholipids but
also the proportion of EPA and docosahexaenoic acid were enhanced,
a result that proves the partial transformation of the linolenic
acid into EPA also in humans (6). In diabetics, however, only
the $\alpha$-linolenic acid was increased, but no transformation into
EPA occurred (12). It is generally known that likewise diabetics
are only to a small degree able to transform linoleic acid into
arachidonic acid (13). There were marked distinctions between the
healthy control group and the diabetics after a 4 weeks diet with
linseed oil with respect to the effects of LDL and HDL on the
$PGI_2$ biosynthesis: LDL and HDL taken from healthy persons under
the linseed oil diet enhanced the $PGI_2$ synthesis (7). In diabetics,
however, the diet had no effect on the action of their LP on $PGI_2$
synthesis. These results can be considered as further confirmation
of close connections between changes in the fatty acid pattern and
altered influence on $PGI_2$ synthesis. The inability to transform
linoleic and linolenic acid into fatty acids with longer chains
deprives the diabetics, though beeing kept on   linseed oil, of
the possibility to use the antiatherogenic effect of the EPA (14)
to prevent the development of macroangiopathies.

Szczeklik et al. (15) had critically discussed our suggestion that
LDL-cholesterol and HDL-cholesterol influence the $PGI_2$ synthesis
by themselves. They proposed the hypothesis that serum lipid
peroxides are concentrated in the LDL fraction and that therefore
LDL inhibit the $PGI_2$ synthesis and are atherogenic (16). We repeated the experiments and obtained the following results: Related
to nmol MDA/mg lipoprotein-cholesterol we found in healthy subjects and in hyperlipidemics of type II and IV only one third of the
amounts of peroxides in the LDL compared with that in HDL. Considering the amounts of LDL and HDL in serum there was no difference in the peroxide content in nmol/ml MDA serum between LDL
and HDL. To prove the dependence of the diminished $PGI_2$ synthesis
on the peroxide content Szczeklik et al. (15) added butylated
hydroxytoluene (BHT) prior to the isolation steps of LP and found
a marked decrease of the peroxide content and a decline of the

inhibitory action on $PGI_2$ synthesis. We repeated these experiments with butylated hydroxytoluene but found under our experimental conditions only a statistically not significant decline in the peroxide content of the LDL. In our experiments LDL from male and female persons with and without addition of BHT were checked for their influence on the $PGI_2$ synthesis. We obtained similar dose-response curves regardless whether they were calculated with respect to cholesterol or lipid peroxides as determined by MDA. The cause of the discrepancies is obviously to be found in the different methodical conditions. We centrifugated with 2oo.ooo g for 7 h, Szczeklik with 1oo.ooo x g for 18-2o h. Besides, we ultrafiltrated our preparations 3 h while Szczeklik et al. dialyzed 48 h. Our total time period for preparation was lo h, that of Szczeklik 66-68 h. This longer preparation procedure for the isolation of LDL makes the enhanced formation of lipid peroxides and their suppression by added BHT understandable.

We conclude that the differing influences on $PGI_2$ synthesis of LDL and HDL from male and female subjects of different age and from diabetics with different duration of the disease, kept on a linseed oil diet or not, are not explainable by their differing content of lipid peroxides, since there are no essential differences in the serum peroxide concentrations. Therefore we hold our hypothesis that there must be still not exactly known mechanisms influencing the $PGI_2$ generation which involve intrinsic actions of LDL- and HDL-cholesterol and which can be influenced by diet. Because we had shown (8) the generation of $PGI_2$ to be linearly dependent on the fatty acid patterns of added cholesterol esters from rat heart and kidney, varied by diet, it seems more probable to us that in a similar way the fatty acid patterns of lipoproteins could be responsible for the differing influences of LDL and HDL on $PGI_2$ generation.

## Acknowledgments

These investigations were carried out together with my coworkers Beitz J., Panse M., Mest H.-J., Department of Pharmacology and Toxicology, Martin Luther University Halle-Wittenberg, Halle, GDR, with Honigmann G., and Schimke E. from the Centre of Diabetes and Metabolic Diseases, Berlin, GDR, and Müller G., II. Clinic of Internal Med., Martin Luther University Halle-Wittenberg, Halle,

674

GDR. The excellent technical assistance of Mrs. Seydlitz A. and Mrs. Adler I. is acknowledged.

References

1. Nordøy A, Svensson B, Wiebe D, Hoak JC (1978) Lipoproteins and the inhibitory effect of human endothelial cells on platelet function. Circulat. Res. 43: 527-534

2. Beitz J, Förster W (1980) Influence of human low density and high density lipoprotein cholesterol on the in vitro prostaglandin $I_2$ synthetase activity. Biochim. Biophys. Acta 62o: 352-355

3. Beitz J, Block H-U, Hoffmann P, Förster W (1981) Influence of fatty acids and lipids from biological sources on the in vitro biosynthesis of prostaglandin $I_2$ ($PGI_2$). Pharmacol. Res. Commun. 13: 363-383

4. Beitz J, Förster W (1981) Differential influence of lipoproteins isolated from women and men on the activity of the $PGI_2$ synthetase activity. Prostaglandins and Med. 6: 515-518

5. Förster W, Beitz J, Hoffmann P (1980) Stimulation and inhibition of $PGI_2$ synthetase activity by phospholipids (PL), cholesterol esters (CE), unesterified fatty acids (UFA) and lipoproteins (LDL and HDL). Artery 8: 494-5oo

6. Beitz J, Mest H-J, Förster W (1981) Influence of linseed oil diet on the pattern of serum phospholipids in man. Acta biol. med. germ. 4o: K31-K35

7. Mest H-J, Beitz J, Heinroth I, Block H-U, Förster W. The influence of linseed oil diet on fatty acid pattern in phospholipids, on prostaglandin plasma level and thromboxane formation in platelets in man. Submitted to Klin.Wschr.

8. Förster W, Beitz J (1982) Regulation of prostacyclin synthetase activity by lipids. Pharmacol. Res. Commun. 14: 227-24o

9. Gordon T, Kannel W, Hjortland MC, McNamara PM (1978) Menopause and coronary heart disease. Ann. Intern.Med. 89: 157-161

1o. Johnson M, Reece AH, Harrison HE (1981) Abnormal arachidonic acid metabolism in diabetes: effect of drugs. In: Förster W (ed) Prostaglandins and Thromboxanes, Pergamon Press, Oxford

11. Halushka PV, Mayfield R, Wohltmann HJ, Rogers RC, Goldberg AK, McCoy SA, Loadholt CB, Colwell JA (1981) Increased platelet arachidonic acid metabolism in diabetes mellitus. Diabetes 30 (Supplement): 44-48

12. Beitz J, Schimke E, Honigmann G, Mest H-J, Förster W (1982) In diabetics linseed oil diet does not change the influence of lipoproteins (LP) on the prostaglandin $I_2$ ($PGI_2$) formation. 4th Dresden Lipid Symposium, June 1o-12

13. Brenner RR, Peluffo RO, Mercuri O, Restelli MA (1968) Effect of arachidonic acid in the alloxan-diabetic rat. Am. J. Physiol. 215: 63-7o

14. Dyerberg J, Bang HO, Stofferson E, Moncada S, Vane JR (1978) Eicosapentaenoic acid and prevention of thrombosis and athero-sclerosis. Lancet i: 117-119

15. Szczeklik A, Gryglewski RJ, Domagała B, Zmuda A, Hartwich J, Wozny E, Grzywacz M, Madej J, Gryglewska T (1981) Serum lipo-proteins, lipid peroxides and prostacyclin biosynthesis in patients with coronary heart disease. Prostaglandins 22: 795-8o7

16. Szczeklik A, Gryglewski RJ (198o) Low density lipoproteins (LDL) are carriers for lipid peroxides and inhibit prostacyclin ($PGI_2$) biosynthesis in arteries. Artery 7: 488-495

# 4.1 Platelet Aggregation and Phospholipid Metabolism

# Effects of Platelet-Derived Growth Factor on the Metabolism of Glycerolipids and Arachidonic Acid in Cultured Cells

A. J. R. Habenicht and J. A. Glomset

Platelets contain a mitogenic protein referred to as platelet-derived growth factor[+]. PDGF is released when blood clots and probably also upon injury to the vascular endothelium. It may act as a "wound healing hormone" by promoting the proliferation of connective tissue cells subjacent to a site of endothelial damage or denudation. It may also contribute to the proliferative response of arterial smooth muscle cells observed in atherosclerosis.

We have been interested in the mechanism by which PDGF initiates cell cycle traverse and have developed a model cell culture response system to study the biochemical changes in lipid metabolism that are induced by PDGF (1, 2). Arterial smooth muscle cells or Swiss 3T3 cells are allowed to become quiescent in culture in the presence of plasma-derived serum. Then PDGF is added to trigger cell cycle traverse. The Swiss 3T3 cell system offers the advantage that more than 95 % of the cells respond to the mitogen as compared with less than 2 % in the control cells as demonstrated by autoradiography.

Recently it has been demonstrated that arterial smooth muscle cells and Swiss 3T3 cells have high affinity receptors for PDGF (3). Upon binding of PDGF to the high affinity receptor a series of changes takes place. These changes resemble those that have been reported to occur in response to epidermal growth factor (4). One of the earliest changes is the phosphorylation of membrane bound proteins (5). We have focussed attention on another early change that involves the metabolism of membrane lipids including Pl and AA (6).

An early change in the metabolism of Pl and AA has been observed in a growing number of agonist-response systems (7). These systems are as varied as secretion, muscle contraction, and mitogenesis. Changes in these lipids during the response of platelets to thrombin have been studied particularly intensively (8 - 10) because of their possible involvement in prostaglandin formation. It has been thought for a number of years that the interaction of thrombin with platelets leads to activation of a phospholipase C that attacks Pl, generating DG, and that the DG is subsequently converted to PA and then back to Pl (see thick arrows in Fig. 1). However, alternate reaction sequences have recently been proposed (see dotted arrows in Fig. 1) (6, 8, 9 - 11, 14).

---

[+] Abbreviations: PDGF - Platelet-derived growth factor; Pl - phosphatidylinositol; DG - diacylglycerol; MG - monoacylglycerol; AA - arachidonic acid; TG - triacylglycerol; PC - phosphatidylcholine; PA - phosphatidic acid; lyso - denotes the respective lyso phospholipids

This work was supported by the Deutsche Forschungsgemeinschaft, FRG, and the Howard Hughes Medical Institute, National Institutes of Health Grants RR00166 and HL18645, R.J. Reynolds Industries, Inc., USA

The focus of controversy has been on the identity of the enzymes that are involved in PI metabolism and particularly on the identity of those enzymes that lead to the release of free arachidonic acid, a question of considerable potential physiological importance. So far no direct evidence has been presented for any one of the possible steps involved (Fig. 1).

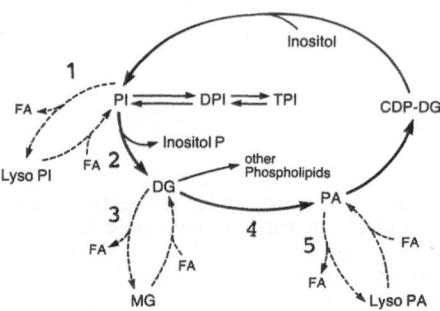

Fig. 1. Proposed mechanisms of PI turnover in different agonist response systems. Thick arrows denote the "classical PI cycle" (7). Dotted arrows denote alternate reactions involving AA hydrolysis and mechanisms of reacylation. CDP-DG: cytidinediphospho-diacylglycerol; DPI, TPI: phosphatidylinositolphosphate and phosphatidylinositoldiphosphate respectively, FA: fatty acid.
Reaction 1: PI specific phospholipase A$_2$ (11); reaction 2: PI specific phospholipase C (6); reaction 3: DG lipase (6, 9, 10); reaction 4: DG kinase (7); reaction 5: PA specific phospholipase A$_2$ (8)

We therefore decided to determine whether the interaction of PDGF with Swiss 3T3 cells induced changes in PI metabolism that are similar to those observed in other systems. Moreover, it seemed critical to isolate the presumed intermediates to obtain evidence--in intact cell experiments--for the molecular events involved. As can be seen in Fig. 2 PDGF induces an early degradation of PI without changing the concentration of lyso PI.

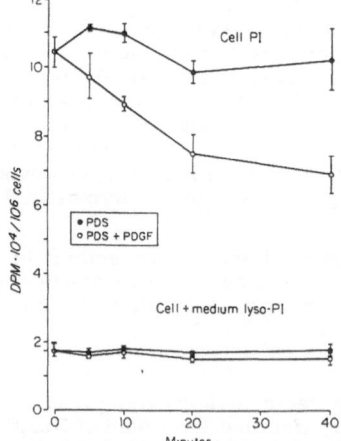

Fig. 2. Effect of platelet-derived growth factor on radioactivity in phosphatidylinositol and lysophosphatidylinositol in Swiss 3T3 cells biosynthetically prelabeled with [³H]myo-inositol (6)

The decrement in Pl becomes measurable within 2 - 5 minutes, and is associated with a transient rise in cell DG (Fig. 3).

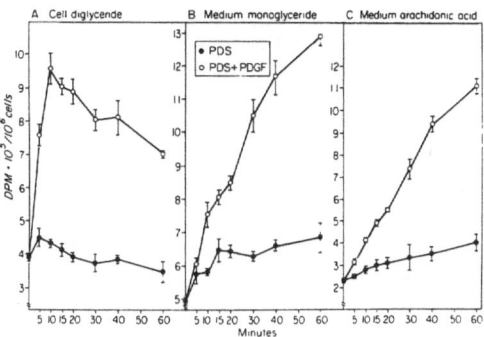

<u>Fig. 3.</u> Kinetics of diacylglycerol formation, monoacylglycerol release, and arachidonic acid release within 60 min. in Swiss 3T3 cells biosynthetically prelabeled with $\left[^{3}H\right]$ glycerol and $\left[^{14}C\right]$ arachidonic acid (6)

The rise in cell DG is detectable within one minute and continues for 10 minutes. Thereafter, cell DG declines. The decline in DG seems to depend at least partially on hydrolysis since PDGF markedly stimulates the generation of MG (Fig. 3), and also stimulates a nearly linear accumulation of AA (Fig. 3). Thus, PDGF seems to stimulate successive action of a phospholipase C and a DG lipase. This interpretation is strengthened by the results shown in Table 1.

<u>Table 1.</u> Radioactivity of various phospholipids, triacylglycerol, diacylglycerol and monoacylglycerol 20 min. after addition of platelet-derived growth factor to Swiss 3T3 cells biosynthetically prelabeled with $\left[^{14}C\right]$ arachidonic acid

| Lipid | Control | PDGF | p value |
|---|---|---|---|
| | \multicolumn{2}{c|}{dpm x $10^4/10^6$ cells} | |
| Pl | 13.8 + 0.7 | 9.4 + 0.8 | < 0.001 |
| DG | 1.7 + 0.1 | 3.1 + 0.4 | < 0.005 |
| MG | 0.5 + 0.1 | 1.1 + 0.1 | < 0.001 |
| CDP-DG | 1.2 + 0.1 | 1.2 + 0.1 | N.S. |
| Free fatty acid | 2.9 + 0.1 | 5.2 + 0.5 | < 0.005 |
| TG | 2.4 + 0.1 | 2.4 + 0.2 | N.S. |
| PC | 21.5 + 1.5 | 22.2 + 2.4 | N.S. |
| PE | 19.3 + 0.8 | 20.2 + 1.5 | N.S. |

They demonstrate that addition of PDGF to AA prelabeled cells leads to a decrease in labeled Pl that corresponds very closely to an increase in radioactivity in DG, MG, and free AA. Furthermore, no major changes occur in TG and PC. Since PDGF not only stimulates the incorporation of myoinositol into Pl but also the incorporation of AA and free glycerol into this lipid, more than simply the reutilization of DG must have been involved (Fig. 1).

A major question that remains to be answered in our system is whether the MG generated in our cells is reutilized for PI synthesis. There is little evidence for or against
such a pathway in the literature. However, we have recently obtained preliminary
evidence that a MG phospholipid pathway indeed exists. We therefore suggest that
PDGF stimulates the successive action of phospholipase C and diglyceride lipase generating DG + MG + AA and that the MG is reincorporated into cell lipids by an acyl-
CoA-MG acyltransferase (see reaction 3 in Fig. 1 and Fig. 4).

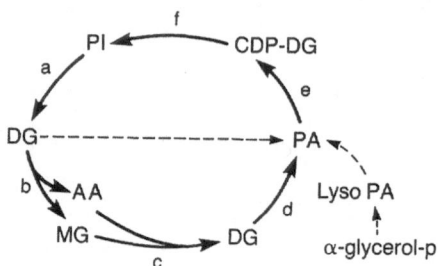

Fig. 4. Possible mechanism of PI turnover in Swiss 3T3 cells stimulated by PDGF.
Letters denote enzymes involved: a) PI specific phospholipase C; b) DG lipase;
c) MG acyltransferase; d) DG kinase; e) PA cytidinediphosphotransferase;
f) cytidinediphosphodiacylglycerol-inositoltransferase. Dotted lines denote pathways not investigated in this study

Although there appears to be resynthesis of PI from MG it is not clear whether other
pathways, including the $\alpha$-glycerolphosphate pathway, also contribute to resynthesis
of PI in PDGF stimulated cells (see Fig. 4). The regulation of the DG lipase-MG acyltransferase pathway would contribute to the amount of free AA in these cells. This
pathway therefore would regulate the availability of AA to cyclooxygenase and lipoxygenase (12, 14), generating a number of biologically extremely active derivatives
of AA.

The DG generated by the phospholipase C reaction and the DG generated by the MG
acyltransferase reaction might be localized at different sites within the cell or within
the affected membrane. This would provide a means to separately regulate DG hydrolysis and DG synthesis. Another question of interest relates to the mechanism of acti-
vation/inactivation of the various enzymes involved in PI turnover (13). Finally the
significance of the dramatic changes in membrane lipids of PDGF-stimulated cells for
cell cycle traverse remains to be investigated.

References

1. Habenicht AJR, Glomset JA, Ross R (1980) J Biol Chem 255: 5134–5140
2. Schmidt RA, Glomset JA, Wight TN, Habenicht AJR, Ross R (1982) J Cell
   Biol, in press
3. Bowen-Pope D, Ross R (1982) J Biol Chem 257, in press
4. Carpenter G, King L, Jr, Cohen S (1979) J Biol Chem 254: 4884–4891
5. Ek B, Westermark B, Wasteson Å, Heldin CH (1982) Nature 295: 419–420
6. Habenicht AJR, Glomset JA, King WC, Nist C, Mitchell CD, Ross R (1981) J Biol
   Chem 256: 12329–12335
7. Irvine RF, Dawson, RMC, Freinkel N (1981) In: Contemporary Metabolism,
   Freinkel N (ed) Vol. 2, in press
8. Lapetina EG, Billah MM, Cuatrecasas P (1981) J Biol Chem 256: 11984–11987

9. Bell RL, Majerus PW (1980) J Biol Chem 255: 1790-1792
10. Rittenhouse-Simmons S (1980) J Biol Chem 255: 2259-2262
11. Hong SL, Deykin O (1981) J Biol Chem 256: 5215-5219
12. Coughlin SR, Moskowitz MA, Zetter BR, Antoniades HN, Levine L (1980) Nature 288: 600-602
13. Kishimoto A, Takai Y, Mori T, Kikkawa U, Nishizuka Y (1980) J Biol Chem 255: 2273-2276
14. Rittenhouse-Simmons S, Deykin O (1981) In: Platelets in Biology and Pathology-2, Gordon (ed) Elsevier/North-Holland Biomedical Press, 349-372

# The Phosphatidylinositol Response and the Activation of Platelets

E. G. Lapedina, M. M. Billah, and P. Cuatrecasas

## A. Introduction

Several platelet stimuli, such as thrombin (1), ADP (2), collagen (3), platelet-activating factor (4) or ionophore A23187 (1), activate the degradation of phosphatidylinositol by a specific phospholipase C activity, initiating in this way the "phosphatidylinositol-cycle" (Fig 1). This response occurs very early during stimulation, is highly sensitive to low levels of agonists and is suggestive of a crucial role in the initial phases of platelet activation. The phosphatidylinositol response could be achieved by the mobilization of intracellular $Ca^{2+}$ with low concentration of the ionophore A23187 (100 nM) (5) and by the interaction of specific agonists with their platelet receptors (1,5). Phosphatidylinositol (as well as phosphatidylcholine or phosphatidylethanolamine) could also subsequently be degraded by phospholipase $A_2$ activity and contribute in this way to the liberation of arachidonic acid (6).

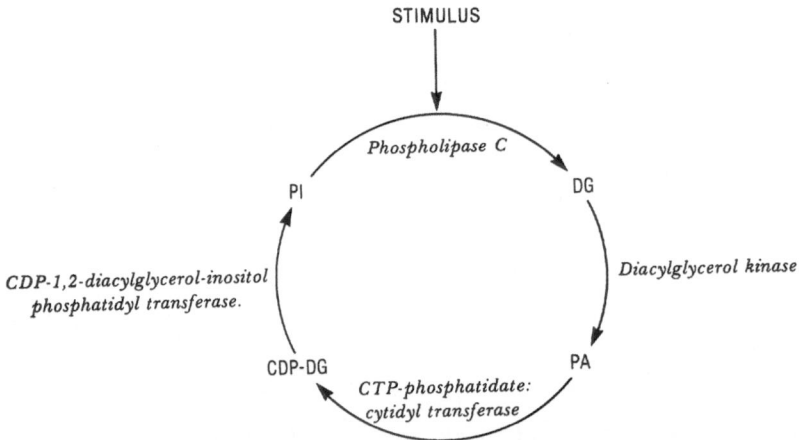

Fig. 1. The phosphatidylinositol cycle. Stimulation of platelets induces the initial degradation of phosphatidylinositol (PI) by the stimulation of a phosphatidylinositol-specific phospholipase C. This degradation of PI leads to the formation of 1,2-diacylglycerol (DG) which is phosphorylated to phosphatidic acid (PA) by the action of 1,2-diacylglycerol kinase. PA could be further transformed to CDP-diacylglycerol (CDP-DG) by CTP-phosphatidate:cytidyl transferase and, finally, to PI by the action of CDP-1,2-diacylglycerol-inositol phosphatidyl transferase

## I - Stimulation of the Phosphatidylinositol Cycle

Platelet-activating factor stimulates the phosphatidylinositol cycle (Fig 1,2) in a similar way as has previously been reported for (4) thrombin (1), collagen (3) and ionophore A23187 (1). There is a rapid degradation of [$^{32}$P]phosphatidylino- sitol and the concomitant appearance of [$^{32}$P]phosphatidic acid. Phosphatidic acid is then decreased as a consequence of its conversion to phosphatidylinositol as shown by a considerable increase of [$^{32}$P]phosphatidylinositol (Fig 2).

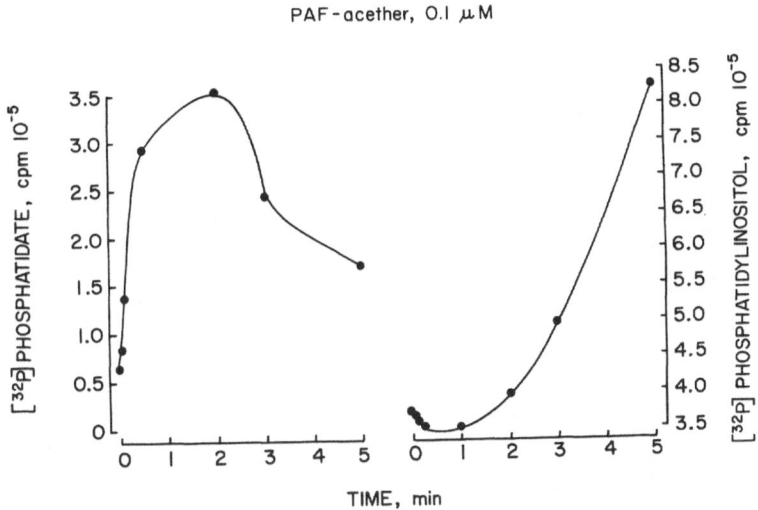

Fig. 2. Platelet-activating factor stimulates the phosphatidylinositol cycle in platelets. Platelets prelabeled with ($^{32}$P)orthophosphate were exposed to PAF-acether (0.1 µM) for different periods of time as indicated and the $^{32}$P-radioactivity in phosphatidic acid and phosphatidylinositol was determined. Details as in reference 4

## II - Receptor-Linked or Ca$^{2+}$-Mediated Degradation of Phosphatidylinositol by Phospholipase C

Thrombin and ionophore A23187 also stimulate the phosphatidylinositol-specific phospholipase C as reflected by the appearance of phosphatidic acid (Fig 3) (1). However, ionophore A23187 is 5-6 times less effective in producing phosphatidic acid than thrombin. It indicates that the mobilization of Ca$^{2+}$ alone is not a sufficient trigger to cause the maximal degradation of phosphatidylinositol by the phospholipase C pathway. Moreover, the addition of thrombin to platelets previously treated with ionophore A23187, still induces a further degradation of phosphatidyl- inositol through the phospholipase C pathway and produces an equivalent amount of phosphatidic acid. These results suggest the existence of an ionophore A23187- insensitive fraction of phosphatidylinositol whose degradation by phospholipase C requires the interaction of thrombin with its receptor. In this regard, a recent study, which combines the use of hirudin and thrombin, has suggested that the continuous occupation of thrombin receptors is essential for the accumulation of phosphatidic acid (7). Phosphatidic acid possesses ionophoretic properties (1,4,6) and its accumulation may, therefore, be involved in the process of amplification of Ca$^{2+}$-mobilization and the release of arachidonic acid from membrane phospholipids (6).

686

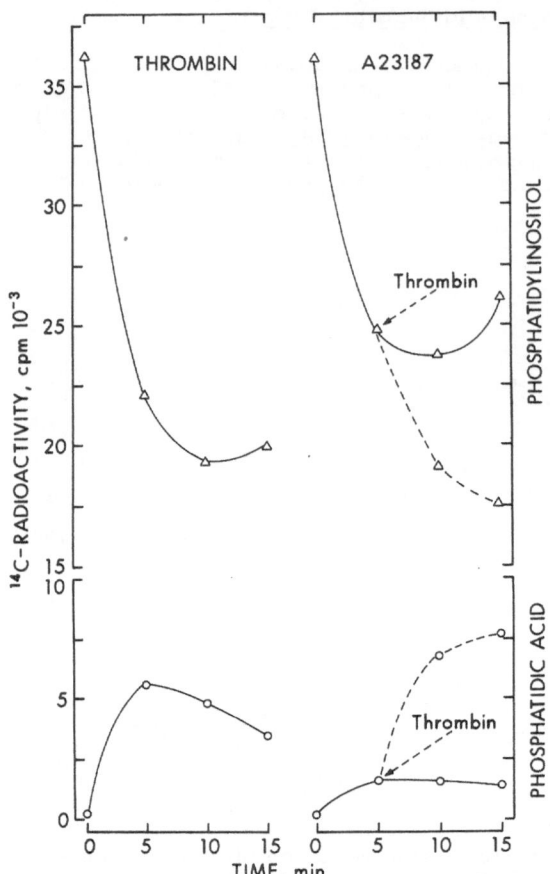

Fig. 3. Degradation of phosphatidylinositol and formation of phosphatidic acid induced by thrombin and ionophore A23187. Platelets prelabeled with [$^{14}$C]arachidonic acid were incubated with thrombin (1 unit/ml) or with ionophore A23187 (10 μM) for different times as indicated. Arrows and broken lines indicate assays in which thrombin (1 units/ml) was added to platelets after these had been incubated for 5 min with ionophore A23187. These concentrations of thrombin and ionophore A23187 produced maximal release of [$^{14}$C]arachidonic acid. Details as in reference 1

### III - Formation of Phosphatidic acid is associated with the release of serotonin

The release of serotonin in stimulated platelets could occur independently of phospholipase $A_2$ activity and of the products of the cyclooxygenase or lipoxygenase pathways (Fig 4). Trifluoperazine, an inhibitor of phospholipases of the $A_2$-type, will abolish the release of arachidonic acid from platelet phospholipids, but will not block the release of serotonin induced by platelet-activating factor (Fig 4). Trifluoperazine, however, does not affect the stimulation by platelet-activating factor of the phosphatidylinositol-cycle, in which phosphatidic acid is an obligatory intermediate (Figs 1,4). The relationship between the formation of phosphatidic acid and the release of serotonin might be based on two important actions of phosphatidic acid. It induces calcium mobilization in platelets and other systems and it is a potent fusogenic agent at low concentration of $Ca^{2+}$ (4).

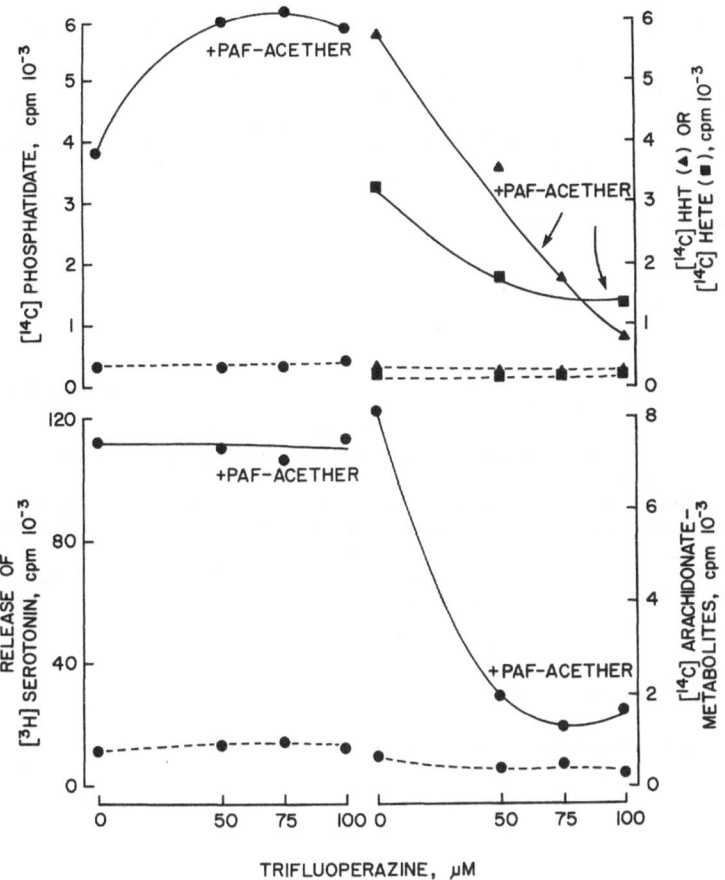

**Fig. 4.** Effect of trifluoperazine on the platelet-activating factor (PAF-acether) induced release of serotonin, arachidonate metabolites and the formation of phosphatidic acid, cyclooxygenase (HHT) and lipoxygenase (HETE) metabolites. Platelets prelabeled with [$^{14}$C]arachidonic acid and [$^3$H]serotonin were preincubated with different concentrations of trifluoperazine for 5 min at 37°C and then with PAF-acether (0.1 µM) for 1 min. The release of [$^3$H]serotonin and [$^{14}$C]arachidonic acid plus [$^{14}$C]arachidonate metabolites was determined in the experiments shown in the lower panels. Formation of phosphatidic acid, 12-L-hydroxy-5,8,10-heptade-catrienoic acid (HHT) and 12-L-hydroxy-5,8,10,14-eicosatetraenoic acid (HETE) was measured in the experiments shown in the upper panels. Broken lines refer to experiments having only trifluoperazine. Other details as in reference 4

## B.  Concluding Remarks

The differential effects of ionophore A23187 and thrombin in platelets allows the identification of different metabolic pools of phosphatidylinositol. A minor fraction of phosphatidylinositol is sensitive to a small rise of cytosolic $Ca^{2+}$, and it is recycled via the phosphatidylinositol cycle. Degradation by phospholipase C of another, quantitatively major, fraction of phosphatidylinositol leads to the accumulation of phosphatidic acid and requires continuous occupation of receptors.

A third fraction of phosphatidylinositol is subsequently degraded by phospholipase $A_2$. This phospholipase $A_2$ activity, in addition to phospholipase $A_2$-degradation of phosphatidylcholine, phosphatidylethanolanine and phosphatidic acid, account for the liberation of arachidonic acid in stimulated platelets.

The information indicates that the stimulation of the phosphatidylinositol-cycle in platelets is a general response to agonists such as thrombin, ionophore A23187, platelet activating factor, collagen and ADP and may be a fundamental step in the initial chain of reactions related to platelet responses.

References

1.  Lapetina, EG, Billah, MM, Cuatrecasas, P (1981) The initial action of thrombin on platelets. Conversion of phosphatidylinositol to phosphatidic acid preceding the production of arachidonic acid. J Biol Chem 256:5037-5040
2.  Lloyd, JV, Mustard, JF (1974) Changes in $^{32}$P-Content of phosphatidic acid and the phosphoinositides of rabbit platelets during aggregation induced by collagen or thrombin. Br J Haematol 26:243-253
3.  Broekman, MJ, Ward, JW, Marcus, AJ (1980) Phospholipid metabolism in stimulated human platelets. Changes in phosphatidylinositol, phosphatidic acid, and lysophospholipids. J Clin Invest 66:275-283
4.  Lapetina, EG (1982) Platelet-activating factor stimulates the phosphatidylinositol cycle. Appearance of phosphatidic acid is associated with the release of serotonin in horse platelets. J Biol Chem 257:7314-7317
5.  Billah, MM, Lapetina, EG (1982) Evidence for multiple metabolic pools of phosphatidylinositol in stimulated platelets. J Biol Chem, in press.
6.  Lapetina, EG (1982) Regulation of Arachidonic acid production: role of phospholipases C and $A_2$. Trends Pharmacol Sci 3:115-118
7.  Holmsen, H, Dangelmaier, CA, Holmsen, H-K (1981) Thrombin-induced platelet responses differ in requirement for receptor occupancy. Evidence for tight coupling of occupancy and compartmentalized phosphatidic acid formation. J Biol Chem 256:9393-9396.

# Platelet Phospholipid Fatty Acids and Platelet Aggregation

S. Renaud, L. McGregor, D. Blache, and M. Lagarde

## A. Introduction

The intake of saturated fats appear to be one of the main risk factors
for coronary heart disease (CHD). In addition to increase serum lipids
and to induce atherosclerosis, saturated fats markedly enhance certain
platelet functions and thereby, predispose to thrombosis (1,2). By contrast, linoleic and linolenic acids, the main dietary polyunsaturated
fatty acids, are known for their hypolipidemic effects, but also, appear
to inhibit the effects of saturated fats on platelet functions (1,2).

Changes in the dietary fatty acids are known to be responsible for
changes in the composition of the platelet phospholipids (3,4). Moreover,
platelet phospholipids are involved in most of the platelet functions by
providing
- a surface for the enzymatic process of clotting, this activity being
frequently referred to platelet factor 3 (a lipoprotein surface) (5).
- arachidonic acid, the precursor of endoperoxides and thromboxane responsible for platelet aggregation (5). Thus, the modification in the
platelet phospholipid fatty acids induced by diet, may play a role in
observed changes in platelet function and eventually, in CHD.

## I - Essential fatty acid (EFA) deficiency and platelet functions

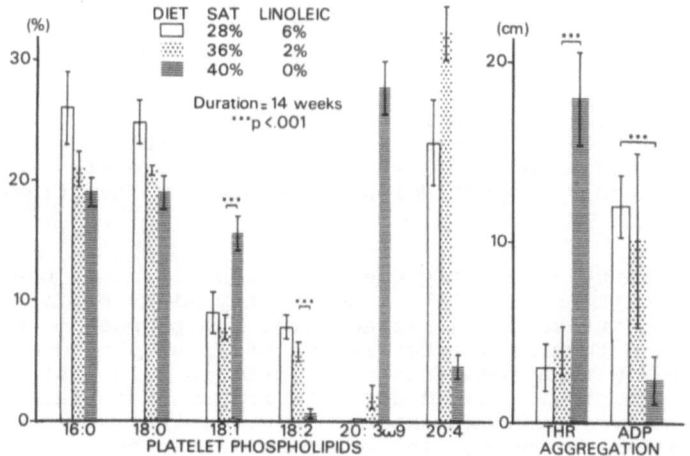

Fig. 1. Fatty acid composition of total platelet phospholipids and
platelet aggregation in EFA deficient rats (linoleic acid 0%) as
compared to rats fed 2 and 6% linoleic acid. Adapted from reference
6 by permission of Thrombosis Research

690

EFA deficiency can be induced in a few weeks (Fig. 1) in rat fed a
purified diet containing trace amounts of linoleic acid, but 40 % in
weight of a saturated fat such as hydrogenated coconut oil. Under
these conditions, the deficiency is not severe enough to cause hemorrhagic renal necrosis and death. However, in platelet rich plasma
(PRP) of these animals, as compared to rats fed 2 or 6 % linoleic
acid, a highly significant (p<.001) increase in the response of platelets to aggregation by thrombin is observed (Fig. 1) (6). Increasing
linoleic acid from 2 to 6 %, does not improve much the platelet response. By contrast, the aggregation of platelets to ADP is markedly
inhibited in the EFA deficient animals.

In the platelet phospholipids, the enormous increase in 20:3ω9 at the
expense of 20:4ω6, known to occur in EFA deficient rat (7), might possibly explain the differences in the response of platelets. However,
it remains to determine the mechanisms involved since 20:3ω9 does not
appear to be a substrate for cyclooxygenase (8).

II - Saturated fats and platelet aggregation in rat

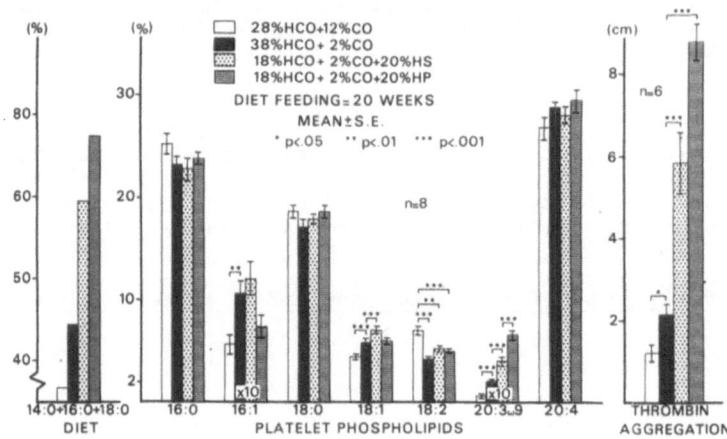

Fig. 2. Fatty acid composition of total platelet phospholipids and
platelet aggregation to thrombin in rats fed increased amounts of saturated (14:0+16:0+18:0) fatty acids. HCO=Hydrogenated Coconut Oil.
CO=Corn Oil. HS=Hydrogenated Sunflower oil. HP=Hydrogenated Palm oil.
Adapted from reference 9 by permission of Laboratory Investigation

Definite EFA deficiency apparently does not occur in adult Western
human populations although a relative deficiency might be feasible in
relation to a high intake of saturated fats. The purpose of our study
in rats (9) was to determine whether increased amounts of dietary saturated fatty acids with a same intake of linoleic acid (1%) sufficient
to prevent EFA deficiency, would modify the response of platelets to
thrombin-induced aggregation. As shown in Fig. 2, the increase in the
response of platelets to aggregation was parallel to the level of the
dietary saturated fatty acids. In the platelet phospholipids, the only
fatty acid which runned parallel to both aggregation and the intake of
saturated fats was 20:3ω9, the fatty acid specifically increased in EFA
deficiency as observed in animals of Fig. 1.

## III - Dietary fats, platelet functions and phospholipid composition in man

Recently, we have reported preliminary results (10,11) of our studies in European farmers, on the relationship between dietary components and platelet functions. Hereafter, are shown the correlations obtained in the 250 male farmers from France and Great Britain, studied in 1977-78. It can be seen in Table 1 that the dietary saturated fatty acids were not correlated with 16:0 or 18:0 in the platelet phospholipids but rather with 20:3ω9, a result corresponding to this reported in Fig. 2. In the diet, 18:3 but mostly 18:2, were significantly inversely correlated with 20:3ω9 in the phospholipids. This confirms the inhibitory effect of the EFA on the level of 20:3ω9 as shown by other investigators in animals (7). Dietary 18:2 was not positively correlated with 20:4ω6 in the phospholipids, but rather with 18:2, and 18:0 (as observed in man on diet enriched in EFA) (4), as well as with 22:4ω6.

Table 1. Univariate correlations (r) between dietary and platelet phospholipid fatty acids in 250 male farmers

| DIET | PLATELET PHOSPHOLIPIDS | | | | | |
|------|------|------|------|------------|------------|------------|
| | 16:0 | 18:0 | 18:2 | 20:3 (ω9) | 20:4 (ω6) | 22:4 (ω6) |
| SAT | -.05 | .11 | ***-.22 | ***.28 | .02 | ***-.39 |
| 18:3 | -.07 | *.13 | ***.28 | *-.15 | .04 | -.05 |
| 18:2 | .10 | ***.29 | ***.52 | ***-.35 | *-.12 | ***.35 |

*p<.05          ***p<.001

SAT = Saturated Fatty Acids (14:0 + 16:0 + 18:0). Diet evaluation was done by chemical analysis of the duplicate portion of a 24 hour period (10). Fatty acid analysis of diet and platelet total phospholipids s were performed as previously reported (10) by GLC, but with 12 foot glass columns packed with 8 % Supelco 2340 on 100/120 chromosorb W-AW and temperature programming 135°-230°C, 2°/min.

Concerning the platelet functions, it is shown in Table 2 that only the clotting activity of platelets ($F_3$-CT) and the thrombin-induced aggregation were significantly correlated with the intake of saturated fats, as was serum cholesterol. The dietary EFA were inversely correlated with the $F_3$-CT and thrombin induced aggregation, but not with the aggregation induced by collagen or ADP. Only 18:2 in the diet was inversely correlated with serum cholesterol. By contrast, 18:2 and 18:3 were positively correlated with ADP-induced aggregation, a result similar to this we observed in rats under the conditions of Fig. 1.

The relationship between the platelet phospholipid fatty acids and some platelet function tests are reported in Table 3. Of interest might be the opposite correlations with 18:2 and 20:3ω9. Similarly, the significant correlation of 20:3ω9, positive with thrombin aggregation (and $F_3$-CT), negative with ADP and opposite results with 18:2 are also concordant with those of Figs 1 and 2.

692

Table 2. Univariate correlation (r) between dietary fatty acids and blood parameters in 250 male farmers

| | PLATELET FUNCTIONS | | | | SERUM |
|---|---|---|---|---|---|
| DIET | $F_3$-CT | THR | ADP | COLL | Chol |
| SAT | .35*** | .21*** | -.14* | .07 | .25*** |
| 18:3 | -.27*** | -.34*** | .21*** | .03 | .00 |
| 18:2 | -.23*** | -.13* | .23*** | .06 | -.35*** |

*p<.05       ***p<.001

Diet evaluation as in Fig. 1. Platelet function tests and serum cholesterol (Chol) were determined as in previous studies (10). Clotting activity of platelets ($F_3$-CT). Platelet aggregation to thrombin (THR), ADP, collagen (COLL), epinephrine (EPI).

Table 3. Univariate correlation (r) between platelet phospholipid fatty acids

| | PLATELET PHOSPHOLIPIDS | | | | | |
|---|---|---|---|---|---|---|
| FUNCTION | 16:0 | 18:0 | 18:2 | 20:3 ($\omega$9) | 20:4 ($\omega$6) | 22:4 ($\omega$6) |
| $F_3$-CT | .08 | .11 | -.18** | .29*** | -.09 | -.12* |
| THR | .11 | -.04 | -.08 | .17** | -.01 | .07 |
| ADP | -.09 | -.04 | .13* | -.13* | .02 | .10 |
| COLL | .07 | .17** | .20*** | -.07 | -.04 | -.01 |

*p<.05       **p<.01       ***p<.001
Abbreviations as in Tables 1 and 2

IV - Incorporation of fatty acids into platelet phospholipids

To determine whether 20:3$\omega$9 and 18:2 in the platelet phospholipids are really responsible for the opposite effects observed on platelet functions, these fatty acids, previously bound to albumin by incubation with incomplete Tyrode containing albumin (3.5 g/l) were incorporated into human platelets collected with ACD. After 2 hours incubation at 37°C, the platelet suspension was acidified (pH = 6.4), centrifuged and resuspended in Tyrode (without calcium) containing gelatin at pH = 7.4. Platelet aggregation was studied in the platelet suspension while fatty acid composition of the phospholipids was determined on an aliquot of platelets. The results indicate that 20:3$\omega$9 increased the response of platelets to thrombin, but decreased this to ADP and to collagen. Opposite effects were observed with 18:2. It seems that the mechanism of the effect of 20:3$\omega$9 is through the lipoxygenase pathway.

## B. Concluding Remarks

The dietary fats known for their predisposing (saturated) or preventive (polyunsaturated) effects on CHD, induce significant modifications in certain platelet phospholipid fatty acids, both in man and
in animals. Those changes in the platelet phospholipids appear to be
responsible for drastic modifications in platelet functions which may
significantly contribute to the susceptibility of populations to
thrombosis and CHD.

*Acknowledgments*  We are greatly indebted to J.L. Martin (CNRS, LP 5440)
for his competent statistical evaluation of the data obtained in farmers, and to R. Morazain, E. Dumont, C. Thevenon, C. Covacho for their
skillful participation to the studies mentioned here.

## References

1. Renaud S, Gautheron P (1973) Dietary fats and experimental (cardiac
   and venous) thrombosis. Haemostasis 2:53-72
2. Hornstra G (1973) Dietary fats and arterial thrombosis. Haemostasis
   2:21-52
3. Gautheron P, Renaud S (1972) Hyperlipemia induced hypercoagulable
   state in rat. Role of an increased activity of platelet phosphatidyl serine in response to certain dietary fatty acids. Thromb Res
   1:353-370
4. Jakubowski JA, Ardlie NG (1978) Modification of human platelet
   function by a diet enriched in saturated or polyunsaturated fat.
   Atherosclerosis 31:335-344
5. Marcus AJ (1978) The role of lipids in platelet function : with
   particular reference to the arachidonic acid pathway. J Lip Res 19:
   793-826
6. McGregor L, Renaud S (1978) Effect of dietary linoleic acid deficiency on platelet aggregation and phospholipid fatty acids of
   rats. Thromb Res 12:921-927
7. Holman RT (1960) The ratio of trienoic-tetranoic acids in tissue
   lipids as a measure of essential fatty acid requirement. J Nutr 70:
   405-410
8. Raz A, Minkes M, Needleman P (1977) Endoperoxides and thromboxanes:
   structural determinants for platelet aggregation and vasoconstriction. Biochim Biophys Acta 488:305-311
9. McGregor L, Morazain R, Renaud S (1980) A comparison of the effects
   of dietary short and long chain saturated fatty acids on platelet
   functions, platelet phospholipids and blood coagulation in rats.
   Lab Invest 43:438-442
10. Renaud S, Morazain R, Godsey F, Dumont E, Symington IS, Gillanders
    EM and O'Brien JR (1981) Platelet functions in relation to diet
    and serum lipids in British farmers. Brit Heart J 46:562-570
11. Renaud S, Dumont E, Godsey F, MacGregor L, Morazain R (1981) Ef-
    fects of diet on blood clotting and platelet aggregation. In:
    Nutrition in the 1980's. Selvey N, White PL (eds), NY, Alan R Liss
    Inc, p 361

# Regulatory Function of the Cellular Thiol-Disulfide Status in the Metabolic Control of Human Blood Platelet Aggregation

U. Till, P. Arese, A. Bosia, B. Hofmann, J. Hofmann, W. Lösche, G. P. Pescarmona, P. Spangenberg, and K. Thielmann

The participation of blood platelets in physiological and pathological events is necessarily preceeded by an activation of the respective cells apparent in the changing of the shape, increasing adhe-
sivenes, aggregation and release. The underlying metabolic reaction
sequences, as well as the changes in structural components, are not
completely understood. The results obtained previously caused us to
think about the possible existence of a regulatory function played
by the cellular levels of reduced glutathione (GSH) and NADPH in the
activation process:
- During the platelet aggregation induced by arachidonic acid (AA),
the cellular levels of both compounds fall rapidly off in the initial
phase, being subsequently normalized by a powerful stimulation of
the hexose monophosphate shunt (HMPS) (1).
- Diminished capacity of the HMPS in platelets genetically deficient
in glucose-6-phosphate dehydrogenase is accompanied by decreased
levels of both compounds and by altered platelet aggregation (2).
- When compounds causing a fast, but reversible fall in platelet GSH
and different aggregation inducers are simultaneously added to platelet rich plasma (PRP), the aggregation trace is influenced in two
ways: (i) accelerated aggregation followed by (ii) a complete deaggregation of these cells, which would otherwise irreversibly aggregate.
Preincubation with the GSH depleting compounds causes the deaggrega-
ting effect or leads to a lack of response to the inducer (3-5, Fig.5).

Different metabolic systems and structural components involved in
the process of platelet activation are tested in regard to their possible contribution to sulfhydryl/disulfide (SH/SS) related changes
in the activation. Diamide (azodicarboxylicacid-bis-dimethylamide)
was choosen to induce perturbation of the platelet SH/SS status by
oxidizing GSH to GSSG (Fig. 1).

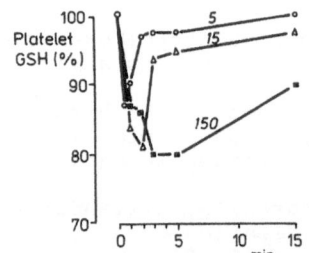

Fig. 1. Time course of platelet GSH
level after addition of diamide (concentrations in µM as indicated beside the
curves) to PRP in concentrations known
to influence platelet aggregation (3)

## Morphology of platelet aggregates

The morphological feature of aggregates after full scale aggregation
in PRP shows striking differences between irreversible and diamide
mediated reversible aggregation (Fig. 2). After irreversible aggregation the single cells are no longer demarcable. The aggregates are
surrounded by loop-like or vesicular structures, respectively, which
probably arise from fusionated plasma membranes. During diamide mediated reversible aggregation at the point of maximum aggregation all
characteristics of cell fusion are completely lacking. The same morphological differences between both types of aggregation are also

obtained with different aggregation stimuli. The results point to a suppression of fusiogenic events in platelet membranes caused by diminished cellular GSH levels.

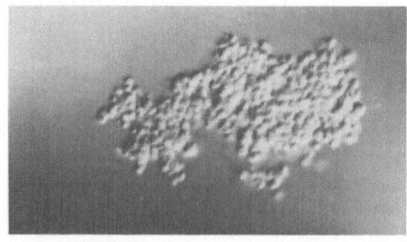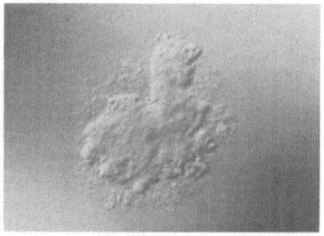

Fig. 2. Interference contrast microscopical pictures of platelet aggregation in PRP induced by 1 mM AA = irreversible aggregation (left side), and by 1 mM AA plus 100 μM diamide = reversible aggregation (right side). The photographs were taken at the point of maximum aggregation. Original magnification: 500 x

## Nucleotides

As shown in Fig. 3 the time course in the levels of both cAMP and cGMP during platelet aggregation can not be used to explain the differences between irreversible and diamide mediated reversible aggregation. The same holds true for changes in the pattern of adenine and related nucleotides (metabolic pool). As, at least during the first minute, the changes are very similar in both types of aggregation, an insufficient energy supply does not seem to be a valid reason for the switch to deaggregation.

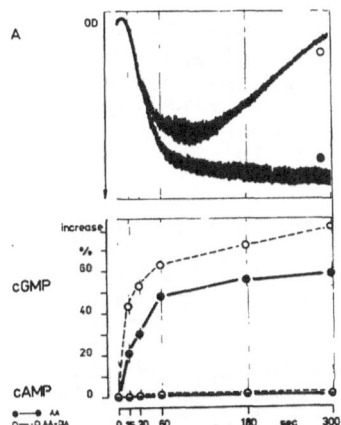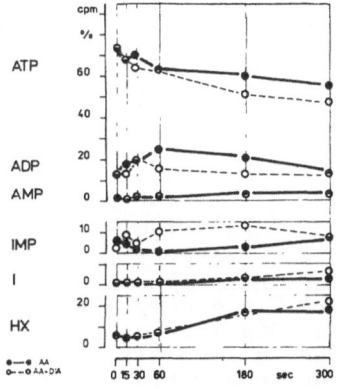

Fig. 3. Time course of cellular levels of cAMP and cGMP during irreversible aggregation induced by 1 mM AA and reversible aggregation induced by 1 mM AA plus 100 μM diamide, respectively, in PRP. Corresponding aggregation traces are given in the upper part
Fig. 4. Changes in the levels of compounds included in the metabolic pool of adenine nuleotides during irreversible and reversible aggregation, respectively. The same conditions as given in Fig. 3 are used. Percents of total radioactivity after prelabelling with 14C-adenine are plotted. I=inosine, HX=hypoxanthine

## Platelet proteins

The diamide mediated perturbation of platelet GSH level and the altered aggregation, also depending on the incubation time and the employed concentration of diamide, is accompanied by a formation of platelet protein polymers.

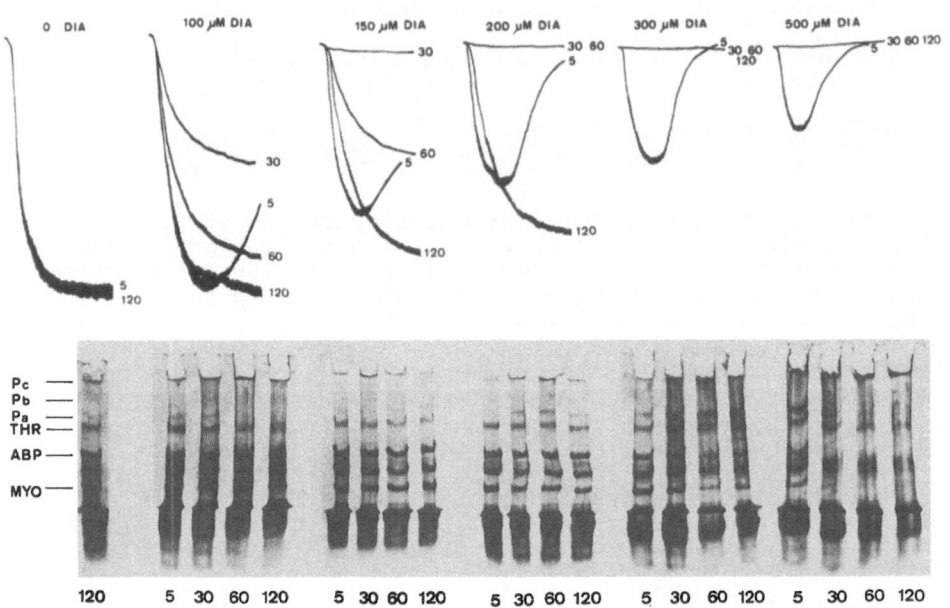

Fig. 5. Diamide mediated changes in the pattern of platelet proteins depending on concentration and incubation time (min), resp., as indicated. SDS polyacrylamide electrophoresis was performed with 3.5 % polyacrylamide plus 0.3 % agarose. MYO=myosin, ABP=actin binding protein, THR=thrombin sensitive protein, Pa-Pc=newly formed polymers. Corresponding aggregation traces at 5 $\mu$M ADP are given in the upper part

The presence of disulfide linkages in the polymers is indicated by their cancellation with dithiothreitol (not shown). The switch from irreversible to reversible aggregation is mainly connected with the occurence of the polymer Pa, whereas a further polymerization (Pb, Pc) is linked to a complete inhibition of aggregation. After some time, at low diamide concentrations, the protein polymerization is reversed, and a recovery of irreversible aggregation appears, most probably due to a restoration of the GSH level through an activation of the HMPS. Proteins involved in the polymer formation are mainly the actin binding protein and myosin, which disappear at high diamide concentrations. Preliminary results from two-dimensional electrophoresis under reduced conditions in the second dimension confirm this suggestion. Glycoproteins were proved to be excluded from the polymerization .

## AA metabolism

Metabolization of AA in the cyclooxygenase (CO) and lipoxygenase (LO) pathway is involved in the reaction sequence leading to platelet activation. As CO is known to be activated by an oxidation of its SH-groups (6), a decrease in cellular GSH level should speed up the formation of thromboxane (TX) A2 – a very potent stimulator of platelet aggregation. This idea is in accordance with an accelerated aggregation and malondialdehyde formation observed by simultaneous administration of diamide and low dosis of aggregation inducers (3). The diamide mediated deaggregation, however, is not stimulated by CO products, because the inhibition of CO with aspirin does not prevent the deaggregation phenomenon (Fig. 6).

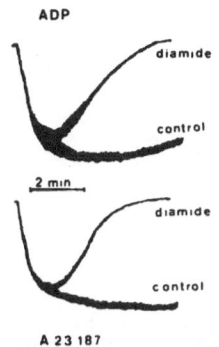

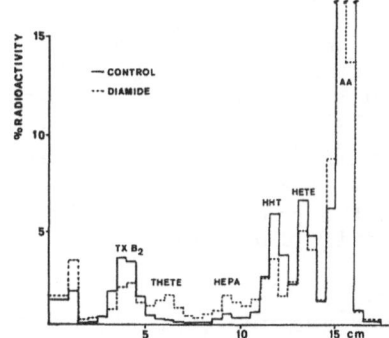

Fig. 6. Aggregation in PRP induced by 10 uM ADP or 5 uM A 23 187, resp., with or without simultaneous addition of 100 uM diamide after preincubation with o.4 M aspirin

Fig. 7. Pattern of AA metabolites in saline suspended platelets after 10 min incubation with or without 500 uM diamide followed by 10 min incubation with 160 uM 14C-AA. TLC according to BRYANT & BAILEY (7)

In the LO pathway GSH is consumed in the conversion of 12-hydroperoxy-eicosatetraenoic acid (HPETE) to the corresponding hydroxide (HETE) (7). In accordance with BRYANT & BAILEY's previous results, the incubation of platelets with diamide results in a diminished formation of HETE from exogenous AA, and the occurence of newly formed compounds: trihydroxy-eicosatrienoic acid (THETE) and hydroxy-epoxy-eicosatetraenoic acid (HEPA), which probably arise from accumulated HPETE (Fig. 7). It was discussed by WILSON et al. (9) that HPETE can bind itself to cell membrane structures and thereby influence cell activation. More direct evidence of a possible contribution of LO products in triggering the diamide mediated deaggregation derives from a simple experimental set-up: It was shown by PORTER et al. (10) that non-enzymic oxidation of AA with air oxygen leads to the formation of different hydroperoxides similar to those formed by LO. Applying air-oxidized AA (about 30 % oxidation) to PRP brings about the same accelerated aggregation and deaggregation as found with the combined addition of non-oxidized AA plus diamide (Fig. 8).

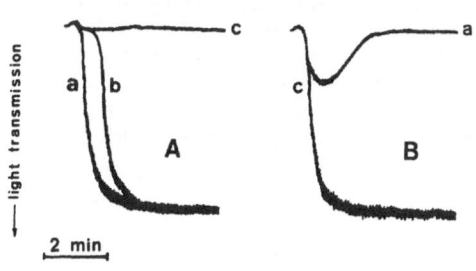

Fig. 8. Aggregation in PRP induced by different concentrations of AA.
A: AA stored under nitrogen.
B: AA exposed to a stream of air for 24 h at 30° and redissolved in the original volume

a - 1.0; b - 0.5; c - 0.25 mM AA

698

## Conclusions

Summing up, close connections between cellular SH/SS status and platelet activation could be evinced. Diminuation of platelet GSH level is very sensitively reflected in changes of the in-vitro aggregation. The observed deviation from normal aggregation suggests alterations in or at the plasma membrane. In accordance with this assumption are the connections between the disturbed aggregation and the polymerization of proteins known to belong to the cytosceleton. It implies effects on the arrangement and mobility of membrane phospholipids which are assumed to be involved in the process of cell fusion. A further system affected by SH/SS changes is the metabolization of AA. Changes in the activity of CO seem to be responsible for the observed acceleration of aggregation, whereas alterations in the LO pathway accompany the deaggregation. Whether the accumulation of HPETE and its derivatives is necessarily linked to changes in the protein pattern, or it is only an alternative mechanism with a comparable effect to the protein polymerizations, is to be cleared up by further investigations which are on work.

## REFERENCES

(1) Pescarmona GP, Bosia A, Hofmann J, Lösche W, Arese P, and Till U (1981) Effect of arachidonic acid on the hexose monophosphate shunt and related coenzymes in human blood platelets. Acta biol. med. germ. 40: K7-K14

(2) Hofmann J, Bosia A, Arese P, Lösche W, Pescarmona GP, Tarzartes O, and Till U (1981) Glucose-6-phosphate dehydrogenase deficiency in human platelets and its effect on platelet aggregation. Acta biol. med. germ. 40: 1707-1714

(3) Hofmann J, Lösche W, Bosia A, Till U, Pescarmona GP, Arese P, and Thielmann K (1980) The effect of decreased GSH level on human blood platelet function. Artery 8: 431-436

(4) Patscheke H, and Wörner P (1978) Sequential effects of the thiol-oxidizing agent diamide on platelets. Thrombos. Res. 12: 609-618

(5) Hofmann J, Lösche W, Hofmann B, Arese P, Bosia A, Pescarmona GP, and Till U (1982) Compounds which cause reversible pertubation of the cellular thiol-disulfide status affect the aggregation behaviour of human blood platelets. Acta biol. med. germ. submitted to publication

(6) Egan RW, Paxton J, and Kuehl FA (1976) Mechanism for irreversible self-deactivation of prostaglandin syntethase. J. Biol. Chem. 251: 7329-7335

(7) Bryant RW, and Bailey JM (1979) Isolation of a new lipoxygenase metabolite of arachidonic acid, 8,11,12-trihydroxy-5,9,14-eicosatrienoic acid from human platelets. Prostaglandins 17: 9-18

(8) Bryant RW, and Bailey JM (1981) Involvement of glutathione peroxidase and hexose monophosphate shunt in the platelet lipoxygenase pathway. International symposium on Leukotrienes and Other Lipoxygenase Products, Florence, June 10-12

(9) Porter NA, Wolf RA, Yarbo EM, and Weenen H (1979) The autoxidation of arachidonic acid: formation of the proposed SRS-A intermediate. Biochem. Biophys. Res. Commun. 89: 1058-1064

(10) Wilson AGE, Kung MW, Anderson MW, and Eling TE (1979) Covalent binding of intermediates formed during the metabolism of arachidonic acid by human platelet subcellular fractions. Prostaglandins 18: 409-422

# 4.2 Prostanoids

# The Formation of Eicosanoids During Inflammation

D. H. Nugteren, E. Christ-Hazelhof, and G. A. A. Kivitis

The discovery in 1971 (1) that non-steroidal anti-inflammatory drugs such as aspirin and indomethacin inhibit prostaglandin biosynthesis, was the first indication of a connection between the enzymic oxygenation of arachidonic acid (20:4) and inflammation. Some years later, it was shown that human adherent rheumatoid synovial cells had a high potency for PG-biosynthesis (2). The detection of an arachidonate-5-lipoxygenase in glycogen-elicited rabbit peritoneal polymorphonuclear leukocytes (PMN's) (3) has recently culminated in the discovery that slow-reacting substances in anaphylaxis and leukotactic factors are also arachidonate metabolites. All these substances are now known under the general name "eicosanoids" and play important regulatory rôles in the cell.

Inflammation is a response of the body to a challenge with an unwanted entity. In its early phase, the resident cells, particularly the mast cells and tissue leukocytes and macrophages, respond by secreting a variety of factors, resulting in alterations in vascular flow, increased permeability of the blood vessels, oedema formation and entry of cells from the circulation. Certain cell types at the site of inflammation, start to proliferate. After about 8 hours, the short-living PMN's dominate. This phase is later on succeeded by a situation, lasting for several days, in which macrophages are the main scavenger cells. If it proves difficult to remove the foreign material, the inflammation more and more acquires a chronic aspect and a number of cell types interact to give a granuloma or an encapsulated area. Depending on the kind of insult, fibroblasts and also the various cells of the immune system, can play a rôle. In a number of chronic aberrations, such as rheuma, the immunological component is predominant.

For a better understanding of the rôle of the various oxygenation products of 20:4, we determined all known prostaglandins, conjugated hydroxy acids and leukotrienes in samples obtained during the successive phases of an inflammation. We used sterile polyester sponges, impregnated with 1 ml of a 2% carrageenin solution in 0.9% saline, which were inserted under the back-skin of rats. In this model, there is a rapid recruitment of PMN's, followed by proliferation of macrophages after some days. Finally, the sponge becomes granulomatous and fully encapsulated. That prostaglandins are involved in carrageenin-induced inflammation appears very likely: anti-inflammatory drugs inhibit swelling of the rat paw and also rats deficient in essential fatty acids (EFA) display a less strong reaction (4).

In order to determine the point of time at which the potency for eicosanoid formation was at its maximum, rats were sacrificed after different periods after insertion of the carrageenin sponge, varying from 4 hours till 7 days. The whole sponge with the inflammatory cells was taken from the animal and incubated with 5 µg [1-$^{14}$C]-arachidonic acid in 2 ml 0.2 M tris. HCl, pH 8.0, in the presence of 10 µg of the Ca$^{2+}$-ionophore A23187 and 300 µg CaCl$_2$.2H$_2$O for 15 min at 37°C. It appeared that the conversion of 20:4 was at its maximum when the sponge had been placed under the rat skin for 8 h.

Thereafter, the kind of products was more closely established in '8 hour-sponges', by comparing the chromatographic properties of the compounds formed from radioactive 20:4 with those of all the known eicosanoids. (Reference prostanoids were

available from own stocks; 5, 8, 9, 11, 12 and 15-hydroxyeicosatetraenoic acids
(5), leukotriene $C_4$ ($LTC_4$) and $LTD_4$ were obtained by organic synthesis (6) and
$LTB_4$ by incubation of 20:4 with rat basophilic leukaemia cells.) Using HPLC on
reversed phase (RP 18) and Partisil 5 ($SiO_2$)-columns in combination with three
different TLC systems, it was possible to separate and identify each radioactive
compound formed. Four major products were found: thromboxane $B_2$ ($TXB_2$), HHT
(12-OH-17:3), 5-HETE (5-OH-20:4) and $LTB_4$ (Z,E,E,Z). Minor products included two
(E,E,E,Z) $LTB_4$-isomers, two (5,6) $LTB_4$-isomers, $LTC_4$, $LTD_4$ and 11, 12 and
15-mono-HETE's.

Because it is assumed that the availability of free arachidonic acid is mostly
rate-limiting in eicosanoid biosynthesis, we developed a HPLC method in which the
products from endogenously liberated fatty acids could be determined without
using radioactivity. The cells (mostly PMN's) from 8 hour carrageenin sponges
were harvested by squeezing the sponge. About $10^8$ cells in 2 ml medium were
incubated for 15 min at 37°C in the absence and presence of A23187 and $Ca^{2+}$.
Thereafter, $PGB_2$, 17-OH- 10,13,15-22:3 and $LTC_4$-methylester (500 ng of each) were
added as internal standards. The solution was acidified and extracted with ether.
The ether phase was subjected to reversed phase HPLC for the determination of HHT
and 5-HETE (at 234 nm with 17-OH-22:3 as internal standard) and $LTB_4$ (at 270 nm
with $PGB_2$ as I.S.). The water phase was treated with Amberlite XAD-8 and the
resin eluted with methanol for the assay of $LTC_4$ and $LTD_4$ (at 280 nm with $LTC_4$-
mono-Me as internal standard). The results of a representative experiment are
given in Table I.

Table I. Product formation by rat PMN's 8 h after carrageenin inflammation
(ng/$10^8$ cells)

| A23187 + $Ca^{2+}$ | HHT | 5-HETE | $LTB_4$ | $LTC_4$ | $LTD_4$ |
|---|---|---|---|---|---|
| - | 150 | 120 | 80 | - | - |
| + | 120 | 570 | 950 | 20 | 20 |

It can be seen that the formation of HHT, and therefore also of $TXB_2$, is independent of the presence of $Ca^{2+}$-ionophore. However, the 5-lipoxygenation and subsequent leukotriene formation is strongly enhanced by $Ca^{2+}$. It is interesting to
note that $LTC_4$ and $LTD_4$ are only minor products; $LTB_4$ is definitely the major
product and its strong leukotactic activity is in all probability an important
aspect in the development of the inflammation.

Experiments were also done with EFA-deficient rats and with rats which had been
fed different vegetable oils with a varying content of linoleic acid (18:2, n-6)
or linolenic acid (18:3, n-3). In the case EFA-deficiency, the 20:4 of the
2-position of the phospholipids is replaced by 20:3 (n-9), while during feeding
with (n-3)-polyunsaturated fatty acids, as present in linseed oil and fish oil,
20:5 (n-3) can be incorporated. The consequences of this for eicosanoid formation
is currently a hot topic. Weaned rats were, for 5 months, put on three different
diets with 35 en% hardened coconut oil, sunflower seed oil or linseed oil. Carrageenin sponges were then implanted for 8 hours in six animals from each group.
Eicosanoid formation, after stimulation with A23187, was determined as described
above, using HPLC.

Table II. Dietary influences on product formation by carrageenin-elicited rat
PMN's stimulated with A23187 (ng/$10^8$ cells, mean of 6 animals per group)

| dietary vegetable oil | 5-OH-20:3 | 5-OH-20:4 (5-HETE) | 5-OH-20:5 | $LTB_3$ | $LTB_4$ | $LTB_5$ | 9+13-OH-18:2 |
|---|---|---|---|---|---|---|---|
| hardened coconut | 810 | 80 | - | - | 80 | - | 60 |
| sunflower seed | - | 1330 | - | - | 330 | - | 430 |
| linseed | - | 830 | 310 | - | 230 | 110 | 250 |

From Table II it can be seen that apart from eicosanoids derived from 20:4, also
5-OH-20:3, 5-OH-20:5, $LTB_5$, 9-OH-18:2 and/or 13-OH-18:2 were found; identification
of these compounds rested on chromatographic behaviour and on GLC-MS of the
trimethyl-silylated methyl esters. We conclude that in the case of EFA-deficiency,
relatively much 5-OH-20:3 but, remarkably enough, hardly any $LTB_3$ is formed and
that 5-OH-20:4 and $LTB_4$-formation are significantly depressed. In the linseed oil
group, 5-OH-20:5 and $LTB_5$ could be detected but 5-OH-20:4 and $LTB_4$ remained the
major products. The formation of considerable amounts of conjugated hydroxy acids
derived from linoleic acid is also noteworthy (7).

Summarizing, the subcutaneous carrageenin-impregnated sponge has proven to be a
suitable model for the study of the participation of eicosanoids in inflammation.
Product formation was at its maximum 8 hours after challenge, so in the acute
phase when many PMN's were present. Two enzymic pathways were then predominant,
leading to the formation of thromboxane + HHT and the leukotactic leukotriene $B_4$.
The slow-reacting substances of anaphylaxis, $LTC_4$ and $LTD_4$, were of much less
importance, at least in regard to mass. The pattern of products (n-6 versus n-3)
could, to a certain extent, be influenced by the type of fat in the diet.

Acknowledgements

The animal experiments were carried out by Messrs. E. Haddeman and J.A. Don.

References

1. Vane, J.R. (1971). Inhibition of prostaglandin synthesis as a mechanism of
   action for aspirin-like drugs. Nature New Biology 231:232-235.
2. Dayer, J.-M., Krane, S.M., Russell, R.G.G., Robinson, D.R. (1976). Production
   of collagenase and prostaglandins by isolated adherent rheumatoid synovial
   cells. Proc. Nat. Acad. Sci. USA 73:945-949.
3. Borgeat, P., Hamberg, M., Samuelsson, B. (1976). Transformation of arachidonic
   acid and homo-γ-linolenic acid by rabbit polymorphonuclear leukocytes. J.
   Biol. Chem. 251: 7816-7820.
4. Bonta, I.L., Bult, H., Van der Ven, L.L.M., Noordhoek, J. (1976). Essential
   fatty acid deficiency: a condition to discriminate prostaglandin and non-
   prostaglandin mediated components of inflammation. Agents and Actions 6:154-158.
5. Boeynaems, J.M., Oates, J.A., Hubbard, W.C. (1980). Preparation and characterization of hydroperoxyeicosatetraenoic acids (HPETE's). Prostaglandins 19:87-97.
6. Corey, E.J., Barton, A.E., Clark, D.A. (1980). Synthesis of the slow-reacting
   substance of anaphylaxis leukotriene C-I from arachidonic acid. J. Am. Chem.
   Soc. 102:4278-4279.
7. Hubbard, W.C., Hough, A.J., Brash, A.R., Watson, J.T., Oates, J.A. (1980).
   Metabolism of linoleic and arachidonic acids in $VX_2$ carcinoma tissue: identification of monohydroxyoctadecadienoic acids and monohydroxy-eicosatetraenoic
   acids. Prostaglandins 20:431-447.

# Prostaglandins, Cyclic Nucleotides and Atherosclerosis

F. Numano

## Introduction

Since the pioneering work of von Euler, Goldblatt and Bergström, the biological effects of prostaglandins have been given increasing attention (1). The discovery of thromboxane $A_2$ (TXA$_2$) in 1974 and clarification of the physiological role together with the discovery of prostacyclin(PGI$_2$) in 1975 have shed light on the important role of prostaglandins in regulation of platelet activity and the vascular wall, as well as on the interrelationship in thrombotic and atherosclerotic disorders (2, 3, 4).

## "Endotheliopathy" and Prostaglandins

Recent studies on atherogenesis have been directed to the function of the endothelial line of the vessel wall, possibly as a key to the solution of initiation and progression of atherosclerosis (5).

Until recently, endothelial lines were thought to be only a boundary between the blood stream and the vessel wall and were regarded as a passive barrier. However, recent studies have made it clear that the endothelial line itself is an independent tissue synthesizing many hormones and substances such as histamine, collagen, factor VIII, plasminogen activator, tissue thromboplastin, heparin, and plays important physiological functions including selective permeability, and the function of repelling platelets in the maintenance of the exquisite balance between the vessel wall and the blood stream (6, 7).

Vascular injury is one of the most important key mechanisms in initiation and progression of atherosclerosis (8). Our group have confirmed that rabbits subjected to risk factors such as stress of painful stimuli, angiotensin II, epinephrine, cholesterol, cigarette smoke etc., there were edematous changes in the aortic wall characterized by acute plasmal infiltration (9). This infiltrate included large molecules such as VLDL and LDL due to the contraction and increased phagocytic activity of the endothelial cells. Furthermore, when such challenges were repeated in laboratory animals, there was a thickening of the intima in the aortic wall followed by formation of atheromatous lesions (10).

TXA$_2$ induces a potent contraction of the vessel wall. Our recent studies confirmed that TXA$_2$ induces edematous changes in the arterial wall (3) and the content of cyclic AMP in the intima of the aorta of animals which is regulated by PGI$_2$ and plays an important role in the modulation of the release of TXA$_2$ in platelets decreased significantly, as compared with findings in healthy controls (Fig. 1).

Table I shows the changes in the levels of TXB$_2$ and 6-keto PGF$_{1\alpha}$ in plasma of rabbits given one dose of TXA$_2$, angiotensin II, adrenaline or cholesterol to induce edematous changes in the aortic wall. It is interesting that not only TXA$_2$ but also angiotensin and adrenaline administration resulted in an increase of TXB$_2$ and 6-keto PGF$_{1\alpha}$. Therefore, TXA$_2$ may play an important role in the induction of edematous changes in the aorta following administration of various substances and the increase in levels of 6-keto PGF$_{1\alpha}$ indicate an antagonistic effect. That is, edematous change, which is thought to be a key phenomenon in the initiation of atherosclerosis, may be due to an unbalance between TXB$_2$ and prostacyclin and be characterized by "endotheliopathy" (7, 11).

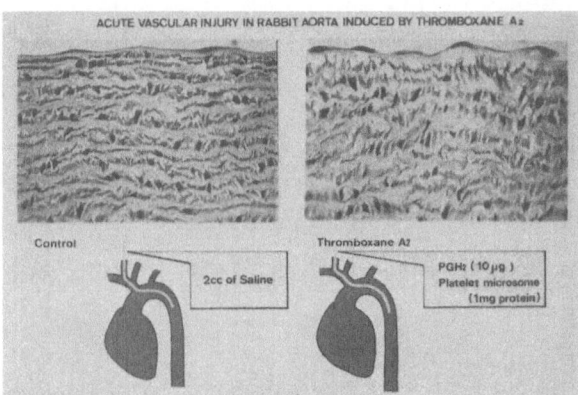

ACUTE VASCULAR INJURY IN RABBIT AORTA INDUCED BY THROMBOXANE A₂

Control

Thromboxane A₂

2cc of Saline

PGH₂ (10 μg)
Platelet microsome
(1mg protein)

Fig. 1

Changes in plasma levels of thromboxane B₂ and 6-keto PGF₁α
in rabbits administered one dose of thromboxane A₂(I.A.),
Angiotensin II (I.A.), Adrenaline (I.A.), and cholesterol(p.o.)

| prostanoids. Groups | TXB₂ (pg/ml) | | 6-keto PGF₁α(pg/ml) | | Vascular injury |
|---|---|---|---|---|---|
| | before | 1min after | before | 1min after | |
| Placebo control saline 1cc | | 284 ± 68 | | 427 ± 23 | (−) |
| thromboxane A₂ PGH₂ 25ug & microsome 4mg protein/ | 216.3 ± 53 | 1234** ± 137 | 380 ± 24 | 4384.3** ± 158 | (卌) |
| Angiotensin II (10⁷/kg I.A.) | | 812* ± 128 | | 3643** ± 189 | (卅) |
| Adrenaline (10⁷/kg I.A.) | | 736 ± 189 | | 1684 ± 317 | (卅) |
| Cholesterol # (1g/kg p.o.) | | 398 ± 101 | | 716 ± 112 | (+) |

\# 30min after   * P<0.05   ** P<0.01   before vs. after

Table I

## Contraction of Endothelial Cells by TXA₂

Thromboxane A₂ contracts the vessel wall (2). The question of whether or not TXA₂
contracts the endothelial cells has been highlighted in an attempt to clarify the
association with edematous change. The existence of contractile protein has been
confirmed in endothelial cells (12) and contraction of endothelial cells has been
much discussed as a main route of vascular permeability and edematous change in
the vessel wall.

Fig. 2 shows scanning electron microscopy of cultured rabbit endothelial cells.
These cells were taken from the aorta of rabbits and cultivated for 10 passages.
Cells proliferated in one layer, as shown in Fig. 2, and the presence of factor
VIII was confirmed in these cells by using antiserum of factor VIII to certify
that these were indeed endothelial cells. A mixture of 50 μg of prostaglandin H₂
and 5 μg of microsomes had been added to the media in which 2000 pg/ml of TXB₂
was found to be synthesized 1 min after mixing. With this addition, these endothelial cells became swollen and ditch-like formations ran in all directions among
the cells. Electron microscopic examination revealed folds, indentation and
pinches in nuclei of these cells, all characteristic features of contraction of
cells (13).

These studies also revealed a concomitant increase in the levels of cyclic AMP in
both tissues and media and of 6-keto PGF₁α in the media, As shown in Fig. 3.
These data suggest that TXA₂ does contract endothelial cells which in turn increases the permeability and initiates vascular injury.

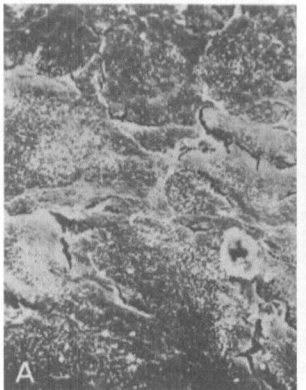

Fig. 2A
(Control)

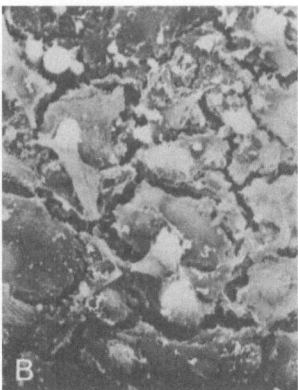

Fig. 2B
(Thromboxane)

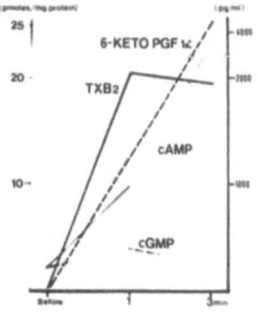

CHANGES IN LEVELS OF THROMBOXANE
B₂ (TXB₂),cAMP,cGMP & 6-KETO-PGF 1α
WITH ADDITION OF TXA₂ TO THE TISSUE
CULTURE MEDIUM

Fig. 3

## Thromboxane-induced Myocardial Infarction

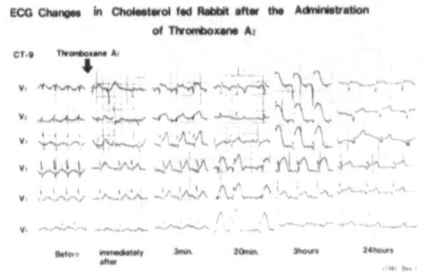

ECG Changes in Cholesterol fed Rabbit after the Administration of Thromboxane A₂

Before  immediately after  3min.  20min.  3hours  24hours

Fig. 4

Thromboxane-induced Myocardial Infarction

in cholesterol-fed rabbits**

| Group | No. | myocardial infarction | Plasma levels of | | | |
|---|---|---|---|---|---|---|
| | | | Thromboxane B₂ (pg/ml) | | 6-keto PGF₁α (pg/ml) | |
| | | | before | immediately after | before | immediately after |
| Chol.-fed | 12 | 12 (7 died) | 380 ± 98 | 2640 ± 450 | 100 ± 10 | 1284 ± 297 |
| Controls | 7 | 0 | 216 ± 48 | 1230 ± 280 | 324 ± 25 | 1870 ± 248 |

\* prostaglandin H₂ 25μg + microsome 4mg protein
\*\* fed 1% cholesterol containing diet for 15 weeks then commercial pellets for 10 weeks

\*\* P<0.01
\* P<0.05  before vs. immediately after

‡‡ P<0.01
‡ P<0.05  Normal vs. cholesterol-fed group

Table II

Fig. 4 demonstrates the ECG changes of a cholesterol-fed rabbit administered TXA₂ into coronary artery through a catheter placed in situ. Immediately after the flush of TXA₂, the ST elevation was remarkable and increased gradually followed by Q waves. That is, typical myocardial infarction could be induced by administration of TXA₂.

We used seven 8 month old male rabbits as control and 12 aged matched rabbits which had been fed a 1% cholesterol containing diet for 15 weeks, then a commercial diet for 10 weeks. TXA₂ was prepared with the mixture of 25 μg of prostaglandin H₂ and 4 mg protein of cow platelet was flushed into the aorta at the orifice of the coronary artery through a Fogarty catheter.

As shown in Table II, all rabbits fed a cholesterol diet exhibited typical ST elevation. These ECG data are shown in Fig. 4. Plasma levels of GOT, GPT and CPK abruptly increased and 7 rabbits died within 48 hours.

Phosphorylase activity in the heart muscle (14) revealed various sized ischemic areas (Fig. 5). Magnified picture shown in Fig. 6 clearly demonstrates the boundary of stained and no stained area in myocardium which suggests the ischemia due to the total occlusion of the supplying branches of coronary artery. Microthrombi were also detected in many intravascular coronary arteries. On the contrary, the control rabbits tolerated well the administration of TXA₂, ECG changes related to myocardial damage were nil and no rabbit died.

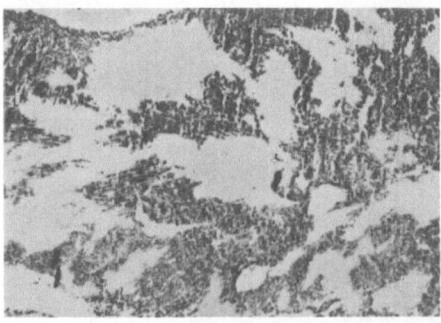

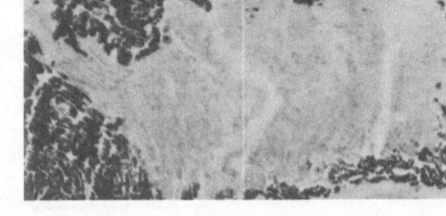

Fig. 5  (×4)          Fig. 6  (×20)
Phosphorylase activity in myocardium

With regard to the differences between normal and cholesterol-fed groups, data are shown in Table II and Fig. 7. Table II shows statistically significant low plasma levels of 6-keto $PGF_{1\alpha}$ and in turn high levels of $TXB_2$ in cholesterol-fed rabbits, as compared with findings in the control rabbits. Furthermore, in the placebo treated rabbits, flush of the mixture was associated with a release of 6-keto $PGF_{1\alpha}$ in the plasma. However, in cholesterol-fed rabbits, the plasma levels of $TXB_2$ were statistically high and in turn the release of 6-keto $PGF_{1\alpha}$ was significantly low after the flush of the mixture, as compared with findings in the control rabbits (Fig. 7).

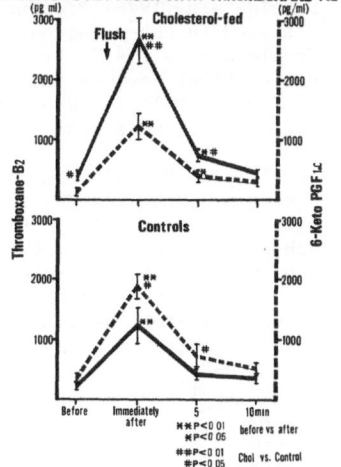

PLASMA LEVELS OF THROMBOXANE B2 AND 6-KETO PGF1α IN CONTROLS AND CHOLESTEROL-FED RABBITS AFTER FLUSH WITH THROMBOXANE A2

Fig. 7

These data suggest that the vessel wall is equipped with an immediate reaction mechanism against the increase of thromboxane and the lack of this factor due to sclerosis results in fatal damage in the myocardium following total occlusion of the coronary sclerosis vessels (15, 16). Actually, we confirmed that the content of cAMP (regulated by $PGI_2$) in the aortic wall in rabbits was decreased with progression of atherosclerosis with cholesterol feeding (17, 18) and Dembińska-Kieć et al reported a decrease in prostacyclin in the arterial wall of rabbits fed a high cholesterol diet (19, 20).

## Concluding Remarks

Our investigations clearly demonstrated the important role of $TXA_2$ in, what we call "endotheliopathy". Prostacyclin and cyclic nucleotides are regulators and an unbalance in the levels of these regulators lead to considerable damage. Chemotherapy to right the unbalance should be most beneficial to prevent/treat atherosclerosis and related disorders.

## Acknowledgement

Gratitude is extended to M. Ohara for pertinent collaboration in these studies.

References

1. Subbiah MTR (1978) Prostaglandins and the arterial wall: An avenue for research in the pathogenesis of atherosclerosis. Mayo Clin Proc 53: 60-62
2. Gryglewski RJ (1980) Prostaglandins, platelets and atherosclerosis. CRC Critical Reviews in Biochemistry 7: 291-338
3. Numano F (1981) Thromboxane $A_2$ and atherosclerosis. In: De Las Heras FG, Vega S (eds) Medicinal Chemistry Advances. Pergamon Press, Oxford, pp 131-140
4. Vane JR, Moncada S (1980) Prostacyclin and vascular disease. In: Bevan JA et al (eds) Vascular Neuroeffector Mechanisms. Raven Press, NY, pp 99-106
5. Harker LA, Schwartz SM, Ross R (1981) Endothelium and arteriosclerosis. Clinics in Haematology 10: 283-296
6. Schwartz CJ, Ross GG, Lewis LJ (1978) Arterial endothelial structure and function with particular reference to permeability. In: Paoletti R, Gotto AM (eds) Atherosclerosis Reviews. Raven Press, NY, Vol.3, pp 109-124
7. Numano F (1980) Chemotherapy of atherosclerosis. Jpn Circul J 44: 55-68
8. Ross R, Glomset J (1976) The pathogenesis of atherosclerosis. New Eng J Med 295: 369-377
9. Shimamoto T (1969) Experimental study on atherosclerosis. Acta Path Jap 19: 15-43
10. Shimamoto T, Kobayashi M, Numano F (1975) Immunofluorescent demonstration of plasma protein entry into arterial wall by cholesterol, epinephrine, norepinephrine and angiotensin II. Acta Path Jap 25: 51-67
11. Numano F, Shimamoto T (1978) Prevention and regression of atherosclerosis. In: Carlson LA, Paoletti R, Weber G (eds) International Conference on Atherosclerosis. Raven Press, NY, pp 631-636
12. Becker CG, Murphy GE (1969) Demonstration of contractile protein in endothelium and cells of heart valves, endocardium, intima, arteriosclerotic plaques and Aschoff bodies of rheumatic heart disease. Amer J Pathol 55: 1-37
13. Majno G, Shea SM, Leventhal M (1969) Endothelial contraction induced by histamine-type mediator. An electron microscopic study. J Cell Biol 42: 647-672
14. Takeuchi T, Kuriaki H (1955) Histochemical detection of phosphorylase in animal tissues. J Histochem Cytochem 3: 153-160
15. Sasagawa S, Moriya K, Sugaya Y, Mitani J, Yajima M (1982) Effect of thromboxane $A_2$ injection on the rabbit coronary artery. I. Physiological effects in healthy animals. Exp Mol Path in press
16. Numano F, Yajima M, Nishiyama K, Shimokado K, Numano Fe, Sasagawa S, Moriya K (1982) Effect of thromboxane $A_2$ injection on the rabbit coronary artery. II. The production of infarcts in cholesterol-fed animals. Exp Mol Path in press
17. Numano F, Maezawa H, Shimamoto T, Adachi K (1976) Changes of cyclic AMP and cyclic AMP phosphodiesterase in the progression and regression of experimental atherosclerosis. Ann N.Y. Acad Sci 275: 311-320
18. Numano F (1979) Cyclic nucleotides and atherosclerosis. In: Cehovic G, Robison GA (eds) Cyclic Nucleotides and Therapeutic Perspectives. Pergamon Press, Oxford, pp 137-146
19. Dembińska-Kieć A, Gryglewska T, Zmuda A, Gryglewski RJ (1977) The generation of prostacyclin by arteries and by the coronary vascular bed is reduced in experimental atherosclerosis in rabbits. Prostaglandins 14: 1025-1035
20. Gryglewski RJ, Szczeklik A (1981) Prostacyclin and atherosclerosis. In: Lewis PJ, Grady JO (eds) Clinical Pharmacology of Prostacyclin. Raven Press, NY, pp 89-95

# Prostacyclin Formation, Plasma Factor, Platelet Sensitivity and Prostacyclin Degradation in Coronary Heart Disease

H. Sinzinger

Atherosclerosis Research Group Vienna (ASF) at the Department of Medical Physiology, University of Vienna and Atherosclerosis and Thrombosis Research Group (ATK) of the Austrian Academy of Sciences, Vienna, Austria.

## A. Introduction

Since the discovery of prostacyclin in 1976 by Moncada and colleagues great interest has been given to this new field of atherosclerosis research. The findings that this new biologically extremely active compound has very strong antiaggregatory and vasodilatory properties supported the early suggestions. Later on, it has been found, that in experimental atherosclerosis (2), experimental diabetes (3), as well as in human atherosclerosis (4) and diabetes mellitus (5) vascular $PGI_2$-formation is severely depressed. At this time it was thought that prostacyclin probably might act as a hemostatic regulator via being a circulating hormone (6).

However, in the recent past, many doubts about this assumption were brought up (7) and it is now more and more accepted, that prostacyclin plays its role working only at a local level at the interaction between the vascular wall and the cellular and plasmatic elements.

It is the goal of this investigation to give a short summary on the results obtained during the last year in my laboratory drawing special attention to the special situation in the coronary vascular bed.

## B. Material and Methods

The methods used are briefly stated. More detailed information is given in original papers dealing with some of the particular topics.

Human coronary artery prostacyclin formation was tested using the platelet aggregation bioassay technique (ADP-induced aggregation) in a Born-type aggregometer.

The "plasma factor" was tested using either the platelet aggregation bioassay or radioimmunoassays for 6-keto-$PGF_1$alpha or 6,15-diketo-$PGF_1$alpha. Material from rat aorta, human coronary artery, swine abdominal aorta and cultured endothelial and smooth muscle cells were used. The plasma factor was expressed as the difference between incubation in buffer or in plasma respectively.

The influence of ß-thromboglobulin was tested using plasma from patients with ß-TG values lower or higher than 50ng/ml. Plasma from patients with hyperlipoproteinemia (types IIa, IIb and IV) and diabetes mellitus ( juvenile onset (JOD) or maturity onset (MOD) diabetes). The platelet derived growth factor was isolated according to Antoniades and co-workers (8) and tested on coronary artery prostacyclin formation (platelet aggregation bioassay).

Leucotrienes $C_4$ and $D_4$ were added in different doses to coronary arteries and their effect on arterial $PGI_2$-generation examined using again the platelet aggregation bioassay technique.

Platelet sensitivity testing to the antiaggregatory prostaglandins ($PGI_2$, $PGE_1$, $PGD_2$) was done by inhibiting the ADP-induced aggregation by various concentrations of these prostaglandins. The platelet sensitivity was given as the dose suppressing the induced aggregation response to the half ($ID_{50}$) in ng/ml platelet rich plasma. The test was done in 600µl samples.

710

C. Results

The prostacyclin synthesis by human coronary arteries is significantly lower than the generation found by unchanged (morphological control) coronary vascular tissue (table 1).

Table 1. Prostacyclin formation by human coronary arteries

| vascular tissue | prostacyclin synthesis | number |
|---|---|---|
| atheroscl. LAD | $3,21 \pm 1,8$ | 12 |
| normal LAD | $7,11 \pm 1,4$ | 6 |

$\bar{x} \pm$ SEM; $PGI_2$ in pg/mg/min
18 - 54 mg tissue wet weight

The platelet sensitivity to $PGI_2$ and $PGE_1$ is in patients with angiographically verified coronary heart disease and patients after myocardial infarction significantly lower than in age and sex matched controls (figure 1).

Figure 1. Platelet sensitivity to $PGI_2$ in patients with angiographically proven coronary heart disease of both sexes

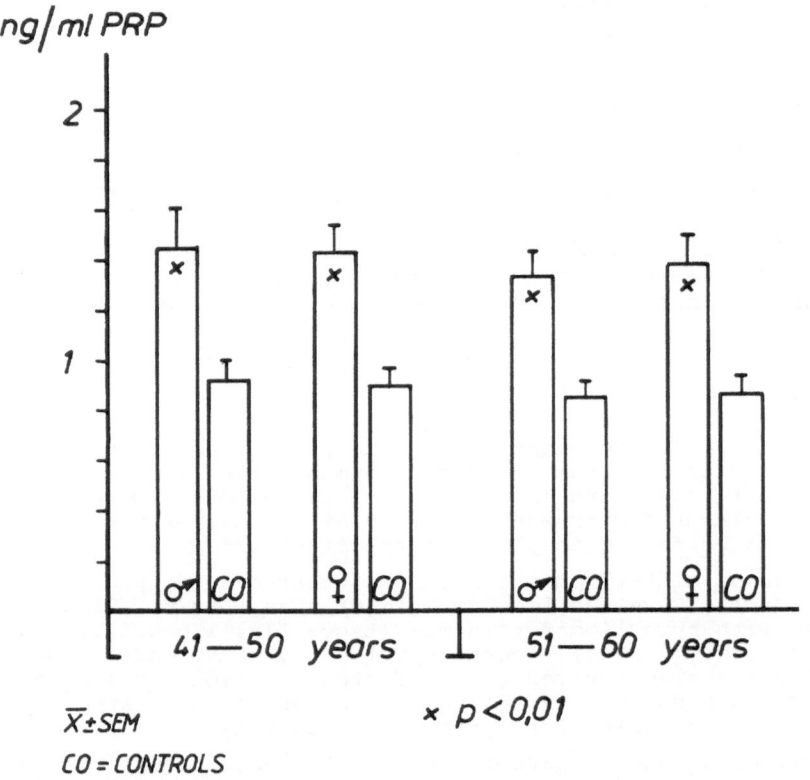

In patients of the same age groups as shown in figure 1 suffering from acute angina pectoris there is a sudden decrease in platelet sensitivity for $PGE_1$ and $PGI_2$ (figure 2) as well. However, neither in coronary heart disease, nor in angina pectoris the sensitivity changes for $PGD_2$ were statistically significant different though the trends were running parallel. The significant findings for $PGI_2$ and $PGE_1$ were always running parallel, showning an r of more than 0,80.

Figure 2. Platelet sensitivity to $PGI_2$ in patients with coronary heart disease of both sexes in acute angina and one hour later (a). ap...angina pectoris

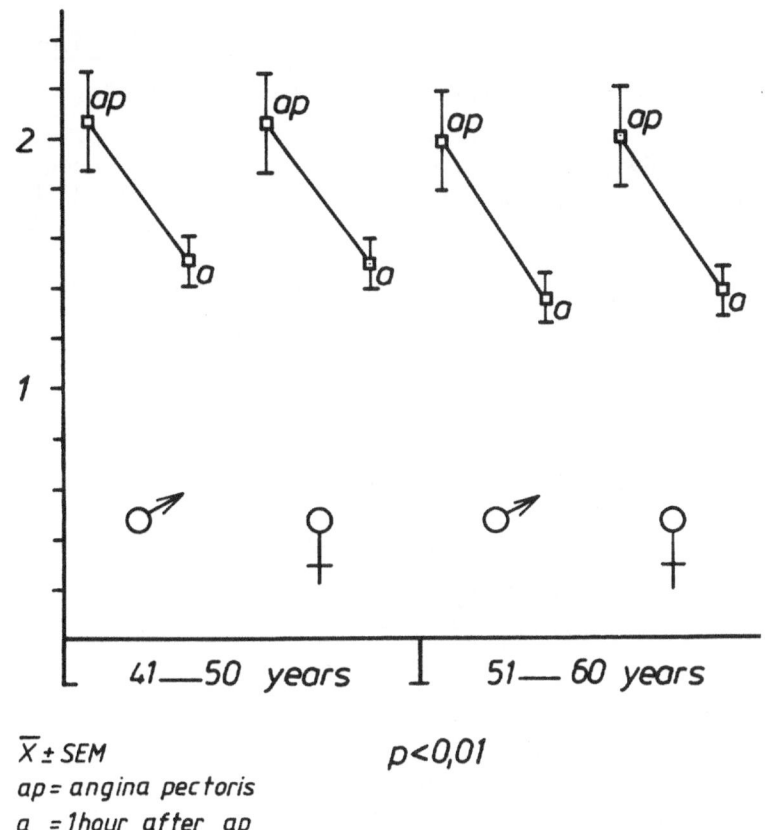

$\overline{X} \pm SEM$    $p<0,01$

ap = angina pectoris

a = 1hour after ap

Human plasma is able to increase significantly the $PGI_2$-formation by different vascular tissue as measured by $PGI_2$-synthesis or 6-keto-PG $F_1$alpha and 6,15-diketo-$PGF_1$alpha respectively. Plasma from patients with coronary heart disease exhibits a trend to a lower stimulatory capacity, however, this trend never reached the level of significance. The same occured with high and low ß-TG plasmas or plasma from MOD and JOD respectively. The involvement of 1, 2 or 3 coronary vessels seen by angiography had no influence. The presence of any type of hyperlipoproteinemia again caused a non-significant decrease in plasma factor activity.

Incubating human coronary arteries with platelet derived growth factor an unexpected extreme increase in $PGI_2$-generation was observed (table 2), which was in general more than the 5-fold of normal synthesis. The most interesting finding is, that the capacity to stimulate $PGI_2$-synthesis is lower in atherosclerotic arteries than in morphologically unchanged coronary vascular bed.

Table 2.  PDGF STIMULATES CORONARY ARTERY PGI$_2$

| MEDIUM | ATHEROSCL. | N | NORMAL | N |
|---|---|---|---|---|
| BUFFER | $3,88 \pm 0,83$ | 8 | $7,76 \pm 1,56$ | 6 |
| 10NG PDGF | $4,17 \pm 0,75$ | 8 | $9,31 \pm 2,01$ | 6 |
| 50NG PDGF | $8,26 \pm 0,94$ | 8 | $25,26 \pm 2,37$ | 6 |
| 100NG PDGF | $10,86 \pm 1,17$ | 8 | $37,63 \pm 3,69$ | 6 |

$\bar{X} \pm$ SEM; PGI$_2$ IN PG/MG/MIN.; 31-65 MG

In a different methodological approach coronary arteries were perfused under addition of various concentrations of leucotrienes, showing that leucotriene C$_4$ (LTC$_4$) - table 3 - as well as LTD$_4$ are very potent stimulators of coronary vascular bed PGI$_2$-formation

Table 3.

LEUCOTRIENE C$_4$ STIMULATES PGI$_2$

| MEDIUM | PGI$_2$ | N |
|---|---|---|
| BU + 1NG | $48,3 \pm 3,7$ | 8 |
| BU + 5NG | $46,7 \pm 4,1$ | 7 |
| BU +10NG | $57,4 \pm 5,6$ | 8 |
| BU +50NG | $86,3 \pm 6,1$ | 9 |
| BU +100NG | $113,7 \pm 6,0$ | 10 |
| BUFFER | $46,7 \pm 3,8$ | 10 |

PG/CM$^2$; $\bar{X} \pm$ SEM

Studying the degradation of PGI$_2$ in plasma of patients with clinically proven atherosclerosis (peripheral vascular disease, coronary heart disease, cerebral vascular disease) no difference between these patients and healthy controls can be found

D. Discussion

Summarizing our findings demonstrate that there exist many factors being capable to influence the complex system of PGI$_2$ regulating the hemostatic balance. Most of these factors, as the vascular PGI$_2$-formation for example have been attributed to be the key regulator of this hemostatic system.

However, we found, that in concentrations occuring most likely in circulation the platelet derived growth factor is the substance have the most significant influence in this system.

The recently reported doubts (7) that prostacyclin is really acting as a circulating hormone stimulated us to present the following hypothesis: If the PDGF is liberated from the platelets alpha-granules it acts extremely stimulating at the local level on the endothelial PGI$_2$-generation. The prostacyclin thus generated (figure 3) elevates the platelet c-AMP and thus inhibits further PDGF liberation. However, PDGF acting on atherosclerotic vascular tissue is able to enhance the PGI$_2$-formation much less (to less sometimes ?). This might promote further PDGF-liberation by a low intraplatelet

Figure 3. Scheme of hemostatic balance in coronary arteries

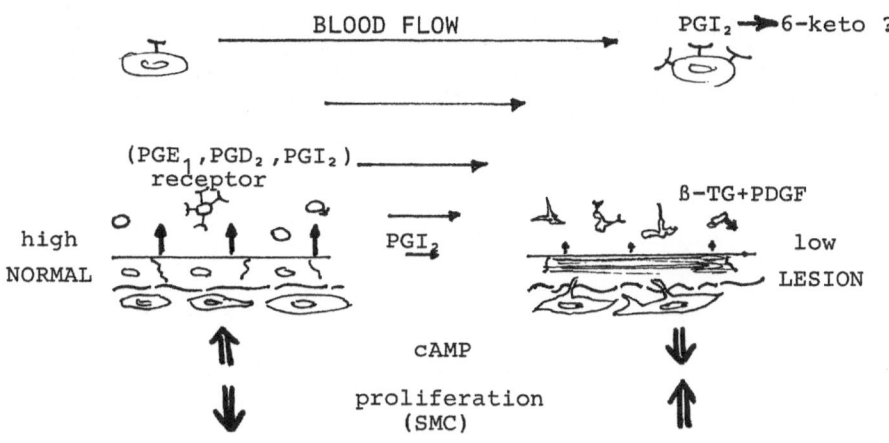

c-AMP and a vitious circle. In addition under these circumstances the vascular smooth muscle cells might be stimulated to proliferate being one of the key events occuring in atherosclerosis (9).

Therefore, we think that a sufficient response of vascular tissue to PDGF in synthetizing $PGI_2$ might be one of the key mechanisms in human atherosclerosis. It should be the goal of further studies to discover why atherosclerotic tissue has a lower responding capacity to PGDF. This might open a new pathophysiological mechanism and probably a new avenue for a treatment of the disease.

Acknowledgements  The helpful cooperation of Christa Hoche,PhD, Josef Kaliman,MD and Achilleus Kefalides,MD,PhD, Beate Rüger, Andrea Gall And Ilse Eisler is kindly acknowledged !

The prostaglandins and leukotrienes used in this study were supplied by Dr.John E.Pike (The Upjohn Company, Kalamazoo, Michigan,USA), Dr. John O'Grady (Wellcome Pharma, Beckenham, UK), Prof.Dr.Cesare A.Gandolfi (Farmitalia Carlo Erba, Milan, Italy) and Merck (Canada).

E. References

1. Moncada S, Gryglewski RJ, Bunting S, Vane JR (1976) An enzyme isolated from arteries transforms prostaglandin endoperoxides to an unstable substance that inhibits platelet aggregation. Nature 271: 663-665.
2. Dembinska-Kiec A, Gryglewska T, Zmuda A, Gryglewski RJ (1977) The generation of prostacyclin by arteries and by the coronary vascular bed is reduced in experimental atherosclerosis in rabbits. Prostaglandins 14: 1025-1034.
3. Harrison HE, Reece A, Johnson M (1978) Decreased vascular prostacyclin in experimental diabetes. Life Sci. 23: 351-358.
4. Sinzinger H, Feigl W, Silberbauer K (1979) Prostacyclin formation by atherosclerotic human arteries. Lancet i: 469.
5. Silberbauer K, Schernthaner G, Sinzinger H, Piza-Katzer H, Winter M (1979) Decreased vascular prostacyclin in juvenile-onset diabetics. The New Engl. J.Med. 300: 366.
6. Gryglewski RJ, Korbut R, Ocetkiewicz, Splawinski J, Wojtaszek B, Swies J (1978) Lungs as a generator of prostacyclin - hypothesis on physiological significance. Arch. Pharm. 304: 45-50.

714

7. Steer ML, McIntyre DE, Levine L, Salzman EW (1980) Is prostacyclin a physiologically important circulating anti-platelet agent ? Nature 283: 194-195.
8. Antoniades HN, Scher CD, Stiles CD (1979) Purification of human platelet derived growth factor. Proc.Nat.Acad.Sci. 76: 1809-1813.
9. Ross R, Glomset JA (1973) Atherosclerosis and the arterial smooth muscle - proliferation of smooth muscle is a key event in the genesis of the lesions of atherosclerosis. Science 180: 1332-1336.

# Vascular Resistance and Platelet Function on Cardiovascular Drugs and Diets Affecting Prostanoid Formation

P.C.Weber

Prostanoids have increasingly been recognized as important physiologic modulators of hemodynamics and haemostasis, and alterations in prostanoid formation have been reported in known risk factors for the development as well as overt hypertensive and arteriosclerotic vessel disease. Therefore, the effects of established antihypertensive, antithrombotic and antianginal treatment on prostanoid formation will be discussed against this background. The literature cited is selective, for detailed reviews regarding platelets and vascular disease, prostanoids and ischemic heart disease, prostaglandins (PG) and the kidney, hypertension and the renin-angiotensin-system, see references (1-5).

As outlined in Table 1, many studies (6-25) have demonstrated an association between cardiovascular risk factors and increased formation of thromboxane (TX)$A_2$ and reduced synthesis of $PGE_2$ and $PGI_2$. This imbalance in prostanoid formation may increase vascular resistance and platelet reactivity contributing to the development of ischemic vascular disease. Beside the factors cited in Table 1, the natural risk indicators such as age (26), and sex (27) are also assumed to operate, at least in part, by shifting the balance between vasodilatory/antiaggregatory $PGE_2/PGI_2$ and vasoconstrictor/aggregatory $TXA_2$. Thus, altered prostanoid formation is not only found in established hypertension (4, 18-21) and advanced arteriosclerotic vessel disease (23, 24, 28) but may precede and may well be causally involved into their natural history.

Table 1. Cardiovascular Risk Factors and Prostanoid Formation

| Risk Factors | Prostanoid Formation | | Effects | Reference |
|---|---|---|---|---|
| | Platelets | Vasculature-Kidney | | |
| Heredity | | $PGE_2\downarrow$, $PGF_{2\alpha}\uparrow$ | VR$\uparrow$ | 6-9 |
| High Salt | | $PGE_2\downarrow$ | BP$\uparrow$,PR$\uparrow$,PRA$\downarrow$ | 10,11 |
| High Cholesterol | $TXA_2\uparrow$ | $PGI_2\downarrow$ | PR$\uparrow$,PF$\uparrow$ | 12-14 |
| Nicotine | $TXA_2(\uparrow)$ | $PGI_2\downarrow$ | NE$\uparrow$E$\uparrow$,HR$\uparrow$,BP$\uparrow$ | 15,16 |
| Contraceptives | $TXA_2(\uparrow)$ | $PGI_2(\downarrow)$ | PF$\uparrow$,BP$\uparrow$,PRA$\uparrow$ | 17 |
| Hypertension | $TXA_2\uparrow$ | $PGE_2\downarrow$,$PGI_2\downarrow$ | VR$\uparrow$,PF$\uparrow$,PRA$\downarrow$ | 18-21 |
| Diabetes Mell. | $TXA_2\uparrow$ | $PGI_2\downarrow$ | PF$\uparrow$ | 22-25 |

VR = vascular resistance; BP = blood pressure; PR = pressure response; PF = platelet function; NE, E = norepinephrine, epinephrine; PRA = plasma renin activity; ( ) = not definitely established.

Consequently, if altered prostanoid formation turns out to be important in hypertensive and ischemic vascular disease, dietary or pharmacological treatment aimed at the correction of the imbalance in prostaglandin formation may prove clinically effective.

Indeed, with the exception of centrally acting hypotensive drugs and, may be β-blockers, antihypertensive treatment that reduces vascular resistance - which is characteristically elevated in hypertension – is associated with increased formation of vasodilator prostaglandins in the kidney and probably the blood vessel wall, leading in parallel also to an increase of renin secretion (Table 2). In addition, some of these antihypertensive drugs seem to inhibit also formation of vasoconstrictive thromboxane in platelets.

Table 2. Effects of Antihypertensive Therapy on Prostanoid Formation

| Treatment | Prostanoid Formation | | Effects | Reference |
|---|---|---|---|---|
| | Vasculature-Kidney | Platelets | | |
| Low Salt | $PGE_2\uparrow$ | | BP$\downarrow$,PRA$\uparrow$ | 10,11 |
| Diuretics | $PGE_2\uparrow$,$PGI_2\uparrow$ | | BP$\downarrow$,VR$\downarrow$,PRA$\uparrow$ | 5,20,29,30 |
| Vasodilators | $PGI_2\uparrow$ | $TXA_2\downarrow$ | VR$\downarrow$,BP$\downarrow$,PRA$\uparrow$ | 31,32 |
| CE Inhibitors | $PGI_2\uparrow$ | | BP$\downarrow$,VR$\downarrow$,PRA$\uparrow$ | 33-35 |
| Beta Blocker | | $TXA_2\downarrow$ | HR$\downarrow$,BP$\downarrow$,VR$\rightarrow\uparrow$ $Ca^{++}\downarrow$,PF$\downarrow$ | 29,36-39 |

BP = blood pressure; VR = vascular resistance; PRA = plasma renin activity; HR = heart rate; $Ca^{++}$ = calcium availability; PF = platelet function.

That these changes of prostanoid formation after antihypertensive drugs may contribute in a "physiological" manner to their blood pressure lowering effect is supported by several findings: Inhibition of prostaglandin formation by non-steroidal antiinflammatory drugs (NSAID) increases vascular resistance (41) and the pressor response to vasoactive hormones (40), and blunts the blood pressure lowering action of many antihypertensive drugs (29, 35, 37). NSAID induce also a decrease of renin secretion (5), compatible with the observation that vasodilator prostaglandins increase renin release (5, 42). In accordance with the findings that a low and unresponsive plasma renin activity in essential hypertension is associated with reduced formation of vasodilator $PGE_2$ and $PGI_2$ (5, 19, 21) and alterations of renal blood flow (43), red cell cation fluxes (44) and with a genetic predisposition for high blood pressure (45), these studies indicate that abnormalities in the spectrum of prostaglandins may have a key position in the development and the natural history of hypertensive vascular disease. Consequently, drugs that reverse these prostaglandin abnormalities may reduce blood pressure by correcting one of the more proximal defects determining the clinical course of this disease.

Increased platelet aggregability has been repeatedly found in hypertensive and ischemic vessel disease, and platelets and arachidonic acid metabolites may contribute to the gradual development and acute clinical events of atherothrombotic disorders (1, 2, 38). Antiplatelet serum and platelet inhibiting drugs that interfere with the metabolism of arachidonic acid have been shown to inhibit experimental arteriosclerosis (46, 47). Various drugs, thought to act primarily by interference with platelet function have been used clinically, although a pathogenetic role of platelet abnormalities in these conditions has not yet been definitely established in humans. As summarized in Table 3, many studies (48-61) demonstrate indeed "beneficial" effects of antithrombotic and antianginal drugs on platelet $TXA_2$ and vascular $PGI_2$ formation, that is an increase of the ratio between $PGI_2$ and $TXA_2$, either by inhibition of $TXA_2$ formation, or by stimulating $PGI_2$ production, or both.

Table 3. Effects of Antithrombotic Treatment on Prostanoid Formation

| Therapy | Prostanoid Formation | | Effects | Reference |
|---|---|---|---|---|
| | Platelets | Vasculature | | |
| Antithrombotic | | | | |
| Aspirin | | | | |
|   low dose | $TXA_2\downarrow$ | $PGI_2(\rightarrow)$ | $PF\downarrow$ | 48–52 |
|   high dose | $TXA_2\downarrow$ | $PGI_2(\downarrow)$ | $PF\downarrow,BP(\uparrow)$ | 53,54 |
| Dipyridamole | | $PGI_2\uparrow$ | $VR\downarrow,PF\downarrow$ | 55 |
| Nicotinic Acid | | $PGI_2\uparrow$ | $VR\downarrow$ | 56 |
| Antioxidants | $TXA_2\downarrow$ | $PGI_2(\uparrow)$ | $PF\downarrow$ | 57,58 |
| Sulfinpyrazone | $TXA_2(\downarrow)$ | $PGI_2(\downarrow)$ | $PF\downarrow$ | 59,52 |
| Antianginal | | | | |
| Nitroglycerin | $TXA_2\downarrow$ | $PGI_2\uparrow,PGE_2\uparrow$ | $VR\downarrow$ | 60,61 |
| Beta Blocker | $TXA_2\downarrow$ | | $HR\downarrow,BP\downarrow$ | 36,38,39 |
| Dietary | | | | |
| Vegetable Oil C18:2ω–6 | $TXA_2(\uparrow)$ | $PGI_2(\uparrow)$ | $PF(\downarrow),Chol\downarrow$ | 62 |
| Recent Developments | | | | |
| Fish Oil C20:5ω–3 | $TXA_2\downarrow TXA_3(\uparrow)$ | $PGI_2(\rightarrow),PGI_3(\uparrow)$ | $PF\downarrow,BP\downarrow$ | 63–65 |
| $TXA_2$-Synthesis Inhibitors | $TXA_2\downarrow,PGE_2\uparrow$ | $PGI_2\uparrow$ | $PF\downarrow$ | 67–70 |
| Pyrazolin-one-derivative (BAY g 6575) | $HPETE(\downarrow)$ | $PGI_2(\uparrow)$ | $PF\downarrow$ | 71,72 |

PF = platelet function; BP = blood pressure; VR = vascular resistance; HR = heart rate; HPETE = hydroperoxy fatty acids; () = not definitely established; Chol = cholesterol.

There has been uncertainty with respect to the optimal dose of aspirin to be used in clinical trials. However, recent experimental (48) and clinical (49-52) studies clearly indicate superiority of low dose aspirin (50-100 mg/day, or less) with respect to already effective inhibition of $TXA_2$ formation at largely unchanged $PGI_2$ production. These recent findings may explain, in part, the relative ineffectiveness of high dose aspirin in previous, large scale clinical trials (53, 54).

718

Besides aspirin, experimental and circumstantial evidence suggest
that dipyridamole (55), nicotinic acid (56), antioxidants such as
vitamine E and C (57, 58) and sulfinpyrazone (52, 59) may operate,
if at all, partly through a normalization of altered prostanoid
formation in the platelet and the blood vessel wall.

Nitroglycerin which is the most effective antianginal drug available at present has also been shown to have profound effects on
prostanoid formation which may contribute to its action. Similarly, the beneficial effects of betablockers may partly be due to
effects on arachidonic acid metabolism due to reduced $Ca^{++}$ availability after binding to cellular phospholipids.

Although a beneficial effect of increased intake of vegetable polyunsaturated fatty acids, in the first line linoleic acid ($C18:2\omega-6$),
on the balance between $PGI_2$ and $TXA_2$ has not been established unequivocally (62), dietary supplementation has been advocated to in-
discriminately elevate the polyunsaturated/saturated fatty acid
ratio in plasma and tissue lipids and to reduce intake and circulating levels of cholesterol.

More recent research areas in this field include nutritional manipulation to influence the spectrum of proaggregatory and antiaggregatory prostanoids and leukotrienes by supplementation of specific
prostaglandin precursor fatty acids, such as $C20:5\omega-3$ (63-65), or
$C20:3\omega-6$ (66), further, pharmacological strategies to develop selective thromboxane synthetase inhibitors, such as imidazol-deriva-
tives (67-69), or azo-analogues of prostaglandins (70), and the
design of pyrazolin-one derivatives, such as nafazatrom, whose antithrombotic (71) and antimetastatic potential (72) may be related,
in part, to its activity as a lipoxygenase inhibitor.


## References

1. Schafer AI, Handin RI (1979). Progr.Cardiovasc.Dis.22:31-52.
2. Hirsh PD, Campbell WB, Willerson JT, Hillis LD (1981). Am.J.Med.
   71:1009-26.
3. Levenson DJ, Simmons Jr CE, Brenner BM (1982). Am.J.Med.72:354-
   74.
4. Weber PC, Siess W, Scherer B et al (1982). Klin.Wochenschr.60:
   479-488.
5. Weber PC, Siess W (1982). Pharmacol.Ther.15:321-37.
6. Ahnfelt-Rønne I, Arrigoni-Martelli E (1978). Biochem.Pharmacol.
   27:2363-7.
7. Scherer B, Weber PC (1980). Klin.Wochenschr.58:1099-1104.
8. Shibouta Y, Terashita ZI, Inada Y et al (1981). Eur.J.Pharmacol.
   70:247-56.
9. Sustarsic DL, McPartland RP, Rapp JP (1981). J.Lab.Clin.Med.98:
   599-606.
10. Weber PC, Larsson C, Scherer B (1977). Nature 266:65-6.
11. Rathaus M, Podjarny E, Weiss E et al (1981). Clin.Sci.60:405-10.
12. Stuart MJ, Gerrard JM, White JG (1980). N.Engl.J.Med.302:6-10.
13. Kawaguchi H, Tshibashi T, Imai Y (1981). Lipids 16:37-42.
14. Rosendorff C, Hoffman JIE, Verrier ED et al (1981). Circ.Res.
    48:320-9.
15. Wennmalm A (1982). Prostaglandins 23: 139-44.
16. Siess W, Lorenz R, Roth P, Weber PC (1982). Circulation 66:
    (in press).
17. Schorer AE, Gerrard JM, White JG, Krivit W (1978). Prostaglan-
    dins and Med.1:5-11.

18. Tan SY, Sweet P, Mulrow PJ (1978). Prostaglandins 15:139-50.
19. Grose JH, Lebel M, Gbeassor FM (1980). Clin.Sci.59:121s-3s.
20. Abe K, Yasujima M, Irokawa N et al (1978). Clin.Sci.Mol.Med.
    55:363s-6s.
21. Weber PC, Scherer B, Held E et al (1979). Clin.Sci.57:259s-61s.
22. Halushka PV, Rogers RC, Loadholt CB, Colwell JA (1981). J.Lab.
    Clin.Med.97:87-96.
23. Butkus A, Skrinska VA, Schumacher OP (1980). Thromb.Res.19:
    211-23.
24. Harrison HE, Reece AH, Johnson M (1978). Life Sci.23:351-6.
25. Silberbauer K, Schernthaner G, Sinzinger H et al (1979). N.Engl.
    J.Med.300:366-367 (letter).
26. Kent RS, Kitchell BB, Shand DG, Whorton AR (1981). Prostaglan-
    dins 21:483-90.
27. Nordoy A, Svensson B, Haycraft D et al (1978). Scand.J.Haema-
    tol.21:177-87.
28. Dembinska-Kiec A, Gryglewska T, Zmuda A, Gryglewski RJ (1977).
    Prostaglandins 14:1025-34.
29. Watkins J, Abbot EC, Hensby CN et al (1980). Br.Med.J.281:702-5.
30. Webster J, Dollery CT, Hensby CN (1980). Clin.Sci.59:125s-128s.
31. Luderer JR, Demers LM, Janson RW et al (1980). Res.Comm.Chem.
    Pathol.Pharmacol.28:43-52.
32. Greenwald JE, Wong LK, Alexander M, Bianchine JR (1980). Adv.
    Prostagl.Thromb.Res.6:293-295.
33. Mullane KM, Moncada S (1980). Europ.J.Pharmacol.66:355-65.
34. Moore TJ, Crantz FR, Hollenberg NK (1981). Hypertension 3: 168-
    73.
35. Witzgall H, Hirsch F, Scherer B, Weber PC (1982). Clin.Sci.62:
    611-615.
36. Weksler BB, Gillick M, Pink J (1977). Blood 49:185-96.
37. Durao V, Prata MM, Goncalves LMP (1977). Lancet iv:1005-7.
38. Mehta J, Mehta P (1981). Am.J.Cardiol.47:331-34.
39. Campbell WB, Johnson AR, Callahan KS, Graham RM (1981). Lancet
    iv:1382-84.
40. Aiken JW, Vane JR (1973). J.Pharmacol.Exptl.Therap.184:678-87.
41. Friedman PL, Brown EJ, Gunther S et al (1981). N.Engl.J.Med.
    305:1171-75.
42. Whorton AR, Misono K, Hollifield et al (1977). Prostaglandins
    14:1095-104.
43. Bianchi G, Cusi D, Gatti M (1979). Lancet i:173-77.
44. Duhm J, Göbel BD, Lorenz R, Weber PC (1982). Hypertension 4:
    in press.
45. Fasola AF, Martz BL, Helmer OM (1968). J.Appl.Physiol.25:410-15.
46. Pick R, Chediak J, Glick G (1979). J.Clin.Invest. 63:158-62.
47. Moore S, Friedman RJ, Singal DP et al (1976). Thromb.Haemost.
    35:70-81.
48. Burch JW, Baenziger NL, Stanford N, Majerus PW (1978). Proc.
    Natl.Acad.Sci.75:5181-4.
49. Patrono C, Ciabattoni G, Pinca E et al (1980). Thromb.Res.17:
    317-27.
50. Masotti G, Galanti G, Poggesi L et al (1979). Lancet iv:1213-16.
51. Harter HR, Burch JW, Majerus PW et al (1979). N.Engl.J.Med.301:
    577-79.
52. Lorenz R, Siess W, Weber PC (1981). Europ.J.Pharmacol.70:511-18.
53. Aspirin Myocardial Infarction Study Research Group (1980). JAMA
    243:661-9.
54. Elwood PC, Sweetnam PM (1979). Lancet iv:1313-15.
55. Moncada S, Korbut R (1978). Lancet ii: 1286-89.
56. Eklund B, Kaijser L, Navak J, Wennmalm A (1979). Prostaglandins
    17:821-30.

720

57. Beetens JR, Claeys M, Herman G (1981). Biochem.Pharmacol.30: 2811-15.
58. Chan AC, Leith MK (1981). Am.J.Clin.Nutr.34:2341-47.
59. The Anturane Reinfarction Trial Research Group (1980). N.Engl. Med.302:250-56.
60. Levin RI, Jaffe EA, Weksler BB, Tack-Goldman K (1981). J.Clin. Invest.67:762-69.
61. Morcillio E, Reid PR, Dubin N et al (1980). Am.J.Cardiol.45: 53-57.
62. tenHoor F, de Deckere EAM, Haddeman E et al (1980). Adv.PG and TX Research 8:1771-81.
63. Dyerberg J, Bang HO, Stoffersen E et al (1978). Lancet ii:117-19.
64. Siess W, Roth P, Scherer B et al (1980). Lancet i:441-44.
65. Murphy RC, Pickett WC, Culp BR, Lands WEM (1981). Prostaglandins 22:613-22.
66. Kernoff PBA, Willis AL, Stone KJ et al (1977). Br.Med.J.(2): 1441-44.
67. Moncada S, Bunting S, Mullane K (1977). Prostaglandins 13:611-18.
68. Tyler HM, Saxton CAPD, Parry MJ (1981). Lancet i: 629-32.
69. Vermylen J, Defreyn G, Carreras LO et al (1981). Lancet ii: 1073-75.
70. Gorman RR, Shebuski RJ, Aiken JW, Bundy GL (1981). Federation Proc.40:1997-2000.
71. Seuter F, Busse WD, Meng K et al (1979). Drug Res.29:54-59.
72. Honn KV, Dunn JR (1982). FEBS LETTERS 139:65-68.

# 5 Epidemiology and Prevention

# Coronary Heart Disease - Geographical Differences and Time Trends

F. H. Epstein

The recognition of striking geographical differences in the frequency of atherosclerosis and its consequences provided a major stimulus
for epidemiological research into the reasons for these variations
during the last 30 years. Secular changes in mortality from ischaemic heart disease have likewise attracted attention since the early
1950ies. It was also recognized that the extent of coronary atherosclerosis and the occurrence of myocardial infarction might not necessarily follow the same time trends.

## Time Trends in Mortality

Until the mid-seventies, the concern over the epidemic proportions
of these disease in industrialized countries and the threat of similar trends in developing countries was so great that a major decline
in coronary heart disease mortality was beyond the imagination of
most atherosclerosis-watchers. Yet, two papers in 1974 and 1975 (1,2)
suggested a dramatic downturn in the United States, having started
5-10 years earlier. The situation was reviewed at a conference held
at the National Institutes of Health in Bethesda in 1978 (3). There
was a consensus that the decline was real, partly due to successful
primary prevention efforts and that better medical care (i.e. secondary prevention) had also made a contribution. The age-adjusted decline between 1968 and 1978 amounted to about 24% in U.S. men, 26%
in white and 31% in non-white U.S. women, the reduction being even
greater at younger that at older ages (4). Remarkably, the downward
trend is continuing in the United States at an annual rate of about
2% (R.J. Havlik, personal communication).

The experiences in the United States provoked a comprehensive look
at the trends in other countries which were presented at the "Bethesda Conference" (5). The decline in Australia approaches that seen in
the United States, with lesser reductions in Canada and New Zealand,
in that order. Two low-mortality countries, Israel and Japan, also
showed major declines (6). Such analyses are necessarily confined to
the more developed countries with adequate mortality statistics.
Small rises or falls are observed in the majority of other countries
with higher or intermediate ischaemic heart disease mortalities, with
rises predominating in countries which ranked low around 1970 (7).
The trends in women generally parallel those amongst men (8). Where a
downward trend in heart disease has occurred in men, it was preceded
by a decline amongst women (9). In the United States, cohort analysis

indicates that the rates for the total category of "heart disease" have been successively declining in women since 1945; for men, the pattern has been less clear-cut, the trend being definitely downward since about 1965 (10). In Australia, however, cohort analysis for ischaemic heart disease deaths showed similar upward and downward trends for men and women (11).

The changes in ischaemic heart disease mortality are becoming common knowledge but no systematic attempt has hitherto been made to relate the trends for cardiovascular diseases to those for other major causes of death. An improvement in heart disease mortality would do no good if it were compensated by an increase in other causes of death. Conversely, it would be gratifying if the practice of preventive cardiology would have a favourable effect on other diseases as well. The data shown (<u>Table 1</u>) represent a preliminary assessment of large numbers of detailed data for selected countries from W.H.O. tapes, analyzed in the United States at the National Center for Health Statistics, in collaboration with the National Heart, Lung and Blood Institute. In order to follow trends for a longer period of time (i.e. prior to 1968), it was necessary to discard the category of ischaemic heart disease which has been periodically redefined, and use "nonrheumatic and hypertensive heart disease" which largely reflects heart disease due to coronary atherosclerosis. Amongst other diseases, "cancer other than lung" was selected for this first approach, since rates for lung cancer increased almost universally and would have obscured the trends for other sites. Trends for "total deaths" are also shown. The findings are arranged according to heart disease trends in the two 10-year time periods. Total mortality is related to mortality from heart disease with a fairly high degree of correspondence. In the 22 countries, 44 comparisons can be made. In the 8 comparisons where heart disease declines, total mortality also declines in 6. When heart disease rises (24 comparisons), total mortality also rises in 6 and stays the same in 17 instances. Heart disease remains unchanged in 12 instances and in 5 of them, total mortality remains the same as well. Therefore, heart disease seems to determine to a large extent what happens to total mortality. This is supported by the fact that cancer mortality shows surprisingly little trend in most countries. To the extent that trends exist, there is no evidence that they go in opposite directions as would be the case if conditions protecting against heart disease caused cancer and vice versa. Thus, in the 8 instances where heart disease declines, cancer stays the same or declines as well in 5 instances. In 24 comparisons where heart disease rises, cancer declines in only 4, whereas in the 12 instances where heart disease does not change, the same happens to cancer in 9 of the 12 comparisons. Simultaneous analysis of secular mortality trends for several diseases is important and monitoring the corresponding international trends may provide new insights into interrelationships between diseases and factors which might protect against more than one disease at the same time.

Time Trends in Incidence and Prognosis

Time trends in mortality can occur because the disease is showing a decline in incidence, because of a decrease in the mortality of persons with the disease or, indeed, a combination of the two. Effec-

tive primary prevention would be responsible mostly for a falling incidence while secondary prevention improves prognosis. Available information is still inadequate to provide a definitive answer to the
question to what relative extent changes in incidence, prognosis or
both are at work in causing the observed changes in overall heart
disease mortality.

Data on changes in coronary heart disease (CHD) incidence are not uniform (Table 2). However, if the Rochester Study is taken as pointing
on the whole toward a decline, 4 of the 6 investigations suggest that
there has been a decrease in incidence. The data from the DuPont Company indicate an overall decline of 18% but it would be hazardous to
extrapolate from one large industrial population to the country as a
whole. Nevertheless, on the balance, the data from the 3 countries
where the decline in mortality has been especially pronounced suggest
that there may have been concomitant changes in incidence (the "hospital separation" data from Canada include hospital deaths which have, indeed, diminished but there is a possibility that this has been
more than compensated by the admission of increasingly milder cases).
Autopsy data from New Orleans are in line with a postulated decrease
in CHD incidence; in that city, the mean extent of coronary atherosclerotic lesions has decreased substantially amongst white though
not black men in the last 10 years (18). Data on prognosis (Table 3)
suggest strongly that survival during the first month after a heart
attack has improved while those on long-term survival show no such
trend (the situation in Göteborg, in a country where national mortality rates have, if anything, increased, may be related to the widespread use of beta-blockers in a community with a tradition of preventive cardiology). It would seem, therefore, that in the United
States at least, both primary and secondary prevention played a role
in reducing overall mortality rates from heart disease. The factors
contributing to downward or upward mortality may not be quantitatively the same in different countries, calling for continuing international collaboration in evaluating the trends over time.


Changes in Risk Factors and Living Habits


If a decline in mortality is due wholly or in part to a decline in
incidence, a parallel change in CHD risk factors and the living habits which determine them should be demonstrable. The necessary comparisons may be made within the same country or between countries.
Between-country comparisons are limited to data on nutrition and
smoking. According to one analysis of food disappearance data published by the Food and Agricultural Organization, change in percent
of calories from saturated fat between 1963-65 and 1954-56 and percent change in heart disease mortality some 10 years later showed
no overall correlation (9). If, however, the combined effect of different dietary fats is expressed in terms of a lipid score, estimated from the formulae of Keys or Hegsted and based on food disappearance data from 20 countries averaged over the years 1954-1965,
this score is found to correlate significantly with CHD mortality during 1969-1973 (23, 24). Given the margins of error involved in such
calculations, it is not surprising that different methods of assessment give divergent results. On the balance, available data are in
accordance with the view that there is a correlation between the
kinds of fat consumed and CHD mortality in different countries and

that any changes in these dietary patterns are associated with concomitant changes in mortality. With regard to smoking habits, there is
no overall correlation between change in cigarette consumption and
change in heart disease mortality between the early 1960ies and 1970
ies in 21 countries (9) which does not mean that such correlations
may not exist in one or more of the separate countries.

In addition to these broad, international comparisons, there are now
more detailed data for several individual countries. The evidence from
the United States is known best (3, 6). The per capita consumption of
saturated fats in the U.S. has decreased by 48 percent and comsump-
tion of vegetable fats has increased by 74% since 1963. These changes
are explained by reduced consumption of dairy products and an increase in the intake of vegetable oils so that the P/S ratio of the average diet is now close to 0.5, compared to former values around 0.2
(6). There has been an average reduction of serum cholesterol between
3 and 8% in all age groups (6). Similarly, since 1963, the per capita
consumption of tobacco has decreased by around 30% (6). The detection
and treatment of hypertension has dramatically improved in the last
decade (6). It can be calculated that the cumulative effect of the
changes in average serum cholesterol, blood pressure and smoking in
the U.S. would be expected to lead to a reduction of coronary heart
disease death rates amongst men of the order of 20% (3, p. 293). Although the mean changes in each individual risk factor level are small,
seemingly minor changes maintained over time go a long way in altering
risk. The fact that the drop in expected coronary heart disease mortality is of the same order of magnitude as the observed decline does
not establish by itself a cause-and-effect relationship but must be
accepted as one piece of strong suggestive evidence that a major part
of the declining trend in the United States is related to progress
in primary prevention. As indicated before, the underlying changes
in life styles started already in the 1960ies and risk factor changes
may also date back further (25). It can be calculated by correlating
the risk factor changes observed in the Seven Country Study (26) with
corresponding national mortality rates that the "incubation period"
between exposure to major risk factors and maximum effects on mortality rates may be around 10 years (27).

In two other countries, changes in life styles and risk factors appear to parallel changes in coronary heart disease mortality. In
Australia, the dietary changes are, in general, similar to those in
the United States. with some levelling off in tobacco use and indications of lower mortality due to hypertension (28). In New Zealand,
diet, serum cholesterol levels and smoking habits appear to have
changed in the same direction (29). In Israel, where the P/S ratio
has already been high for some time, changes in total fat consumption
between 1949 and 1977 are correlated with CHD mortality (30).

Alterations in living habits and health practices have to be seen
within their social setting. Secular mortality trends differ by social class, particularly well documented in Britain (9), and there
are also distinct differences in risk factor levels by income and
education. Social class and CHD risk are inversely related, independent of the major risk factors (31, 32). International "transeconomic" trends of arterial diseases in the 1970ies were recently analyzed; moving from low to high GNP (gross national product) in 48 de-

veloping and industrialized countries, a sinusoidal relationship to change in mortality was observed, rising, falling and then slightly rising again (33). The biological mechanisms responsible for these differences are still unknown. However, shifts in social structure must be taken into account in assessing secular trends.


## Mortality Trends: Impact of Primary and Secondary Prevention


An attempt may now be made to reconstruct the present situation and ask to what relative extent primary and secondary prevention might contribute to mortality trends, based on the data which have been reviewed. Where a decrease in incidence, referable to primary prevention, has been observed, it would amount conservatively to at least 10% in 10 years. The short- and longterm improvement in mortality amongst survivors of myocardial infarction in the population may be estimated to be at least 10-20%. How much change in CHD mortality might be "explained" by putting these percentages into a theoretical model (Table 4)? In a base population of 1,000 "middle-aged" men free of CHD and disregarding the already existing pool of myocardial infarction survivors, 100 new events of heart attacks may be expected over the next 10 years, with 30 dying in the first month and another 30 of the 70 survivors over the following 10 years. The impact of a 10% reduction in incidence or a similar reduction in mortality amongst survivors on the total death rate may now be calculated, amounting to 10% and 7%, respectively. If both incidence and mortality were reduced by 10% each, the death rate would decline 17%, while a combination of a 10% reduction in incidence and a 20% reduction in mortality would cause the death rate from CHD to decline 23% which is in the range actually observed in the United States.


This model can be varied by changing the incidence rate which is lower in many countries, chosing different rather than the same mortality rates for short- and longterm survival and allowing for the fact that population averages take no account of the existence of subgroups which respond to preventive and curative measures better or worse than the average. The usefulness of such a model lies in its ability to answer the question what different mixes, as it were, of preventive and curative medicine can "explain" a given change in CHD mortality. Both lines of attack can evidently have a profound effect and it would be most unfortunate to play one approach against the other since both approaches are needed. Various new treatments will continue to influence the outlook for heart disease patients. New diagnostic methods play an increasingly important role in selecting patients for the most suitable treatment. Primary prevention has been making and will continue to make great strides. The outlook, therefore, is bright.

728

## Conclusions and the Task Ahead

The recognition of major recent changes in CHD mortality has brought a new dynamic element into research and its applications toward reducing the burden of this disease in the community. The urgent task is to understand the causes of these trends in order to take or intensify preventive action. An essential prerequisite for an effective strategy is the development of a coordinated, international monitoring and surveillance system, now being created through the joint efforts of the W.H.O. and the National Heart, Lung and Blood Institute, U.S. Public Health Service. Such a system will not only check on progress in prevention or lack of it, but provide indispensable information on changes in risk factors and associated life styles, as well as currently missing data on incidence, survival rates and their changes over time. These problems concern not only countries where trends are already declining and requiring reinforcement but those in which the disease is on the increase. The total endeavour includes many aspects of cardiovascular and atherosclerosis research.

Acknowledgment  Great appreciation is expressed to Mr. Thomas J. Thom who collaborated and helped with the preparation of Table 1.

## References

1. Walker WJ (1974) Coronary mortality: what is going on? J Am Med Ass 227: 1045-46
2. Gordon T, Thom T (1975) The recent decrease in CHD mortality. Prevent Med 4: 115-25
3. Havlik R, Feinleib M, eds (1979) Proceedings of the Conference on the Decline in Coronary Heart Disease Mortality. US Department of Health, Education and Welfare, PHS, DHEW, Publication No. (NIH) 79-1610
4. Feinleib M, Havlik RJ, Thom TJ (1982) The changing pattern of ischaemic heart disease. Cardiovasc Med 7: 139-146
5. Epstein FH, Pisa Z (1979) International comparisons in ischaemic heart disease mortality. In ref 3, pp. 55-88
6. Levy RI (1981) Declining mortality in coronary heart disease. Arteriosclerosis 1: 312-325
7. Epstein FH (1980) Recent international changes in coronary heart disease mortality. Nutr and Metabol 24 (Suppl 1) 45-49
8. Epstein FH (in press) International mortality trends and secular changes. In: Internat.Symp on Epidemiology and Prevention of Atherosclerotic Disease (M. Mancini, ed), Academic Press
9. Marmot MG, Booth M, Beral V (1981) Changes in heart disease mortality in England and Wales and other countries. Health Trends 13: 33-38
10. Patrick CH, Palesch YY, Feinleib M, Brody JA (1982) Sex differences in declining cohort death rates from heart disease. Am J Pub Health 72: 161-166
11. Dobson AJ, Gibberd AW, Wheeler DJ, Leeder SR (1981) Age-specific trends in mortality from ischaemic heart-disease and cerebrovascular disease in Australia. Am J Epid 113: 404-12

12. Pell S, Fayerweather WE (1982) Morbidity trends in myocardial infarction in a large employed population, 1957-1979. CVD Epidemiol Newsletter, Am Heart Ass 31: 56
13. Elveback LR, Connolly DC, Kurland LT (1981) Coronary heart disease in residents of Rochester, Minnesota. II. Mortality, Incidence and Survivorship, 1950-1975. Mayo Clin Proc 56: 665-672
14. Kannel WB, Thom T (1979) Implications of the recent decline in cardiovascular mortality. Cardiovasc Med 4: 983-997
15. Friedman GD (1979) Decline in hospitalizations for coronary heart disease and stroke: The Kaiser-Permanente experience in Northern California, 1971-1977. In ref 3, pp. 109-114
16. Hobbs MST, Martin CA, Armstrong BK (submitted for publ) An analysis of trends in mortality from ischaemic heart disease and hospital admission rates for acute myocardial infarction and other ischaemic heart disease in Perth, Western Australia 1968-1979
17. Chronic Disease in Canada (1981) 2: 9-12 (Health and Welfare, Canada)
18. Strong JP, Guzman MA (1980) Decrease in coronary atherosclerosis in New Orleans. Laboratory Invest 43: 297-301
19. Nanas S, Mansour M, Liu K, Stamler J et al (1982) Changes in pattern of sudden death over the last two decades. CVD Epidemiol Newsletter, Am Heart Ass 31: 47
20. Weinblatt E, Goldberg JD, Ruberman W, Frank CW, Monk MA, Chaudhary BS (1982) Mortality after first myocardial infarction. J Am Med Ass 247: 1576-1581
21. Goldberg R, Szklo M, Tonascia JA, Kennedy HL (1979) Time trends in prognosis of patients with myocardial infarction: a population-based study. Johns Hopkins Med J 144: 73-80
22. Vedin A, Wilhelmsson C, Bergstrand R, Johannson S, Ulvenstam G, Wedel H, Wilhelmsen L, Aberg A (1982) Secular trends in survival after myocardial infarction? CVD Epidemiol Newsletter, Am Heart Ass 31: 53
23. Liu K, Stamler J, Trevisan M, Moss D (submitted for publ) Dietary lipids, sugar, fiber and mortality from coronary heart disease: a bivariate analysis of international data
24. Arteriosclerosis 1981. Report of the Working Group on Arteriosclerosis of the National Heart, Lung and Blood Institute, Volume 2. NIH Publ No 82-2035 Sept 1981, pp 313-314
25. Feinleib M, Garrison RJ, Stallones L, Kannel WB, Castelli WP and McNamara PM (1979) A comparison of blood pressure, total cholesterol and cigarette smoking in parents in 1950 and their children in 1970. Am J Epid 110: 291-303
26. Keys A (1970) Coronary heart disease in seven countries. Circulation Suppl I, 1-211
27. Rose G (submitted for publ) The incubation period of coronary heart disease
28. Dwyer T and Hetzel BS (1980) A comparison of trends of coronary heart disease mortality in Australia, USA and England and Wales with reference to three major risk factors - hypertension, cigarette smoking and diet. Int J Epidemiol 9: 65-71
29. Beaglehole R, Hay DR, Foster FH, Sharpe DN (1981) Trends in coronary heart disease mortality and associated risk factors in New Zealand. New Zealand Med J 685: 371-5.
30. Palgi A (1981) Association between dietary changes and mortality rates: Israel 1949 to 1977; a trend-free regression model. Am J Clin Nutr 34: 1569-1583
31. Holme I (1980) Paper presented at 8th European Congress of Cardiology, Paris, June 1980

32. Rose G, Marmot MG (1981) Social class and coronary heart disease. Brit Heart J 45: 13–19
33. Ionnidis PJ, Efthymiopoulou GD (1982) International transeconomic trends of arterial diseases in the mid-1970s. Am J Epidemiol 115: 278–297

Table 1. TRENDS FOR HEART DISEASE (HD*), TOTAL MORTALITY (TM) AND CANCER (OTHER THAN LUNG) IN DIFFERENT COUNTRIES DURING TWO TIME PERIODS (I:1955-1965; II:1965-1975); MEN AGED 45-64

| HD | | TM | | CA (excl. lung) | | COUNTRIES |
|---|---|---|---|---|---|---|
| I | II | I | II | I | II | |
| ↓ | ↓ | ↓ | ↓ | o | ↓ | JAPAN |
| o | ↓ | ↓ | ↓ | ↑ | ↑ | FRANCE |
| | | ↓ | o | o | o | CANADA |
| | | o | ↓ | o | o | USA (white men) |
| ↑ | ↓ | o | ↓ | o | ↑ | AUSTRALIA |
| | | o | o | o | ↑ | NEW ZEALAND |
| | | o | ↓ | o | o | SWITZERLAND |
| ↑ | o | ↑ | ↓ | o | o | F.R. GERMANY |
| | | ↑ | o | o | o | DENMARK |
| | | o | ↓ | ↑ | o | BELGIUM |
| | | o | ↓ | o | o | AUSTRIA |
| | | o | o | ↑ | o | ITALY |
| | | o | o | o | o | SCOTLAND |
| | | o | ↓ | ↓ | ↓ | FINLAND |
| o | ↑ | o | ↑ | o | ↑ | CZECHOSLOVAKIA |
| | | ↓ | ↑ | ↑ | ↑ | POLAND |
| ↑ | ↑ | o | ↓ | ↓ | o | ENGLAND & WALES |
| | | o | o | ↓ | o | NORTHERN IRELAND |
| | | o | o | o | o | IRELAND, SWEDEN |
| | | ↑ | o | o | o | NETHERLANDS |
| | | ↑ | o | ↓ | o | NORWAY |

* HD: non-rheumatic heart disease and hypertension

Nat. Center for Health Statistics; National Heart, Lung & Blood Institute, NIH; DHHS; prelimin. data

Table 2.  DATA ON CHANGES IN CORONARY HEART DISEASE INCIDENCE

| Study | Time Period | Measure | Decline | Reference |
|---|---|---|---|---|
| DuPont Co., USA | 1957-1964/1973-9 | Incidence of MI | Yes | (12), 1982 |
| Rochester, Minnesota | 1955-9/1970-5 | Incidence of MI | No | (13), 1981 |
| | | Incidence of CHD | Yes | |
| | | Incidence of SD | Yes | |
| Framingham, Mass. | 1962-6/1968-72 | Incidence of MI | No | (14), 1979 |
| Kaiser-Permanente, Cal. | 1971/1977 | Hospital Admissions | Yes | (15), 1979 |
| Perth, Australia | 1968/1979 | Hospital Admissions | Yes | (16), 1982 |
| Canadian Provinces | 1969/1979 | Hospital Separations | No | (17), 1981 |

MI: Myocardial Infarction; CHD: coronary heart disease; SD: sudden death

Table 3.  DATA ON CHANGES IN CORONARY HEART DISEASE PROGNOSIS

| Time after Attack | Study | Time Period | Improvement | Reference |
|---|---|---|---|---|
| First Month | Kaiser-Permanente, Cal. | 1971/1977 | No | (15), 1979 |
| | DuPont Co., USA | 1957-64/1973-9 | Yes | (12), 1982 |
| | Rochester, Minnesota | 1965-9/1970-5 | Yes | (13), 1981 |
| | Framingham, Massachusetts* | 1962-6/1968-72 | Yes | (14), 1979 |
| | Chicago, Illinois | 1955-65/1975-9 | Yes | (19), 1982 |
| | Canadian Provinces | 1969/1977 | Yes | (17), 1981 |
| Past First Month | H.I.P., New York | 1960ies/1970ies | No | (20), 1982 |
| | Rochester, Minnesota | 1965-9/1970-5 | No | (13), 1981 |
| | Baltimore, Maryland | 1966-7/1971 | No | (21), 1979 |
| | Göteborg, Sweden | 1968/1977 | Yes | (22), 1982 |

* not specified what time interval after attack covered by analysis

732

Table 4.     ESTIMATING THE EFFECT OF PRIMARY AND SECONDARY PREVENTION ON CHD DEATH RATES

| Reduction in: | | New Events | Deaths: | | | Decline in: | |
| Incidence | Mortality | | In first Month | Amongst Survivors | Total | Incidence | Death Rate |
|---|---|---|---|---|---|---|---|
| - | - | 100* | 30* | 30* | 60 | - | - |
| 10% | - | 90 | 27 | 27 | 57 | 10% | 10% |
| - | 10% | 100 | 27 | 29 | 56 | - | 7% |
| 10% | 10% | 90 | 24 | 26 | 50 | 10% | 17% |
| 10% | 20% | 90 | 22 | 24 | 46 | 10% | 23% |

* see text

# Coronary Disease Risk Factors: A Population View

H. Blackburn and D. Jacobs

The evidence is strong that levels of blood cholesterol, arterial blood
pressure and cigarette smoking influence the risk of coronary atherosclerosis and heart disease (CHD).  The inference that they are causal
is based on the strength, consistency and independent predictive power
of the associations found in populations and the congruence of the
epidemiological with clinical and experimental evidence.  Most informed
investigators have accepted this evidence as providing a strong
rationale for preventive practice and public policy.  Nevertheless,
much work remains for effective translation of this evidence into public
health action.  In addition, much detail remains to be elaborated in the
risk factor-disease relationships and the mechanisms of their causal
effects.  Moreover, new findings beg explanation, such as the possible
inverse association between an individual's blood lipoprotein levels and
risk of colon cancer, and the varied relationship of obesity to cardiovascular (CVD) disease risk.  We believe that we can most constructively
treat here those issues which are inconsistent or controversial.
Therefore, we will consider the shape of the risk factor relationships
to disease, certain departures from prediction, touch on underlying
mechanisms, and discuss the implications of these newer findings for
research and strategies of primary prevention.

## Detailed Risk Factor-Disease Relationships

Systematic population studies indicate that a positive, continuous,
probably exponential relationship exists between systolic and diastolic
blood pressure (BP) and future CHD risk.  This is apparent in plots of
incidence against the simple distributions and as well in the least
squares solutions.  Currently the details of the BP-CHD relationship are
being less avidly pursued than those for the blood lipoproteins,
presumably because control of hypertension reduces risk, and because of
the strength and consistency of the relationship, for which plausible
mechanisms are established.  These, in turn, are compatible with the
theory of pathogenesis in atherosclerosis which holds that lipid insudation occurs according to lateral wall pressure and arterial injury.
The cigarette smoking relationship to CHD risk is understood and studied
even less.  This may be due in part to the other nocent influences
of smoking, particularly lung disease, and in part from absence of an
objective measure of smoke exposure.  Though quantitative measures are
now available, it is conjectural whether it would be worth the cost to
re-examine all the relationships of smoking and disease using these new
chemical methods and repeating the longitudinal population studies.
Additionally, pathogenetic mechanisms for smoking in atherosclerosis are
not established, and hardly well formulated.  Despite these remarkable
deficiencies, it is interesting that few if any investigators call for
more evidence, through controlled trials, or suggest that health action
about smoking be postponed.  Similarly, most consider the favorable
metabolic effect of weight loss in our society a sufficient rationale to
recommend weight control and prevention of obesity for the whole population despite the evidence that overweight is little related to CHD or
mortality risk.  In great contrast is the doubt, still publicly

734

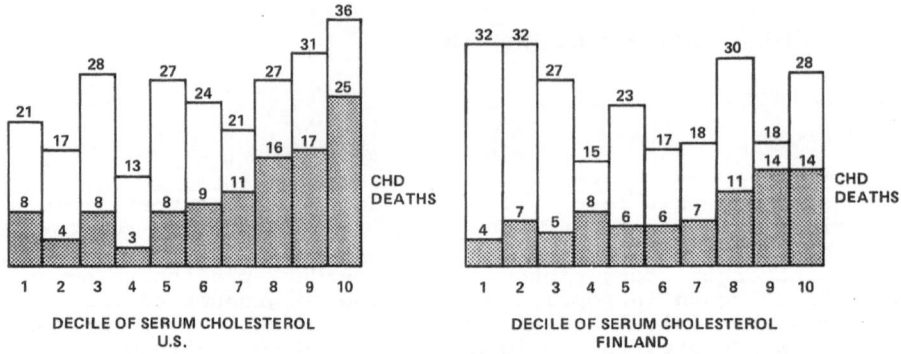

<u>Fig. 1.</u> Ten year CHD incidents and deaths (Keys A, 1980)

expressed by some investigators, about the validity of the extensive
diet-lipid-atherosclerosis evidence or the wisdom of population-wide
changes in composition of the habitual diet. Here we speculate on the
causes of the uncertainty and of the considerably renewed interest and
activity in the field.

Let us consider first the shape of the TC-CHD relationship in some of
the Seven Countries Study populations in Figure 1 (1). In U.S. rail
workers and in Finland (and in the pooled Northern European countries),
CHD rates tend to meander below the 6th or 7th decile. They appear to
increase regularly and rapidly from the 7th to the 10th decile. There
is even an occasional suggestion of lower rates in middle deciles of the
distribution though statistical tests comparing them do not approach
significance. In fact, no monotonic model, either linear or exponential, fits these data in the lower deciles better than any other. Each
fits relatively well. A model with a zero slope for deciles 1 to 6
would be just as accurate as the other models. However, a priori
assumption of a threshold model denies what we call "the principle of
biological continuity," i.e., that underlying mathematical behavior in
the lower deciles is a less obvious version of the sharply increasing
rates in the upper deciles. Actually we believe to have demonstrated
that it is not possible in these or most data to distinguish in this
part of the distribution between zero relationships and small positive
slopes (2). Thus, though these findings do not support a strong effect
of TC in the lower part of the distribution, neither do they support
strongly no effect at all. Of course it is a philosophical matter
whether to put "faith" in a model which averages out the variation and
adheres to "biological continuity" or to trust only the observed data,
subject as they are to random variation. A model which would average
the 1st and 2nd deciles, 3rd and 4th, etc., would declare the lower
deciles as a whole at lower risk than the higher, and conclude there is
a continuous gradient of risk. Because attributable risk is great of
even small gradients in risk by TC level, so must be the public health
implications. Therefore, we consider that these direct observations
should not be treated casually or in isolation from other population
data or from the clinical and experimental evidence which suggests a
continuous dose-effect of TC level on CHD risk. An increasingly
shallow risk gradient from 5 to 10 to 15 year follow-up in the Seven
Countries data suggests the possibility that the TC-CHD gradient gets
smaller as a cohort ages (as was also demonstrated in Framingham) and as
follow-up is more remote from the initial TC measurement.

Table 1. Aha pooling project serum cholesterol standardized incidence ratio first CHD event

| Q | TC | POOL 5 | ALB | CH-GAS | CH-WE | FRAM | TECUM | LA | MN CVD | MN RR |
|---|---|---|---|---|---|---|---|---|---|---|
| I | ≤194 | 72 | 72 | 100 | 62 | 74 | 10 | 37 | 64 | 47 |
| II | 194-218 | 61 | 67 | 61 | 57 | 50 | 83 | 46 | 78 | 50 |
| III | 218-240 | 78 | 72 | 89 | 70 | 88 | 56 | 116 | 117 | 77 |
| IV | 240-268 | 129 | 129 | 124 | 99 | 160 | 145 | 73 | 117 | 96 |
| V | >268 | 158 | 177 | 118 | 159 | 167 | 242 | 143 | 189 | 194 |
| RR | | 2.4 | 2.5 | 1.5 | 2.7 | 2.7 | 4.9 | — | — | 4.0 |
| # | | 647 | 156 | 123 | 142 | 177 | 49 | 72 | 28 | 112 |

POOLING PROJECT RESEARCH GROUP, 1978

The next interesting finding, seen in Table 1, is the possible excess risk at the lower end of the TC distribution seen in 4 of 8 studies in the Pooling Project and elsewhere (3, 4). Is it real and universal and what might be its explanations and implications? The risk findings for both CHD and non-CHD deaths associated with a low relative position in the TC distribution, without regard to absolute TC value, suggests to us the possibility of a general phenomenon of excess risk in "hypocholesteremic" individuals. It is speculated that individuals found toward the lower end of any distribution might be as distinctive as those at the upper end in their departure from heterogeneity or at least a genetic admixture with evolutionary survival value. Details about the lipoprotein subfraction composition of such individuals at the lower end of the TC distribution might be useful. The Framingham data suggest that much of the excess overall mortality in men at the lower TC values is accounted for by excess cancer deaths. The new, though inconsistently found relationships between diet, TC and colon cancer risk are mentioned because they are influencing discussions on preventive strategy (5, 6). The subject is given a thoroughgoing consideration elsewhere in this symposium. An inverse relationship of individual TC level to colon cancer may exist within some populations. This may be in part due to a relationship of HDL levels to risk of cancer (7). On the other hand, mean TC levels in populations are unrelated or inversely related to colon cancer death rates (6, 8). In fact, the higher are reported national CHD death rates the lower are the colon cancer deaths (6).

When such paradoxes appear between correlations found in populations (ecological correlations) and those for individual relationships within populations, several phenomena need to be considered. Case 1: When population and individual risk correlations are consonant and positive: When both individuals and populations with higher risk factor values have a higher observed disease incidence, would this not speak strongly for a significant environmental influence? If the population correlations are strong, genetic susceptibility must be widespread, with intrinsic differences contributing importantly to the range of the population distribution, whether that range is "set" high or low. Case 2: When individual and population findings are not consonant: a) Where the risk factor is significantly related to risk within but not between populations, would it not be likely that an individual intrinsic factor is more powerfully operative than a mass, ecological one? An example might be the relationship of TC and colon cancer: Population TC means and distributions differ, as do the habitual population diets which are primarily responsible for them. Dietary patterns which result in low population TC distributions appear compatible with lower population risk of colon cancer. Findings within some populations suggest that individual colon cancer risk is related to low TC level. This might be

predominately genetic or interactive with habitual diet; plausible
mechanisms exist for either influence. For example, a low TC might
depend on an individual eating pattern low in a co-factor such as carotenes. On the intrinsic side, metabolic adaptations responsible for a
low personal TC level might also result in greater bile acid secretion
and concentration as co-carcinogens in the colon. Though a common
dietary factor has not emerged, the inverse relationship of plasma TC
level and fecal steroids is likely. b) Where significantly positive
individual correlations exist but a given population's values deviate
from the ecologic regression line. The example reported in this
symposium by Richard has risk factor profiles in France predicting
individual risk but population CHD rates there are below those expected
from wider population correlations. Does not this case suggest the
presence of a possible <u>protective</u> environmental factor operating at the
population level? c) Where weak correlations are found for individuals
and strong relationships between populations, a powerful environmental
force may yet be operative but not easily demonstrable due to attenuated
individual correlations when: 1) the whole population distribution of
the risk variable is set high or exceeds some "threshold" effect; 2)
when the environment or social behavior related to that variable is
homogeneous 3) when intra-individual variation is virtually equal to
inter-individual variation, 4) or when the measurement is unreliable for
individual characterization though valid for characterizing populations.
A well known example of this phenomenon is habitual dietary fatty acid
intake, generally so strongly related to population TC values and CHD
rates but significantly related to individual TC levels and CHD risk in
U.S. populations only when great care is taken to minimize individual
variability and reduce technical error (9).

Such apparent paradoxes between the correlations computed between
populations - ecological correlations - and those computed between
individuals - individual correlations - are not contradictory. The two
correlations may in fact be completely different; one reflects the ecologic factors which affect all individuals in the population more or
less equally and are different between populations; the other reflects
individual factors which specify the usual state for each person. The
"ecologic fallacy" is to interpret one set of associations as the
other.* Stated otherwise, individual differences most determine indi-

---

*The distinction between ecologic and individual correlations is
expressed mathematically in the model

$$CA_{ij} = M_{CA} + E_{i,CA} + I_{ij,CA} + error$$

$$TC_{ij} = M_{TC} + E_{i,TC} + I_{ij,TC} + error$$

where CA refers to colon cancer (presence or absence) and TC to total
serum cholesterol. The index i refers to the population, j to the individual. M is the term for the grand mean; E is the term for the ecologic factor and it sums to zero across populations. I is the term for
the individual factor, and sums to zero within each population. The
ecologic correlation is computed between CA and TC using population wide
data from which individual variations have been removed. The individual
correlation is computed between CA and TC using individual data within
each population; it may be averaged across populations, if this is
justified, to get a composite estimate. The computation of the individual correlation therefore does not involve the terms in E, and the
ecological correlation does not involve the terms in I. Presumably both
CA and TC have multiple determinants, some of which may coincide. The
factors which determine the usual levels for populations - the E terms
- may be different from those which determine the usual levels for in-

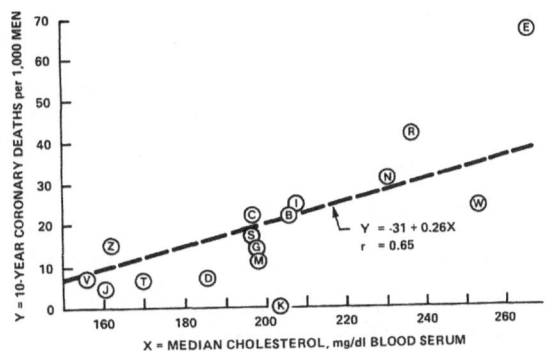

Fig. 2. Serum cholesterol versus 290 coronary deaths (no cardiovascular disease at entry) age-standardized death rate

vidual risk when the ecologic influence is similarly distributed. Ecologic differences most determine population risk when individual susceptibility is similarly distributed.

## A Population View

Thus insights can be gained by looking at population data in the mass, along with individual data and by explaining or reconciling their discordance. Each of these views, population and individual, is valid within its own context. But the failure to look at population findings along with individual is, we believe, responsible for much of the unnecessary professional controversy in the diet-heart matter. Those concerned only with individual variations find it difficult to see the population issue or recognize its implications for the public health, in contrast to individual health. Those who look mainly at the population picture need reminding that any useful model for risk has to account for individual uniqueness and wide human variation. Can we put these two aspects together and resolve a balanced individual-population view?

It is accepted now that large population differences, age and sex-specific, exist in CHD incidence and mortality. The Framingham, Honolulu, Puerto Rico (10) and the Seven Countries Study (1, 11) are highly relevant to this issue because of their attention to standardization. Established differences in 10-year CHD incidence range from near zero to almost 66 per thousand, per decade, between fourteen areas of the Seven Countries. The ecological correlations are strong between mean values of TC and average fatty acid and cholesterol composition of the population diet, between mean TC and CHD incidence (Figure 2) and finally, between habitual diet and CHD rates (1). The ecological coefficients of correlation found between TC, diet and CHD may be somewhat greater than the true correlation because initially the populations were selected by purported (but quite undocumented) differences in CHD rates and eating patterns. However, this triangular connection of Diet-TC-CHD is well established and clearly set forth elsewhere. We only reiterate the preventive implications of such large disparities in disease rates, risk factor levels and population behavior

---

*dividuals - the I terms. Thus, the ecologic and individual correlations are distinct mathematical entities and may bear no resemblance to one another.

(keeping in mind the ecological fallacy). These findings lead us to the concept that hyperlipidemia is relative, that statistical norms are deficient, and that some external criterion of reference is more appropriate for optimal lipid levels, such as population disease risk. If whole populations are relatively hyperlipoproteinemic and at relatively excess CHD risk, the disparate disease rates and population risks are not likely to be explained by population differences in frequency of monogenic lipid disorders or even of those polygenic determinants of blood lipid responses to diet (12). Population geneticists do not speculate that disease differences of such magnitude derive from large genetic differences, if the populations are sizable and heterogeneous. We have previously developed speculative and illustrative models for the impo-tance of intrinsic factors in determining individual TC levels and of environment (diet) in determining the average population TC levels and of distribution (12). All these observations have had a profound effect on our thinking about mass diseases, their causes and the strategies needed for prevention. We believe the evidence allows us to extend the classic concept that all disease is an interaction of host and environmental factors to the idea that mass diseases (such as atherosclerosis and hypertension) are the interaction of powerful cultural factors with widespread susceptibility in human populations. The corollary is that a favorable environment should encourage the minimal exhibition of susceptible phenotypes and lower manifest disease.

But apparent departures from prediction occur in both the individual and population relationships. Some are apparent in the Seven Countries, as in Figure 2 on TC values and CHD risk which is greater than expected in East Ⓔ over West Finland Ⓦ . In Finland, genetic differences as well as significant differences in the distribution of smoking and blood pressure may apply, as well as unknown metabolic differences. The phenomenon of Crete ( Ⓚ in Figure 2) with its high fat, olive oil intake is an equally fascinating natural experiment from which more might be learned.

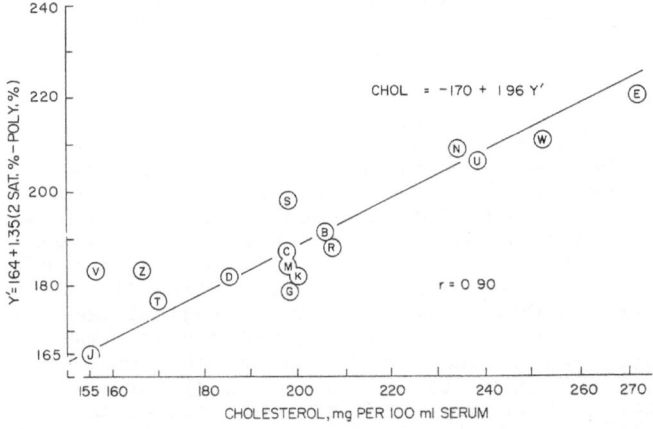

Fig. 3. Population mean cholesterol values versus diet fatty acids

Interesting speculation arises on considering Figure 3 in which the ecologic relationship between dietary fatty acid intake and TC levels in the Seven Countries Study departs from the Keys-Minnesota individual correlations (1, 13). In individuals studies for weeks in metabolis ward conditions, TC increases 1 mg/dl for every unit increase in the score 1.35 (2S - P) where S and P are the percent of daily calories consumed from saturated and polyunsaturated fatty acids respectively. Ecologic regression of TC on this score indicates a slope of 1.96 where the metabolic ward experiments in small groups would have predicted a slope of only 1. Countries as units are apparently twice as "responsive" to habitual diet as are individuals. The mean TC of populations increases 2 mg/dl for every unit increase in the dietary fat score. This suggests an ecologic factor affecting TC approximately equally in most individuals, and causing TC to be higher than expected based on short-term experiments of fatty acid change. The response to a lifetime of different fat intake may result in metabolic adaptations which raise TC, or the dietary fat score for countries carries "information" on other dietary constituents which affect TC, e.g., fiber and vegetable protein. The greatest discrepancies claimed between diet, TC and CHD rates are from investigations among small, isolated, primitive cultures. Important as they may be, the Eskimo, Samburu, and Masai experiences provide, in our view, insufficient evidence of discrepant relationships, chiefly because their field epidemiological methods and sample sizes are inadequate. However, a much better documented discrepancy between observed diet and expected blood lipid values (predicted by the Keys-Minnesota equation) is in the South Pacific Islanders on Tokelau and Pukapuka (14). Based on fatty acid composition of their diets, TC values are some 60-80 mg/dl lower than predicted, yet differences between the islands confirm to prediction. Little to nothing is known about CHD incidence in these small populations. But the findings suggest that physiologic, metabolic, and cultural adaptations may indeed occur more rapidly in such isolates than in larger, more heterogeneous populations and that these in turn may affect the relationship between diet, blood lipid response and disease. However, it may also be that other factors operate in the diet of these islanders including the normally different metabolic routes by which the short-chain fatty acids of coconut oil are handled.

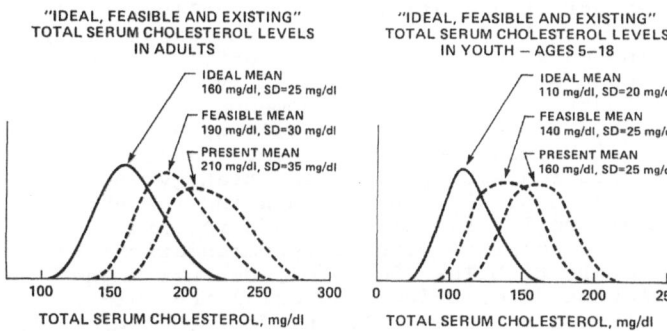

Fig. 4

## Risk Factors in Children

Information is increasing on the distribution of risk characteristics in youth which are widely disparate between populations. In the examples summarized by epidemiologists in Figure 4, mean TC values in children parallel the mean values in adults with an adjustment of about 50 mg/dl (2). Relative hyperlipidemia in youth, and its related mass eating behavior, is considered a likely precursor of mass adult atherosclerosis.

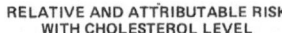

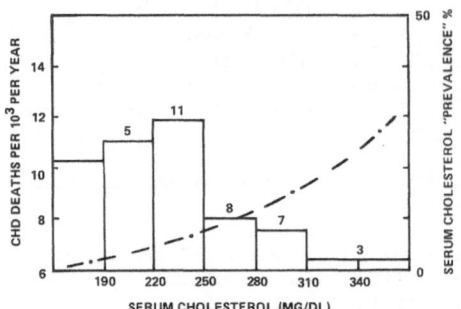

ATTRIBUTABLE OR EXCESS CHD
DEATHS/1000/10 YEARS*
(EXCESS RISK X EXPOSURE)

| TC | % POPULATION | %XS DEATHS |
|---|---|---|
| < 220 | 45 | 10 |
| > 310 | 5 | 15 |
| 220-310 | 50 | 75 |

*ROSE: FRAMINGHAM, 26: 1970;
WHO EXPERT COMMITTEE REPORT, 1982

Fig. 5. Serum cholesterol

## Attributable Risk

Geoffrey Rose has composed the display in Figure 5 of relative and
attributable risk from Framingham distributions of TC and CHD risk (15).
Against a background histogram of Framingham TC distributions is
displayed the familiar curvilinear relationship between TC level and
individual CHD risk based on the Framingham logistic solution. The
numbers imposed on the columns are the excess CHD cases attributable to
TC level. These are obtained by multiplying the relative risk at that
level by the population exposed. We have added the table next to the
figure to show the proportion of excess cases deriving from the several
parts of the TC distribution. This analysis within populations also
contributes to a population view of primary CHD prevention. It shows
that relatively few excess CHD cases occur in the upper or lower
extremes of the distribution, either because of the low population exposure or low relative risk. Rather it illustrates dramatically that 75%
of the excess cases attributable to TC level come from the large central
part of the distribution having only "moderately elevated" TC values
(220 to 310 mg/dl). The Gothenburg experience reported by Wilhelmsen in
this symposium differently illustrates the same phenomenon. Half the
population is clearly too great a proportion to be dealt with in a
screening, medical care model with individual follow-up. Rather this
mass phenomenon requires a population-wide prevention strategy and
program. Failure to consider these population findings and thereby
making extrapolations from individual correlations leads to unnecessary
controversy and sometimes to inappropriate general recommendations such
as to reduce individual TC levels to below 220 mg/dl, but not much
below. An hypothetical population TC distribution reflecting this
desirable state for individuals but an infeasible one for populations is
displayed in Figure 6. In fact, nature does not present such distorted
distributions. The advice to achieve a specific value is difficult to
achieve for individuals and clearly is unattainable for populations. The
population distributions appropriate to optimal public health are more
likely, we think, to resemble the lefthand curves for adults in Figure 4;
these are also compatible with the reasonable advice for individuals to
seek values "below 220 mg/dl." But finally, these models consider only
physiological risk factors. There is, of course, a parallel distribution
of health behaviors which are socially determined-socially learned.
Attempts to approach only those individuals identified at any specified
risk factor level or estimated high risk must have less than optimal
effect on community behavior or risk. The population norms and determinants of health behavior are much more universal. In many modern
cultures there is insufficient social support for change in these norms,
even when the individual is persuaded and motivated to try.

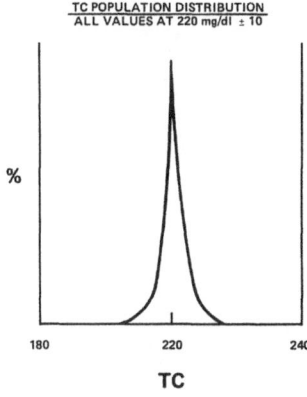

TC **Fig. 6**

## Duration of Exposure

Of the several alternative explanations for discrepant population data, one of the least-known factors is the duration of exposure to risk. One can hardly know from a single measure, or even a short-term series, the true individual or population exposure to a risk factor. Similarly, slopes of the time trends in population exposures, whether stable, ascending or descending, can usually only be surmised. Risk predictions from the long-term observations on which we base estimates of risk, and of the preventability of CHD, might well depend on whether the measures were constant or on an ascending or descending limb at the moment they were taken. Exposure may be more crucial in youth. On the other hand, age-specific national changes in reported CHD mortality are, in historical terms, remarkably rapid, both upward and downward. Similarly, time trends in population TC levels are documented to change quickly and in different directions (1). More standardized data from population-based samples are needed for men, women and children, with detailed lipoprotein fractions, collected over extensive periods. A "new epidemiology" is needed for the simultaneous monitoring of trends in death, disease, risk factors and risk related behaviors (16). Moreover, our understanding of the interactions of risk characteristics is about as limited as that on duration of exposure. Though we and others have suggested that a particular luxurious diet leading to mass hyperlipidemia is a necessary factor for mass atherosclerosis and high CHD incidence rates (17), in fact, the evidence is equally compatible with no high CHD incidence population occurring where any of the three major risk characteristics is missing or relatively low. Thus, it may be that diet, mass elevated lipids, and frequent high blood pressure and cigarette smoking may all be necessary to mass atherosclerosis. Obviously, there are conceptual and factual deficiencies in all these observations and syntheses. Presumably the only solution to these is more and better data.

Table 2. A model for population risk reduction

| Percentage of the population declared "at risk" and educated in risk factor lowering | Modelled linear percentage risk reduction achievable in individuals | Estimated percentage reduction in population risk | Modelled percentage risk reduction achievable in individuals (without social supports) | Modelled percentage reduction in population risk | Estimated percentage risk reduction achievable in individuals (with social supports) | Estimated percentage reduction in population risk |
|---|---|---|---|---|---|---|
| (a) | (b) | (a) x (b) | (c) | (a) x (c) | (d) | (a) x (d) |
| < 1 | 25 | < 0.1 | 25 | 0.1 | N/A | N/A |
| 10 | 23 | 2.3 | 23 | 2.3 | N/A | N/A |
| 25 | 20 | 5.0 | 15 | 3.8 | N/A | N/A |
| 50 | 15 | 7.5 | 10 | 5.0 | N/A | N/A |
| 100 | 5 | 5.0 | N/A | N/A | 10 | 10 |

## A Population Strategy to Shift Risk Factor Distributions

In a quantitative model of prevention in Table 2, a first assumption is
that risk can be lowered by 25% with intensive counselling in a high
risk individual (effectively 0% of the population) but that effectiveness of direct strategies decreases linearly thereafter, to give 23%
risk reduction in the top decile, 15% in the top half of the population
risk and perhaps 5% risk lowering only for the whole community. People
not in the prevention program are assumed to achieve no risk reduction.
The decrease in risk in the whole population is the product of the
columns and is smallest for intervention only in the higher risk groups.
A refinement is shown in column (c) in which half the community is
labelled as "high risk," but the considerable cost and inefficiencies of
screening and putting 50% of the population on a special program is
modelled to achieve the risk reduction in column (c) with the product of
columns (a) and (c) showing the population effect. Finally, column (d)
embodies the idea that a community-wide, multiple strategy program
diffuses the ideas and social support for change and achieves more and
wider effect than the linear model of column (b). The product of
columns (a) and (d) suggests that the population-wide strategy changes
community norms and values significantly and is an efficient strategy
for reducing population risk.

## Other Questions

What may be wrong with these data and these interpretations? We and
many others suggest that taken together the evidence provides a firm
base for a successful population approach to primary prevention. It is
conceivable, however, that both the data and our interpretations of them
are off the mark. For example, the continuous model of relative risk
may be questioned. We find it difficult to believe that nature acts
with absolute thresholds; rather we incline to "the principle of biological continuity" and are not now prepared to reject the idea that
risk is multifactorial and continuous. However, if exponential or other
monotonic models are not the best solutions for the true relationships,
and the risk is not smoothly rising, then the basic idea of a continuum
of risk is challenged. In turn, an important preventive concept also
might not hold: that various combinations of moderate elevations of risk
produce similar absolute individual risk. However, nature does not
usually present us with risk dichotomies and it is difficult to arrive
at logical mechanisms for discontinuous risk. But as we have discussed
here, the data are actually compatible with any of these models and we
must consider whether the discontinuous model, if widely confirmed, would
affect strategies to shift entire risk factor distributions downward.

For the nonce, it seems to us that such a population strategy holds, in the presence of safety and feasibility, though the case is admittedly less arguable if we were to be concerned only with the upper tertile of TC levels in the U.S. population. It appears that substantial numbers of people in high risk societies need to be involved in behavioral change to prevent individual incident cases and to reduce the population disease burden, whatever the risk model used or educational strategy adopted. Finally, the models we suggest here for the estimated effects of downward shifts in population risk factor distributions are quite untested as are the educational strategies which lead communities of free people to make more informed and healthier choices. The three NIH-sponsored research and demonstration projects in CHD prevention in the U.S. are perhaps the closest to experimental tests of the population strategies likely to be carried out in this century (18).

REFERENCES

1.  Keys A (1980) Seven countries:  Death and coronary heart disease in ten years.  Harvard University Press, Cambridge
2.  Blackburn H, Berenson G, Christakis G, et al (1979) Conference on the health  effects of blood lipids:  Optimal distributions for populations.  Workshop report:  epidemiology section.  Prev Med 8: 612-678
3.  The Pooling Project Research Group (1978) Relationship of blood pressure, serum  cholesterol, smoking habits, relative weight and ECG abnormalities to incidence of major coronary events:  Final report of the pooling project.  J Chronic Dis 31: 201
4.  Kagan A, McGee D, Yano K, et al, (1981) Serum cholesterol and mortality in a, Japanese-American population.  The Honolulu Heart Program.  Am J Epidemiology 114:  11-20
5.  Epstein F (1982) Cholesterol, coronary heart disease, cancer and diet.  Atherosclerosis Rev (in press)
6.  Sidney S, Farquhar J (1982) Cholesterol, cancer and public policy.  N Engl J Med  (in press)
7.  Keys A (1980) Alpha lipoprotein (HDL) cholesterol in the serum and risk of coronary heart disease and death.  Lancet 2: 603-606
8.  Rose G, Blackburn, H et al (1974) Colon cancer and blood cholesterol.  Lancet i: 181-183
9.  Shekelle RB, MacMillan Shryock A, Paul O, Lepper M, Stamler J, Liu S, Raynor W  (1981) Diet, serum cholesterol and death from coronary heart disease.  N Engl J Med 304: 65-70
10. Gordon T, Garcia-Palmieri MR, Kagan A, Kannel WB, Schiffman J (1974) Differences in coronary heart disease mortality in Framingham, Honolulu and Puerto Rico.  Chronic Dis 27: 329
11. Keys A (ed) (1970) Coronary heart disease in seven countries.  Circulation 41: Suppl 1
12. Blackburn H (1980) Diet-lipid-atherosclerosis relationship: Epidemiological evidence and public health implications.  In: Gotto AM, Smith LC, Allen B (eds) Atherosclerosis V (Proceedings of the Fifth International Symposium on Atherosclerosis), Springer-Verlag, New York
13. Keys A, Parlin, RW (1966) Serum choelsterol response to changes in dietary lipids.  Am J Clin Nutr 19: 175-181

14. Prior IA, Davidson F, Salmord CE, Czochanska Z (1981) Cholesterol, coconuts and diet on Polynesian Atolls; a natural experiment. Am J Clin Nutr 34: 1552-1561
15. Report of a WHO Expert Committee (1982) Prevention of Coronary Heart Disease WHO Technical Report, series no. 678, Geneva
16. Gillum RF, Prineas RJ, Luepker RV, Taylor HL, Jacobs Jr DR, Kottke TE, Blackburn H (1982) Decline in coronary death. A search for explanations. Minn Med 65: 235-238
17. Blackburn, H (1979) Diet and mass hyperlipidemia: a public health view. In: Levy R, Rifkind B, Dennis B, Ernst, N (eds) Nutrition, Lipids, and Coronary Heart Disease, Raven Press, New York
18. Report of the NIH-sponsored community research and demonstration programs in primary prevention of coronary heart disease (1982) submitted to Circulation

# Pediatric Precursors of Atherosclerosis

C. J. Glueck, P. M. Laskarzewski, J. A. Morrison, M. J. Mellies, and P. R. Khoury

From the Lipid Research Clinic, General Clinical Research Center, and CLINFO Centers, University of Cincinnati, College of Medicine, Departments of Medicine and Pediatrics

## Introduction

Clinical manifestations of coronary heart disease (CHD), cerebrovascular disease (CVD), and peripheral vascular disease (PVD) as well as the clinical sequellae of hypertension, are generally not present in children. However, the evidence that the atherosclerotic lesion has its anatomic origins in childhood and adolescence is both broad-based and persuasive. The presence of anatomically and hemodynamically advanced coronary artery occlusion in young war victims unselected for coronary heart disease risk factors indicates that occlusive atherosclerosis is well underway in young American men by their late teens and early twenties.

Therapeutic intervention in adults designed to ameliorate CHD risk factors after a morbid event (myocardial infarction, stroke, peripheral vascular insufficiency, hypertensive cerebral and cardiovascular disease) has not been notably successful. Conversely, primary prevention of atherosclerosis through amelioration of CHD risk factors appears to have much more promise. As summarized by Figure 1, there is now extensive and significant evidence that primary intervention for CHD risk factors will have major longitudinal benefit.

1) Hypertension detection and therapy will unequivocally reduce sequellae of hypertensive vascular disease, including hypertensive cardiovascular disease, cerebrovascular disease and renal vascular disease.

2) As recently demonstrated in the Oslo Study, a 13% diet-induced reduction in mean plasma total cholesterol reduced coronary heart disease event rates (morbidity and mortality) by as much as 47% in a group of high risk men whose fasting serum cholesterols were over 300 mg/dl before therapy.

3) Cessation of cigarette smoking will reduce subsequent risk for coronary heart disease and lung cancer.

4) Successful therapy for obesity will reduce hypertension, sharply reduce triglyceride, moderately reduce LDL cholesterol, and significantly increase HDL cholesterol.

5) Increase in aerobic exercise is generally associated with an increase in HDL cholesterol and habitual long-term exercise or job-related physical activity may be related to relative protection against coronary heart disease.

6) As recently shown in the Oslo Study, significant reduction of dietary cholesterol and saturated fat reduces total and LDL cholesterol, with a resultant reduction in CHD morbidity and mortality.

There is no magic about detection of precursors for coronary heart disease in children; the methodology does not differ appreciably from adults if one takes in account dynamic changes in lipids, lipoproteins, body mass, and blood pressure

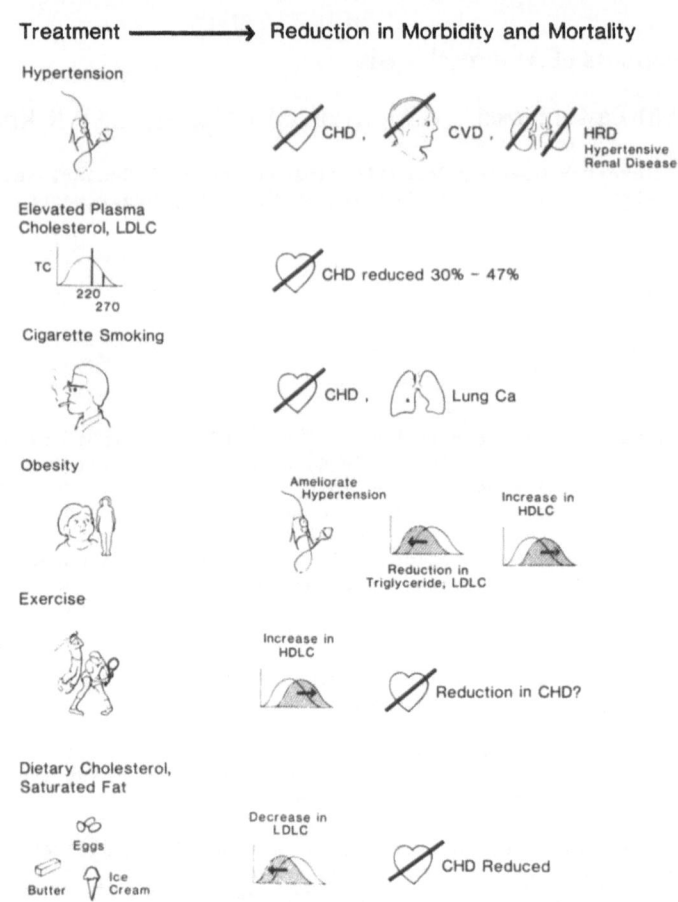

Figure 1. Does therapeutic, primary amelioration and treatment of risk factors for coronary heart disease, stroke, and hypertension, reduce morbidity and mortality from these diseases in adults?

which occur during adolescence (Figure 2). What has, in the past, hindered both the study of pediatric precursors of atherosclerosis and intervention has been the absence of "smoking pistol evidence" that primary prevention of coronary heart disease risk factors in adults would ameliorate atherosclerosis. This evidence, which is now increasingly available, is convincing (Figures 1,2). Within this frame of reference, the purpose of this chapter is to assess understanding of pediatric precursors of atherosclerosis and indicate the state of the art relative to intervention for these risk factors.

Pediatric Precursors of Atherosclerosis

An extensive series of population studies in the United States (Cincinnati, Ohio, Princeton School District; Muscatine, Iowa; Bogalusa, Louisiana; Rochester, Minnesota; Miami, Florida; and New York City) and throughout Europe, Japan, and South America, have now documented the prevalence of CHD risk factors in children of variegated socioeconomic status, race and country of national origin, and have

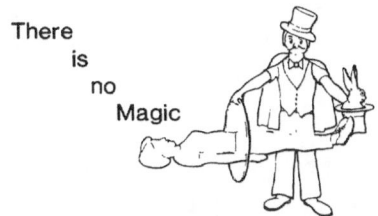

There
is
no
Magic

about detection of pediatric precursors for atherosclerosis and hypertension in children; the methodology does not differ appreciably from adults if one takes into account dynamic changes which occur during adolescence

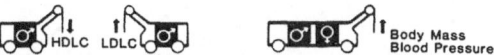

What has in the past hindered both the study of pediatric precursors for atherosclerosis/hypertension and appropriate intervention has been the absence of

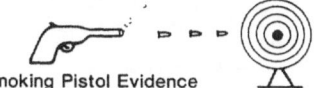

Smoking Pistol Evidence

that primary prevention of coronary heart disease risk factors

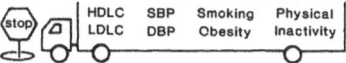

in adults would ameloriate atherosclerosis

This evidence is rapidly being accrued

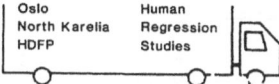

**Figure 2.** Diagnosis and relevance of pediatric precursors of atherosclerosis and hypertension.

provided useful "normal" distributions for total cholesterol, high and low density lipoprotein cholesterols (HDLC, LDLC), systolic and diastolic blood pressure, measures of body mass index, cigarette smoking, and alcohol intake. In addition to these studies, very extensive work has been completed on parent-child and sibling aggregations for coronary heart disease risk factors, studies which should markedly facilitate identification of children and adolescents at high risk for coronary heart disease, cerebrovascular disease, and hypertension.

Armed with extensive information about the ease and efficiency of diagnosis of pediatric precursors for atherosclerosis, extensive data for localization of children within risk factor distributions, and family studies outlining the ramifications of risk factor abnormalities in children, investigators and clinicians now have a unique opportunity to initiate primary prevention of atherosclerosis at a period when either the atherosclerosis is reversible or can be prevented.

Figure 3 displays major pediatric precursors for adult coronary, cerebral, and peripheral vascular disease, and sequellae of hypertension. As indicated in Figure 3, the major CHD risk factors in children are highly interrelated, as they

748

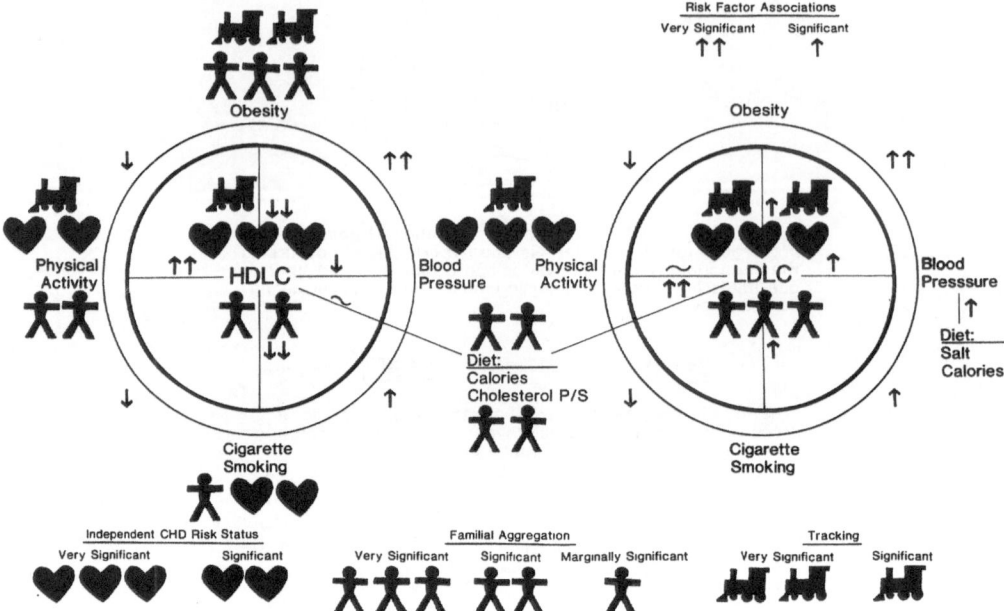

<u>Figure 3.</u> Coronary heart disease, stroke, and hypertension risk factors: interrelationships, independent risk factor status, familial aggregation, and maintenance of rank order over time, "tracking".

are in adults, and identification of, and intervention for any given risk factor in childhood without simultaneous consideration of other risk factors is inappropriate.

Low Density Lipoprotein Cholesterol

As displayed in Figure 1, a major pediatric coronary heart disease risk factor is low density lipoprotein cholesterol (LDLC). LDLC is known in adults to have very significant independent CHD risk factor status and its aggregation in families is very significant (Figure 2). Hence, early family history of coronary heart disease or stroke, and/or knowledge of parental elevation of LDLC should mandate sampling of fasting serum or plasma for LDLC levels in children from such affected kindreds. Of additional importance is the observation that LDLC in children tends to "track", i.e., to maintain its rank order over time (Figure 3). Thus, children with elevated total cholesterol and LDLC are likely to remain in the upper part of the cholesterol-LDLC distribution, and remain at high CHD risk as young adults. Hypercholesterolemic children predict hypercholesterolemic parents and predict coronary heart disease morbidity and mortality in first degree relatives (Figure 4). Conversely, pediatric progeny of young adults sustaining myocardial infarction themselves are likely to have hypercholesterolemia (Figure 5).

LDLC levels are highly related to dietary cholesterol and the ratio of polyunsaturated to saturated fatty acids both in normal children and in children with elevated total and LDL cholesterol (Figure 3). Multiple studies in normal children have demonstrated that easily achievable reductions of dietary cholesterol and reductions of saturated fat and/or increases of polyunsaturated fat will produce up to a 30% reduction of LDL cholesterol. In infants and children (ages 2-5 yrs) heterozygous for familial hypercholesterolemia, therapy with a low cholesterol, low saturate, polyunsaturate rich diet reduces LDL cholesterol to

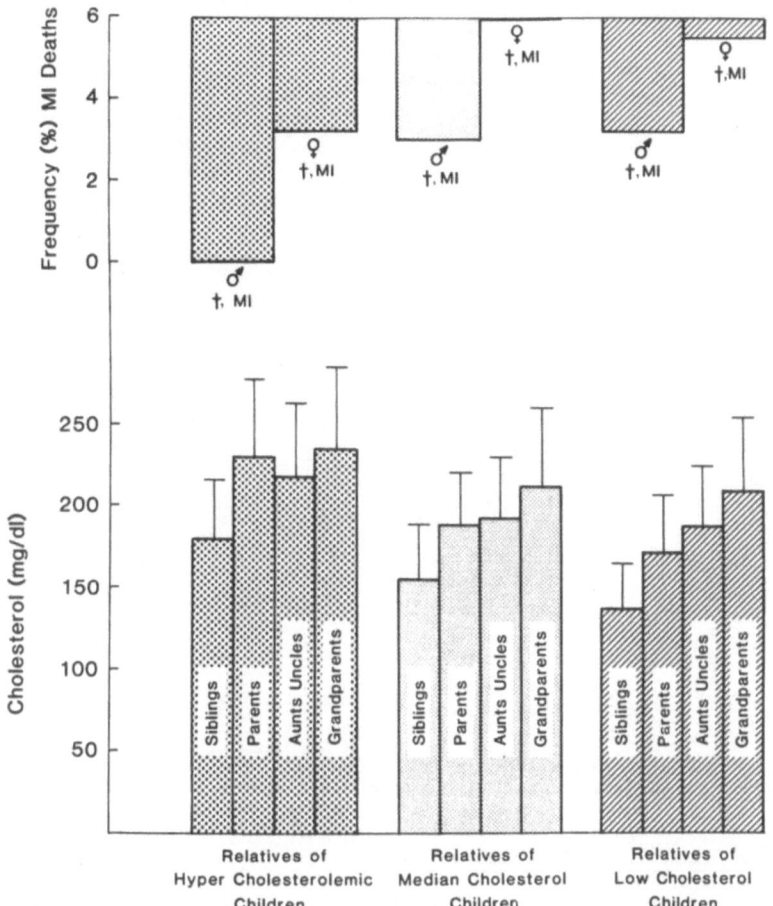

Figure 4. Hypercholesterolemic children predict hypercholesterolemic adult family members who have increased frequency of death from myocardial infarction. (Taken from Schrott, H.G. et al (1979). Circulation 59:320-326, 1979

normal levels in approximately 60% of subjects. Where diet alone does not suf-, fice to lower LDL cholesterol to the normal range, diet plus added cholestyramine and/or colestipol resin will reduce LDL cholesterol to the normal range in approximately 75% of heterozygous FH children.

In children, LDL cholesterol is significantly related to blood pressure, both in unselected population groups and in children from families selected by probands with essential hypertension (Figure 3). There is a positive association between LDLC and body mass index in children, and a weak positive association between cigarette smoking and LDLC in children (Figure 3). There is no significant association between LDLC and physical activity in children (Figure 3).

During adolescence in males, and concurrent with sexual maturation, LDL cholesterol rises. This increment is positively correlated with the increase in endogenous testosterone production. Conversely, in females there is no consistent change in LDL cholesterol levels during adolescence. Moreover, during adolescence, racial differences in LDL become more apparent. For any given total cholesterol level, black children have lower LDLC and lower triglyceride levels than white children; this is somewhat more marked in boys than in girls.

750

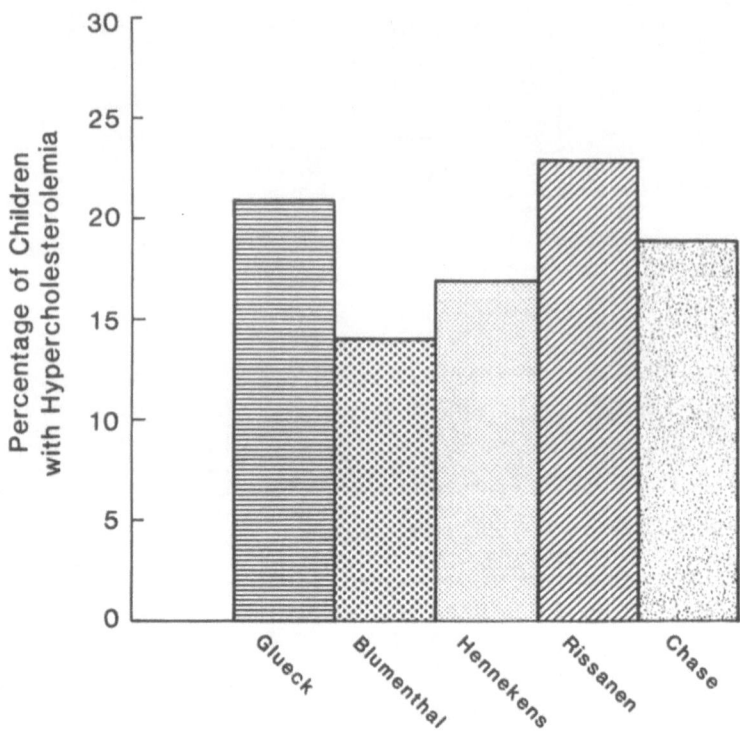

Figure 5. Percentage of children with hypercholesterolemia from families where their parent(s) sustained premature myocardial infarction

High Density Lipoprotein Cholesterol (HDLC)

A second major coronary heart disease risk factor in children is HDL cholesterol (HDLC). As summarized by Figure 3, HDLC has very significant independent CHD risk factor status, is significantly aggregated within families, and exhibits significant tracking in children. Hence, familial clustering of low HDL cholesterol is (not surprisingly) associated with increased risk of coronary heart disease and stroke, particularly ischemic stroke in children, while familial hyperalphalipoproteinemia is associated with protection from coronary heart disease morbidity and mortality.

Of considerable importance in children with hypercholesterolemia is the observation that nearly 20% have elevations of HDLC, not LDLC which accounts for their hypercholesterolemia. Such children would putatively be at reduced risk for coronary heart disease rather than increased risk. As displayed in Figure 3, HDLC is very significantly and inversely associated with relative obesity and cigarette smoking, and is strongly and positively associated with habitual physical activity. In free-living population groups and in progeny of probands with essential hypertension, HDLC is significantly and inversely related to blood pressure (Figure 3). In contrast to LDLC, the relationship of dietary intake to HDLC levels in childhood is much less significant; there is an inverse association between dietary sucrose and total carbohydrate and HDLC, and a weak positive correlation between dietary cholesterol and HDLC. HDLC is strongly and inversely related to triglyceride, and this probably accounts for the failure of triglyceride to be an independent coronary heart disease risk factor, since hypertriglyceridemia appears to be primarily a marker for low HDL and/or abnormalities of HDLC metabolism.

In boys, during adolescence, HDL cholesterol falls sharply, and triglycerides rise, concurrent with sexual maturation. This male decrement in HDLC during adolescence is apparently correlated with testosterone production, with an inverse correlation between endogenous testosterone and HDLC. Conversely, in girls, there are no consistent changes in HDLC during adolescence. Thus, at the conclusion of adolescence, in regards to lipoprotein status, males are at higher risk than females, having lower levels of HDL cholesterol, higher levels of LDL cholesterol, and higher levels of triglyceride.

## Obesity

Although obesity clearly has its origins in childhood, strongly tracks throughout childhood and adolescence, and exhibits very significant familial aggregation, it does not have independent coronary heart disease risk factor status (Figure 3). More likely, relative ponderosity in childhood and adulthood affects coronary heart disease through its influence on other CHD risk factors, particularly a strong inverse association with HDLC, a strong positive association with blood pressure, and a moderate positive association with LDLC (Figure 3).

## Habitual Physical Activity

In adults, epidemiologic studies suggest that habitual physical activity, either at work or during leisure time, may be inversely related with coronary heart disease risk and may have an independent coronary heart disease risk factor status (Figures 1,3). Habitual physical activity in children and young adolescents appears to track significantly and has significant familial aggregation (Figure 3). Whether or not habitual physical activity has risk factor protective status independent of other coronary heart disease risk factors is not well known, but we do know that habitual physical activity is positively related to HDL cholesterol, inversely related to obesity, and inversely related to cigarette smoking both in adults and in children (Figure 3).

## Cigarette Smoking

Cigarette smoking has independent CHD risk factor status and has marginally significant familial aggregation. Its effects on CHD are, in part, mediated through its strong inverse association with HDL cholesterol, positive association with blood pressure, and inverse association with habitual physical activity (Figure 3).

## Blood Pressure

Both systolic and diastolic blood pressure have significant independent CHD risk factor status, significant familial aggregation, and moderately significant tracking in childhood (Figure 3). Hypertensive children are likely to share attributes of hypertension, particularly obesity, with their parents and are more likely to be relatively hypertensive than are offspring of normotensive parents. Familial aggregation of hypertension can be discerned in infancy, reflecting a substantial genetic component to familial aggregation of hypertension. Hypertension's positive association with CHD risk is probably, in part, mediated through its inverse association with HDLC and positive association with obesity (Figure 3).

## Which Children Should be Evaluated

Short of sampling all children for the major coronary heart disease risk factors, a topic which will be discussed below, evaluation for CHD risk factors should be carried out in children from all families with the disorders displayed in Figure 6. Thus, all children from kindreds exhibiting parental and sibling myocardial infarction and/or stroke before age 55 should be sampled, since they are at greatly increased risk for familial hypercholesterolemia, familial combined

752

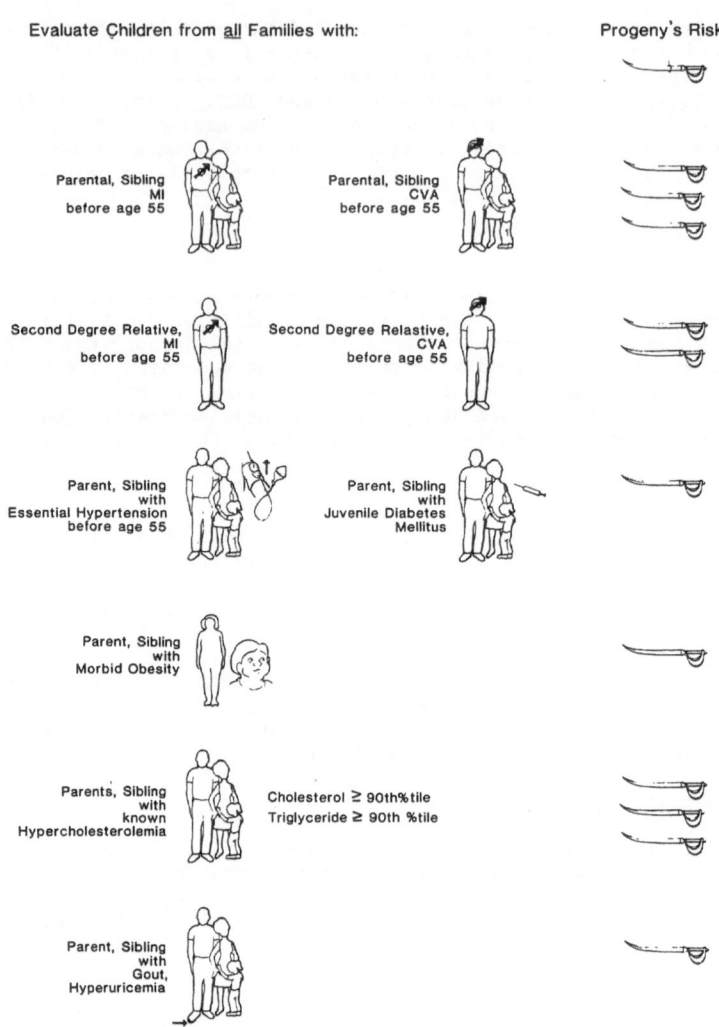

Evaluate Children from all Families with:                    Progeny's Risk

Parental, Sibling
MI
before age 55

Parental, Sibling
CVA
before age 55

Second Degree Relative,
MI
before age 55

Second Degree Relastive,
CVA
before age 55

Parent, Sibling
with
Essential Hypertension
before age 55

Parent, Sibling
with
Juvenile Diabetes
Mellitus

Parent, Sibling
with
Morbid Obesity

Parents, Sibling
with
known
Hypercholesterolemia

Cholesterol ≥ 90th%tile
Triglyceride ≥ 90th %tile

Parent, Sibling
with
Gout,
Hyperuricemia

Figure 6. Evaluation of children guided by family history


hyperlipidemia, and familial hypertriglyceridemia as well as for hypertension
and obesity. In adddition, in kindreds characterized by parental-sibling CVA
before age 55, there is a high degree of probability that siblings and/or progeny
of affected parents may have as their sole lipoprotein defect, low HDL cholesterol. As displayed in Figure 6, it also seems reasonable to assess children
from families where a second degree relative has sustained a myocardial infarction or CVA before age 55.

Risk factor sampling should also be carried out in kindreds where a parent or
sibling has essential hypertension before age 55, and/or juvenile onset diabetes
mellitus. Within-family clustering of hypertension is associated with high LDL,
high triglyceride, low HDL, and obesity, and families with juvenile onset diabetes mellitus often have first degree relatives with high triglyceride, higher LDL
cholesterol, and low HDL.

Children from kindreds having parents or siblings with morbid obesity should be sampled since they are likely themselves to be obese, and as such are more likely to have hypertension, low HDL cholesterol, higher triglyceride, and higher LDL cholesterol (Figure 6).

As displayed in Figure 6, children from kindreds where a parent or sibling has known hypercholesterolemia, known elevations of LDL cholesterol, known reductions of HDL cholesterol, or known elevations of triglyceride should be sampled, since there is a greatly increased chance that children from such kindreds will themselves have dyslipoproteinemias (Figure 6).

Children from kindreds whose parents and siblings suffer from gout or hyperuricemia should be sampled, since they are more likely to have lower HDL, high triglyceride, obesity, and hypertension (Figure 6).

Should CHD Risk Factors be Assessed Routinely in all Children

We do not yet know the cost effectiveness of sampling for CHD risk factors in selected children (Figure 6), as compared to sampling in all children (Figure 7). In addition, it is unlikely that any, as yet unpublished, prospective studies will provide us with enough cost-effectiveness information to adequately answer the question of who should be sampled, families already thought to be at risk vs sampling of all children. However, since sampling for CHD risk in all children is relatively inexpensive, and since prevalence of pediatric precursors of atherosclerosis is very high, particularly in Westernized industrialized

1. Blood Pressure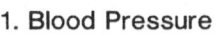

2. Relative Ponderosity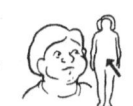

3. Regular Aerobic Exercise Status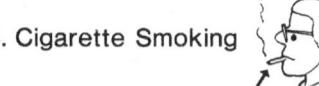

4. Cigarette Smoking

## At Least Once in <u>All</u> Children Measure

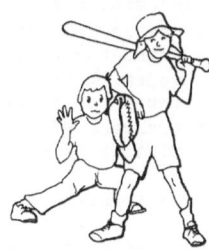

→ Total Plasma Cholesterol
→ HDL Cholesterol
→ Triglyceride
→ LDL Cholesterol

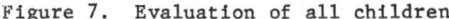

Figure 7. Evaluation of all children

countries, our current recommendation is that all children be routinely assessed for the following at healthy child care visits: measurement of blood pressure, relative ponderosity, determination of regular aerobic exercise status, and cigarette smoking (Figure 7). We would also strongly recommend that at least once, in all children, a measurement be obtained in fasting plasma of total plasma cholesterol, triglyceride, and HDL cholesterol, along with calculation, possible in most cases, of LDL cholesterol [LDLC=total cholesterol – HDLC-TG/5] (Figure 7).

### Secondary, Primary, and Familial Hypercholesterolemia, Hypertriglyceridemia, Hypertension, and Obesity

As a result of sampling strategies, be they limited to high risk families (Figure 6), or generalized for all children (Figure 7), it is necessary to differentiate secondary from primary hypercholesterolemia, hypertriglyceridemia, hypertension, and obesity, and where possible, to identify familial (monogenic) dyslipoproteinemia (Tables 1 and 2). As summarized in Table 1, the estimated proportion of affected children with identifiable secondary causes of hypercholesterolemia is 90-95%; of hypertriglyceridemia, 70-90%; of hypertension, only 0.2%, and of obesity, 99+%.

By far the most common cause of acquired (secondary) hypercholesterolemia in children is excessive intake of dietary cholesterol and saturated fat; there is also an extensive list of diseases, drugs, and metabolic states which can produce acquired hypercholesterolemia, as displayed in Table 1.

In our experience, the most common causes of acquired hypertriglyceridemia in children are excessive alcohol intake (in adolescence), uncontrolled juvenile diabetes mellitus, and oral contraceptives (Table 1). There are also, however, multiple other causes of secondary hypertriglyceridemia in children which need to be ruled out (Table 1).

In contrast to hypercholesterolemia and hypertriglyceridemia, where a great majority of affected cases reflect secondary, acquired disorders, the overwhelming majority of children with persistent hypertension rarely have identifiable diseases, drugs, metabolic states which account for their hypertension, as summarized in Table 1. Whether excessive salt intake by itself can account for hypertension in children remains a matter of controversy, although it appears that excessive salt intake in children genetically susceptible for essential hypertension may lead to an expression of the hypertensive phenotype (Table 1).

For obesity, in our experience, diseases, drugs, or metabolic states accounting for juvenile obesity are exceptionally rare, with a great preponderance of obesity directly related to an excess of caloric intake over caloric expenditure (Table 1).

As summarized in Table 1, the Princeton School District, Cincinnati LRC Family Studies, in those children identified with hypercholesterolemia, from 4% to 13% could be shown to have primary and familial hypercholesterolemia defined by the presence of hypercholesterolemia in the pediatric proband and at least one similarly affected first-degree relatives, and exclusion of secondary hyperlipidemias. Also from the Princeton Family Study, approximately 7% to 29% of subjects recalled because of hypertriglyceridemia could be shown to have primary hypertriglyceridemia (absence of secondary causes), and familial hypertriglyceridemia defined by the presence of primary hypertriglyceridemia in the proband, and at least two other similarly affected first-degree relatives (Table 1).

Table 2 summarizes data relative to familial (monogenic) dyslipoproteinemias and familial aggregation of hypertension and obesity in childhood. As displayed in Table 2, familial hypercholesterolemia is transmitted as an autosomal dominant trait, is completely penetrant by childhood, has a relatively high prevalence of heterozygosity, and can be diagnosed in infancy. Risk of coronary heart disease

TABLE 1

Causes of Secondary Hypercholesterolemia, Secondary Hypertriglyceridemia,
Secondary Hypertension, and Secondary Obesity in Children

| Hypercholesterolemia | Hypertriglyceridemia |
|---|---|
| Excessive cholesterol, saturated fat | Alcohol |
| Hypothyroidism | Hypothyroidism |
| Nephrotic Syndrome | Nephrotic Syndrome |
| Uncontrolled Diabetes | Uncontrolled Diabetes |
| Obstructive Hepatic Disease | Obstructive Hepatic Disease |
| Hepatitis, Porphyria | Hepatitis |
| Cushing's Syndrome | Cushing's Syndrome |
| Uremia | Uremia; Glycogen storage disease |
| Dysglobulinemias, Myeloma | Dysglobulinemia, Myeloma, Systemic Lupus |
| Exogenous Corticosteroids | Exogenous Corticosteroids |
| Exogenous Androgenic Steroids | Oral Contraceptives |
| Oral Contraceptives | Diuretic Antihypertensives |
| Diuretic Antihypertensives | Beta Blockers |
| Pregnancy | Acute Metabolic Stress (Trauma, Fever) |
| | Pregnancy |

| Hypertension | Obesity |
|---|---|
| Excessive salt intake, only in Genetically Susceptible? | Excessive Caloric Intake (above caloric expenditure) |
| Coarctation of Aorta | Hypothyroidism |
| Renal Artery Sterosis | Cushing's Syndrome |
| Chronic Pyelonephritis, Glomerulonephritis | |
| Obesity, only in Genetically Susceptible? | |
| Uremia | |
| Exogenous Corticosteroids | Exogenous Corticosteroids |
| Oral Contraceptives | Oral Contraceptives |
| Pregnancy (Toxemia) | |

Estimated proportion of affected children with identifiable secondary causes of:

Hypercholesterolemia - 90-95%
Hypertriglyceridemia - 70-90%
Hypertension     -  0.2%
Obesity          -  99+%

Estimated % of subjects recalled because of hypercholesterolemia with Familial
Hypercholesterolemia 4%-13%

Estimated % of subjects recalled because of hypertriglyceridemia with Familial
Hypertriglyceridemia 7%-29%

TABLE 2

Familial Dyslipoproteinemias, Hypertension, and Obesity in Childhood

| Familial Dyslipoproteinemia | Prevalence Heterozygote (†=Homozygote) | Age of Earliest Diagnosis | Age when Phenotypic Expresion is Thought to be Complete |
|---|---|---|---|
| Hypobetalipoproteinemia | .7% | Infancy | Young childhood |
| Hyperalphalipoproteinemia | .8% | Infancy | Young childhood |
| Hypercholesterolemia | .1-1% | Infancy | Young childhood |
| Hypertriglyceridemia | 1% | Childhood | Young adulthood |
| Combined hyperlipidemia | .1-1.8% | Childhood | Young adulthood |
| Type III hyperlipoproteinemia | .1%† | Childhood | Young Adulthood |
| | 40% | Childhood | Childhood |
| Hypertension | | Infancy | Young adulthood |
| Obesity | | Childhood | Young Adulthood |

| | Mode of Inheritance | Risk of CHD Increased | Risk of CHD Reduced |
|---|---|---|---|
| Hypobetalipoproteinemia | Autosomal Dominant | | XX |
| Hyperalphalipoproteinemia | Autosomal Dominant | | XX |
| Hypercholesterolemia | Autosomal Dominant | XXXX | |
| Hypertriglyceridemia | Autosomal Dominant | XX | |
| Combined Hyperlipidemia | Autosomal Dominant | XX | |
| Type III Hyperlipoproteinemia | Autosomal Recessive | XX | |
| Hypertension | Probably Polygenic? | XX | |
| Obesity | Probably Polygenic? | X | |

| | Penetrance of Phenotype |
|---|---|
| Hypobetalipoproteinemia | Complete by childhood |
| Hyperalphalipoproteinemia | Complete by childhood? |
| Hypercholesterolemia | Complete by childhood |
| Hypertriglyceridemia | Rare in childhood, incomplete in adulthood |
| Combined Hyperlipidemia | Incomplete in childhood, complete in adulthood |
| Type III Hyperlipoproteinemia | Very rare in childhood, incomplete in adulthood |
| Hypertension | Relatively uncommon in childhood, incomplete in adulthood? |
| Obesity | Common in childhood, complete in adulthood? |

| | Longevity Increased | Longevity Reduced |
|---|---|---|
| Hypobetalipoproteinemia | XX | |
| Hyperalphalipoproteinemia | XX | |
| Hypercholesterolemia | | XXXX |
| Hypertriglyceridemia | | XX |
| Combined Hyperlipidemia | | XXX |
| Type III Hyperlipoproteinemia | | XX |
| Hypertension | | XX |
| Obesity | | X |

with familial hypercholesterolemia is dramatically increased, and longevity is reduced. Conversely, familial hypertriglyceridemia, also apparently inherited as an autosomal dominant trait, is rarely penetrant in childhood, and is not fully penetrant in adulthood. Although the prevalence of the heterozygous state (for familial hypertriglyceridemia) is estimated to be as high as 1%, phenotypic expression is not complete until young adulthood. Whether or not familial hypertriglyceridemia is associated with an increased risk of coronary heart disease and reduced longevity is a matter of controversy; estimates range from no increased associated CHD risk to extensively increased CHD risk (Table 2).

The third major and common familial dyslipoproteinemia, familial combined hyperlipidemia, is also apparently transmitted as an autosomal dominant trait, but the penetrance of the phenotype is incomplete in childhood; phenotypic expression is thought to be complete in young adulthood. Because it is thought that one genotype can account for three different phenotypes (Type IIA, IIB and IV lipoprotein phenotypes) the clinical differentiation in small kindreds between familial combined hyperlipidemia, familial hypercholesterolemia, (types IIA and IIB phenotypes), and familial hypertriglyceridemia is difficult to impossible.

Familial Type III hyperlipoproteinemia, transmitted as an autosomal recessive, is phenotypically very rare in childhood and not completely expressed in adulthood. The homozygous phenotype is relatively rare, while the heterozygote, abnormal for apolipoprotein E isoform III, has an astonishing prevalence of 40% of the population. Cardiovascular ramifications of these normolipidemic heterozygotes for apolipoprotein E genotypic deficiency (for familial Type) III are totally unknown.

As displayed in Table 2, familial hyperalpha- and familial hypobetalipoproteinemia are common in childhood, apparently inherited as autosomal dominants diagnosable in infancy and phenotypically completely expressed in young childhood. These disorders are (fortunately) associated with increased longevity and reduced coronary heart disease event rates.

Neither hypertension nor obesity are thought to exhibit monogenic inheritance. Their inheritance is probably polygenic. Phenotypic prevalence of hypertension and obesity, age of earliest diagnosis, and age when phenotypic expressions are thought to be complete, are summarized in Table 2.

## SUMMARY

Pediatric precursors for atherosclerosis are easily identifiable in children and adolescents, and because they track well, children at high risk to myocardial infarction, stroke, and hypertension are likely to mature to become high risk adults, with the morbid and lethal consequences of these diseases. We do not yet know whether identification of pediatric precursors for atherosclerosis in childhood and appropriate longitudinal intervention will reduce future risk, although the results of primary prevention studies in adults for treatment of hypercholesterolemia and suggest that primary prevention, initiated in childhood, would be associated with the significant reduction of eventual risk. Of particular importance, given the psychological and social implications of identification of pediatric precursors for atherosclerosis, risk factors which were thought to be present must be repetitively demonstrated using accurate, reproducible methodology, and with a careful differentiation between primary (familial) disorders, and disorders secondary to diseases, drugs, or diet. Since atherosclerosis has its genesis in childhood, and since pediatric precursors for atherosclerosis are usually fully expressed and easily diagnosed in childhood, better understanding of the pathophysiology of these risk factors in childhood should provide the optimal approach to preventive medicine.

758

REFERENCES

1. Glueck CJ, Laskarzewski P, Rao DC, Morrison JA (1982)  In press.  Familial
aggregation of coronary risk factors.  In Complications in Coronary Heart
Disease.  Eds, Connor W, Bristow D.  Lippincott Co.

# Intervention on Single Risk Factors: Hyperlipoproteinemia

R. I. Levy

The evidence on the association between levels of blood cholesterol and risk of coronary artery disease (CAD) is extensive and unequivocal (1-4). The cumulative supportive data include (a) animal studies in which a hypercholesterolemic diet produces atherosclerotic lesions (b) biological studies of the atherosclerotic plaque (c) epidemiologic studies of populations which vary in levels of blood cholesterol and extent of CAD (d) the prevalence of hypercholesterolemia in individuals with clinically diagnosed atherosclerotic disease and (e) research on genetic hypercholesterolemia which almost always manifests itself in premature CAD.

## Lipoproteins As Risk Factors

The major plasma lipids do not circulate free in the plasma, but circulate as lipid-protein complexes. Because each of the lipoproteins contains varing amounts of cholesterol and because each has differing associations with CAD, measurement of individual lipoprotein levels offers more information than that of total cholesterol alone.

It is clear that more clinically useful information can be obtained by measuring the carriers of blood cholesterol - the lipoproteins - than by a simple measurement of total cholesterol. Low density lipoproteins (LDL) are the major carriers of cholesterol and have been directly associated with increased risk of vascular disease. On the other hand, high density lipoproteins (HDL) are independently and inversely related to CHD risk, so that higher levels of HDL are associated with lower cardiovascular event rates. Nevertheless, until long-term data accumulate on lipoprotein levels in relation to CHD, the definition of CAD risk will continue to be based on evidence from the past three decades relating to levels of total cholesterol. The association between cholesterol and CAD is linear so that the risk increases proportionately to the cholesterol level, although no encountered level seems to be risk-free.

Plasma LDL concentrations correlate closely with plasma cholesterol levels because 60-75% of the total plasma cholesterol is normally transported by this lipoprotein. LDL has been directly and strongly associated with CAD and atherosclerosis. Data from the Framingham Study show that LDL remains a predictor of risk even in the oldest age group surveyed. LDL levels have been positively associated with a high intake of dietary fat - in particular the saturated fatty acids - and to a lesser extent, dietary cholesterol.

HDL, on the other hand, accounts for only 20-25% of the total plasma cholesterol and has a strong inverse relationship to CAD that is independent of other risk factors. Thus higher levels of HDL correlate with less cardiovascular disease. This association has been further confirmed in post-mortem studies and coronary angiography, which show that the degree of coronary atherosclerosis and the increased risk for vascular events are inversely linked to HDL levels in both young and older age groups.

HDL levels have been positively associated with exercise and moderate alcohol consumption, and negatively related to obesity, cigarette smoking and poor diabetes control (5).

## Influence of Diet on Lipids and Lipoproteins

The level of blood cholesterol at birth is low in man. This level rises during infancy - a rise partly explicable by changes in the diet. Although the levels of lipids and lipoproteins are influenced by a myriad of nutrients and nutrient components of the diet, in most instances, the greatest dietary influence is imposed by the amount and type of fat, cholesterol, and calories consumed (6).

## Effects of Dietary Cholesterol

The effect of dietary cholesterol on blood cholesterol levels has been measured and characterized by closely controlled metabolic investigations which have studied changes in serum cholesterol by changing cholesterol intake. The KEYS formula ($\Delta$ cholesterol = 6.77 $\Delta$ C - 0.5) predicts about a 6 mg change in serum cholesterol when the diet changes in cholesterol content by 100 mg (7). According to the formula by MATTSON et al ($\Delta$ cholesterol = 1.6 + 0.118 $\Delta$ dietary cholesterol/1000 K cal) serum cholesterol changes about 12 mg/dl for each 100 mg of dietary cholesterol per 1000 K cal (8). A third formular derived by HEGSTED et al (9) predicts that a change of 100 mg dietary cholesterol will lead to a change of about 5 mg/100 ml in serum cholesterol.

Up to the present time, repeated demonstrations of an effect of dietary cholesterol on blood cholesterol have not stilled controversy. For although the "average" effect of dietary cholesterol is predictable, the variation in an individual's response - which is probably regulated by several other factors, many of them genetic in origin - cannot be predetermined. Dietary cholesterol appears to have much less effect on the plasma cholesterol than the saturated fatty acids. The effect of cholesterol is also nonlinear; apparently daily intakes up to 300-600 mg contribute to the greatest change in levels of blood cholesterol (10).

Furthermore, clinical investigations indicate a wide range of individual variations (probably regulated by genetic predisposition). The extremes of this variability in response have been characterized as a hyper- and hypo-response to cholesterol.

In the daily American diet the intake of cholesterol is supplied primarily by egg yolks. Organ meats - although concentrated sources of cholesterol - occur less frequently in the general dietary pattern. Another important contribution is from foods of animal origin e.g., meats, milk - which are even more important as concentrated sources of saturated fatty acids.

The daily intake of saturated fatty acids is most often derived from animal fats e.g., lard, well marbled meats (top grades and certain cuts), meats not trimmed of fat, sausages, cold cuts, whole milk and cream products (cheeses, butter, sweet and sour cream and ice cream). Other sources of saturated fatty acids may be: a) vegetable fat so hydrogenated that it becomes as saturated as animal fats and b) palm oil, palm kernel oil and coconut oil - vegetable fats that are composed pre-dominantly of saturated fatty acids.


## Type of Fat

The predictability of the differing influences of dietary fatty acids on blood cholesterol levels was quantified in the KEYS formula (11) that is:  saturated fatty acids have twice the per-gram effect in increasing levels of blood cholesterol as do polyunsaturated fatty acids in de-creasing these levels.  This cholesterol-raising effect of the saturated fatty acids appears to be specific to those fatty acids which contain fewer than 12, but more than 18 carbon atoms (12).  In terms of usual intake, this primarily includes palmitic fatty acid and lauric fatty acid, the first coming from foods of the animal kingdom and the latter from the vegetable oils - palm oil and coconut oil.  Subsequent clinical studies have demonstrated that the important lowering which comes from decreasing the saturated fatty acids can be increased by an intake of polyunsaturated fatty acids as partial replacement for the saturated fatty acid removed.


## Genetics vs. Environment

Confusion in interpreting the influence of diet on lipoproteins and lipids is caused by individual (genetic) response, but also is mitigated by other factors.  These include the initial serum cholesterol and lipo-protein level, the body weight, the quality and quantity of fat and fatty acids in the diet, the level of dietary cholesterol in the diets compared and the experimental design, that is, whether the study is carried out in a free or controlled environment.

Both genetic and environmental factors influence each person's lipid and lipoprotein levels.  This can be readily shown on review of available study data.  Individuals within a country or community often have widely divergent blood lipid and lipoprotein levels.  When given the same diet in a maximally controlled environment, individuals within the group attain and maintain different average levels of lipids and lipoproteins. Such individual responses are affected by large, nondietary intrinsic factors which are probably genetic (13).

On the other hand, the effect of diet on lipid and lipoprotein levels has been clearly demonstrated.  First, while holding constant other predisposing factors in the environment, it is possible to lower levels of lipids and lipoproteins in almost everyone by changing the diet.

Second, multifactorial population studies leave little doubt of the role of diet (especially the intake of total fat, saturated fat and choles-terol) in determining the average level of lipids and lipoproteins in different countries (4,14).  Such dietary influences are demonstrated by studies comparing Japanese populations on the mainland and in Hawaii and California (15).  The increased frequency of elevated cholesterol values among Japanese migrants in Hawaii and in California compared to those living in Japan suggests that hyperlipidemia is strongly affected by dietary factors.  For example, the prevalence of hypercholesterolemia (> 260 mg/dl) in Hawaii and California is 4 and 5 times, respectively, the rate of Japanese men living in Japan.

In populations surveyed in the Seven Countries Study, most of the dif-

ferences in average serum cholesterol levels among the populations were
consonant with differences in the amount and kind of dietary fat consumed (16). Populations manifesting high average cholesterol levels and
higher levels of LDL (and high rates of atherosclerotic disease) have
saturated fat intakes of 15% or more of calories. In contrast, populations with low average serum cholesterol levels have saturated fat intakes of 10% or less of calories.

These dietary relationships are evident when we contrast the countries
of Japan and Finland. In Japan, where the studies were performed, the
saturated fat intake was about 3% of calories and the average cholesterol was below 160 mg% (while the CHD rate was among the lowest of
industrial countries). In comparison, in East Finland, where 22% of
calories are from saturated fatty acids, the average cholesterol level
is above 240 mg% (and the Finns have one of the highest atherosclerotic
disease rates of any culture) (17). In a 1981 report (Western Electric
Study) of a single country study (18), it was concluded that the intake
of saturated fatty acids and dietary cholesterol were prospectively
positively related to change in the level of serum cholesterol and risk
of coronary death in middle-aged American men.

Thus an individual's level of lipids and lipoproteins is determined both
by the environment (diet is a major factor) as well as by intrinsic,
genetically determined variables. When the level of lipids and lipoproteins (LDL) are elevated because of intrinsic or dietary causes, the
incidence of the clinical sequellea of atherosclerosis is higher.

## Influence of Drugs on Lipoproteins

To achieve additional lipid-lowering, drug therapy may be added to diet.
A variety of powerful and effective hypolipidemic drugs are now available. They may be classified into three basic categories: a) those
that affect lipoprotein production; b) those that affect intravascular
lipoprotein catabolism; c) and those that affect lipoprotein removal
(19,20).

It can be demonstrated that nicotinic acid affects the outflow of VLDL
from the liver. When one uses nicotinic acid, the synthesis and release
of VLDL decreases markedly. Nicotinic acid is thus very effective for
the subject with excess VLDL or IDL. Other drugs have no effect on the
release of VLDL from the liver, (while still others, such as cholestyramine and colestipol, actually appear to increase the synthesis of
VLDL). The bile acid sequestrants seem to work by enhancing the rate of
removal of the LDL remnant form from the plasma apparently by increasing
peripheral LDL receptor activity. The mode of action of clofibrate is
unclear. It may affect lipoprotein production but clearly enhances the
breakdown of the VLDL and intermediates to LDL in the plasma. In fact,
treatment of VLDL excess with clofibrate will often raise LDL levels.
Nicotinic acid consistently increases levels of HDL. The other lipid
lowering drugs have only minimal effects on HDL and, in fact, probucol
lowers HDL levels.

With this knowledge, we can now explain why nicotinic acid is effective,
whether the problem is too much VLDL or its ultimate remnant form LDL.
One can also explain why the bile acid sequestrants are effective when
the problem is too much LDL but are ineffective in controlling VLDL
excesses (20). Understanding the mode of action of these lipid lowering
drugs then clearly allows one to tailor one's therapy to specific lipoprotein excesses and explains why some drugs work in some types of hy-

perlipoproteinemia but not in others. All of the currently available lipid lowering drugs, however, are associated with real and/or potential side effects. Thus they must be used circumspectly while we seek to determine directly in man whether aggressive alteration of cholesterol and lipoprotein levels will alter cardiovascular risk (20).

## Evidence for Regression of Atherosclerosis

Animal Data

The most direct evidence for the regression of atherosclerosis comes from animal studies (that cannot be readily duplicated in man). Animal studies employing nonhuman primates accumulated over the last 10 years not only show that the progression of atherosclerosis can be stopped, but they clearly demonstrate that regression of atherosclerosis can be produced by lowering the levels of circulating cholesterol. A limitation of these studies, obtained by at least eight different research groups, is that extreme cholesterol levels were tested. However, CLARKSON'S study (21) reported in 1979, suggests that regression of coronary lesions in the species closest to man can be achieved by lowering and maintaining a cholesterol level of 200 mg/100 ml. This experiment included a group of Rhesus monkeys fed a cholesterolrich diet for 19 months. Serum cholesterol levels reached almost 800 mg/100 ml when one-third of the cohort were sacrificed. Thereafter, a remaining one-third were placed for 24 months on a diet to maintain cholesterol at 300 mg/100 ml.

The final group was fed, for a further 24 months, a diet to maintain their cholesterol levels at approximately 200 mg/100 ml (a level that we can hope to achieve in most freeliving Americans). In the animals sacrificed at cholesterol levels of 800 mg/100 ml, extensive coronary atherosclerosis was found (luminal narrowing, internal thickening and fat in the vessels). When sacrificed, those animals whose cholesterol levels had been maintained for an additional two years at 300 mg/100 ml showed more advanced coronary stenosis as determined by serial sections. Conversely, animals which had been maintained at a cholesterol level of 200 mg/100 ml showed statistically significant decreases in coronary artery stenosis, fat in vessels, medial and internal elastic lamina damage. There was no doubt that over the two year period when serum cholesterol was lowered to 200 mg/100 ml in these animals, regression of lesions occurred.

There is some presumptive evidence that regression of atherosclerosis can occur in man. Reduction in incidence rates of atherosclerosis has been reported in groups who have undergone extremes of calorie (and dietary fat) deprivation such as during periods of starvation and wartime. However, it is not possible to identify which of several potential factors explains this apparent regression in atherosclerosis.

Several caveats must be remembered in attempting to relate the evidence from animal studies to that from studies of humans: the human atherosclerotic lesions may develop differently from the experimentally induced atherosclerosis in animals. Consequently, the finding of regression in animals cannot be generalized to man. Secondly, the lesions that regress are foamy rather than the classical fibrous calcified plaque. Thirdly, atherosclerosis in man may be due to a multiplicity of causes and not just to hypercholesterolemia, as in the experimental atherosclerosis induced in animals. Future studies will need to focus on the interaction of other cardiovascular risk factors in the reversal of the atherosclerotic process.

Clinical Trial Data

The evidence on the reversibility of the atherosclerotic process in
humans is ambiguous, in part because of the difficulties in collecting
this type of information.  Perhaps the main problem is to determine the
extent and degree of atherosclerosis in living man.  If one relies on
secondary prevention trials of lipid lowering, it is necessary for a-
symptomatic arteriosclerosis first to become symptomatic - a process
that may take many years.  As the data from the Coronary Drug Project
(22) show, an enormous number of subjects must sustain a sufficient
number of coronary events before the efficacy of the lowering of cholesterol can be assessed meaningfully.

Between 1955 and the present, about two dozen single factor prevention
trials of diet-induced or drug-induced cholesterol lowering in primary
or secondary coronary heart disease prevention trials have been reported.

All of the investigations, whether performed on a double blind basis or
not, showed that some lowering of serum cholesterol could be achieved.
The average cholesterol reduction was approximately 10% to 15% in free-
living populations.  But in none of these studies was there a statistically significant difference in terms of the "hard" endpoints (heart
attack and death).  In those studies that were not double blinded there
were some changes in "soft" end-points such as angina, but such endpoints are difficult to evaluate, especially when a non-blind design is
used (23).

The recent report of the Oslo Study Group of 1200 high risk, but otherwise healthy (normotensive) men that a 13% reduction in serum cholesterol achieved by open (non-blind) dietary change in the intervention
group was associated at the end of a five year study period with a 47%
lower incidence of myocardial infarction (fatal and non-fatal) and sudden death (p=0.03) in the intervention group as compared to the control,
is most hopeful (24).  An associated 45% greater decrease in mean tobacco consumption in the intervention group as well as their overall more
intensive follow-ups makes it difficult, however, to clearly define the
contribution of cholesterol lowering to the reduced incidence of death
and disease.

All of the above studies do provide two important answers:  that cholesterol can be lowered by diet and that a lowering of at least 10% can
be achieved in a freeliving population.  A key question remains to be
definitely answered, however: will cholesterol-lowering alone (lowering
LDL) delay or prevent the development of premature atherosclerosis?  The
results of current studies such as the NHLBI's Lipid Research Clinics
Coronary Primary Prevention Trial are expected to clarify the issue
(25).

Evidence of Risk Factor Modification

Until there is conclusive proof of the long-term benefits of lipid-lowering, some interesting and encouraging observations on risk factor
modification can be made now.  Significant changes in food consumption
patterns are occurring in the United States.  Consumption of milk and
cream, butter, eggs, fats and oils of animal origin is decreasing, while

the consumption of vegetable fats is increasing. Health nutrition surveys (HANES) conducted in 1960-1962 and 1971-1974 suggest a modest lowering of cholesterol levels in the population during the 10-year period
(26). The population studies conducted by the Lipid Research Clinics in
1972-1976 suggest a 4-8% drop in plasma cholesterol levels in the U.S.
over the past decade, with the most striking changes occurring in the
most educated and higher socioeconomic groups (27). These dietary changes have coincided temporarily with a dramatic decline in mortality from
cardiovascular disease in the U.S.

It thus appears that the facts on hand today clearly establish the level
of blood cholesterol (and more specifically LDL cholesterol) as a major
coronary artery disease risk factor.

It is also clear that diet (especially the amount and kind of fat and
cholesterol) is a major determinant of the level of cholesterol (and
LDL) in the bloodstream. Though direct clinical trial evidence of the
value of reducing cholesterol (LDL) in man is still deficient, presumptive epidemiologic and animal data on hand would strongly support lowering the content of saturated fat and cholesterol in the diet while we
await more definitive information.

References

1.  Dawber, T. R., Kannel, W. B., Revotskie, N., and Kagan, A. (1962).
    The epidemiology of coronary heart disease. The Framingham Enquiry.
    Proceedings of the Royal Society of Medicine 551, 265
2.  Report of the 1977 working group to review the 1971 report by the
    National Heart, Lung, and Blood Institute Task Force on Arterio-
    sclerosis: Arteriosclerosis. (1977). Washington, D. C., DHEW Pub-
    lication No. (NIH) 78-1526
3.  Kannel, W. B., Castelli, W. P. and Gordon, T. (1979). Cholesterol
    in the prediction of atherosclerotic disease. New perspectives
    based on the Framingham Study. Annals of Internal Medicine 90, 85
4.  Stamler, J. (1979). Population studies. In Nutrition, Lipids, and
    Coronary Heart Disease - A Global View, p. 25, R. I. Levy, B. M.
    Rikfind, B. H. Dennis and N. Ernst (eds.), New York, New York, Raven
    Press
5.  Tyroler, H. A. (ed). (1980). Epidemiology of plasma h-density lipo-
    protein cholesterol levels. The Lipid Research Clinics Program
    Prevalence Study. Circulation 62 (Suppl. IV) 1-135
6.  Schonfeld, G. et al (1982). Effects of dietary cholesterol and
    fatty acids on plasma lipoproteins. Journal of Clinical Investi-
    gations 69, 1072
7.  Keys, A., Anderson, J. T. and Grande, F. (1965). Serum cholesterol
    response to changes in the diet II. The effect of cholesterol in
    the diet. Metabolism 14, 759
8.  Mattson, F. H., Erickson, B. A. and Kligman, A. M. (1972). Effect
    of dietary cholesterol on serum cholesterol in man. American Jour-
    nal of Clinical Nutrition 25, 589
9.  Hegsted, D. M., McGandy, R. B., Myers, M. L. and Stare, F. J.(1965).
    Quantitative effects of dietary fat on serum cholesterol in man.
    American Journal of Clinical Nutrition 17, 281
10. McGill, H. C. (1979). The relationship of dietary cholesterol to
    serum cholesterol concentration and to atherosclerosis in man.
    American Journal of Clinical Nutrition 32, 2664
11. Keys. A., Anderson, J. T. and Grande, F. (1957) Prediction of
    serum-cholesterol responses of man to changes in fats in the diet.
    Lancet 2, 959

12. Keys, A., Anderson, J. T. and Grande, F. (1965). Serum cholesterol response to change in the diet. Part III. Differences among individuals. Metabolism 14, 776.

13. McGandy, R. B., Hegsted, D. M., Myers, M. L. and Stare, F. J.(1966). Dietary carbohydrate and serum cholesterol levels in man. American Journal of Clinical Nutrition 18, 237

14. Keys, A. (1975). Coronary heart disease - The global picture. Atherosclerosis 22, 149

15. Kato, H., Tillotson, J., Nichaman, M., Rhoades, G. and Hamilton, H. (1973). Epidemiologic studies of coronary heart disease and stroke in Japanese men living in Japan, Hawaii, and California: Serum lipids and diet. American Journal of Epidemiology 97, 372

16. Keys, A. (ed.). (1970). Coronary heart disease in seven countries. Circulation 41, Suppl. I

17. Blackburn, H. (1979). Diet and mass hyperlipidemia: Public health considerations - A point of view. In Nutrition, Lipids, and Coronary Heart Disease - A Global View, p. 309, R. I. Levy, B. M. Rifkind, B. H. Dennis, and N. Ernst (eds.). New York, New York, Raven Press

18. Shekelle, R. B., Shryock, A. M., Paul, O., Lepper, M., Stamler, J., Liu, S. and Raynor, W. J. (1981). Diet, serum cholesterol and death from coronary heart disease. The Western Electric Study. New England Journal of Medicine 304, 648

19. Levy, R. I. (1980). Hyperlipoproteinemia and its management. J Cardiovascular Med 5:435 - 452

20. Levy R. I. (1980). Drugs used in the treatment of hyperlipoproteinemia. In Goodman and Gilman's The Pharmacologic Basis of Therapeutics. 6th Ed. New York, McMillan 834, 847

21. Clarkson, T. B., Lebner, D. M., Wagner, W. D., St. Clair, R. W., Bond, M. G. and Bullock, B. C. (1979). A study of atherosclerosis regression in macara mulatta. I. Design of experiment and lesion induction. Experimental and Molecular Pathology 30, 360

22. The Coronary Drug Project Research Group. (1973). The Coronary Drug Project. Initial findings leading to modification of its research protocol. Journal of the American Medical Association 226, 652

23. Levy, R. I. (1980). Dietary prevention of coronary artery disease - A policy overview. In Atherosclerosis V. Proceedings of the Fifth International Symposium on Atherosclerosis. p. 199, A. M. Gotto, L. C. Smith, and B. Allen (eds.). New York, New York, Springer-Verlag

24. Hjermann, I., et al. (1981). Effect of diet and smoking intervention on the incidence of coronary heart disease. Report from the Oslo Study Group of a Randomized Trial in Healthy Men. The Lancet 2, 8259: 1303-1310

25. The Lipid Research Clinics Program. (1979). The coronary primary prevention trial: design and implementation. Journal of Chronic Disease 32, 609

26. Abraham, S., Johnson, C. I., and Carroll, M. D. (1977). A comparison of levels of serum cholesterol of adults 18-74 years of age in the United States in 1960-72 and 1971-74. Advance data from Vital and Health Statistics of the National Center of Health Statistics. U. S. Department of Health, Education and Welfare, No. 5:1-4

27. The Lipid Research Clinics Population Studies Data Book. (1980). The Prevalence Study. Aggregate distributions of lipids, lipoproteins, and selected variables in 11 North American populations. NIH Publication No. 80-1527

# Intervention on Single Risk Factor: Hypertension

A. Zanchetti and F. Magrini

A. The choice of the most suitable drug. Pathophysiological or empirical approach?

The corollary to the conception of high blood pressure as a risk factor is that reduction of raised blood pressure will be of benefit in preventing or reversing cardiovascular disease, and that the means - mostly pharmacologic - lowering high blood pressure must not necessarily be specific, i.e. interfering with the causes of hypertension, but they must simply reduce arterial pressure significantly.

Now that there is a large range of antihypertensive drugs available, the problem has naturally arisen how the most suitable drug should be chosen for any single patient. Should the physician follow a pathophysiological or an empirical approach (1)? There is no doubt that the most rational approach would consist in matching the pharmacological properties of the drug with the pathophysiological alterations of the patient. But in doing that, two sets of difficulties are met, one relating to the patient, the other to the drug.

As to the physiopathologic profile of the patient this is certainly complex and variable. Arterial pressure is regulated through a multiplicity of factors, and measuring of even the main factors is hardly conceivable. Inferring the whole physiopathologic picture from a single variable or marker is unwarranted and misleading. Some of these markers are of dubious significance, and indeed it is uncertain whether they really mean what we want them to mean (1).

The measurement of renin was introduced for profiling the vasoconstriction-volume spectrum of the hypertensive patient, and for predicting the antihypertensive efficacy of either beta-blockers or diuretics (2). However. to limit ourselves to only the practical side of the matter, plasma renin activity has shown itself to be quite an approximate, and unfaithful index in the choice between beta-blockers and diuretics (3), and in uncomplicated hypertensives it is also a poor index for the effectiveness of an angiotensin converting enzyme inhibitor, such as captopril, as we shall see soon.

Plasma catecholamines have recently become increasingly popular as markers of sympathetic activity in hypertension. It seems rational, however, before applying these indices in the rational approach to antihypertensive treatment, to ask ourselves whether plasma noradrenaline or adrenaline are sufficiently sensitive indices of that mild increase in tonic sympathetic activity that might be hypothetized to occur in essential hypertension or might differentiate the various hypertensive patients among themselves. The well known observation that plasma catecholamines increase during tilting upright or exercise simply means that they can signal the tremendous sympathetic activation occurring physiologically under these conditions. The point is, however, whether plasma catecholamines can also reveal slight changes in sympathetic activity (3).

Our findings cast doubt on this possibility (4). In a group of hyper
tensive patients tilting caused a two-fold increase in plasma noradrenaline, and plasma adrenaline also rose. In the same subjects
sympathetic activity was modulated in both ways by stimulating or
deactivating the carotid sinus baroreflex by means of the neck pres-
sure-chamber. Reduction in baroreceptor activity caused a high signi
ficant increase in mean arterial pressure and in heart rate, but
only a minor and nonsignificant increase in plasma noradrenaline.
Stimulation of the baroreceptors caused a significant reduction in
mean arterial pressure, but only a transient and nonsignificant decrease in plasma noradrenaline and adrenaline. This suggests that,
if differences in sympathetic activity among hypertensives are
rather small, they may not be adequately evaluated by using plasma
catecholamines as markers of sympathetic activity.

Finally, and obviously, the measurement of multiple variables with
refined techniques, even more refined and reliable than the ones
available now, contrasts with the requirement for simplified evaluation of the hypertensive patient  especially the mild and moderate
one, in view of the large number of patients and the public health
problems involved.

If there are difficulties in correctly profiling the physiopathologic pattern of the individual patient, there are also uncertainties
on the side of the drug. "No single drug with a single action": this
well-known axiom means that we are still confused about the mechanism of action of several antihypertensive drugs.

Diuretics have been used in treating hypertension for more than
twenty years, and still the real mechanism of their antihypertensive
action is being discussed. Beta-adrenergic receptor blockers are
also a splendid example of uncertain interpretation of certain thera
peutic effects. Their variable or dubious relations with renin, cate
cholamines, central or peripheral sympathetic mechanisms, and with
the hemodynamic pattern of hypertension need not be reminded here in
detail (1).

Captopril is the latest example of our problems of interpretation
(5). This interesting compound has recently been introduced as a
specific agent for converting enzyme inhibition  and its excellent
antihypertensive action has been interpreted as a direct consequence
of a decreased vasoconstrictive effect of angiotensin and to a reduced aldosterone secretion. The antihypertensive action of captopril, however, might also depend on interference with another scarce
ly appreciated property of angiotensin, facilitation of sympathetic
activity. We have recently shown that, when administered to patients
with essential hypertension, captopril stimulates baroreflexes (6).
Furthermore, other peptides, like bradykinin and other kinins, can
be substrates to the action of angiotensin converting enzyme, and
part of the hypotensive activity of captopril might result from an
increased systemic or renal concentration of these vasodilating substances. Whatever the various action mechanisms of captopril may be,
there is increasing consensus on the observation that the relation
between pretreatment plasma renin and hypotensive response to capto
pril, particularly in prolonged administration, is not so strict as
it was originally maintained. For instance, our group has shown that
captopril can be equally effective in lowering arterial pressure before and after administration of a beta-blocker in doses that had
largely suppressed plasma renin levels (7).

These difficulties for a pathophysiological approach do not mean that a pragmatic approach to treatment of hypertension should be an irrational one  However, rather than applying doubtful rational assumptions to uncertain prediction of the outcome of therapy, rational correction of insufficient or unwanted responses once occurred seems a more rewarding approach  and can take advantage of the increasing understanding of the physiopathology of hypertension and the mechanisms of action of antihypertensive drugs. Examples of this approach are addition of a beta-blocker to a diuretic in patients with poor hypotensive response to diuretics, where the beta-blocker can dampen an excessive renin stimulation; and the triple association of a vasodilator, beta-blocker and diuretic in order to take advantage of the mutual interference between the various pharmacologic properties of these drugs.

## B. Can hypertension be prevented?

The last question into the future og hypertension is whether time is ready for thinking of primary prevention of hypertension  rather than simply thinking of prevention of vascular damage caused by hypertension. Is sufficient knowledge of causes of hypertension available today, or foreseeable tomorrow. such as to make intervention on these causes possible? If that derangement of blood pressure control that we define hypertension is due, as is generally believed. to an interaction between genetic and environmental factors, do we know sufficiently well both categories of factors as to be able to influence them? The investigators who have embraced the theory that essential hypertension results from a primary disturbance in renal sodium excretion have been preaching to drastically reduce dietary salt intake. waving the attractive image of the bon sauvage, the good savage, who does not eat salt and is free of hypertension (8).

The hypothesis that salt plays a critical importance in the pathogenesis of hypertension has undoubtedly received great impetus recently from the numerous reports that transport of sodium across the membrane of erythrocytes (9-12), leucocytes (13) and lymphocytes (14) is altered in essential hypertension, and from the hypothesis that reduced sodium extrusion might lead to increased intracellular concentration of both sodium and calcium ions. The claim that these membrane alterations would only occur in subjects with essential hypertension and in normotensive subjects with a familial history of hypertension (15,16) has led to the suggestion that measurement of ion fluxes across the erythrocyte membrane may represent a useful marker of genetic predisposition to essential hypertension. In the frame of this interpretation limitation in dietary sodium intake might be used as a preventive measure in predisposed subjects.

There are reasonable doubts, however. that prevent us from reaching hasty conclusions, especially conclusions having a not negligible impact on our present life style. Firstly, there is no general agreement about which of the described abnormalities is the pathophysiologically important marker. The various groups of investigators have described and do stress different abnormalities, which involve the ouabain sensitive sodium-potassium pump (13) the furosemide sensitive sodium-potassium co-transport (15,16) the sodium-sodium (or lithium) counter-transport (12). It is not yet clear whether these transport abnormalities would progressively lead to hypertension by increasing vascular smooth muscle contractility, or by increasing peripheral or central neural excitability (in

770

particular by increasing transmitter availability at postganglionic
sympathetic endings or elsewhere), or rather by interfering with
renal sodium excretion. Indeed it is hardly known whether the abnormalities found in blood cells really occur in those tissues the involvement of which could be responsible for hypertension. It is also
unclear why and how the same abnormality from an "innocent" stage of
concealed hypertension (as that found in normotensive children of
hypertensives) should at given time lead to "overt" hypertension.
Finally, it has recently been maintained that these ion flux abnorma
lities would not be primary in origin, would not be markers of a dif
fuse genetic membrane alteration, but would rather be secondary consequences of the action of a so-called natriuretic hormone  the secretion of which would be secondary to a primary renal abnormality.
An even more crucial question is in my opinion  as to whether membrane abnormalities are uniformly spread to the entire population of
essential hypertensive subjects, and really and clearly limited to
this population without involving normotensive subjects without a
familial background of hypertension. Should this be true  it would
represent a definite contradiction with the quatitative hypothesis
advanced by Pickering. We should remember, however  that the relative difficulty of the methods employed has limited the measurements of trans-membrane fluxes to small and highly selected groups
of subjects. There have been many previous instances in which introduction of a new methodology led the experts to believe that some
biological abnormality was specific and characteristic of hypertension; instances in which these hopes were subsequently found
delusive. This is not to deny that the measurement of ion fluxes
across membranes has opened an extremely interesting new approach
to the pathogenesis of hypertension· indeed the concepts and hypotheses advances are too important to be dismissed by superficial
criticism. However, clinical and preventive application of these
concepts must wait until an answer is provided to the many questions
unsolved.


References

1. Zanchetti A (1980) Rational approaches to clinical therapy of
   hypertension. In Turner P. (ed.): Clinical Pharmacology &
   Therapeutics. Pp 270-274, London  Macmillan.
2. Laragh J H  (1973) Vasoconstriction-volume analysis for understanding and treating hypertension. The use of renin and aldosterone profiles. Am J Med 55: 261-274.
3. Zanchetti A, Mancia G  Leonetti G (1979) Humoral markers of hyper
   tension. In Albertini A, Da Prada M, Peskar BA (eds.): Radioimmunoassays of Drugs and Hormones in Cardiovascular Medicine. Pp
   3-15, Amsterdam, Elsevier.
4. Mancia G, Leonetti G  Picotti GB, Ferrari A, Galva MD  Gregorini
   L, Parati G, Pomidossi G. Ravazzani C, Sala C, Zanchetti A (1979)
   Plasma catecholamines and blood pressure responses to the carotid
   baroreceptor reflex in essential hypertension. Clin Sci 57, Suppl
   5: 156-167.
5. Zanchetti A, Tarazi RC (eds.): Angiotensin Converting Enzyme Inhibition. Am J Cardiol, Suppl, in press.
6. Mancia G, Parati G, Pomidossi G, Grassi G, Bertinieri G, Buccino
   N, Ferrari A, Gregorini L, Rupoli L  Zanchetti A: Modification of
   arterial baroreflexes by captopril in essential hypertension. In
   Zanchetti A, Tarazi RC (eds): Angiotensin Converting Enzyme Inhibition. Am J Cardiol, Suppl, in press.

7. Leonetti G, Bianchini C, Terzoli L, Gradnik R, Tusa M, Bramati E, Zanchetti A: Acute hypotensive and renin stimulating actions of captopril before and during treatment with a beta-blocking drug. In Zanchetti A, Tarazi RC (eds): Angiotensin Converting Enzyme Inhibition. Am J Cardiol, Suppl, in press.
8. Freis ED (1976) Salt volume and the prevention of hypertension. Circulation 53: 589-595.
9. Wessels F, Junge-Hulsing G, Losse M (1967) Untersuchungen zur Natriumpermeabilität der Erythrozyten bei Hypertonikern und Normotonikern mit familiarer Hochdruckbelastrung. Z Kreislaufforsch 56: 374-380.
10. Postnov Y, Orlov S, Shevchenko A, Adler A (1977) Altered sodium permeability, calcium binding and $Na^+$, $K^+$-ATPase activity in the red blood cell membrane in essential hypertension. Pflügers Arch 371: 263-264.
11. Garay RP, Meyer P (1979) A new test showing abnormal net $Na^+$ and $K^+$ fluxes in erythrocytes of essential hypertensive patients. Lancet 1: 349-353.
12. Canessa M, Adragna N, Solomon HS, Connolly TM, Tosteson DC (1980) Increased sodium, lythium countertransport in red cells of patients with essential hypertension. N Engl J Med 302: 772-776.
13. Edmondson RPS, Thomas RD, Hilton PJ, Patrick J, Jones NF (1975) Abnormal leucocyte composition and sodium transport in essential hypertension. Lancet 1: 1003-1005.
14. Ambrosioni E, Tartagni L, Montebugnoli L, Magnani B (1979) Intra lymphocytic sodium in hypertensive patients: a significant correlation. Clin Sci 57: 325-327.
15. Garay RP, Dagher G. Pernollet MG Devynck MA Meyer P (1980) Inherited defect in $Na^+$ $K^+$ co-transport system in erythrocytes from essential hypertensive patients. Nature 284: 281-283.
16. Garay RP, Elghozi JL, Dagher G, Meyer P (1980) Laboratory distinction between essential and secondary hypertension by measurement of erythrocyte cation fluxes. N Engl J Med 382: 769-771.

# Intervention of Single Risk Factors of Atherosclerosis: Thrombosis

H. K. Breddin

## Introduction

While it is well established, that secondary thrombosis is an important factor for the propagation of atherosclerotic lesions, it is
still undecided whether platelets and coagulation factors play a role
in the developement of the initial atherosclerotic lesions. In atherosclerotic plaques platelet material and fibrin are often found and
arterial thrombi contain platelets and fibrin. Platelet adhesion and
aggregation at damaged arterial vessel walls are primary steps in the
formation of arterial thrombi. Apparently both hemostatic systems,
namely primary hemostasis, which is mainly influenced by platelets
and their function and plasmatic coagulation are involved in secondary
arterial thrombosis at established atherosclerotic lesions.

## I. Coagulation Factors and Fibrinolysis in Atherosclerosis

What do we know about the role of platelet function, coagulation factors or fibrinolysis in the developement of arterial thrombi on atherosclerotic lesions ?

Abnormalities of hemostatic parameters found in patients with coronary
heart disease or with cerebral or peripheral vascular occlusions may
be cause or consequence of atherosclerotic or thrombotic processes.
Abnormalities of platelet function, coagulation factors and fibrinolysis parameters may be correlated with other risk factors and they may
be a secondary phenomenon following thrombotic processes as they are
regularily found in acute venous thromboses.

There are two ways to establish whether changes in platelet function,
coagulation or fibrinolysis are correlated with an enhanced or reduced risk of atherosclerosis and arterial thrombosis.

1. If in patients with arterial occlusive disease characteristic changes in platelet function or coagulation parameters are found it can be
established in prospective trials, if these changes are correlated
with an enhanced incidence of vascular occlusions.

2. It can be investigated if atherosclerosis and thrombosis in patients or animals with defined defects of platelet function, coagulàtion
or fibrinolysis,are less frequent than in the general population.

## II Correlations between Changes in Platelet Function and Coagulation and the Risk for Atherosclerosis and Thrombosis

Apparently some of the risk factors which enhance venous thrombosis are
of much less importance for the progredience of atherosclerosis or of
arterial thrombosis. In patients with antithrombin-III-deficiency, who
have a high risk of venous thrombosis, arterial thrombosis has only
rarely been observed.

Many investigators have tried to develop methods measuring platelet
function or coagulation factors which allow the detection of an enhanced risk of thrombosis, specially in patients with vascular disease.

## 1. Platelet Adhesiveness

All methods to detect enhanced platelet adhesion are still relatively unreliable. A number of investigators observed an enhanced platelet adhesiveness in patients with peripheral atherosclerosis, with diabetes or with coronary heart disease. Usually glassbead filters have been used for such investigations. But increased platelet adhesiveness has been found only in groups of patients and there not consistently. In the individual patient it has not been possible with the methods used so far to predict an enhanced risk of thrombosis.

## 2. ADP-, Collagen- and Adrenalin-induced Aggregation

With these methods many investigators observed an enhanced platelet aggregability in patients with diabetes (1 - 7). Such changes were also found in patients with recent myocardial infarction (8 - 12). No differences between healthy subjects and MI-patients could be observed by others (13 - 15). Only few and small prospective studies have been performed to evaluate if in individual patients enhanced platelet aggregation is an indicator of an enhanced risk of thrombosis or of recurrent reinfarction.

## 3. Spontaneous Platelet Aggregation

Vreeken and van Aken (16) described a patient who showed spontaneous aggregation in the usual aggregometers without addition of an aggregation inducing substance. Similar cases with enhanced spontaneous aggregation have been reported by Wu and Hoak (17), in patients with intermittent ischemic cerebral attacks, with acute myocardial infarction or acute periperal vascular occlusions.

With a method which measures spontaneous platelet aggregation (18, 19) we found an age dependent increase of spontaneous platelet aggregation in healthy individuals. In about 1000 patients with diabetes mellitus, an increase of spontaneous aggregation was found in all age groups compared with the healthy persons. In patients with coronary heart disease, no age dependent increase of spontaneous aggregation was found. But spontaneous aggregation was enhanced in all age groups compared to the healthy persons (20).

In 1978 a study has been initiated in Frankfurt a.M., which was named PARD-study (Platelet Aggregation as Risk Factor in Diabetes). In this study 330 diabetics are investigated at 3 month's intervals. Spontaneous aggregation, other platelet functions and coagulation parameters are measured. It is the primary goal of this prospective study to clarify, if enhanced platelet aggregation is an individual risk factor of thrombotic vascular occlusions in diabetic patients.

Other platelet function tests as platelet survival time, β-TG-levels, platelet factor 4 or the presence of in vivo formed platelet aggregates have been used to identify patients with an enhanced risk of thrombosis but no prospective studies on the predidive value of these methods have been published so far.

## 4. Coagulation Factors and Atherosclerosis

Increased levels of fibrinogen have been described in patients with recent myocardial infarcts by Pilgeram (21) and by Renny and Ogston (22). Pola und Savi (23) found increased fibrinogen levels in patients with vascular occlusions. Low antithrombin III-levels have been reported by Yue et al. (24) in patients with ischemic heart disease. In the prospective Northwick Park Heart study (25), 1510 persons aged 40 - 60

years have been investigated and followed for 1 1/2 - 7 years. Patients
who later died from cardiovascular causes when entering the study had
significantly higher factor VII-, factor VIII- and fibrinogen-levels
than the surviving population. Patients in whom two of the risk factors
were present, had a 5 x higher risk of cardiovascular death than the
surviving population.

Table 1. Coagulation factors and risk of cardiovascular death (Meade
et al. 1980)

|  | Cardiovascular deaths | Survivors | p |
|---|---|---|---|
| F. VII-activity % | 116 ± 32 | 102 ± 24 | <0.01 |
| F. VIII : C % | 114,5 ± 18 | 97.7 ± 34 | <0.05 |
| Fibrinogen mg % | 332 ± 85 | 293 ± 60 | <0.01 |
| Cholesterol mmol/l | 6.64 ± 1.3 | 6.02 ± 1.1 | <0.05 |

Elevated factor VII-activity was a relevant prospective risk factor in
this study. Actually the coagulation changes were stronger associated
with cardiovascular death then high blood cholesterol levels. Further
prospective studies are needed to confirm these results.

The higher values of factor VII and factor VIII found in the patients
of high risk in this study were within the normal range and therefore
detection of individual patients with a high risk would not be possible
using these parameters.

In this study no significant correlation has been found between antithrombin III levels, platelet number, platelet adhesiveness, factor
VIII related antigen or Ristocetin cofactor and cardiovascular death.

The identification of patient groups with a higher risk of arterial
thrombosis could facilitate new clinical trials of antithrombotic
drugs. The chances to detect drug effects in different treatment
groups would probably increase markedly if a relative large group of
patients with a low risk of new arterial thromboses could be excluded
in secondary prevention studies.

## 5. Platelet and Coagulation Defects and the Risk of Atherosclerosis and Arterial Thrombosis

It seems possible that patients with inborn or acquired defects of
platelet function or coagulation factors have a reduced risk of atherosclerosis or its thromboembolic complications. Some data on patients
with hemophilia A and B have been reported (26). In patients with severe hemophilia A myocardial infarcts and cerebral thrombosis or peripheral arterial thrombosis have not been observed. But the number of
patients with hemophilia of higher age is rather small in all centers.
Patients with severe hemophilia A or B, on whom autopsies had been
performed showed atheromatous plaques in different vascular regions
(26, 27). In patients with mild hemophilia A or B, myocardial infarctions have been repeatedly described and coronary thrombosis has been
frequent at autopsies. Whether the risk of arterial thrombosis in
these patients is reduced is not yet known. Clinical studies with long
term anticoagulant treatment in patients with myocardial or cerebral
occlusions and also in patients with peripheral arterial occlusions
have not made it likely that this treatment reduces the progredience

of atherosclerosis. Da Silva et al. in the Basel-Study (28) showed, that anticoagulants did not influence the developement of arterial stenoses but reduced the frequency of arterial occlusion.

Two plasmatic factors are closely related with platelet function: Fibrinogen and the von Willebrand factor. Both factors play an important role in the primary reactions of hemostasis and thrombogenesis. New experimental animal studies have shown that the total lack of von Willebrand factor markedly reduces the risk of atherosclerosis (29, 30, 31). In pigs with severe von Willebrand factor deficiency (homocygotes) the extent of spontaneous and dietary induced atherosclerosis of the aorta was markedly reduced. In pigs with slight von Willebrand deficiency (heterocygotes), the extent of spontaneous and dietary induced atherosclerosis of the aorta was not reduced.

The extent of dietary induced atherosclerosis of the coronaries was reduced in von Willebrand pigs. The developement of atherosclerosis after balloon induced denudation of the coronaries was not inhibited in homocygote von Willebrand pigs but myocardial infarcts were less frequent (31).

In patients with mild forms of von Willebrand disease, atherosclerosis and coronary thrombosis have been observed about as frequently as in the normal population. Investigations in patients with severe von Willebrand's disease are under way (Rokitansky-Duguid-project of ETRO).

It seems likely that systemic changes of coagulation factors are of slight relevance for the developement of atherosclerosis but may play a larger role in the pathogenesis of secondary thrombosis.

The findings that animals with severe von Willebrand's syndrome have reduced atherosclerosis may imply that atherosclerosis and its thrombotic sequelae could be reduced if platelet function as well as the activity of coagulation factors are inhibited simultaneously.

## III. Secondary Prevention of Thrombosis in Patients with Atherosclerotic Lesions

### 1. Anticoagulants

Oral anticoagulants reduce the incidence of recurrent myocardial infarction but not of total death. This has been shown in a number of prospective clinical studies. In a recent Dutch study (32) a group of 493 patients over 60 years of age, who had been on anticoagulant treatment after a myocardial infarction, and who received anticoagulants for another 2 years was compared with 439 patients who were treated with placebo. Total death was reduced in the anticoagulant group from 13.4 to 7.6 %. The incidence of myocardial infarcts was reduced from 15.9 - 5.7 %. The intensity of anticoagulant treatment was well controlled. This study has shown that intensive anticoagulant treatment at least in MI-patients which have been on anticoagulant treatment before is of objective value. Such results can probably not be obtained in other countries, who do not posess instruments similar to the well organized Dutch thrombosis services.

### 2. Longterm Studies with Acetylsalicylic Acid (ASA) in Patients with Recent Myocardial Infarction

Soon after the long lasting aggregation inhibiting effect of ASA became known in 1967, several clinical studies on the possible antithrombotic effect of this seemingly well known drug have been started. It

was the general assumption of investigators as that time that the inhibition of platelet aggregation corresponds with or at least goes a-
long with an antithrombotic effect.

During the following years eight larger clinical trials on the effect
of ASA in the secondary prevention of myocardial infarction have been
performed. These trials were the Elwood I and II (33, 34), the American Coronary Drug Project (CDP) (35), the Aspirin Myocardial Infarction
Study (AMIS) (36), the Persantin Aspirin Reinfarction Study (PARIS)
(37), the French EPSIM Study (38), the German-Austrian Myocardial Infarction Study (39) and the DDR-Aspirin Study (40). The Aspirin dose
in these studies varied between 300 and 1500 mg/day.

In none of these studies a significant effect of acetylsalicylic acid
on total mortality was found. In the French EPSIM-Study no significant
difference between anticoagulant treatment and Aspirin-treatment was
observed. In 6 of the remaining 7 studies there was a trend in favour
of Aspirin. But in the largest of these studies, the Aspirin Myocardial Infarction Study (AMIS) total mortality was higher in the ASA-group.

The CDP-Study, in which patients were included, who after their qualifying myocardial infarct had been on other treatment regimes showed a
marked trend in favour of ASA. Also the second Elwood trial, in which
patients in the treatment groups received 900 mg ASA/day showed a 17 %
reduction of total mortality in the ASA-treated group compared with the
placebo group and a 22 % reduction of coronary death. These differences were not significant (Tab. 2).

Table 2. ASA - MI - Studies

| Study | Year | N | total mortality | | |
| | | | Placebo % | ASA % | Reduction % |
|---|---|---|---|---|---|
| Elwood I | 1974 | 1239 | 10.9 | 8.3 | -25 |
| CDP | 1976 | 1529 | 8.3 | 5.8 | -30 |
| Elwood II | 1979 | 1682 | 14.8 | 12.3 | -17 |
| AMIS | 1980 | 2267 | 9.7 | 10.8 | +11 |
| PARIS | 1980 | 1216 | 12.8 | 10.5 | -18 |
| German-Austrian | 1980 | 626 | 13.4 | 11.5 | -18 |

On the other hand survived reinfarctions were reduced by 22 - 40 % in
5 studies including the AMIS trial (Tab. 3).

Three studies should be discussed in more detail. In the AMIS-Study
patients received either placebo or 1 g of Aspirin in 2 daily doses
of 500 mg each. In the PARIS-Study patients were treated with 3 x
324 mg/day and in the German-Austrian reinfarction study patients received 3 x 500 mg of microencapsulated ASA/day. An important difference between the studies was the time between the qualifying infarct
and inclusion into the study. In the AMIS-Study a mean of 25 months
had elapsed and in the PARIS-Study this time was similarily long. In
the German-Austrian Study the time between infarction and inclusion

Table 3. ASA - MI - Studies

| Study | N | survived reinfarctions | | |
| | | Placebo % | ASA % | Reduction in % |
|---|---|---|---|---|
| CDP | 1529 | 4 | 4 | - |
| Elwood II | 1682 | 10.9 | 7.1 | -34 |
| AMIS | 4524 | 8.1 | 6.3 | -22 |
| PARIS | 1216 | 9.9 | 6.9 | -30 |
| German-Austrian | 626 | 7.1 | 4.1 | -42 |
| DDR | 1340 | 6.7 | 3.6 | -46 |

into the study was relatively short with a mean of 40 days. In the AMIS-Study no difference in total mortality, lethal reinfarctions or sudden death was observed between the ASA and placebo group. These events were slightly more frequent in the ASA-groups. A retrospective analysis showed that the risk distribution between the two treatment groups was not identical. If this was taken into consideration there was a minimal advantage in favour of the ASA-group. In the Persantin-Aspirin-Study which was planned in a very similar way as the AMIS-Study, a larger difference in favour of the ASA-group was found, which also was not significant. In a subgroup of patients in the PARIS-Study, which had been included into the study during the first six months after the qualifying infarct, total mortality in the ASA-group was 9.2 % compared to 10.6 % in the group treated with ASA + Di-pyridamole and 18.9 % in the placebo group. The number of patients in that subgroup consisted of 20 % of the total study population. In the retrospective analysis the difference between Persantin-Aspirin and placebo for coronary death after 3 years of treatment was significant. The incidence of survived reinfarctions in the three studies was lowest in the Phenprocoumon group of the German-Austrian Study. AMIS and PARIS showed that the incidence of stroke was markedly reduced compared to the placebo groups.

## 3. Sulfinpyrazone Studies in Patients with Recent Myocardial Infarct

Two trials with Sulfinpyrazone in patients with recent myocardial infarctions have been published so far (41, 42). In the American Study a significant reduction of sudden death was observed during the first six months of treatment in patients, who received 4 x 200 mg of Sulfinpyrazone per day. In the Italian study patients received 2 x 400 mg/day. In the American study total mortality was reduced by 28 %, in the Italian study by 12 %.

Non fatal reinfarctions were reduced by 23 % in the American Sulfin-pyrazone study, which was not significant and by 57 % in the Italian study which was a significant difference. On the other hand in the American study sudden deaths were reduced by 40 %, while there was an increase in sudden deaths in the Italian study. Death by reinfarction, which was not affected in the American study was reduced by 50 % in the Italian study. Although both studies showed positive effects these differing results make evaluation of this drug still very difficult.

4. Prevention of Thrombosis in the Cerebral Circulation.

Anticoagulants have shown some effect in preventing cerebral thrombosis but in general this treatment is not propagated because of the high incidence of intracerebral bleedings, which often are fatal. Since several studies (43, 44, 45, 46) have shown acetylsalicylic acid to be effective in the reduction of recurrent ischemic attacks and stroke, this treatment has become accepted for patients with recent transient ischemic attacks. A Canadian study in which Sulfinpyrazone has been compared with ASA showed no positive effects of Sulfinpyrazone wheras a significant reduction of TIA and stroke was observed in the Aspirin group compared with the placebo group.

5. Anticoagulants and Platelet Active Drugs in the Long Term Prevention of Thromboses in Peripheral Atherosclerosis

An interesting study has been published by Bollinger et al. (47). Patients were treated after thrombendarterectomy or after bypass-surgery of peripheral vascular occlusions for 2 years either with coumarines or with acetylsalicylic acid alone or in combination with Dipyridamole. In this study the treatment with platelet function inhibitors resulted in 80 % of nonoccluded vessels in the group which was treated after thrombendarterectomy compared to 58 % in the coumarine treated group, which was a significant difference. In the patient group in which a bypass-operation had been performed, oral anticoagulants performed better then platelet function inhibitors, but here the difference was not significant.

6. Is there a Different Antithrombotic Effect of ASA in Men and in Women

In the Canadian study on patients with transient intermittent cerebral attacks (45), ASA was effective in men only. Similar results have been reported in other studies as in the German-Austrian Reinfarction Study (39). In this trial the difference in coronary mortality was significant in the retrospective analysis if men alone were considered. But these findings are not consistant. No such difference was observed in the PARIS-trial (37).

The proportion of women compared with men in all studies was relatively small. In the Canadian TIA-study some women also had lesser endpoints than men. The reduced effect of platelet function inhibitors may have been influenced in this study mainly by this fact and not so much by a different reaction of females to antiplatelet drugs. Although some animal experiments seem to conform a sex difference in reaction to antiplatelet function inhibitors, this problem will have to be further investigated.

IV. On the Mechanism of the Antithrombotic Effect of Platelet Function Inhibitors

Acetylsalicylic acid (ASA) was the first drug to be tested in a variety of diseases for its antithrombotic effect. In man single doses of 100 mg ASA and more inhibit platelet aggregation for several days by inhibiting platelet cyclooxygenase. This effect leads to the inhibition of thromboxane $A_2$-formation in the platelets.

Following the concept of an important role of the prostaglandin metabolism in the regulation of blood-vessel wall interactions, Moncada and Vane (48) suggested the use of very small doses of ASA - in the range of 100 - 200 mg/day - in future clinical trials of the antithrombotic effect of this drug. It was their hypothesis that in higher

doses ASA inhibits prostacyclin formation in the vessel wall as well
as thromboxane $A_2$ formation in the platelets and that the antithrombotic effect of ASA is closely related with the inhibition of thromboxane $A_2$ formation in the platelets and therefore with the inhibition
of platelet aggregation.

Several animal thrombosis studies by different investigators are not
compatible with this concept (49, 50, 51). In these studies ASA doses
of 1 - 10 mg/kg, which are sufficient to inhibit cyclooxygenase in the
platelets, had little if any antithrombotic effect, but higher doses
up to 100 mg/kg more effectively inhibited experimental thromboses.

New experimental and pharmacokinetic studies have made it likely that
ASA inhibits other platelet functions as shape change and adhesion besides aggregation dose dependently and for hours only (52).

## V. Primary Prevention Studies

No primary prevention studies with antithrombotic drugs have been published so far  Such a study has been initiated by Peto and Doll in
healthy male doctors with 500 mg of Aspirin/day.

Antithrombotic treatment could be more effective if patients who are
at high risk to get new vascular occlusions could be selected by sufficiently reliable tests of platelet function or coagulation. Some
prospective trials are underway with the aim to define such test systems.

Considering the results of the different secondary prevention, trials
with antithrombotic drugs it seems unlikely that a positive effect of
these drugs can be established in primary prevention studies if it will
not be possible to preselect patient groups, who are at higher risk of
coronary, peripheral or cerebral thrombotic occlusions. The chances to
find such parameters or a combination of such tests, is not small. But
more prospective studies with newly devised techniques will have to
establish their value and may then enhance the chances of further clinical trials to establish the effects of old and more effective new
antithrombotic drugs.

## References

1. Heath H, Bridgen WD, Canever JV, Pollock J, Hunter PR, Kelsey J,
   Bloom A (1971) Platelet adhesiveness and aggregation in relation to
   diabetic retinopathy. Diabetologia 7: 308-315
2. Hassanein AA, El-Garf TA, El-Baz Z (1972) Platelet aggregation in
   diabetes mellitus and the effect of insulin in vivo on aggregation.
   Thrombos Diathes Haemorrh (Stuttg) 27: 114-120
3. Kwaan HC, Colwell JA, Cruz S, Suawanwela N, Dobbie JG (1972) Increased platelet aggregation in diabetes mellitus. J Lab Clin Med
   80: 236-247
4. Bensoussan D, Levy-Toledano S, Passa P, Caen J, Canivet J (1975)
   Platelet hyperaggregation and increased plasma level of von Willebrand factor in diabetics with retinopathy. Diabetologia 11:307-312
5. Colwell JA, Halushka PV, Sargi K, Levine L, Sagel J, Raghavani ChB,
   Nair MG (1976) Altered platelet function in diabetes mellitus.
   Diabetes 25 (Suppl 2): 826-831
6. Colwell JA, Halushka PV, Sarji KE, Lopes-Virella MF, Sagel J (1979)
   Vascular disease in diabetes. Pathophysiological mechanisms and
   therapy. Arch intern Med 139: 225-230
7. Matsuo T, Ohki Y (1977) Classification of platelet aggregation pat-

terns with two ADP solutions (the double-ADP method) and its clinical application to diabetes mellitus. Thromb Res 11: 453-461
8. O'Brien JR, Path FC, Heywood JB, Heady JA (1966) The quantitation of platelet aggregation induced by four compounds: A study in relation to myocardial infarction. Thrombos Diathes Hemorrh (Stuttg) 16:752-767
9. Zahavi J, Dreyfuss F (1969) An abnormal pattern of adenosine diphosphate-induced platelet aggregation in acute myocardial infarction. Thrombos Diathes haemorrh (Stuttg) 21: 76-88
10. Sano T, Motomiya T, Yamazaki H (1979) Platelet release reaction in vivo in patients with ischemic heart disease after isometric exercise and its prevention with dipyridamole. Thrombos Haemostas 42: 1589-1597
11. Zahavi J (1977) The role of platelets in myocardial infarction, ischemic heart disease, cerebrovascular disease, thromboembolic disorders and acute idiopathic pericarditis. Thromb Haemostas 38: 1073-1084
12. Gormsen J, Nielsen JD, Andersen LA (1977) ADP-induced platelet aggregation in vitro in patients with ischemic heart disease and peripheral thromboatherosclerosis. Acta Med Scand 201: 509-513
13. Rozenberg MC, Stormorken H (1967) Comparison of glass adhesiveness and rate of aggregation of blood platelets. Scand Clin Lab Invest 19: 82-85
14. Steele PP, Weily HS, Davies H, Genton E (1973) Platelet function studies in coronary artery disease. Circulation 48: 1193-1200
15. Davis JW, Phillips PE, Yue KTN, Lewis D, Hartman LR (1978) Platelet aggregation in adult onset diabetes mellitus and coronary artery disease. J Amer Med Ass 239: 732-734
16. Vreeken J, van Aken WG (1971) Spontaneous aggregation of blood platelets as a cause of idiopathic thrombosis and recurrent painful toes and fingers. Lancet II: 1394-1397
17. Wu KK, Hoak JC (1976) Spontaneous platelet aggregation in arterial insufficiency: Mechanism and implications. Thromb Haemostas 35: 702-711
18. Breddin K (1965) Über die gesteigerte Thrombozytenagglutination bei Gefäßkrankheiten. Schweiz med Wschr 95: 655-660 (1965)
19. Breddin HK, Grun H, Krzywanek HJ, Schremmer WP (1976) On the measurement of spontaneous platelet aggregation. The platelet aggregation test III. Method and first clinical results. Thromb Haemostas 35: 669-691
20. Krzywanek HJ (1981) Änderung der Plättchenfunktion bei Gefäßkrankheiten. in: Breddin HK (Ed.): Thrombose und Atherogenese, Pathophysiologie und Therapie der arteriellen Verschlußkrankheit, Bein- und Beckenvenenthrombose. G.Witzstrock, Baden Baden, Köln, New York 59-70
21. Pilgeram LO (1961) Relation of plasma fibrinogen concentration changes to human arteriosclerosis. J Appl physiol 16: 660-664
22. Rennie JAN, Ogston D (1976) Changes in coagulation factors following acute myocardial infarction in man. Haemostasis 5:258-264
23. Pola P, Savi L: Fibrinogenemia determined immunnephelometrically as a possible parameter in the evaluation of peripheral atherosclerotic arteriopathy (1978) Atherosclerosis 29: 205-216
24. Yue RH, Gertler MM, Starr T, Koutrouby R (1976) Alteration of plasma antithrombin III levels in ischemic heart disease. Thrombos haemostas (Stuttg) 35: 598-606
25. Meade TW, Chakrabarti R, Haines AP, North WRS, Stirling Y, Thompson SG, Brozovic M (1980) Haemostatic function and cardiovascular death: early result of a prospective study. Lancet : 1050-1054
26. Lechner K, Ehringer H, Holzner HJ, Möslacher H, Pokiser H (1972) Thrombotische Herzinfarkte bei hereditären Minus-Koagulopathien (Faktor I - XIII) und hereditären Plättchenanomalien. In: Marx R, Thies HA: Herzinfarkt und Blutgerinnung, Schattauer, Stuttgart,

New York 79-87
27. Lechner K, Resch F (1981) Blutgerinnungs- und Fibrinolyseverände-
    rungen bei Patienten mit Gefäßerkrankungen. In: Breddin HK: Throm-
    bose und Atherogenese. Risikofaktoren bei gefäßchirurgischen Ein-
    griffen, Beckenvenenthrombose. Witzstrock Baden Baden, Köln, New
    York 79-85
28. DaSilva A, Widmer LK, Martin H, Ramseier L (1974) Long-term anti-
    coagulation in occlusion of peripheral arteries. In: Deutsch E,
    Lechner K, Brinkhous KM, Hinnom S: Thrombosis, pathogenesis and
    clinical trials. Schattauer Stuttgart, New York 253-261
29. Fuster V, Bowie W, Lewis JC, Fass DN, Owen CA, Brown AL (1978) Re-
    sistance to arteriosclerosis in pigs with von Willebrand's disease.
    J clin Invest 61: 722-730
30. Fuster V, Fass DN, Bowie EJW (1973) Resistance to atherosclerosis
    in pigs with genetic and therapeutic inhibition of platelet func-
    tion (Abstr) Thrombos Haemostas 42: 270
31. Griggs TR, Sulzer DL, Reddick RL, Brinkhous KM (1979) Induced co-
    ronary and aortic atherosclerosis in pigs with von Willebrand's
    disease. (Abstr) Thrombos Haemostas 42: 270
32. Sixty plus Reinfarction Study Research Group (1980) A double blind
    trial to assess longterm oral anticoagulant therapy in elderly
    patients after myocardial infarction. Lancet II: 989-994
33. Elwood PC, Cochrane AL, Burr ML, Sweetnam PM, Williams G, Welsby E,
    Hughes SJ, Renton R (1974) a randomised controlled trial of acetyl-
    salicylic acid in the secondary prevention of mortality from myo-
    cardial infarction. Brit med J 2: 436-443
34. Elwood PC, Sweetnam PM (1979) Aspirin and secondary mortality
    after myocardial infarction. Lancet II: 1313-1315
35. Coronary Drug Project Group (1976) Aspirin in coronary heart di-
    disease. J chron Dis 29: 625-642
36. Aspirin Myocardial Infarction Study Research Group (1980) A rando-
    mised controlled trial of aspirin in persons recovered from myocar-
    dial infarction. J Amer med Ass 243: 661-669
37. Persantin-Aspirin Study Research Group (1980) Persantin and aspi-
    rin in coronary heart disease. Circulation 62: 449-461
38. Boissel JP, Leizorovicz A, Schbath J, Destors JM, Gillet J (1981)
    E.P.S.I.M., the french oral anticoagulant-Aspirin trial in post
    myocardial infarction patients: design organisation and quality
    control procedures. Scand J Haematol Suppl 38: 47-69
39. Breddin HK, Loew D, Lechner K, Überla K, Walter E (1980) Secondary
    prevention of myocardial infarction. A comparison of acetylsali-
    cylic acid, placebo and phenprocoumon. Haemostasis 9: 325-344
40. Vogel G, Fischer Ch, Huyke R (1981) Prevention of reinfarction with
    acetylsalicylic acid. In: Breddin HK, Loew D, Überla K, Dorndorf W,
    Marx R: Prophylaxis of venous, peripheral, cardiac and cerebral
    vascular diseases with acetylsalicylic acid. F.K.Schattauer, Stuttg,
    New York 122-128
41. Anturane Reinfarction Trial Research Group (1980) Sulfinpyrazone in
    the prevention of sudden death after myocardial infarction. New
    Engl J med 302: 250-256
42. Anturan Reinfarction Italian Study Group (1982) Sulfinpyrazone in
    post myocardial infarction. Lancet I: 237-242
43. Fields WS, Lemak, NA, Frankowski RF, Hardy RJ (1977) Controlled
    trial of aspirin in cerebral ischemia. Stroke 8: 301-316
44. Fields WS, Lemak NA, Frankowski RF, Hardy RJ (1978) Controlled tri-
    al of aspirin in cerebral ischemia Part II. Surgical group. Stroke
    9: 309-319 (1978)
45. Canadian Cooperative Study Group (1978) A randomised trial of aspi-
    rin in threatened stroke. New Engl J med 299: 53-59
46. Reuter R, Dorndorf W (1978) Aspirin in patients with cerebral ische-
    mia and normal angiograms or non surgical lesions. In: Breddin HK,
    Dorndorf W, Loew D, Marx R (Eds.): Acetylsalicylic acid in cerebral

ischemia and coronary heart disease. Schattauer Stuttg, New York 97-106

47. Bollinger A, Schneider E, Pouliadis G, Brunner U (1981) Thrombozytenfunktionshemmer und Antikoagulantien nach gefäßrekonstruktiven Eingriffen im femoro-poplitealen Bereich. Resultate einer prospektiven Studie. In: Breddin K,(Ed.): Thrombose und Atherogenese, Risikofaktoren bei gefäßchirurgischen Eingriffen, Beckenthrombose. Witzstrock Baden Baden, Köln, New York 276-279

48. Moncada S, Vane JR (1979) Arachidonic acid and metabolites and the interaction between platelets and blood vessel walls. New Engl J med 300: 1142-1147

49. Meng K, O'Dea K (1974) The protective effect of acetylsalicylic acid on laser-induced venous thrombosis in the rat. Naunyn-Schmiedebergs Arch.Pharmacol 283: 379-388

50. Haarmann W (1981) Erfahrungen mit Azetylsalizylsäure, Dipyridamol und Sulfinpyrazon in verschiedenen Tiermodellen. In: Breddin HK, Gross D, Rotter W (Eds): Thrombosemodelle am Tier. Prostaglandine und Thrombogenese. Schattauer Stuttg. New York 173-188

51. Busse WD, Seuter F (1981) Erfahrungen mit Azetylsalizylsäure, Dipyridamol und Sulfinpyrazon in verschiedenen Tiermodellen. In: Breddin HK, Gross D, Rotter W (Eds): Thrombosemodelle am Tier. Prostaglandine und Thrombogenese. Schattauer Stuttg New York 157-172

52. Pietsch U, Lippmann M, Scharrer I, Breddin HK (1977) Neue Befunde zur Wirkung von Azetylsalizylsäure. Die Hemmwirkung auf den Formwandel der Thrombozyten und ihre Bedeutung für die Dosierung als Antithrombotikum. In: Alexander K, Cachovan M Diabetische Angiopathien. Witzstrock Baden Baden 348-351

53. Breddin HK, Rheinfelder J, Sehrbrock M, Trautmann KO, Kirchmaier CM (1981) Infarktprophylaxe mit Aggregationshemmern. In Gross R, Holtmeier HJ (Eds): Blutgerinnung und Fibrinolyse Thieme Stuttg, New York 79-87

# Intervention on Smoking: An Individual and Collective Challenge

F. Gutzwiller and W. Schweizer

## 1. Introduction

The World Health Organization notes in a recent report: "The control
of cigarette smoking could do more to improve health and prolong life
in (developed) countries than any other single action in the whole
field of preventive medicine".

Cigarette smokers have a 70 per cent greater rate of death from all
causes than non-smokers; detailed reviews on all aspects of smoking
and its hazards are available (Royal College of Physicians, 1977,
The Surgeon General 1979, Kannel 1981).

Moreover, a large portion of smoker's excess risk for heart diesease
disappears within two years after quitting - and within 10 to 15 years
an ex-smoker's chance of an early coronary death is no greater than a
non-smoker's.

The per capita consumption of tobacco has, in the U.S., declined
steadily since 1973 and it is now on the lowest level of the century.
Today there are over 30 million ex-smokers in the U.S. alone
(DHHS 1980).

95 percent of smokers who successfully quit do so on their own. Four
factors seem to be of major importance in their success: health concerns (including symptoms); a desire to set an example for others; a
desire for self-control; and aesthetic reasons (such as breath odor
and loss of taste for food).

A large share of the decline in smoking rates is due to a drop in the
proportion of men who smoke, but the percentage of women who smoke has
decreased negligibly. However, in most countries, there has been a
doubling of the rate at which adolescent women (12 to 18 years) smoke.

On this background, this review attempts to discuss the approaches to
the problem of smoking cessation, i.e. the possible interventions on
an individual level (traditional health education), on the level of
whole population groups (community health education), and of whole
societies.

## 2. Cessation of Smoking I: Individual Approaches

Traditional approaches to smoking cessation include hypnosis, individual and group counseling and strategies derived both from learning
theory and behavioral science (SHEWCHUK et al. 1977; WYNDER et al.
1979). Although most of these efforts have moderately high initial

success rates (40 to 89 per cent), long-term success rates are less impressive (BERNSTEIN 1969; SCHWARTZ 1977); only about 20 to 25 per cent of those who quit smoking are still abstinent one year after seeking treatment.

A similar general pattern of results, in which one year success rates (per cent non-smoking) above 30 per cent are highly respectable and rates above 50 per cent are extraordinary, has been observed over a broad range of smoking cessation programs (National Cancer Institute 1977). On the background of these results, five problem areas need specific discussion.

## 2.1. Behavioral Science Techniques

Progress in the behavioral sciences has been relatively slow in this area. MARSTON and MCFALL (1971) conducted a rigorous experimental comparison of several techniques developed by behavioral scientists and found that all produced immediate success followed by almost total relapse. However, in recent programs some break-throughs may have been made. Major aspects of those behavioral components are briefly outlined below.

## 2.2. Social Influence

Success in giving up smoking is often dependent on the complex influence provided by the individual offering assistance and other significant persons in the smoker's social environment. Very powerful counter-conditioning programs have been shown to lose their effectiveness if the "social climate" in which they are applied lacks non-specific supportive qualities (HARRIS and LICHTENSTEIN, 1974).

But engineering optimal social influence is difficult. BRENGELMANN (1974) found e.g. that face-to-face treatment was no more effective in the long run than treatment administered through the mail.

## 2.3. Maintenance

However, since long-term success is the most desirable outcome, the key to improving the results of smoking-cessation approaches is the development of methodes that help smokers stay off cigarettes permanently.

One successful maintenance technic involved "booster" messages by telephone. In a pilot study successful quitters who were given this telephone number were twice as likely to be abstinent one month after stopping than those who were not given access to these messages (DUBREN 1977).

## 2.4. Drug Therapy, Aversion, and Fear Arousal Techniques

Drugs have been tested against placebos in various smoking cessation programs. Evaluations found generally that participants who were given drugs such as lobeline or a tranquilizer had about the same success rates as those on placebos (SCHWARTZ 1976). A nicotine

chewing-gum developed in Sweden showed early promising results.
Follow-up studies are now being conducted in several European countries (RUSSELL et al. 1980).

Aversion therapy utilizes techniques such as over-exposure to smoke,
rapid-smoking, breath-holding, and electric shock. In addition to
health concerns regarding rapid smoking (MILLER et al. 1977; SACHS
et al. 1978), aversion techniques do not show  promise as a widely
applicable cessation method (SCHWARTZ 1975). Yet in selected groups,
there have been impressive results (SCHMAHL et al. 1972; LICHTENSTEIN
1973a). With rapid smoking, after 5 to 6 years nearly 40 per cent of
the original subjects were still abstinent (LICHTENSTEIN et al. 1977).
The same holds true for fear arousal techniques (LEVENTHAL 1971);
on the contrary, people who smoke to reduce anxiety often smoke more
after receiving a strong health threat in order to reduce their anxiety and fear (LICHTENSTEIN et al. 1973).

## 2.5. Social and Psychologic Approaches to the Adolescent Smoker

Most of these approaches attempt to discourage smoking by providing
specific behavioral training about possible smoking situations and
how to cope with such pressures, rather than teaching about the
effects of smoking on health only (EVANS 1976).

So-called "Life Skills Training Programs" (American Health Foundation) are usually conducted by the regular classroom teacher and
use a combination of group discussion, modeling and behavior re-
hearsal to teach students the kind of basic life skills that will
enable them both to resist direct social pressure to smoke and decrease their susceptibility to indirect social influences (by promoting greater autonomy, self-esteem and self-confidence). Thus,
the problem of cigarette smoking is addressed indirectly within
the context of self-development (WILLIAMS et al. 1977).

## 3. Cessation of Smoking II: Interventions in Whole Population Groups

All individual efforts to change life-styles are, in a sense, limited by the fact that also social norms, the "social climate" ought
to be changed to really develop effective large-scale programs. Individual changes, without support from environmental changes, are
difficult to maintain. This is one of the central arguments for
community (or population group oriented) wide health education programs.

Since the beginning of the seventies, a number of so-called "comprehensive cardiovascular community control programs" have been developed and evaluated. One such program, recently completed, is the
Swiss National Research Program 1 (National Research Program Collaborative Group 1978, 1981, 1982).

The National Research Program 1 on "Primary Prevention of cardiovascular diseases in Switzerland" was designed to determine whether
community health education can reduce cardiovascular risk factors in
the population. Two communities (12,000 inhabitants each) in the
French speaking and two (16,000 inhabitants each) in the German

speaking part of the country were selected either for intervention or comparison.Following baseline screening in 1977 (stratified random samples, n = 2,000 for each community, age 16-69 years) and the community intervention program (1978-1980), a final assessment on the initial participants was performed at the end of 1980. Amongst the regular smokers, 26 per cent have stopped during this period in the intervention communities whereas 18 per cent did so in the control areas. 5 per cent of non-smokers began to smoke during the same period in the intervention communities whereas 8 per cent did so in the control areas. There was also significant reduction of smokers amongst young people aged 14 to 16 in the intervention communities.

Table 1 shows the results obtained so far in the framework of multifactorial intervention programs. The "Net-Effect" on the total population in most programs does not seem too impressive. However, considering the quantity of persons concerned in these publications, and the few resources necessary for community oriented health education, this certainly represents a promising approach.

Table 1. Smoking Results of multifactorial intervention programs

| Study | Population | | % change smokers[1] | | Publication |
|-------|------------|------|------|------|------|
| | | | High Risk | Total Pop. | |
| Stanford | communities | USA | + 1 | $-10^2$ | Farquhar et al., 1977 |
| North Karelia | communities | SF | ... | $-13(m)^2$ $- 8(f)^2$ | Puska et al., 1979 |
| Oslo | communities | NR | -45 | ... | Hjermann et al., 1981 |
| Oberperfuss | communities | A | - 8 | ... | Rhomberg, 1981 |
| Nat. Research Program 1 | communities | CH | ... | - 8 | NRP Collab. Group, 1982 |
| HDPP | 24 Factories | U.K. | -12 | - 7 | Rose et al., 1980 |
| WHO Project | Factories | U.K. | -19,8 | $-16,9^3$ | Marmot et al., 1979 |
| WHO Project | Factories | B | - 6,5 | 0 | Kornitzer et al., 1980 |
| WHO Project | Factories | I | 0 | 0 | Mariotti et al., 1981 |

1 Difference in prevalence of smokers between intervention and control groups
2 Mean reported daily smoking
3 Excluding high risk group

Source: Epstein F.H., 1982, modified

## 4. Cessation of Smoking III: Societal Interventions; The Impact of Anti-Smoking Campaigns on Consumption

On a societal level, smokers seem to have reacted quite strongly to the scientific evidence linking smoking to disease. The Terry Report was credited with having caused a decrease of cigarette demand in the U.S. of 5 to 7 per cent (WARNER 1977). British Researches have estimated that the first two reports of the Royal College of Physicians, published in 1962 and 1971, have temporarily decreased cigarette consumption by roughly 5 per cent each (ATKINSON et al. 1973). For Switzerland, a permanent reduction of cigarette demand by 8 to 12 per cent through publicity was estimated (LEU 1980). For the U.S., it was concluded that "in the absence of any campaign, per capita consumption in the U.S. likely would have exceeded its actual 1975 value by 20 to 30 per cent" (WARNER 1981).

Only speculations are possible on the effects of a continued anti-smoking campaign. The sharp downturn in per capita consumption of cigarettes in 1967-1969 provides an interesting lesson, however (STAMLER 1978). During those years, "equal time" messages were presented on radio and television. With the 1970 congressional legislation banning cigarette advertising on radio and TV, these messages disappeared. Since then cigarette advertising has been switched to magazines, newspapers and billboards, at a cost of about $ 400 million per year in the U.S. alone; and consumption rose again.

However, some of the important indirect effects of publicity have to be acknowledged, too.

First, anti-smoking publicity, together with heavy commercial promotion campaigns, has stimulated an overwhelming majority of smokers to switch to filter cigarettes (Royal College of Physicians 1977), has contributed to the substantial lowering of the average "tar" and nicotine content per cigarette (HAMMOND et al. 1976), and has induced smokers to smoke less of each cigarette.

Furthermore, publicity has stimulated the militancy of non-smokers and has changed attitudes about the "rights of non-smokers". This is reflected by the founding of non-smoker associations, pressing for non-smoking sections in restaurants, increasing demand for larger sections for non-smokers in public transport systems, non-smoking areas on the job, smoking restrictions in public buildings, etc., and for legislative anti-smoking efforts.

Alle these factors may have intensified the pressures on smokers to quit (EISINGER 1971). In addition, the recent increases in success rates of smoking cessation programs may well be due to such changes in the social environment multiplying the effectiveness of previously unsuccessful programs.

Finally, evidence on the impact of smoking reduction on the observed mortality decline in U.S. CVD death rates is mounting (KLEINMAN et al. 1978).

788

## 5. Conclusions: Obstacles to Prevention

Cessation of smoking is still a very difficult undertaking for most individuals. But some definite progress in health education methods and materials has been made, to assist individuals and groups.

On the level of communities, there are now convincing data, that community health education is both feasible and cost-effective. On the level of our societies, however, there are still formidable obstacles to more effective anti-smoking intervention.

This is not surprising. The U.S. for instance is a leading producer of tobacco leaf and utilizes a price support system which is designed to protect tobacco growers (SAPOLSKY 1980). The six major manufacturers produce over 145 brands of cigarettes, with retail sales of over $ 15 billion and profits exceeding $ 1 billion (Institute of Medicine 1982).

However, eleven countries have banned all tobacco advertising. Norway, Sweden and Finland have central government advisory bodies on action to curtail smoking. In Finland 0,5 per cent of all tobacco revenue is channelled into public education on smoking.

Smoking and health remain one of the great challenges to the field of public health. However, the experience of the past two decades showed remarkable progress on all levels. Smoking and its associated diseases are not constantsof modern life. Both lifestyles and disease patterns can be changed.

## References

1. Atkinson AB, Skegg JL (1973) Anti-Smoking Publicity and the Demand for Tobacco in the U.K. The Manchester School of Economic and Social Studies 41: 265
2. Bernstein DA (1969) Modification of smoking behavior: an evaluative review. Psychol Bull 71: 418
3. Brengelmann JL (1976) Experimente zur Behandlung des Rauchens. Verlag W. Kohlhammer, Stuttgart
4. Dubren R (1977) Self-reinforcement by recorded telephone messages to maintain non-smoking behavior. J Consult Clin Psychol 45: 358
5. Eisinger EA (1971) Psychological Predictors of Smoking Recidivism. J Hlth Soc Behav 12: 355
6. Epstein FH (1982) Personal communication
7. Evans RI (1976) Smoking in children: developing a social psychological strategy of deterrence. Prev Med 5: 122
8. Farquhar JW, Maccoby N, Wood D et al. (1977) Community Education for Cardiovascular Health. Lancet 1: 1192
9. Hammond EC, Garfinkel L, Seidman H et al. (1976) "Tar" and Nicotine Content of Cigarette Smoke in Relation to Death Rates. Environm Research 12: 263

10. Harris DE, Lichtenstein E (1974) Contribution of non-specific social factors to a successful behavioral treatment of smoking. Directory of research in smoking and health (No. 661), N.C.S.H., Bethesda, MD
11. Hjermann I, Velve Byre K, Holme I et al. (1981) Effect of Diet and Smoking Intervention on the Incidence of Coronary Heart Disease. Lancet 2: 1303
12. Institute of Medicine (1982) Perspectives on Health Promotion and Disease Prevention in the United States. National Academy of Sciences, Washington, D.C.
13. Kannel WB (1981) Update on the role of cigarette smoking in coronary artery disease. Am Heart J 101: 319
14. Kleinman JC, Feldman JJ, Monk MM (1978) Trends in Smoking and Ischemic Heart Disease Mortality. Proceedings of the Conference on the Decline in Coronary Heart Disease Mortality, NHLBI, Bethesda, Md., p.195
15. Leu RE (1980) Modifying Risk Taking Behavior Through Public Policy: The Case of Cigarette Smoking. Discussion Paper No. 49, Inst. for Social Sciences, University of Basel, Switzerland
16. Leventhal H (1971) Fear Appeals and Persuasion: The Differentiation of Motivation Construct. Am J Publ Health 61: 1208
17. Lichtenstein E, Deutzer CS (1973) Implications of Psychological Research for Smoking Control Clinics. Health Serv Reports 88: 535
18. Lichtenstein E, Harris DE, Birchler GR et al. (1973a) Comparison of rapid smoking, warm, smoky air, and attention placebo in the modification of smoking behavior. J Consult Clin Psychol 40: 92
19. Lichtenstein E, Rodrigues MRP (1977) Long-term effects of rapid smoking treatment for dependent cigarette smokers. Addict Behav 2: 109
20. Mariotti S et al. (1981) Europ. Heart J 2 (Suppl A): 47
21. Marmot MG (1979) WHO collaborative project. Bull World Hlth Org 57: 331
22. Marston AR, McFall RM (1971) Comparison of behavior modification approaches to smoking reduction. J Consult Clin Psychol 36: 153
23. Miller LC, Schilling AF, Logan DL et al. (1977) Potential Hazards of Rapid Smoking as a Technic for the Modification of Smoking Behavior. N Engl J Med 297: 590
24. National Cancer Institute (1977) The Smoking Digest: Progress Report on a Nation Kicking the Habit. U.S. Department of Health, Education and Welfare, NCI, Bethesda, MD.
25. National Research Program Collaborative Group (1978) Planning and Organization. Soz Präv Med 23: 280
26. National Research Program Collaborative Group (1981) Die Epidemiologie der Risikofaktoren für kardiovaskuläre Krankheiten in der Schweiz. Schweiz med Wschr 111 (Supplementum 12)
27. National Research Program Collaborative Group (1982) Prophylaxe von Herz-Kreislauf-Krankheiten in der Schweiz. Paul Haupt, Bern
28. Puska P, Tuomilehto J, Salonen J et al. (1979) Changes in coronary risk factors during comprehensive five year community programme to control cardiovascular diseases (North Karelia Project). Br Med J 2: 1173
29. Rhomberg HP (1981) Risikofaktoren in Oberperfuss. Wiener Klin Wschr 93 (Suppl. 127)

790

30. Rose G, Heller RF, Tunstall Pedoe H, Christie DGS (1980) Heart Disease Prevention Project: A randomized controlled trial in industry. Brit Med J 1: 747
31. Royal College of Physicians (1977) Smoking or Health, Pitman Medical, London
32. Sapolsky HM (1980) The Political Obstacles to the Control of Cigarette Smoking in the United States. J Health Politics, Policy and Law 5: 277
33. Schmahl DP, Lichtenstein E, Harris DE (1972) Successful treatment of habitual smokers with warm, smoky air and rapid smoking. J Consult Clin Psychol 38: 105
34. Schwartz JL (1976) A Critical Review and Evaluation of Smoking Control Methods. Public Health Reports 84: 483
35. Schwartz JL (1977) Research Methodology in Smoking Cessation: a critique. Proceeding of the Third World Conference on Smoking and Health (DHEW Publ. No (NIH) 77-1413), Vol. 2, Washington D.C., Government Printing Office, p. 665
36. Shewchuk LA, Wynder EL (1977) Guidelines on smoking cessation clinics. Prev Med 6: 130
37. Stamler J (1978) Lifestyles, Major Risk Factors, Proof and Public Policy. Circulation 58: 3
38. The Surgeon General's Report on Health Promotion and Disease Prevention (1979) Healthy People. DHEW (PHS) Publication No. 79-55071, Washington D.C.
39. U.S. Department of Health and Human Services (1980) Health United States 1980. DHHS Publication No (PHS) 81-1232, Hyattsville, MD. p. 294
40. Warner KE (1977) The Effects of the Anti-Smoking Campaigns on Cigarette Consumption. Am J Publ Health 67: 645
41. Warner KE (1981) Cigarette Smoking in the 1970's: The Impact of the Anti-Smoking Campaign on Consumption. Science 211: 729
42. Williams CL, Arnold CA, Wynder EL (1977) Primary prevention of chronic diesease beginning in childhood: the "know your body" program: design of study. Prev Med 6: 344
43. Wynder EL, Hoffmann D (1979) Tobacco and Health: A Societal Challenge. N Engl J Med 300: 894
44. Kornitzer M, De Backer G, Dramaix M et al. (1980) The Belgian Heart Disease Prevention Project. Circularion 61: 18
45. Russell MAH, Raw M, Jarvis MJ (1980) Clinical use of nicotine chewing-gum. Brit Med J 281: 481
46. Sachs PL, Hall RG, Hall SM (1978) Effects of Rapid Smoking: Physiologic Evaluation of a Smoking Cessation Therapy. Ann Int Med 88: 639

# Multiple Risk Factor Intervention Trials

O. Paul

I have had the opportunity over the past thirteen years to participate
in the discussions, proposals, plans and execution of one large multiple
risk factor trial intended to contribute to our knowledge of the control
and prevention of coronary heart disease. The subject at the time of
our earliest consideration seemed complex. With the passage of years
with experience, there has been ample confirmation of this initial impression. Now as I discuss this with you, I realize that such an investigative undertaking is indeed complicated and there are many opportunities for incorrect assumptions and inadequate execution and less than
optimal interpretation of the results. Perhaps it is admirable, or some
might say, less charitably, astonishing, that anyone would want to un-
dertake one. Nonetheless, I have found that the pleasures and the sat-
isfactions and the excitement and the yield in terms of knowledge have
greatly outweighed the pains and concerns.

I should like to mention first some of the problems which must be recognized. That I start with problems is a reflection of course of their
importance. But as we shall see later, they are not the whole story.

With a multi-factorial trial, it is hoped to be able to conclude that a
two, three, four, or more pronged attack has had a decisive effect on
reducing mortality and morbidity from coronary heart disease. Regret-
fully, it is unlikely that at the end, one can with considerable assurance say exactly how much each phase of intervention has contributed to
the presumably positive result. I always recall a conversation I had
with the late Professor Jerome Cornfield, a statistician whom I greatly
admired for his sagacity and honesty and common sense. Professor Cornfield said at the end of a multi-factorial trial, such as ours, it
might be possible to arrive at some general indication of the effectiveness of a single intervention technique, but that was about as far
as it would be safe to go. This kind of limitation must be accepted at
the outset when the trial is being planned. I have heard the Multiple
Risk Factor Trial[1] often described as being able to provide the answer
to the diet-heart controversy. Such is not the case and this expecta-
tion has never existed in our minds.

Another problem to be recognized early is that with several risk factors to be identified in a given population and when identified modified or limited or eliminated by intervention, there are multiple opportunities for difficulties in trial design. How reasonable are the expectations regarding the ability of the intervention to reduce coronary
risk, how valid are the determinations of the numbers of months or
years required to achieve a change in mortality rates, how accurate are
the predictions regarding changes in the control population, and what
about the estimates of dropout and non-compliance in a population so
diversely composed? Each of these considerations is formidable enough
with a trial limited to one factor. Multiply each of these considerations by three or more and one has a situation ripe for errors in prediction. Such errors if substantial usually compromise the ability of
the trial to arrive at a successful conclusion because of a reduction
in power. In the Multiple Risk Factor Intervention Trial, it was assumed early in the 1970's on the basis of reasonable evidence that min-

imal change would occur in the blood lipids and hypertensive status and smoking habits of the men in the Usual Care population over an average of six years. As has been described in our published material[2], such has not been the case. It may be pertinent here to quote from a report on design considerations in the Trial published in 1977:[3] "The preceding discussion may well induce extreme doubt about the relevance of the design assumptions and the complex calculations based on those assumptions. It should be noted, however, that difficulties of this sort are inherent in any design problem with imperfect information but generally are not emphasized. We felt it worthwhile to make abundantly clear, in this instance, the difficulties of realistic modeling."

Sometimes forgotten is the possibility that there may be important interactions between the several intervention techniques. Today in pharmacologic therapy, this problem is well recognized and constitutes an ever-expanding field of new knowledge. Does one technique used against one risk factor have a favorable or an unfavorable effect on another risk factor; and have these interactions been projected in the design? As one example, in our study, we observed that the use of thiazide diuretics in the management of high blood pressure not only was associated with a lowering of blood pressure but also reduced the diet-lowering effect on serum cholesterol by about one half, while at the same time being associated with a rise in serum triglycerides. As a second example, is the weight gain seen in individuals who stop smoking cigarettes significantly detrimental to the control of hypertension and hyperlipidemia?

In our study, we talked at length about how intervention should be handled. Would we combat all these factors simultaneously. or only one at a time, and if the latter, in what sequence? This is rather like the dilemma facing those in cancer chemotherapy. It was our decision to initiate intervention efforts with approximately ten group sessions covering all risk factors, even though not every participant possessed all three factors. Subsequently, we continued to try to modify all the factors present, although with time and experience, in individual cases it was often found necessary to concentrate particularly on one unfavorable influence, such as cigarette smoking.

With a multiple attack to modify several unfavorable health influences, one recognizes that especial expertise and perhaps technical resources may be required in each area. We did encourage a broad range of knowledge in our staffs so that every member was reasonably conversant with each scientific problem. However, much of the leadership in the cigarette smoking program was properly accepted by staff members trained in psychology or psychiatry. In the field of diet, our nutritionists were the experts, backed up by the Principal Investigators. In hypertension, physicians and nurses were those chiefly involved. One might execute a trial only with generalists, but it seemed to us--and I believe in retrospect correctly--that generalists were not enough. Such special talents of course require budgetary commitments, and they also complicate the process of hiring personnel, and working out training activities which must be received by minds variously prepared.

Such diversity of staff background has the potential of fragmenting the intervention effort unduly, of allowing domination by the group which becomes more powerful, and of discouraging effective communication between members of the several disciplines. While it would be untrue to say that none of these problems occurred in our Trial, it is my impression that they were well handled. Probably the most powerful and positive force was the influence of our clinic, regional and national meetings; in the latter two, staff members had invaluable opportunities to meet and talk with their counterparts from other centers. There was a great deal of cross-fertilization, of mutual education, and perhaps most important of all of achievement of a fine staff morale.

One fairly minor difficulty which may arise in a multiple risk factor trial and which we encountered is the need members of each of these disciplines and groups expressed to be represented at every level of decision making. Does one place on every committee a Principal Investigator, a nutritionist, a behaviorist, a hypertension nurse-specialist, an intervention director, etc.? I cannot say that this was the invariable practice in the Multiple Risk Factor Intervention Trial, but it was the usual policy. This did mean that committees tended to be larger than might be considered optimal, and larger committees usually meant larger travel expense. It also entailed careful selection of committee chairpersons to try to make sure that the committees worked usefully and not merely windily or contentiously.

Finally an issue which can be very important to certain of the investigators and staff members is that of institutional credit for the time and effort devoted to the research. With a staff of nearly 500 people involved including over fifty Principal Investigators, how is there enough individual glory and visibility and credit to go around? Not everyone is going to be a lead author of an important publication. Not everyone is going to present a paper such as this in Boston, London, Berlin or Milan. Yet the research results presented would be impossible without the collaboration of all investigators and staff, and most in the group were not laboratory technicians but individuals with professional careers seeking advancement. We had no perfect answer here either, but our Committee on Publications and Presentations did an admirable job in distributing the many opportunities for authorship and lecture equitably. Further, a large roster of credits accompanied most of our published articles.

I should now like to discuss the favorable aspects inherent in a multiple risk factor trial.

It is clear that the major reason such trials are undertaken in the area of a chronic disease such as coronary heart disease, in which overall annual incidence rates in adults for fatal disease are less than one percent, is to increase the yield of events by permitting selection of a very high risk population. The findings from the Framingham Study[4] and the Pooling Project[5] have illustrated with clarity and consistency how the existence of one risk factor such as hypertension predisposes to an excess of deaths from coronary heart disease above that expected in the absence of such a finding; but this excess is greatly magnified if two or three risk factors are present. Therefore, it makes sense in terms of economy in numbers of participants, duration of the study, and costs to select that population which is at very high risk. Clearly this effort to locate and recruit such individuals can be counterproductive in time and costs if the presence of so many factors was required that millions of persons must be screened to identify the chosen few. In the Multiple Risk Factor Trial in which coronary risk was calculated using up to three variables, we found it necessary to screen 360,000 men aged thirty-five to fifty-seven in order to recruit at the end 12,000 eligible subjects--a sizable but not overwhelming task. The group which recommended to the National Institutes of Health that the Multiple Risk Factor Intervention Trial be conducted[6] concluded that a definitive study limited to diet alone might cost up to one billion dollars, approximately ten times the cost of MRFIT. In good part, this was because of the large size of the study population which would be required. Today with research funds in short supply, costs are carefully scrutinized and chances of funding are reduced for those projects bear-

ing too large a price tag.  Further, in an era in which dynamic changes
in the lifestyle and specific diagnosis and treatment of coronary heart
disease are occurring in the general population, it is critical that the
projected duration of the trial not be so long that the original assumptions regarding the urgency of the health problem and relative stability
of the control population are totally invalid.

The choice of a multi-factor intervention study may also be made because
of its comparability to what the practicing physician does or may do in
the office, clinic or hospital.  The doctor finding high blood pressure
in a middle-aged male who smokes thirty cigarettes a day should not limit his role to treating the hypertension with diet and/or drugs or giving strong--we hope strong--advice regarding stopping smoking.  He
should do both.  There may thus be a distinct advantage in conducting
the research study in a fashion having direct comparability and application to clinical practice.  One of the lessons we learned in the Multiple Risk Factor Intervention Trial, which has clear implications for the
medical profession and for community health bodies, is the usefulness of
group education sessions in the attack on the several health problems we
attempted to modify.

One dividend of such a type of investigative effort is the invaluable
learning experience for representatives of the several disciplines involved.  In our study, we were a pioneer in enlisting not only the physicians, epidemiologists, nutritionists, lipid specialists and statisticians, but also men and women trained in psychology and having expertise
in behavior analysis and modification.  Whereas initially, some of the
physicians and other scientists were inclined to view members of this
last group with a wary attitude, it was not long before mutual respect
and understanding developed.  The very breadth of the investigation and
the necessity for the involvement of the several disciplines were positive influences for all concerned.  We have also regarded the opportunity to train many younger people in the sciences represented in this
Trial to be one very valuable return for the monies invested.

It is also true that a multi-factorial study offers a substantial by-
product in terms of varied ancillary studies.  When three variables are
under study and several types of experts are involved, the possibili-
ites for productive and usually inexpensive ancillary investigations are
multiple.  We certainly found this to be the case.  Such ancillary projects are to be encouraged, providing they do not conflict with or complicate unduly the main purposes of the trial, for they offer promise
of contributing new knowledge at minimal expense, and equally important, they elevate the level of interest and enthusiasm of the investigators and staff.

In conclusion, I have commented upon certain of the very great opportunities, and some of the important problems, existing in a multiple
risk factor intervention trial.  I have given certain examples from the
Multiple Risk Factor Intervention Trial conducted in the United States,
but I believe such examples are applicable to other investigations
elsewhere.  Certainly, such scientific studies require most careful
planning; and execution with very competent investigators of varied
backgrounds and concern for high-level quality control; and final detailed analysis of the results to present the findings in a fashion
which makes biological sense.  Is all this difficult?--yes.  Is it after all really worthwhile?--also yes.

References

1.  Zukel WJ, Paul O, and Schnaper HW (1981) The Multiple Risk Factor
    Intervention Trial (MRFIT). Preventive Medicine 10:387-401
2.  Caggiula AW, Christakis G, Farrand M, Hulley SB, Johnson R, Lasser
    NL, Stamler J, and Widdowson G (1981) The Multiple Risk Factor In-
    tervention Trial (MRFIT). IV. Intervention on Blood Lipids. Preven-
    tive Medicine 10:443-475
3.  The Multiple Risk Factor Intervention Trial Group (1977)
    Statistical Design Considerations in the NHLI Multiple Risk Factor
    Intervention Trial (MRFIT). J. Chron, Dis. 30:261-275
4.  Kannel WB, Gordon T eds (1971). The Framingham Study - An Epidemi-
    ological Investigation of Cardiovascular Disease, Section 27. U.S.
    Dept. of Health, Education and Welfare, PHS, NIH, Washington, D.C.
5.  The Pooling Project Research Group (1978) Relationship of Blood
    Pressure, Serum Cholesterol, Smoking Habit, Relative Weight and ECG
    Abnormalities to Incidence of Major Coronary Events:  Final Report
    of the Pooling Project.  American Heart Assoc. Monograph No. 60
6.  National Heart and Lung Institute Task Force on Arteriosclerosis
    (1971) Arteriosclerosis.  Dept. of Health, Education and Welfare
    Publication No. (NIH) 72-137

# Pharmacological Approach to the Prevention of Atherosclerosis

G. Crepaldi, G. Baggio, and E. Manzato

The prevention of Atherosclerosis (ATS) is generally divided into pri=
mary and secondary. Primary prevention is the set of interventions car=
ried out on the asymptomatic patient before the appearance of athero=
sclerotic complications (angina, myocardial infarction, stroke, etc.),
whereas by secondary prevention it is usually indicated any interven=
tion after a clinical event has already occurred(1). Thus, pharmaco=
logical studies for the prevention of ATS should be divided into pri=
mary and secondary, even though this division is not always present
in all the epidemiological trials.

Pathogenetic agents of ATS are unfortunately unknown. For this reason
prevention of ATS means all the interventions to find out and fight
the so called risk factors connected with the incidence of the disease.
However, only few of these risk factors are modifiable by drugs.

## Primary prevention of Atherosclerosis

The risk factors modifiable by drugs in the primary prevention of ATS
are: hyperlipidemia , hypertension and diabetes.

The lipid lowering drug trials in primary prevention are listed in Tab.
1 (2-5). The Krasno & Kidera's study(2) reports that cumulative dis=
tribution of fatal and non fatal myocardial infarction during 39 months
in men, initially free from coronary heart disease, is significantly
lower in treated vs untreated groups. In the W.H.O. trial(3) the treat=
ment does not affect any fatal heart attack, whereas it significantly
reduces non fatal ischemic heart disease(IHD) incidence in comparison
with placebo. The Dörr trial(4) demonstrates a decrease in total mor=
tality rate as well as in the coronary heart disease deaths. But this
result is significant only for male patients. Results from the Lipid
Research Clinics(5) are expected by 1984. The results of these trials
with lipid lowering drugs are achieved with a mean percent cholesterol
decrease from 9 to 15%.

The primary prevention trials with lipid lowering drugs show a definite
result for non fatal IHD. Non conclusive or indifferent results are re=
ported for fatal IHD and total mortality (with the exception of the
Dörr trial in men). There is also an increased total mortality in the
treated group of the W.H.O. trial.

The first aim of all the trials concerning the prevention of ATS by
drug treatment of hypertension was the control of high blood pressure.
For this reason patients with atherosclerotic lesions were not always
excluded from these trials. Therefore, it is often difficult to assign
such trials to primary or secondary prevention of ATS. We thought it
correct to consider them all in the primary prevention.

Since HAMILTON report(6), several studies on this topic have been per=
formed (Tab. 2)(7-17). Many different drugs, a great number of subjects,
different protocols were used. After the dramatic incidence of mortal=
ity in the Veterans study(18) during the treatment of severe hyperten=
sion with placebo, only patients with mild hypertension were admitted

Table 1. Lipid lowering drug trials in primary prevention of ATS

| | number | follow up yrs | dose day gr | effect on total mortality | fatal IHD | non fatal IHD |
|---|---|---|---|---|---|---|
| Clofibrate (Krasno,1972)(2) | 3,219 | 1-5 | 2.0 | n.r. | n.r. | pos |
| Clofibrate (W.H.O.,1978)(3) | 15,745 | 5.3 | 1.6 | neg | ind | pos |
| Colestipol (Dörr,1978)(4) | 2,278 | 1-3 | 10 | ♂ pos<br>♀ ind | pos<br>ind | pos<br>ind |
| Cholestyramine (CPPT,1979)(5) | 3,810 | ongoing | 24 | ? | ? | ? |

pos : treated significantly better than placebo group
neg : placebo significantly better than treated group
ind : no significant difference between treated and placebo group
n.r.: not reported

to the subsequent trials. In the Veterans Administration Cooperative Study Group on Anti-Hypertensive Agents (VACSG)(7), some differences on morbidity and mortality, especially for cerebrovascular events, are found. However, these figures do not reach statistical significance. This trial was restricted entirely to males. In the Beevers Study(8), the incidence of stroke is statistically related to the adequacy of the control of blood pressure. In the Public Health Service Hospital Trial (PHSHT)(9), the treatment is most effective in preventing hyper= tensive complications, but the incidence of myocardial infarction and sudden death is similar in the treated and in the untreated subjects. The Göteborg Study(11) shows a significant effect of treatment on total mortality, while the morbid events due to coronary heart disease are not significantly affected by the treatment, even though a positive trend is present. The data of Hypertension Detection and Follow-up Pro= gram (HDFP)(12,13) indicate a great reduction in total mortality with systematic management of hypertension; a positive effect on stroke and IHD, but not a statistical evaluation, is also reported. The Australian Trial(14) definitely demonstrates a decrease (more than 50%) in cere=

Table 2. Hypertension treatment trials in primary prevention of ATS

| | number | follow up yrs | effect on total mortality | stroke | IHD |
|---|---|---|---|---|---|
| VACSG 1970(7) | 523 | 3.2 | ind | ind | ind |
| Beevers 1973(8) | 499 | 2+12 | n.r. | pos | ind |
| PHSHT 1977(9) | 389 | 7.0 | n.r. | ind | ind |
| Beevers 1978(10) | 1,247 | 1.0 | pos | pos | ind |
| Göteborg Study 1978(11) | 1,026 | 4.3 | pos | ind | ind |
| HDFP 1979(12,13) | 10,940 | 5.0 | pos | pos ? | pos ? |
| Australian T. 1980(14) | 3,427 | 4.0 | pos | pos | ind |
| Oslo Study 1980(15) | 785 | 5.5 | ind | pos | ind |
| Brighton Study 1981(16) | 961 | 5.0 | pos | pos | pos |
| WHO-Rome Group 1981(17) | 603 | 4.0 | ? | ? | ? |

brovascular disease in the treated group. Total mortality and morbidity
from cardiovascular events in the Oslo Study on Hypertension(15)do not
show differences between control and treated group, however, cerebro=
vascular events occurred only in the control group. In the Brighton
Study(16) the good control of hypertension results in a significantly
lower incidence of morbidity and mortality, both for cerebrovascular
and IHD. Preliminary results from the Roman project of W.H.O.(17) dem=
onstrate a trend in reducing cardiovascular events in the treated group
in comparison with controls.

To summarize, it is evident that the treatment of mild hypertension has
beneficial effects on cerebrovascular disease and total mortality, while
it is generally indifferent towards IHD.

The main mortality cause of **diabetes** in the pre-insulin era was diabetic
coma; after the introduction of insulin, the leading mortality cause
has been cardiovascular disease. However, the prevalence of cardiovas=
cular mortality was much higher in the 1936-1945 period, when long-act=
ing insulin was introduced, in comparison with the 1922-1936 period,
when multiple injections of regular insulin were used for the control
of diabetes(19).

In poor controlled diabetes many factors may be related to cardiovas=
cular disease. Hyperglycemia, lipid and lipoprotein abnormalities, in=
sulin, microangiopathy, neuropathy, hyperviscosity are specific causes
of endothelial injury. A strict relationship even between abnormal glu=
cose tolerance test and increased mortality from cardiovascular disease
has recently been reported(20). However, in respect to the high number
of risk factors for macroangiopathy present in diabetes, it is diffi=
cult to relate a decrease in the incidence of ATS complications to dif=
ferent drug treatment. An increased mortality for myocardial infarction
has been reported in diabetics treated with Tolbutamide(21). While this
study has raised much criticism in a few not randomized studies(22,23).
Tolbutamide seemed to protect against cardiovascular death.

Thus, the best way of protecting diabetics from the increased cardio=
vascular complications is the excellent metabolic control of the dis=
ease obtained with diet and physical exercise in patients with type II
diabetes and with regular insulin multiple injections in type I dia=
tes.


Secondary prevention of Atherosclerosis

As for the primary, for the secondary prevention of ATS the risk fac=
tors modifiable by drugs are: **hyperlipidemia, hypertension and diabetes**. For
the reasons explained before, we considered hypertension and diabetes
only in the primary prevention. After a clinical complication of ATS
has occurred, other factors are traditionally taken into account, par=
ticularly thrombosis, ischemia, arrhythmias. In this view, we shall
consider trials with lipid lowering drugs, beta-blockers and platelet
active drugs.

The **lipid** lowering drug trials in the secondary prevention of ATS are
listed in Tab. 3(24-30). They started almost 10 years before the pri=
mary prevention trials, when hyperlipidemias were clearly recognized
as important risk factors for atherogenesis. Nevertheless, it is now
established that the prognosis of myocardial infarction is not related
only to the presence of risk factors, but it is strongly determined by
the extent of the damage of the myocardium(31).

In the Coronary Drug Project (CDP) a statistically significant decrease

Table 3. Lipid lowering drug trials in secondary prevention of ATS

| | number | follow up months | dose day | effect on | | |
|---|---|---|---|---|---|---|
| | | | | total mortality | fatal IHD | non fatal IHD |
| Estrogen (24) | | 56 | 2.5 mg | neg | n.r. | n.r. |
| Estrogen (25) | | 21 | 5.0 mg | ind | n.r. | neg |
| Dextrothyroxine (26) | | 36 | 6.0 mg | neg | neg | neg |
| Clofibrate (27) | | 74 | 1.8 gr | ind | ind | neg |
| Nicotinic Acid (27) (CDP,1970-1975) | 8,341 | 74 | 3.0 gr | ind | ind | pos |
| Clofibrate (Newcastle T.,1971)(28) | 497 | 43 | 1.5÷ 2.0 gr | n.r. | pos | pos |
| Clofibrate (Scottish T.,1971)(29) | 717 | 40 | 1.6÷ 2.0 gr | ind | ind | pos |
| Clofibrate + Nicotinic Acid (Carlson,1980)(30) | 558 | 36÷ 48 | 2.0 gr 3.0 gr | ind | ind | pos |

in the incidence of definite non fatal myocardial infarction is found
only in the group treated with nicotinic acid(27). The total cardiovas=
cular death rate in the treated group of the Newcastle Trial(28) de=
creases significantly, while this is not true for the Scottish Trial
(29). In the Stockholm IHD Study(30), after 5 years of follow up, IHD
mortality difference between placebo and the treated group is not sig=
nificant, whereas the incidence of non fatal myocardial infarction is
lower in the drug treated group. The hypocholesterolemic effect of these
trials ranges from 7 to 20%.

Conclusive evaluations from lipid lowering drug trials in secondary
prevention of ATS (excluding hormonal treatment) are partially posi=
tive for non fatal IHD, while the difference between placebo and the
treated group is mostly indifferent for total mortality and fatal IHD.
Anyway, up to now secondary prevention trials have shown consistent
results only with the use of clofibrate and nicotinic acid.

The effect of **beta-blockers** after myocardial infarction has been studied
by several authors (Tab. 4)(32-37). Of these trials we have considered
only those which started beta-blocker treatment at least 7 days after
myocardial infarction, since their use in the first week does not
strictly aim at the prevention of reinfarction. Beta-blockers in sever=
al trials seem to reduce mortality and sudden cardiac death, even if
some negative side effects are also reported.

**Platelet active** drugs seem to modify the mechanisms (mediated by prostacy=
clins, tromboxane, growth factors, etc.) involved in atherogenesis and
in initiating the clinical event. This is the basis for the use of these
drugs in ATS prevention (Tab. 5)(38-45). The first drug taken into ac=
count a quarter of century ago was aspirin. Afterwards most of the
trials used aspirin in different doses or an association of aspirin +
dipyridamole, two trials, instead, used sulfipyrazone. Among trials
of platelet active drugs in secondary prevention of ATS, positive and
significant results are reported by Elwood(40) for non fatal IHD and
from ARIS(45) for fatal and non fatal IHD. However, in several of these
studies a clear trend in reducing ATS complications is observed.

Table 4. Beta-blocker trials in secondary prevention of ATS

| | number | follow up months | dose day mg | effect on | | |
|---|---|---|---|---|---|---|
| | | | | total mortality | sudden cardiac death | reinfarc= tion |
| Alprenolol (Wilhelmsson,1974)(32) | 230 | 24 | 400 | pos | pos | n.r. |
| Practolol(Mult Intern Study,1977)(33) | 3,030 | 14 | 400 | pos | pos | ind |
| Propranolol (Baber,1980)(34) | 720 | 9 | 120 | ind | ind | ind |
| Timolol(Norw Mult Group,1981)(35) | 1,884 | 17 | 20 | pos | pos | pos |
| Propranolol (BHAT,1981)(36) | 3,837 | 24 | 180+ 240 | pos | pos | n.r. |
| Propranolol(Norw Mult Trial,1982)(37) | 560 | 12 | 160 | ind | pos | ind |

Table 5. Platelet active drug trials in secondary prevention of ATS

| | number | follow up months | dose day mg | effect on | | |
|---|---|---|---|---|---|---|
| | | | | total mortality | fatal IHD | non fatal IHD |
| Aspirin (Elwood,1974)(38) | 1,239 | 12 | 300 | ind | n.r. | n.r. |
| Aspirin (CDPA,1976)(39) | 1,529 | 22 | 972 | ind | ind | ind |
| Aspirin (Elwood,1979)(40) | 1,682 | 12 | 900 | ind | pos | n.r. |
| Aspirin (AMIS,1980)(41) | 4,524 | 40 | 1,000 | ind | ind | ind |
| Aspirin (Germ-Aust,1980)(42) | 1,060 | 24 | 1,500 | ind | ind | ind |
| Aspirin Aspirin+dipyridamole (PARIS,1980)(43) | 2,026 | 41 | 972 972+ 225 | ind | ind | ind |
| Sulfinpyrazone (ART,1980)(44) | 1,629 | 16 | 800 | (pos) | (pos) | (pos) |
| Sulfinpyrazone (ARIS,1982)(45) | 727 | 19 | 800 | pos | pos | pos |

(pos): treated better than placebo group during the first six months

Table 6. Platelet active drug trials in treatment of transient isch=
emic attacks

|  | number | follow up months | dose day mg | effect |
|---|---|---|---|---|
| Aspirin   Med (46) | 189 | 24 | 1300 | ind |
| Aspirin   Surg(47) | 125 | 24 | 1300 | ind |
| (Fields,1977,1978) | | | | |
| Aspirin | 144 | 26 | 1300 | ♂pos,♀ind |
| Aspirin+Sulfinpyrazone | 146 | 26 | 1300+800 | ind |
| Sulfinpyrazone | 156 | 26 | 800 | ind |
| (Canadian Study,1978)(48) | | | | |

Med : only aspirin
Surg: aspirin after carotid reconstructive surgery

Also in the treatment of transient ischemic attacks (Tab. 6)(46-48)
not significant results are reported within treated and controls both
with aspirin and aspirin + sulfinpyrazone. A benefit of aspirin is
obtained only in a male group(48).

Conclusions

The pharmacological approach to the prevention of ATS is very complex.
The list of drugs and trials concerning this topic is longer than the
one here presented. Several problems lie under all the clinical trials
(31): randomization, statistical evaluation, follow-up length, side
effects, monitoring of commonly occurring diseases, etc. Such problems
have not been considered here because of space limits. Moreover, the
mechanisms of drugs used for the prevention of ATS should be thoroughly
investigated in order to assess clearly which ones are to be used on
patients already affected by clinical events, on asymptomatic patients
with parietal lesions and on normal patients with one or more risk
factors of ATS. Among all the problems, one is particularly important:
up to now all the primary prevention trials have not been able to dis=

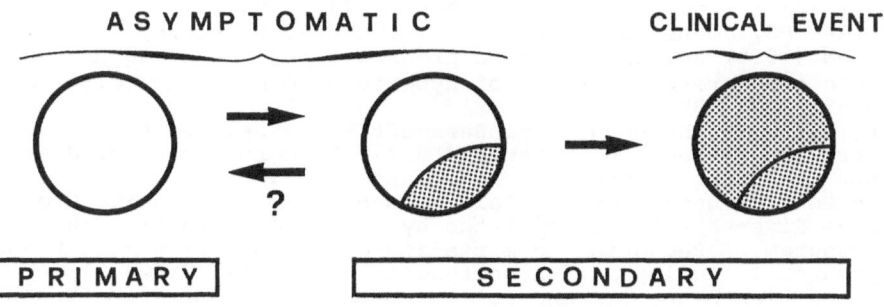

Fig. 1. A proposal for a new definition of primary and secondary pre=
vention of ATS

tinguish exactly whether the treatment was performed on completely nor=
mal subjects already affected by parietal lesions. From the studies
on regression(49), we now know that some of these parietal lesions
could be healed (or at least repaired).

In the next future it could be worthwhile to change the generally ac=
cepted definitions of primary and secondary prevention of ATS. The real
primary prevention should be restricted to the asymptomatic subject
with normal arterial wall and with one or more risk factors. If this
is not possible, we should then operate the secondary prevention on
patients with parietal lesions in order to prevent clinical events
and, if possible, to obtain regression of the lesion.

References

1. Levy RI (1980) Dietary prevention of coronary artery disease-A pol=
   icy overview. In: Gotto AM Jr, Smith LC, Allen B(eds) Atheroscle=
   rosis V, Springer-Verlag, New York Heidelberg Berlin, pp199-208
2. Krasno LR, Kidera GJ (1972) Clofibrate in coronary heart disease.
   Effect on morbidity and mortality. JAMA 219: 845-851
3. Committee of Principal Investigators (1978) A co-operative trial
   in the primary prevention of ischaemic heart disease using clofi=
   brate. Br Heart J 40: 1069-1118
4. Dörr AE, Gundersen K, Schneider JC Jr, Spencer TW, Martin WB (1978)
   Colestipol hydrochloride in hypercholesterolemic patients. Effect
   on serum cholesterol and mortality. J Chron Dis 31: 5-14
5. Lipid Research Clinics Program (1979) The coronary primary preven=
   tion trial: design and implementation. J Chron Dis 32: 609-631
6. Hamilton M, Thompson EN, Wisniewski TKM (1964) The role of blood-
   pressure control in preventing complications of hypertension.
   Lancet i: 235-238
7. Veterans Administration Cooperative Study Group on Antihypertensive
   Agents (1970) Effect of treatment on morbidity in hypertension.
   II. Results in patients with diastolic blood pressure averaging
   90 through 114 mmHg. JAMA 213: 1143-1152
8. Beevers DG, Fairman MJ, Hamilton M, Harpur JE (1973) The influence
   of antihypertensive treatment over the incidence of cerebral vas=
   cular disease. Postgrad Med J 49: 905-907
9. Smith WMCF (1977) Treatment of mild hypertension. Results of a
   ten-year intervention trial. U.S. Public Health Service Hospitals
   Cooperative Study Group. Circ. Res. 40(1): 98-105
10. Beevers DG, Johnston J, Devine BL, Dunn FG, Larkin H, Tittering=
    ton DM (1978) Relation between prognosis and the blood pressure
    before and during treatment of hypertensive patients. Clin Sci Mol
    Med 55: 333s-336s
11. Berglund G, Wilhelmsen L, Sannerstedt R, Hansson L, Andersson O,
    Sivertsson R, Wedel H, Wikstrand J (1978) Coronary heart disease
    after treatment of hypertension. Lancet i: 1-5
12. Hypertension Detection and Follow-up Program Cooperative Group
    (1979) Five-year findings of the hypertension detection and follow-
    up program. I.Reduction in mortality of persons with high blood
    pressure, including mild hypertension. JAMA 242: 2562-2571
13. Hypertension Detection and Follow-up Program Cooperative Group
    (1979) Five-year findings of the hypertension detection and follow-
    up program. II.Mortality by race, sex and age. JAMA 242: 2572-2577
14. Management Committee (1980) The Australian therapeutic trial in
    mild hypertension. Lancet i: 1261-1267
15. Helgeland A (1980) Treatment of mild hypertension: a five year
    controlled drug trial. The Oslo Study. Am J Med 69: 725-732

16. Trafford JAP, Horn CR, O'Neal H, McGonigle R, Halford-Maw L, Evans R (1981) Five year follow-up of effects of treatment of mild and moderate hypertension. Br Med J 282: 1111-1113
17. Gruppo di Ricerca del Progetto Romano di Prevenzione della Cardio= patia Coronarica (1981) La prevenzione di alcune complicanze car= diovascolari mediante trattamento multifattoriale degli ipertesi. G Ital Cardiol 11: 164-169
18. Veterans Administration Cooperative Study Group on Antihypertensive Agents (1967) Effects of treatment on morbidity in hypertension. Results in patients with diastolic blood pressures averaging 115 through 129 mmHg. JAMA 202: 1028-1034
19. Johnsson S (1960) Retinopathy and nephropathy in diabetes mellitus (comparison of the effects of two forms of treatment) Diabetes 9: 1-8
20. Jarrett RJ, Mc Cartney P, Keen H (1982) The Bedford survey: ten year mortality rates in newly diagnosed diabetics, borderline dia= betics and normoglycaemic controls and risk indices for coronary heart disease in borderline diabetics. Diabetologia 22: 79-84
21. University Group Diabetes Program (1970) A study of the effects of hypoglycemic agents of the vascular complications of patients with adult-onset diabetes. Diabetes 19(2): 747-830
22. Paasikivi J, Wahlberg F (1971) Preventive tolbutamide treatment and arterial disease in mild hyperglycaemia. Diabetologia 7: 323-327
23. Paasikivi J (1971) Long-term tolbutamide of survivors from myocar= dial infarction. Acta diabet lat 8(1): 437-443
24. Coronary Drug Project Research Group (1973) Findings leading to discontinuation of the 2.5 mg/day estrogen group. JAMA 226:652-657
25. Coronary Drug Project Research Group (1970) Initial findings lead= ing to modifications of its research protocol. JAMA 214: 1303-1313
26. Coronary Drug Project Research Group (1972) Findings leading to further modifications of its protocol with respect to dextrothy= roxine. JAMA 220: 996-1008
27. Coronary Drug Project Research Group (1975) Clofibrate and niacin in coronary heart disease. JAMA 231: 360-381
28. Newcastle upon Tyne Region Group of Physicians (1971) Trial of clofibrate in the treatment of ischaemic heart disease. Br Med J 4: 767-775
29. Scottish Society of Physicians Research Committee (1971) Ischaemic heart disease: a secondary prevention trial using clofibrate. Br Med J 4: 775-784
30. Rosenhamer G, Carlson LA (1980) Effect of combined clofibrate-nic= otinic acid treatment in ischemic heart disease. Atherosclerosis 37: 129-138
31. Oliver MF (1981) Coronary heart disease prevention. Trials using drugs to control hyperlipidaemia. In: Miller NE, Lewis B (eds) Lipoprotein, atherosclerosis and coronary heart disease, Elsevier Amsterdam, pp165-195
32. Wilhelmsson C, Vedin JA, Wilhelmsen L, Tibblin G, Werkö L (1974) Reduction of sudden deaths after myocardial infarction by treat= ment with alprenolol. Lancet ii: 1157-1160
33. Multicentre International Study (1977) Reduction in mortality af= ter myocardial infarction with long-term beta-adrenoceptor block= ade. Br Med J 2: 419-421
34. Baber NS, Wainwright Evans D, Howitt G, Thomas M, Wilson C, Lewis JA, Dawes PM, Handler K, Tuson R (1980) Multicentre post-infarc= tion trial of propranolol in 49 hospitals in the United Kingdom, Italy, and Yugoslavia. Br Heart J 44: 96-100
35. Norwegian Multicenter Study Group (1981) Timolol-induced reduction in mortality and reinfarction in patients surviving acute myocar= dial infarction. N Engl J Med 304: 801-807

36. Beta-blocker Heart Attack Trial Research Group (1982) A random=
    ized trial of propranolol in patients with acute myocardial infarc=
    tion. JAMA 247: 1707-1714
37. Hansteen V, Møinichen E, Lorentsen E, Andersen A, Strøm O, Søiland
    K, Dyrbekk D, Refsum AM, Tromsdal A, Knudsen K, Eika C, Bakken J
    jun, Smith P, Hoff PI (1982) One year's treatment with propranolol
    after myocardial infarction: preliminary report of Norwegian Multi=
    centre trial. Br Med J 284: 155-160
38. Elwood PC, Cochrane AL, Burr ML, Sweetnam PM, Williams G, Welsby
    E, Hughes SJ, Renton R (1974) A randomized controlled trial of
    acetyl salicylic acid in the secondary prevention of mortality
    from myocardial infarction. Br Med J 1: 436-440
39. Coronary Drug Project Research Group (1976) Aspirin in coronary
    heart disease. J Chron Dis 29: 625-642
40. Elwood PC, Sweetnam PM (1979) Aspirin and secondary mortality af=
    ter myocardial infarction. Lancet ii: 1313-1315
41. Aspirin Myocardial Infarction Study Research Group (1980) A ran=
    domized, controlled trial of aspirin in persons recovered from
    myocardial infarction. JAMA 243: 661-669
42. Breddin K, Loew D, Lechner K, Überla K, Walter E (1980) Secondary
    prevention of myocardial infarction. A comparison of acetylsali=
    cylic acid, placebo and phenprocoumon. Haemostasis 9: 325-344
43. Persantine-Aspirin Reinfarction Study Research Group (1980) Per=
    santine and aspirin in coronary heart disease. Circulation 62:
    449-461
44. Anturane Reinfarction Trial Research Group (1980) Sulfinpyrazone
    in the prevention of sudden death after myocardial infarction. N
    Engl J Med 31: 250-256
45. Anturan Reinfarction Italian Study (1982) Sulphinpyrazone in post-
    myocardial infarction. Lancet i: 237-242
46. Fields WS, Lemak NA, Frankowski RF, Hardy RJ (1977) Controlled
    trial of aspirin in cerebral ischemia. Stroke 8: 301-316
47. Fields WS, Lemak NA, Frankowski RF, Hardy RJ (1978) Controlled
    trial of aspirin in cerebral ischemia. Part II. Surgical group.
    Stroke 9: 309-319
48. Canadian Cooperative Study Group (1978) A randomized trial of as=
    pirin and sulfinpyrazone in threatened stroke. N Engl J Med 299:
    53-59
49. Stary HC (1979) Regression of atherosclerosis in primates.Virchows
    Arch (Pathol Anat) 383: 117-134

5.1 Epidemiology

# Role of Lipid Profiles in Assessing Atherogenesis

W. B. Kannel and W. P. Castelli

Atherosclerosis is a multifactorial process with blood lipids playing a central role. The concept of the role of blood lipids in atherogenesis has undergone a metamorphosis from an initial focus on the serum total cholesterol, to other lipids, then to the lipoproteins which transport them and now on the distribution of the serum total cholesterol in the low, high and very low density lipoproteins (1).

It is now recognized that the established positive relationship of the serum total cholesterol to coronary heart disease incidence derives from the LDL cholesterol component. The HDL-cholesterol component is <u>inversely</u> related to risk (1,2). The VLDL and its cholesterol or triglyceride components appear to make no direct contribution to atherogenesis (1,2).

At any given level of serum total cholesterol, risk varies widely depending on the ratio of LDL or total cholesterol to HDL-cholesterol (Fig. 1). This provides a practical, efficient means for assessing the joint effect of the two-way traffic of cholesterol entering and leaving the tissues (Fig. 2).

Figure 1

Figure 2

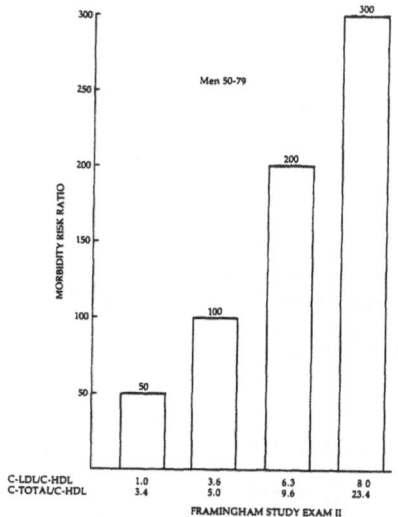

Four-Year Risk of Coronary Heart Disease According to Ratio of Cholesterol Lipoprotein Fractions

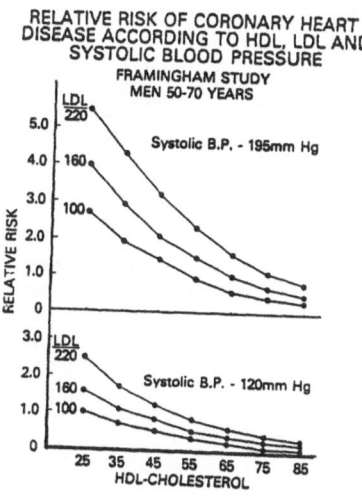

Addition of VLDL or its triglyceride to the LDL and HDL information does not enhance prediction of coronary heart disease as judged from likelihood ratio analysis (Table 1).

Table 1. Likelihood ratios for risk of coronary heart disease according to lipid profiles. Framingham Study. 7 year follow-up. Men & Women 50-80

|  | LIKELIHOOD RATIOS | |
| --- | --- | --- |
| HDL + LDL CHOLESTEROL | MEN | WOMEN |
| WITH TRIGLYCERIDE | 18.90*** | 24.73*** |
| WITHOUT TRIGLYCERIDE | 18.66*** | 23.70*** |

*** P < .001

However, further refinements in the lipid profile may be forthcoming because there are several HDL and LDL subfractions which appear to have differenc atherogenic potential, possibly determined by their apoprotein make-up. The protective effect of HDL-cholesterol is at least as strong as the LDL-cholesterol atherogenic effect, as judged by regression coefficients for coronary heart disease incidence standardized for the different range of values so as to allow a direct comparison on an equal footing (Table 2).

Table 2. Strength of coronary heart disease predictions according to lipoprotein partition of cholesterol. Persons 50-79

|  | LIKELIHOOD RATIOS | |
| --- | --- | --- |
| LIPID | MEN | WOMEN |
| TOTAL CHOLESTEROL | 1.98 | 2.26 |
| HDL-CHOLESTEROL | -14.0** | -21.2** |
| LDL-CHOLESTEROL | 4.4* | 4.5* |
| VLDL CHOLESTEROL | 1.03 | 5.04* |

*P < .05        **P < .001

Every 10 mg/dl variation in HDL-cholesterol is associated with a 50% change in risk. (Table 3)

Table 3. Efficiency of Cholesterol-Lipoprotein ratios comprised of LDL-C, HDL-C and Total Cholesterol. Framingham Study. 8 year Follow-Up. Men & Women 50-80

|  | LIKELIHOOD RATIOS | |
| --- | --- | --- |
| RATIOS | MEN | WOMEN |
| LDL/HDL-C | 17.54*** | 17.97*** |
| TOTAL/HDL-C | 16.76*** | 21.41*** |
| LINEAR COMBINATIONS | MEN | WOMEN |
| LDL-C + HDL-C | 20.06*** | 18.01*** |
| TOTAL-C + HDL-C | 18.56*** | 20.58*** |

***P$ < .001

Linear combinations of LDL and HDL-cholesterol provide only a marginal improvement over the theoretically lessdesirable ratio of the two cholesterol components (Table 3). It is also of interest that the LDL/HDL cholesterol ratio predicts coronary heart disease no more efficiently than the more practical total cholesterol/HDL-cholesterol ratio (Table 3). This is not suprising, since the bulk of the total cholesterol is carried in the LDL fraction, insuring a reasonably high correlation.

Coronary heart disease risk associated with any LDL/HDL ratio is also affected by age, sex, and the level of other cardiovascular risk factors. In particular, the risk associated with any combination of LDL and HDL-cholesterol is markedly affected by the associated blood pressure (Fig. 2).

Whereas coronary heart disease is clearly related to blood lipids, their relationship to other atherosclerotic disease and to overall mortality is less clear (2). The partition of the total cholesterol into LDL and HDL fractions fails to restore the predictive capacity of cholesterol beyond age 50 for stroke as it does for coronary heart disease (Table 4). For LDL cholesterol, there is even a paradoxical significant _inverse_ relationship in women.

Table 4. Regression of Incidence of Specified Events on HDL, LDL, and VLDL Cholesterol: The Framingham Study. 4-Year Follow-Up

| CARDIO-VASCULAR MORBIDITY | STANDARDIZED MULTIVARIATE REGRESSION COEFFICIENTS | | | | | |
|---|---|---|---|---|---|---|
| | HDL CHOLESTEROL | | LDL CHOLESTEROL | | VLDL CHOLESTEROL | |
| | MEN | WOMEN | MEN | WOMEN | MEN | WOMEN |
| STROKE | -.118 | -.173 | .009 | -.621*** | .076 | -.055 |
| CARDIAC FAILURE | -.486* | -.740** | .061 | -.106 | .129 | .034 |
| INTERMITTEMT CLAUDICATION | -.037 | +.010 | .224 | -.014 | .042 | .084 |

*P ＜ .05    **P ＜ .01    ***P ＜ .001

Epidemiologic data also indicate a possible excess overall mortality at low as well as high values, despite a strong favorable relationship of low cholesterol values to CHD mortality, the leading cause of death (Fig. 3).

Figure 3

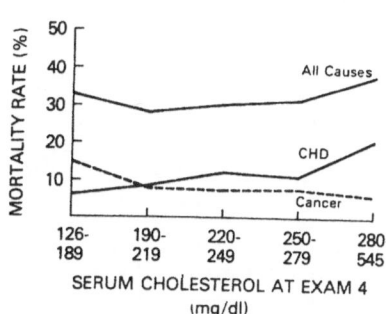

Age adjusted mortality rates (20 years) for all causes, coronary heart disease (CHD) and cancer, by serum cholesterol measured at Exam 4 of the Framingham Study in men aged 35-64 years.

In contrast to LDL and total cholesterol, the expected inverse relation of HDL-cholesterol to virtually all atherosclerotic end points as well as to total mortality is consistently observed (Table 4). Recent reports also suggest an excess of colon cancer mortality at extremely low (126-189) serum total cholesterol values (3). Curiously, no relationship has been noted for women. This anomaly and the paradoxical finding that high fat diets predispose to colon cancer tends to discredit a causal association. Average population total cholesterol values of 140/180 mg/dl are consistently associated with the lowest rates of atherosclerosis and coronary heart disease, and those in the 190-200 mg/dl range are also associated with a favorable overall health status (4). Total cholesterol values exceeding 200 mg/dl are generally suboptimal as regards cardiovascular health. The most favorable response to anti-lipemic therapy or prophylaxis would appear to be to achieve a total/HDL ratio well below the 5.0 standard ratio and possible the optimal values approximate a ratio of 3.5, which corresponds to half the standard risk for men in the U.S.A. Fortunately, many of the measures advocated for coronary heart disease prophylaxis, including weight reduction, exercise, quitting cigarettes and moderate alcohol intake, also raise HDL. There is obviously more to be learned about the role of blood lipid profiles in predicting atherosclerosis and in assessing the efficacy of treatment. However, recognizing the incomplete stage of knowledge is no excuse for failure to apply what is known more effectively.

REFERENCES

1.  Kannel WB, Castelli WP, Gordon T: (1979) Cholesterol in the prediction of atherosclerotic disease. New perspectives based on the Framingham Study. Ann Intern Med 90:85-91.

2.  Gordon T, Kannel WB, Castelli WP, Dawber TR: (1981) Lipoproteins, cardiovascular disease and death. The Framingham Study. Arch Intern Med 141:1128-1131.

3.  Feinleib M: (1981) On a possible inverse relationship between serum cholesterol and cancer mortality. Am J Epidemiol 114:5-10.

4.  Conference on the Health Effects of Blood Lipids: (1979) Optimal Distributions for Populations. Workshop Report: Epidemiologic Section. Prev Med 612-678.

# Plasma Lipids and Lipoprotein Cholesterol Distributions and US-USSR Steering Committee for Cardiovascular Area I: Pathogenesis of Atherosclerosis

A. N. Klimov

## A. Introduction

The roles of plasma lipids and lipoproteins in the development of atherosclerotic heart disease have been investigated extensively. Epidemiologic studies, clinical case series, and animal experiments all implicate plasma total cholesterol as a risk factor for coronary heart disease (1). Studies have indicated that high density lipoprotein (HDL) cholesterol may be a protective factor in contrast to the risk associated with elevated low density lipoprotein (LDL) cholesterol levels (2-6). The current interest in HDL cholesterol as an anti-atherogenic risk factor for heart disease has stimulated epidemiologic investigations of its correlates (7).

The Joint US-USSR Lipid Research Clinics (LRC) Program studied cardiovascular disease and such related factors as lipids and lipoproteins and their correlates in selected US and USSR subpopulations. In 1972, the governments of the United States and the Soviet Union signed a five-year cooperative agreement in the areas of health and medical sciences. This agreement was renewed in 1977 for a five-year period. One component of this agreement, known as Cardiovascular Area I--Pathogenesis of Atherosclerosis, led to the establishment of LRCs in Moscow and Leningrad (8, 9).

## B. Methods

The data presented here were collected in the Joint US-USSR Program Prevalence Study. Participants were selected from nine well-defined target subpopulations in the US and two in the USSR. These subpopulations covered a broad range of geographic, cultural, socioeconomic, demographic, and ethnic groups.

The Prevalence Study involved two sequential examinations. The first was a brief screening (Visit 1). The more extensive Visit 2 examination included lipoprotein quantification, a 24-hour dietary recall, personal and family histories relevant to vascular disease, a detailed medication history, blood pressure and anthropometric measurements, resting and exercise ECGs, and nonlipid clinical chemistries. Average daily ethanol intake was calculated from a 7-day recall consisting of questions specifically addressing ethanol use during the previous week. Data collection methods, including lipid laboratory procedures and nutrition assessment, were standardized according to a common protocol and personnel were trained and certified (10).

The data base for this study is restricted to white males, aged 40 to 59 years, randomly selected from the Visit 1 participants who also participated in Visit 2. Participants who had fasted less than 12 hours were excluded. Data on lipid and lipoprotein distributions are presented for samples of 1,045 US males and 1,002 USSR males by age groups 40-49 and 50-59 years.

## C.  Results

The US and USSR distributions of triglyceride, HDL cholesterol, and the ratios of HDL to plasma total cholesterol and LDL to HDL cholesterol differ significantly.  The two USSR age groups have significantly higher mean values for plasma total cholesterol, HDL cholesterol, and the HDL to plasma total cholesterol ratio and significantly lower mean values for plasma triglyceride and the LDL to HDL cholesterol ratio than the respective US age groups.  In addition, for the 40 to 49 year age group, the US and USSR distributions of plasma total cholesterol and LDL cholesterol differ significantly and the USSR sample has significantly higher mean levels of LDL cholesterol.  The VLDL cholesterol distributions were strikingly similar.  See Table 1.

Table 1.  Distribution Comparison of Plasma Lipids, Lipoproteins and HDL Cholesterol Between the US and USSR Sample.  White Males Ages 40-49 and 50-59

| | N | Chol mg/dl | Trig mg/dl | HDL mg/dl | LDL mg/dl | VLDL mg/dl | HDL/ Chol | LDL/ HDL |
|---|---|---|---|---|---|---|---|---|
| 40-49 years | | | | | | | | |
| US | 549 | 212* | 149* | 45* | 142§ | 25 | .22* | 3.5* |
| USSR | 576 | 225 | 125 | 52 | 149 | 24 | .24 | 3.1 |
| 50-59 years | | | | | | | | |
| US | 495 | 215† | 143§ | 46* | 145 | 25 | .22* | 3.4* |
| USSR | 422 | 222 | 127 | 52 | 146 | 24 | .24 | 3.1 |

*p<.01 for two sample t-tests and Kolmogorov-Smirnov test
†p<.01 for two sample t-test
§p<.01 for Kolmogorov-Smirnov test

Multiple regression models of the association of HDL cholesterol with demographic and other characteristics and with triglyceride levels were developed, controlling for subpopulation differences.  The characteristics selected for the two countries by stepwise multiple regressions were similar (Table 2).  For both samples, Quetelet Index, ethanol consumption, cigarette smoking, education, saturated fatty acids (SFA), and carbohydrate were selected.  Physical activity and

Table 2.  Pearson Product Moment Correlations Between HDL Cholesterol and Triglyceride and the Demographic and Other Characteristics Included in the Regression Models for the US and USSR Samples

| Variables | US | USSR |
|---|---|---|
| Ethanol (gm/day) | .273* | .389* |
| Quetelet Index (gm/cm$^2$) | -.197* | -.332* |
| Smoking (cigarettes/day) | -.119* | .031 |
| Carbohydrate (% kcal) | -.142 | -.073 |
| SFA (% kcal) | -.051 | -.183* |
| Age | .095* | --- |
| Kilocalories | --- | -.012 |
| Triglyceride | -.291* | -.300* |

*p<.014.  Correlations with p<.014 are significant at the experiment-wide Type I error level of $\alpha=.1$.

age also were selected for the US sample, while kilocalories was
selected for the USSR sample. Quetelet Index and ethanol consumption associated significantly with HDL cholesterol in both countries,
Quetelet Index negatively and ethanol consumption positively. For
the US sample, cigarette smoking and age also associated significantly with HDL cholesterol, cigarette smoking negatively and age
positively. For the USSR sample, SFA was negatively correlated with
HDL cholesterol. Triglyceride was negatively correlated with HDL
cholesterol in both countries.

Excluding triglyceride the multiple regression model (Table 3) for
the US sample indicates partial regression coefficients largest for
Quetelet Index and smallest for smoking; the standardized regression
coefficients for ethanol consumption and Quetelet Index were similar
in magnitude. For the USSR sample, the partial regression coefficients are largest for Quetelet Index and smallest for total kilocalories. As for the US sample, the standardized regression coefficients of ethanol consumption and Quetelet Index were similar.

**Table 3.** Stepwise Multiple Regression Analyses with HDL Cholesterol
as the Dependent Variable and the Demographic and Other Characteristics as the Independent Variables

| Variables | Partial Regression Coefficient | | Standardized Regression Coefficient | |
|---|---|---|---|---|
| | US | USSR | US | USSR |
| Quetelet (gm/cm$^2$) | -9.587† | -16.681† | -3.302 | -5.390 |
| Ethanol (gm/day) | .148† | .222† | 2.815 | 5.081 |
| Carbohydrate (% kcal) | -.214† | -.232† | -2.093 | -2.194 |
| Smoking (# cig/day) | -.134† | -.152* | -2.072 | -1.635 |
| SFA (% kcal) | -.222* | -.350* | -.913 | -1.730 |
| Education | 1.322* | 3.616† | --- | --- |
| Kilocalories | --- | -.002* | --- | -1.520 |
| Age | .162* | --- | .914 | --- |
| Physical Activity | 2.563† | --- | --- | --- |
| $R^2$ | .249 | .310 | | |
| $R^2$ (with subpopulation | .182 | .306 | | |

*.01 $\leq$ p < .05
†p < .01

For the US sample, the multiple correlation coefficient for the full
model was .249. After adjusting for subpopulation differences, the
proportion of the variation in HDL cholesterol levels accounted for
by the remaining chracteristics was .182. For the USSR sample, the
multiple correlation coefficient for the full model was .310, which
is higher than that for the US. Adjusting for subpopulations, this
decreased slightly to .306.

Including triglyceride in the multiple regression model (Table 4)
shows that although triglyceride has a stronger association with HDL
cholesterol than any other characteristic, each variable, except SFA
and total kilocalories in the USSR sample, remained significantly
associated with HDL cholesterol. The directions of the associations
remained unchanged from the first model.

814

The proportion of variation of HDL cholesterol explained in the US
sample increased with the addition of triglyceride to the model from
.249 to .299. This decreased to .237 when subpopulation effects were
controlled for. Controlling for subpopulation and triglyceride, the
proportion of the variability of HDL cholesterol accounted for by the
other characteristics was .159. Controlling for subpopulation and
the other characteristics, the proportion of variability of HDL
cholesterol accounted for by triglyceride was only .066.

Table 4. Stepwise Multiple Regression Analyses with HDL Cholesterol
as the Dependent Variable and with Triglyceride and the Demographic
and Other Characteristics as the Independent Variables

| Variables | Partial Regression Coefficients | | Standardized Regression Coefficients | |
|---|---|---|---|---|
| | US | USSR | US | USSR |
| Triglyceride (mg/dl) | -.026† | -.045† | -2.984 | -4.619 |
| Ethanol (gm/day) | .154† | .252† | 2.919 | 5.770 |
| Quetelet (gm/cm$^2$) | -7.179† | -12.390† | -2.472 | -4.003 |
| Carbohydrate (% kcal) | -.194† | -.230† | -1.898 | -2.179 |
| Smoking (# cig/day) | -.121† | -.106 | -1.865 | -1.144 |
| SFA (% kcal) | -.237* | -.363* | -.974 | -1.798 |
| Education | 1.229* | 3.512† | --- | --- |
| Kilocalories | --- | -.001 | --- | -1.098 |
| Age | .153* | --- | .863 | --- |
| Physical activity | 2.099† | --- | --- | --- |
| $R^2$ | .299 | .387 | | |
| $R^2$ (with subpopulation) | .237 | .383 | | |
| $R^2$ (with subpopulation, triglyceride) | .159 | .321 | | |
| $R^2$ (with subpopulation, other characteristics) | .066 | .112 | | |

*.01 ≤ p < .05
†p < .01

The multiple regression coefficient for the USSR sample also increased, to .387. Controlling for subpopulation effects reduced
this slightly, to .383. Controlling for subpopulation and triglyceride, the proportion of variation of HDL cholesterol explained
by the other characteristics was .321, higher than that for the US
sample. The proportion of the variation in HDL cholesterol accounted
for by triglyceride when subpopulation and the other characteristics
were controlled for is .112.

D.  Summary

In this study, the distributions of the lipids and lipoprotein cholesterol fractions in samples from the US and USSR are compared, and
selected demographic and other characteristics are evaluated multi-
variably as potential determinants of HDL cholesterol levels. It
must be stressed that the samples selected for this study were not
designed to be representative of the entire populations of either the
US or USSR. The analyses reported here, based on common survey
methods and highly standardized laboratory measurements, disclose
contrasts in population distributions of lipids and lipoproteins in

middle-aged men in US and USSR LRC samples.  Despite these differences, the present report indicates that ethanol consumption, a lean
body, and abstinence from cigarette smoking are associated with
increased levels of HDL cholesterol in both the US and USSR samples.

*Acknowledgments*   This manuscript was prepared at the Central
Patient Registry and Coordinating Center for the Lipid Research
Clinics Program, a part of the Department of Biostatistics, School
of Public Health, University of North Carolina at Chapel Hill, by
D. Ingram, R. Mills, and M. Maciolowski with assistance from
D.B. Shestov, V.F. Trufanov, V.A. Polessky and G.A. Zhukovsky.

# References

1.  Klimov AN:  Reasons and conditions for development of athero-
    sclerosis.  In:  Preventive Cardiology (GI Kosoitzky, Ed.)
    Medisina, Moscow, 1977
2.  Miller GJ, Miller NE:  Plasma high density lipoprotein concen-
    tration and development of ischemic heart disease.  Lancet 1:16-
    19, 1975
3.  Heiss G, Johnson NJ, Reiland S, Davis CE, Tyroler HA:  The
    epidemiology of plasma high-density lipoprotein cholesterol
    levels.  Circ 62 (suppl IV):IV-116-IV-136, 1980
4.  US-USSR Steering Committee for Problem Area I (The Pathogenesis
    of Atherosclerosis):  Collaborative US-USSR study on the preva-
    lence of dyslipoproteinemias and ischemic heart disease in
    American and Soviet populations.  Am J Card 40:260-268, 1977
5.  US-USSR Steering Committee for Problem Area I (The Pathogenesis
    of Atherosclerosis):  The collaborative US-USSR study on the
    prevalence of dyslipoproteinemias and ischemic heart disease in
    the Soviet and American populations.  Ter Arkh  4:26, 1977 (in
    Russian)
6.  US-USSR Steering Committee for Problem Area I (The Pathogenesis
    of Atherosclerosis):  Population Descriptions and Methodology
    for the Collaboration in Problem Area I.  Presented at the First
    Joint US-USSR Lipoprotein Symposium; 1981 May; Leningrad, USSR
    (in press)
7.  Albers JJ, Warnick GR, Johnson N, Bachorik PS, Muesing R, Lippel
    K, Williams OD:  Quality control of plasma high-density lipo-
    protein cholesterol measurement methods.  The Lipid Research
    Clinic Program Prevalence Study.  Circ 62 (suppl IV): IV-9-IV-
    18, 1980
8.  US-USSR Steering Committee for Problem Area I (The Pathogenesis
    of Atherosclerosis):  Nutrition assessment methods and basic
    intake levels.  Presented at the First Joint US-USSR Lipoprotein
    Symposium; 1981 May, Leningrad, USSR (in press)
9.  Hulley S, Ashman P, Kuller L, Lasser N, Sherwin R:  HDL cho-
    lesterol levels in the Multiple Risk Factor Intervention Trial
    (MRFIT) by the MRFIT Research Group.  Lipids 14:119, 1979
10. The Lipid Research Clinics Program:  Protocol of the Lipid
    Research Clinics Program Prevalence Study.  Central Patient
    Registry and Coordinating Center, Department of Biostatistics,
    UNC at Chapel Hill, 1974

# The Belgian Heart Disease Prevention Project: Six Years Coronary Risk Factor Evolution

M. Kornitzer, G. De Backer, M. Dramaix, and C. Thilly

In the early 1970's several controlled multifactorial prevention trials were launched that used a wide variety of methods and intervention techniques. Both the Multiple Risk Factor Intervention Trial (1),in the United States, and the Oslo Study (2) were aimed at modifying the coronary risk profile in high-risk men by means of face-to-face counseling. The Goteborg Study (3) involved the random allocation of 10,000 subjects into an intervention group and 20,000 subjects into two control groups; both face-to-face advice and group dynamics were used in the intervention group with the cooperation of specialised clinics. All the above mentioned studies were based on individual randomization. A controlled, non randomized, multifactorial study was conducted in North Karelia (Finland), a neighbouring province was used as control (4). Counseling was mainly provided through mass media.

The Belgian Heart Disease Prevention Project, which forms part of the World Health Organization (WHO) European Collaborative Trial (5) used both face-to-face and mass media techniques. It has been carried out in an industrial population, the random allocation being one of occupational units. Prevention is aimed at male subjects age 40-59. Thirty factories were paired off according to type of industry and one member of each pair was randomly allocated into the intervention group, with the other serving as a control. Nineteen thousand four hundred sixty three subjects were listed : 83.7% of those took part in the base-line examination. In the intervention group, all subjects were initially screened for risk factors (systolic blood pressure, weight and height, serum cholesterol and smoking habits). In the control group, 10% of the subjects, in each occupational unit, were randomly selected to undergo the same thorough initial examination, the other 90% were only subjected to a resting ECG. For all subjects who underwent the same thorough initial examination risk profiles were established on the basis of the initial results, according to a risk score. The subjects who belonged to the top 21% of the risk score distribution in the intervention units were placed in the high-risk group and accordingly received at least twice a year individual advice for the first two years, and yearly thereafter. In addition, 5% of the subjects in the intervention group were randomly selected for annual examinations. Finally, the 10% subjects in the control group who underwent the complete base-line examination were reexamined after 2 and 4 years. All subjects still at work after 5.5-6 years follow-up were invited to the final examination and around 70% accepted.

## Results

When high-risk group are compared, the coronary risk profile, defined by means of the multiple logistic function, was significantly decreased in the intervention group throughout the trial, although less so at end-screening (Fig.1).

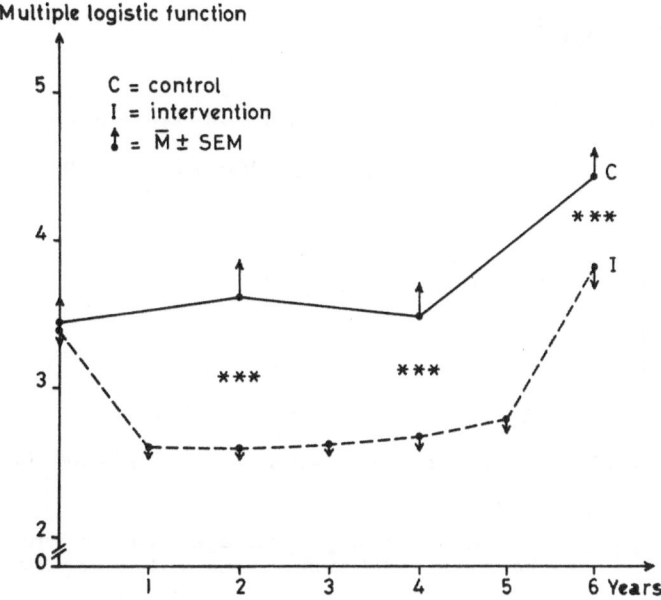

Fig. 1.  Evolution of the coronary risk profile (Multiple Logistic
         Function) in the high-risk groups

Another way of presenting the results is based on the formula :

$$Change(\%)=\frac{(change\ in\ intervention\ group-change\ in\ control\ group)\times100}{initial\ grand\ mean\ intervention\ group}$$

Whereas change expressed in % is 28.6% at two years it is decreased
to 11.4% at end-screening (Fig.2).

818

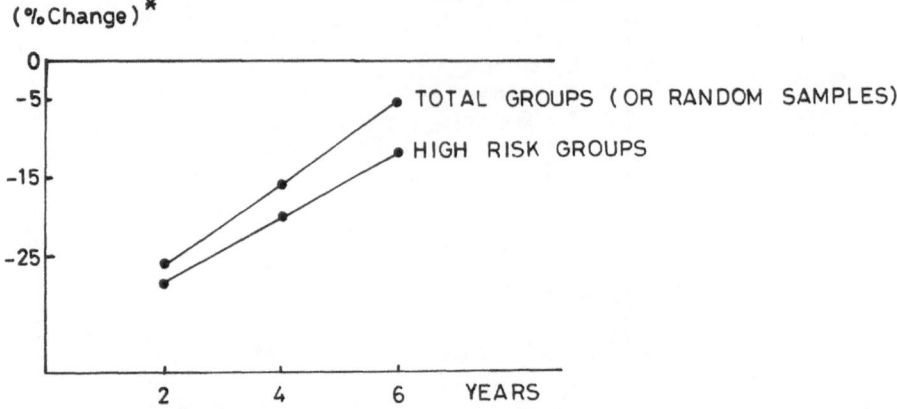

(%Change)*

∗ %Change=(Δ Intervention − Δ Control) 100/Initial Grand Mean Intervention

Fig. 2. Net change (in percentage) in the coronary risk profile in the high-risk groups and total groups or random samples

For the random samples or total groups were 79% had essentially received advice by means of booklets and posters, the coronary risk profile was not permanently modified. Whereas at 2 and 4 years, we observed a significant difference between intervention and control groups, no such difference was observed at end-screening. This was due to a lessening of influence on blood pressure and smoking (Fig.3). Whereas change expressed in % was 26.3% at 2 years, it dropped to a trivial 5.3% at end-screening (Fig.2).

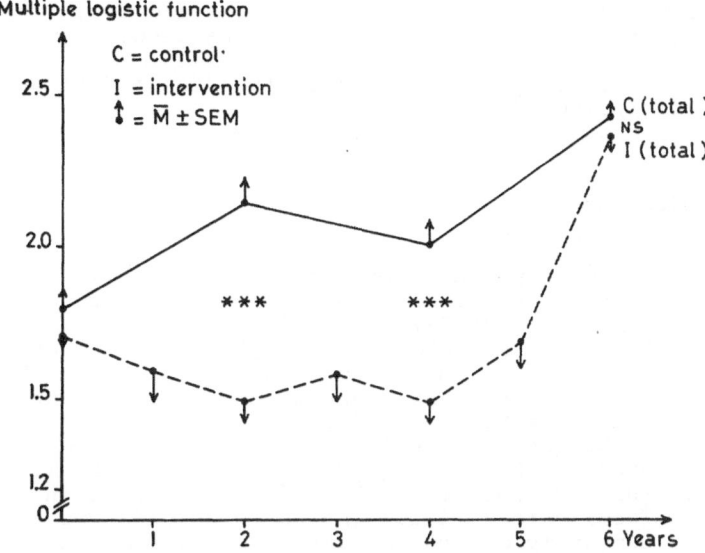

**Fig. 3.** Evolution of the coronary risk profile (Multiple Logistic
Function) in the total groups or random samples

Comments

These results show clearly that the intervention program had a
major and during impact, although less so after 6 years, on the coronary risk profile of the high-risk subjects who received individually
tailored advice by two physicians attached to the Project. On the
other hand, the part of the intervention programme introduced during
the first year by way of posters and booklets aimed at 79% of the
intervention group, did not result in a permanent modification of
the coronary risk profile. It seems that the favorable effect of
the intervention programme obtained in the high-risk group has been
"diluted" by the lack of permanent effect on the rest of the intervention group. It has been initially estimated that, without any
intervention, 30% to 40% of new coronary events will be observed in
the high risk group (21% of the intervention group). Thus, a risk
reduction of 40% in that group reduce coronary heart disease (CHD)
incidence by 12-16% in the whole of the intervention group.
If, at the same time, the intervention programme achieved a risk
reduction of 10% in the "lower-risk" group, the overall effect would
yield a meaningful 20 to 24% net reduction in the incidence of CHD.
The modification of the coronary risk profile achieved in the intervention group at 2 and 4 years of follow-up falls short of the initially estimated targets.

From the Laboratory of Epidemiology and Social Medicine, Free
University of Brussels and the Department of Cardiology, State
University of Ghent, Belgium.
Supported by grant N°20202 of the "Fonds National de la Recherche
Scientifique."

## References

1.  The Multiple Risk Factor Intervention Trial (MRFIT)(1976) A
    national study of primary prevention of coronary heart disease.
    JAMA 235: 825-827.
2.  Leren P, Askevold EM, Foss OP, Frøili A, Grymyr D, Helgeland A,
    Hjerman I, Holme I, Lund-Larsen PG, Norum KR (1975) The Oslo
    Study - Cardiovascular disease in middle-aged and young Oslo
    men. Acta Med Scand 588: 1-38
3.  Wilhelmsen L, Tibblin G, Werko L (1972) A primary preventive
    study in Gothenburg, Sweden. Prev Med 1: 153-160.
4.  Puska P, Koskela K, Pakarinen H, Puumalainen P, Soininen V,
    Tuomilehto J (1976) The North Karelia Project : A programme for
    community control of cardiovascular diseases. Scand J Soc Med
    4: 57-60.
5.  World Health Organization European Collaborative Group (1974)
    An international controlled trial in the multifactorial preven-
    tion of coronary heart disease. Int J Epidemiol 3: 219-224.

# Pecularities of Coronary Heart Diseases in the French Population

J. L. Richard

The relatively low death rates from Coronary Heart Disease (CHD) in the specified rubric (A 83) of the International classification for death statistics is a stable phenomenon in France and has often been questioned. A gross underestimation has been suggested. Certainly a misclassification of deaths from CHD in less specified rubrics like rubric A 84 (other forms of heart disease) or even rubric A 136–137 (ill-defined and unspecified causes) could lead to an underestimation of the coronary mortality. An estimation of the true corrected French mortality from CHD can be proposed between the rates of the specific rubric A 83 and the sum of the 3 rubrics A 83, A 84 and A 136–137. In any case this sum gives undoubtedly the maximum possible rate of the French coronary mortality, as all other deaths are attributed to causes clearly well specified as non coronary.

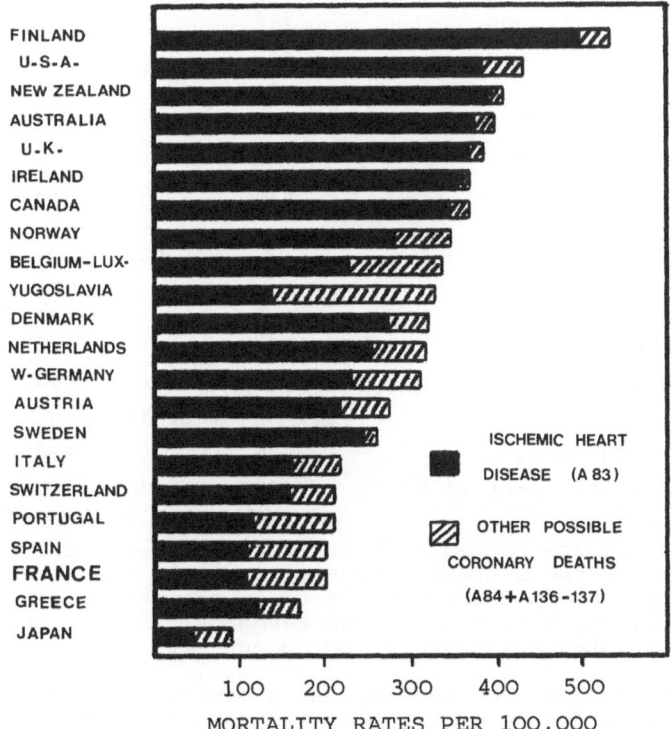

Figure 1. Estimation of CHD mortality among the 22 countries of OECD. Men 35–64 years – Age standardized rates

The age standardized rates among men 35-64 years old are given on figure 1 for rubric A 83 and the sum mentioned above in the 22 countries of the Organisation for Economic Cooperation and Development (OECD) : the maximum estimated French rates are still relatively low but in agreement with the geographic location of France, taking into account the increasing CHD mortality gradient from the south to the north of Europe.

Morbidity surveys lead to similar conclusions. Table 1 gives age and follow-up standardized incidences in different cohorts of the Seven Countries Study or in the Pooling Project and in the Paris Prospective Study (1). Paris incidence rates are in the middle of European Incidences classified by geographic location. After adjustment on the levels of classical risk factors, the incidence of the American cohort of the Seven Countries Study and that of the Pooling Project are respectively 1.5 and 2.2 times higher than the Paris Study incidence.

Table 1. Standardized incidence of coronary heart disease in 3 prospective studies

| Study | Sample size | Number of CHD | Standardized rates per 1000 |
|---|---|---|---|
| I. 5 year incidence - Age at entry 40-59 | | | |
| Seven Countries Study | | | |
| East Finland | 775 | 31 | 43.0 |
| United States | 2454 | 79 | 32.6 |
| Holland | 864 | 28 | 31.1 |
| Slavonia | 694 | 10 | 17.0 |
| Rural Italy | 1665 | 28 | 16.6 |
| West Finland | 845 | 13 | 14.9 |
| Rome | 758 | 9 | 12.3 |
| Dalmatia | 671 | 8 | 10.3 |
| Greece | 1208 | 10 | 8.2 |
| Serbia | 1545 | 8 | 5.3 |
| Paris Prospective Study | 7434 | 165 | 16.8 |
| II. 8.6 year incidence - Age at entry 45-49 | | | |
| Pooling Project | 2066 | 194 | 93.9 |
| Paris Prospective Study | 7434 | 165 | 29.7 |

In the French myocardial infarction registers conducted in Normandy and in the south of the country incidence rates are lower than rates reported by the WHO Study using the same methodology (2). It is very unlikely that a gross under-registration of cases could explain such low rates which are in agreement with national mortality (Figure 2).

The reasons for that relative protection towards CHD are not well known. The levels of the main coronary risk factors are not very low in the French population but seem to be in the same range as in other countries of middle Europe. Diet, as far as main nutrients are concerned, does not provide a likely explanation : in particular, mean consumption of animal products and of saturated lipids is very high in France (Figure 3). On the other hand, French nutrition seems

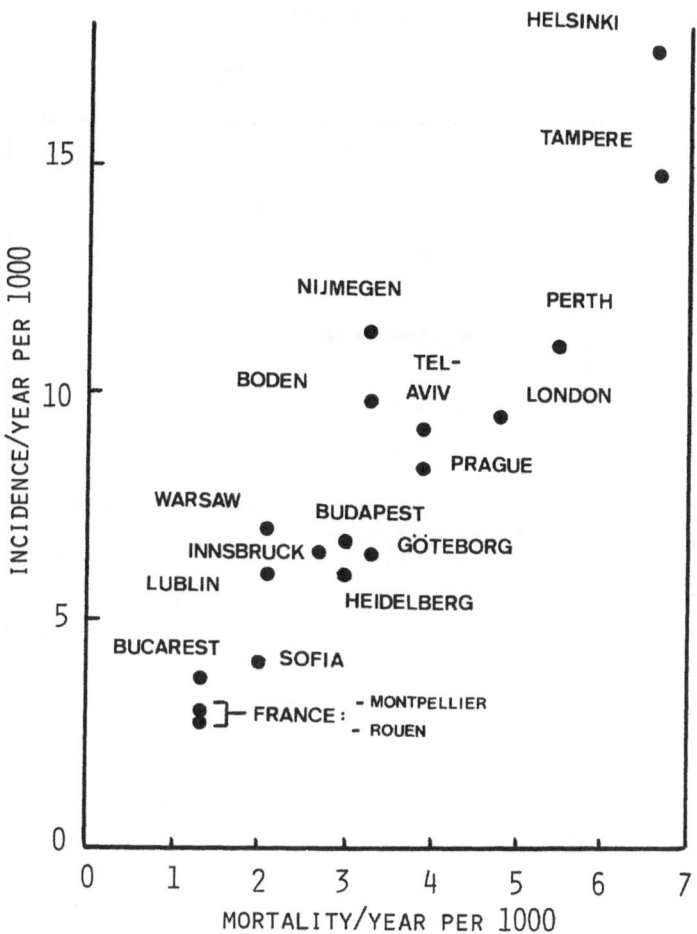

Figure 2. Annual mean incidence of acute myocardial infarction (WHO Registers) and national male mortality from CHD. Men 45-64 years

really different from that of Mediterranean countries in spite of the similarity of their coronary mortality at variance with diet heart hypothesis.

Recently, a 20% increase of HDL-cholesterol has been reported with regard to levels usually observed in Western male population (3). Such a high level could account for, at least partly, the low French incidence or mortality rates. These high levels seem partly independent of alcohol consumption and their mechanisms are not explained. But the mean national high alcohol consumption could also account for low mortality rates from CHD by other mechanisms than HDL-cholesterol increase.

In fact the relationships of alcohol and alcoholism with cardiac pathology are complex and need careful examination in the community.

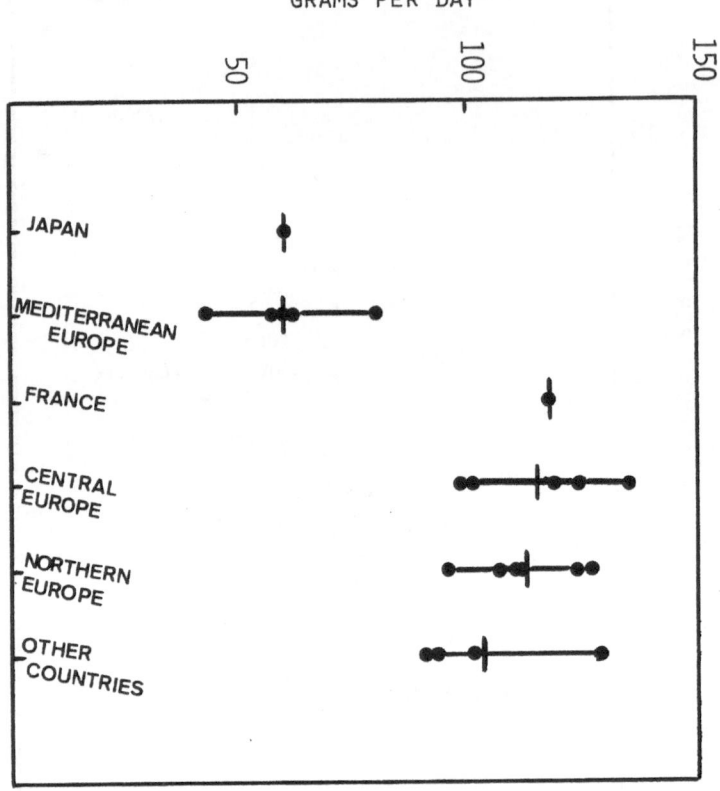

GRAMS PER DAY

**Figure 3.** Food consumption statistics OECD among 22 countries - Fat animal products

Heavy drinkers have cardiac deaths possibly independent of coronary atherosclerosis. Such an acute myocardial pathology has often no recognized etiology and could explain the positive association obser-ved among French regions between alcohol consumption and coronary mortality, at variance with the negative-relationship observed between countries in international comparisons. Such a discrepancy could also reflect a higher lethality of acute coronary events among heavy drinkers. Data from the French registers are in agreement with this hypothesis : the global incidence of acute events is similar in both registers, but the mortality is higher in Normandy where alcohol consumption is more important. In the Paris Prospective Study well-defined sudden deaths are associated with classical coronary risk factors, but unexpected deaths with cardiac symptoms and without the precise criteria of sudden death are significantly linked only to alcoholism in a multivariate analysis taking into account other main risk factors.

The relatively low incidence and mortality rates from CHD in France must be reasonably accepted as roughly true, but clearly their causes remain unexplained and are probably complex.

References

1. Ducimetière P, Richard JL, Cambien F, Rakotovao R, Claude JR
   (1980) Coronary heart disease in middle-aged frenchmen. Comparisons between Paris Prospective Study, Seven Countries Study and
   Pooling Project. Lancet 1:1346–1349
2. World Health Organisation, Regional Office for Europe : Myocardial Infarction Community Registers (1976) WHO Publications –
   Copenhagen
3. Debonder-Decoopman E, Fievet-Desreumaux C, Campos E, Moulin S,
   Dewailly P, Sezille G, Jaillard J (1980) Plasma levels of VLDL+
   LDL, cholesterol, HDL-cholesterol, triglycerides and apoproteins
   B and A[1] in a healthy population. Atherosclerosis 37:559–568

# The Fate of the Patient with OPAD Detected at an Early Stage. Preliminary Data on an 11-year Follow-up of 239 Men with OPAD and 239 Controls

L. K. Widmer, A. Delley, M.-T. Widmer, L. Biland, A. Da Silva, and A. Braun

In the prospective epidemiological Basle study a
5-year follow-up yielded a low amputation rate but
a high incidence of concomitant vascular disease
and a high mortality for men with OPAD (1). In order
to check these rather surprising results, a 10-year
follow-up was planned for this subgroup and age-matched
healthy men of the same population.

## METHODS

Population: The OPAD group consisted of 239 men mostly
detected at an early stage (70% without claudication,
44% presenting with only stenoses) age at entry 57,3 $\pm$
7.1, observation interval 11.3 $\pm$ 3.7 years. For each
patient an age-matched control without signs and
symptoms of OPAD was randomly selected from the same
industrial sub-population; age at entry 57.0 $\pm$ 7.8
years.

Re-examination of the surviving subgroup (drop-out 1.8%):
(a) Interview on the state of health, concomitant cardiac
and cerebrovascular disease, interval treatment and socio-
medical consequences; (b) non-invasive examination of
peripheral, coronary and extracranial arteries, analysis
of risk-profile.

Analysis of the non surviving group: Information on cause of death could be obtained for all patients who had
died during the observation interval. Statistical analysis by $\chi^2$-test and Fisher-test resp. (n < 20).

RESULTS

1. Surviving subgroup

The following validated anamnestic data were
reported at follow-up.
- Peripheral circulation: Only 1/3 of OPAD subjects suffered from intermittent claudication.
  The incidence of "local complications" acute
  occlusion, trophic lesions, amputation was low
  in the OPAD (40%) and, as was to be expected,
  very low in the control group (6%) (p< 0.001),
  table 1.

table 1. Peripheral circulation surviving subgroup

|  | controls | OPAD | p |
|---|---|---|---|
| n | 199 | 129 | |
| Signs/symptoms acute occlusion | 1,5% | 7.8 | <0.01 |
| Trophic lesions | 3.5 | 7.6 | n.s. |
| Amputation | 0.5* | 2.4 | n.s. |

* motorcycle accident

- Concomitant coronary and extracranial artery
  disease
  were reported by 37% of the OPAD subjects vs
  10% of the controls (p < 0.001).

table 2. Concomitant vascular disease surviving
subgroup

|  | controls | OPAD | p |
|---|---|---|---|
| n | 199 | 129 | |
| Myocardial infarction | 5.5% | 15.5% | <0.05 |
| Angina pectoris | 3.5 | 17.8 | <0.001 |
| Stroke | 4.0 | 12.4 | <0.05 |

- The state of health: Diminished well-being was
  reported by 32% of the OPAD group and 17% of the
  controls(p < 0.05), treatment with cardio-vascular
  drugs by 69% vs 37% (p < 0.01).

- Social consequences: i.e. incapacity to work, change of place of work and/or premature retirement were reported by 12.4% of OPAD patients and 0% of the controls (p < 0.001); 3/4 of those with social consequences reported OPAD as the single reason for this.

2. Mortality

The 11-year mortality was 36.8 in the OPAD group compared with 12.6% for controls (p < 0.001), with an average age at death of $66.3 \pm 7$ vs $71.4 \pm 6$ years. In OPAD patients 53% of deaths were due to cardiovascular disease; 39% to coronary heart disease, 4.5% to cerebrovascular and 9% to other vascular diseases.

table 3. Cause of death according to death certificate

|  | controls | OPAD | p |
|---|---|---|---|
| n | 239 | 239 | |
| Cardiovascular disease | 3.3% | 19.7% | < 0.001 |
| Coronary heart disease | 1.3 | 14.2 | < 0.001 |
| Cerebrovascular | 1.3 | 1.7 | n.s. |
| Peripheral artery | 0.8 | 3.3 | < 0.05 |
| Tumor | 5.0 | 11.3 | < 0.1 |

The correlation between the risk profile at entry (cigarettes, systolic blood pressure, diabetes, cholesterol level) and mortality will be reported in a separate paper (2).

CONCLUSION

The fate of men with OPAD detected at an early stage was characterized by
- a low incidence of local complications,
- a high incidence of coronary and cerebroarterial disease,
- considerable social consequences (capacity to work and requirement of medical care).
- a considerable excess mortality on coronary heart desease.
- tentative conclusions as to the indication of aggr. treatment are drawn.

SUMMARY

The fate of 239 men with OPAD detected at an early
state (Basler Studie (1)) was compared in an 11-year
follow-up to that of 239 controls, men of the same
industrial population. age at entry 57 ± 7.

In the surviving OPAD group a few (acute occlusion
7.8%, amputation 2,4) local complications, a high incidence of concomitant cardio-vascular disease and
frequent social consequences were observed (p < 0.001
for all 3 parameters).

The 11-year mortality, significantly higher in OPAD
with 36.8% than in controls 12.6% (p < 0.001) was mainly
due to coronary heart disease and cerebro-arterial
disease (19.7) followed by tumor in 11.3%; controls 29%
and 5% respectively (p < 0.001).

The fate of OPAD patients is considerably worse, than
that of controls, even when OPAD is detected at an
early asymptomatic or oligo-symptomatic stage. Are risk
factors and the condition of coronary circulation
adequatly considered, especially when planning aggressive
treatment of OPAD?

LITERATUR

1) A. DA SILVA, L.K. WIDMER, Occlusive peripheral artery
   disease - A prospective epidemiological study of 2630
   men - Basle Study I-III, 1959-1976, Huber, Berne 1980

2) A. VOGT, A. DELLEY, in press, Diss. Basle 1982

# Population Attributable Events – Implications for Prevention

L. Wilhelmsen, K. Svärdsudd, and H. Wedel

## A. Introduction

Epidemiologists and statisticians have greatly improved the ability
to predict the risk of suffering coronary heart disease (CHD) events
in various populations over the recent decade. Clinicians have also
begun to adopt the high risk concept in their practices. The most wide-spread example is treatment of a symptomless person with a blood
pressure (BP) in the uppermost part of the distribution. Similarly
"patients" with high blood lipids may be put on diet or lipid-lowering
drugs due to their expected high risk of suffering a CHD event. However, the responsibility of the physicians should not only be confined to patients or to definitely high risk individuals. The problem
of CHD, which is a mass disease in many countries, has to be considered from a population point of view. The question is whether the present attitudes and practice are optimal in this respect.

It should also be kept in mind that epidemiological studies have had
to use end points which are clinically detectable such as non-fatal
or fatal myocardial infarction (MI) or sudden coronary death (SD).
The occurence of these diseases does certainly mirror the prevalence
of atherosclerosis in the group, but in the single individual with
CHD it might not be the case. It is also possible that the occurence
of clinical MI or SD is associated with additional causative factors
which precipitate the event in an individual with enough atherosclerosis. In recent years the possibility of coronary spasm precipita-
ting an MI or SD has also been shown. Thus, risk factors for MI and
SD should not be confused with risk factors for atherosclerosis if
this specific entity has not been studied.

## B. Population Attributable Events - Definition

It has been found in several studies that CHD victims are not always
burdened with extensive elevations of the conventional risk factors
high BP, high total serum cholesterol or abberations of the lipo-protein pattern, and many patients have not been heavy smokers. On the
contrary it is common to see patients who have a combination of moderately disturbed factors. Furthermore, the disease incidence in the
population is not only dependent upon the risk, but also on the prevalence of subjects in the population afflicted with that risk.

The individual attributable risk is defined as the excess risk in an
individual above the risk in an individual without the factor. An example: if the risk for a CHD event during a period is 2 % in a non-
smoker, and 5 % in a smoker of 15-24 cig./day, the excess risk - or
attributable  - risk of smoking that amount is 3 %. The population
attributable events, defined as the number of events due to the factor in the population, depends on the product of individual attributable risk and the number of individuals afflicted with the factor in
the population. Thus, contrary to what is commonly used in for example insurance statistics, we are concerned with absolute rather than
with relative terms.

ROSE (1981) has recently referred to the high (relative) risk of elevated BP in young individuals, but the even higher absolute risk in older people with similar BP elevations because of the high prevalence of such subjects in the community. SVÄRDSUDD (1978) and WILHELMSEN et al. (1980) have discussed the relative benefits of treating definitely hypertensive subjects versus primary prevention of BP increase over almost the entire BP distribution.

In the present paper the three most important risk factors for MI and SD - elevated BP, Abberations of blood lipids, tobacco smoking, and the combination of them - will be discussed from the concept "population attributable events".

## C. Study Populations and Methods

The present paper deals with results from two prospective studies in random population samples of men living in Göteborg, Sweden.

The Study of Men Born in 1913 started in 1963 when all the men were exactly 50 years old. One third of all men in the city were invited and 855 (88 %) participated in the initial examination. They have been re-examined in 1967, 1973, and 1980-81. Non-fatal MI and stroke, and cause-specific mortality have been followed carefully during the entire period. The autopsy rate is high in the city - close to 90 % of all fatal cases. This population sample has not been subjected to any special intervention measures, but hypertension andclinical diseases have been treated according to general routines in the community.

The second series consists of a random third of all men born during the years 1915-1922 and 1924-1925. Out of about 10,000 invited men 75 % participated in the initial examination during 1970-73. They constituted the intervention group in a primary preventive trial, and the remaining two thirds of the population in these age-groups were controls. All men have been followed by special registers for MI, stroke and cause-specific mortality including SD. Re-examinations of the the whole samples or random subsamples have been performed in 1974-1977 and 1980-1983. The intervention has mainly concerned the high risk subjects with high BP, high serum cholesterol, or smoking more than 15 cigarettes per day, but those with high risk according to a multivariate risk prediction estimated from the previously menthioned population sample of 50-year-old men have also been intervened upon (WILHELMSEN et al. 1973).

## D. Results

### 1. Serum Cholesterol

The distribution curves for subjects who suffered CHD during follow-up, and those men who did not suffer CHD, were similar in shape, but the curve for those men suffering CHD was, as expected, displaced to the right. Thus, most of the CHD victims had rather "normal" levels if the Swedish general population is used as standard for normality. If HDL-cholesterol estimations or other determinations of lipo-proteins had been available in 1963 a better separation between the CHD and non-CHD groups had probably been possible.

The incidence of MI+SD during 17 years follow-up of the Men Born in 1913 was strongly associated with cholesterol at entry to the study.

However, most of the CHD cases occurred among subjects with relatively moderately elevated levels in this population - between cholesterol levels 5.5 and 7.5 mmol/l. Various methods of calculating the number of events attributable to cholesterol elevation can be adopted. We calculated the number of events that would have occurred if the events in subjects with cholesterol above 5.25 mmol/l were attributed to hypercholesterolemia. Most of the attributable cases occurred below cholesterol 7.5 mmol/l, and subjects with very high levels contributed only a minor amount of the total number of events. An approach to possibilities in prevention would be to calculate the number of potentially preventable events if serum cholesterol could be decreased over a major part of the distribution. Such an attempt would also theoretically give a greater benefit than treating only those with the highest levels.

The above mentioned results were taken from the Study of Men Born in 1913. The analysis of the results from the preventive trial gives similar results,but the intervention against those with the highest cholesterol levels partly influences the picture. Among those with total serum cholesterol above 7.8 mmol/l alpha-lipoproteincholesterol was measured and related to MI or SD during follow-up, but was of no predictive value in addition to that of total serum cholesterol (WIKLUND et al. 1980).

## 2. Blood Pressure

As for serum cholesterol there was the expected displacement to the right of the distribution curve for the CHD group among the 50-year-old men at entry, and this is mirrored by an increasing relative risk with increasing BP. Furthermore, analogous with the previous variable most CHD cases occurred among subjects with relatively normal BP:s.

This finding was even more evident in the preventive trial in which a comprehensive anti-hypertensive treatment programme has been in operation. The curve for incidence showed a down-ward trend for the highest BP:s presumably due to the treatment. In this population sample the events attributable to increased BP occurred among subjects with BP:s below to-days cut-off points for anti-hypertensive drug treatment, and only a minority occurred among those on treatment. A shift to the left of the major part of the BP distribution curve by some type of non-pharmacological intervention (decreased sodium intake, body weight decrease, etc.) would be the intervention of choice if any further effect on morbidity should be achieved (SVÄRDSUDD 1978, WILHELMSEN 1979, WILHELMSEN et al. 1980).

## 3. Tobacco Smoking

In the Study of Men Born in 1913 a strong rising incidence of CHD with increasing smoking habits was seen. Non-smokers and ex-smokers had the same incidence. However, in accordance with the findings for the two previously discussed risk factors the highest absolute number of events was seen among the moderate smokers - 50 events among those smoking 1-14 grams tobacco per day, 31 events among those smoking 15-24 grams, and only 9 among those smoking 25 grams or more a day. If events attributable to smoking are calculated by subtracting the incidence among non-smokers and ex-smokers the respective numbers are 27, 20 and 6 events.

In the Primary Preventive Trial the incidence did not rise with increasing tobacco consumption above 1-14 grams per day, and consequently the number of events among the moderate and heavý smokers at entry

to the trial and before intervention was even lower than in the prospective study without intervention against smoking.

## 4. Multivariate Risk Prediction

With the aid of various multivariate statistical methods it has been
possible to improve the prediction considerably, so that close to 50%
of all MI and SD cases can be found among the 20% of the population
with the highest risk (WILHELMSEN et al. 1973, and others). By using
non-linear functions such as isotonic regression an even better fit
can be achieved. Thus, a small number of subjects with 100% risk of
suffering MI or SD during 13 years follow-up could be selected (WIL-
HELMSEN et al. 1979). A better prediction will probably be achieved
by using more modern methods of lipoprotein analysis. In a case-control study we used a multivariate analysis and found that out of several serum apolipoproteins, serum apo A II increased the predictive
power significantly, and these results indicate that 50% of MI cases
can be found among the 10% with highest multiple risk (FAGER et al.
1981). Even with these methods, however, a great number of events will
occur among subjects who have not been assigned a particularly high
risk. However, for the individual the high relative risk is certainly
of utmost importance.

## E. Concluding Remarks

The high risk concept has been valuable for preventive actions, and
various clinics created for the care of high risk subjects such as
hypertension clinics, lipid clinics, anti-smoking clinics, and so forth
have certainly been of benefit for these individuals, but these measures
offer only limited answers to the community problem of CHD, which has
to be attacked with more general preventive actions. In many instances
it might also be easier to change a major part of the population than
to affect only a selected high risk group, in which healthy individuals
have to be converted to "patients".

Acknowledgments   We thank many colleagues in Göteborg who have been
active in the studies, and especially G. Tibblin, L. Welin, D. Elmfeldt, G. Berglund, O. Samuelsson and M. Hagmann. The studies were
supported by grants from the Bank of Sweden Tercentenary Fund and
the Swedish National Organization against Heart and Chest Diseases.

## References

1. Rose G (1981) Strategy of prevention: lessons from cardiovascular
   disease. Brit Med J 282: 1847-1851
2. Svärdsudd K (1978) High blood pressure. A longitudinal population
   study of men born in 1913, with special reference to development
   and consequences for health. Ph D Thesis. Göteborg, Sweden
3. Wilhelmsen L, Svärdsudd K, Berglund G (1980) Development of high
   blood pressure and its consequences for health. In: Kesteloot H,
   Joossens JV (ed) Epidemiology of high blood pressure. Martinus
   Nijhoff Publ. The Hague, Boston, London, pp 311-324
4. Wilhelmsen L, Wedel H, Tibblin G (1973) Multivariate analysis of
   risk for coronary heart disease. Circulation 48: 950-958
5. Wiklund O, Wilhelmsen L, Elmfeldt D, Wedel H, Valek J, Gustafson A
   (1980) Alpha-lipoprotein cholesterol concentration in relation to
   subsequent myocardial infarction in hypercholesterolemic men. Atherosclerosis 37: 47-53

6. Wilhelmsen L (1979) Salt and hypertension. Clin Sci 57: 455s–458s
7. Fager G, Wiklund O, Olofsson S-O, Wilhelmsen L, Bondjers G (1981) Multivariate analysis of serum apolipoproteins and risk factors in relation to acute myocardial infarction. Arteriosclerosis 1: 273–279

# Risk Factors in Insulin Dependent Diabetics

H. Haller and M. Hanefeld

Diabetics treated with insulin exhibit excessive cardiovascular mortality. Therefore we analysed:
1. The prevalence of cardiovascular risk factors in a representative group (n = 33o) of diabetics and compared the parameters with randomly selected probands. 2. In a follow up study (time intervall 4 years) we reexamined 156 diabetics 55 died. The relations of risk factors to cardiovascular complications were investigated. All prevalence factors are higher in females than in males, specially HTG.

Prevalence factors (observed/expected) in comparison with the control-population, age standardized

|        | m   | f    |
|--------|-----|------|
| Obesity | 1.2 | 1.9  |
| HTG    | 2.o | 27.4 |
| HCH    | 1.8 | 2.3  |
| HLP    | 1.9 | 5.4  |

After 4 years follow up we see a remarkable decrease of prevalence particularly HTG in females.

| Risk factors | | at entry (n = 33o) | at reexamination (n = 23o) | significance (p) |
|--------------|-------|------|------|---------|
| Obesity | total | 21.3 | 4.3 | < 1 % |
|         | m     | 13.3 | o   | < 1 % |
|         | f     | 27.6 | 4.3 | < 1 % |
| HTG     | total | 23.1 | 12.2 | < 1 % |
|         | m     | 16.o | 14.6 | n.s. |
|         | f     | 28.9 | 9.6 | < 1 % |
| HCH     | total | 1o.6 | o.4 | <1 % |
|         | m     | 5.3  | o   | <5 % |
|         | f     | 15.o | o.9 | <1 % |
| HLP     | total | 28.o | 14.o | <1 % |
|         | m     | 18.7 | 14.6 | n.s. |
|         | f     | 35.6 | 13.2 | <1 % |

expressed as percent of frequency

The mortality factors IHD and stroke in comparison with risk factors show convinced confirmity. The frequency of HLP was in females who died by IHD 8 times higher than in males. The death rate in all diabetics was 16.6 % and 56 % of them died by cardiovascular diseases, 42 % were suffering from IHD and 12 % from peripheral occlusions.
Conclusions: Insulin dependent diabetics particularly females exhibit a high level of coronary risk factors. During follow up risk factors are diminished. Out of the influence of therapy it can be explained by the high levels of risk factors in the patients group which died.

# Contribution to the Discussion

E. Nüssel

The results of the reported epidemiologic studies raise the question how risk factors can be tackled in the sense of interventive prevention on a large scale.

The mass communicative intervention - with the help of television, radio and press and the structural intervention - based on law and order - are relatively well developed in many countries.

The interpersonal intervention, based on communication between human beings, however, is underdeveloped.

In the so-called Eberbach/Wiesloch-Study some experience was gathered in developing this form of intervention:

-   It is necessary and possible to motivate the local physicians, Kindergartens, schools, factories, clubs and the local administration to collaborate in partnership.

-   In nearly all social groups we find citizens developing intervention measures on their own initiative and creativity. They are also responsible for the practical application. All activities are carried out in an honorary capacity, possibly supported by private donations.

-   All preventive activities are co-ordinated by a steering group comprising representatives of all social groups, as well as the local physicians.

This model - we call it "Kommunale Prävention" - was initiated in Eberbach. In the meantime it has stood the test in Wiesloch. 98 % of the population in both towns took part in the first screening for detecting risk factors. We presume that the high participation is due to the characteristic of the model.
A similarly high participation at a 10% random sample examination was recently reached in Eberbach. There we found that from men aged 30 to 45, classified as smokers in 1976, 30 % have given up smoking in the ensuing five years. This observation is in contrast to the prevailing trend in the FRG. How far this remarkable change in smoking behaviour is directly related to our activities remains to be proven.

# Cardiovascular Epidemiology and Preventive Community Programmes in Austria

H. P. Rhomberg

In 1977 a coronary risk factor survey was carried out in the village of Oberperfuß, Tyrol. Adults aged between 20 and 64 years (295 men and 316 women) corresponding to 70 and 75% of the population participated in the basic survey. In subsequent years the attempt was made in a community orientated intervention programme to lower the three major risk factors: smoking, hypertension and hypercholesterinaemia. After three years significant results were obtained as far as cholesterol and blood pressure reductions were concerned. However, no significant changes in smoking habits were observed (1).

Based on the experience of this pilot study a further study was started in the neighbouring village of Zirl (population approx. 4500). Under the Austrian health service system all adults are entitled to one free preventive medical examination per year as well as minimum urine, blood and cholesterol laboratory tests and women are also entitled to a Pap test. During the first year of our study all persons aged 19 and above and resident in Zirl were invited to make an appointment with their general practitioners for a medical check up (each month 10% were invited but in the two sommer months no invitations were sent out). More than a quarter of those invited took advantage of the offer. By the end of the second year 35 % of the target population had been examined once or twice. Dietary counselling for those requiring it was also provided by trained hospital dieticans visiting Zirl. Data analysis was centralised.

In the entire Land of Vorarlberg (population 270 000) a preventive programme aiming at early detection of coronary risk factors and cancer started 10 years ago and is still in progress. An evaluation of mortality and morbidity in recent years as compared to other Austrian Länder where such an intense programme did not take place, is under way.

Reference

1. Rhomberg, H.P. (1981) Koronare Risikofaktoren in einer ländlichen Bevölkerung und deren Beeinflußbarkeit innerhalb von 3 Jahren - Wien. klin.Wschr. 93, Suppl. 127

## 5.2 Hypocholesterolemia – A Risk Factor?

# Clinical Associations of Hypocholesterolaemia

B. Lewis and M. Mancini

There is cogent evidence to justify the treatment of hypercholesterol-aemia in individuals with elevated levels of low density lipoprotein (LDL), and to reduce the mean plasma cholesterol of populations at high risk of coronary disease (1,2). However cholesterol and its precursor hydroxymethylglutaryl CoA are important metabolic inter-mediates, and unesterified cholesterol is an obligatory component of the plasma membranes of all cells. As circulating LDL is a major source of the cholesterol of extrahepatic cells, it may be hypothe-sized that very low plasma levels of this lipoprotein may have un-toward effects. The hypothesis merits critical examination, for it has bearing on recommendations to the population to restrict intake of saturated fatty acids and cholesterol, and on the use of lipid-lowering drugs in clinical practice.

Five sets of data are relevant to this issue:
   i. the epidemiological associations of low plasma cholesterol
  ii. the effects of fat intake in experimental carcinogenesis
 iii. clinical and metabolic findings in genetic hypolipidaemic states
  iv. studies of mechanisms that could account, directly or indirectly, for an association between low cholesterol levels and non-cardio-vascular diseases
   v. the effects of plasma cholesterol reduction on non-cardiovascular disease rates.

## i Epidemiology

This is addressed by three contributors to the Workshop. Of 27 longi-tudinal studies in several countries reviewed by Feinleib (3), 15 showed evidence that men in the lowest quintile of plasma cholesterol were at increased risk of developing cancer. The reason for the inconsistency between these surveys is unclear but may be due in part to the relatively small size of many surveys in the context of cancer epidemiology, particularly interpreting organ-specific data. Dr.Feinleib reports on a 24 year follow-up of the Framingham cohort. Multivariate analysis showed a significant inverse relationship between cholesterol level and cancer risk in men, but not in women (the association has been confined to males in all studies except the Finnish Social Insurance Institution data reported by Dr. Pyörälä).

Men with low cholesterol levels are at low risk of coronary heart disease, and Dr. Feinleib has examined the extent to which increased cancer risk might be a consequence of competing mortality; no support for this explanation was obtained in an analysis of men 55-64 years with cholesterol levels <6 or >6 mmol/l.

One of the difficult obstacles to understanding a cholesterol-cancer association, the "chicken-egg problem" is whether low cholesterol levels are a precondition of cancer risk or whether they merely reflect

early undiagnosed cancer or a precursor disease such as benign colonic
neoplasms.  In the Framingham data exclusion of cancer cases presenting
in the first 6 years of follow-up slightly attenuated but did not
abolish the inverse relationship between cholesterol levels and risk.
Dr. Pyörälä discusses the very extensive pooled data on 54000 men
analysed by the International Collaborative Group: the low plasma
cholesterol was chiefly a feature of cases dying within 1 year of
measurement, much less evident at 2-5 years and minuscule at 6-10 years;
this favours the view that undiagnosed cancer is largely responsible
for the low cholesterol levels.  However, in one of the 10 participating groups a significant inverse relationship remained at 6-10 years.
He also reported that in the Seven Countries Study no relationship
was observed between serum cholesterol and cancer mortality.

Dr. Tyroler's 20-year follow-up study in Evans County is discussed in
part in section iv.  This is one of the investigations in which cancer
mortality was inversely related to plasma cholesterol; but the association proves to be a complex one in which risk was highest in the upper
and lower tertiles of the cholesterol distribution (increased by 53%
and 42% respectively).  Thus the relationship was U-shaped, rendering
it difficult to envisage any simple causal interpretation.

In contrast with longitudinal studies within single populations, cross-
cultural data reveal strong direct, not inverse, associations between
mortality rates from several common malignancies (colon, breast, pancreatic and ovarian cancers and leukaemia) and the main dietary determinants of plasma cholesterol level, i.e. dietary fat and cholesterol
(4-8). The index of fat intake has been, perforce, its availability
for consumption. These findings are consonant with experimental data
referred to in section ii, and with several case-control studies (7).
Nevertheless, within the low-fat consuming, low mean plasma cholesterol
population of Hiroshima-Nagasaki an inverse relationship was still
apparent.

## ii Experimental data

Interactions between nutrition and the response to organ-selective
carcinogens have been extensively studied over 50 years (e.g. 5-11).
A high fat intake appears to act as a promoter rather than an inducer
in a variety of models of breast and colon carcinogenesis, when chemical carcinogens, radiation or tumour transplantation are employed. Fat
intake of the magnitude typical of Western diets increases the tumour
yield 2-12 fold compared with low fat diets.

Secular changes in dietary habits provide some indication of relationships between fat consumption and noncardiovascular disease rates in
man. In the past 3 decades animal fat intake has increased some 4-fold
in Japan. During this period age-standardised cancer mortality has
risen by 28% (12), despite a decline in gastric cancer. Breast cancer
mortality has risen by 30% during this period, and colon cancer by 135%.

## iii Genetic hypolipidaemias

In abetalipoproteinaemia and homozygous hypobetalipoproteinaemia
LDL and other apo B-containing lipoproteins are absent from plasma,
the total cholesterol level of which is about 1 mmol/l. Such patients
have, i.a., severe neurological deficits, retinopathy and abnormal red
cell morphology.  Dr. Illingworth discusses the evidence suggesting
that impaired absorption and transport of α-tocopherol in these
disorders is responsible for the neurological and retinal lesions,

which did not deteriorate over an 8 year period in patients receiving supplements of the vitamin. (It should be recalled that in Dr.Kane's patient with abetalipoproteinaemia due to absence of apo B100, in whom fat absorption was not impaired, the typical neurological deficits were present; hence a defect of transport of α-tocopherol appears more important than malabsorption.) He also reviews the possibility that the lack of LDL and hypocholesterolaemia, by depriving peripheral cells of their major source of cholesterol, lead to increased sterol synthesis and increased LDL receptor activity in such cells. Though evidence of enhanced synthesis was obtained this was attributable to cholesterol malabsorption. Tissues with a high requirements for LDL-derived cholesterol, i.e. adrenal cortex and corpus luteum, which utilise cholesterol for steroid hormone synthesis, do show some evidence of functional impairment in abetalipoproteinaemia. Dr. Illingworth observed normal basal production of cortisol and adrenal androgens, but a reduced response to ACTH infusion. In this situation of very high demand for cholesterol, absence of LDL is associated with impaired cellular function.

## iv Explanatory hypotheses for a cholesterol-cancer relationship

The biological significance of epidemiological associations is enhanced by the existence of plausible mechanisms to account for them. Two hypotheses are discussed by Dr. Marenah. One concerns the association between retinoids, cholesterol and cancer; if tenable it would imply that low cholesterol levels are merely a confounding variable. In the Evans County study reported by Dr. Tyroler, low plasma retinol was predictive of high cancer risk. (Other studies have shown an inverse relationship between dietary availability of the provitamin, β-carotene, and cancer risk.) Kark (13) has noted that plasma retinol and cholesterol concentrations are directly related; and he has demonstrated by multivariate analysis that while low retinol level is independently predictive of cancer mortality, cholesterol is not predictive if retinol is controlled for.

Dr. Marenah has confirmed, by simultaneous measurements, that plasma retinol and cholesterol levels are positively correlated. She showed that this was attributable to relationships with LDL and very low density lipoproteins. The molar ratio of retinol to retinol-binding protein was independent of cholesterol level. β-carotene levels were directly related to cholesterol and LDL, and also to high density lipoprotein concentration. The metabolic basis of retinol-cholesterol relationships is obscure. Both substances are carried from the small intestine in chylomicrons, but their subsequent transport is separate. Wald (14) has proposed that common dietary factors may determine plasma levels of both retinol and cholesterol; relevant experimental support for this has not been advanced as yet. In Dr. Tyroler's analysis of the Evans County study a striking interaction is demonstrated between social class and cholesterol-cancer associations: using multivariate analysis to control age, smoking and obesity, it was shown that plasma cholesterol was significantly related to cancer mortality only in the lower social class. This is not readily explained. Speculatively, dietary intake of β-carotene, retinol and saturated fat are limited in some members of this lower-income group, resulting in a predisposition to cancer and to hypocholesterolaemia. Also, social class differences may have contributed to the inconsistencies between the published longitudinal studies of cholesterol-cancer associations. Dr. Laskarzewski suggests that familial factors may influence the relationships between dietary cholesterol and plasma LDL, and that these may be associated with cancer risk.

Dr. Marenah also tested the hypothesis that hypocholesterolaemia
alters the chemical and physical properties of cell membranes by
depleting them of unesterified cholesterol; it has been suggested
that abnormal membrane fluidity might predispose to neoplastic change
(15). The composition and membrane fluidity of freshly harvested
lymphocytes was measured in normal men whose LDL cholesterol ranged
from <2 to >7 mmol/l. No significant relationships between membrane
properties and plasma lipoproteins were present. Hence homeostatic
mechanisms appear to be efficient in stabilising cell free cholesterol
content except in extreme circumstances.

A striking relationship between hypocholesterolaemia (<3 mmol/l) and
terminal illness is documented by Dr. Oster. In acute hospital
admissions with a variety of pathology persisting low cholesterol
levels were associated with a high mortality rate. This may be
analogous to the poor prognostic implication of low plasma cholesterol
in protein - energy malnutrition in infants, in which impaired lipoprotein synthesis may account for the hypolipidaemia and the fatty
liver (16).

## v Plasma cholesterol change and non-cardiovascular disease

The incidence of and mortality from non-cardiovascular diseases have
been recorded in several studies involving the reduction of plasma
cholesterol by dietary means or drugs. Such studies have in all
cases been designed for other purposes, e.g. trials of primary or
secondary prevention of coronary heart disease; they were not intended
for, and in many cases their size does not justify drawing conclusions
concerning relationships between cholesterol changes and non-cardiovascular disorders such as cancer. Probably because of small-number
effects the trends in non-cardiovascular mortality are often inconsistent. While the WHO primary prevention trial of clofibrate
suggested an excess cancer risk in the intervention group, the
Coronary Drug Project secondary prevention trial showed similar
cancer mortality rates in the clofibrate and placebo groups. If,
in the WHO study, the excess of cancer in the clofibrate group were
due to the fall of plasma cholesterol, it would be expected that
mortality rates would be higher in the subgroup who responded to the
drug with a reduction in cholesterol level than in those in whom
plasma cholesterol did not fall. In fact total mortality was no
higher, and tended to be lower, in the former subgroup (17).

The outcome of three major dietary primary prevention trials, in
which noncardiovascular mortality was reported, are shown in Table 1.
In one, lipid reduction was associated with increased mortality, in
one there was essentially no change and in the third noncardiovascular
mortality was lower.

## Conclusion

The possible relationship between hypocholesterolaemia and cancer has
been under justifiably close scrutiny. The balance of evidence summarised in this Workshop provides no reason to believe that hypocholesterolaemia is causally associated with cancer in general, nor with
cancer in specific sites. While further studies are desirable, no
evidence has been adduced to suggest that the momentum of coronary
heart disease prevention efforts, by reduction of lipoprotein-mediated
risk, should be reduced.

Table 1. Dietary primary prevention trials, annual rates per cent

|  |  | CHD morbidity | CHD mortality | non-cardio-vascular mortality |
|---|---|---|---|---|
| Finnish Mental Hospital | diet | 0.12 | 0.72 | 2.44 |
| Study (male + female) | control | 0.65 | 1.42 | 2.36 |
| Los Angeles          all | diet | 3.00 | 1.24 | 3.69 |
| Veterans Study | control | 4.13 | 1.50 | 3.08 |
| < 65 y. | diet | 2.63 |  |  |
|  | control | 4.75 |  |  |
| Oslo Heart Study | diet | 0.63 | 0.20 | 0.17 |
|  | control | 1.15 | 0.45 | 0.25 |

References

1. Grundy SM (chairman). Rationale of the diet-heart statement of the American Heart Association. Report of Nutrition Committee. Circulation 1982, 65: 839A-854A

2. Lewis B. Ischaemic heart disease: the scientific bases of prevention. In Progress in Cardiology 10. Eds JF Goodwin, PN Yu, 1981. Philadelphia: Lea and Febiger

3. Feinleib M. Workshop on cholesterol and noncardiovascular mortality. Prev Med 1982, 11: 360-67

4. Armstrong B, Doll R. Environmental factors and cancer incidence and mortality in different countries with special reference to dietary practices. Int J Cancer 1975, 15: 617-31

5. Carroll KK. Lipids and carcinogenesis. J Env Path Toxicol 1980, 3: 253-71

6. Liu K, Stamler J, Moss D, Garside D, Persky V, Soltero I. Dietary cholesterol, fat, fibre and colon cancer mortality: an analysis of international data. Lancet 1979, ii: 782-85

7. Reddy BS, Cohen LA, McCoy GD, Hill P, Weisburger JH, Wynder EL. Nutrition and its relationship to cancer. Adv Cancer Res 1980, 32: 237-343

8. Doll R, Peto R. The causes of cancer. J Nat Cancer Inst 1981, 66: 1191-1308

9. Watson AF, Mellanby E. Tar cancer in mice. The condition of the skin when modified by external treatment or diet. Brit J Exp Path 1930, 11: 311-22

846

10. Weisburger JH, Reddy BS, Wynder EL. Colon cancer: its epidemiology and experimental production. Cancer 1977, 40: 2414-20

11. Chan PC, Head JF, Cohen LA, Wynder EL. Influence of dietary fat on the induction of mammary tumours by N-nitrosomethylurea. J Nat Cancer Inst 1977, 59: 1279-83

12. Department of Statistics and Information. Japanese Ministry of Health and Welfare, 1982.

13. Kark JD, Smith AH, Hames CG. Serum retinol and the inverse relationship between serum cholesterol and cancer. Brit Med J 1982, 284: 152-54

14. Wald NJ. Vitamin A and cancer in humans. In Disease and the Environment. Eds Rees, Purcell. New York: Wiley

15. Oliver MF. Diet and coronary heart disease. Brit Med Bull 1981, 37: 49-58

16. Lewis B, Hansen JDL, Wittman W, Krut LH. Plasma free fatty acids in kwashiorkor and the pathogenesis of the fatty liver. Am J Clin Nutrit 1964, 15: 161-68

17. Committee of Principal Investigators Report on a WHO Cooperative Trial on Primary Prevention of Ischaemic Heart Disease using Clofibrate to lower Serum Cholesterol - Mortality Follow-up. Lancet 1980, ii: 379-384

# On a Possible Inverse Relationship Between Plasma Cholesterol and the Risk of Cancer. The Framingham Study

M. Feinleib

Hypercholesterolemia has been clearly established as a risk factor for cardiovascular disease through innumerable laboratory, clinical, and epidemiological studies. In the last few years, however, some epidemiologic studies have presented evidence that hypocholesterolemia may be a risk factor for non-cardiovascular diseases. The evidence from these studies were presented at a workshop convened at the National Heart, Lung, & Blood Institute in May of 1981. A summary of this workshop has recently been published (1). The evidence is by no means totally consistent. About half of the studies including those in Framingham, Stockholm, Evans County, Hiroshima-Nagasaki, and Honolulu showed an inverse relationship between blood cholesterol and total cancer mortality in men. On the other hand, studies such as those in Tecumseh, the Western Collaborative Study, the Chicago Gas Light Company study, and the Western Electric Study failed to show any relationship. None of the studies has reported any significant relationships between cholesterol and non-cardiovascular diseases in women. A summary of the findings from the Framingham Study (2-4) will serve to illustrate the types of data which have been reported by those that found an inverse relationship.

The Framingham study of cancer consisted of a review of the accumulated records of all 5,209 people who participated in the Framingham Heart Study. Six hundred and ninety-one confirmed cases of cancer were found over a 24 year follow-up period. Ninety-four percent of these malignancies were histologically confirmed. The site distribution of malignancies was similar to that found in the third national cancer survey in the United States. All cancer cases occurring before the fourth biennial examination were excluded and mortality rates were measured starting with the fourth biennial examination because that was the exam for which the most complete data was available on other cofactors which might influence mortality trends. The age-adjusted 20-year mortality from all causes, from coronary heart disease, and from cancer among men in the Framingham Cohort is shown in Figure 1. The denominator populations at risk in the five strata of serum cholesterol consisted of about 250 men in each of the lowest and the highest groups, and 500 men in each of the three middle groups. (Prior to 1970 serum cholesterol was measured. Plasma cholesterol has been measured since then.) A significant direct relationship between cholesterol level and coronary heart disease is evident with the highest stratum having about three times the risk of death from CHD as the lowest stratum. For cancer mortality there is a significant inverse relationship with the lowest stratum having about twice the risk of the highest stratum. The overall trend in mortality from all causes tends to be U-shaped.

848

A number of artifacts may account for these findings and several of them will be discussed here. A major potential bias that has been stressed by many of the investigators is that those who are destined to die from malignancies during the follow-up period already had early malignancies when first examined. Their baseline cholesterols may have been depressed due to the presence of an already existing cancer. The mortality data were therefore reexamined excluding all deaths during the first 4 years after exam 4 and the results are shown in Figure 2. The trends for both CHD and for cancer mortality are almost identical to those shown in Figure 1 where deaths between exam 4 and exam 6 are included. It is, of course, possible that the elimination of the first 4 years' experience does not compensate for the effects of early or occult malignancies and that their effect may last for many years before the tumor is diagnosed or results in death. A similar analysis was therefore performed in relation to the incidence of cancer in contrast to the previous data on mortality. Figure 3 shows that the incidence of cancer during the 18 years after exam 4 parallelled the mortality rate.

**Table 1.** Number of cancer cases occurring in the early and later follow-up

| Serum cholesterol at exam 4, mg/dl | Years of follow-up | | | % in first 6 years |
|---|---|---|---|---|
| | 0–6 | 7–18 | 1–18 | |
| 126–189 | 9 | 32 | 43 | 21% |
| 190–219 | 12 | 46 | 58 | 21% |
| 220–249 | 5 | 57 | 62 | 9% |
| 250–279 | 10 | 33 | 43 | 23% |
| 280–545 | 3 | 16 | 19 | 16% |

Framingham Study, men 35–69 years

Table 1 shows the number of incident cancer cases occurring within the first 6 years of follow-up and also in the subsequent 12 years by baseline level of serum cholesterol. It is seen that there were no significant differences in the proportion of cases occurring during the first 6 years of follow-up in each stratum of cholesterol. If all cancer cases occurring in the first 6 years following exam 4 are excluded from the analysis, we get the trends shown in Figure 4 are obtained. It is seen that there is an inverse relation between the incidence of cancer from the period 6 to 12 years after baseline and the level of serum cholesterol. This would make the hypothesis that an existing malignancy was causing the inverse relationship somewhat more tenuous.

Still another way of examining this issue was to compare the cholesterol levels among cancer cases with those of controls for different durations prior to the diagnosis of the cancers. This is shown in Table 2. The control group consisted of 912 individuals that had cholesterol measurements taken for every exam between exam 4 and 11. It is seen that for all of the intervals the cancer cases had lower cholesterols prior to the diagnosis of the cancer than did the control series. Although the numbers are small for the earlier periods, there is a clear trend for up to 10 years prior to diagnosis for the cancer cases to have lower cholesterols.

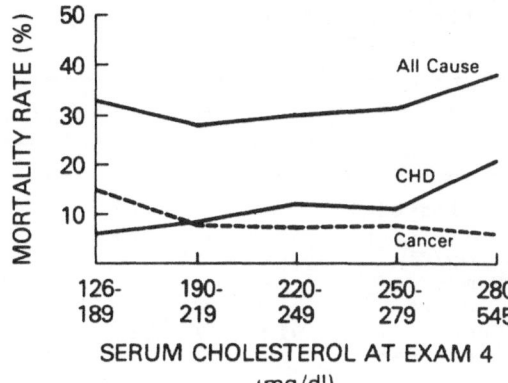

Fig. 1. Age-adjusted mortality rates (20 years) by serum cholesterol measured at Exam 4 of the Framingham Study in men aged 35-64 years

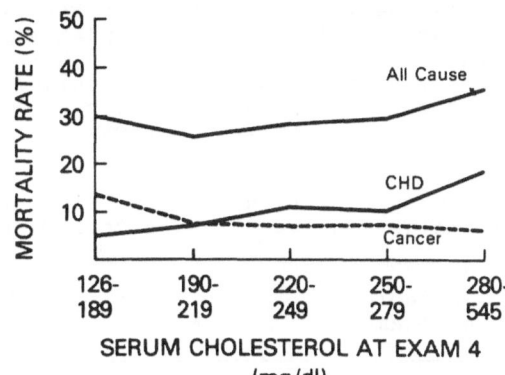

Fig. 2. Age-adjusted mortality rates (20 years) excluding deaths within first four years after Exam 4

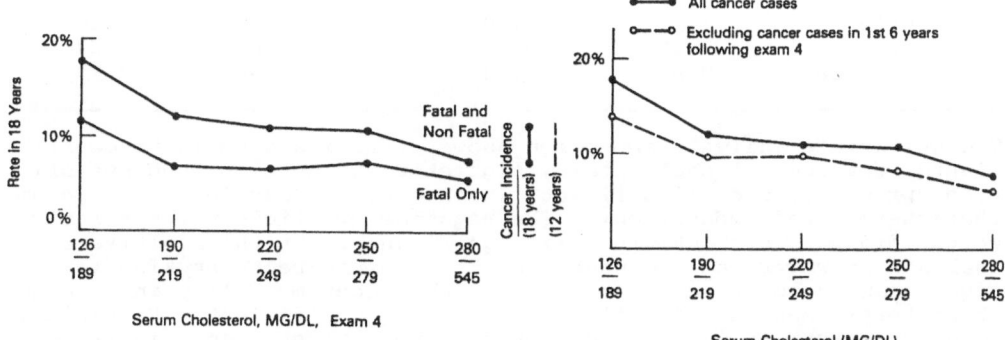

Fig. 3. Age-adjusted mortality and morbidity rates (18 years) for cancer by serum cholesterol measured at Exam 4 of the Framingham Study in men aged 35-69 years

Fig. 4. Age-adjusted incidence rates for cancer by serum cholesterol measured at Exam 4 of the Framingham Study in men aged 35-69 years

Table 2. Difference in serum cholesterol for cancer cases
and noncases

| | Years prior to cancer diagnosis | | | | | | |
| | 14-12 | 12-10 | 10-8 | 8-6 | 6-4 | 4-2 | 2-0 |
|---|---|---|---|---|---|---|---|
| Cholesterol difference mg/dl | -5.5 | -4.0 | -9.1 | -11.3 | -5.1 | -6.6 | -15.8 |
| Number of cases | 28 | 49 | 64 | 80 | 92 | 103 | 113 |
| Number of noncases | 912 | 912 | 912 | 912 | 912 | 912 | 912 |

Framingham Study men 40-69, age-adjusted

It is possible that the inverse relationship between cancer and
cholesterol level can be explained by confounding variables that is,
other risk factors which were associated with both low cholesterol
and the occurrence of cancer. The multiple logistic function was
used to look at the role of several other factors acting simultaneously. The results are shown in Table 3.

Table 3. t-values for logistic function coefficients for cancer
mortality during 20 years following exam 4. Framingham Study

| Variable at exam 4 | Multivariate Analyses | | Univariate Analyses | |
| | Men | Women | Men | Women |
|---|---|---|---|---|
| Ca/Pop | (151/1836) | (146/2242) | (151/1836) | (146/2242) |
| Age | 6.05 | 4.28 | 6.60 | 5.12 |
| Alcohol | 4.27 | 0.84 | 4.82 | 0.19 |
| Serum chol. | -3.10 | -1.09 | -3.25 | 0.88 |
| Cigarettes | 2.80 | -0.38 | 2.17 | -1.52 |
| Education | -1.21 | -0.80 | -3.95 | -2.20 |
| Met. Rel. Wt. | -1.26 | 0.28 | -1.69 | 1.67 |
| Systolic BP | 0.85 | 0.23 | 2.34 | 2.75 |

The univariate analysis among men shows significant positive coefficients for age, alcohol intake, cigarette consumption, and systolic
blood pressure, and significant inverse relationships for serum
cholesterol and education. The negative coefficient for relative
weight did not reach statistical significance. In the multivariate
analysis, however, age, alcohol intake, and cigarette smoking remain
significantly positively associated with cancer mortality and serum
cholesterol had a significant negative coefficient. Education,
relative weight, and systolic pressure no longer had significant
coefficients. Although among women several of the cofactors had
significant coefficients in the univariate analysis, only age
remained significant in the multivariate analysis. It should be
stressed here, however, that the covariables available for analysis
were those that were collected in relation to studies of cardiovascular disease. Other covariables which may be more strongly related
to cancer occurrence were not available in this data base.

Table 4.  Comparison of cancer mortality adjusting for competing risk
of coronary heart disease, men 55-64.  Framingham Heart Study

|  | Cancer mortality 20 years Chiang's life table method | |
| --- | --- | --- |
| Baseline cholesterol at Examination 4 | Crude rate | Rate, eliminating CHD death |
| Low  < 240 mg/dl | 19.7% | 20.0% |
| High > 240 mg/dl | 14.3% | 14.5% |

Another possible explanation for the inverse association between
cholesterol level and cancer mortality is that of competing risks
from other diseases.  In particular, since coronary heart disease
has a positive association with cholesterol level it is possible
that there is a greater chance for people with low cholesterol to
die of non-coronary causes.  This issue was explored by using a
competing risk analysis based on a life table method described by
C. L. Chiang (5).  The population was dichotomized at a level of 240
mg/dl of cholesterol into a low and high cholesterol group as shown
in Table 4. The cancer mortality rate over 20 years was observed to
be 19.7% in the low cholesterol group versus 14.3% in the high
cholesterol group.  When deaths due to CHD were eliminated and
adjustments made using the competing risk life table method, the
estimated net cancer mortality rate was 20% in the low cholesterol
group and 14.5% in the high cholesterol group.  Thus, it does not
seem likely that competing risk of death has produced the inverse
relationship between cancer and cholesterol levels.

There are still other factors that might be considered in assessing
the epidemiologic relationship of serum cholesterol to cancer
occurrence.  As stated previously, data from other studies are not
entirely consistent with that from Framingham.  About fifteen other
studies have findings roughly similar to that of Framingham but
about a dozen others find no significant relationship.  At the
Workshop it was concluded that there is probably not a causal
relationship between low cholesterol and cancer mortality or incidence but rather that low cholesterol may serve as a marker for some
predisposition to cancer.  Thus, the role of other confounding
factors remains to be explored.  Among these, the leading current
hypothesis is that a deficiency of Vitamin A may be linked to cancer
occurrence and may also be linked to low serum cholesterol levels.
This possibility, as well as numerous others, remains to be explored
by further research.

References
1. Feinleib M (1982) Summary of a workshop on cholesterol and non-
   cardiovascular disease mortality.  Prev Med 11:360-367
2. Williams RR, Sorlie PD, Feinleib M, McNamara PM, Kannel WB,
   Dawber TR (1981) Cancer incidence by levels of cholesterol. JAMA
   245:247-252
3. Feinleib M (1981) On a possible inverse relationship between
   serum cholesterol and cancer mortality. Amer J Epidemiol 114:5-10
4. Sorlie PD, Feinleib M (To be published) The serum cholesterol-
   cancer relationship: An analysis of time trends in the Framingham
   Study
5. Chiang CL (1961) On the probability of death from specific causes
   in the presence of competing risks.  Fourth Berkeley Symposium on
   Mathematic Statistics and Probability, Vol. IV.  Berkeley CA:
   University of California Press.  Pp. 169-180

# Cholesterol and Steroid Hormone Metabolism in Abetalipoproteinemia

D. Illingworth, N. A. Alam, and E. E. Sundberg

Phenotypic abetalipoproteinemia (ABL) may occur on the basis of two genotypically distinct disorders in which affected patients are homozygotes. The classic form of ABL is inherited as an autosomal recessive trait and obligate heterozygote parents have normal concentrations of plasma cholesterol. In contrast, homozygous hypoabetalipoproteinemia (HHBL) is transmitted by an autosomal dominant mode of inheritance and heterozygotes have reduced levels of total and LDL cholesterol. The biochemical and clinical features of ABL and HHBL are similar and both disorders are characterised by a total absence of all apoprotein B containing lipoproteins from plasma, hypocholesterolemia (plasma cholesterol 25-30 mg/dl), acanthocytes and fat malabsorption with steatorrhea. These features are present from birth whereas in untreated patients the development of progressive neurological symptoms and pigmentary retinal degeneration develop insidiously and first become clinically evident in childhood. The present report aims to briefly review three areas: 1) What is the basis for the acquired neurological changes in ABL? 2) Does an absence of plasma LDL result in increased rates of cellular cholesterol synthesis (such as occurs in vitro when cultured cells are grown in LDL depleted media)? and 3) Is steroid hormone production impaired in patients with phenotypic ABL?

## Neurological and retinal dysfunction

Current evidence supports the view that the progressive retinal and neurological symptoms (areflexia, ataxia) which develop insidiously in untreated patients with phenotypic ABL represent a manifestation of vitamin E deficiency. Patients with ABL have a dual deficit in both the absorption and transport of vitamin E. Impaired formation of chylomicrons in the intestinal mucosa results in malabsorption of dietary fats and the fat soluble vitamins whereas the inability to form hepatic VLDL and LDL results in an impaired ability to transport vitamin E in plasma. Recent studies have shown a striking similarity between the neurological lesions which develop in vitamin E deficient rhesus monkeys (Nelson et al 1981) and those which occur in untreated patients with ABL (Miller et al 1980). Several recently discovered cases of phenotypic ABL have also shown neurological improvement following therapy with high doses of vitamin E (Malloy et al 1981). We have documented a lack of progression in neurological and retinal changes in three patients with ABL treated with high dose vitamin E

(200-250 I.U. per kg per day) plus vitamins A and K for a period of 4-8 years. These observations support the view that these acquired degenerative changes are attributable to vitamin E deficiency. Although high dose vitamin E supplements will not raise the serum levels above 2 μg/ml the concentrations of vitamin E in adipose tissue from one patient maintained on 10,000 I.U. per day have recently been shown to be normal (Kayden HJ, Illingworth DR, unpublished).

## Regulation of cholesterol biosynthesis

The concept that an absence of plasma LDL may result in increased rates of cellular cholesterol biosynthesis has been examined in vitro and in vivo. The rate of incorporation of $^{14}C$ acetate into cholesterol by skin biopsies (Brown et al 1975) and freshly isolated mononuclear cells (Ho et al and Table 1) from patients with ABL are 3-6 fold higher than those in normal lipidemic controls. In contrast LDL

Table 1. Cholesterol synthesis in freshly isolated mononuclear cells from patients with abetalipoproteinemia and control subjects

| Subjects | Acetate → cholesterol (pm/$10^7$ cells/5 hr) |
|---|---|
| Abeta  28 M | 218 |
| Abeta   8 M | 120 |
| Homozygous Hypobeta 18 F | 54 |
| Controls (± SEM, n=5) | 38 ± 14 |

degradation by freshly isolated mononuclear cells from patients with ABL appears to be normal (Reichl et al 1978). Total body synthesis of cholesterol (estimated by the sterol balance technique) is twice normal in ABL but in adult patients this increase can be adequately explained on the basis of malabsorption of endogenously secreted biliary cholesterol (Illingworth et al 1980). These studies suggest that despite an absence of LDL the number of LDL receptors and, to a lesser extent, the rates of cellular cholesterol biosynthesis are much lower than would be anticipated from the results of in vitro studies with cells grown in LDL-free culture media.

The lipoprotein particles in the HDL fraction of ABL plasma have an unusual density distribution in which the $HDL_2$:$HDL_3$ ratio is 3 to 1. Most of the apo E in HDL is present in the $HDL_2$ density range and the possibility arises that binding of these particles to cellular receptors may serve to regulate cholesterol synthesis in ABL. To test this hypothesis, cultured human fibroblasts were grown to confluence, derepressed for 24 hrs in lipoprotein-free media and then

854

incubated for 24 hrs in the presence of increasing concentrations of
HDL$_2$ or HDL$_3$ isolated from the plasma of normal and ABL subjects as
well as with LDL and HDL$_2$ from a patient with Type III hyperlipidemia
and apo E III deficiency. Sterol synthesis was determined after
incubation of the cells for a further 5 hrs in the presence of $^{14}$C
acetate (Figure 1). HDL$_3$ from both normal and ABL plasma stimulated

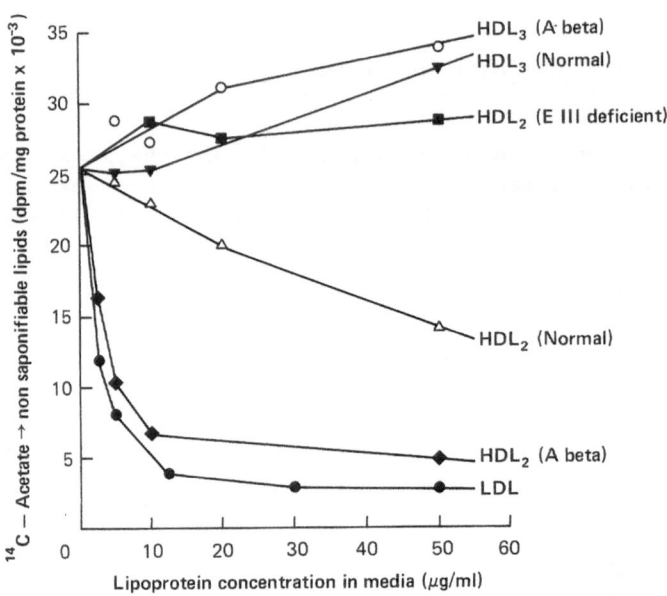

FIG. 1. The effects of plasma lipoproteins from normal subjects and
patients with abetalipoproteinemia on sterol synthesis by cultured
human fibroblasts. Confluent cells were derepressed for 24 hr in 10%
LDS, incubated for 24 hr in the presence of purified lipoproteins and
then incubated for a further 5 hr with 2-$^{14}$C acetate. Each point
represents the mean of duplicate incubations. Lipoprotein concentration is expressed in µg protein/ml

cholesterol synthesis in a concentration-dependent manner whereas incubation of the cells with the HDL$_2$ fraction from a patient with
apo E III deficiency caused a smaller increase. In contrast incubation
of the cells with either LDL or HDL$_2$ from ABL plasma resulted in a
marked inhibition of cholesterol synthesis. The inhibition observed
with HDL$_2$ from ABL plasma was several-fold greater than that seen with
normal HDL$_2$ and, when expressed in terms of the cholesterol content
of the lipoproteins, HDL$_2$ from ABL was a more effective inhibitor than
normal LDL. These results suggest that the apo E rich HDL$_2$ present in
the plasma of patients with ABL may serve to regulate cholesterol
homeostasis in this disorder.

Steroid hormone production in abetalipoproteinemia

Receptor mediated uptake of LDL appears to be most important in
tissues which actively synthesize steroid hormones such as the corpus
luteum and adrenal cortex (Carr et al 1981a,b). These tissues possess
the greatest number of LDL receptors in vivo and, when cultured in
vitro, secrete significantly larger amounts of progesterone or cortisol
when the culture medium contains LDL. If cellular uptake of LDL cholesterol is indeed critical for optimal rates of steroid hormone biosynthesis, then steroidogenesis should be impaired in patients with
phenotypic ABL. Such an impairment would be expected to be most
evident for those hormones with the highest specific rates of production per gram of tissue. Recent studies have documented normal
basal rates of production of adrenal corticosteroids in 3 patients
with phenotypic ABL (Illingworth et al 1982a,b) but have provided
evidence for an impaired response to prolonged stimulation with ACTH
(Figure 2). This was manifest by lower serum concentrations of

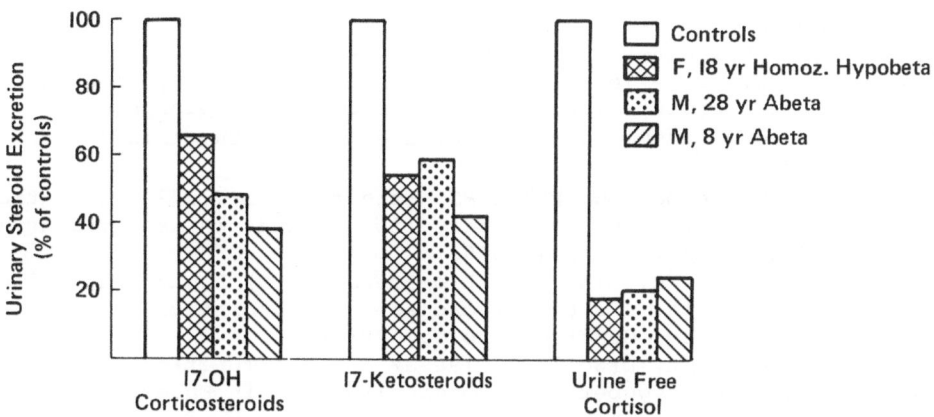

FIG. 2. Rates of excretion of 17 hydroxycorticosteroids, 17 keto-
steroids and urine free-cortisol during ACTH infusion (24-36 hr) in
three patients with phenotypic abetalipoproteinemia and control
subjects

cortisol as well as by reduced rates of excretion of 17 OHCS, 17 KS,
and urine-free cortisol. Serum concentrations of progesterone during
the mid-luteal phase of the ovarian cycle in one young woman with HHBL

were also reduced (maximal 1.6 ng/ml; normal 5-10 ng/ml). Taken together these studies suggest that a complete lack of LDL does not impair steroid hormone production in the basal state but does lead to an impairment when the rates of steroid secretion are high (e.g. ACTH stimulation or luteal phase of the ovarian cycle). Thus, despite the ability of $HDL_2$ from ABL plasma to inhibit cholesterol synthesis in vitro the rate of in vivo uptake of these particles by the adrenal cortex appears to be insufficient to meet the increased demands for cholesterol which result from ACTH stimulation.

Acknowledgements  The cooperation of our patients and the care provided by the staff of the Clinical Research Center is appreciated. This work was supported by USPHS Grant HL28399 and by the General Clinical Research Center Program (RR334). DRI is a recipient of a Research Career Development Award (HL00953).

## References

Brown MS, Brannan PG, Bohmfalk HA, Brunschede GY, Dana SE, Helgeson J, Goldstein JL (1975) Use of mutant fibroblasts in the analysis of the regulation of cholesterol metabolism in human cells. J Cell Physiol 85: 425-436.

Carr BR, Simpson ER (1981a) Lipoprotein utilization and cholesterol synthesis by the human fetal adrenal gland. Endocrine Rev 2: 306-326.

Carr BR, Sadler RK, Rochelle DB, Stalmach MA, MacDonald PC, Simpson ER (1981b) Plasma lipoprotein regulation of progesterone biosynthesis by human corpus luteum tissue in organ culture. J Clin Endocrinol Metab 52: 875-881.

Ho YK, Faust JR, Bilheimer DW, Brown MS, Goldstein JL (1977) Regulation of cholesterol synthesis by low density lipoproteins in isolated human lymphocytes. J Exp Med 145: 1531-1549.

Illingworth DR, Connor WE, Lin DS, DiLiberti J (1980) Lipid metabolism in abetalipoproteinemia: a study of cholesterol absorption and sterol balance in two patients. Gastroenterology 78: 68-75.

Illingworth DR, Kenny TA, Orwoll ES (1982a) Adrenal function in heterozygous and homozygous hypobetalipoproteinemia. J Clin Endocrinol Metab 54: 27-33.

Illingworth DR, Kenny T, Connor WE, Orwoll ES (1982b) Corticosteroid production in abetalipoproteinemia: evidence for an impaired response to ACTH. J Lab Clin Med (in press).

Malloy MJ, Kane JP, Hardman DA, Hamilton RL, Dalal KB (1981) Normotriglyceridemic abetalipoproteinemia. J Clin Invest 67: 1441-1450.

Miller RG, David CJF, Illingworth DR, Bradley W (1980) The neuropathy of abetalipoproteinemia. Neurology 30: 1286-1291.

Nelson JS, Fitch CD, Fisher VW, Brown GO, Chou AC (1981) Progressive neuropathologic lesions in vitamin E deficient rhesus monkeys. J Neuropath Exp Neurol 40: 166-186.

Reichl D, Myant NB, Lloyd JK (1978) Surface binding and catabolism of low density lipoprotein by circulating lymphocytes from patients with abetalipoproteinemia. Biochim Biophys Acta 530: 124-131.

# Associations Between Plasma Cholesterol, Cell Membrane Composition and Fluidity, and Retinoid Concentrations in a Normal Male Polulation

C. B. Marenah, B. Lewis, D. Hassall, N. E. Miller, D. Mitchell, K. Bruckdorfer, B. Slavin, C. Cortese, A. La Ville, and P. Turner

Reduction of plasma cholesterol levels by diet and, when appropriate, by other means is a widely accepted component of programmes to reduce coronary heart disease risk[1]. In preventive medicine risk/benefit considerations are even more exacting than in therapy[2]; hence any suggestion that low cholesterol levels might have adverse effects deserves close scrutiny. Some prospective studies have shown an increased risk of total cancer mortality[3] or colon cancer deaths[4] in the lowest quintile of plasma cholesterol, though this was not observed in other studies[5,6].

Cholesterol is a ubiquitous component of animal cells functioning as a constituent of plasma membranes[7] and a precursor of biologically-important steroids. Extrahepatic cells, though capable of cholesterol synthesis, appear to obtain this sterol largely by internalisation of low density lipoprotein (LDL), in situ synthesis being largely repressed[8]. The key precursor of cholesterol, HMGCoA, is also required for production of non-steroid intermediates important in cell function: isopentenyladenine, dolichol and ubiquinone[9].

Many hypothetical bases may be considered for a low cholesterol-cancer association, if one exists. These include an effect of competing mortality or a hypocholesterolaemic effect of undiagnosed cancer[10] or of a precursor lesion. Plasma retinol[11], and dietary intake of β carotene[12], are inversely related to cancer mortality, and the predictive power of low cholesterol levels has been attributed to a direct association between plasma levels of cholesterol and retinol[13]. Other hypotheses imply a causal role of low cholesterol levels in cancer. Thus it has been proposed that reduction of plasma cholesterol depletes cells of cholesterol, leading to deleterious changes in fluidity of the plasma membrane[14], alternatively that low plasma cholesterol may be associated with increased bile acid excretion (bile acids being promoters of colon cancer in experimental models).

In the present study we have investigated two of these hypotheses, relating to plasma membrane fluidity and associations between cholesterol and retinoid transport. Plasma cholesterol was measured in a population sample of 300 men aged 25-55 years, free from overt illness and not taking therapeutic diets or drugs known to influence lipid metabolism. Of these a sample of 150 representing the lowest, modal and highest quintiles of plasma cholesterol were recalled in the fasted state. No subject had xanthomas or xanthelasmas. Blood samples were obtained for measurement of lipoproteins (by preparative ultra-centrifugation and enzymatic lipid analyses) and of retinol and β carotene (by high pressure liquid chromatography) and for isolation of lymphocytes (centrifugation through Ficoll-Hypaque). Fluidity of lymphocyte plasma membranes was measured at 37°C using the fluorescent probe diphenylhexatriene, and their free cholesterol and phospholipid contents measured enzymatically and by colorimetry respectively.

Due to regression to the mean some redistribution of plasma cholesterol
levels was seen in the second sampling; plasma membrane studies and
retinoid levels were therefore related to the distributions of plasma
lipids and lipoproteins at the time of recall (very low density lipo-
protein=VLDL, low density lipoprotein=LDL, high density lipoprotein=
HDL).

## Results and discussion

The lymphocyte observations are compared in Table 1 with distributions
of plasma and lipoprotein cholesterol concentrations.

Table 1. Free cholesterol/phospholipid molar ratio (FC/PL) and relative
microviscosity (RMV) of lymphocytes (mean±SD), by quintile of plasma
and lipoprotein cholesterol (ranges in mmol/l)

| Quintile | I | II | III | IV | V |
|---|---|---|---|---|---|
| Plasma chol | 3.2-5.0 | 5.1-5.5 | 5.6-6.3 | 6.4-7.3 | 7.4-10.0 |
| FC/PL | 0.46±0.30 | 0.52±0.28 | 0.52±0.38 | 0.61±0.40 | 0.57±0.32 |
| RMV | 0.90±0.05 | 0.89±0.05 | 0.90±0.05 | 0.89±0.04 | 0.90±0.04 |
| VLDL chol | 0.01-0.18 | 0.19-0.30 | 0.31-0.52 | 0.53-0.77 | 0.78-2.78 |
| FC/PL | 0.47±0.35 | 0.44±0.33 | 0.54±0.28 | 0.64±0.37 | 0.68±0.35 |
| RMV | 0.91±0.05 | 0.90±0.04 | 0.90±0.04 | 0.89±0.04 | 0.88±0.04 |
| LDL chol | 1.45-3.10 | 3.11-3.60 | 3.61-4.11 | 4.12-5.01 | 5.02-7.55 |
| FC/PL | 0.58±0.32 | 0.49±0.27 | 0.53±0.42 | 0.68±0.40 | 0.50±0.28 |
| RMV | 0.88±0.04 | 0.90±0.04 | 0.88±0.05 | 0.91±0.04 | 0.89±0.04 |
| HDL chol | 0.87-1.33 | 1.34-1.47 | 1.48-1.66 | 1.67-1.79 | 1.80-2.55 |
| FC/PL | 0.57±0.35 | 0.50±0.33 | 0.53±0.43 | 0.60±0.25 | 0.50±0.36 |
| RMV | 0.91±0.05 | 0.88±0.04 | 0.91±0.04 | 0.92±0.05 | 0.89±0.04 |

The lymphocyte free cholesterol/phospholipid ratio showed a non-significant trend to higher values in the higher quintiles of plasma cholesterol; this was attributable to a relationship between the FC/PL ratio
in lymphocytes and VLDL-cholesterol in plasma. There was no relationship between the lymphocyte FC/PL ratio and either LDL cholesterol or
HDL-cholesterol. There were no discernable relationships between lymphocyte microviscosity at 37ºC and levels of cholesterol in plasma or in
any lipoprotein class; correlation coefficients between these variables
ranged from -0.16 to 0.018. There were no statistically-significant
differences between the FC/PL ratios or RMVs in Quintile I and those
of other quintiles of cholesterol or lipoprotein fractions.

The direct relationship between plasma cholesterol and retinol levels[13]
was confirmed ( Table 2 ). It was attributable to correlations
between plasma retinol and VLDL-and LDL-cholesterol levels, while HDL
cholesterol showed no relationship with retinol. Retinol-binding
protein levels showed similar associations. The molar ratio of retinol
to retinol-binding protein showed no evident relationships with
cholesterol or lipoprotein levels, and was less than unity in all

groups. Plasma β-carotene levels showed a direct relationship with cholesterol in plasma and its constituent lipoproteins, which was most pronounced with LDL and HDL cholesterol.

Relationships between the distributions of plasma lipoproteins and levels of plasma retinoids are shown in Table 2.

Table 2. Plasma retinol (μg/l), retinol-binding protein (RBP, mg/l), β-carotene (μg/l) as means±SD, and retinol/RBP molar ratio, by quintile of plasma and lipoprotein cholesterol (ranges in mmol/l)

| Quintile | I | II | III | IV | V |
|---|---|---|---|---|---|
| Plasma cholesterol | 3.2-5.0 | 5.1-5.5 | 5.6-6.3 | 6.4-7.3 | 7.4-10.0 |
| retinol | 602±177 | 682±150* | 749±167** | 749±150*** | 776±252** |
| RBP | 59±13 | 65±11 | 70±12** | 71±17** | 73±18** |
| β carotene | 368±177 | 433±227 | 429±176 | 584±278*** | 505±278* |
| ret/RBP | 0.74±0.13 | 0.76±0.07 | 0.78±0.12 | 0.79±0.12 | 0.77±0.11 |
| | | | | | |
| VLDL chol | 0.01-0.18 | 0.19-0.30 | 0.31-0.52 | 0.53-0.77 | 0.78-2.78 |
| retinol | 625±169 | 693±180 | 746±167** | 708±137* | 804±253** |
| RBP | 60±12 | 67±16* | 71±15** | 66±11* | 75±19*** |
| β carotene | 495±239 | 447±264 | 510±259 | 478±207 | 389±223 |
| ret/RBP | 0.75±0.11 | 0.76±0.11 | 0.77±0.12 | 0.79±0.13 | 0.78±0.11 |
| | | | | | |
| LDL chol | 1.45-3.10 | 3.11-3.60 | 3.61-4.11 | 4.12-5.01 | 5.02-7.55 |
| retinol | 621±199 | 672±140 | 737±162* | 787±244** | 742±163* |
| RBP | 61±14 | 64±11 | 68±13* | 73±20** | 72±14** |
| β carotene | 362±175 | 456±228* | 446±242 | 536±252** | 524±247** |
| ret/RBP | 0.75±0.13 | 0.76±0.11 | 0.79±0.13 | 0.78±0.08 | 0.76±0.12 |
| | | | | | |
| HDL chol | 0.87-1.33 | 1.34-1.47 | 1.48-1.66 | 1.67-1.79 | 1.80-2.55 |
| retinol | 702±183 | 729±222 | 710±161 | 712±225 | 712±170 |
| RBP | 66±13 | 71±17 | 67±14 | 68±17 | 66±14 |
| β carotene | 383±225 | 387±164 | 508±244* | 500±216* | 549±294** |
| ret/RBP | 0.78±0.10 | 0.74±0.13 | 0.78±0.07 | 0.77±0.13 | 0.79±0.13 |

*$P<0.05$; **$P<0.01$; ***$P<0.001$, compared with Quintile 1.

The mean of the highest quintile of plasma cholesterol was almost two-fold greater than that of the lowest quintile; for VLDL there was a 12-fold difference and for LDL it was more than two-fold. Despite the considerable range of lipoprotein levels, the lymphocyte microviscosity measurements showed complete independence between membrane fluidity and plasma cholesterol and lipoprotein levels. The ratio of free cholesterol to phospholipid is a major determinant of membrane fluidity. There was no discernable correlation between this ratio and LDL cholesterol concentration ($r=-0.017$), this lipoprotein being of greatest interest because its internalisation is the major source of cholesterol in extrahepatic cells[8] and because LDL cholesterol is closely correlated with total plasma cholesterol in man. The ratio was greater in cells from subjects in the highest quintile of VLDL-cholesterol. The biological significance of this is uncertain, and it was not reflected in differences in fluidity. Despite the evidence that HDL can function as an acceptor of cell free cholesterol, there was no evidence of an inverse relationship between HDL cholesterol levels and lymphocyte free cholesterol content or free cholesterol/phospholipid ratio; nor did lymphocyte microviscosity show any association with HDL cholesterol.

Lymphocytes were employed as a model of cell membrane composition
and structure in the present study not only because of their access-
ability but because they could be harvested in sufficient numbers
to permit analyses in their native state, and because they possess
the homeostatic mechanisms of the LDL pathway regulating their free
cholesterol content[15]. To the extent that lymphocytes are representative of other cells possessing a regulated high-affinity receptor-
mediated mechanism for uptake of LDL cholesterol, it may be inferred
that the ranges of LDL cholesterol and of total plasma cholesterol
seen in normal British men are not determinants of cell membrane
fluidity or cholesterol/phospholipid ratio in such cells. The LDL
pathway appears ubiquitous in nucleated extrahepatic cells which have
been investigated[16], and is also demonstrable in hepatocyte membranes
under certain circumstances[17]; presumably this highly regulated mechanism effectively stabilises cell free cholesterol content except in
extreme situations such as abetalipoproteinaemia. One reservation must
be expressed. While the cells of solid tissues are exposed to interstitial fluid concentrations of LDL, the circulation of lymphocytes
between lymph nodes and plasma exposes them, for a small proportion of
their life span, to full plasma concentrations of LDL. Work is therefore in progress to study the homeostasis of cell membrane fluidity in
cells other than lymphocytes.

The observations on retinol concentrations confirm the finding of a
direct association with plasma cholesterol level[13]. They show, furthermore, that this association reflects direct correlations with LDL
cholesterol and VLDL cholesterol levels,.but not with HDL cholesterol.
The mechanism of this relationship is unclear; retinol and cholesterol,
though both lipophilic, have distinct transport proteins except after
intestinal absorption when they share carriage in chylomicrons and
chylomicron remnants. Impressive evidence has been presented that
plasma retinol and cholesterol have common dietary determinants[18].
However the known correlations between diet and plasma cholesterol
within single populations, though significant, account for a relatively
small part of the variance of the latter; and dietary preformed retinol
intake is not closely related to plasma levels of the vitamin except
in previously malnourished persons. The correlation between β carotene
and cholesterol levels is explicable on the basis of its transport in
the apolar core of LDL and HDL. Whatever the basis of the direct
relationship between retinol and cholesterol levels, our findings are
similar to those made by Kark and his colleagues (on stored serum) and
are compatible with their conclusion from multivariate analysis of
Evans County, Georgia data that plasma retinol, but not cholesterol,
is independently predictive of cancer mortality[13].

We gratefully acknowledge the help of the Medical Department of the
Greater London Council.


References

1. Lewis B (1980) Dietary prevention of ischaemic heart disease: a
   policy for the 80's. Brit Med J 281:177-80

2. Rose G (1981) Strategy of prevention: lessons from cardiovascular
   disease. Brit Med J 282:1847-51

3. Williams RR, Sorlie PD, Feinleib M, McNamara PM, Kannel WB, Dawber TR
   (1981) Cancer incidence by level of cholesterol. J A M A 245:247-52

4. Rose GA, Blackburn H, Keys A, Taylor HL, Kannel WB, Paul O, Reid DD,
   Stamler J (1974) Colon cancer and blood cholesterol. Lancet i:181-83

5. Dyer AR, Stamler J, Paul O, Shekelle RB, Schoenberger JA, Berkson DM, Lepper M, Collette P, Shekelle S, Lindberg H (1981) Serum cholesterol and risk of death from cancer and other causes in three Chicago epidemiological studies. J Chron Dis 34:249-60

6. Cambien R, Ducimetiere P, Richard J (1980) Total serum cholesterol and cancer mortality in a middle-aged male population. Am J Epidem 112:388

7. Cooper RA (1977) Abnormalities of cell-membrane fluidity in the pathogenesis of disease. New Eng J Med 297: 371-77

8. Brown MS, Faust JR, Goldstein JL (1975) Role of the low density lipoprotein receptor in regulating the content of free and esterified cholesterol in human fibroblasts. J Clin Invest 55:783-93

9. Fears R (1981) The contribution of the cholesterol biosynthetic pathway to intermediary metabolism and cell function. Biochem J 199:1-7

10. Rose G, Shipley MJ (1980) Plasma lipids and mortality: a source of error. Lancet i: 523-26

11. Wald N, Idle M, Boreham J, Bailey A (1980) Low serum vitamin A and subsequent risk of cancer: preliminary results of a prospective study. Lancet ii: 813-15

12. Shekelle RB, Lepper M, Liu S, Maliza C, Raynor WJ, Rossof AH, Paul O, Shryock AM, Stamler J (1981) Dietary vitamin A and risk of cancer in the Western Electric Study. Lancet ii:1186-89

13. Kark JD, Smith AH, Hames CG (1982) Serum retinol and the inverse relationship between serum cholesterol and cancer. Brit Med J 284:152-54

14. Oliver MF (1981) Diet and coronary heart disease. Brit Med Bull 37:49-58

15. Ho YK, Brown MS, Bilheimer DW, Goldstein JL (1976) Regulation of low density lipoprotein receptor activity in freshly isolated human lymphocytes. J clin Invest 58:1465-1474

16. Goldstein JL, Brown MS (1977) The low-density lipoprotein pathway and its relation to atherosclerosis. AnnRev Biochem 46:897-930

17. Mahley RW, Hui DY, Innerarity TL, Weisgraber KH (1981) Two independent lipoprotein receptors or hepatic membranes of dog, swine and man. Apo-B, E and apo-E receptors. J Clin Invest 68: 1197-1206

18. Wald NJ (1981) Vitamin A and cancer in humans. In Disease and the Environment. Eds Rees, Purcell. Wiley, New York

# The Prognostic Significance of Hypocholesterolemia in Hospitalized Patients

P. Oster, M. Kohlmeier, F. Nold, and G. Schlierf

It has been a uniform finding of prospective and cross sectional studies that the plasma cholesterol level is a potent risk factor for coronary heart disease (1). In the last years, however, a discussion has emerged, whether low cholesterol levels (especially below 180 mg/dl) could be associated with an increased risk of cancer (2). Several papers of this workshop deal with this relationship. We performed two studies in freshly hospitalized patients in order to evaluate the clinical prognosis of severe hypocholesterolemia. The results emphasize the variety of causes for hypocholesterolemia and the poor prognosis of these patients.

## Study 1

Serum cholesterol determinations were performed in patients admitted consecutively to the medical department of the University of Heidelberg by means of the SMA-12 Autoanalyzer. In 200 of 3,700 patients hypocholesterolemia below 120 mg/dl was found, which, on the next day, could be confirmed in 91 patients. From the remaining 109 patients 65 had now levels above 120 mg/dl, 24 had died and 20 patients were discharged or transfered to other hospitals. In the 91 patients with two hypocholesterolemic values ultracentrifugation analysis of lipoproteins was performed according to LRC procedures, phospholipids were determined with a test kit from Boehringer Mannheim, FRG (3). The results are expressed as medians.

The mortality of the 91 patients with two consecutive serum cholesterol values below 120 mg/dl was 32 %, compared to a mortality of 7.3 % in all 3,700 patients. From the original group of 200 hypocholesterolemic patients at least 53 died (26.5 %). The patients were grouped into 5 disease categories (Table 1).

Table 1. Disease groups associated with hypocholesterolemia

|  | n | Deaths | % Deaths |
|---|---|---|---|
| 1. malignancies | 18 | 6 | 33 |
| 2. liver disease | 29 | 9 | 31 |
| 3. malabsorption | 10 | 1 | 10 |
| 4. heart disease | 22 | 8 | 36 |
| 5. miscellaneous | 12 | 5 | 42 |

The mortality was lowest in the malabsorption and highest in the miscellaneous group (4 sepsis, 2 tubelculosis, 2 Guillain Barre paralysis, 1 hyperthyroidism, 1 malaria, 1 acute renal failure, 1 hemorrhagic gastritis). Two characteristics were common in many patients regardless of the grouping. These were anemia (hemoglobin < 12 g/dl for men and < 10.5 g/dl for women), and the need for parenteral nutrition (40 % glucose and amino acid solutions). Of the latter group the mortality rate was 18.2 %, of the former it was 27.6 %. 30 % of the patients were kachectic ( < 90 % of ideal body weight) 10 of them died (33 %). The mortality of the 91 hypocholesterolemic patients was equally distributed in all age groups; in total serum (0.66) and especially in the LDL and HDL fractions the cholesterol/phospholipid ratio was markedly decreased.

## Study 2

Serum lipid determinations were performed in 100 patients, consecutively admitted to a geriatric hospital (mean age 77 years), with enzymatic methods and test kits from Boehringer Mannheim, FRG.

In 11 patients hypocholesterolemia below 120 mg/dl was found. Four of these patients (36 %) died (leukemia, stroke and CHD, pneumonia, metastatic carcinoma) in contrast to 8 % of the whole group. Five of the 11 patients had serum cholesterol levels below 100 mg/dl, 3 of them died, 2 had to have emergency surgery (sepsis, ileus). The diagnoses of the remaining hypocholesterolemic patients, who were discharged from the hospital in relatively good condition, were plasmacytoma, chronic schizophrenia and diabetes mellitus, pneumonia, TIA and a suspected intraabdominal tumor and stroke.

The lipid values of the elderly patients are given in Table 2.

Table 2. Serum lipid values (mg/dl) in 100 geriatric patients and in a subgroup of 11 hypocholesterolemic patients ( < 120 mg/dl)

|  | Triglycerides | Cholesterol | HDL–Chol. | Free chol. | Phospholipids |
|---|---|---|---|---|---|
| n = 100 |  |  |  |  |  |
| median | 130 | 199 | 34.6 | 62 | 200 |
| range | 30 – 669 | 79 – 402 | 0.5 – 86.5 | 28 – 133 | 97 – 440 |
| n = 11 |  |  |  |  |  |
| median | 114 | 103 | 16.8 | 40 | 188 |
| range | 86 – 288 | 83 – 115 | 10.1 – 25.6 | 28 – 49 | 125 – 280 |

Half of the patients had serum cholesterol values below 200 mg/dl, the median of HDL cholesterol was low. The patient with the highest HDL cholesterol level also had the highest total cholesterol; the correlation between total and HDL cholesterol was positive (p < 0.05). The most striking finding in the hypocholesterolemic patients was a markedly decreased cholesterol/phospholipid ratio (0.55) of whole serum lipids.

## Discussion

Severe hypocholesterolemia as defined by total plasma cholesterol levels below 120 mg/dl existed in 2.5 % of patients admitted to a university hospital and in 11 % of patients admitted to a geriatric hospital. In a health and nutrition survey of 20 – 40-year-old Heidelberg men (4) 0.6 % of the subjects had hypocholesterolemia (108 – 119 mg/dl). One had an acute viral illness prior to cholesterol determination, two had chronic gastrointestinal disease and two reported strenuous physical activity.

Hypocholesterolemia in hospitalized patients is associated with a 5-fold increased mortality. The key to the pathophysiological understanding of this finding might be the markedly decreased cholesterol/phospholipid ratio; the relation of cholesterol to phospholipids being important for membrane function and platelet aggregation (5, 6). On the other hand, hypocholesterolemia can be found in a variety of conditions without indicating a poor prognosis (3). Together with the poor reproducibility of low cholesterol values (91 from 200 in study 1) on the next day, which may be explained by regression to the mean or spontaneous course of disease) epidemiological data about the prognostic significance of hypocholesterolemia should include at least two cholesterol measurements and take into account the health status of the person at the time of cholesterol determination; then possibly existing correlations would become much stronger.

## Abstract

Hypocholesterolemia below 120 mg/dl in two studies was associated with a 5-fold increased mortality when measured after admission to the hospital. A variety of diseases was associated with low cholesterol levels, a uniform finding being a markedly decreased cholesterol/phospholipid ratio. The fact that low cholesterol levels could be confirmed in less than 50 % of the patients on the next day may be a cautionary note for epidemiological studies with single cholesterol determinations.

## References

1. Kannel, WB, Castelli WP, Gordon T, McNamara PM (1971) Serum cholesterol, lipoproteins and the risk of coronary heart disease. The Framingham Study. Ann. Intern. Med. 74: 1-12
2. Peterson B, Trell E, Sternby NH (1981) Low cholesterol level as risk factor for noncoronary death in middle-aged men. JAMA 245: 2056-2057
3. Oster P, Muchowski H, Heuck CC, Schlierf G (1981) The prognostic significance of hypocholesterolemia in hospitalized patients. Klin. Wochenschr. 59: 857-860
4. Arab L, Schellenberg B, Schlierf G (1981) Ernährung und Gesundheit. Eine Untersuchung bei jungen Frauen und Männern in Heidelberg. Karger, Basel
5. Cooper RA, Shatill SJ (1980) Membrane cholesterol - is enough too much? New Engl. J. Med. 302: 49-51
6. Stuart MJ, Gerrard JM, White JW (1980) Effect of cholesterol on production of thromboxane $B_2$ by platelets in vitro. New Engl. J. Med. 302: 6-10

# The Association of Low Serum Cholesterol Level to the Risk of Cancer. Significance with Respect to Dietary Modification for Coronary Heart Disease Prevention

K. Pyörälä

Within the multifactorial etiological framework of atherosclerotic
vascular disease, a high population average level for plasma total
cholesterol, mainly reflecting the level of low density lipoprotein
cholesterol, is a key characteristic of those "western" or
"westernized" populations which have a high incidence of coronary heart
disease (CHD). In these populations the large majority of people have
elevated plasma cholesterol levels as compared with "biologically
normal" values. Elevation of plasma cholesterol level often clusters
with the presence of other CHD risk factors, like elevated blood pressure and cigarette smoking, and in fact the large majority of CHD events
occur among people with mild or moderate elevations of these risk
factors and not among the small group of individuals with markedly
elevated risk factor levels. Therefore, an approach aiming to a general
lowering of risk distribution in the population is needed in the
primary prevention of CHD. Diets of populations having high average
levels of plasma cholesterol have a high content of saturated fats and
cholesterol, and concomitantly, consumption of complex carbohydrates is
often low and the total intake of calories excessive in relation to
energy expenditure. Therefore, a population approach aiming to a
lowering of the population distribution of plasma cholesterol requires
progressive changes in the national diets with respect to above factors.

An association between a low plasma cholesterol level and an increased
risk of death from cancer recently observed in several prospective
population studies has lead to extensive efforts for a further clarification of this question having potential relevance with respect to
attempts to lower plasma cholesterol for CHD prevention. At a Workshop on Cholesterol and Non-cardiovascular Disease Mortality, held in
May 1981 at the National Institutes of Health in the U.S.A., 17 studies
addressing this question were reported and, furthermore, data were
available from 9 other studies reported in the literature (1). The
results of these studies were far from consistent; an inverse association between plasma cholesterol and total cancer mortality was observed in 14 studies, but was not found in 12 studies. In those
studies which shoved an increased cancer risk at the lowest plasma
cholesterol level the risk was, on an average, 1.7 times higher than
at the population's average plasma cholesterol level. In 5 studies
a significant inverse association was found between plasma cholesterol
and mortality from colon cancer. The panel of experts reviewing these
reports concluded that despite inconsistencies among the findings from
various studies there was in some of them a weak association between
very low plasma cholesterol level and colon cancer and, if present,
this association did not disappear, while adjustment was made for
potential confounding variables. The panelists considered that the
data available did not substantiate any direct cause and effect relationship between low plasma cholesterol and cancer. After giving recommendations for further research the panelists expressed as their
unanimous opinion that "the data did not preclude, countermand or
contradict the current public health message which recommends that those
with elevated cholesterol levels seek to lower them through diets lower
in saturated fat and cholesterol".

A small number of cancer deaths has been a problem in many of the
previously published studies, particularly in analyses concerning
specific sites of cancer.  The International Collaborative Group recently completed an analysis on the association between plasma
cholesterol and the risk of cancer death among 60,000 middle-aged men
from 10 population studies in 7 countries, (Denmark, 1 study; Finland,
2 studies; France, 1 study; Japan, 1 study; U.K., 2 studies; and
U.S.A., 3 studies) (2).  Standardized plasma cholesterol levels of
nearly 1,500 persons dying of cancer were compared with those of remaining men.  In analyses of combined results of these studies, men
dying of cancer within 1 year of the cholesterol determination had mean
plasma cholesterol levels 25-30 mg/dl lower than the rest of the men.
This inverse association between plasma cholesterol and cancer death,
however, diminished markedly with time.  For 2-5 years after baseline
the mean cholesterol for cancer decedents was only 4-5 mg/dl lower than
for others and for 6-10 years after baseline the corresponding difference was less than 2 mg/dl.  These differences were highly significant
for the first year (p < 0.001), less significant for years 2-5
(p < 0.05), and no more significant for years 6-10.  As to cancer at
specific sites, lung cancer mortality was inversely associated with
plasma cholesterol in the first year, but thereafter no significant
association was observed.  No significant association was found between
plasma cholesterol level and colon cancer mortality.  The individual
studies generally followed the above pattern, with only one exception.
In the Finnish Social Insurance Institution's study, the difference in
the mean plasma cholesterol level of cancer decedents and others increased with the follow-up time, being -8 mg/dl for years 6-10
(p < 0.05).  Analyses on the plasma cholesterol-cancer relationship in
this study population have been extended also to female participants
of the study and to the total incidence of colon cancer within a 10-
year follow-up period based, in addition to death certificates, to
hospital discharge data (3).  In women a statistically significant,
inverse association was found between baseline plasma cholesterol and
incidence of colon cancer in years 5-10.  In men this association was
not statistically significant.

The main result of the International Collaborative Group analyses - an
inverse association between plasma cholesterol and mortality from all
cancers during the first year, diminishing and disappearing thereafter
- is consistent with the hypothesis that this association is due to an
effect of undetected cancer on plasma cholesterol level, rather than to
an increase of cancer risk caused by a low plasma cholesterol.  The
question concerning the association between plasma cholesterol level
and incidence of colon cancer appears to be more complicated, some
studies, like the Finnish Social Insurance Institution's study, showing
an increased cancer risk appearing several years after the measurement
of plasma cholesterol.  Further studies are needed for a better delineation of this association in different populations and such studies
should examine the total incidence of colon cancer, including non-fatal
cases.  Further research should also be directed to possible biological
explanations of the association between hypocholesterolemia and colon
cancer, in case this association becomes repeatedly confirmed in
epidemiological studies.

Although there is some evidence for an association between a low plasma
cholesterol level and the risk of colon cancer, this risk, if true,
does not appear to be large.  The position of the individual at the
low end of the population distribution of plasma cholesterol may be a
"marker" of colon cancer risk, rather than a low plasma cholesterol
level as such.  With respect to the safety of dietary modification
recommended for lowering population distribution of plasma

cholesterol in populations with high plasma cholesterol mean values, it is important to note that many populations with traditional diets compatible with low plasma cholesterol levels, like Japanese and some Southern European populations, have an excellent life expectancy and no particular increase in the incidence of colon cancer.

In conclusion, on the basis of available evidence there appears to be reasonable assurance of safety concerning a dietary lowering of the population distribution of plasma cholesterol in populations with a high incidence of CHD.

References

1. Feinleib M (1982) Summary of a workshop on cholesterol and non-cardiovascular mortality.  Prev Med 11:360-367
2. International Collaborative Group (1982) Cancer and cholesterol: inverse association?  IX World Congress of Cardiology, June 20-26, 1982, Moscow, USSR, Abstracts, Volume II, 333
3. Aromaa A, Reunanen A, Knekt P, Maatela J, Unpublished results

# Serum Cholesterol and Cancer Mortality in White Males: Social Class Effects, Evans County Twenty Year Follow-Up Study

H. A. Tyroler, M. G. Knowles, C. E. Davis, J. Kark, I. Peleg, S. Heyden, and C. G. Hames

## A.  Introduction

Recent studies of the relationship between cholesterol and noncardio-vascular disease, particularly cancer, have produced inconsistent results.  The association of cholesterol with cancer, when present, appears stronger (or present only) for males than females (1).  Several investigators report no association between cholesterol and cancer (2); others suggest that inverse associations are attributable to subclinical disease at time of cholesterol determination (3, 4).  Kark et al. (5) reported an inverse association between cholesterol and cancer incidence, in the Evans County study population, followed for a period of fourteen years.  Davis et al. (6) demonstrated that the association in the Evans County Study was curvilinear over a 20 year period. We extend the Evans County analyses testing the hypothesis that rural, lower social status, farming occupations modify the cholesterol cancer association.

## B.  Materials and Methods

The Evans County Study included a 50% random sample of residents ages 15-39 and 100% ages 40 and older, 92% of whom were examined in 1960-62. Serum cholesterol was determined using a modified Abell-Kendall method (7) with quality control established by the Center for Disease Control, Atlanta, Georgia (CDC).  For the present analysis, 2,654 persons aged 25 and older were studied over a 20 year follow-up period.  Three persons who died of cancer within one year of intake, and 57 persons missing intake cholesterol values were excluded.  Nine hundred and eighty-seven deaths occurred over the 20 years; 177 had mention of cancer present at time of death.

Age, race, sex specific cholesterol tertiles were constructed.  Survival time was calculated from date of intake examination until death, loss of follow-up, or end of follow-up period, when 1,615 persons were alive and 52 of unknown vital status.  Social class was measured by the McGuire White method (8) and the white male population dichotomized on median score into upper and lower social class strata.  Kaplan-Meier survival curves were constructed separately for each social class. The proportional hazards model (9) was used to assess the relation between cancer mortality and cholesterol controlling for potential confounders.

## C.  Results

Sixty-three of the 177 cancer deaths occurred among white males.  Kaplan-Meier survival function curves were used to estimate the life table adjusted cumulative percent deaths within race-sex-age specific cholesterol tertiles (see Table 1).

Table 1.  Evans County Twenty Year Cancer Mortality Study, Cumulative Percent Dead* by Cause, Cholesterol Tertile and Social Class - White Males

| Social Class | Cholesterol Tertile | | | |
| --- | --- | --- | --- | --- |
| | Low | Mid | High | Total |
| *All Cause Mortality* | | | | |
| Upper (147/391)** | 26 | 35 | 49 | 38 |
| Lower (191/425) | 46 | 43 | 50 | 46 |
| Total (338/816) | 39 | 39 | 49 | 42 |
| *All Non-CVD, Non-Cancer, Non-Violent Mortality* | | | | |
| Upper (23/391) | 6 | 7 | 8 | 7 |
| Lower (37/425) | 17 | 7 | 9 | 11 |
| Total (60/816) | 12 | 7 | 8 | 9 |
| *Cancer Mortality* | | | | |
| Upper (24/391) | 7 | 4 | 11 | 8 |
| Lower (39/425) | 16 | 6 | 14 | 12 |
| Total (63/816) | 12 | 5 | 13 | 10 |

*Based on Kaplan-Meier analysis:  % Mortality = (1-% survival)
**Number deaths
 Number at risk

Mortality risk from all causes combined increased stepwise with increasing cholesterol for upper social class white men.  There was a slight suggestion of a curvilinear relation of all causes mortality to cholesterol in lower social class men who had higher mortality than upper social class men, particularly at the lowest cholesterol levels.  The risk of dying from non-cardiovascular, non-cancer causes, excluding violent deaths, was unrelated to cholesterol among upper class white males; however, the risk was twice as high for the low cholesterol compared to the other tertiles among lower social class males.  Cancer mortality was increased for men with both highest and lowest cholesterol values.  The excess was particularly prominent in the lowest cholesterol tertile for low social class men.

Survival differences among groups stratified by cholesterol levels were apparent early in the follow-up and persisted over twenty years.  Men with mid-level serum cholesterol had greatest survival free of cancer.  Men with both high and low cholesterol levels exhibited increasingly greater cancer mortality with passage of time.

870

Multivariable regression analyses of the relation of cholesterol to
time to cancer death, controlling for the possible confounding effects
of age, smoking, and body mass (Quetelet Index) were performed for
white males stratified by social class (see Table 2).

Table 2. Evans County Twenty Year Cancer Mortality Study, Multivariate
Analysis* of Factors Predicting Time to Death from Cancer by Social
Class - White Males

|  | Upper Social Class (USC) | | Lower Social Class (LSC) | |
|  | β | (p) | β | (p) |
| --- | --- | --- | --- | --- |
| Age | 0.088 | (0.000) | 0.118 | (0.000) |
| Cholesterol | -0.023 | (0.599) | -0.062 | (0.001) |
| Cholesterol$^2$ | 0.006 | (0.524) | 0.015 | (0.001) |
| Smoking | 1.644 | (0.005) | 0.279 | (0.431) |
| Quetelet Index | -0.695 | (0.135) | 0.154 | (0.568) |
| Farm | 0.446 | (0.374) | -0.019 | (0.956) |

*Cox Proportional Hazard Model
Smoking:  0 = No, 1 = Yes
Farm:     0 = Farm Occup., 1 = Non-Farm Occup.
Death:    Cancer (140-209, 8th ICDA)

There was a highly statistically significant curvilinear association
of cholesterol with cancer mortality in LSC men; this relationship
was present, but was not statistically significant in the USC.  Farming
occupations were not associated with cancer mortality in either social
class.

D.  Discussion

The twenty year follow-up in the Evans County Heart Study cohort confirms the earlier report of an association of cancer mortality with
baseline cholesterol levels, but presents a more complex set of findings than that simply of an inverse linear association.  The risk of
cancer mortality among males varied in a curvilinear manner with serum
cholesterol.  The association, in Evans County, was demonstrable excluding all cancer deaths occurring during the first year, was present
over the entire period of follow-up, and appeared to increase with
duration since cholesterol determination.

The findings for white men persisted controlling for smoking and weight.
The possibility of pre-existant occult, latent malignancy with subtle
effects on lipid metabolism cannot, of course, be addressed in this
study.

The statistically significant curvilinear relationship of cholesterol
with cancer in white men was contributed primarily by LSC men.  In
Evans County these were predominantly blue collar laborers and farmers,
in contrast to men of professional, business and white collar occupations in USC.

Fifty percent of USC vs 2% of LSC males were in professional, white collar occupations. Approximately 35% of both USC and LSC persons were in farming occupations. Blue collar and service workers represented 60% of the LSC occupations vs 13% of USC.

The social class attribute which exposes the cholesterol cancer association would appear not to be related to farming occupations exposures per se. The proportion in farming occupations was similar in USC and LSC and farming per se was not a significant predictor of cancer mortality in the proportionate hazards model.

Kark et al. (10) have reported on the inverse association of serum retinol and cancer risk in the Evans County Study, a finding replicated by Wald (11). More recently Kark et al (12) have reported a correlation between serum cholesterol and retinol which may provide an explanation for the observed cholesterol cancer association. The analysis of findings in Evans County suggests that regardless of the explanation ultimately derived for the associations detected, appreciable elevation in cancer mortality risk was associated only with the extremes of the cholesterol distribution and increase in cancer mortality risk with low cholesterol was marked only in lower social class men. A similar increase was present for all non-cancer, non-CVD, non-violent deaths among low social class, low cholesterol white men. This was reflected in the association of all cause mortality with cholesterol levels in low social class white men. The markedly different cholesterol - cancer mortality relation in upper and lower social class men residing in the same community, i.e., Evans County, suggests the possibility of different physiologic meaning of low cholesterol in different environments. This may shed light on the differences in the cholesterol cancer association reported from diverse population studies (1, 13, 14, 15) and points to the need to explicate possibly different determinants of low cholesterol in different social and environmental circumstances.

## References

1.  Feinleib M (1981) On a possible inverse relationship between serum cholesterol and cancer mortality. Am J Epidemiol 114: 5
2.  Dyer AR, Stamley J, Paul O, Shekelle RB, Schoenberger JA, Berkson DM, Lepper M, Collette P, Shekelle S, Lindberg HA (1981) Serum cholesterol and risk of death from cancer and other causes in three Chicago epidemiological studies. J Chronic Dis 34: 249
3.  Combian F, Dulcimetiere P, Richard J (1980) Total serum cholesterol and cancer mortality in a middle-aged male population. Am J Epidemiol 112: 388
4.  Rose G, Shipley MJ (1980) Plasma lipids and mortality: A source of error. Lancet 1: 523
5.  Kark JD, Smith A, Hames CG (1980) The relationship of serum cholesterol to the incidence of cancer in Evans County, Georgia. J Chronic Dis 33: 311
6.  Davis CE, Knowles M, Kark J, Heyden S, Hames CG, Tyroler HA (1982) chapter in *Dietary Fats and Health*. Serum cholesterol levels and cancer mortality: Evans County Twenty-Year Follow-Up Study (in press)

7.  Tyroler HA, Heyden S, Bartel AG, Cassel J, Cornoni JC, Hames CG, Kleinbaum D (1971) Blood pressure and cholesterol as coronary heart disease risk factors.  Arch Intern Med 128: 907
8.  McGuire C, White GD (1955) The measurement of social status. Research paper in Human Development No. 3, Department of Educational Psychology, The University of Texas
9.  Cox DR (1972) Regression models and life tables (with discussion). J Royal Stat Soc B 34: 187
10. Kark J, Smith A, Switzer BR, Hames CG (1981) Serum vitamin A (retinol) and cancer incidence in Evans County, Georgia.  J Natl Cancer Inst 66: 7
11. Wald N, Idle M, Boreham J, Batley A (1980) Low serum vitamin A and subsequent risk of cancer:  Preliminary results of a prospective study.  Lancet 2: 813
12. Kark J, Smith A, Switzer BR, Hames CG (1981) Retinol, carotene, and the cancer/cholesterol association.  Lancet 1: 1371
13. Kagan A, McGee DL, Yano K, Rhoads GG, Nomura A (1981) Serum cholesterol and mortality in a Japanese-American population: The Honolulu Heart Program.  Am J Epidemiol 114: 11
14. Kozarevic Dj, Penezica S, McGee D, Vojvodic N, Gordon T, Racic Z, Zukel W, Dawber T (1981) Serum cholesterol and mortality:  The Yugoslavia Cardiovascular Disease Study.  Am J Epidemiol 114: 21
15. Garcia-Palmieri MR, Sorlie PD, Costas R Jr, Havlik RJ (1981) An apparent inverse relationship between serum cholesterol and cancer mortality in Puerto Rico.  Am J Epidemiol 114: 29

# 5.3 Smoking and Atherosclerosis

# Carbon Monoxide and Atherosclerosis

P. Astrup

There is clear evidence that moderately elevated carboxyhemoglobin levels are associated with various changes of the cardiovascular system. Those changes occur at carboxyhemoglobin levels of 5-2o %, often found in inhaling smokers.

## Physiological effects of carbon monoxide of possible atherogenic significans

A very significant change is the increased vascular permeability. Carbon monoxide exposure (2o-25 % COHb) of men for 3 hours leads to a 5o % increase in disappearance rate from the blood of injected serum $I^{135}$-albumin (1), and to an increase in capillary filtration rate measured plethysmographically on the calf (2).

The occurence of increased permeability during exposure to carbon monoxide could also be demonstrated in dogs, where the lymph flow and the protein flux in the thoracic duct increased considerably. It was of interest that the increase in protein flux was more pronounced for the high molecular proteins than for the low molecular ones (3).

Carbon monoxide exposure also leads to hyperlipemia (4,5). The induced elevation of serum cholesterol has usually led to 15 % higher levels for the first 2 to 3 weeks of exposure in comparison to the groups not exposed to carbon monoxide, after which the levels have been approximately the same in the two groups. Hypoxia has a similar effect.

Finally, acut exposure of human individuals to carbon monoxide leading to about 15 % carboxyhemoglobin levels leads to a decrease in bleeding time, to an increase in circulating aggregates of thrombocytes, and to a decreased aggregability of thrombocytes stimulated with ADP or collagen, with a normalisation of all parameters after 1 1/1 hours, when the carboxyhemoglobin level is considerably elevated of 2 cigarettes with high nicotine content, leading to carboxyhemoglobin levels of only 3 %, the effects were 2-3 times greater, while the inhalation of nicotine-free cigarettes did not have any effects (6).

## Atherogenic and arterial wall injuring effects of carbon monoxide

The mentioned effects on vascular permeability and on serum cholesterol are clearly atherogenic, and were related to our previous findings in 1967 (4), that moderately elevated carboxyhemoglobin levels for 8-10 weeks were associated with an up to 15o % increased accumulation of cholesterol in the arterial walls of cholesterol-fed rabbits. However, when keeping serum cholesterol concentration on the same level in two groups of animals, exposed or not exposed to

CO, by individual cholesterol feeding, no enhancement of the cholesterol accumulation in the arterial walls occurs (7). Further, the cholesterol uptake rate in the arterial intima of carbon monoxide exposed animals, measured by using a sophisticated double isotope technique, was not increased either, except in the aortic arch where a slight increase was demonstrated. The perhaps more important coronaries were not investigated.

Since the hypercholesterolemic effect of carbon monoxide exposure is observed only in the first weeks of exposure, this explains that the enhancement of arterial accumulation of cholesterol has been difficult to observe in long-lasting experiments, 40-60 weeks or more, with serum cholesterol levels highly increased in both the exposed and the non-exposed groups of animals for a long period.

The pathologists in our group observed microscopical changes in the arterial intima of non-cholesterol fed rabbits exposed to 180-200 ppm carbon monoxide (14-16 % COHb) for a few weeks (9). The injuries were first of all characterized by an increased subendothelial edema and other lesions indistinguishable from what by experienced investigators have been described as early atherosclerotic intimal changes. However, other pathologists of the team (9) were later unable to repeat findings of intimal damage caused by carbon monoxide exposure by using a blind technique. The experiments were repeated by using carbon monoxide concentration from 200 up to 4000 ppm, with the same lack of evidence of a direct histotoxic effect of carbon monoxide on the intima/subintima of coronary arteries and aortas. Therefore, our conclusions are today, that moderate carbon monoxide exposure does not lead to morphological changes of the vascular wall.

The well documented higher prevalence of atherosclerosis in smokers in comparison to non-smokers is clearly correlated to their carboxyhemoglobin levels, since it can be calculated, that smokers with carboxyhemoglobin levels of 5 % or more have a 21 times higher prevalence of atherosclerosis than smokers with a carboxyhemoglobin level of 3 % or less (10). This does not mean, however, that a causal relationship exists. To my knowledge no evidence has so far been documented for a clear, unambigious atherogenic effect of carbon monoxide, neither in epidemiological studies nor in animal experiments. This has not been the case either with animal experiments with nicotine exposure or tobacco smoke exposure.

It would be of great importance if the atherogenic components of tobacco smoke and the involved pathological effects could be identified, since this might give us a better understanding of the atherogenic process itself, and also might lead to a better prevention of the vascular diseases caused by tobacco smoking.

877

*References*

1. Parving. H.-H. 1972.  The effect of hypoxia and carbon monoxide on plasma volume and capillary permeability to albumin.  *Scand. J. clin. Lab. Invest.* 3o: 49-56.
2. Siggaard-Andersen J., K. Kjeldsen, F. Bonde Petersen and P. Astrup. 1967.  A possible connection between carbon monoxide exposure, capillary filtration rate, and atherosclerosis.  *Acta Med. Scand.* 182: 397-399.
3. Parving, H.-H., K. Ohlsson, H.J. Buchardt-Hansen and M. Rørth. 1972.  Effect of carbon monoxide exposure on capillary permeability to albumin and alfa$_2$-macroglobulin.  *Scand. J. clin. Lab. Invest.* 29: 381-388.
4. Astrup, P., D. Trolle, H.M. Olsen and K. Kjeldsen.  1975.  Effects of moderate hypoxia exposure on fetal development.  *Arch. environm. Health.* 3o: 15-16.
5. Kjeldsen, K. 1969.  Smoking and Atherosclerosis.  Thesis. pp. 145. Munksgaard, Copenhagen.
6. Madsen, K., J. Dyerberg and P. Astrup:  Unpublished results.
7. Stender, S., P. Astrup and K. Kjeldsen. 1977.  The effect of carbon monoxide on cholesterol in the aortic wall of rabbits. *Atherosclerosis.* 28: 357-367.
8. Armitage, A.K., R.F. Davies and D.M. Turner. 1976.  The effects of carbon monoxide on the development of atherosclerosis in the white carneau pigeon. *Atherosclerosis.* 23: 333-344.
9. Hugod, C., L.H. Hawkins, K. Kjeldsen, H.K. Thomsen and P. Astrup. 1978.  Effect of carbon monoxide exposure on aortic and coronary intimal morphology in the rabbit. *Atherosclerosis.* 333-342.
1o. Wald, N., S. Howard, P.G. Smith and K. Kjeldsen. 1973.  Association between atherosclerotic diseases and carboxyhaemoglobin levels in tobacco smokers.  *Brit. Med. J.* 1: 761-765.

# The Influence of Smoking on Plasmalipoproteins

J. Augustin, B. Beedgen, L. Buchholz, A. Gnasso, W. Haberbosch, U. Spohr, and
G. Schettler

## Introduction

In several studies over the past decades a high incidence of coronary heart disease
in smokers has been demonstrated (1). But it is still unclear how tobacco components
are related to the development of atherosclerosis. A variety of mechanisms have been
hypothesized for hypercholesterolemia and hypertension regarding the etiology of
coronary heart disease. No information is available regarding the molecular basis of
the smoking effect on atherogenesis. In addition there is little experimental evidence
to explain epidemiological data. Recently in a number of studies a correlation between
smoking and certain plasma lipids has been reported (2, 3). HDL cholesterol as a
negative risk factor for coronary heart disease was found to be lower in cigarette
smokers (4-6). Acute effects of cigarette smoking or nicotine on lipoprotein metabolism
had not been reported so far. For this reason we designed studies on the effect of
acute smoking and orally absorbed nicotine on intravascular lipolytic activities, lipids
and apoproteins in different plasmalipoproteins. In addition epidemiological data
support the finding that smoking and especially nicotine have a profound influence on
lipoprotein metabolism.

## Methods

To investigate acute effects of cigarette smoking on plasma lipids and lipoproteins,
20 fasting, young smokers between the age of 23 - 28 inhaled the smoke of two cigarettes
(nicotine content 1.84 mg/cigarette) within 15 min. Ten sham smokers served as
controls. Blood samples were taken before, during and up to 60 min. after the procedure. To test the influence of nicotine, 16 healthy, young volunteers chewed nicotine-containing gums (16 mg) for 30 min. Sequential separation of lipoproteins from
EDTA plasma into density classes $< 1.006$ g/ml (VLDL), $1.006 - 1.063$ g/ml (LDL)
and $> 1.063$ g/ml (HDL) was achieved in duplicates with the Beckman airfuge. For
apoprotein quantification plasma samples were centrifuged in the Beckman L8-70 centri -
fuge with a 70.1 TI rotor. Separation of lipoproteins was monitored by lipoprotein
electrophoresis. Zonal ultracentrifugation was performed with the Beckman 40 TI
rotor with a discontinuous gradient. Cholesterol, triglycerides and phospholipids
were determined with Boehringer Mannheim kits; free fatty acids were measured with
the method of Nowack (7); lipases immunochemically according to Greten et al. (8);
plasma nicotine levels were determined by gaschromatography according to Hengen et
al. (9) Catecholamines were measured by the method of DaPrada et al. (10), densitometric quantification of apo C-peptides was performed after ultrathin flatbed isoelectric focussing. Statistics with levels of significance ($p < 0.05$) were evaluated
according to Wilcoxon-Wilcox (11).

## Results

During smoking plasma nicotine levels rose from 46 ($+$ 4) to 148 ($+$ 5) nmol/l, free
fatty acids from $972.5 + 126.7$ to $1303.4 + 147.6$ $\mu$mol (Fig. 1). Hepatic triglyceride
lipase and lipoprotein lipase were considerably activated without intravenous injection
of heparin (Fig. 2a). Plasma triglycerides fell from $149 + 7.4$ to $123.3 + 7.6$ mg%,
VLDL-triglycerides from $79.7 + 6$ to $57.4 + 5.4$ mg%. In addition, LDL-triglycerides,

**Fig. 1**

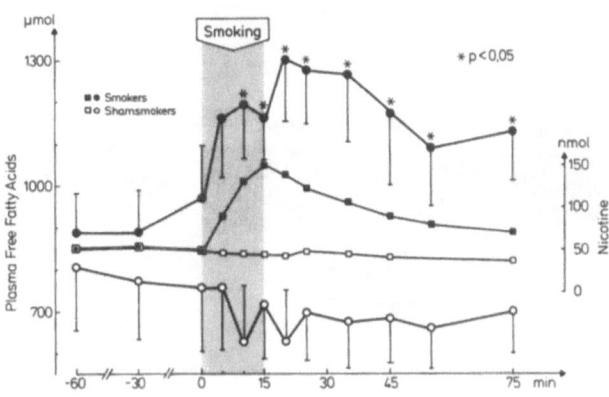

Smoking and Lipids
Free Fatty Acids [●○] and Nicotine [■□]

**Fig. 2a and 2b**

**A**  Acute effects of
SMOKING ON PLASMA LIPOPROTEINS

SMOKING results in

| | | | |
|---|---|---|---|
| ↑ | Plasma nicotine | 46 → | 148 nM |
| | Free fatty acids | 0.97 → | 1.3 mM |
| | HTGL | 323 → | 444 U |
| | LDL - TG | 36 → | 48 mg% |
| | LDL - PL | 66 → | 81 mg% |
| | LDL - Chol. | 95 → | 103 mg% |
| ↓ | VLDL - TG | 80 → | 57 mg% |
| | HDL - PL | 138 → | 119 mg% |
| | HDL - Chol. | 60 → | 55 mg% |

**B**  Acute effects of
NICOTINE ON PLASMALIPOPROTEINS

CHEWING NICOTINE GUMS results in

| | | | |
|---|---|---|---|
| ↑ | Plasma nicotine | 42 → | 159 nM |
| | Free fatty acids | 0.96 → | 1.12 mM |
| | HTGL | 185 → | 344 U |
| | LDL - TG | 23 → | 26 mg% |
| | LDL - PL | 72 → | 76 mg% |
| | LDL - Chol. | 108 → | 112 mg% |
| ↓ | VLDL - TG | 61 → | 54 mg% |
| | HDL - PL | 105 → | 100 mg% |
| | HDL - Chol | 49 → | 45 mg% |

-phospholipids and -apo B considerably increased. This was accompanied by a decrease in HDL-phospholipids from $138.4 + 9.4$ to $118.7 + 8.5$ mg%. HDL-cholesterol was
also influenced and fell from $59.6 + 4.7$ to $55.2 + 4.5$ mg%. However, this value was
slightly above the level of significance. In summary, these data demonstrate a fundamental influence of acute cigarette smoking on lipoprotein metabolism (Fig. 3). Stimulation of the intravascular lipolytic activities probably leads to an increase of the inter-
conversion of triglyceride-rich lipoproteins to cholesterol-enriched LDL. In addition,
the structure of HDL is influenced, possibly with HDL-LDL-interaction. It has to be
evaluated whether a smoker's HDL is as protective as an HDL from a nonsmoker. The
considerable decrease in HDL-phospholipids with a simultaneously substantial increase
in LDL-phospholipids could be understood as a direct transfer of HDL-phospholipids
to LDL-particles. In a further study we wanted to elucidate whether nicotine is a
component and cigarette smoke responsible for the observed effects on lipoprotein metabolism. A summary of the data is given in Fig. 2b. After oral absorption of nicotine,
again an increase of plasma free fatty acids from 960 ($+ 230$) to 1120 ($+ 35$ μmol/l)
was found. Hepatic triglyceride lipase was again stimulated in this study. A concomitant increase in lipoprotein lipase was not significant. The activation of lipases was

Fig. 3

The Influence of Smoking on Plasma Lipoproteins

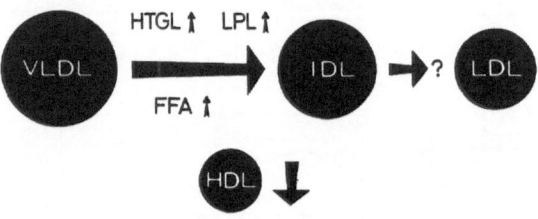

accompanied by a decrease in plasma triglycerides and phospholipids. VLDL-triglycerides fell from 61 (+ 60) to 54 (+ 61). The increase in LDL-cholesterol and -phospho-
lipids was comparable with the data from the study with acute smoking. HDL-cholesterol
fell from 49 (+ 11) to 45 (+ 10) (Fig. 4), HDL-phospholipids from 105 (+ 24) to 100 (+ 27)
mg%.

Fig. 4

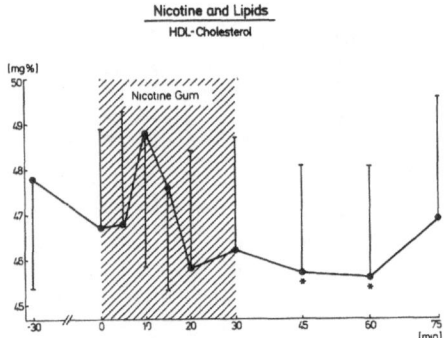

During the absorption of nicotine, a slight increase in epinephrine could be observed
with no change or even a slight decrease in plasma norepinephrine levels (Fig. 5).

Fig. 5

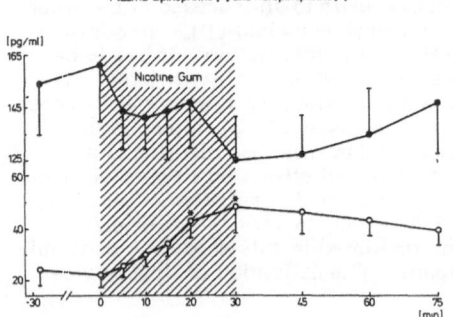

Recently it has been demonstrated that changes in plasma epinephrine levels, as observed in our experiments, are unlikely to explain the considerable increase in plasma free fatty acids found in our study (12). The data indicate that the influence of smoking on lipoprotein lipids is due to the effect of nicotine with activation of intravascular lipolysis and degradation of triglyceride-rich lipoproteins, which are then found in the LDL-density range. In addition, important changes in the HDL-composition could be demonstrated. Simultaneous measurement of plasma epinephrine and norepinephrine revealed that under these conditions circulating catecholamines are of minor importance in the regulation of intravascular lipolysis. Only a nicotine-mediated release of norepinephrine at local sympathetic synapsis with an adipose tissue might stimulate intracellular lipolysis. However, it is impossible to estimate the contribution of this mechanism for intravascular free fatty acid levels. The release of lipases into the blood stream during the smoking experiments is unlikely to be a result of direct interactions between enzyme receptors at the capillary endothelial wall and the strongly alkaline nicotine. Sympathetic synapsis at the vascular wall with a nicotine-depending norepinephrine release could induce the displacement of the enzymes from the endothelium (Fig. 6).

Fig. 6                 THE POSSIBLE ROLE OF NICOTINE ON PLASMA LIPOPROTEINS

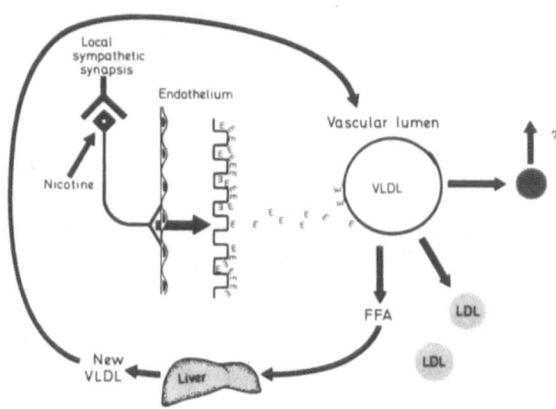

In addition to the stimulation of intracellular hormone-sensitive lipolysis in adipose tissue another sympathetic effect, activation and release of plasma lipases, may therefore be responsible for the increase in plasma free fatty acids during smoking. This mechanism would provide a further regulation of plasma free fatty acid levels. The substrate of this system, triglyceride-rich lipoproteins, is generally available. The activation of plasma lipolytic activities is accompanied by a decrease in VLDL-trigly-cerides and -cholesterol after nicotine exposure. Released free fatty acids are taken up by the liver and incorporated into newly synthesized VLDL. Therefore VLDL-turnover may be appreciably stimulated in smokers. The net effect on VLDL-catabolism may be much more pronounced than detectable in plasma in this study. The intra-vascular hydrolysis of VLDL is accompanied by a transfer of surface components to HDL. This effect can also be seen during nicotine application with a slight increase in HDL-cholesterol during the smoking or chewing procedure. This however is followed by a significant decrease in both parameters, especially HDL-cholesterol. HDL-metabolism in plasma is considered to be rather slow. Besides differences in lipid- and protein degradation of HDL, a second, more dynamic pathway, influenced by nicotine, should be discussed. Zonal ultracentrifugation demonstrates that the decrease in total HDL is accompanied by a change in the ratio of $HDL_2$ to $HDL_3$ in favor of $HDL_2$ (Fig. 7).

ZONAL ULTRAZENTRIFUGATION
HUMAN PLASMA

Fig. 7

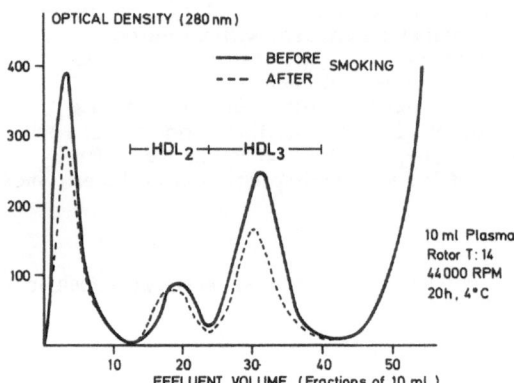

The results suggest that lower HDL-cholesterol levels in smokers are due to the effect of nicotine. Whether this mechanism explains the relation between smoking and arterio-sclerosis, however, requires further investigations.

## References

1. Doyle JT, TR Dawber, WB Kannel, AS Heslin and HA Kahn (1962) New Engl. J. Med. 266: 796
2. Konttinen A and M Rajasalmi (1963) Brit. Med. J. 30: 850
3. Bellimoria JD, H Pozner, B Metselaar, FW Best and DCO James (1975) Athero-sclerosis 21: 61
4. Bradby GVH, AJ Valente and KW Walton (1978) Lancet 8103: 1271
5. Williams P, D Robinson and A Bailey (1979) Lancet 8107: 72
6. Førde OH, DS Thelle, NE Miller and OD Mjøs (1978) Acta Med. Scand. 203: 21
7. Nowack M (1965) J. Lipid Res. 6: 431
8. Greten H, V Laible, G Zipperle and J Augustin (1977) Arteriosclerosis 26: 563
9. Hengen N and M Hengen (1978) Clin. Chem. 24: 50
10. DaPrada M and G Züricher (1976) Life Sci. 19: 1161
11. Wilcoxon F and RA Wilcox (1964) Lederle Laboratories, New York
12. Galster AD (1981) J. Clin. Invest. 67: 1729-1738

# Smoking and Atherosclerotic Disease. The Oslo Study

I. Holme, I. Hjermann, L. A. Solberg, and P. Leren

The Oslo Study is a combined epidemiological and preventive study in
middle aged men(1).In the following, both epidemiological findings
and preventive efforts with relation to smoking and atherosclerotic
disease will be discussed.

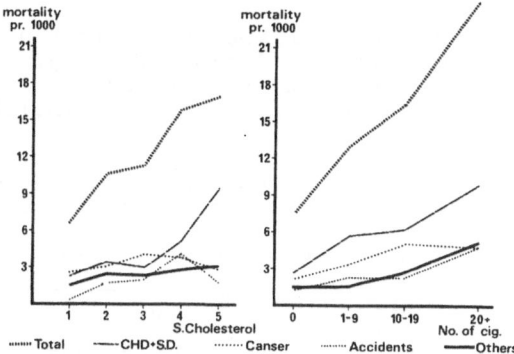

<u>Fig.1.</u>  Cause-specific mortality rates per thousand by serum cholesterol
in quintiles and number of cigarettes

This figure presents total and cause-specific 4½ year mortality by
increasing serum cholesterol (in quintiles) and by number of ciga-
rettes(2).It is shown that cigarette smoking is a strong risk factor
for both total mortality, cancer mortality and for coronary heart
disease (CHD) and sudden death (SD) as previous shown in many other
studies.  A clear "dose-response" curve is present both for total
mortality and for CHD+SD.  This picture contrasts with the 4½ year
follow-up of acute myocardial infarction (AMI) incidence,

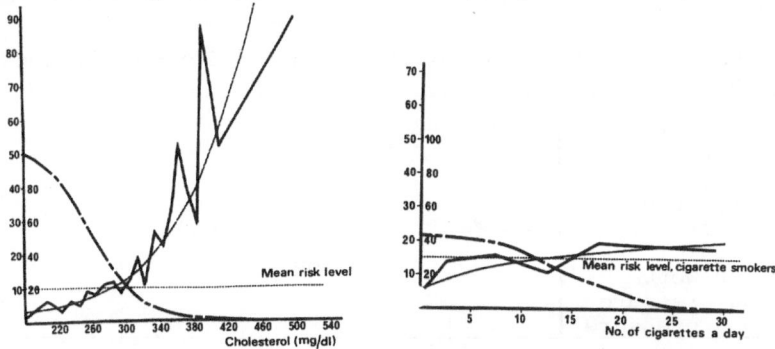

<u>Fig.2.</u>  Four and two-thirds years of AMI acute myocardial infarction by the risk
factors serum cholesterol and number of cigarettes smoked per day, together with

1 minus cumulative distribution function of risk factors, in healthy men, aged 40-49 years at entry, in the Oslo Study, 1972-1973. Note: Vertical axis represents AMI per thousand to the left of ordinate and 1 minus distribution function (in per cent) to right of ordinate

showing the same "dose-response" curve for cholesterol, while for the cigarette factor, the AMI-incidence levels off from 5-10 cigarettes per day. Thus, as far as AMI-incidence is concerned, a very weak "dose-response" relationship exists for cigarette smoking. Only a 50 per cent higher risk exists between those smoking 25 cigarettes per day compared to those smoking 1-4 cigarettes daily. Thus, the AMI-incidence in relation to smoking indicate that the important question is wether you smoke or not.

If, however, cigarette smokingwas a clear-cut etiologic factor related to AMI-incidence, one might have expected a"dose-response"relationship with increasing amounts of cigarettes smoked.

It is of course difficult to evaluate the reason for this discrepancy between the mortality- and incidence-findings for cigarette smoking. One reason might be that the effect of smoking on CHD is more hazardous after the angina or the infarction has been established.

The next table shows that the per cent of daily cigarette smokers is about 4 times as high in the lowest social stratum as compared with the highest stratum, as defined from education and income (3).

Table 1. Risk factors and social socioeconomic classes. Healthy men. Age 50-49. n=14677

| n | I<br>186 | II<br>2592 | III<br>1571 | IV<br>9485 | V<br>843 |
|---|---|---|---|---|---|
| Syst BP | 132.1 | 133.1 | 133.8 | 135.7 | 135.3 |
| Diast BP | 85.8 | 85.5 | 85.7 | 86.5 | 87.2 |
| Cholesterol | 259.7 | 261.1 | 264.5 | 269.0 | 272.6 |
| Smokers (%) | 17.7 | 29.6 | 38.0 | 50.2 | 65.7 |
| Risk score | 5.7 | 7.7 | 9.0 | 10.8 | 13.3 |

The cigarette smoking factor reveals by far the greatest social class gradient compared to the other risk factors, although the cholesterol gradient is of significant magnitude.

This unequal distribution of smoking in different social classes might to some extent modify the relationship between smoking and CHD+SD-mortality.

Table 2. Factors possibly related to atherosclerotic lesions n=129

| Tot.cholesterol<br>Tot.triglycerides<br>HDL cholesterol<br>Cholesterol ratio<br>No. of cigarettes<br>Phys.act. at leisure<br>Phys.act. at work<br>Syst. blood pressure<br>Diast. blood pressure | ⟶ | raised<br>atherosclerotic<br>lesions |
|---|---|---|

In a pathological prospective study of atherosclerotic lesions in coronary and cerebral arteries we collaborated with the International Atherosclerosis center in New Orleans (dr.Strong), where blind, standardized estimations of raised atherosclerotic lesions were made. We related the extent of lesions to the risk factors observed,from a few weeks to 6 years prior to death.(4).

Table 3. Partial correlations coefficients. Study of raised atherosclerotic lesions (RL) in relation to risk factors

|  | Coronary RL | Cerebral RL |
|---|---|---|
| Cholesterol | .28 ** | .23 ** |
| Systolic BP | .23 *** | .45 *** |
| HDL | − .31 ** | − .11 ** |

Triglycerides and smoking habits:  Not    signif.

   *p<.05         **p<.01         ***p<.001

In the multivariate analysis the most potent predictors of coronary and cerebral atherosclerotic lesions were cholesterol ratio (defined as the ratio of HDL cholesterol to non-HDL cholesterol) the total cholesterol and the blood pressure. No. of cigarettes were among the variables that did not come out significantly in the analysis.

The lack of association in this analysis between smoking and atherosclerotic lesions was surprising. The observation might be explained by methodological limitations of the study: First of all the analysis is based on only one observation of the risk factor at screening and nothing is known of the time course of the risk factor for the individual. Next, the method of measuring atherosclerosis is not very exact, and other diseases before death may have been confounding variables in the atherosclerotic process.

However, in spite of these limitations the lipid factors and the blood pressure came out as significant predictors for degree of atherosclerosis in coronary and cerebral arteries. Therefore, the possible causal relationship between smoking and atherosclerosis at least seems to be much weaker than for blood pressure and lipids.

Thus, the most likely explanation for the classical, strong association between smoking and coronary heart disease, is the possible influence of smoking on other factors, as the platelet function, on coagulation and fibrinolysis, on the induction of arrythmias and other possible direct effects on the myocardium. If such causal effects from smoking on CHD exists, one would expect that controlled trials on the effect of antismoking, might reduce CHD incidence.

However, only one monofactorial intervention study on the smoking factor has been carried out, and this study was negative with respect to total mortality. What we really need, is a controlled trial, showing a significant preventive effect on CHD from antismoking advice.

Table 4. Comparability of study groups before trial.
Diet-antismoking trial, Oslo Study

| — | Intervention group (n=604) | Control group (n=628) |
|---|---|---|
| Sex | Male | Male |
| Age (mean and range; yr) | 45·2 (40–49) | 45·2 (40–49) |
| History/symptoms of CHD | None | None |
| Mean daily cigarette consumption | 13·0 | 12·5 |
| Smokers (%) | 79·1 | 79·6 |
| Body weight* (kg) | 77·3±10·3 | 78·2±9·8 |
| Height (cm) | 177·4±6·0 | 176·9±6·3 |
| Serum cholesterol* (mg/dl) | | |
| Screening examination | 328·2±26·9 | 329·2±27·5 |
| 1st re-examination | 322·7±27·6 | 322·5±28·9 |
| Range (mean of these 2 examinations) | 290–379 | 290–379 |
| Serum triglycerides* (mmol/l) | | |
| Screening examination | 2·80±1·5 | 2·84±1·5 |
| 1st re-examination | 2·21±0·9 | 2·25±1·1 |
| SBP (mm Hg) | <150 | <150 |
| % with SBP⩾150 mm Hg and/or DBP⩾98 mm Hg at screening | 23 | 20 |
| Sedentary workers (%) | 50 | 48 |
| Diet score* | 14·8±6·1 | 14·1±6·1 |

*Value ±1 SD. Subjects were non-fasting at the screening examination and fasting at the 1st re-examination. SBP=systolic blood pressure; DBP=diastolic blood pressure.

We have performed a two-factorial controlled trial on the effect of diet and antismoking advice in middle aged healthy, coronary high risk men (5). This table shows that there were more than 600 men in each of the two groups after randomization. Cholesterol values ranged from 290 to 380 mg per cent and 80 per cent of the men were daily cigarette smokers.

Only eating and smoking were subject to intervention, and as you see from this figures:

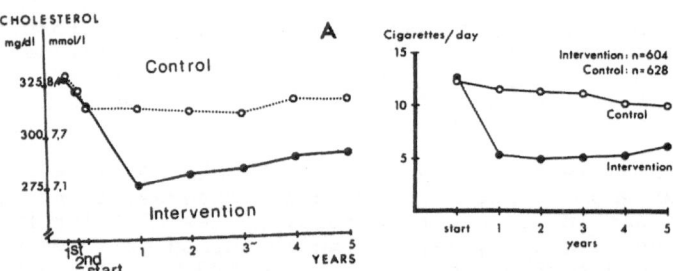

Fig. 3. Intervention effects on serum cholesterol and smoking. Pipe smoking is included; 50 g pipe tobacco/week equals 7 cigarettes/day

a considerable difference was obtained between the two groups in total serum cholesterol and daily consumption of cigarettes (about 13 per cent and 45 per cent respectively).

This resulted in a significant difference between the groups in 5-year incidence of AMI+SD, as shown in the following slide.

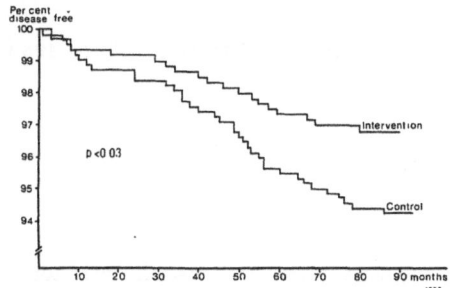

Fig. 4. Life table analysis of CHD (fatal and non-fatal myocardial infarction and sudden death) in intervention and control groups

In an attempt to separate the effects of cholesterol lowering and cigarette reduction in this study, a statistical analysis (based on the Cox proportional hazard model) has been carried out).

It revealed that at least 60 per cent of the difference could be explained by the change in serum cholesterol factor only, whereas the per cent explanation amounted to (most optimistically) 23 per cent (26 per cent among cigarette smokers) with regard to change in cigarette consumption.

With respect to risk reduction the dietetic program has been the most successful. Although cigarette consumption was reduced be 45 per cent in the intervention group as compared to controls, this was not by far enough to produce a significant reduction in risk.

Thus, it is not possible to conclude from the Oslo Study findings that smoking definitely is causally related to atherosclerosis although probably causally related to coronary heart disease.

References

1. Leren P, Askevold EM, Foss OP, Frøli A, Grymyr D, Helgeland A, Hjermann I, Holme I, Lund-Larsen PG, Norum KR (1975) The Oslo Study. Cardiovascular disease in middle-aged and young Oslo-men. Acta med scand Suppl 588:1-38.
2. Holme I, Helgeland A, Hjermann I, Leren P, Lund-Larsen PG (1980) 4 2/3 years' incidence of coronary heart disease in middle-aged men. The Oslo Study. Amer J Epidem 112, No 1:149-160.
3. Holme I, Helgeland A, Hjermann I, Leren P, Lund-Larsen PG (1976) Coronary risk factors in various occupational groups: the Oslo Study 1977 Brit J prev soc Med 31:96-100.
4. Holme I, Enger SC, Helgeland A, Hjermann I, Leren P, Lund-Larsen PG, Solberg LAa, Strong JP (1981) Risk factors and Raised Atherosclerotic Lesions in Coronary and Cerebral arteries. Arteriosclerosis 1:250-256.
5. Hjermann I, Byre K Velve, Holme I, Leren P (1981) Effect of diet and smoking intervention on the incidence of coronary heart disease. Lancet II:1303-1310.

# Epidemiology of Cardiovascular Disease in Different Countries in Relation to Smoking

M. G. Marmot

The relation between smoking and cardiovascular disease has long been recognised. International epidemiological studies have helped to define more precisely the nature of this relationship, the circumstances under which it holds, to give clues to the mechanisms by which smoking exerts its effects, and to give a guide to the possibilities of prevention.

## I.  Smoking and Coronary Heart Disease (CHD) in Different Countries

In countries where CHD is common, smoking is related to CHD incidence and mortality.  The relationship is strong, shows a dose-response pattern and is independent of other factors.  For example, in Great Britain, in the Whitehall study of civil servants(1) social class, represented here by grade of employment, and smoking are related independently to CHD mortality in 10 years (Fig.1).

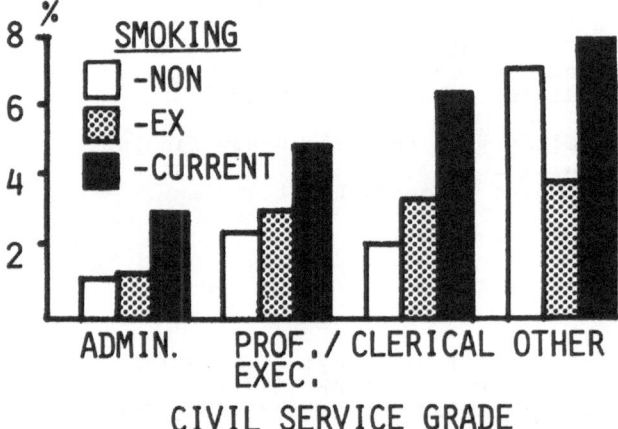

Fig. 1.  Ten-year CHD mortality (%) according to grade of employment and cigarette smoking (Whitehall Study)

The relation between smoking and CHD is less strong or non-existent in countries where CHD rates are low, such as Puerto Rico(2) and Japan.  In the NiHonSan study of men of Japanese ancestry living in Japan, Hawaii and California(3), smoking was not associated with CHD incidence in Japan, but was among Japanese men in Hawaii(4).  A possible explanation is that plasma cholesterol levels (and CHD rates) are lower in Japan than Hawaii.  As Fig. 2 shows, in Hawaii at higher levels of plasma cholesterol ( $\geqslant$5.18 mmol/l), smoking was more strongly associated with CHD incidence than at lower levels.  The lack of association between smoking and CHD in Japan at higher cholesterol levels may result from the fact that in Japan the overall cholesterol distribution is shifted to the left compared to Hawaii.  It may also reflect the necessity for potentiating factors other than elevated plasma cholesterol to be present for smoking to increase the risk of CHD.

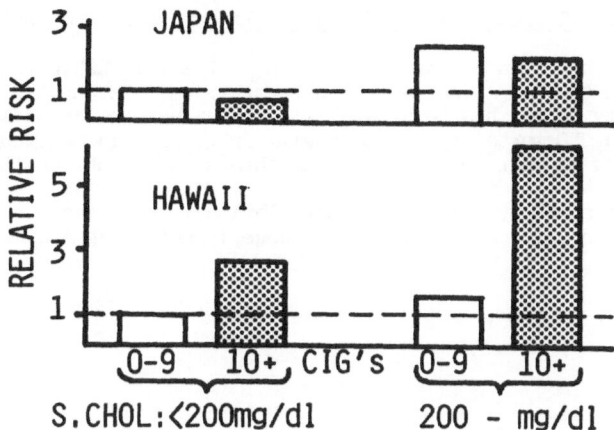

Fig. 2. Relative risk of developing CHD in men of Japanese ancestry in Japan and Hawaii according to plasma cholesterol and smoking

Similarly in their study of CHD in seven countries, Keys and colleagues found the slope of the regression of CHD incidence rate on cigarette use to be steepest where CHD is most common(5).

Perhaps because smoking is a predictor of CHD only within high rate populations, the correlation between cigarette consumption and smoking internationally is weak (Fig.3). Heart disease mortality figures from twenty-one countries come from data published by W.H.O., and have been standardised for age.

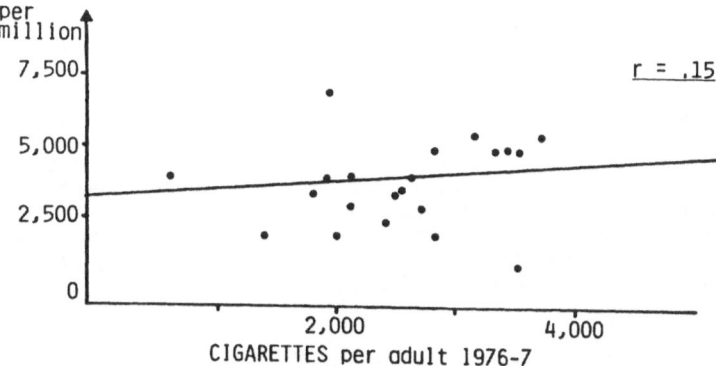

Fig. 3. Correlation between heart disease (A83, A84) mortality in men 45-64 and cigarette consumption per capita in twenty-one countries

The weak correlation (r = .15) may be a reflection of inaccuracies in the data as the correlation between lung cancer mortality and smoking was also not strong (r = .3) and there is little doubt as to the strength and consistency of this latter association.

## II. Trends in Heart Disease - Explained by Smoking?

Much prominence has been given to the remarkable recent decline in CHD mortality in the U.S.A. and some other countries. In the U.S.A., the decline in CHD mortality in men has been paralleled by a decrease in smoking(6). In women, the decline in CHD mortality has been similar to that in men, but in middle-aged women, smoking has not decreased. This throws some doubt on the possibility that the decrease in smoking was the major cause of the male decrease in CHD. Further doubt is shown by the lack of correlation in twenty-one countries between change in cigarette consumption and change in heart disease mortality (Fig.4).

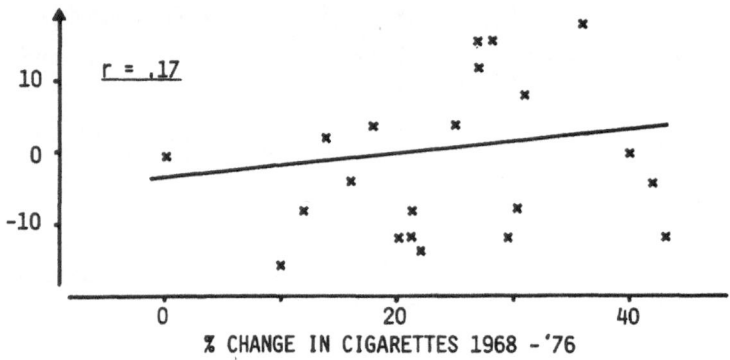

Fig. 4. % change in heart disease mortality (1968-1977) in men 45-64 and % change in per capita cigarette consumption 1968-1977 in twenty-one countries

The possible limitation of this form of analysis is again shown by the lack of correlation between changes in cigarette consumption and changes in lung cancer mortality over the same period (r = .13). Allowing for a 10-year lag period, i.e. correlating changes in mortality with changes in smoking 10 years previously did not strengthen the correlations. These attempts at associations are fraught with difficulties. Types of cigarette and tobacco content may change and cigarette consumption figures in different countries are not generally available for age-sex-social class groups. In England and Wales such figures are available. Analyses have shown that as CHD mortality changed from being more common in higher (I & II) social classes to being more common in lower (IV & V) classes, smoking also became relatively more common in classes IV & V(7).

## III. Smoking and Type of Vascular Disease

In the Whitehall study, smoking was associated with mortality from CHD and cerebrovascular disease. The relation of smoking to incidence of various types of vascular disease is shown in Fig. 5(8).

In general, the relation of smoking to cardiovascular disease incidence is weaker in older men. Smoking is strongly related both to sudden cardiac death and myocardial infarction but weakly, or not at all, to angina pectoris. The division on clinical grounds of cerebrovascular disease into cerebral thrombosis (in Framingham, labelled atherothrombotic brain infarction) and cerebral haemorrhage, is often dubious. Nevertheless, smoking appears to be related more strongly to cerebral thrombosis than to cerebral haemorrhage.

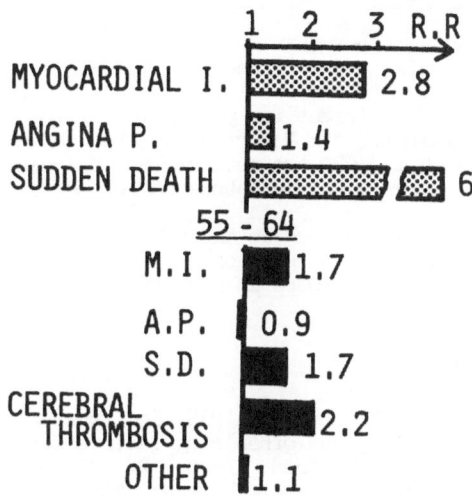

Fig. 5. 16-year incidence of cardiovascular disease in men in the Framingham Study, expressed as relative risk in heavy smokers ( ⩾20/day) vs non-smokers(8)

If we think of these cardiovascular diseases as having a chronic atheromatous component and an acute component leading to myocardial infarction, sudden death or cerebral thrombosis, then these findings would be consistent with smoking affecting the acute component primarily. This may, for example, be an effect of smoking on clotting factors or an effect on myocardial irritability. The lack of association with angina would indicate a lack of association between smoking and atheroma - assuming that this is the pathological process underlying most cases of angina pectoris.

The finding that within one year of giving up smoking, ex-smokers have a reduced risk of CHD (9, 10) is in favour of smoking exerting an acute effect. In favour of an additional chronic effect, is the failure of the CHD rates in ex-smokers to decline to those in never-smokers until five years have elapsed. Also Auerbach et al have reported that in post-mortem examinations, advanced coronary atheroma and hyaline thickening in myocardial arterioles is greater in heavy smokers than in non-smokers (11). It seems likely, therefore that smoking may affect both the acute and chronic component of CHD, but not in the absence of other atherogenic factors, most probably elevated plasma cholesterol.

IV. Type of Smoking

In their follow-up study of British Doctors, Doll & Peto found that men who reported they inhaled cigarette smoke had higher mortality from ischaemic heart disease than non-inhalers(10). This was true also in the Whitehall study(12), but the relative risk were small (less than 1.6).

The type of cigarette is also of interest. A change to filter-tip cigarettes in the U.K. appears to have accounted for no decrease in CHD mortality(13). Among inhalers in the Whitehall study, tar content of cigarettes was strongly related to CHD mortality only in light smokers. Among heavy smokers, the CHD mortality in men smoking low-tar cigarettes was 84% of that of men smoking high-tar brands (12). This figure is similar to that reported by Hammond et al(14).


## V. Implications for Prevention

Factors other than smoking are responsible for international differences in CHD mortality and for trends in mortality. In the presence of these other factors leading to atherosclerosis, smoking increases the risk of heart disease and stroke. The ideal target for prevention is to encourage young people not to take up the smoking habit. Nevertheless, the data on ex-smokers suggest the risk of lung cancer and CHD are reversible. Changing to low tar cigarettes is likely to have only a marginal influence on CHD mortality.

In countries such as the U.K. smoking is now much more common in lower social classes(7). Current strategies to decrease smoking have been ineffective in diffusing through all groups in society.


## References

1. Reid DD, Hamilton PJS, McCartney P, Rose G, Jarrett RJ, Keen H (1976) Smoking and other risk factors for coronary heart disease in British Civil Servants. Lancet 2: 979-984
2. Gordon T, Garcia-Palmieri MR, Kagan A, Kannel WB, Schiffman J. (1974) Differences in coronary heart disease in Framingham, Honolulu and Puerto Rico. J Chron Dis 27: 329-344
3. Syme SL, Marmot MG, Kagan A, Kato H, Rhoads GG (1975) Epidemiologic studies of coronary heart disease and stroke in Japanese men living in Japan, Hawaii, and California: Introduction. Am J Epidem 102: 477-480
4. Robertson TL, Kato H, Gordon et al (1977) Epidemiologic studies of coronary heart disease and stroke in Japanese men living in Japan, Hawaii and California: Coronary heart disease risk factors in Japan and Hawaii. Am J Cardiol 39: 244-249
5. Keys A (1980) Seven Countries. Harvard University Press, Cambridge, Mass
6. Kleinman JC, Feldman JJ, Monk MA (1979) Trends in smoking and ischaemic heart disease mortality in Havlik RJ and Feinleib M.Ed. Proceedings of the conference on the decline in coronary heart disease mortality. U.S.D.H.E.W. N.I.H. Publ. No. 79-1610
7. Marmot MG, Adelstein AM, Robinson N, Rose GA (1978) Changing social class distribution of heart disease. Brit Med J 2: 1109-1112
8. Shurtleff D (1970) The Framingham Study. An epidemiological investigation of cardiovascular disease (ed Kannel WB and Gordon T) Section 26. U.S.Govt. Printing Office. Washington DC
9. Hammond EC, Garfinkel L (1969) Coronary heart disease, stroke and aortic aneurysm. Arch Environmental Health 19: 167
10. Doll R, Peto R (1976) Mortality in relation to smoking: 20 years' observations on male British doctors. Brit Med J 2: 1525-1536
11. Auerbach O, Carter HW, Garfinkel L, Hammond EC (1976) Cigarette smoking and coronary artery disease. Chest 70: 697-705
12. Higenbottam T, Shipley M, Rose G (1982) Cigarettes, lung cancer and coronary heart disease: The effects of inhalation and tar yield. J. Epidemiol Community Health 36: 113-117
13. Wald N (1976) Mortality from lung cancer and coronary heart disease in relation to changes in smoking habits. Lancet 1: 136-138
14. Hammond EC, Garfinkel L, Seidman H, Lew EA (1977) Some recent findings concerning cigarette smoking in Hiatt HH, Watson JD, Winston JA eds. Origins of human cancer ... Book A. Cold Spring Harbor Laboratory, New York, pp 101-113

# Smoking and Atherosclerosis: Risk Factor Reduction

M. A. H. Russell

Atherosclerosis causes more deaths in developed societies than any other disease. It is a disease that has no cure, and it is unlikely that one will ever be found. While it is true that certain drugs and surgical procedures have some very limited palliative use, the real answer lies in prevention. Few would deny that giving up smoking (or better still never starting it) is an essential part of any preventive strategy. It is, moreover, an important factor at all stages of prevention; primary, secondary and tertiary.

It is my brief to consider how the smoking factor in atherosclerotic cardio-vascular disease can be more effectively reduced. I shall consider first why it is that people find it so difficult to give up smoking. Secondly, I shall consider two new approaches which give reason to hope for better results in the future. These are nicotine chewing-gum and the concerted efforts of family doctors. Thirdly, I shall consider the limitations of switching to lower yield cigarettes, or to a pipe or cigars. Finally, I shall suggest a new approach to the design of less harmful cigarettes and why snuff use could prove a satisfactory substitute for smoking.

## Smoking as an addiction

The main reason why people find it so difficult to give up smoking is that it is a form of drug dependence, the drug of course being nicotine. The modern cigarette is a highly effective device for getting nicotine to the brain. After each inhaled puff, nicotine gets into the blood and the brain with intravenous-like rapidity and smokers tend to modify the way they puff and inhale to regulate the amount they take in. Twenty cigarettes a day mounts up to 7,300 a year, each puffed about ten times. This is more than 70,000 intravenous-like shots of nicotine hitting the smoker's brain each year. Nicotine has many pharmacological effects that may be rewarding and, like most other addictive drugs, it induces tolerance and physical as well as psychological effects can occur when it is withdrawn.

Surveys have shown that less than one in four smokers in Britain succeed in stopping permanently before the age of sixty. This is not for want of trying. 70% of smokers would like to stop and 50% have made two or more unsuccessful attempts. Thus most people smoke not because they really want to, but because they cannot easily stop. In other words, they smoke mainly because they are hooked, and for the great majority cigarette smoking is first and foremost a drug-taking activity.

## Anti-Smoking Campaigns

It is not appropriate here to review all the traditional measures that have characterised the anti-smoking campaigns of the past twenty years. These measures include health education in schools, campaigns on mass media, restrictions on cigarette advertising, health warnings on cigarette packs, restrictions on smoking in public places, high taxation on tobacco, withdrawal clinics and other smoking cessation programmes. It has to be admitted that the combined effect of all these approaches has been rather limited. In Britain, for example, the 20% reduction between 1960 and 1980 in the per capita consumption of manufactured cigarettes among men has been offset by the 30% increase among women over the same period. Despite all the efforts that have been made to reduce smoking, there are still 18 million people in Britain who continue to smoke cigarettes.

894

The reasons for this failure are complex. The various approaches have not been sufficiently coordinated or sustained. Promotion of cigarettes has gone largely unfettered and there has been a lack of political will to provide the funds and legislation necessary to implement an adequate policy. But the main obstacle to success is the addictive nature of smoking. Thus the campaigns have succeeded in making the majority of smokers want to stop and try to stop but success has been blocked by their addiction. There is nothing new about this. Historical examples abound of the failure of laws, excommunication, death and torture to prevent the spread of tobacco use over the past five centuries.

## Treatment for Smokers

Physicians, psychologists and other health professionals have devised all kinds of methods in the search for a successful treatment method for smokers. Tranquillisers, lobeline, hypnosis, acupuncture, aversion therapy and other psychological methods have all failed to achieve more than a placebo effect. None of these methods give better results than simple attention and support which produces success rates ranging from about 15% to 25% still abstinent at one year follow-up.

More encouraging results are beginning to emerge with the use of a brand of nicotine chewing-gum developed in Sweden some ten years ago[1] but now considerably refined and improved. Nicotine is released slowly over 20-30 minutes as the gum is chewed and is absorbed through the buccal mucosa. It reduces craving and eases withdrawal symptoms by providing an alternative source of nicotine and, in addition, a substitute oral activity. It also appears to reduce the tendency for people to gain weight after giving up smoking. In a comparative study at our clinic[2], those treated with the gum had a success rate of 38% at one year follow-up compared to only 14% for intensive psychological treatment. More recently, in a double-blind placebo-controlled trial[3], we obtained a success rate of 47% not smoking at one year follow-up compared to 21% for those on placebo gum (table 1). We believe that, after more than twenty years of unsuccessful research into all kinds of treatment methods for smokers, nicotine chewing gum is the first treatment to have been developed that has a specific effect over and above that attributable to an attention-placebo response.

Table 1. Treatment with nicotine chewing-gum (% Abstinent)

| Time from start of treatment | Placeo Gum (n=58) | Active Gum (n=58) | Statistical Significance |
|---|---|---|---|
| One month | 33% | 62% | P <.01 |
| One year | 21% | 47% | P <.01 |

## Family Physician Intervention

One of the problems with specialised smoking withdrawal clinics has been the reluctance of smokers to attend. Few clinics in Britain have been able to attract more than 200 to 300 clients a year. Another problem has been the tendency to attract the more difficult and highly dependent cases who are less likely to succeed. While it is probable that the availability of a more effective treatment, viz nicotine gum, will enable the clinics to attract more smokers, they are unlikely to prove the most cost-effective route for direct intervention with a target population that runs to many millions of smokers, a substantial proportion of whom would never attend. One way to overcome this problem would be to apply intervention through family physicians.

Some 95% of the British population visit their General Practitioners (GPs) at least once over a five-year period, and about 75% attend at least once over the course of a year. In GPs then we have a system already available that has face-

to-face contact with the majority of the 18 million smokers in Britain.    Unlike
the clinics their access is not limited to a selected sample of highly dependent
smokers.    They also have access to the mass of less educated smokers who have
responded least to the traditional health education approaches.

In a recent study[4], we showed that when GPs gave simple but firm advice against
smoking together with a leaflet and warning of follow-up, they achieved a one-year
success rate of 5.1% compared to only 0.3% in non-intervention controls (table 2).

Table 2.  Effect of family physician advice (% abstinent)

|              | Control (n=340) | Question-naire only (n=430) | Advice (n=389) | Advice and Leaflet (n=408) | Statistical Significance |
|--------------|-----------------|------------------------------|----------------|-----------------------------|---------------------------|
| One month    | 3.0%            | 3.0%                         | 4.6%           | 7.5%                        | P<.001                    |
| One year     | 0.3%            | 1.6%                         | 3.3%           | 5.1%                        | P<.001                    |

At first glance 5.1% may not seem impressive, but this was achieved with a procedure that took up no more than 1-2 minutes of the physician's time.    More ex-
smokers can be created by minimal intervention with many smokers than by more
intensive work with a few.    We calculated that any GP who adopted such a procedure
as a routine could expect to achieve about 25 long-term successes a year.    This
is about the same number achieved per year by the average clinic in Britain.    The
potential effect of the 20,000 plus GPs in Britain acting in this way is considerable.

We have just completed a further study among GPs and their patients.    Preliminary
analysis shows that when GPs offer nicotine gum to their patients and prescribe it
for those who agree to try it the one-year success rate is boosted to 10.8%.
This figure is based on all the smokers who attended, including those who never
accepted or took the gum.    A higher success rate can be expected when the analysis
is completed based on those who actually used the gum.

The potential efficacy of widespread intervention by family physicians is very
great and will be enhanced when the nicotine chewing-gum is more freely available.
We believe that these two new approaches, used in combination as part of a co-
ordinated programme at a national level, could in time lead to a substantial
reduction in the prevalence of smoking.

Lower Yield Cigarettes

Even if success is achieved in lowering the prevalence of cigarette smoking, it is
unlikely that it will be eliminated altogether.    In Britain, 13% of doctors still
smoke cigarettes[5].    It would, therefore, seem unrealistic to expect the general
population to get below this before a very long time, and a 13% prevalence rate
for Britain would still mean almost 6 million smokers.    So, what can be done to
lower the risks for those who continue to smoke cigarettes?

One approach presently pursued in many countries is to encourage smokers to switch
to lower yield cigarettes.    But this is subject to two limitations.    First, there
comes a point where acceptability is lost so that smokers will simply not smoke
cigarettes if the yields are too low.    The curves for sales-weighted tar and
nicotine deliveries of cigarettes sold to the public and the proportion of smokers
who smoke low yield cigarettes have tended to flatten in many countries as the
acceptability limits of their smoking populations are reached.

The second limitation to the use of low-tar, low-nicotine cigarettes is the tendency
for smokers to regulate their smoke intake.    By taking larger puffs, smoking to
a shorter butt length, blocking the ventilation holes and inhaling more deeply

they are able to get as much out of lower yield cigarettes as they formerly got from high yield brands. In a recent study we measured the blood nicotine and carboxyhaemoglobin (COHb) levels of 326 smokers who were smoking their usual brands in their usual way[6]. Those smokers who had switched to lower yield cigarettes had similar levels to those who were still smoking higher yield brands (table 3). It is, therefore, unlikely that their health risks were substantially different.

Table 3. Blood nicotine and COHb levels in smokers of high, middle and low yield cigarettes

|  | Men | | | Women | |
|  | Plain (n=17) | Filter (n=82) | Ventilated F. (n=25) | Filter (n=150) | Ventilated F. (n=52) |
|---|---|---|---|---|---|
| Tar yield(mg) | 25.9 | 17.9 | 9.3 | 17.7 | 9.7 |
| Nicotine yield(mg) | 1.9 | 1.3 | 0.8 | 1.3 | 0.8 |
| No.cigs/day | 40 | 35 | 38 | 33 | 32 |
| Blood nicotine(ng/ml) | 36.2 | 33.8 | 29.5 | 32.6 | 30.9 |
| COHb (%) | 6.3 | 8.0 | 7.8 | 8.8 | 8.0 |

The study above was concerned with natural switching, ie smokers who had themselves chosen to switch to lower yield brands. Smaller scale studies of experimental switching have tended to show different results. Smokers who are required by the conditions of an experiment to switch to lower yield cigarettes do show some reduction in blood nicotine levels albeit proportionately less than the reduction in yields. In other words they show some tendency to regulate their intake to compensate for the reduction in yields but, as a group, do not compensate completely. Table 4 shows the results of one such study[7]. Intake measures are shown for two occasions when smoking their usual brand and then after 2 days and up to 10 weeks on a low-tar low-nicotine brand.

Table 4. Average blood nicotine and COHb levels of 12 subjects before and after switching to low yield cigarettes

|  | Usual Brand (Tar 17.4, Nic 1.3, CO 17.0mg) | | Low-tar Low-nicotine Brand (Tar 10.9, Nic 0.7, CO 12.9mg) | | |
|---|---|---|---|---|---|
|  | Occ 1 | Occ 2 | 2 days | 8 weeks | 10 weeks |
| Cigs/day | 24 | 20 | 21 | 23 | 24 |
| Blood nicotine(ng/ml) | 32.4 | 33.2 | 20.8 | 22.7 | 22.8 |
| COHb (%) | 7.4 | 7.0 | 6.9 | 7.6 | 7.8 |

It will have been noted that after switching to lower yield cigarettes under natural conditions compensation was virtually complete and smoke intake was not appreciably reduced, whereas under experimental conditions compensation was on average only partial and smoke intake was reduced appreciably. The discrepancy could arise from the fact that the natural switchers were self-selected, whereas all subjects switched in the experimental study. It is possible that, under natural conditions, switching to lower yield cigarettes is maintained only by those who compensate fully and that those who fail to do so revert to a higher yielding brand. However, the results of the experimental study suggest that if smokers could be persuaded to persist longer in their attempt to switch they might in time adapt to a lower intake. Furthermore, it is possible that those who experience the greatest initial difficulty in switching are the ones whose smoke intake is most reduced and who would therefore obtain the greatest benefits to their health.

## Switching to a pipe or cigars

Epidemiological evidence of the relative safety of pipe and cigar smoking is based on older studies of predominantly primary smokers of pipes and cigars who had not been cigarette smokers. There is now much evidence suggesting that when cigarette smokers switch to pipe or cigar smoking they tend to inhale, especially if they smoke heavily and use milder tobaccos or smaller milder cigars. Smokers who continue to inhale will not reduce their health risk and may even increase it[8]. The risks will only be reduced if inhalation is avoided. This is something that is easily checked non-invasively by a simple breath-test of the expired-air carbon monoxide level.

## Low-tar, low-CO, medium-nicotine cigarettes[9]

The limitations of low-tar low-nicotine cigarettes have been mentioned above. It is indeed somewhat illogical to expect people who cannot stop smoking because they are addicted to nicotine to switch to cigarettes which deliver hardly any nicotine. On the premise that people smoke mainly for nicotine but die mainly from the tar, CO and other substances they inhale with the nicotine, it would seem logical to develop cigarettes having low-tar, low-CO and low deliveries of all components known to be harmful but delivering sufficient nicotine to maintain acceptability and to prevent excessive compensatory changes in the smoking pattern. There are encouraging signs that the Tobacco Industry is turning its attention ever so slightly to this approach. Nicotine yields of some brands are now reduced proportionally less than tar yields in an effort to improve the acceptability of low-yield brands.

## Snuff as a substitute for cigarettes

Historical evidence suggests that snuff might prove a satisfactory substitute for smoking. The history of tobacco use over the past 500 years includes no example of a society in which its use once established has been abandoned. This does not bode well for plans to eliminate its use in our society. However, there are examples of switching from one form of tobacco use to another. In the 18th Century the British population switched to snuffing for almost a hundred years before going back again to smoking. Nicotine intake is the obvious common factor in all forms of tobacco use. We have been particularly impressed by the rapid absorption of nicotine after taking dry snuff into the nose[10]. Within ten minutes after taking snuff, blood nicotine concentrations are obtained that are comparable to those after the ten minutes or so it takes to smoke a cigarette. Absorption of nicotine from snuff is far more rapid than from nicotine chewing-gum or the non-inhaled smoking of a large cigar. All this suggests that it might prove acceptable to smokers as a long-term alternative to continued smoking.

There is little doubt that snuff use would be far less harmful than smoking. It produces no tar, CO or other harmful gases. Switching to snuff would substantially reduce the risk of lung cancer, bronchitis and emphysema at the cost of a slight increase in the risk of cancer of the nasopharynx. The position is less clear regarding the risk of cardiovascular disease, for it is still not known whether nicotine, CO or some other component is the major aetiological factor. Clarification of this issue should be a major concern of epidemiologists. There are sufficient numbers of wet snuff users in Scandinavia and the United States to make such study feasible.

## Summary and Conclusions

1) Preventive measures to reduce the risk factors due to smoking are probably the most important part of any strategy to reduce premature death and disability from atherosclerotic cardiovascular disease.
2) Previous failures to deal more successfully with the smoking problem stem mainly from a failure to recognise it as a predominantly drug-taking activity.
3) At the individual level, the availability of a new form of treatment with nicotine chewing-gum has greatly enhanced success rates.

4)  Brief intervention by physicians during all contacts with their patients is an
effective measure that could substantially reduce the prevalence of smoking throughout the population if it were widely adopted as a routine part of medical practice.
5)  Switching to a pipe, cigars or conventional low-tar, low-nicotine cigarettes
does not in general lead to the expected reduction in the intake of harmful smoke
components and is consequently likely to have little benefit to health.
6)  Since it is unlikely that the prevalence of cigarette smoking will fall below
15-20% before a very long time, safer forms of nicotine intake should be explored.
Two of the most promising are snuff and the development of low-tar, low-CO and
medium-nicotine (rather than low-nicotine) cigarettes.

## References

1.  Ferno,O. et al. (1973) Psychopharmacologia.31:201-204.
2.  Raw,M. et al. (1980) Brit.Med.J. 281:481-482.
3.  Jarvis, MJ. et al. (1982) Brit.Med.J. In Press.
4.  Russell, MAH. et al. (1979) Brit.Med.J. 2:231-235.
5.  Hallett, R. (1982) J.Roy.Coll.Gen.Practit. In Press.
6.  Russell, MAH. et al. (1980) Brit.Med.J.280:972-975.
7.  Russell, MAH. et al. (1982) Brit.J.Addict.77:145-158.
8,  Gyntelberg,F. et al. (1982) Lancet 1:987-989.
9.  Russell, MAH. (1976) Brit.Med.J. 1:1430-1433.
10. Russell, MAH. et al. (1981) Brit.Med.J. 283:814-817.

# Nicotine and Atherosclerosis

H. Schievelbein and G. Heinemann

Since the 1964 Surgeon General's Report, many epidemiological investigations have confirmed that, besides high blood cholesterol and hypertension, cigarette smoking is a main risk factor for the development of coronary heart disease (CHD) (1). Cigarette smoke consists of a mixture of thousands of different compounds, among which nicotine is regarded as the most pharmacologically-active component (2). The pharmacologic and toxicologic effects of nicotine are well-known, and should only be mentioned briefly. The main pharmacological action of nicotine is its stimulation of sympathetic ganglia and of the adrenal medulla, resulting in the release of catecholamines from sympathetic nerves and chromaffine tissues in different organs, thereby influencing fat metabolism, carbohydrate metabolism, thrombocytes, and blood coagulation (3). Furthermore, nicotine is known to release antidiuretic hormone from the pituitary (4) and to increase corticosteroid secretion (5). In higher doses of nicotine, stimulation is followed by paralysis of the central and peripheral nervous system and rapid death (6).

The pronounced positive inotrop and chronotrop action of nicotine on the heart consequently leads to the question whether nicotine contributes to the pathogenesis of atherosclerosis and myocardial infarction. One possible mechanism for the development of atherosclerosis is the action of nicotine on the coagulation pathway and platelet function. The studies pertaining to coagulation changes have resulted in conflicting data without leading to an unanimous understanding (7). The same holds true for investigations of the influence of nicotine on platelet aggregation. While in most in vitro studies a potentiation of platelet aggregation could be observed (8), it has repeatedly been shown in clinical investigations that smokers have a decreased incidence of postoperative deep vein thrombosis (9-11), thus contradicting the significance of the above mentioned effects.

Acceleration of the development of atherosclerosis may also be a consequence of the effect of nicotine on fat metabolism. Besides the well-known release of free fatty acids it has recently been shown by Augustin et al. that nicotine itself might be able to increase LDL-cholesterol and to decrease VLDL-triglycerides, HDL-cholesterol and HDL-phospholipids (12). However, the results of these experiments have not yet been confirmed so far, and if they hold true the question will arise whether chronic effects on the cardiovascular system can be derived.

In individuals, already suffering from CHD, it has been hypothesized that nicotine may aggravate ischemia by increasing cardiac oxygen demand and by increasing platelet adhesiveness (13). Furthermore, it has been speculated that nicotine may favour the development of arrhythmias by lowering the cardiac threshold to ventricular fibrillation (14), by depressing conduction, and enhancing automaticity (15). Both the nicotine-dependent ischemia and the nicotine-dependent arrhythmia may finally result in myocardial infarction.

In the past, many experiments have dealt with the possible effects of nicotine administration on the development of arterial wall injuries in animals, some of which should be mentioned briefly. One of the purposes of a long-term experiment, performed by our group, was to investigate, whether atherosclerosis in rabbits can be induced by administration of nicotine alone (16). After 20 months treatment, all animals had developed atherosclerotic lesions in the aorta and in the coronary arteries without any difference between the control and the experimental group. Similarly, Fisher et al. reported that nicotine failed to affect atherosclerosis of aorta and both extramural and intramural coronary arteries in rabbits (17). Furthermore, Liu et al. showed that nicotine alone was unable to produce atherosclerotic lesions in Rhesus monkeys (18). So, as an overall impression the '79 Surgeon General Report' has stated that nicotine does not affect atherogenesis in animals.

When evaluating the outcome of the long-term studies, a main deficiency of many chronic animal experiments should not be overlooked. The administration of nicotine by means of intraperitoneal or subcutaneous injections or by oral application may lead to acute nicotine poisoning of the animals and is unlikely to simulate chronic nicotine exposure. Moreover, it should not be forgotten that the daily dose of nicotine used in the animal studies, in general, was several times higher per kilogram bodyweight than the daily amount of nicotine absorbed by cigarette smokers.

Recently, investigations were published which seem to confirm the hypothesis that nicotine has no atherogenic effects. Wald et al. measured the level of cotinine and COHb in the blood of cigarette-, cigar-, and pipe smokers (19). The authors found that pipe smokers had a considerably higher level of cotinine, the main metabolite of nicotine degradation, than cigarette smokers. Based on well-known epidemiological data that pipe smokers have little, if any, extra risk of death from CHD, the authors conclude that nicotine is unlikely to be a major cause of CHD-mortality in cigarette smokers. Investigations of Russell et al. (20) as well as of Gritz et al. (21) on nicotine levels in snuff users and habitual smokeless tobacco users (dipped snuff and chewing tobacco users) seem to confirm the hypothesis of Wald et al. (Table 1).

Table 1. Mean serum cotinine and nicotine levels in tobacco users

| Tobacco product | Serum cotinine (ng/ml) | Serum nicotine (ng/ml) | Authors |
|---|---|---|---|
| Cigarettes | 306 ± 13 | | Wald et al. 1981 |
| Cigars | 121 ± 17 | | |
| Pipe-tobacco | 389 ± 34 | | |
| Cigarettes | 335 ± 146 | 36.2 ± 14 | Russell et al. |
| Snuff | 411 ± 305 | 35.6 ± 21 | 1981 |
| Dipped snuff and chewing tobacco | 197 ± 48 | 21.6 ± 5 | Gritz et al. 1981 |

## Concluding Remarks

Although nicotine may theoretically play a role in the etiology of atherosclerosis and myocardial infarction, there is no established evidence which supports the hypothesis that nicotine has any influence on the development of atherosclerosis. Bearing in mind the cardiovascular action of nicotine via release of catecholamines it has to be mentioned that physical exercise and mental stress may result considerably higher increase in plasma catecholamine concentrations compaired to cigarette smoking (22, 23). Summarizing the presented evidence we conclude that the contribution of nicotine to the development of atherosclerosis is an open question. Properly designed and conducted animal experiments in which nicotine is chronically administered in realistic doses are necessary. In our opinion there are many other substances in tobacco smoke which could be more responsible for the excess CHD-mortality in smokers than nicotine is, but are not investigated yet.

## References

1. The Health Consequences of Smoking (1979) U.S. Department of Health and Welfare, Washington
2. Wynder EL, Hoffmann D, Gori GB (1975) Smoking and Health. Proceedings of the 3rd World Conference. Modifying the Risk for the Smoker. DHEW Publ. No. (NIH) 76-1221
3. Schievelbein H (1977) The evidence for nicotine as an etiological factor in cardiovascular disease (CVD). In: Schettler G, Goto Y, Hata Y, Klose G (eds) Atherosclerosis IV, Springer Verlag Berlin-Heidelberg-New York, p 167
4. Burn HH, Truelove LH, Brun J (1945) The antidiuretic action of nicotine and of smoking. Brit Med J 1: 403-406
5. Kershbaum A, Pappajohn DL, Bellet S, Hirabayaschi M, Shafiha H (1968) Effect of smoking and nicotine on adrenocortical secretion. J Amer Med Assoc 203: 275-277
6. Petty FA (1963) Industrial Hygiene and Toxicology, Vol. 2. In: Fassett DW, Irish DD (eds) Toxicology. Interscience Publishers New York
7. Mehta P, Mehta J (1981) Effect of smoking and nicotine on platelet - endothelial cell activity. In: Mehta J, Mehta P (eds) Platelets and Prostaglandins in Cardiovascular Disease, Futura Publishing Company, p 289
8. Saba SR, Mason RG (1975) Some effects of nicotine on platelets. Thromb Res 7: 819-822
9. Handley AJ, Teather D (1974) Influence of smoking on deep vein thrombosis after myocardial infarction. Brit Med J 3: 230-231
10. Marks P, Emerson PA (1974) Increased incidence of deep vein thrombosis after myocardial infarction in non-smokers. Brit Med J 3: 232-234
11. Clayton JK, Anderson JA, McNicol GP (1978) Effect of cigarette smoking on subsequent postoperative thromboembolic disease in gynaecological patients. Brit Med J 2: 402
12. Augustin J, Beedgen B, Spohr U, Winkel F (1982) The influence of smoking on the plasmalipoproteins. Innere Med 9: 104-106
13. Levine PH (1973) An acute effect of cigarette smoking on platelet function. A possible link between smoking and arterial

thrombosis. Circulation 48: 619-620

14. Bellet S, Deguzman NT, Kostis JB, Roman L, Fleischmann D (1972) The effect of inhalation of cigarette smoke on ventricular fibrillation threshold in normal dogs and dogs with acute myocardial infarction. Amer Heart J 83: 67-68

15. Greenspan K Edmands RE, Knoebel SB, Fish C (1969) Some effects of nicotine on cardiac automaticity, conduction, and inotrophy. Arch Inter Med 123: 707-709

16. Schievelbein H, Londong V, Londong W, Grumbach H, Remplik V, Schauer A, Immich H (1970) Nicotine and arteriosclerosis. Z Klin Chem Klin Biochem 8: 190-196

17. Fisher ER, Rothstein R, Wholey MH, Nelson R (1973) Influence of nicotine on experimental atherosclerosis and its determinants. Arch Path 96: 298-301

18. Liu LB, Taylor CB, Peng SK, Mikkelson B (1979) Experimental atherosclerosis in Rhesus monkeys induced by multiple risk factors: cholesterol, vitamin D, and nicotine. Arterial Wall V: 25-30

19. Wald NJ, Idle M, Boreham J, Bailey A, Van Vunakis H (1981) Serum cotinine levels in pipe smokers: evidence against nicotine as cause of coronary heart disease. The Lancet 2: 775-777

20. Russell MAH, Jarvis MJ, Devitt G, Feyerabend C (1981) Nicotine intake by snuff users. Brit Med J 283: 814-818

21. Gritz ER, Baer-Weiss V, Benowitz NL, Van Vunakis H, Jarvik ME (1981) Plasma nicotine and cotinine concentration in habitual smokeless tobacco users. Clin Pharmacol Therap 30: 201-204

22. Vecht RJ, Graham GWS, Sever PS (1978) Plasma noradrenaline concentrations during isomeric exercise. Brit Heart J 40: 1216-1217

23. Danner SA, Endert E, Koster RW, Dunning AJ (1981) Biochemical and circulatory parameters during purely mental stress. Acta Med Scand 209: 305-308

# Smoking: A Pediatric Disease

T. Strasser

## Atherosclerotic Lesions and Smoking

The epidemiologic associations of smoking with atherosclerosis, especially that of the peripheral and coronary arteries are well known and often quoted. Less frequently are references made to morphological population studies, such as the WHO Cooperative Study of Atherosclerosis of the Aorta and Coronary Arteries in Five Towns (1), although it has clearly demonstrated the grave anatomical consequences of smoking.

Fig. 1 shows the prevalence of atherosclerotic lesions - fatty streaks, fibrous plaques, complicated and calcified lesions - in the abdominal aorta in smokers and non-smokers. There is little difference in the prevalence of fatty streaks and fibrous plaques, but complicated lesions and, particularly, calcified lesions are considerably more frequent in heavy and even in light smokers, than in non-smokers. This difference is even more conspicuous when comparing the surfaces these lesions cover in the abdominal aorta (Fig. 2) (2) and in the coronary arteries (Fig. 3) (3).

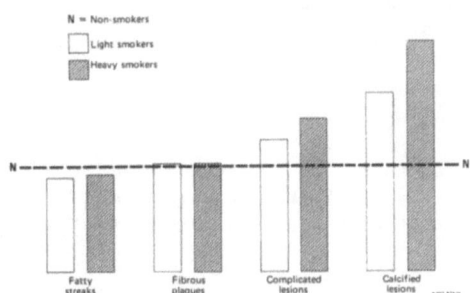

**Fig. 1.** Prevalence of atherosclerotic lesions in abdominal aorta in smokers compared with non-smokers

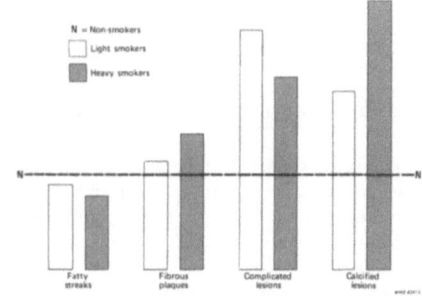

**Fig. 2.** Extent of atherosclerotic lesions in the abdominal aorta in smokers, compared with non-smokers

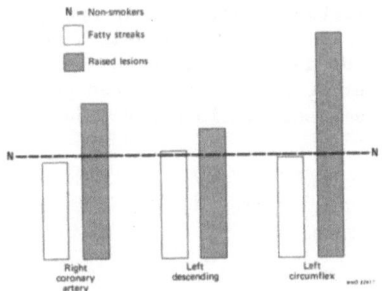

**Fig. 3.** Surface of atherosclerotic lesions in coronary arteries of heavy smokers, compared with non-smokers

## The Early Onset of Atherosclerosis

As well known today, the first atherosclerotic lesions may start in childhood.
The statement that atherosclerosis is a paediatric disease has almost become a
cliché.   Fig. 4 shows how rapidly the proportion of the population <u>free</u> of fibrous
plaques in the coronary arteries declines with age (1).    Since there are still
few data available in children, the lines between birth and adolescence are
tentative (though plausible) extrapolations.    The early onset of atherosclerotic
changes in the studied populations is remarkable.

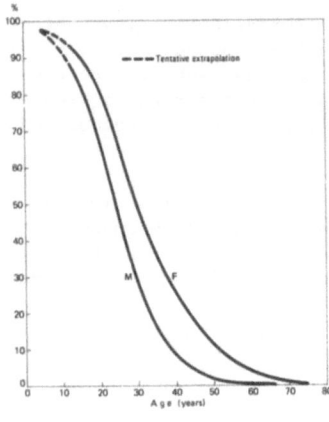

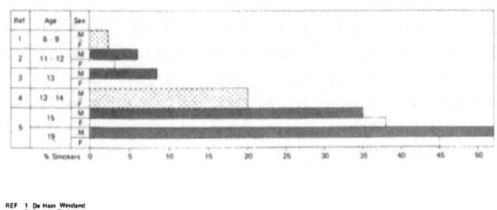

**Fig. 5.** Prevalence of smoking in
children and adolescents - selected
samples

**Fig. 4.** Proportion of population
free of fibrous plaques in
5 European towns

## Smoking: A Paediatric Disease

It is, on the other hand, all too often forgotten that - as a matter of course -
the atherogenetic noxae may start at least as early as atherosclerosis itself.
The contention of the present paper is to show that smoking, too, is a paediatric
disease.

Is smoking, indeed, <u>a disease</u>?   A "destructive process in the organism" (4), a
disease results in impaired function of one or several organs; it may cause a
feeling of ill-health; may lead to various complications; and shortens life expectancy.   Diseases are a burden to society; they may inflict suffering on the family;
they are unwanted phenomena and people usually would like to get rid of them.   All
of these statements apply to smoking.

Is smoking a <u>paediatric</u> disease?   In Fig. 5 (5) information has been compiled from
5 studies (6-9).   In terms of the first cigarette smoked, smoking in the population starts soon after the 6th year of life.   The prevalence of smoking then
rises rapidly in both girls and boys and at the end of adolescence reaches the
rates seen in middle aged men and women.   The number of cigarettes smoked per day
increases after adolescence, but the smoking disease itself is in general fully
established in youth.

There are, of course, considerable differences on the world scene, as shown by a recent WHO report (10). In developing countries, such as Ethiopia and India, smoking seems to start somewhat later (Fig. 6), than in a developed country such as Australia. Regrettably, information on smoking at young ages is available only from few countries (11). The great concern that should cause the high prevalence of smoking at young age may be mitigated to some extent by the fact that in some countries the trend of adolescent smoking is declining. The example of Sweden (Fig. 7) (10), a country with a particularly vigorous antismoking programme would be reconforting, but on the global level such improvements are cancelled out by the fact that the smoking disease is in rapid ascension in developing countries, the 3/4 majority of the world's population.

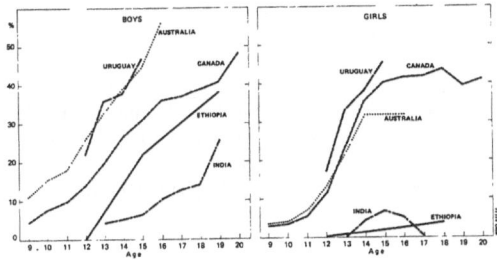
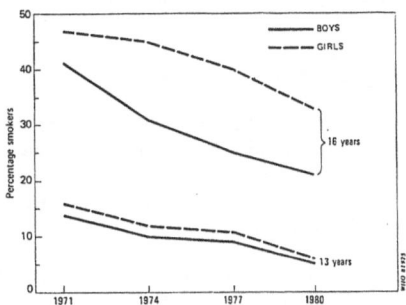

Fig. 6. Approximate percentage of smokers in selected countries by age and sex

Fig. 7. Trends in prevalence of cigarette smoking for boys and girls aged 13 and 16 years in Sweden

The Epidemiology of Smoking

The great secular epidemic of cigarette smoking started around the beginning of this century in men, and in the thirties in women. Today smoking has the characteristics of a pandemic, spreading from the developed to the developing world where it is steeply rising.

Considerable literature is available on the very complex sociological, behavioural, psychological, economic, marketing and historical aspects of smoking. The contagious nature of smoking is, however, rarely realized, perhaps because the phenomenon itself has insufficiently been conceptualized by (and for) the medical profession as a disease. For instance, according to a study by the Netherlands Heart Foundation, 65% of Dutch general practitioners smoke, and 25% smoke in front of their patient (12). The situation is better in some countries (e.g. the United Kingdom, where physicians smoke considerably less than a few decades ago) but it also may be worse in many others. (Some reports from Finland (13), France (14), and New Zealand (15) indicate that smoking in physicians is steadily declining, e.g. from 66% to 43% in French doctors - still a high proportion. Thirty-four % of staff of a medical school in England still smoke (16)).

Children and adolescents are contaminated with the smoking behaviour of adults, either directly, or indirectly through their peers. The prevention of smoking in children calls for concerted action along many lines; i.a. action across generations is needed, such as the Swedish "Smoke Free Generation" Programme (16).

Smoking prevention includes many non-medical types of intervention (e.g. educational, behavioural, administrative action) but still the medical profession is bound to play a prominent role in it.    The attitude and behaviour of physicians regarding smoking control and prevention is essential.    Unless completely adopted and fully endorsed by the medical profession, the prevention of smoking may in fact be jeopardized by physicians.    As long as it is considered a mere habit, though unhealthy, medical doctors may not be sufficiently motivated to combat vigorously enough the further spread of the epidemic.    However, if smoking were conceptualized and percieved as an important contagious disease, the medical and other health professions may become more aware of the gravity of the problem. The association between atherosclerotic lesions and smoking itself, even without the respiratory and cancer aspects, sufficiently justifies that smoking be categorized as a disease, primarily a disease of childhood and adolescence.

## Reference

1.    Kagan AR, Sternby NH, Uemura K et al. (1976)  Atherosclerosis of the aorta and coronary arteries in five towns.  Bull. World Health Organ. 53: 485-645

2.    Lifsic AM (1976)  Atherosclerosis in smokers.  Bull. World Health Organ. 53: 631-638

3.    Vihert AM, Zdanov VS, Lifsic AM (1976)  Atherosclerosis in males doing manual and brain work.  Kardiologija 16: 119-123 (in Russian)

4.    Garmonsway GN (1980)  The Penguin English Dictionary

5.    Strasser T (1981)  Erforschung und bekämpfung der Vorstadien der Atherosklerose im Kindesalter.  Die Rolle der Weltgesundheitsorganisation.  Wiss. Tagung d.  Deutschen Kinderärzte, Düsseldorf, 21-24 September 1981

6.    de Haas JH (1978)  Risk factors of CHD in children – a retrospective view of the Westland study.  Postgraduate Medical Journal 54: 187-189

7.    Bewley BR (1978) Smoking in childhood.  Postgraduate Medical Journal 54: 197-198

8.    Laaser U (1977)  Risikofaktoren bei Jugendlichen.  Indikatoren des Kardiovaskulären Risikos bei Schülern der Obsertufe in Köln.  Fortschritte der Medizin 95 (5), 256-262

9.    WHO/ISFC Meeting on Precursors of Atherosclerosis in Children.   Geneva, 12-14 October 1977 (CVD/78.1)

10.   World Health Organization (Geneva, February 1982) Tobacco Report

11.   Masironi R, Roy L (1982)  Cigarette smoking in young age groups.  Geographic prevalence.  WHO document SMO/82.3

12.   Dekker E (1981)  Smoking behaviours in dutch general practitioners, in: Tobacco e Giovani, Conferenzia Internazionale, Venezia

13.   Rimpelä M, Kantanen M, Kokko S, Vuori H (1976)  A study of the health behaviour of physicians.  Suomen Lääkärilehti 31: 2639-2648 (in Finnish)

14. Freour P, Tessier JF, Gachie JP et al. (1980)  Le tabagisme chez les prati- ciens girondins et son évolution en dix ans.  Comparaison avec la population générale.   Bordeaux médical 13: 253-260

15. Hay DR (1980)  Cigarette smoking in New Zealand doctors: results from the 1976 population census.  New Zealand Med. Journal 91: 285-288

16. Elind AK (1979)  Smoking among the staff of a medical school.  Medical Education 13: 163-171

# Smoking and Lipid Metabolism

## S. Heyden

Smokers have elevated LDL and/or decreased HDL cholesterol levels in comparison to non-smokers. The Israeli Incidence Study showed that the HDL cholesterol levels of ex-smokers approach those of non-smokers in all age groups (Goldbourt and Medalie):

| Age | Smokers | HDL Cholesterol in mg/dl<br>Ex-smokers | Non-smokers |
|---|---|---|---|
| 40-64 | 35.6 | 37.2 | 37.6 |

Morrison et al (1979) reported in the Lipid Research Clinic Princeton School Study that lower HDL and higher LDL cholesterol levels were found in 12 to 19 year old smoking teenagers as compared to non-smoking teenagers.

The four-year interim report from the MRFIT study[*] (Caggiula et al, 1981) has documented for the first time the confounding factors which may influence HDL levels among smokers. "At baseline, smokers as a group reported higher intakes of total calories, saturated fat, dietary cholesterol, and alcohol, and lower intakes of polyunsaturated fat than non-smokers." The authors presented a table where substantial increases in HDL cholesterol were evident only in the nonhypertensive subgroups, and the greatest increase was noted in the smokers who quit during the first four years:

| Weight change: | Loss ≥10 lb | Loss 5-9 lb | Little change | Gain ≥5 lb |
|---|---|---|---|---|
| N. of participants | 1,391 | 922 | 1,899 | 1,096 |
| | | Mean change in plasma HDL cholesterol (%) | | |
| **Nonhypertensive** | | | | |
| Nonsmokers | +8.6 | +6.6 | +1.7 | +1.4 |
| Ex-smokers | +9.0 | +7.7 | +7.6 | +5.0 |
| Smokers | +5.3 | +7.3 | +1.2 | -2.9 |
| **Hypertensive** | | | | |
| Nonsmokers | +2.9 | -0.1 | -1.4 | -5.7 |
| Ex-smokers | +5.2 | +4.9 | -0.2 | -3.9 |
| Smokers | +5.3 | +2.1 | -2.4 | -6.8 |

## Smoking and Coffee Consumption

In two studies (Heyden, et al, 1979) involving a randomized group of 360 adults in Evans County, we were able to show that heavy coffee consumption per se (5 or more cups of coffee per day) neither elevates LDL values nor lowers HDL values. However, there are relatively few heavy coffee drinkers who do not smoke heavily at the same time - the two habits are associated in the vast majority of people. Our observational study demonstrated a significant interaction effect between caffeine and nicotine for total serum cholesterol and LDL-cholesterol levels, i.e., the combination of smoking and coffee drinking revealed significantly higher LDL and total cholesterol levels than in coffee drinkers who did not smoke. A similar trend, but statistically insignificant interaction effect, was shown on HDL-cholesterol levels in this population.

[*] Abbreviated table from: Caggiula, A.W. et al: The Multiple Risk Factor Intervention Trial. IV. Intervention on Blood Lipids. Prev. Med. 10:443, 1981.

# The Influence of Smoking on Systolic and Diastolic Blood Pressure

Sp. Kritsikis, and Sp. Bafaloukos

Within a group of 846 males of age 30 - 59 (mean 46.97), selected from
a representative sample of 6.000 individuals (three generations) from
the native population of Salamis Island (Athens area), the influence
of smoking on systolic and diastolic blood pressure was studied.

The percentage of smokers varied from 55.1% to 65.6% between equal
size age clusters (5 years each). The sample mean of systolic blood
pressure for smokers was found to be 136.64 mm Hg, while for nonsmokers
was found to be 145.98 mm Hg. The difference between these means is
highly statistically significant (t = -7.92, p<0.0001). Also the sample
mean of the diastolic blood pressure for smokers was found to be
83.93 mm Hg, while for non-smokers was 88.11 mm Hg. This difference
is also highly statistically significant (t = -7.86, p<0.0001). The
difference in systolic blood pressure was much more significant for
the age clusters 30-34, 45-49, and 50-54 years. The difference in
diastolic blood pressure was much more significant for the age clusters
30-34 and 45-49. In the remaining clusters a less significant difference for both types of blood pressure was detected.

These results reveal that long term smoking has a negative effect on
the levels of systolic and diastolic blood pressure, a fact which is
in agreement with recent bibliographical findings (1). Several interpretations (2, 3, 4), have been proposed as precise explanations of
this phenomenon and its connections with the mechanisms causing a
high frequency of atherosclerosis. However, a more detailed etiological
investigation is still required.

## References

1. Perloff DMD (1977) Symposium on Hypertension. The Medical Clinics
   of North America, V 61, no 3
2. Russel CS, Taylor R, Law CE (1968) Smoking in pregnancy maternal
   blood pressure, pregnancy outcome, baby weight and growth related
   factors, A prespective study. Brit J Prev Soc Med 22: 119
3. Seltzer CC (1974) Effect of smoking on blood pressure. Amer Heart
   J 87: 558
4. Stebbings JH (1973) Two observed associations between respiratory
   allergies and hypertension in non-smokers. Amer J Epidemiol 97: 4

**TABLE I.** Difference of the mean values of the systolic blood pressure in men, smokers and non smokers correlated with age

| A. SYSTOLIC BLOOD PRESSURE (mm Hg) – Mean Values | | | | | | | |
|---|---|---|---|---|---|---|---|
| Age | 25 – 29 | 30 – 34 | 35 – 39 | 40 – 44 | 45 – 49 | 50 – 54 | 55 – 60 |
| Smokers | 123.41 | 122.12 | 126.11 | 126.38 | 127.79 | 134.87 | 140.63 |
| Non smokers | 132.50 | 131.16 | 127.87 | 129.48 | 136.28 | 142.96 | 147.45 |
| D$\bar{x}$ | 9.09 | 9.04 | 1.76 | 3.10 | 8.49 | 8.09 | 6.82 |
| p | <0.103 | <0.0001 | <0.422 | <0.194 | <0.0001 | <0.005 | <0.017 |

| B. DIASTOLIC BLOOD PRESSURE (mm Hg) – Mean Values | | | | | | | |
|---|---|---|---|---|---|---|---|
| Smokers | 77.17 | 76.75 | 79.22 | 81.05 | 80.82 | 85.08 | 85.87 |
| Non smokers | 78.25 | 82.00 | 81.06 | 82.40 | 86.87 | 88.55 | 89.91 |
| D$\bar{x}$ | 1.08 | 5.25 | 1.84 | 1.35 | 6.05 | 3.47 | 4.04 |
| p | <0.753 | <0.002 | <0.260 | <0.420 | <0.0001 | <0.032 | <0.024 |

**Figure 1.** Frequency of men smokers correlated with age N = 1319

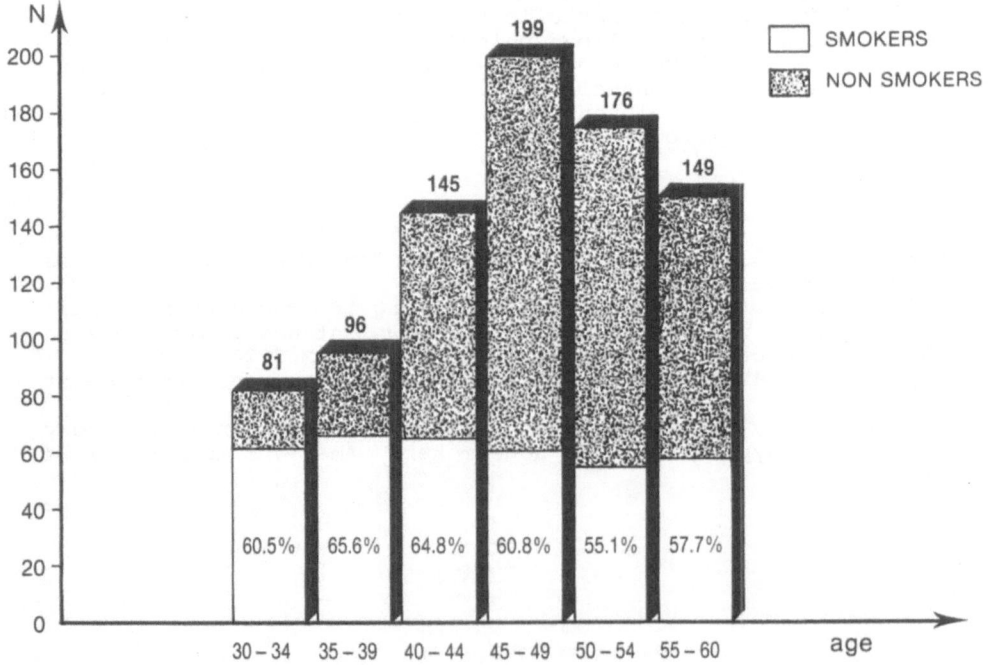

## 5.4 Serum Lipid Lowering in Secondary Prevention

# Current Japanese Situations on Secondary Prevention and Lipid Lowering Drugs

S. Hatano

There are multi-center cooperative studies on the evaluation of lipid lowering effects of various drugs, such as clofibrate, pantethine, niceritrol, gamma-oryzanol and probucol. These were carried out with a double-blind design, monitoring the effects for 4 months or longer. All of these drugs were effective in reducing plasma lipid levels with negligible side effects. There are a few small scale primary prevention trials using lipid lowering drugs. The one with anabolic steroid and tocopherol was concluded with encouraging results. The second one used clofibrate. The third one with dextran sulfate is continuing. There is, however, no secondary prevention trial in Japan (Table 1).

Table 1. Studies with lipid lowering drugs in Japan

**1. Evaluation of effectiveness**

| (Drugs) | (Authors) | (Reported in:) |
|---------|-----------|----------------|
| Clofibrate | M. Murakami et al. | 1978 |
| Pantethine | Y. Goto et al. | 1980 |
| Niceritrol | Y. Hata et al. | 1981 |
| γ-Oryzanol | Y. Hata et al. | 1981 |
| Probucol | Y. Hata et al. | 1981 |

**2. Primary prevention**

| | | |
|---------|-----------|----------------|
| Ethylnandrol and Tocopherol | M. Tsushima et al. | 1977 |
| Clofibrate | H. Miyashita et al. | in press |
| Dextran Sulfate | Y. Goto et al. | on going |

**3. Secondary prevention**

None

We may count some possible reasons for a smaller number of research work in this important area. Ischemic heart disease has been paid less attention because it is still a less common disease in Japan. Hyperlipidemia or smoking did not appear to be a significant risk factor of ischemic heart disease, compared with the role played by high blood pressure in Japan. It is considered to be a protective factor against cerebral hemorrhage in many epidemiological studies. The main reason for this must be because of general low blood lipid levels of the Japanese population (Table 2).

Table 2. Possible reasons for less researches on prevention of ischemic heart disease with lipid lowering drugs in Japan

---

1. Low mortality and morbidity from IHD

2. Low blood lipids level

3. Low contribution  of lipids as risk factor

---

Crude death rate for ischemic heart disease was only 6.6% of all cause death rate and a fourth that for stroke. Age-sex specific death rates for men were one sixth to one seventh those in Sweden or in the United States.

Incidence rate of myocardial infarction in Hiroshima and Nagasaki, Japan, appeared to be roughly one half that of ethnical Japanese in Hawaii according to the Ni-Hon-San Study on NIH (1), one third that in Göteborg or one fourth that in London in the WHO community study (2).

Number of patients with ischemic heart disease under medical care was estimated to be about 100,000 in the whole country and the rate was about 1 per 1,000 according to a national one-day survey (3). It was about half of stroke patients, but hospitalized patients at an acute consisted much less part in cardiovascular patients.

The notion that Japanese has low prevalence of ischemic heart disease may be supported by objective observations such as low prevalence of ECG abnormalities suggesting ischemic heart disease. Frequency of definite Q and QS, i.e., 1-1 and 1-2 according to Minnesota Code in the middle-aged population was less than 0.5% (4), and much lower than Western populations such as observed in the Tecumseh Study (5).

Further to note is epidemiological observations on risk factors of ischemic heart disease. The most potent risk factor for ischemic heart disease is high blood pressure. Hyperlipidemia and cigarette smoking appeared as less significant risk factors in Japanese populations. Cholesterol generally appeared to have a negative association with cerebral hemorrhage in geographical and between-population comparisons and between-individual comparisons in one study area (6-10).

The level of serum cholesterol was lower than in Western countries in most age groups except those at the fourth decade of age or among children. Levels reported by the Lipid Research Clinic group were lower than those in preceding reports (11), but Japanese data based on a nation-wide random sample reported by the Ministry of Health and Welfare showed much lower figures (4). Mean cholesterol in those aged 30 and over was 189 mg/dl in men and 191 mg/dl in women. All the measurement of cholesterol was carried out in Osaka Center for Adult Disease, which has been standardized by CDC, Atlanta, USA. When hypercholesterolemia is defined as serum cholesterol of 260 mg/dl and over, its frequency was less than 5% at nearly all age groups in men and women (4).

The relative low level of blood lipids stemmed from diet. Japanese government has been conducting a national survey of nutrition on a stratified national sample every year (12). According to a recent report in 1979, average total calory consumption for adult was 2,200, no greater than that of the American people. Total fat intake was 52 g, and was 21% of total caloric intake, while 39% of calory was taken from fat in one American Study (13). The P/S ratio of fat from some Japanese nutrition studies was between 1 and 2, while it was 0.24 in USA. Average Japanese situations on diet were therefore much better with regard to fat intake, than dietary goals for the Americans, except high salt consumption. Under these circumstances, the needs for lipid lowering drugs are limited in Japan for the time being, and this is applicable also to patients with ischemic heart disease, mortality and morbidity of which is not high in spite of rapid economic development. These may explain the not-yet-ready situation on embarking upon secondary as well as primary prevention trials using lipid lowering drugs in Japan.

Table 3. Dietary intake in Japan and USA

| | JAPAN[12] national 1975 | USA[13] Singman et al 1952 | USA[14] dietary goals |
|---|---|---|---|
| Tot.Calory | 2,188 (100) | 2,356 (100) | avoid overweight |
| Carbohydrate (g) | 337 (62) | 237 (40) | 48% cal |
| cereal | 95 (17) | — | |
| sugar | 1 (0.2) | 62 (11) | 10% |
| Fat (g) | 52 (21) | 102 (39) | 30% |
| saturated | — | 41 (16) | 10% |
| unsaturated | — | 10 (4) | 10% |
| cholesterol | — | 590 | 300mg |
| p/s ratio | [>1.0] | 0.24 | 1.0 |
| NaCl (g) | 14 | — | 5 |

In addition to these medical situations, I may count liberal and free medical services in Japan as a disturbing element. Physicians are paid on the basis of fee for the service. Patients prefer to receive drugs from physicians. These tend to invite overtreatment.

Nearly 100% of Japanese population is covered by social health insurance, which provides almost free medical services. Patients are free to choose any doctor at any place at any time, if he so wishes. Mass health screening for cardiovascular diseases has been practiced in firms and communities. Determination of serum cholesterol is one of the favorite screening items. Subjects who are found to have moderate hyperlipidemia may often be advised to consult a physician who would then start and continue to give a lipid lowering drug. Even when a patient agrees to be enrolled into a controlled trial using a lipid lowering drug, certain length of wash-out time is required before putting him into the trial.

This generous system no doubt helped improve general health of the nation but may also have added difficulty to implementing a prevention study of sufficient scale and duration.

References

1. Robertson TL, Kato H, Rhoads GG et al.: Epidemiologic studies of coronary heart disease and stroke in Japanese men living in Japan, Hawaii and California. Am J Cardiol 39: 239-243, 1977

2. WHO Regional Office for Europe: Myocardial infarction community registers. Public Health Report 5. WHO, Copenhagen, 1977
3. Office of Statistics and Information, Jpn Ministry of Health and Welfare ed: Patients Survey 1979. Kosei Tokei Kyokai, Tokyo, 1981 (in Japanese)
4. Bureau of Tuberculosis and Chronic Disease: Jpn Ministry of Health and Welfare: An outline of results from the basic survey on cardio-vascular disease. J Jpn Ass for Cerebro-Cardiovascular Dis Control 17: (1) Suppl 1-33, 1982 (in Japanese)
5. Higgins ITT, Kannel WB, Dawber TR: The electrocardiogram in epi-demiological studies, reproducibility, validity, and international comparison. Brit J Prev Soc Med 19: 53-68, 1965
6. Hirota Y et al: A multivariate analysis of risk factors for cerebro-vascular disease in Hysayama, Jyushu Island, Japan. Behaviormetrika No 2, 1-11, 1975
7. Matsuzaki T: Risk factors for stroke and myocardial infarction. In: R. Shigiya, Y. Komachi and T. Watanab eds: Nutrition and cardio-vascular disease in Japanese. Hoken Dojin Sha, Tokyo, 1976. (in Japanese)
8. Tanaka H, Ueda Y, Date C et al: Epidemiological analysis on the stroke risk factors in the rural Japanese. Jpn J Geriatrics 13: 98-107, 1976
9. Shimamoto T, Komachi Y: Risk factors for cerebral stroke. Sogo Rinsho 27: 47-53, 1978. (in Japanese)
10. Konishi M, Iida M, Shimamoto T et al: Epidemiological and patho-logical studies of cerebral infarction and myocardial infarction in Japan. J Jpn Atheroscl Soc 8: 455-465, 1980. (in Japanese with English summary)
11. The lipid Research Clinic Program Epidemiology Committee: Plasma lipid distributions in selected North American populations: The Lipid Research Clinic Program Prevalence Study. Circulation 60: 427-429, 1979
12. Bureau of Nutrition, Jpn Ministry of Health and Welfare ed: Current status of national nutrition 1957. Daiichi Shuppan, Tokyo, 1978
13. Singman HS, Berman SN, Cowell C et al: The Anti-Coronary Club: 1957-1972. Am J Clin Nutr 33: 1183-1191, 1980

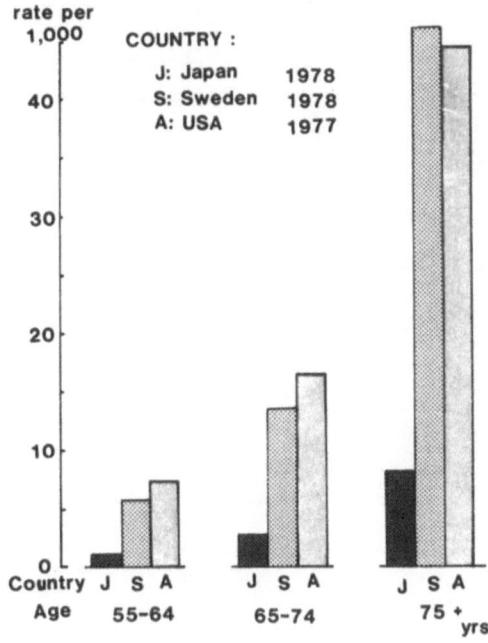

Fig. 1. Death rate from ischemic heart disease in three age-groups of men in three countries

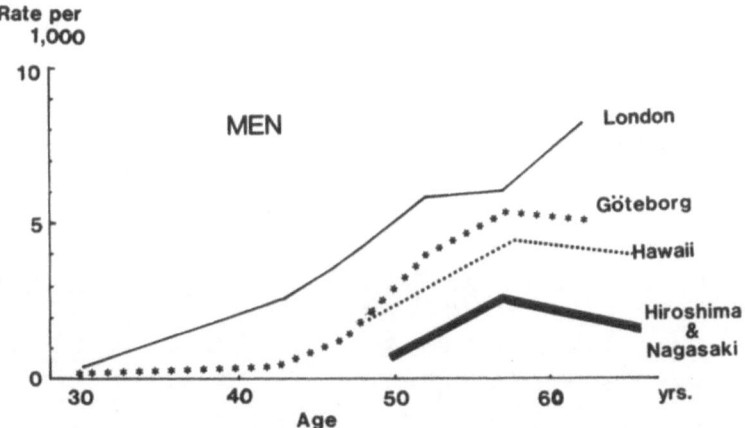

Fig. 2. Age-specific incidence rate of myocardial infarction (Ni-Hon-San study[1] and WHO study[2])

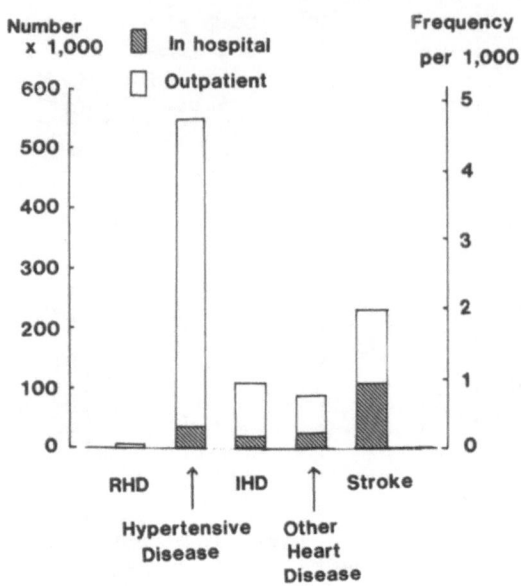

<u>Fig. 3.</u> Estimated number and frequency of patients with major
cardiovascular diseases (National 1-Day Patients Survey 1979)[3]

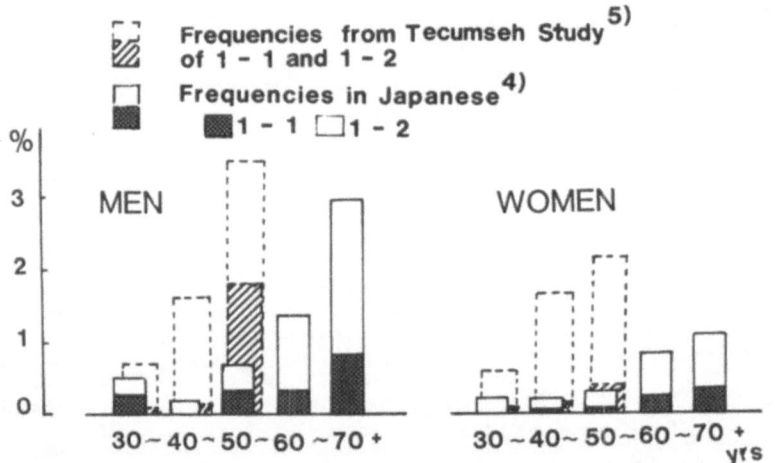

<u>Fig. 4.</u> Frequency of abnormal Q/QS in Japanese and Tecumseh,
USA population according to Minnesota Code

( Minnesota Code)

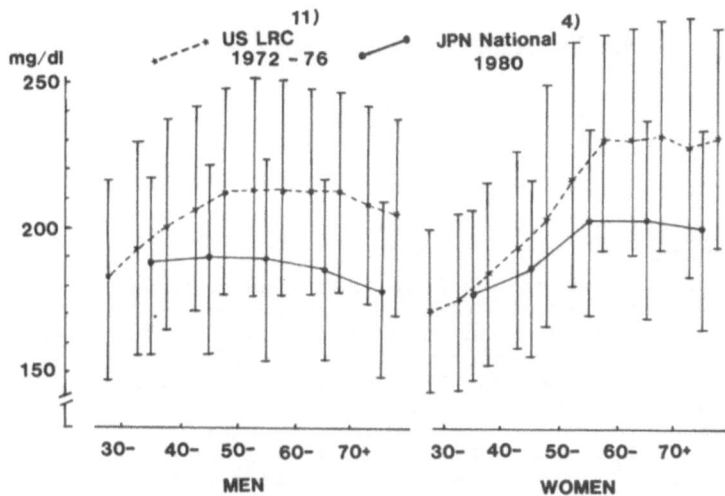

**Fig. 5.** Mean and standard deviation of total cholesterol in USA[11] and Japan[4]

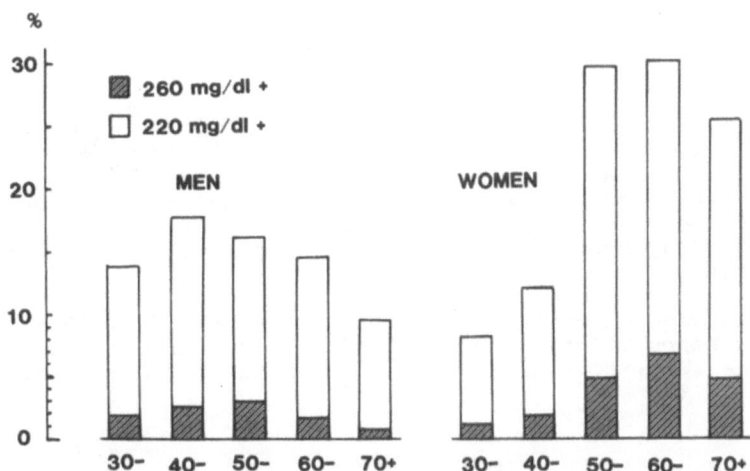

**Fig. 6.** Prevalence of hypercholesterolemia in Japanese population (National CVD Survey 1980)[4]

# Serum Lipid Lowering in Secondary Prevention: A Review

G. Lamm

## A. Introduction

Few people would contest the fact that atherosclerosis in general
and coronary heart disease (CHD) in particular is less frequent
in populations with low mean serum lipid levels. The wide gap
between this basic fact and the high expectations implied in the
title become even more conspicuous when one considers the two
jumps in logic separating the two. The first jump implies that
reduction of elevated lipids restores the protection against CHD
to the same level as would be linked with a low-lipid level a
limine. The second jump assumes that lipid correction acts as
forcefully after the manifestation of CHD as during its pro-
tracted development. Both assumptions are poorly proven - if at
all - and this fact should be kept in mind before reviewing the
secondary preventive trials performed up to now.

## B. Overview

This review will deal only with the major controlled trials. Observational studies and trials with meaningless numbers will not be
considered. Twelve such trials were found to qualify for these
criteria and they are listed in the literature reference under 1-11
(The Coronary Drug Project was considered separately for Clofibrate
and for Niacin).

The time-span covered by these trials is 20 years, from 1961 to 1980.
One could be happy if this would be the only difference between the
trials. There were, however, many other substantial differences, as
shown in Table 1.

Table 1. Overview of 12 trials

| Lipid lowering agent | | Time since AMI | |
|---|---|---|---|
| Diet | 5 | 1 - 3 months | 3 |
| Clofibrate Drug | 7 | 3 - 6   " | 3 |
| | | 6 -12   " | 0 |
| | | 1 year or more | 6 |
| **Length of trial** | | **Numbers treated** | |
| > 2 years | 1 | > 50 | 1 |
| 2 - 5 years | 10 | 51 - 100 | 3 |
| 5 - 12  " | 1 | 101 - 300 | 5 |
| | | 301 - 500 | 2 |
| | | 501 -1000 | 1 |

Five trials applied dietary means to reduce cholesterol - and practically each dietary approach was different from the others: low-fat diet, addition of corn or soybean oil. Out of the seven drug trials three were conducted with Clofibrate, one with Nicotinic-acid, one with their combination, one with oestrogen and another with (colestipol.

Even if one assumes - with little justification - that the method of lipid - lowering is irrelevant, the differences remain worrying. In six trials patients were enrolled in the study more than one year after their qualifying infarction. There are only three trials where this was reduced to 1 to 3 months. In addition to this in the two British Clofibrate Trials (Scottish and New Castle) angina alone was also a criterion of eligibility. In the largest trial, the Coronary Drug Project, 50 % of the patients had their qualifying infarction more than two years prior to enrollment!

Numbers of enrolled and followed patients in the treatment group also vary widely from 50 to over 600. But at least the majority - 8 - deals with more than 100 patients - even though this is also insufficient for meaningful analysis. There is more uniformity in the length of the trial , which in most cases is five years.

In five of the twelve trials one cannot speak of clinically manifest hypercholesterolaemia although epidemiologists frown upon levels between 230-260 mg% (Table 2).

Table 2. Cholesterol

| Initial levels mg% | | Reduction % | | |
|---|---|---|---|---|
| 230 - 259 | 5 | 6 - | 10 | 4 |
| 260 - 289 | 7 | 11 - | 15 | 5 |
| | | 16 | | 3 |

The overall reduction achieved from these initial levels also showed great variation: only in three trials did the reduction exceed 15 %, while in four it stayed below 10 %. It is worth to note that diet trials did not fare worse in this respect than the drug ones.

C. Specific aspects

Each one of the reviewed trials has already been scrutinized and criticized in the literature. It is therefore proposed to discuss them under a few general headings, instead of going through their merits and shortcomings one by one.

1. Patient selection and sampling frame

Wide differences between trials with regard to time elapsed since qualifying infarctions were already mentioned. Variations in the preselection of possible candidates are much less conspicuous. In the Oestrogen-trial of Oliver e.g. "all men between 35 and 64 years admitted to two medical wards of the Edinburgh Royal Infirmary within 48 hours of the first acute myocardial infarct (AMI)" were eligible. From 182 such men 82 were excluded on the ground of various criteria, i. e. 45 %. In the New-Castle Clofibrate trial 22 consultants were asked to apply the selection criteria to an unspecified universe of patients. There is no indication about the sampling frame, i. e. the total number of subjects scrutinized for inclusion, nor about the percentage rejected - although the rejection criteria are known.

These facts do not necessarily weaken the results.of the individual trials: the question there being to detect a difference between intervention and control groups. However, secondary prevention should mean the application of measures of proven benefit to the whole postmyocardial infarction population. In this perspective exact information on the sampling frame and on the proportion of patients rejected becomes essential. Otherwise no interference can be made from the trial to the general AMI population.

## 2. Initial cholesterol levels

This was not a selection criteria in most trials, hence the trials were lowering cholesterol both in low or medium level and in high cholesterol patients. E.g. 20 % of the patients in Oliver's Oestrogen trial had initial cholesterol below 200 mg%, and only 40 % above 250 mg %. In the largest trial, the Coronary Drug Project, 50 % of the patients had entry levels below 250 mg%. Only two studies used cholesterol levels as selection criteria: the Colestipol study of Dorr et al. had an entry mean of 313 mg% - but only 1/3 of its subjects had a coronary heart disease at entry and their entry values are not published. The only trial where initial cholesterol values in patients with AMI were used for selection is that of Rosenhamer and Larson, with a mean starting value of 260 mg%. In the remaining trials the mean initial cholesterol was also around 260 mg%, with the exception of the Oslo study (Leren) where it was 296 mg%.

This wide variation could help to draw farfetching conclusions to the whole AMI population - it is also in line with the concept of secondary prevention. On the other hand it weakens the results of some trials: what benefit could be expected from lowering "low" cholesterol levels?

## 3. Treatment effect

Reduction of cholesterol was modest in most of the trials: around 12 %, although initial response after start of treatment was regularly more expressed. Interestingly enough, the lowest response was observed in the largest trial, the Coronary Drug Project. Here the reduction amounted only to 6 % with Clofibrate and 9 % with Niacin. Although caution was expressed for using retrospectively created subgroups in randomized trials (12), it might be enlightening to have a look at the relation of mean final cholesterol values and the observed mortality in the various subgroups (both Placebo and Clofibrate) in this trial.

Table 3

| Final Cholesterol mg% | Mortality % |
|---|---|
| 196 | 16 |
| 202 | 21.2 |
| 236 | 25.5 |
| 239 | 18.7 |
| 248 | 18.1 |
| 260 | 20.2 |
| 311 | 21.3 |
| 311 | 15.5 |

The two lowest mortalities were observed in the two Clofibrate subgroups with a)starting level below 250 mg% and subsequent fall and b)starting level above 250 mg% and subsequent rise. There is no detectable correlation between the two values in this table. In most of the other trials as well there was little or no correlation between cholesterol response and outcome.

Between-trial comparisons - as far as this is permitted - also tell the same story. There are trials with a fairly good cholesterol reduction and negative outcome and vice versa.

Table 4

| Mean Cholesterol reduction % | | Outcome |
|---|---|---|
| Oestrogen (Oliver) | 18 % | negative |
| Corn-oil (Rose) | 11 % | negative |
| Low-fat (Middlesex Hospital) | 15 % | negative |
| Soya-bean oil (MRC) | 12 % | aequivocal |
| Modified fat diet (Bierenbaum) | 10 % | positive |
| Oslo-Diet Heart Study (Leren) | 17 % | aequivocal |
| Clofibrate (Scottish Soc. Physicians) | 16 % | aequivocal |
| Clofibrate (New-Castle) | 8 % | aequivocal |
| Clofibrate (Coronary Drug Project) | 6 % | negative |
| Niacin (Coronary Drug Project) | 9 % | negative |
| Colestipol (Dorr) | 11 % | positive |
| Clofibrate-Niacin (Rosenhamer) | 14 % | positive |

4. Outcome

We will consider here three outcome criteria: total mortality, IHD mortality and non-fatal IHD events. Classification into positive (favourable), negative (unfavourable or no benefit) and aequivocal categories was done by taking each trial as a whole. Results in subgroups are not considered.

Table 5

| Outcome | Total mortality | IHD mortality | Non-fatal events |
|---|---|---|---|
| Positive | 2 | 4 | 3 |
| Negative | 4 | 6 | 4 |
| Aequivocal | 2 | 2 | 4 |
| Missing information | 4 | 0 | 1 |

Total mortality is the most important criterion. Only the two most recently reported trials were positive in this category. However the Colestipol-trial (Dorr) is a mixture of primary and secondary prevention and lacks the clear definition of patients with coronary heart disease (176 men and 109 women). From the Clofibrate-Niacin trial (Rosenhamer and Carlson) we have only - a highly encouraging - interim report. Even lumping together the positive and aequivocal results, the balance with negative outcome remains 50:50. The picture does not change much in the other two outcome groups, although a favourable trend in non-fatal events was reported in seven trials, in three of them significantly so. The balance should become more favourable if one would consider subgroup results as well, e.g. the angina subgroup in the two Clofibrate trials from the UK. Drug trials seem to fare off somewhat better, but one has to take into account that the five diet trials were conducted about twenty years ago and many of them would not stand present-day criticism.
Summing up the trial-evidence , one is compelled to say that up to the present moment there is no prima facie scientific evidence for lipid lowering as a general tool in secondary prevention. The evidence still has to come in.

924

## D. Conclusion

Trial results however are not the only and exclusive rationale in medicine. Other evidence should also be considered.
High cholesterol levels continue to imply higher risk of death and relapse after the first manifestation of CHD. This was clearly shown by the Framingham Study (13) and the Coronary Drug Project (14), among others.
Correction of high cholesterol was shown to lead to the regression of atherosclerotic lesions in animal experiments. (15)
Lately the Oslo-Study demonstrated distinct benefits of dietary treatment of hypercholesterolaemia in very high-risk subjects. (16)
There is little reason to doubt that this applies also to patients with already manifest IHD, although other factors related to this manifestation, e.g. infarct size, left ventricular impairment, etc. might obscure this effect.
Further incoming evidence will hopefully clarify which patients, from what kind and extent of lipid lowering benefit the most. Much was learnt from the weaknesses of the trials in the past to foster this optimism. But it is unlikely that all the new knowledge will abolish the carefully balanced recommendations of the three councils of the International Society and Federation of Cardiology (Epidemiology, Arteriosclerosis and Rehabilitation) formulated in 1980 (17) and quoted here in the form of a condensed extract: ... "In patients with established coronary heart disease, some but not all studies indicate that the level of plasma cholesterol continues to be a risk factor for recurrent myocardial infarction, albeit a weaker one than for the first attack. The controlled-trial evidence justifying plasma lipid reduction in secondary prevention is limited, but ....
....the possible benefits of reasonable dietary modification, including obesity control, should not be withheld from myocardial infarction patients or from the elderly. The value of antihyperlipidaemic drug therapy in coronary heart disease prevention has not been demonstrated, and its potential for untoward effects must be borne in mind. Such therapy is justified in patients with gross hyperlipidaemia and/or where there is a major risk of vascular or other serious complications...."

References

1. Oliver MF and Boyd GS: Influence of reduction of serum lipids on prognosis of coronary heart disease. Lancet, 1961, ii 499
2. Rose GA, Thomson WB, and Williams RT,: Corn oil in treatment of ischaemic heart disease. Brit. Med. J.1, 1965, 1531
3. Research Committee: Low-fat diet in myocardial infarction. Lancet, 1965, ii 501
4. Research Committee MRC: Controlled trial of soya-bean oil in myocardial infarction. Lancet, 1968, ii 693
5. Bierenbaum ML, et al.: The 5-year experience of modified fat diets on younger men with coronary heart disease. Circulation, XLII, 1970, 943
6. Leren P,: The Oslo Diet-Heart Study. Eleven year report. Circulation, XLII, 1970, 935
7. Research Committee of the Scottish Society of Physicians: Ischaemic heart disease: A secondary prevention trial using Clofibrate. Brit. med. J. 4, 1971, 775
8. Study group of physicians of the New-Castle upon Tyne region: Trial of Clofibrate in the treatment of ischaemic heart disease. Brit. Med. J. 4, 1971, 767
9. The Coronary Drug Project Research Group: Clofibrate and Niacin in coronary heart disease. Jama, 231, 1975, 360
10. Dorr AE, et al.: Colestipol hydrochlorid in hypercholesterolemic patients - Effect on serum cholesterol and mortality. J. Chron.Dis. 31, 1978, 5

11. Rosenhamer G, and Carlson LA.: Effect of combined Clofibrate-Nicotinic acid treatment in ischaemic heart disease. Atherosclerosis 37, 1980, 129
12. Coronary Drug Project Research Group: Influence of adherence to treatment and response of cholesterol on mortality in the Coronary Drug Project. N.Engl. J. Med. 303, 1980, 1038
13. Kannel WB, Sorlie PD, and McNamara PM.: Prognosis after initial myocardial infarction: The Framingham Study. Am. J. Cardiol.44, 1979, 53
14. Coronary Drug Project Research Group: Factors influencing long-term prognosis in the Coronary Drug Project. J. Chron. Dis.27, 1974, 267
15. Vesselinovitch O, Wissler RW, et al.: Reversal of advanced atherosclerosis in rhesus monkeys. Atherosclerosis 23, 1976, 155
16. Hjerman J, et al: Effect of diet and smoking intervention on the incidence of coronary heart disease. Lancet, 1981 ii 1303
17. ISFC Scientific councils on arteriosclerosis, epidemiology and prevention and rehabilitation: Secondary prevention in myocardial infarction survivors. Circulation 65, 1982, 216A

# A Controlled Trial of Substantial Reduction of Plasma Lipids in Symptomatic Atherosclerosis: An Angiographic Study

R. G. M. Duffield, B. Lewis, N. E. Miller, and C. W. Jamieson

Hypercholesterolaemia, low HDL cholesterol levels and hypertriglyceridaemia are predictive of increased risk of atherosclerotic diseases.
To establish that these associations represent cause and effect,
however, it is necessary to show that control of these risk factors
favourably affects the natural history of atherosclerosis and its
consequences. Three forms of intervention study have been carried out
in man, in which plasma lipoprotein levels have been modified by diet,
drugs or other therapeutic measures[1]. Most trials of primary prevention
of coronary heart disease (CHD) have suggested that its incidence is
reduced[1]; in the most rigorously-designed trial a lipid lowering diet
together with anti-smoking counselling was employed[2]. Of the CHD
secondary prevention trials some have achieved a reduction in events
while others have had negative outcomes.

The third category, arteriographic assessment of the progression or
regression of atherosclerosis has the advantages of a direct approach
and of requiring far fewer subjects; but it has been limited until
recently by problems of quantitation and reproducibility. Many, but
not all case reports have described regression[3,4]. The use of serial
quantitative arteriography in a group of hyperlipidaemic patients
with early asymptomatic atherosclerosis by Barndt et al[5] was a major
advance. This was an uncontrolled study; those subjects in whom diet
and drugs effectively reduced plasma lipids showed regression of
lesions, while those in whom treatment of hyperlipidaemia was unsuccessful showed progressive atherosclerosis.

We here report the interim results of a controlled arteriographic
study of the course of femoral atherosclerosis in hyperlipidaemic
patients. To our knowledge this is the first such trial in which the
participants were randomised into an intervention group and a usual
care group, permitting comparison between the evolution of atherosclerosis in treated patients and its natural history as assessed in
the controls. This was necessary as regression can occur without
intervention against risk factors; and it permitted us to investigate
the possibility that differing rates of progression might occur in
the two groups. The second major feature of the trial was the intention
to achieve large changes in plasma lipoprotein levels, by using the
treatment or treatment combination appropriate to the type of hyperlipidaemia. Inadequacy of the changes in plasma lipids is likely to
have been a partial explanation of negative or equivocal results in
some trials of CHD prevention, for the outcome of such trials more
often indicated a reduction of events in those in which the fall in
plasma cholesterol level was extensive[6]. The third feature of the
present study was the selection of subjects with intermittent
claudication; thus they had extensive atherosclerosis.

## Methods, Subjects and Intervention Protocol

Patients were invited to participate on the basis of hyperlipidaemia (cholesterol >6.5 mmol.l$^{-1}$ and/or triglyceride >2 mmol.l$^{-1}$) associated with stable intermittent claudication due to superficial femoral atherosclerosis, without haemodynamically-significant aorto-iliac disease. Informed consent was obtained. Subjects aged >64 years, those with diastolic blood pressure >100 mm Hg, diabetics and patients requiring prompt surgical treatment were excluded. After baseline observations, 24 patients were randomised into intervention and usual-care groups, which were closely matched (Table 1).

Table 1. Baseline characteristics

|  | Treatment | Usual care |
|---|---|---|
| Mean age | 54.8 | 56.1 |
| Males | 10 | 11 |
| Females | 2 | 1 |
| Mean duration of symptoms (months) | 14 | 12 |
| Hyperlipoproteinaemia: |  |  |
| IIa, IIb | 8 | 8 |
| III | 3 | 1 |
| IV | 1 | 3 |
| cholesterol, mmol.l$^{-1}$ | 8.05±0.41 | 7.72±0.26 |
| triglyceride, mmol.l$^{-1}$ | 3.25±0.80 | 3.10±0.50 |
| HDL-cholesterol, mmol.l$^{-1}$ | 1.23±0.12 | 1.20±0.07 |
| Cigarette use per day: |  |  |
| 0 | 4 | 4 |
| 1-10 | 2 | 4 |
| 11-20 | 3 | 2 |
| >20 | 3 | 2 |

Lipoproteins were separated by preparative ultracentrifugation and heparin-MnCl$_2$ precipitation. Lipid measurements were by manual enzymatic procedures. Biplanar transfemoral arteriography was performed at baseline and after 15-24 months (mean 19). By use of a restraining jig and careful measurements of bony landmarks reproducible localisation of the limb was achieved. A single Xray machine was used, with standard intensifying screens, 0.6 mm focal spot diameter, focus-film distance 135 cm and relatively short film-object distance. To synchronise the 20 msec exposure with the cardiac cycle the exposure was triggered by the R wave of the ECG (with an 0.4 sec delay). Through a Paul New 18 guage arteriogram needle 30 ml meglumine iothalamate was injected at an identical pressure on both occasions.

Patients in both groups received repeated anti-smoking advice and a reducing diet as appropriate. The intervention group were instructed in a fat-modified diet (fat providing 30% of energy, cholesterol intake <250 mg.d$^{-1}$, polyunsaturated fatty acid: saturated fatty acid ratio 1.0). All received one or two lipid lowering drugs. Type II was treated with cholestyramine 12-24 g.d$^{-1}$, supplemented in some patients with nicotinic acid 3-6 g.d$^{-1}$, Type III hyperlipoproteinaemia was treated with clofibrate 1.5 or 2 g.d$^{-1}$; Type IV was treated with nicotinic acid. The mean reduction in plasma cholesterol in the treated group was 25%, and that in plasma triglyceride was 42%; mean HDL-cholesterol increased by 26%. Minor lipoprotein changes occurred in the usual-care group (Table 2).

Arteriograms were read visually and by computerised scanning. The extent and severity of atheroma were similar in the intervention and control groups at baseline. Two independent observers, blinded as to the treatment group, read the coded pairs of films. In 1 cm segments, vessel edge irregularity was assessed, using a magnifying lens and vernier calipers. Cross-sectional plaque area was measured at 1 mm intervals assuming a nominal vessel wall sleeve. Computer-based assessment was performed using the Magiscan programmable image analyser. Input was by a high performance videocamera, the signal being digitized by an analogue converter. Comparable 2.5 cm segments of paired arteriograms were scanned at 0.8 mm intervals. We here report interim analyses based upon an index of edge irregularity.

Results and Discussion

Table 2 shows the mean responses of plasma lipids and smoking during the study, and visual and computer-scanning assessment of changes in arteriographic measurements after 15-24 months.

Table 2. Lipid, smoking and arteriographic changes

|  |  | Treatment | Usual care |
|---|---|---|---|
| Cholesterol, mmol.$1^{-1}$ |  | 6.06±0.32 | 7.48±0.25 |
| Triglyceride, mmol.$1^{-1}$ |  | 1.80±0.20 | 2.81±0.48 |
| HDL cholesterol, mmol.$1^{-1}$ |  | 1.55±0.08 | 1.10±0.09 |
| Cigarettes smoked, mean±S.E.M. |  | 16±2.7 | 14±3.2 |
| Visually assessed segments, n |  | 144 | 156 |
| Segments showing progression, n |  | 10 | 27 |
| % segments showing progression |  | 6.9 | 17.3 |
| Increase in plaque area ($mm^2$ per year per segment) | mean | 0.58 | 1.72 |
|  | range | 0-12 | 0-14 |
| Edge irregularity index |  | 0.019±0.062 | 0.047±0.076 |

In the intervention group the proportion of segments showing progression was reduced by 60% compared with the usual care group ($P<0.01$, chi-square) and the rate of increase in cross-sectional area of plaques was one-third of that in the controls ($P=0.057$, Mann-Whitney U test). This assessment was greatly facilitated by the availability of biplanar radiographs. The edge irregularity index also suggested a greater rate of progression in the usual care group ($P<0.05$, Mann-Whitney U test).

Relating this study to other trials of lipid reduction, a major difference was the more advanced vascular disease in our patients than in some other investigations in which regression could be observed. It is well documented that severe experimental diet-induced atheroma in primates regresses[7,8] when cholesterol levels are reduced to 5.5 mmol.$1^{-1}$ for 24 months[9]. The size and duration of the present study permit only tentative conclusions. Substantial reduction of hyperlipidaemia favourably affected the natural history of symptomatic atherosclerosis of the femoral artery, considerably retarding its further progression. The findings favour the view that hyperlipidaemia in our subjects was causally related to their arterial disease, and that vigorous treatment of lipid risk factors may slow the atherogenic process even when it is advanced. It is already evident that early

plaques are more likely to regress than advanced lesions. The present
trial is continuing, to establish whether severe atheroma in man will
regress after prolonged therapy.

The computer programmes were developed with the assistance of
Drs JMH Brunt and A Colchester at Manchester University. The trial was
supported by a grant from Bristol Laboratories.

## References

1. Lewis B (1981) Ischemic heart disease: the scientific bases of
   prevention. In Progress in Cardiology 10: 21-44. Eds PN Yu,
   JF Goodwin. Philadelphia: Lea and Febiger

2. Hjerrman I, Byre KV, Holme I, Leren P (1981) Effect of diet and
   smoking intervention on the incidence of coronary heart disease.
   Lancet ii: 1303-10

3. Zelis R, Mason DI, Braunwald E, Levy RI (1970) Effects of hyperlipoproteinemias and their treatment on the peripheral circulation.
   J Clin Invest 49: 1007-15

4. Malinow MR (1981) Regression of atherosclerosis in humans: fact or
   myth? Circulation 64: 1-3

5. Barndt R Jr, Blankenhorn DH, Crawford DW, Brooks SM (1977) Regression
   and progression of early femoral atherosclerosis in treated hyperlipoproteinemic patients. Ann Intern Med 86: 139-46

6. Lewis B (1980) The LDL theory and the HDL hypothesis. In Diet and
   Drugs in Atherosclerosis, p 1-8. Eds G Noseda, B Lewis, R Paoletti.
   New York: Raven

7. Armstrong ML, Megan MB (1972) Lipid depletion in atheromatous coronary
   arteries in Rhesus monkeys after regression diets. Circ Res 30:
   675-80

8. Wissler RW, Vesselinovitch D (1976) Studies of regression of advanced
   atherosclerosis in experimental animals and man. Ann N Y Acad Sci
   275: 363-78

9. Wagner WD, St Clair RW, Clarkson TB (1980) A study of atherosclerosis
   regression in Macaca Mulatta II. Am J Pathol 100: 633

# Program of the Surgical Control of the Hyperlipidemias (Posch).
# A Secondary Intervention Trial – 4-Year Lipid Results

J. M. Long, R. B. Moore, J. P. Matts, R. L. Varco, H. Buchwald, and the POSCH Group

## Overview

The Program on the Surgical Control of the Hyperlipidemias (POSCH) is a randomized secondary intervention clinical trial of the effects of lipid modification on atherosclerotic cardiovascular disease. All participants must have experienced one well documented myocardial infarction (MI), have coronary atherosclerosis, and be relatively free of other health problems. Up to 1000 patients are being enrolled in four clinical centers in the United States of America (USA), half receiving the partial ileal bypass (PIB) operation to reduce their plasma total cholesterol by an average of 30% and LDL cholesterol by an average of more than 40%, with the other half serving as controls. Participants are followed intensively for five years and less intensively thereafter. The primary endpoint for POSCH is death from any cause. A number of secondary endpoints and variables are also followed, including serial coronary arteriography. POSCH is funded by a grant from the National Heart, Lung, and Blood Institute of the USA.

## Trial Design

The study's design, standard for clinical trials, is based on the hypothesis that there is no difference in mortality between the intervention group and the control group or that there is a difference. The assumption was made that, for the difference to be clinically significant, the mortality would be reduced by 50% or from 4% per year to 2% per year. Using the assumptions and the design parameters of a two-sided alpha of .05 and a power of .95 the minimum required sample size allowing for a minimal dropout and nonadherence, was calculated to be 800 patients. For the clinical trial, this number was increased to 1000 (500 control, 500 surgical intervention) in order to provide an adequate sample size (i.e., with a contingency factor). POSCH has the ability to enroll about 200 patients per year with over 600 patients enrolled in June 1982.

Participants must have had one, and only one, enzymatically and electrocardiographically documented MI within the last six to 60 months. They must have a cholesterol level of at least 220 mg/dl or at least 200 mg/dl if the LDL cholesterol is 140 mg/dl or greater. Atherosclerosis of the coronary arteries must be demonstrated by coronary angiography. The participants have to be relatively free of hypertension, diabetes mellitus, a number of other major cardiovascular risks (e.g., serious arythmia, heart failure, enlarged heart), and other conditions having a high mortality risk (such as cancer) during the five or more years of their participation in the trial. Thus, POSCH is a unifactorial trial: there is one intervention modality and the participants have essentially a single health problem.

Individuals who meet these extensive eligibility requirements are recruited by four clinical centers covering the North, East, South and
West quadrants of the USA. Eligible individuals who are willing to participate in the trial are randomly assigned to either the control group
or to the intervention group. All participants remain under the care of
their personal physician and receive conventional medical care provided
patients with known coronary heart disease. Those assigned to the surgical (intervention) group have their cholesterol lowered permanently
and maximally by the PIB surgery developed at the University of Minnesota
by Buchwald et al. (1). The PIB operation involves bypassing the distal
one-third or 200 cm (whichever is greater) of the small bowel, and has
been extensively reported since 1963. It is important to clearly distinguish the PIB from the much more drastic jejunal ileal bypass (JIB)
operation. The JIB, developed as a means of reducing body weight in
morbidly obese patients, bypasses 90% of the small bowel in contrast to
the 33% bypassed in the PIB. The JIB has a number of serious side effects including liver failure, arthritis, and electrolyte imbalance,
and is no longer widely used. The PIB does not have these side effects,
nor is there any significant permanent weight loss.

Randomization assignments are made by the Coordinating Center and are
totally unpredictible in advance. However, once randomized, it is obviously not possible to blind either the patient or the clinic staff
as to who received the surgery. The two groups, control and surgery,
are followed carefully for five years, and after five years are followed
less intensively for an indefinite period of time. Every effort is made
to give equal attention to both groups after entry into the study. Both
groups are contacted by phone monthly for three months, bi-monthly for
the remainder of the first year and quarterly thereafter. During the
first five years each participant undergoes an annual intensive three
day examination, similar to the examination done at the baseline period
prior to enrollment in the study. This examination includes: history
and physical examination, including angina and smoking history; a three
day lipid profile, after a 14-hour fast; a 3-hour oral glucose tolerance
test after a 14-hour fast; a battery of other blood chemistry tests;
pulmonary function tests; a graded treadmill exercise ECG stress test;
chest X-ray; and arm and leg blood pressures. At baseline, and at the
third and fifth year of follow-up, the participants undergo heart ca-
therization, including left ventriculography and coronary arteriography,
along with peripheral angiography.

All major study data are processed by the Coordinating Center, a separate
unit of POSCH responsible to an external group of scientific experts
(Data Monitoring Committee) who monitor its operations as well as the
interim results including participant safety. The results are blinded
to everyone else including the trial clinical staff, participants, and
the principal investigators. Three central laboratories assess all data
related to the three major variables of our study: lipids, ECG, and arteriography; without knowledge of the patient's clinic or group assignment.

The primary endpoint in this trial is total mortality. In addition there
are a number of secondary and serial assessment endpoints: cause specific mortality; another myocardial infarction; serial assessment of the
ECG stress test data; and peripheral occlusive disease assessed using
doppler arm and leg blood pressure measurements. Perhaps the most important secondary variable under study is the serial coronary arteriography assessment. This is a feature unique to POSCH, and permits the
documentation of the extent and severity of the atherosclerotic disease
process over time in living subjects and the relationship of the disease process to clinical manifestations of the disease. The control
group provides insights regarding the natural history of the disease.

The intervention group in comparison to the control group provides information regarding the effect of the maximal lowering of plasma cholesterol: Will it retard, arrest or even regress the disease process?

## Results

As is customary and required for such studies, results are kept confidential until the study ends in order to avoid possible bias. At the current time baseline data and the effect of the PIB surgery on the patient's lipid profile can be reported (2).

*Baseline Characteristics.* The average age of participants is 50.6 ± 7.4 (SD) years. Most subjects (91.8%) are males and Caucasian (97.2%). Many (38.2%) have a family history of heart disease, i.e., a family member having premature effect of coronary heart disease (before age 60). Most (56.4%) have a history of angina pectoris, and 43.1% have positive exercise ECG tests. The average weight is 81.9 ± 11.8 kg, average height is 173.9 ± 7.1 cm, average systolic blood pressure is 121.6 mm ± 14.5 mm Hg, and average diastolic blood pressure is 78.8 mm ± 9.4 mm Hg. At baseline 11.8% have never smoked, 48.8% had previously smoked tobacco but stopped prior to baseline, and 39.4% are current tobacco smokers.

*Plasma Total Cholesterol.* The plasma total cholesterol values (mg/dl ± SD) for the control and the surgery groups at baseline, 3-months, 1-year, 2-years, 3-years, and 4-years, with the number of subjects at each time period are given in Table 1. There were no clinically significant differences in the plasma total cholesterol in the controls for the entire period of evaluation. The plasma total cholesterol was reduced significantly (p<.01) and in a sustained manner in the surgery group: 34.5% at 3-months, 29.6% at 1-year, 26.9% at 2-years, 30.2% at 3-years, and 27.3% at 4-years in comparison to the mean baseline value. There was no statistically significant difference between the groups at baseline but there were highly significant (p<.01) differences at each subsequent period of assessment.

*Plasma LDL-Cholesterol.* The LDL-cholesterol values are presented on line two of the Table, in a manner comparable to that used for the plasma total cholesterol. Again, there were no clinically significant differences in the controls over the four years of analysis. In the surgery group, LDL-cholesterol showed an ever greater relative reduction than the total cholesterol; which was significant (p<.01) and sustained: 47.4% at 3-months, 42.2% at 1-year, 41.0% at 2-years, 43.4% at 3-years, and 39.8% at 4-years in comparison to the mean baseline value. The difference between control and the surgery groups was significant (p<.01) at each time interval of assessment after baseline.

*Plasma HDL-Cholesterol.* The plasma HDL-cholesterol values are presented in the Table. In the controls, the HDL-cholesterol level tended to decrease with time: 0.4% at 3-months, 2.1% at 1-year, 3.4% at 2-years, 7.2% at 3-years, and 7.3% at 4-years. In the surgery group, the HDL-cholesterol increased with time: 2.4% at 3-months, 6.8% at 1-year, 4.0% at 2-years, 1.7% at 3-years, and 0.8% at 4-years. At 1-year, 2-years, and 3-years the difference between the control and surgery groups is statistically significant (p<.05). The number of subjects at 4-years is currently too small to declare the observed difference between the control and surgery groups as statistically significant.

*Plasma HDL-Cholesterol/LDL-Cholesterol Ratio.* The HDL-cholesterol to LDL-cholesterol ratios are given in the Table. The control group's LDL-cholesterol changed only slightly and the HDL/LDL ratio in the controls did not change significantly over the 4-year period. However,

Table 1. POSCH Lipid Results (mean mg/dl ± S.D.)

| | Baseline (n=254,236) | 3 Months (n=216,210) | 1 Year (n=168,155) | 2 Years (n=110,111) | 3 Years (n=67,80) | 4 Years (n=35,38) |
|---|---|---|---|---|---|---|
| **Total Cholesterol** | | | | | | |
| Controls | 255.1 ± 35.5 | 248.2 ± 38.4 | 248.9 ± 37.7 | 251.2 ± 31.0 | 243.5 ± 31.8 | 252.2 ± 40.9 |
| % Change | | -2.7 | -2.4 | -1.5 | -4.5 | -1.1 |
| Surgery | 255.0 ± 33.9 | 167.0 ± 28.0 | 179.5 ± 31.3 | 186.4 ± 34.8 | 178.0 ± 30.7 | 185.3 ± 30.2 |
| % Change | | -34.5 | -29.6 | -26.9 | -30.2 | -27.3 |
| **LDL Cholesterol** | | | | | | |
| Controls | 182.7 ± 36.6 | 177.0 ± 35.4 | 176.0 ± 38.6 | 179.5 ± 32.2 | 170.8 ± 36.0 | 173.5 ± 47.4 |
| % Change | | -3.1 | -3.6 | -1.7 | -6.5 | -5.1 |
| Surgery | 182.3 ± 35.0 | 95.8 ± 25.2 | 105.3 ± 29.1 | 107.6 ± 30.3 | 103.2 ± 24.6 | 109.8 ± 30.0 |
| % Change | | -47.4 | -42.2 | -41.0 | -43.4 | -39.8 |
| **HDL Cholesterol** | | | | | | |
| Controls | 41.3 ± 10.0 | 41.1 ± 9.0 | 40.4 ± 10.5 | 39.9 ± 8.8 | 38.3 ± 8.3 | 38.3 ± 9.0 |
| % Change | | -0.4 | -2.1 | -3.4 | -7.2 | -7.3 |
| Surgery | 40.9 ± 9.6 | 41.8 ± 10.1 | 43.6 ± 10.6 | 42.5 ± 10.5 | 41.6 ± 9.5 | 41.2 ± 8.7 |
| % Change | | +2.4 | +6.8 | +4.0 | +1.7 | +0.8 |
| **HDL/LDL Cholesterol Ratio** | | | | | | |
| Controls | .2331 ± .0696 | .2401 ± .0663 | .2404 ± .0843 | .2285 ± .0611 | .2328 ± .0736 | .2308 ± .0614 |
| % Change | | +3.0 | +3.1 | -2.0 | -0.1 | -1.0 |
| Surgery | .2307 ± .0668 | .4614 ± .1466 | .4423 ± .1715 | .4184 ± .1399 | .4211 ± .1224 | .4070 ± .1444 |
| % Change | | +100.0 | +91.7 | +81.4 | +82.5 | +76.4 |
| **VLDL Cholesterol** | | | | | | |
| Controls | 30.3 ± 18.8 | 28.0 ± 16.9 | 29.6 ± 20.5 | 29.5 ± 18.8 | 32.0 ± 22.5 | 36.9 ± 26.0 |
| % Change | | -7.5 | -2.3 | -2.7 | +5.6 | +22.1 |
| Surgery | 30.4 ± 18.0 | 28.6 ± 21.1 | 29.6 ± 21.5 | 34.7 ± 29.1 | 32.0 ± 24.7 | 33.1 ± 18.6 |
| % Change | | -6.2 | -2.7 | +13.9 | +4.9 | +8.6 |
| **Triglycerides** | | | | | | |
| Controls | 194.3 ± 89.3 | 183.2 ± 104.0 | 189.5 ± 104.4 | 198.7 ± 102.8 | 208.3 ± 118.2 | 222.9 ± 146.1 |
| % Change | | -5.7 | -2.4 | +2.3 | +7.2 | +14.7 |
| Surgery | 197.0 ± 91.9 | 195.0 ± 111.4 | 211.1 ± 124.2 | 230.1 ± 169.3 | 212.4 ± 136.9 | 216.3 ± 85.0 |
| % Change | | -1.0 | +7.1 | +16.8 | +7.8 | +9.8 |

* Number of subjects at time interval: first value controls, second surgery group
** Percent change is calculated from baseline

933

since the surgery group's LDL-cholesterol was markedly decreased following partial ileal bypass and the HDL-cholesterol increased slightly with time, there was a very marked increase in the HDL/LDL ratio following surgery which ranged from 100% at 3-months to 76.4% at 4-years. There were very significant (p<.001) differences between control and surgery groups at all follow-up time periods.

*Plasma VLDL-Cholesterol and Plasma Triglycerides.* The plasma VLDL-cholesterol values are given in the Table. There were no statistically significant trends with time in either the control or the surgery group. The plasma triglycerides values are given in the Table. Similar to the VLDL-cholesterol findings, there are no statistically significant trends in either the control or the surgery group.

## Discussion and Conclusions

Coronary heart disease (CHD) is the leading cause of death in the USA and other Western countries. Atherosclerosis is the primary underlying pathology for nearly all coronary heart disease. The plasma cholesterol level is a primary independent risk factor. This has been further refined to be primarily the cholesterol carried in low density lipoproteins, with high density lipoprotein cholesterol levels acting in a presumably "protective" manner. The lipid (or cholesterol) theory of atherogenesis states that atherosclerosis is a disease of multiple causes in which altered lipid (cholesterol) metabolism plays a crucial and operant role. A very large body of evidence from a variety of scientific disciplines supports this theory. However, the corollary to this theory, "Does a reduction in plasma cholesterol level result in a reduction in the incidence and/or severity of atherosclerotic cardiovascular disease?" remains to be conclusively documented.

During the past 25 years there have been a number of clinical trials reporting the effect of plasma cholesterol reduction, by dietary or drug therapy, on atherosclerotic dardiovascular disease. All of the trials except POSCH employed either diet, drug therapy, or a combination of diet and drug therapy as the intervention modality. The net average cholesterol reduction achieved in the completed trials ranged from 7% to 16% (3). The maximum net cholesterol reduction currently reported for the on-going diet or drug trials ranges from 7.4% to the 15-20% range (3). The completed trials have shown no convincing evidence for disease retardation, arrest or reversal associated with the very modest degrees of plasma cholesterol reduction achieved. POSCH is currently achieving an average of about 30% reduction in plasma total cholesterol concentration sustained over 4 years, with more than a 40% reduction in LDL-cholesterol, and a higher HDL-cholesterol level. This study is the only clinical trial of plasma cholesterol reduction using serial coronary and peripheral arteriography to document the extent and severity of atherosclerotic vascular disease and its rate of change during the course of the trial. Thus, POSCH is a clinical trial of the effect of maximum plasma cholesterol modification on atherosclerotic cardiovascular disease itself, as well as on its clinical manifestations (i.e., myocardial infarction, death, etc.). We conclude that POSCH will provide a definitive answer to the corollary of the lipid-atherosclerosis theory for secondary intervention, namely, does plasma lipid lowering result in a reduction in the atherosclerosis cardiovascular risk in man? Should this answer be in the affirmative for total plasma and LDL-cholesterol lowering, the logical extension of these conclusions to primary intervention would be strongly suggested.

References

1. Buchwald H, Moore RB, Varco RL: Surgical treatment of the hyperlipidemia. Circulation 49 (Suppl 1): 1-37, 1974
2. Moore RB, Buchwald H, Varco RL, POSCH Group: The effect of partial
   ileal bypass on plasma lipoproteins. Circulation 62: 469-76, 1980
3. Buchwald H: Overview of Randomized Clinical Trials of Lipid Intervention for Atherosclerotic Cardiovascular Disease. J Chronic Disease, in press

*Members of the POSCH Clinical Trial Study Group.* H Buchwald, RL Varco,
GS Campbell, M Pearce, J Bissett, DH Blankenhorn, A Yellin, ME Sanmarco,
S Brooks, WL Holmes, RD Smink, HS Sawin, N Tuna, K Amplatz, WR Castaneda,
J Stevenson, J Karnegis, JM Long, JP Matts, CM White, LF Fitsch, RB Moore,
B Hansen, J Allen, C Walters, B Kuhn, H Brooks, JC Speech, P Curry,
J Rindal, K Wood, J Carlson, M Stuenkel, M Morris, MJ Masteller, F Russell,
M Huenergardt, R Finley, P Peters, P Gladu, *Data Monitoring Committee.*
TC Chalmers, JE Bearman, CR Conti, G Cooper, L Friedman, SW Greenhouse,
P Meier, CL Meinert, DE Strandness. *Mortality Review Committee.*
JE Edwards, AJ Moss, LCS Griffith, D Spain.

# Platelet-Vessel Wall Interactions in Human and Experimental Hypercholesterolemia

E. Tremoli, C. Galli, and R. Paoletti

Institute of Pharmacology and Pharmacognosy, University of Milan, Milan, Italy.

## INTRODUCTION

The natural history of the atherosclerotic processes depends on a sequence of critical events, resulting from the interaction between blood components, lipids and the arterial wall (1,2,3). Blood platelets may interact directly or _via_ their released products with vessel walls and therefore are considered important in the pathogenesis of the disease (4,5,6).

In this paper the modifications of platelet function and biochemistry in human and experimental hypercholesterolemia are discussed.

## PLATELET STUDIES IN TYPE IIa HYPERCHOLESTEROLEMIA

The main objective of this study was to assess whether platelet function and platelet prostaglandin biosynthesis is altered in a large group of selected type IIa hypercholesterolemic subjects, originating from the same geographic area and with the same dietary habits, in comparison to a group of age and sex matched normocholesterolemic subjects.

150 type IIa hypercholesterolemic subjects were selected in our Lipid Clinic according to WHO criteria (mean cholesterol levels $313.9\pm9$ LDL $241.3\pm8$, VLDL $28.3\pm1$, HDL $44.3\pm3$). The results of platelet studies were compared with those obtained from 80 sex and age matched normocholesterolemic subjects.

Platelet aggregation studies were performed in platelet rich plasma samples (PRP), according to Born turbidimetric technique (7), using ADP, Epinephrine and Collagen as aggregating agents.

As previously reported (8,9,10,11), although in a smaller number of patients, platelets from type IIa subjects required significantly lower amounts of ADP, Epinephrine and Collagen to aggregate, as compared with platelets from normocholesterolemic subjects ($p < 0.0001$).

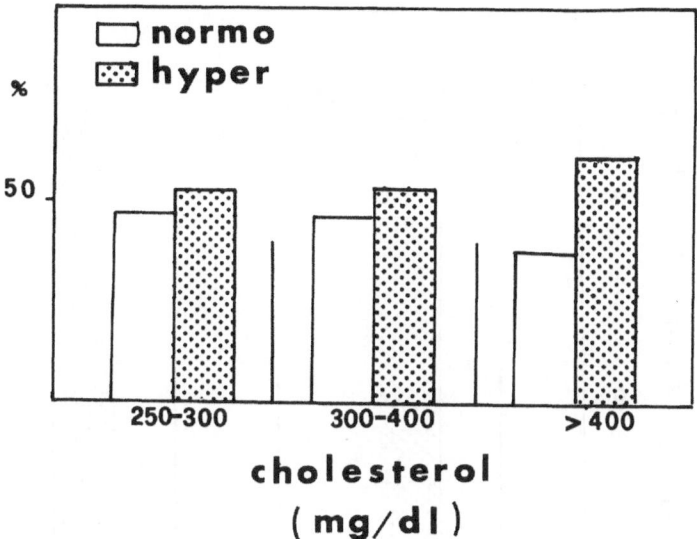

**Fig. 1.** Responses to aggregation in type IIa subjects

A great number of type IIa subjects, however, showed a response to platelet aggregation within the range of that recorded for normal subjects. Type IIa patients were therefore divided in two groups accordingly to their aggregation pattern. Fig. 1 represents the percentage of patients with normal and "hyperreactive" platelets, in relation to serum cholesterol levels. 45% of the patients with cholesterol levels between 250-400 mg/dl had an increased platelet response to aggregation (threshold concentration of ADP 0.25 $\mu$M, Epinephrine 0.06 $\mu$g/ml, Collagen 0.25 $\mu$g/ml). This percentage increased to 61 in those patients with cholesterol levels higher than 400 mg/dl.

No statistically significant correlation was found between age, sex, total and HDL cholesterol levels and platelet response to aggregating agents, confirming previous findings from our laboratory (11).

Malondialdehyde production (MDA) measured in stimulated platelets by the spectrophotometric technique described by Smith et al. (12) and thromboxane $B_2$ production by platelets stimulated with collagen were significantly increased in all the subjects studied.

These results indicate that platelets from type .IIa subjects produce increased amounts of arachidonic acid metabolites, via the cyclooxygenase pathway, and this increase production is not always associated with an abnormal response to the in vitro aggregation.

938

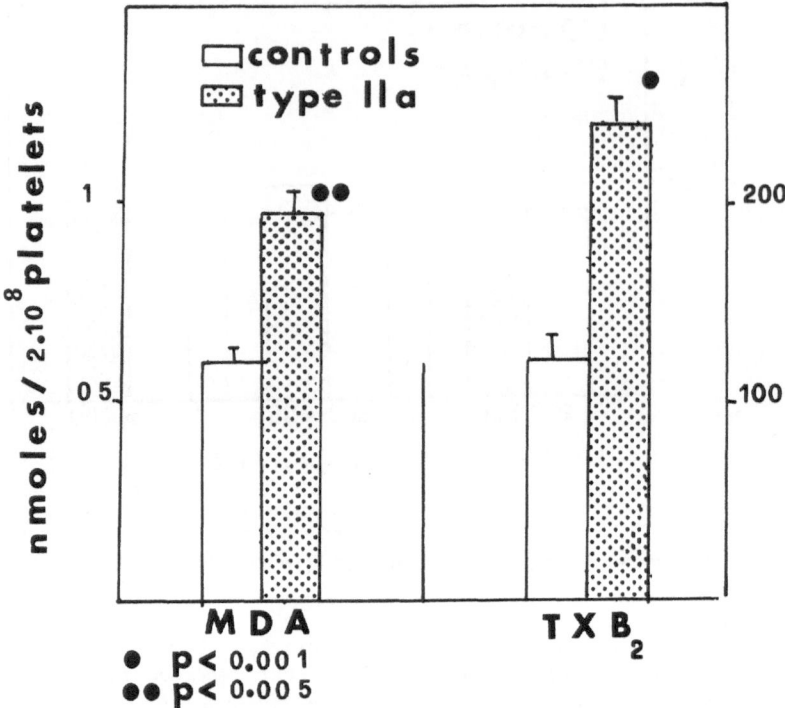

Fig. 2. MDA production by platelets stimulated with 30 ug/ml collagen and Thromboxane B$_2$ (TXB$_2$) formation after collagen stimulation
(10 ug/ml) in type IIa subjects and controls

## PLATELET-VESSEL WALL STUDIES IN EXPERIMENTAL HYPERCHOLESTEROLEMIA

Dietary induced hyperlipidemia has been shown to alter the blood
clotting systems and to predispose to thrombus formation (13).

A study was carried out in our laboratory to evaluate the effects
of experimentally induced hypercholesterolemia on the thromboxane-pro-
stacyclin balance in platelets and aortic tissue in the rabbit.

New Zealand male rabbits were fed either normal or 2% cholesterol
enriched diet for 1 month. At the end of the dietary period animals
were sacrified, blood was collected from the carotid artery for platelet studies and segments of aortic tissue were carefully removed and
kept in crushed ice until use. Platelet sensitivity to arachidonic
acid' induced aggregation (AA) and TXB$_2$ formation were measured. To
investigate the overall effects of dietary induced hypercholesterolemia
on the platelet-vessel wall system, an experimental model based on
the perfusion of platelet rich plasma samples through isolated segments

of thoracic aorta was used (14). PRP samples from normal and hypercholesterolemic animals (HC) were perfused, using a perfusion apparatus, through segments of thoracic aortas of the same animal. In the perfusates the sensitivity of platelets to aggregation induced by arachidonic acid (AA) and 6 KetoPGF$_{1\alpha}$ levels were measured.

As shown in Table 1, platelets from HC animals required lower concentrations of AA to aggregate, as compared to those from normal animals. The aggregation of platelet rich plasma samples perfused through aortic tissue was significantly reduced in both animal groups, as shown by the higher amounts of AA necessary to stimulate platelet aggregation.

|  | Before | After | A/B |
|---|---|---|---|
| Normals (n=8) | 0.31±0.06 | 0.51±0.08 [a] | + 64% |
| HC (n=8) | 0.16±0.01 [d] | 0.34±0.05 [b,c] | +112% |

Table I. AA(mM) concentrations inducing aggregation of PRP samples before and after perfusion through aortas (0.3 mm./min.) in normal and HC rabbits. a) $p < 0.05$ versus values before. b) $p < 0.01$ versus values before. c) not significant difference between the two groups after perfusion. d) $p < 0.02$ between values before perfusion in the two groups

The % increase in the threshold of AA, however, was higher in the HC group, in respect to controls, indicating that the antiaggregatory capacity of the vessel wall was not reduced by the hyperlipidemic state. 6 KetoPGF$_{1\alpha}$ levels measured in the perfused samples were also significantly higher in the HC group (data not shown), suggesting that the observed inhibition of platelet aggregation was mainly due to the production of prostacyclin by the vessel wall. TXB$_2$ levels measured in PRP after stimulation with collagen were similar in the two groups.

On the basis of these results it is possible to conclude that during experimental hypercholesterolemia platelet sensitivity to aggregation is profoundly modified, whereas prostacyclin production by vascular tissue is increased.

940

## CONCLUSIONS

In conclusion our studies in human type IIa hypercholesterolemia show a marked alteration of both platelet function and platelet biochemistry, in terms of aggregation and production of arachidonic acid metabolites. No information is available on the prostacyclin formation by vascular tissue, because of the inconsistency of blood measurements of prostacyclin metabolites.

The experimental model, based on the acute induction of hypercholesterolemia in the rabbit, is comparable, as far as platelet sensitivity to aggregation is concerned, to the human pathological state, but the thromboxane producing capacity appears to be affected to a less extent.

## REFERENCES

1. R. Ross, Atherosclerosis: A problem of the biology of arterial wall cells and their interactions with blood components. Arteriosclerosis, 1:293 (1981).
2. M.B. Stemerman and R. Ross, Experimental atherosclerosis. Fibrous plaque formation in primates, an electron microscopy study. J. Exp. Med., 136:769 (1972).
3. J.F. Mustard, M.A. Packham, The role of blood platelets in atherosclerosis and the complications of atherosclerosis. Thromb. Diath. Haemorrh., 33:444 (1975).
4. H. Holmsen, Biochemistry of the platelet release reaction, Biochemistry and Pharmacology of platelets, Ciba Foundation Symposium, Elsevier North Holland Biomedical Press, Amsterdam, 175 (1975).
5. H. Holmsen, The platelet, its membrane physiology and biochemistry, "Clinics in Hematology", WB Sanders Co, London, 2:235 (1972).
6. R. Ross, J. Glomset, B. Kariya and L. Harker, A platelet-dependent serum factor that stimulates the proliferation of arterial smooth muscle cells in vitro. Proc. Natl. Acad. Sci. USA, 75:4001 (1975).
7. G.V.R. Born, Aggregation of blood platelets by adenosine-diphosphate and its reversal, Nature, Lond. 194:927 (1962).
8. A.C.A. Carvalho, R.W. Colman and R.S. Lees, Platelet function in hyperlipoproteinemia, N. Engl. J. Med., 290:434 (1974).
9. A. Nordoy and J.M. Rodset, Platelet function and platelet phospholipids in patients with hyper-betalipoproteinemia: effect of nicotinic acid and clofibrate. Circulation, 50:570 (1974).
10. R. Fabrizewski and K. Worowski, Enhancement of platelet aggregation and adhesiveness by lipoproteins. J. Ather. Res. 8:988 (1968).
11. E. Tremoli, P. Maderna, M. Sirtori and C.R. Sirtori, Platelet aggregation and malondialdehyde formation in type IIa hypercholesterolemic patients. Haemostasis, 8:47 (1979).
12. J.B. Smith, C.M. Ingerman and M.J. Silver, Malondialdehyde formation as an indicator of prostaglandin production by human platelts. J. Lab. Clin. Med., 88:167 (1976).

13. A. Suehiro, E. Kakishita and K. Nagai, The role of platelet hyper-
    function in thrombus formation in hyperlipidemia. _Thrombosis
    Research_, 25:331 (1982).
14. E. Tremoli, C. Galli, A. Socini and R. Paoletti, Prostaglandins
    in the cardiovascular system: dietary lipid modulation, in
    publication.

# Secondary Prevention of Ischaemic Heart Disease by the Combined Treatment with Clofibrate and Nicotinic Acid

G. Rosenhammer and L. A. Carlson

Two recent large studies, one secondary prevention - the Coronary Drug Project (CDP) (1) - and one primary prevention study - the cooperative clofibrate trial (CCT) (2) - have led to much discussion on the value of serum lipid lowering in general, and of clofibrate in particular. In the CDP clofibrate has no significant effect on IHD, but effects on serum lipids were also modest, only a 6 per cent reduction of cholesterol. In the CCT, where serum cholesterol lowering was somewhat better, a significant reduction of non-fatal infarcts was achieved. However, an excess of deaths in the clofibrate treated group compared to the placebo has caused concern.

Over a three and a half year period beginning in December 1972, 555 survivors of myocardial infarction (442 men and 113 women) under the age of 70 years were recruited from one hospital into a therapeutic trial aimed to reduce serum lipids and to study the effect on subsequent morbidity and mortality. A preliminary report covering the period up to April 1979 has been published (3). Following a stabilization period of three months after infarction, patients were given a dietary programme to reduce serum lipids. Patients were then randomly divided into a) a treatment group which received a combined regimen of nicotinic acid (up to 3 g daily) and 2 g of clofibrate daily, and b) a control group on diet alone. Treatment was not "blinded" owing to the impossibility of conducting a blinded study with nicotinic acid, because of its side effects. All smokers were advised to quit, obese subjects were recommended to reduce weight. Other medical problems such as hypertension were treated according to the routine of the hospital.

The groups were comparable with regard to sex, age, weight, height, smoking habits, blood pressure and previous cardiovascular history. The maximal ASAT-value indicating the size of the infarction did not differ between the groups. There were 73 patients withdrawn from the trial in the drug group and 33 from the control group, the former primarily for subjective side effects or unwillingness to continue. Among those patients who remained in the study and completed the five year trial alive serum cholesterol and triglycerides in the drug treated group showed mean falls of 13 and 23% respectively in comparison with the control group.

Mortality and reinfarction data were assigned to the control and drug treated groups disregarding withdrawals, i e analyses were performed according to the intention-to-treat principle. The results are shown in Table 1.

There were 82 and 61 deaths from all causes in the control and drug treated groups respectively (p < 0.05). For the age group over 60 years, the corresponding figures were 53 and 38 respectively (p < 0.05).

Table 1. Number of clinical "hard" end points in the Stockholm
IHD study

|  | Controls | Drug thearpy | % reduction | P |
|---|---|---|---|---|
| Deaths total | 82 | 61 | 26 | <0.05 |
| Deaths IHD | 73 | 47 | 36 | <0.01 |
| Reinfarction | 25 | 24 | – | – |
| Major IHD (death + reinfarction) | 98 | 71 | 28 | <0.01 |

Initial, non-fatal reinfarcts occurred at rates of 4.1 and 2.8 (p <
0.05) per 100 man-years in control and drug groups respectively.
Combined major IHD expressed as the sum of deaths and initial non-
fatal reinfarctions among patients who were still alive at the end
of the five year trial were, again respectively, 8.1 and 5.7 per
100 man-years (p < 0.01). There were no significant differences in
number of other causes of deaths between the groups.

When analysed according to initial serum cholesterol and triglycerides the difference in total deaths between the control and
drug treated groups was most pronounced among patients with elevated triglycerides and normal cholesterol.

The differences observed between this study and the CDP, in which
clofibrate neither affected IHD mortality nor the incidence of non-
fatal reinfarctions, may be due to the fact that serum cholesterol
reduction on clofibrate in the CDP was very modest, 6% compared to
our 13%. With nicotinic acid treatment in the CDP, which resulted in
a 10% lowering of serum cholesterol, there was a 30% lower incidence
of non-fatal reinfarction than in the control group (p < 0.001).
Likewise in the CCT, where healthy men had been selected on account
of a "high" serum cholesterol, cholesterol was reduced by 9% and
non-fatal infarcts by 25% (p < 0.05).

Two other secondary prevention studies, the Scottish (4) and the
Newcastle (5), have used clofibrate as a lipid lowering drug. In
the former clofibrate reduced mortality in the subgroup having
angina and produced an average serum cholesterol lowering over 4
years of 12% for men and 24% for women. In the Newcastle study death
rates from IHD were significantly reduced and rate of non-fatal reinfarcts was lowered (p = 0.055). The mean reduction in serum
cholesterol in men was 17% over 4 years. These two studies thus
support our hypothesis (6) that a sufficient lipid lowering effect
has to be achieved for obtaining effects on the development of IHD.

References

1. The Coronary Drug Project Research Group (1975) Clofibrate and
   Niacin in coronary heart disease. J Amer Med Ass 231: 360-381
2. Oliver MF, Heady JA, Morris JN, Cooper J (1978) A co-operative
   trial in the primary prevention of ischaemic heart disease using
   clofibrate. Br Heart J XL: 1069-1118
3. Rosenhamer G, Carlson LA (1980) Effect of combined clofibrate -
   - nicotinic acid treatment in ischemic heart disease. Atherosclerosis 37: 129-318

4. Ischaemic heart disease: A secondary prevention trial using clofibrate (1971) Br Med J 4: 775-784
5. Trial of clofibrate in the treatment of ischaemic heart disease (1971) Br Med J 4: 767-775
6. Carlson LA, Rössner S (1975) Results of the coronary drug project - an interpretation. Atherosclerosis 22: 316-323

# 6 Risks of Obesity

# Introduction

F. A. Gries

Before entering the program may I shortly call your mind on the
confounding public discussion about the impact of obesity on general
health and in particular on atherosclerosis, which indeed urged us
to discuss the risks of obesity at this congress.
Obesity is a phenomenon that can be traced back to early periods of
mankind, when it appeared as fertility symbol. But even until the
last century it was - if at all - a problem only for upperclass
people and show monsters (1). Obesity as a public health problem was
brought up only during the last decades of our century. I need not
recall the pioneer work of the American life insurance companies,
which alarmed the public.
The Build and Blood Pressure Study from 1959 (2) and its numerous
interpretations had enormous consequences (3).

The term ideal body weight was created with the intention to define
highest life expectancy. It was described as being considerably
lower than the average weight thus putting the majority of people
of developed societies into an increased risk category. Popular
slogans like "The slimmer the better" were at hand. The interpretation that each kg of body fat may decrease life expectancy  resulted in an enormous psychological and social stress on those individuals who did not present the ideal slim figure.
Public opinion culminated in the statement, that obesity indeed is
the major health problem of our societies.

This is apparently an overinterpretation as pointed out by Epstein
(4) Björntorp (5) and many others.
However, the confusion of the public as well as the medical society
resulted from more recent studies which seemed either to disproved
the health risk of mild obesity or even favoured a moderate overweight of some 20-30 % as desirable body weight. At least in our
country conclusions from these studies were eagerly picked up by
the media and a new ideal of mild obesity was propagated.
This change in public opinion had a desastrous impact on the credi-
bility of medical science and health advices.

More important from a scientific point of view is an apparent problem that has basically questioned the concept of risk and risk
factors: If indeed moderate overweight were beneficial - as concluded from the Chicago Peoples Gas Company Study (6) and the recent Framingham data - we are confronted with the embarrassing
fact, that in this same population generally accepted risk factors
such as hypertension, impaired glucose tolerance, low HDL-levels,
as well as associated other diseases (gallstones etc.) are significantly more frequent. Thus, there would be increased longevity
inspite of increased prevalence of risk factors. Does this mean,
that risk factors have different relevance in obese people as compared with the general population, that risk factors are compen-

948

sated for by other obesity related conditions, or does the recent
discussion simply proceed on false assumptions?

These questions have stimulated much speculation. From studies with
genetically obese animals the concept has been developed, that the
obesity gene is a thrifty gene which allows better adaptation to
changing environmental conditions. In the some direction go recent
reflections of Bradley (7) who discussed, that the increasing frequency of obesity is a beneficial adaptation to changed environmental and nutritional conditions of modern life. This then would mean
that obesity, if only moderate, might not need therapy.

I have raised these few questions in order to give a frame and a
stimulation for the further discussion and we shall now proceed to
the first lecture.

References

1) Scheugel H (1975) Show freaks and monster. M Du Mont Schauberg
      Köln 2. Aufl
2) Soc of Actuaries (1959) Build and blood pressure study Chicago
3) Berger M, Berchtold P, Gries FA, Zimmermann H (1980) Indications
      for the treatment of obesity. Björntorp P, Cairelly M, Howard
      AN (eds) Rec Adv in Obesity Res III John Libbey London
4) Epstein FH (1979) Estimating the effect of preventing obesity in
      total mortality and hypertension. Int J Obesity 3: 163
5) Larsson B, Björntorp P, Tibblin G (1981) The health conse-
      quences of moderate obesity. Int J Obesity 5: 97
6) Dyer AR, Stamler J, Berkson DM, Lindberg HA (1975) Relationship
      of relative weight and body mass index to 14-year mortality in
      the Chicago Peoples Gas Company study. J chronic Dis 28: 109
7) Bradley PJ (1982) Is obesity an advantageous adaptation? Int J
      Obesity 6: 43

# Diabetes Mellitus and Obesity

E. L. Bierman

One of the ways obesity increases the risk of atherosclerosis is through its association with diabetes mellitus, a potent cause of premature, accelerated, and severe atherosclerotic cardiovascular disease. There is an intimate relationship between these two disorders, since most diabetics are obese (1). In terms of the new Diabetes Data Group classification of diabetes, more than three quarters of Western diabetic populations are obese type II diabetics. Data from the Joslin Clinic for almost 5,000 diabetics over the age of 20, suggests that at least 50% of males and 60% of females are more than 20% overweight defined by standards applied to the nondiabetic population. Furthermore, epidemiologic studies have shown that the prevalence of diabetes in a population is a direct function of the average weight of that population (2). Genetic susceptibility appears to play a major role in this relationship since obesity appears to unmask diabetes in those susceptible individuals with a family history of diabetes. Although the degree of obesity in an individual subject appears to influence the severity of glucose intolerance and hyperglycemia in a population, the duration of obesity rather than its degree appears to be the more closely related determinant (1). The reason becomes clear from an examination of the pathophysiological basis for the relationship between obesity and diabetes.

Obesity is associated with hyperinsulinemia, both in the basal state and in response to stimuli for insulin secretion (3). Hyperinsulinemia results from a compensatory increase in insulin secretion, in response to insulin resistance in extrahepatic cells. This insulin resistance appears to be a direct function of fat cell size and is associated with impaired glucose metabolism by cells. Insulin resistance is manifested at both the receptor level (as a consequence of feedback down-regulation of the insulin receptor due to hyperinsulinemia) and at the postreceptor level of glucose metabolism (4).

The obese diabetic maintains hyperinsulinemia compared to thin normal or diabetic individuals both in the basal state and after oral or intravenous glucose stimuli. However, insulin responses are impaired compared to obese nondiabetic controls (3). A deficiency of the acute insulin response to an intravenous glucose pulse is the hallmark of glucose intolerance in the hyperglycemia in the obese diabetic; in fact diabetics with fasting plasma glucose levels above 125 mg/dl uniformly have lost their acute insulin response (5). These results suggest a scheme whereby increasing adiposity leads to insulin resistance and compensatory hyperinsulinemia, which in so-called "simple obesity" does not culminate in hyperglycemia and diabetes. In individuals who are genetically prone, the pancreatic beta cell will fail to keep up with the increased demand for insulin secretion, insulin responses fail and hyperglycemia ensues. This situation is analogous to "high output failure" of the heart.

Hyperinsulinemia per se associated with obesity may play a role in atherosclerosis. There have been three recent population studies

950

demonstrating that high plasma insulin levels, both basal and after
a glucose load, are associated with increased incidence of atherosclerotic coronary heart disease (6).

What are the mechanisms associated with the hyperinsulinemia in the
type II obese diabetic related to the development of atherosclerosis?
From recent insights into the cell biology of atherogenesis, there
are several places in the reaction to injury hypothesis for atherogenesis where insulin excess might play a role.  For example, insulin
in physiologic concentrations in cell culture studies has been shown
to enhance primate arterial smooth muscle cell proliferation (7) and
increase cholesterol flux into extrahepatic cells by directly enhancing low density lipoprotein receptor activity and endogenous cellular
cholesterol synthesis (8).

Low HDL levels have been uniformly observed in obese type II diabetics (9) which could confer an additional risk for atherosclerosis.
The low HDL is characterized by low HDL cholesterol, with partial
substitution of cholesterol by triglyceride in the particle, without a reduction in     HDL particle number (9)(Figure 1).

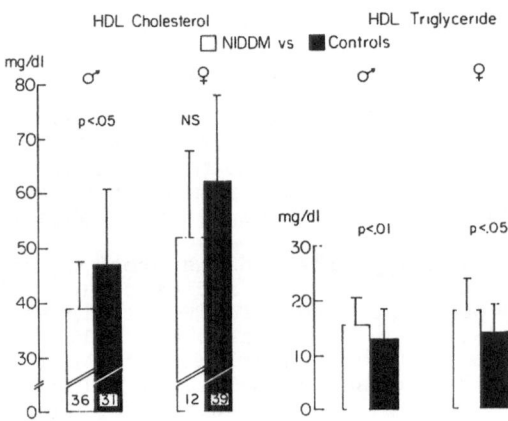

Fig. 1.  Plasma HDL cholesterol and triglyceride levels in non-insu-
lin dependent diabetic (NIDDM) and control males and females.  Numbers of subjects indicated within bars.  Data from Biesbroeck et al.
(9)

951

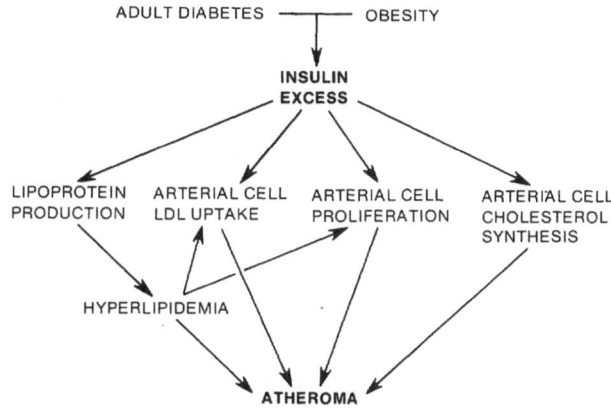

Fig. 2. Some of the multiple mechanisms by which the "diabesity" disorder might be associated with atherogenesis is summarized in Figure 2

## References

1. Bierman EL, Bagdade JD, Porte D Jr (1968) Obesity and diabetes: the odd couple. Am J Clin Nutr 21: 1434-1437
2. West KM, Kalbfleisch JM (1971) Influence of nutritional factors on prevalence of diabetes. Diabetes 20: 99-108
3. Bagdade JD, Bierman EL, Porte D Jr (1967) The significance of basal insulin levels in the evaluation of the insulin response to glucose in diabetic and nondiabetic subjects. J Clin Invest 46: 1549-1557
4. Olefsky JM, Kolterman OG (1981) Mechanisms of insulin resistance in obesity and noninsulin-dependent (type II) diabetes. Am J Med 70: 151-168
5. Brunzell JD, Robertson RP, Lerner RL, Hazzard WR, Ensinck JW, Bierman EL, Porte D Jr (1976) Relationships between fasting glucose levels and insulin secretion during intravenous glucose tolerance tests. J Clin Endocrinol Metab 42: 182-189
6. Stout RW (1981) Blood glucose and atherosclerosis. Arteriosclerosis 1: 227-234
7. Stout RW, Bierman EL, Ross R (1975) The effect of insulin on the proliferation of culture primate arterial smooth muscle cells. Circ Res 36:319-327
8. Chait A, Bierman EL, Albers JJ (1979) Low density lipoprotein receptor activity on cultured human skin fibroblasts: mechanism of insulin-induced stimulation. J Clin Invest 64: 1309-1319
9. Biesbroeck RC, Albers JJ, Wahl PW, Weinberg CR, Bassett ML, Bierman EL (1982) Abnormal composition of high density lipoproteins in non-insulin-dependent diabetics. Diabetes 31: 126-131

# Hypertension in Obesity

P. Björntorp

Having the choice for a lifelong therapy of chronic disease between on the one side changes of life style by diet therapy and advice of exercise and on the other drug treatment the first alternative is preferable. Chronic drug treatment of lifelong diseases has recently been the subject of medical controversy in the conditions of diabetes mellitus and hyperlipidemia. The side effects of this treatment have been discussed and the treatment by diet and exercise reemphasized.

The drug treatment of essential hypertension has experienced a dramatic improvement during the recent past decades, and a wide selection of effective drugs are now available. Side effects have, of course, been reported. In addition, this chronic drug treatment has as yet not been evaluated as strictly as the drug treatment in diabetes mellitus and hyperlipidemia, and in addition has not been controlled in longitudinal studies.

With this background it seems desirable to explore the possibilities available to treat essential hypertension with non-drug therapy. The problem of salt has here attracted a great attention, and intervention studies with salt restriction are going on.

There is, however, another alternative available which should be systematically tested, restrictions of energy intake combined with increased exercise. As will be seen in the following this might be valid particularly in the form of hypertension which often is combined with obesity.

## The Association between Blood Pressure Regulation and Energy Metabolism

There are at least two ways whereby energy metabolism and blood pressure regulation can be thought to be associated. De Fronzo et al (1) have shown that insulin increases the sodium retention in the kidney via an effect on the distal tubuli. The hyperinsulinemia often seen with obesity might give a tendency to sodium retention and therefore hypertension. It is easy to imagine how both the restriction of energy intake and increased exercise would be able to give a blood pressure decrease via such a mechanism, because both are effective ways to lower high plasma insulin levels.

An alternate explanation is the relation between carbohydrate metabolism and catecholamine sensitivity in several different catecholamine sensitive systems (2). It is possible that diet and exercise effects the catecholamine sensitivity to decrease the blood pressure. Particularly with mild early hypertension the catecholamine sensitivity has often been in focus for the discussion of pathogenesis.

## Hypertension in Obesity, a Separate Entity of Essential Hypertension?

Regarded in this way it is possible that the blood pressure elevation often seen in obesity is another symptom among the already previously wellknown metabolic disturbances such as hyperinsulinemia and hyper-triglyceridemia as well as decreased glucose tolerance. It appears likely that the hyperinsulinemia is the earliest and most central symptom. It is then possible to see how this secondarily can lead to a decreased glucose tolerance and diabetes mellitus, to hypertriglyceridemia, and now also to hypertension.

## Diet and Exercise as Therapeutic Alternatives in Hypertension in Obesity

It is wellknown that the blood pressure is decreasing when obesity is treated by diet. Usually this has been considered to be a consequence of the fact that when the energy intake is decreased, the salt intake is also decreased; salt follows calories. A recent study (3) indicates, however, that calory restriction without salt restriction products a considerable decrease of blood pressure in hypertensive obese subjects.

Another study (4) has recently shown that exercise gives a blood pressure decrease in obese subjects. The blood pressure decrease was independent of changes in body weight. Instead there were several statistical associations between the blood pressure decrease and improvements of the metabolic variables, such as decrease of insulin and triglycerides in plasma and an improvement of glucose tolerance. In both these studies the blood pressure decrease was apparently not associated with the salt intake but instead to variables in the energy metabolism.

Diabetes mellitus type II and hypertriglyceridemia, which both often are associated with obesity, are both treated with diet and exercise as a first alternative, and then, if not sufficient, drug treatment is added. It is entirely possible that another obesity associated complication, viz. essential hypertension should be treated along the same principles.

## Research needed

There is now so much background data available that these ideas should be interesting enough to test in practice and on a larger scale in comparison with effective drug treatment. Such trials should be ethically possible if patients with mild hypertension are examined. What we need to know is exactly how effective this treatment is and if the effect is remaining, and how feasible the therapy is. Treatment of obesity in general is difficult, but the type of obesity in patients with essential hypertension seems to have comparably good prognosis for treatment.

Obesity is a prevalent condition and so is elevated blood pressure in obesity. Non-selected hypertensive patients found at random in a population often are obese and have deranged energy metabolism (6). The problem discussed above is thus of considerable quantitative importance.

## References

1. Berglund G, Larsson B, Andersson O, Larsson O, Svärdsudd K, Björn-torp P, Wilhelmsen L (1976) Body composition and glucose metabolism in hypertensive middle-aged males. Acta Med Scand 200: 163-169

2. Björntorp P, de Jounge K, Sjöström L, Sullivan L (1970) The effect of physical training on insulin production in obesity. Metabolism 19: 631-638
3. de Fronzo RA, Cooke CR, Andres R, Faloona GR, Davis PJ (1975) The effect of insulin on renal handling of sodium, potassium, calcium and phosphate in man. J Clin Invest 55: 845-855
4. Krotkiewski M, Mandroukas K, Sjöström L, Sullivan L, Wetterquist H, Björntorp P (1979) Effect of long-term physical training on body fat, metabolism and blood pressure in obesity. Metabolism 28: 650-658
5. Landsberg L, Young JB (1978) Fasting, feeding and regulation of the sympathetic nervous system. N Engl J Med 298: 1295-1301
6. Reisin E, Abel R, Silverberg DS, Eliahou HE, Modan B (1978) Effect of weight loss without salt restriction on the reduction of blood pressure in overweight hypertensive patients. N Engl J Med 298: 1-6

# Surgical Risks in Obese Patients

J. G. Kral

## Introduction

Obesity, commonly defined as increased body weight for height compared to the general population, is associated with significantly greater morbidity compared to normal (1). There is a greater prevalence of surgical diseases in the obese and, other diseases associated with obesity increase the prevalence of surgical complications in over-weight patients (see table). It follows that the increased morbidity in the obese is accompanied by an elevated mortality rate. Since non-surgical treatment is disappointingly unsuccessful, various surgical methods for treating this serious condition have been developed (2) on the assumption that the concomitant weight loss will reduce the morbidity and mortality associated with the obesity, even taking into consideration the morbidity and mortality of the surgery (3).

Table. Surgical diseases and surgical complications in obese patients

| Surgical diseases | Surgical complications |
|---|---|
| Metabolic | Anesthesia |
|    Cholelithiasis | Respiratory |
|    Thromboembolism | Pulmonary |
|    Urolithiasis |    atelectasis |
|    Neoplasia |    pneumonia |
| | Circulatory |
| Physical | Healing |
|    Osteoarthritis |    infection |
|    Caesarian section |    hernia (secondary) |
|    Hernia (primary) | Technical |

It is difficult to assess the risk of surgery in the obese. Selection biases make it practically impossible to interpret such statistics. On the one hand patients considered poor surgical risks due to their obesity have been selected away from elective procedures. This leaves candidates with either more serious primary conditions indicating the surgery, or ones with less serious conditions thus considered to have a lower risk of complications. One the other hand, patients who have been selected away from elective procedures may require emergency operation, in which case they are at still greater risk for complications. Some might even have died prior to surgery and by thus being "selected away" leave patients at less risk, thus improving the surgical statistics.

This review will identify surgical diseases and surgical complications more prevalent in the obese, and will suggest methods for preventing the complications.

956

## Surgical Diseases

### Metabolic

The most common obesity-related surgical disease is cholelithiasis, due in part to increased secretion of lithogenic bile (4). Such bile is supersaturated with cholesterol thus influencing its solubility. Several factors may be responsible for the increased secretion of biliary cholesterol: diet is important, as has been shown in studies of bile composition before and after dietary intervention mainly focussing on the carbohydrate content of the diet (5). Since insulin stimulates hepatic HMG CoA-reductase activity, the rate-limiting enzyme in cholesterol synthesis, it is conceivable that the hyper-insulinemia in obesity increases hepatic secretion of cholesterol. Furthermore, the enlarged adipose tissue compartment represents a substantial pool of cholesterol in obese patients (6).

The most important metabolic complication of obesity is thromboembolism since it is the major cause of spontaneous and post-operative death. Elevated levels of free fatty acids (FFA) due to adipose tissue lipolysis in the obese influence hemostatic variables such as clotting factors and fibrinolysis, as well as prostaglandin and thromboxane synthesis. Furthermore, FFA may have a direct effect on the vessel wall (7). The prevalent hypertriglyceridemia in obesity is similarly associated with significant effects on hemostatic variables which are favorably influenced by dietary management (mainly carbohydrate reduction)(8). The incidence of thromboembolic disease in obesity is potentiated by other factors known to increase the risk of such disease such as smoking and/or oral contraceptives.

Several studies have revealed an increased incidence of urolithiasis in the obese, though the mechanism has not been fully elucidated (9). Here again deranged carbohydrate metabolism may be involved. A rise in urinary calcium after glucose ingestion has been described (10). Insulin dependent glucose uptake in the renal tubular cell has been suggested as a cause of hypercalciuria (11). Body weight has been shown to be an important determining factor in renal handling of calcium and phosphorous (12).

Another group of obesity-related surgical diseases of metabolic origin is neoplasia, particularly in women. Cancer of the uterus=endometrial cancer, and breast cancer are more prevalent in the obese. Benign neoplastic conditions such as myoma and fibroma of the uterus and ovarian cysts are more frequent in overweight women (13). The mechanism for development of these endocrine tumors seems to be conversion of androstenedione to estriol in the enlarged adipose tissue mass (14), thus acting as a metabolic stimulus for malignant and benign neoplasia.

### Physical

The sheer load of excess weight increases the prevalence of osteoarthritis in weight-bearing joints and the spine of obese patients. Most orthopedic surgeons will refuse to perform hip replacement or knee surgery in the morbidly obese until they have lost a substantial amount of weight. The osteoarthritic condition, however, precludes one of the main adjuncts of weight management: physical activity. Severely obese patients are limited to weight-supported activity such as swimming, some types of gymnastics and possibly rowing.

An increased incidence of Cesarian sections in the obese may be con-

sidered a mechanical obstetric disease caused by a physical impediment
to normal delivery causing prolonged labor. Furthermore, a greater
frequency of toxemia of pregnancy, diabetes mellitus and hypertension
during pregnancy influence the rate of cesarian section.

Obesity is associated with a greater frequency of primary herniae,
particularly umbilical herniae. It is probable the overweight creates
chronic increase in intraabdominal pressure which also participates
in causing a greater prevalence of incisional herniae compared to
patients of normal weight.

## Surgical Complications

There are three groups of surgical complications more prevalent in
the obese population: those pertaining to anesthesia, wound healing
and surgical-technical difficulties.

The most common anesthetic complications are related to respiratory
function. Hypoventilation with $CO_2$-retention necessitates post-operative use of respirators more often than in lean or normal weight
patients. Atelectasis and pneumonia are more prevalent in the obese
due to a restrictive ventilatory pattern. The hypoventilatory syndrome combined with decreased general mobility participate in causing
a hypokinetic circulation predisposing to post-operative thrombosis,
further aggravated by the metabolic disturbances mentioned previously.

Would healing is generally recognized as being impaired in overweight
patients. This is most likely due to an increased frequency of wound
infections. Such infections may be caused by serous and sanguinous
secretion from the thick layer of subcutaneous adipose tissue, creat-
ing a rich substrate for bacterial growth. Hypothetically, increased
glucose levels in the blood contribute to this enhanced substrate.
Elevated levels of corticosteroids found in the obese may also impair
wound healing. The (pre) diabetic state of these patients may similarly disturb healing through compromised microcirculation. According to one report, morbidly obese patients have a defect lymphocyte
function (15) with thus might make them more susceptible to post-
operative infections. Wound infections are the single most important
factor causing incisional hernia, closely followed by chest infection
(16). Thus, it is obvious that obese patients are at great risk for
herniation (17).

The last group of surgical complications, technical problems are related to poor access due to obstructing fat, as well as difficulties
in handling the tissues due to their fat content. This high fat
content may also cause the tissues to be more friable, thus more
easily traumatized and more difficult to suture. In a group of 25
morbidly obese surgical patients, 3 (12%) had decreased levels of
connective tissue in biopsies from different organs, possibly reflecting an impaired collagen synthesis, as has been described in
patients with hernia, varicose veins and hemmorrhorids, all of which
are more prevalent in the obese.

## Prevention

It is obvious that great care must be exercised in selection of obese
patients for surgery. Awareness of the many risks of complications
will influence this selection. Efforts must be made to achieve
optimal preoperative conditions in the individual case by regulating

958

diabetic control and normalizing blood pressure. In elective surgery the obese patient must be urged to discontinue smoking at least two months prior to surgery. Similarly, discontinuation of oral contraceptives should be encouraged. Diet management, mainly reducing carbohydrate intake, would seem logical though there is no data defining an appropriate minimum duration of such a diet. Though drastic weight reduction might be the wish of many surgeons, it must be kept in mind that a catabolic state at the time of surgery might be more detrimental than the obesity would have been.

Preoperative physical therapy with respiratory training can help to improve pulmonary function and should be utilized routinely. Physical therapy will also facilitate early post-operative mobilization of the patient—a very important measure for preventing thrombosis, atelectasis and pneumonia. The use of low-dose heparin has been questioned (17) due to the risk of wound hematoma. The use of intermittent compression stockings is probably as effective as low-dose heparin and does not seem to be encumbered by any complications. Such stockings counteract the hypokinetic circulation and seem to activate and release endogenous venous fibrinolytic substances. So-called prophylactic antibiotics have helped to cut the rate of wound infections in the obese. Attention to surgical technique would seem to be more important in obese patients than otherwise and efforts should be made to bring down operating times by using well-manned teams of surgeons familiar with operating on obese patients.

Conclusions

It is necessary to recognize that surgery of the obese patients needs special attention and expertise, though the principles employed are characteristic of all types of surgery. Experience with performing operations for obesity has improved the quality of care in treating obese patients requiring surgery for other diseases. By demonstrating the feasibility of operating on morbidly obese patients, the indications for surgery of such patients have widened, and thus may favorably change the morbidity and mortality in that population.

References

1.  Van Itallie, Theodore B  (1979) Obesity: adverse effects on health and longevity.        Am. J. of Clin. Nutr. 2723-2733
2.  Kral, J G (1982) Surgical Therapy.  In: Obesity. (ed) MRC Greenwood. Contemporary Issues in Nutrition
3.  Van Itallie, Theodore B, Kral, John G (1981) The Dilemma of Morbid Obesity. JAMA 9: 999-1003
4.  Shaffer, Eldon A, Small, Donald M (1977) Biliary Lipid Secretion in Cholesterol Gallstone Disease: The effect of cholecystectomy and obesity. J. Clin. Invest. 59:828-840
5.  Bennion, Lynn J, Grundy, Scott M. (1975) Effects of Obesity and Caloric Intake on Biliary Lipid Metabolism in Man. J. Clin. Invest. 56:996-1011
6.  Schreibman, P H, Dell, R B (1975)  Human adipocyte cholesterol. Concentration, localization and turnover. J. Clin. Invest. 55: 986-993
7.  Mjös, O D (1971) Effect of free fatty acids on myocardial function and oxygen consumption in intact dogs. J. Clin. Invest. 50:1386-1389

8.  Elkeles, R R, Chakrabarti, R, Vickers, M, Stirling, Y, Meade, T W
    (1980) Effect of treatment of hyperlipidaemia on haemostatic
    variables. British Med. J. 281:973-974
9.  Ljunghall, S, Hedstrand, H (1978) Glucose metabolism in renal
    stone formers. Urol. Int. 33:417
10. Lemann, J Jr, Adams, N D, Gray, R W (1979) Urinary calcium
    excretion in human beings. N. Engl. J. Med. 301:535
11. Lindeman, R D, Adler, S, Yiengst, M J, Beard, E S (1967) Influence
    of various nutrients on urinary divalent cation excretion. J. Lab.
    Clin. Med. 70:236
12. Ulmann, A, Aubert, J, Bourdeau, A, Cheynel, C, Bader, C (1982)
    Effects of weight and glucose ingestion on urinary calcium and
    phosphate excretion: Implications for calcium urolithiasis.
    J. Clin. Endocrin. Met. 54:1063-1068
13. Pitkin, R M (1976) Abdominal hysterectomy in obese women. Surg.
    Gynecol. Obstet. 143:532-536
14. Nimrod, A, Ryan, K J (1975) Aromatization of androgens by human
    abdominal and breast fat tissue. J. Clin. Endocrinol. Metab. 40:
    367
15. Hallberg, D, Nilsson, B S, Backman, L (1976) Immunological
    function in patients operated on with small intestinal shunts
    for morbid obesity. Scand. J. Gastroenterol. 11:41-48
16. Bucknall, T E, Cox, P J, Ellis, Harold (1982) Burst abdomen and
    incisional hernia: a prospective study of 1129 major laparotomies.
    British Med. J. 284:931
17. Printen, K J, Miller, E V, Mason, E E, Barnes, R W (1978) Venous
    thromboembolism in the morbidly obese. Surg. Gyn. Obstet. 147:63-64

# Obesity and Lipoprotein Metabolism

## G. Steiner

### Lipoprotein Concentrations, Obesity, and Diet

There is a general, but not universal correlation between the plasma levels of VLDL-triglyceride and obesity (1-3). Similar, though weaker links have been seen in the case of LDL. This probably reflects the fact that in general LDL is the product of VLDL degradation (4). HDL cholesterol levels are also generally acknowledged to be lower in obese than in lean individuals. This may reflect, in part, the inverse relationship between plasma levels of triglyceride and those of HDL cholesterol. However, even after correcting for the impact of this relationship, obesity still is associated with decreased levels of HDL-cholesterol (5). Each of these alterations may account for some of the increase in atherosclerosis associated with obesity.

When considering the effect of changes in body mass, as induced by a variety of diets on lipoproteins, the validity of some common clinical generalizations must also be examined. It is clear that weight reduction will tend to normalize plasma cholesterol and triglyceride levels in many obese hyperlipidemics (6,7). However, this is not always the case. Even as drastic as a procedure as total fasting in morbidly obese individuals produces little change in plasma cholesterol or triglyceride, and that which occurs is not significant until after two weeks (8). The reverse situation, overfeeding, has also produced inconsistent responses in plasma lipids. Some have found slight increases in both cholesterol and triglycerides (8), others have found no changes (9). One aspect which must be considered in interpreting such data is the nature of the diet fed to these individuals. As will be discussed later, there may be significant differences in the kinetics of the lipoproteins as a consequence of the relative proportions of the diet's various nutrients.

### VLDL Kinetics -General Considerations

To this point, the data has all been concerned with concentrations of plasma lipids and lipoproteins. As best, these are are an imprecise reflection of changes in lipoprotein metabolism. At worst, as will be indicated below, major changes in kinetics can occur with no change in concentrations. In general, the Sf 60-400 (i.e. VLDL) particle is the precursor for the Sf 12-60 (i.e. IDL) particle and that in turn for the Sf 0-12 (i.e. LDL) particle (4). Exceptions to this may be seen in type III hyperlipoproteinemia in which there is also direct input of IDL (11); and in type II hyperlipoproteinemia (12), and perhaps in obese type IV hyperlipidemics (13) in whom there is also direct input of LDL. Although we have found evidence of direct transfer of triglyceride to pre-existing VLDL particles in the circulation (14), we have noted a linear relationship between the production rates of VLDL B apolipoprotein and triglyceride (15). Melish et al failed to observe a similar linear relationship (16). However, rather than studying individuals on balanced diets as we had, they studied the effects of a high carbohydrate diet. The effect changes in triglyceride concentrations produced by such a diet on both triglyceride kinetics and VLDL morphology is quite variable and is very different from that seen in a population of individuals, while on a balanced diet, each of whom, has a different triglyceride concentration (15,17,18).

### VLDL Kinetics In Obesity

The total rate of triglyceride production in grossly obese individuals on a weight-maintaining balanced diet is greater than that in lean individuals. However, the obese demonstrate a normal hyperbolic relationship between their plasma triglyceride concentration and their triglyceride production rate per kg (8). When these obese individuals fast, their rates of triglyceride production fall. Despite this decrease in VLDL triglyceride production, there is little change in their plasma triglyceride concentrations (8). This would lead one to predict that, as the production rates fall in these individuals, so also do their rates of triglyceride removal. Indeed, on examining the relation between the triglyceride kinetics to concentrations during fasting, it is apparent that the triglyceride removal is indeed impaired (8). This is consistent with both the well described decrease in adipose tissue lipoprotein lipase on fasting (19) and our observation that the fractional catabolic rate of VLDL B apolipoprotein is linearly related to the activity of lipoprotein lipase (20).

## Role of Hyperinsulinemia

These changes in VLDL triglyceride kinetics are linearly related to the levels of insulin in the plasma (8). This is in accord with the observations that obese humans are insulin-resistant and that, if their pancreatic B cells are sufficiently responsive, they are hyperinsulinemic (21). It is also consistent with other findings in humans in which both rates of triglyceride production and concentrations of plasma triglyceride are also directly related to plasma levels of insulin (22,23). Even in vitro, insulin has been shown to increase VLDL triglyceride production by perfused livers (24).

To determine whether these changes could result from the hyperinsulinemia alone, or from some other phenomenon in the obese, we reproduced a previously described rat model of massive hyperinsulinemia (25). This was done by injecting rats with insulin, up to 6 units per day, for two weeks. At the end of that period there was little difference in body weight, but there was an eight-fold increase in serum insulin compared to controls (26). The hyperinsulinemic rats' adipose tissue showed a diminution in the enhancement of glucose oxidation produced by insulin in vitro. This was accompanied by a decrease in the insulin binding capacity of these adipocytes. However, this was not sufficient to account for the insulin resistance for glucose oxidation was reduced even when normal adipocytes were compared to "hyperinsulinemic" adipocytes which had bound the same amount of insulin per cell (27). Thus, even in the absence of obesity, hyperinsulinemia induced both a receptor and a post-receptor defect.

The hyperinsulinemia induced in these rats was not accompanied by hypertriglyceridemia (26). This contrasts with observations in obese humans and resembles observations in patients with islet adenomas (26). Does it mean that the increase in triglyceride production seen in obese humans does not result from their hyperinsulinemia, but is due to some other aspect of obesity? Does it mean that plasma FFA levels in the presence of massive, but not minor hyperinsulinemia are too low to support VLDL triglyceride production? Does it relate to the amount and, or route of insulin delivery? Does it mean that triglyceride removal is sufficiently elevated to overcome an increase in production?

We are only beginning to get some of the answers to these questions. The plasma levels of FFA do fall 50 percent. However, in spite of this, the production of VLDL triglyceride, as determined by the Triton WR 1339 method (28) rises 160 percent. Hence, the failure of these hyperinsulinemic rats to develop hypertriglyceridemia is not due to a decrease in VLDL triglyceride secretion. The implication of these observations is that triglyceride removal is also greatly accelerated. This is consistent with the observations of others about the influence of insulin on lipoprotein lipase (29).

## Implications in relation to other lipoproteins

The production of LDL as a catabolic product of VLDL allows one to recognize the potential impact of alterations in VLDL kinetics on LDL. Into this consideration must be drawn the data discussed earlier about the direct input of LDL. Ultimately, as in the case of VLDL, the concentration of LDL will depend on the balance between production from these two routes and LDL removal.

The relationship between HDL production, LPL activity and the catabolism of triglyceride rich lipoproteins has been reviewed (30). Certainly the alterations in HDL concentrations observed in obesity can be easily understood in terms of these relationships.

## Acknowledgments

This work was supported by grants from the Medical Research Council of Canada and the Ontario Heart Foundation.

## References

1. Lewis B, Chait A, Wootton IDP, Oakley CM, Krikler DM, Sigurdsson G, February A, Maurer B, Birkhead J (1974) Frequency of risk factors for ischemic heart disease in a healthy British population Lancet i:141

2. Abrams ME, Jarrett RJ, Keen H, Boynes DR, Crossley JN (1969) Oral glucose tolerance and related factors in a normal population sample. II Interrelationships of glycerides, cholesterol and other factors with the glucose and insulin response. Brit. Med. 1:599

3. Lewis B, Chait A, Oakley C, Krikler D, Carlson L, Eriksson M, Boberg J, Mancini M, Oriente P, Paggi E, Michelli H, Malczewski B, Weisswange A, Pometta D (1974) Plasma lipoprotein abnormalities in normal and atherosclerotic subjects in four cities. In: Atherosclerosis III p 839 Schettler G, Weizel A, (Eds) Springer-Verlag, Berlin

4. Reardon MF, Steiner G (1982) The use of kinetics in investigating the metabolism of very low and intermediate density lipoproteins. In: Lipoprotein Kinetics and Modeling. Berman M, Grundy SM, Howard B (Eds) Academic Press

5. Glueck CJ, Taylor HL, Jacobs D, Morrison JA, Beaglehole R, Williams OD (1980) Plasma high-density lipoprotein cholesterol: Association with measurements of body mass. Circulation 62 (IV); 62

6. Blacket RB, Woodhill JM, Leelarthaepin B, Palmer AJ (1975) Type-IV hyperlipidemia and weight-gain after maturity. Lancet ii: 517

7. Leelarthaepin B, Woodhill JM, Palmer AJ, Blacket RB (1974) Obesity diet and type-II hyperlipidemia. Lancet ii: 1217

8. Streja D, Marliss EB, Steiner G (1977) The effects of prolonged fasting on plasma triglyceride kinetics in man. Metabolism 26: 505

9. Sims EAH, Goldman RF, Gluck CM, Horton ES, Kelleher PC, Powe DW (1968) Experimental obesity in man. Trans. Ass. Am. Physicians 81: 153

10. Goldrick RB, Havenstein N, Carroll KF, Reardon M (1972) Effects of overfeeding on lipid and carbohydrate metabolism in lean young adults Metabolism 21:176

11. Reardon MF, Poapst ME, Steiner G (1982) The independent synthesis of intermediate density lipoproteins in type III hyperlipoproteinemia Metabolism (in press)

12. Soutar AK, Myant NB, Thompson GR (1977) Simultaneous measurement of apolipoprotein B turnover in very low and low density lipoproteins in familial hypercholesterolemia. Atherosclerosis

13. Ginsberg H, Le N-A, Gibson J, Mays C, Brown WV (1982) Effect of weight reduction on very low density lipoprotein and low density lipoprotein apoprotein-B metabolism Clin. Res. 30:393A

14. Steiner G, Reardon MF (1982) A model of VLDL metabolism based on its heterogeneity. In: Lipoprotein Kinetics and Modeling. Berman M, Grundy SM, Howard B (Eds) Academic Press

15. Poapst M, Reardon MF, Steiner G (1982) Type IV hyperlipoproteinemia - the relative contributions of increased particle number and expanded particle size. In: Proc. VI Int. Symp. on Atherosclerosis.

16.    Melish J, Ngoc-Anh L, Ginsberg H, Steinberg D, Brown WV. (1980) Dissociation of apolipoprotein B and triglyceride production in very low density lipoproteins. Amer. J. Physiol. 239:E354

17.    Ruderman MB, Jones AL, Krauss RM, and Shafrir, E. (1971) A biochemical and morphologic study of very low density lipoproteins in carbohydrate-induced hypertriglyceridemia. J. Clin. Invest 50:1355-68

18.    Steiner G, Murase T (1975) Triglyceride turnover: A comparison of simultaneous determinations using the radioglyceride and the lipolytic rate procedure. Fed. Proc. 34: 2258

19.    Hollenberg CH (1959) Effect of nutrition on activity and release of lipase from rat adipose tissue. Am. J. Physiol. 197:667

20.    Reardon MF, Sekai H, Steiner G (1980)  The roles of lipoprotein lipase and hepatic triglyceride lipase in the catabolism of triglyceride-rich lipoproteins.  Circulation 62 (Suppl III): 194

21.    Vranic M, Morita S, Steiner G (1980) Insulin resistance in obesity as analyzed by the response of glucosekinetics to glucagon infusion. Diabetes 29: 169

22.    Cattran DC, Steiner G, Wilson DR, Fenton SSA (1979)  Hyperlipidemia after renal transplantation: natural history and pathophysiology. Ann. Int. Med. 91: 554

23.    Olefsky JM, Farquhar JWR, Reaven GM (1974) Reappraisal of the role of insulin in hypertriglyceridemia. Am. J. Med. 57:551

24.    Topping DL, Mayes PA (1972) The immediate effects of insulin and fructose on the metabolism of the perfused liver. Biochem J. 120:295

25.    Kobayshi M, Olefsky JM (1978) Effect of experimental hyperinsulinemia on insulin binding and glucose transport in isolated rat adipocytes. Am. J. Physio. 235: E53

26.    Steiner G, Vranic M (1982) Hyperinsulinemia and hypertriglyceridemia, a vicious cycle with atherogenic potential. Int. J. Obesity 6 (Suppl 1) (in press).

27.    Steiner G, Martin CM, Desai KS (1982) Unpublished observations.

28.    Risser TR, Reaven GM, Reaven EP (1978)  Intestinal contribution to secretion of very low density lipoproteins into plasma. Am J Physio. 234:E277

29.    Garfinkel AS, Nilsson-Ehle P, Schotz MC (1976) Regulation of lipoprotein lipase: Induction by insulin. Biochim. Biophys. Acta 424:264

31.    Nikkila EA, Kuusi T, Harro K, Tikkanen M, Taskinen MR (1980) Lipoprotein lipase and hepatic endothelial lipase are key enzymes in the metabolism of plasma high density lipoproteins, particularly $HDL_2$ in Atherosclerosis V p 387 Gotto AM, Smith LC, Allen B (eds) Springer-Verlag Berlin

# Another Look at Body Weight, Health and Longevity

T. B. VanItallie and A. P. Simopoulos

The adverse effects of "overweight" on health and longevity are
widely acknowledged. However, there has been considerable debate recently about the role of overweight (obesity) as an "independent"
risk factor for premature mortality. In addition, there has been
disagreement about the range beyond which excess weight is associated with a significantly increased mortality ratio (1).

It is clear that overweight persons have an enhanced risk of developing diabetes, hypertension, hyperlipidemia and a host of other
disorders. In general, the risk increases, indeed accelerates, as
obesity becomes more severe. Thus, one would anticipate that obese
persons are more likely than nonobese persons to have a shortened
life span.
Studies of pooled insured lives support the contention that obesity
predisposes to premature death. The Society of Actuaries has reported two large studies (Build and Blood Pressure Study, 1979)
which indicate that the mortality ratio rises as weight increases
above the "desirable" range. The desirable weight range is defined
as the range of weights associated with the greatest life expectancy,
based on life insurance statistics.

Life insurance policies are not readily issued  to persons with
hypertension, diabetes or some other known illness (i.e. rheumatic
heart disease) that is likely to shorten life. However, insurance
examinations conducted prior to 1972 rarely if ever screened subjects for smoking or hyperlipidemia. Thus, one is left with a single weight recorded at the time of the insurance examination and
the probable elimination as policy holders of subjects with overt
diabetes and significant hypertension.

Americans who posses individual life insurance policies are mostly
men and are generally rather affluent. Therefore, policy holders
are not typical of the general population. For these and other
reasons, life insurance statistics have been criticized as being
inaccurate and irrelevant to the population as a whole. Similarly,
the Metropolitan Life (ML) Insurance Company's Tables of Desirable
Weights (1959) have been charcterized by some workers as being
inappropriately and unreasonably stringent.

The disenchantment experienced by some observers with the 1959 ML
tables has had a number of sources but two types of observations
have been given particular attention recently. First, a number of
studies like that of the employees of the Chicago Peoples Gas Company (1264 subjects) have shown that mild obesity was associated with

a lower mortality than "ideal" weight (2). Also, a large survey by Keys et al. (3) showed that when age, blood pressure, serum cholesterol, and smoking were taken into account neither relative weight nor degree of obesity made a significant contribution to predicting risk of future heart disease. Second, the Framingham Heart Study and some other studies have shown a "U-shaped" or "J-shaped" univariate relationship between mortality and relative weight. This means that at both the underweight and the overweight ends of the curve, mortality ratios rise well above the average. The sharp increase in mortality observed among subjects somewhat under desirable weight has given birth to the notion that it may be as hazardous to be underweight as it is to be substantially overweight.

Nevertheless, when the sources of dissatisfaction with the 1959 ML tables are considered in the light of recent evidence, particularly from Framingham, the case for remaining within or near to the ML 1959 desirable weight range is strengthened. Although there are a number of lines of evidence supportive of the concept that "slimmer is better", two deserve particular emphasis. First, there is the recent observation that among Framingham men there was a nearly complete confounding of leanness and cigarette smoking (4). The proportion smoking cigarettes at the time of the first biennial examination ranged from about 55 % in the most overweight group of men to over 80 % in the men who were below desirable weight. Second, when the Framingham men were followed-up for 26 year mortality, it was demonstrated that the ML 1959 standards are appropriate. Of six age- and smoking-specific groups of Framingham men, only one failed to show minimum mortality in the Metropolitan Relative Weight (MRW) 100-109 class. Twenty-six years mortality in women also showed a statistically significant direct relationship with MRW in each age group.

The recent Framingham data suggest that the "U-shaped" or "J-shaped" univariate relationship between mortality and relative weight results from the mortality risks associated with cigarette smoking. As pointed out by Garrison et al. (4) "caution will need to be used in interpreting the results of studies that attempt to estimate the relationship between mortality and levels of relative weight without taking smoking into account". Also, as suggested by many workers (5) both the age of onset of obesity and its duration (severity apart) play important roles in determining the extent to which obesity serves as an "independent" risk factor.

## References

Andres R (1981) Aging, diabetes, and obesity: Standards of normality. Mt Sinai J Med 48: 489-495
Dyer AR, Stamler T, Berkson DM, Lindberg HA (1975) Relationship of relative weight and body mass index to 14-year mortality in the Chicago Peoples Gas Company Study. J Chronic Dis 28: 109-123
Keys A (1980) Seven Countries. A multivariate analysis of death and coronary heart disease.Harvard Univ Press, Cambridge MA

Garrison RJ, Feinleit M, Castelli WP, McNamara PM
    Cigarette smoking as a confounder of the relationship between
    relative weight and long-term mortality in the Framingham
    Heart Study (in press)
Gassow JS (1979) Weight penalties. Brit  Med  J  2: 1171-1172

# 6.1 Addendum

# Status of a Computerized, Angiographic Regression Trial (CLAS)

S. P. Azen, D. H. Blankenhorn, R. H. Selzer, and M. E. Sanmarco

The Cholesterol Lowering Atherosclerosis Study (CLAS) is a prospective randomized clinical trial to test the hypothesis that changes in serum lipids may result in regression of atherosclerosis. The importance of this trial is that it provides a feasible test of this hypothesis since it utilizes a direct measure of atherosclerosis based on computer processing of angiograms.

This paper reports on the study design, analytical methodology and operational aspects of the CLAS study. In addition, results of the first 25 months of the trial are presented.

## Study Design

### Population

The population under study consists of male, non-smoking subjects aged 40 - 59 years, who have progressive atherosclerosis and who have had coronary bypass surgery not involving valve replacement. Entry cholesterol levels must be in the range of 185 - 350 mg%. Eligibility criteria were chosen a) to produce a relatively homogeneous group with respect to the outcome measures, and b) to produce a group expected to have a good response to lipid lowering medication. Atherosclerosis is confirmed through review of the angiogram taken prior to the bypass surgery or at the first angiogram. The bypass surgery must have been performed at least three months prior to the study admission date, and subjects must not have had bilateral femoral artery surgery. Exclusion critera include: diabetes mellitus, hypertension, thyroid disease, renal insufficiency, triglyceride levels of 500 mg% or greater, congestive heart failure, major arrhythmia, ventricular conduction defects, and weight exceeding 1.5 times the ideal weight.

### Screening and Pretrial Visits

There are a total of five screening visits before subjects are randomized into the study. The purpose of the first three screening visits is to ascertain the willingness of the participant to join the research study, to determine baseline lipid levels and nutritional information, to evaluate the patient's health status and to begin nutritional counseling. In addition, the patient is given a complete explanation of the trial.

Two pretrial study visits determine patient compliance and response to the cholesterol lowering drugs: Colestipol and niacin. To be randomized to the study, percent plasma cholesterol drop from baseline during a six week period should be $\geq$ 15%, although patients in 10 - 15% range are reviewed by the clinic staff as possible candidates for the study. The clinic staff and the participant are blinded to the actual lipid values and changes. Eligible candidates are randomized to one of two treatment groups by the project statistician and scheduled for the first angiogram. The use of a long screening process incorporating a drug pretrial has been adopted in hopes of reducing post-randomization dropout.

## Treatment Groups

A total of 180 participants are to be randomized into one of two treatment groups - Control group: Diet intervention + placebo (30 g Avicell and 3 g lactose, daily), Drug group: Diet intervention + drug (30 g Colestipol + 4 - 12 g niacin daily). The dose of niacin is chosen on the basis of the desired cholesterol reduction. Cholesterol reduction goals are 7 - 8 percent for the control group and 30 - 40 percent for the drug group. The randomization process includes balancing on drug and placebo within blocks of age groups: 40 - 44, 45 - 49, 50 - 59 years. The angiographer and staff performing the computer processing of the angiograms are blinded to the treatment assignment. The interval between initial and final angiogram is two years. After randomization, patients are treated and evaluated by the clinical staff at two months intervals.

## Endpoint

The primary endpoint is the change of the degree of atherosclerosis in the femoral arteries as estimated using an algorithm involving digital image processing of the femoral angiogram. Femoral angiography is performed as described by Barndt (1). The computer estimate of atherosclerosis (CEA) follows the procedures described by Brooks (2). The annual progression rate (APR) in CEA is given by

$$APR = \frac{100}{127Y} (CEA_2 - CEA_1) \tag{1}$$

where $CEA_i$ is the $i^{th}$ estimate of atherosclerosis (i = 1,2) and Y is the inter-angiogram interval (= 2 years).

Secondary endpoints are determinations of APR in the coronary and carotid arteries.

## Results

During the first 25 months of clinic operation, 2194 persons have been identified who have coronary bypass surgery. Of these, 1346 possible eligibles have been contacted to ascertain eligibility with respect to age, sex, and smoking status. Of these, 351 presented to the clinic for medical and drug pre-trial evaluation. To date 79 patients have been randomized (38 in drug group, 41 in diet group). Five patients have dropped from the study (4 in drug group, 1 in diet group) for the following reasons: control group - smoking metabolites found in urine; drug group - personal reasons, medications after second bypass incompatible with study medications, medications for uncontrolled blood pressure incompatible with study medications, and unwilling to resume medications after gall bladder surgery.

The following table summarizes treatment progress for forty patients who have had at least one post-randomized follow-up visit

| Variable | Group | Base | Current | % Change | Difference |
|---|---|---|---|---|---|
| CHOL (mg/dl) | drug + | 250 | 189 | − 24* | 18 |
| | diet | 245 | 231 | − 6 | |
| TG (mg/dl) | drug | 149 | 112 | − 20 | 14 |
| | diet | 184 | 172 | − 6 | |
| HDL (mg/dl) | drug | 43 | 57 | 33* | 35 |
| | diet | 43 | 42 | − 2 | |
| HDL 3 (mg/dl) | drug | 16 | 17 | 11 | 0 |
| | diet | 15 | 16 | 11 | |
| LDL (mg/dl) | drug | 176 | 110 | − 36* | 31 |
| | diet | 165 | 153 | − 5 | |
| Weight (lbs) | drug | 186 | 180 | − 3* | 2 |
| | diet | 178 | 176 | − 1 | |
| Diastolic Blood Pressure (mmHg) | drug | 79 | 74 | − 5 | 1 |
| | diet | 79 | 76 | − 4* | |

+ n = 28 (drug), n = 32 (diet)
* percent change is different from 0 when tested at the .01 level.

In addition, analysis of initial data has demonstrated a marked drug effect on several apolipoproteins (significant decrease in Apo B and significant increase in CIII ratio).

Troublesome symptoms observed during the randomized stage include: drug group - rectal bleeding (1), gout (1) skin rash (1), abdominal pain (2); control group - rectal bleeding (1).

Review of the angiograms have revealed that 70% of the patients have clearly visible femoral atheromas, 27% showed ≥ 50% stenosis in the ungrafted coronary arteries, 18% showed ≥ 50% stenosis in the grafts. Computer analysis of 45 femoral angiograms resulted in mean ± sem (range) values of $CEA_1$ equal to: proximal - 54.4 ± 3.6 (25.1 - 130.6); and distal - 59.0 ± 3.2 (27.8 - 102.8). These values indicate a greater level of disease than those from a previously reported series of 54 men with myocardial infarction (2) (mean ± sem = 43.6 ± 2.3).

## Discussion

The demonstrated lipid changes and prevalence of lesions are in accordance with the projections made in planning the design of the CLAS trial. If the treated group were to show a favorable response to therapy, this would suggest that treatment of atherosclerosis through lipid lowering is effective.

## References

1. Barndt R Jr, Blankenhorn DH, Crawford DW et al: Regression and progression of early femoral atherosclerosis in treated hyperlipoproteinemic patients. Ann Int Med 86:139-146, 1977
2. Brooks SH, Blankenhorn DH, Chin HP et al: Design of human atherosclerosis studies by serial angiography. J Chron Dis. 33:347-357, 1980

# Subject Index

# Atherosclerosis V

Proceedings of the Fifth International Symposium

Editors: **A. M. Gotto, Jr., L. C. Smith, B. Allen**

1980. 250 figures, 183 tables. XXXIX, 843 pages
ISBN 3-540-90473-5

**Contents:** Cardiovascular Surgery. – Coronary Bypass Surgery. – Epidemiology of Atherosclerosis Lesions. – Drug Treatment of Hyperlipidemia. – The Arterial Wall – Lipid, Apoprotein and Lipoprotein Origin and Synthesis. – Lipoprotein Structure. – Dietary Prevention of Coronary Heart Disease. – Hyperlipidemia: Prevalence and Inheritance. – Risk Factors in Children. – Diet Treatment of Atherosclerosis. – Immunology. – Animal Models. – Enzymes of Lipoprotein Metabolism. – The Vessel Wall in Atherosclerosis. – Non-Dietary, Non-Pharmacological Treatment of Hyperlipidemia – HDL: Negative Risk Factor for Coronary Heart Disease. – Clinical Trials. – The Arterial Wall – II. – Vessel Wall – Platelet Interaction. – Catabolism of Lipids, Apolipoproteins and Lipoproteins. – Plasma Lipids, Lipoproteins and Atherosclerosis. – Mutants Affecting Lipoproteins and Apoproteins. – Hypertension. – Regression. – The Interrelationship Between Lipid and Prostaglandin Metabolism. – Cellular Metabolism of Lipoproteins. – Apoproteins Quantification. – Index.

Atherosclerosis research has undergone a period of dynamic growth to become an interdisciplinary field involving the activities of a large number of basic and clinical scientists. The advances they have achieved in the last three years towards elucidating the causes of atherosclerosis are reviewed in this book. It contains the contributions of epidemiologists, biochemists, nutritionists, cardiologists and cardiovascular surgeons (among them M. E. DeBakey) to the Fifth International Symposium on Atherosclerosis. The first symposium to be held under the auspices of the new International Atherosclerosis Society, it is an important forum for the exchange of ideas and a source of stimulation for further work in this field.

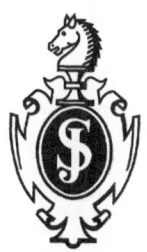

Springer-Verlag
Berlin
Heidelberg
New York

## Arterial Hypertension
Pathogenesis, Diagnosis, and Therapy
Editor: J. Rosenthal
With contributions by numerous experts
Foreword by I. H. Page
1982. 209 figures. XV, 529 pages. ISBN 3-540-90611-8

## Cardiovascular Surgery
Proceedings of the 29th International Congress of the European Society of Cardiovascular Surgery, 1980
Editors: W. Bircks, J. Ostermeyer, H. D. Schulte
1981. 300 figures, 271 tables. XXII, 767 pages.
ISBN 3-540-10929-3

## Hypertrophic Cardiomyopathy
The Therapeutic Role of Calcium Antagonists
Editors: M. Kaltenbach, S. E. Epstein
1982. 172 figures. XIV, 334 pages. ISBN 3-540-11065-8

## Microcirculation of the Heart
Theoretical and Clinical Problems
Editors: H. Tillmanns, W. Kübler, H. Zebe
1982. 177 figures. XIV, 353 pages. ISBN 3-540-11346-0

## Myocardial Infarction at Young Age
International Symposium Held in Bad Krotzingen,
January 30 and 31, 1981
Editor: H. Roskamm
1981. 83 figures. XII, 228 pages. ISBN 3-540-11090-9

## Transluminal Coronary Angioplasty and Intracoronary Thrombolysis
Coronary Heart Disease IV
Editors: M. Kaltenbach, A. Grünzig, K. Rentrop,
W.-D. Bussmann
With contributions by numerous experts
1982. 210 figures. XVIII, 442 pages. ISBN 3-540-11219-7

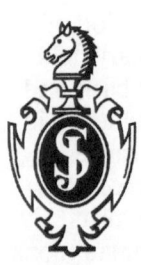

Springer-Verlag
Berlin
Heidelberg
New York

## Vessel Wall in Athero- and Thrombogenesis
Studies in the USSR
Editors: E. I. Chazov, V. N. Smirnov
With contributions by numerous experts
1982. 112 figures. VIII, 224 pages. ISBN 3-540-11384-3